BLACK'S
VETERINARY DICTIONARY

BLACK'S VETERINARY DICTIONARY

BY

WILLIAM C. MILLER

M.R.C.V.S., F.R.S.E.

LATELY DIRECTOR OF THE EQUINE RESEARCH STATION OF
THE ANIMAL HEALTH TRUST, NEWMARKET
FORMERLY COURTAULD PROFESSOR OF ANIMAL HUSBANDRY IN
THE ROYAL VETERINARY COLLEGE, LONDON

AND

GEOFFREY P. WEST

M.R.C.V.S.

TENTH EDITION

WITH 36 PHOTOGRAPHS

AND OVER 250 FIGURES IN THE TEXT

ADAM & CHARLES BLACK

LONDON

A. AND C. BLACK LTD.
4, 5 AND 6 SOHO SQUARE LONDON W.1

FIRST PUBLISHED 1928
SECOND EDITION 1935
THIRD EDITION, ENTIRELY RE-SET, 1953
REPRINTED 1953 AND 1955
FOURTH EDITION 1956
FIFTH EDITION 1959
SIXTH EDITION 1962
SEVENTH EDITION 1964
EIGHTH EDITION 1967
NINTH EDITION 1970
TENTH EDITION 1972

ISBN 0 7136 1335 1

MADE AND PRINTED IN GREAT BRITAIN BY
MORRISON AND GIBB LIMITED, LONDON AND EDINBURGH

PREFACE TO THE TENTH EDITION

THE revision for this new edition covers several developments in veterinary medicine, animal husbandry, public health matters and techniques of interest to farmers. The results of the Swann Committee's recommendations have been incorporated and will be found in the section on additives. The sections on brucellosis and salmonellosis in cattle have been extended, as have those dealing with rabies and diseases of cats. New entries include those on metabolic profile tests, L-forms of bacteria, pheromones, dog ticks, ' oulou fato ' and ulcerative spirochætosis of pigs. Two new photographs have replaced others, and additional tables have been included. The prevention of disease as well as first-aid has received attention, and the purpose of the book as indicated by the Preface to the First Edition has been kept in mind.

1972 G. P. W.

PREFACE TO THE FIRST EDITION

This book has been modelled upon the plan and general design of *Black's Medical Dictionary*, in the hope that it may fill a similar position for those who own, or have under their charge, domesticated animals. It is hoped that it may serve as a work of reference for those who, having no access to technical books upon veterinary subjects, find insufficient information in those numerous popular works intended merely for the domestic treatment of the commoner animal ailments.

An endeavour has accordingly been made to give information in simple language, and to use terms which, while not invariably scientifically correct, do not include the multitude of colloquialisms too frequently associated with animal diseases. Definitions are given of the terms commonly used in veterinary science, but no attempt has been made to include all the compound and often hybrid words which have been introduced during the last two decades. Notes upon anatomy and physiology, giving the most salient features, precede descriptions of the diseases of the various organs of the body. They are intended to make clear to the reader what are the normal functions, and how they may be altered under the influence of disease. The chief contagious and specific diseases have been described in such a way that, while established facts connected with them have been given in some detail, theories and controversies have been rigidly excluded, except in some few cases where practically the whole of our knowledge of a disease is built upon a foundation of surmise.

The systematic diseases have been described for the most part in sufficient detail to enable the practical owner to recognise the symptoms of the commoner of them, and to initiate a species of 'first-aid' treatment which will be rational and free from the mistakes so often encountered in general practice, and to apply measures which will prepare the way for that skilled attention which is to be given later by the veterinary practitioner. Certain diseases which, while strictly speaking systematic, are sufficiently well known by particular names to be considered almost as entities, are described under the heading by which they are most commonly known. In the case of surgical conditions, the principles upon which measures for relief are based have been briefly mentioned, but operative technique is quite foreign to the scope of the book.

Proprietary medicines and foods have been mentioned as seldom as possible, and then only where experience has shown them to be valuable.

To avoid encumbering the text with names, authorities are seldom given, except in those cases where a particular discovery or condition is specifically associated with the name of a particular authority.

With regard to etymology, the nearest word in the original language, together with its English equivalent, has in most cases been given. Words printed simply in italics belong to the Latin tongue, unless otherwise stated. In cases where the original Greek or Latin only is placed in brackets, this indicates that it was used by the writers of antiquity in the sense that it possesses at the present day.

It is hoped that the book will prove of use to the farmer and stock-owner, who depends to a large extent for his living upon the health of his animals; to the owner of a domestic pet, who may find no assistance available during an emergency; to the student, either of veterinary science or of agriculture, who desires to obtain information rapidly and without consulting numerous books or periodicals; and it is hoped that even the busy practitioner may find it useful during the exigencies of his calling. To the police inspector whose work brings him into contact with animal diseases, and to the inspector of the Royal Society for the Prevention of Cruelty to Animals, it should be useful to facilitate the recognition of the nature of the commoner animal ailments.

Dr. J. Comrie of Edinburgh kindly consented to the inclusion in this book of a number of illustrations from *Black's Medical Dictionary*, of which he is editor, and offered much valuable advice and kindly criticism, thereby rendering the task of its preparation considerably lighter; to him the author wishes to extend his thanks and his gratitude.

To Dr. O. Charnock Bradley, the Principal of the Royal (Dick) Veterinary College, the author desires gratefully to acknowledge his indebtedness for much kind advice and assistance; to his colleagues on the staff of the College, and to the contributors, he tenders his sincere thanks; while he desires to take this opportunity to express his gratitude to the publishers for their unfailing kindness and patience during the years this book has taken to prepare.

Wm. C. M.

EDINBURGH, 1927.

LIST OF PLATES

A

ABDOMEN is the middle portion of the trunk. It lies between the thorax, anteriorly, and the pelvis, posteriorly. Its main boundaries are the diaphragm in front, part of the spinal column and its muscles above, the pelvis behind, and the muscles of the abdominal wall form its sides and floor. The entrance to the pelvis is only an arbitrary division posteriorly, since there is no separation between the two cavities in the living animal. The posterior edge of the rib-cage forms part of the wall on either side, and protects the more anteriorly situated organs. The muscles of the abdomen are arranged as broad sheets with their fibres running in four distinct directions. The fibres of the recti muscles run antero-posteriorly, those of the external oblique run mainly downwards, outwards, and backwards, those of the internal oblique run downwards, forwards, and inwards, while the fibres of the transverse abdominal muscles run across the body.

These four muscles, accordingly, give the abdomen the maximum of support, but at the same time they allow of considerable distension without risk of rupture. Forming, as they do, the walls and the floor of the cavity, they are attached to the rib-cage on the one hand (or to some structure connected with it), and to the bones of the pelvis and vertebræ on the other; an arrangement which enables them to take considerable part in the movements of respiration.

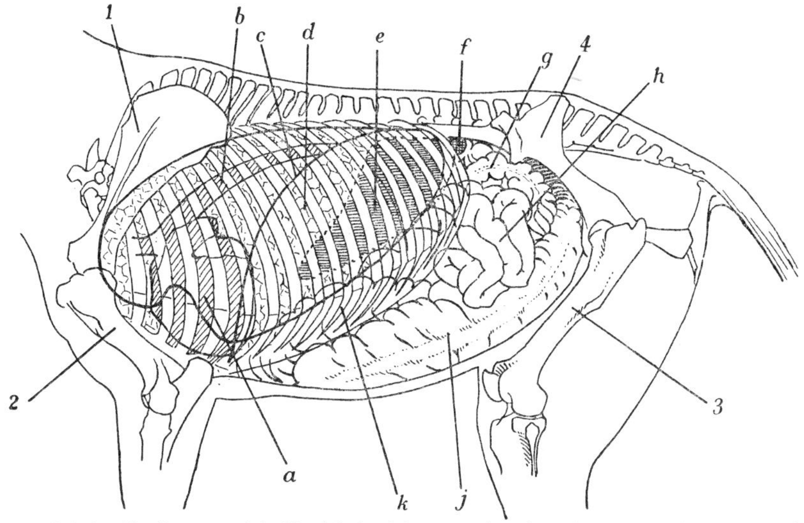

Relationship of organs to left side of body of horse. 1, Scapula; 2, humerus; 3, femur; 4, pelvic; bones. *a*, Heart; *b*, aorta; *c*, line of diaphragm; *d*, left lung; *e*, spleen; *f*, left kidney *g*, small colon; *h*, small intestines; *j*, left ventral colon; *k*, left dorsal colon.

CONTENTS.—The principal contents of the abdomen are the digestive organs, *i.e.* stomach, intestines, and the associated glands — liver and pancreas, and the kidneys and spleen. Each of these organs has a different position in each of the domestic animals, and it is necessary to consider each separately.

Horse.—In the horse the digestive organs in the abdomen are situated mainly towards the lower part of the cavity. The stomach lies towards the upper part of the abdomen behind the diaphragm and liver, and to the left of the middle line. Its position changes to some extent with each respiration, but its average level is between the 13th and 17th ribs. The small intestine (which connects the stomach with the large intestine) has an average length of about 70 feet and a calibre of 2 to 3 inches. Part of it is fixed, and balled the duodenum, and the remainder is only loosely attached by its mesentery. The mesentery of the small intestine—a fold of peritoneum attached to the roof of the abdomen under the 1st and 2nd lumbar vertebræ. The large intestine in the horse consists of the cæcum, large and small colon, and the rectum. The base of the cæcum lies in the right upper flank, and from there the organ curves downwards and forwards, and to a small extent inwards, something like a reversed comma, to end on the lower abdominal floor a little behind the posterior (*i.e.* xiphoid) cartilage of the sternum. It is a cul-de-sac, having its entrance and its exit towards the upper end, but not actually at the end. From

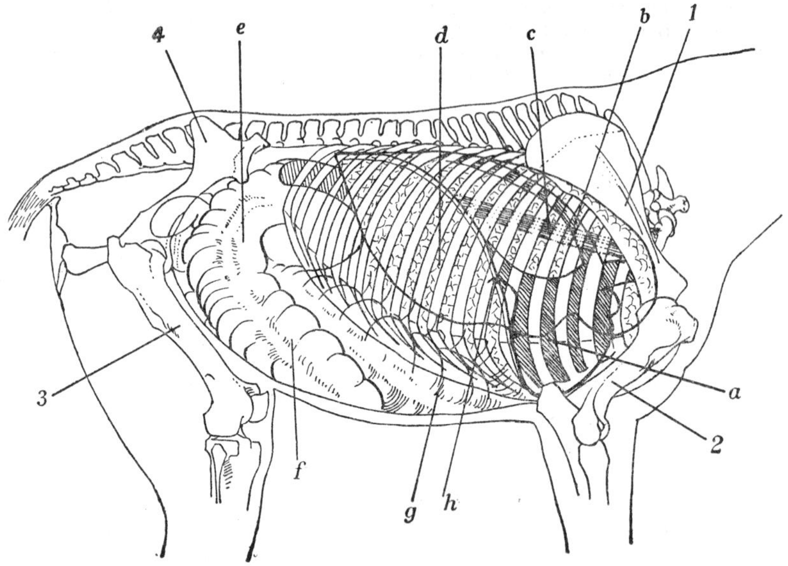

Relationship of organs to right side of body of horse. 1, Scapula; 2, humerus; 3, femur; 4, pelvic bones *a*, Heart; *b*, aorta; *c*, œsophagus; *d*, right lung; *e*, base of cæcum; *f*, cæcum; *g*, right ventral colon *h*, line of diaphragm, with termination of caudal vena cava immediately beyond end of indicating line.

duodenum is about 3½ feet long and begins at the pylorus of the stomach; from here it passes in a double curve to the right kidney, crosses towards the middle line of the body at the head of the last rib, and, turning forwards and to the left, it reaches the left kidney and becomes free. The free part of the small intestine—called the jejunum and ileum—varies so much in position that its general situation only can be given. Its complicated folds and coils lie mainly in the left half of the abdomen from the stomach to the pelvis, insinuated between the other organs which have a more fixed position. It ends at the ileo-cæcal valve, where it empties its contents into the cæcum. It is supported by the the cæcum the large colon takes its origin. It is divided into four parts. The first, known as the right ventral colon, leaves the base of the cæcum at the cæco-colic valve, and runs along the lower right side of the abdomen to the diaphragm immediately above the xiphoid cartilage; from here the tube turns sharply over to the left side of the body at the ventral diaphragmatic flexure, and becomes the left ventral colon; running backwards to the pelvic inlet along the lower left part of the abdomen it again turns, this time upwards, at the pelvic flexure, and becomes the left dorsal colon; this travels forwards to the region of the stomach and once more turns across the body to the right

ABDOMEN

side at the dorsal diaphragmatic flexure, and is now called the right dorsal colon. The right dorsal colon is directed backwards and inwards to the level of the base of the cæcum, and at about the level of the left kidney it becomes constricted to form the small colon. The small colon lies between the large colon and the rectum. It measures from 10 to 12 feet long, and is situated in the space between the stomach and the entrance to the pelvis, its coils being mingled with those of the small intestine. The rectum lies within the pelvis.

The other organs of the abdomen of the horse that require notice are the liver, pancreas, kidneys, and spleen. The liver is situated obliquely on the abdominal surface of the diaphragm; it reaches to the right kidney dorsally, while behind it lie the stomach and the flexures of the great colon, and the duodenum passes along its right lower surface. The pancreas lies in the first curve of the duodenum, and is attached to the liver and stomach. It lies between the 16th and 17th thoracic vertebræ, mainly to the right of the middle line, and high up against the roof of the abdomen. The kidneys of the horse do not lie opposite each other on either side of the abdomen. The right occupies a position under the last two or three rib heads and the first lumbar transverse

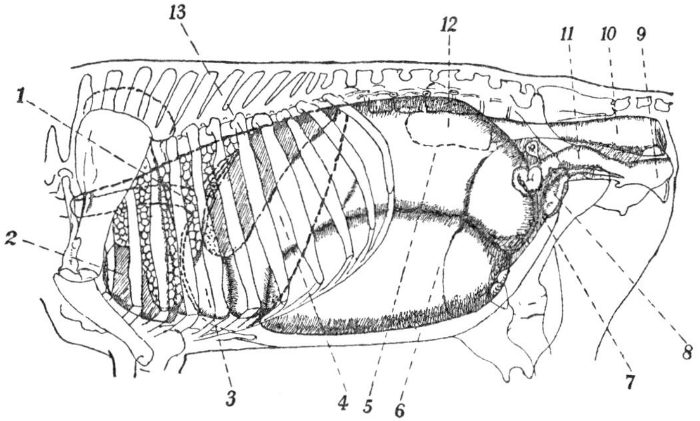

Diagram of the relations of the internal organs to the left side of the surface of the body of the ox (female). 1, Lung; 2, heart; 3, reticulum; 4, rumen; 5 and 6, upper and lower sacs of the rumen; 7, horn of uterus; 8, urinary bladder; 9, vagina; 10, rectum; 11, body of uterus; 12, position of left kidney; 13, spleen.

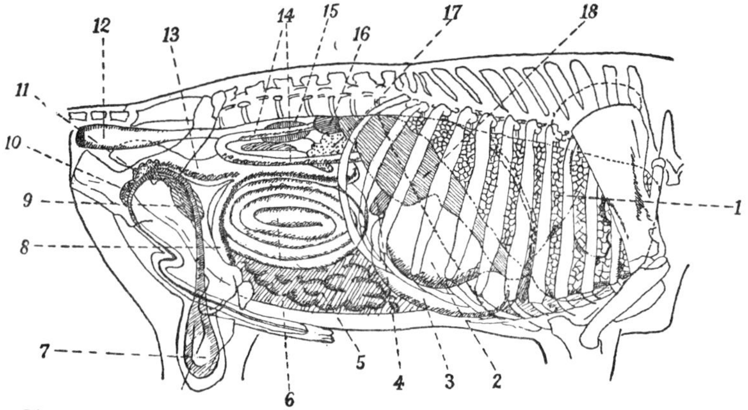

Diagram of the relations of the internal organs to the right side of the surface of the body of the ox (male). 1, Lung; 2, omasum; 3, abomasum; 4, gall-bladder; 5, small intestines; 6, spiral colon; 7, testis; 8, ileum, which opens into the cæcum; 9, urinary bladder; 10, bulbo-urethral glands; 11, seminal vesicles; 12, rectum; 13, cæcum; 14, duodenum; 15, left kidney; 16, right kidney; 17, pancreas; 18, liver.

process. The left is situated farther back, being under the last rib and the first two or three transverse processes of the lumbar vertebræ. Each lies slightly to its own side of the middle line of the body. The spleen is placed in close relationship to the longer and convex surface of the stomach, in the left upper part of the cavity.

In addition to these more important and large structures there are present in the abdomen the main blood-vessels—aorta and vena cava—the nerve and lymph trunks, and numerous glands, as well as vestiges of fœtal tissues. In the female when pregnancy is advanced the abdomen contains the pregnant uterus and its associated structures.

and lateral wall of the abdomen. The 4th stomach, or abomasum, is an elongated flask-shaped sac lying on the right lower wall of the abdomen between it and the right face of the rumen. It opens into the duodenum, which is the first part of the small intestine, and which has a length of about 130 feet, and lies to the right of the cavity, occupying the position between the right face of the rumen, behind the omasum and abomasum, and below the coils of the colon. It terminates in the pear-shaped cæcum, which lies partly in the pelvis and partly in the upper posterior part of the right side of the abdomen. From the cæcum the digestive tube is continued as the colon, which is arranged in a double spiral manner, some

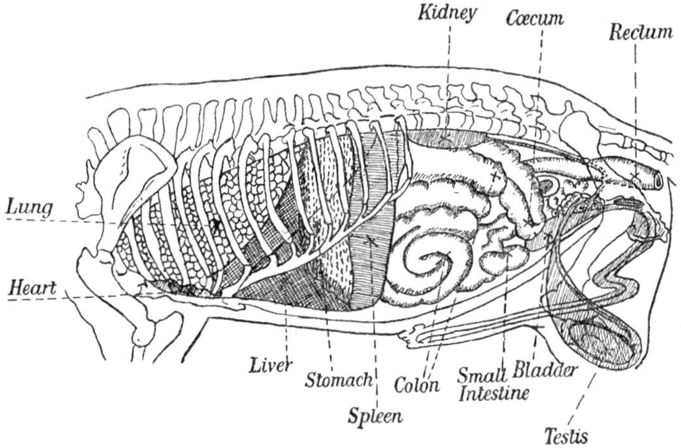

Diagram of the relations of the internal organs to the left side of the surface of the body of the pig (male).

Ox.—Ruminants, possessing four stomachs, have a somewhat modified arrangement in their abdominal cavities. The 1st stomach, or rumen, lies along the whole of the left side of the abdomen from the diaphragm back to the pelvis and, in fact encroaches across to the right side of the body to some extent. The spleen lies on its outer and upper surface, and, with the exception of the left kidney and a part of the 2nd stomach, is the only organ present in the left half of the abdominal cavity. The 2nd stomach, or reticulum, lies low down and to the front of the rumen, and between it and the diaphragm and liver, almost in the middle line. The more or less globular 3rd stomach, or omasum, lies on the right of the median plane about opposite the 7th to 11th ribs. It is in relation to the diaphragm, liver,

of the coils passing to the centre, and others passing out from the centre. Its bulk is in the right flank, about half-way between the spinal column and the floor of the abdomen. The rectum leads from the colon to the outside and is placed in the pelvis. The liver of the ox lies between the right half of the diaphragm and the omasum and reticulum, and presents a gall-bladder which is absent in the horse. The pancreas lies high up between the duodenum and the liver, close against the pillars of the diaphragm. The kidneys are large, irregular, lobed organs with a more or less elliptical outline. The right is situated below the last rib and the first 2 or 3 lumbar transverse processes. The left is peculiar. When the rumen is full it becomes pushed over to the right side of the middle line, to a point behind and below the right kidney. At other times it lies just on the left side of the body. Each kidney is lobulated. The spleen is placed between the left upper part of the rumen and the left abdominal wall.

between the liver and diaphragm and the mass of the intestines. The small intestines (50 to 60 feet long) are arranged in small coils chiefly on the left side and floor of the abdomen from the stomach to

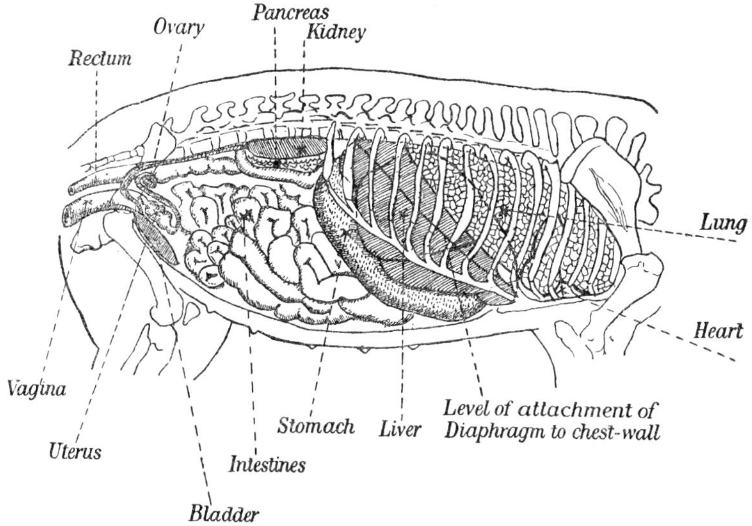

Diagram of the relations of the internal organs to the right side of the surface of the body of the pig (female).

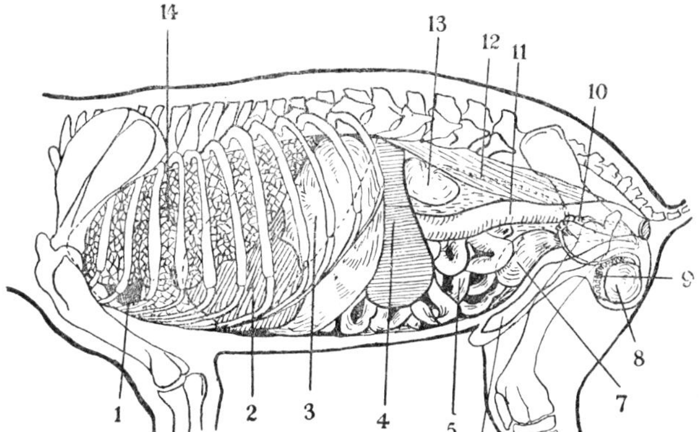

Relations of organs to surface of left side of body of dog (male). 1, Heart; 2, liver; 3, stomach; 4, spleen; 5, small intestines; 6, penis; 7, bladder; 8, testicle; 9, epididymis; 10, prostrate; 11, large colon 12, ureter; 13, kidney; 14, lung.

Sheep.—The main relations of the contents of the abdomen of the sheep are similar to those of the ox, with certain small variations.

Pig.—The arrangement of the contents of the abdomen of the pig differs markedly from the other animals. The stomach is of considerable size, and is situated the pelvis. The large intestines lie high up on the left side except for the cæcum, which is found towards the right flank, often lying amongst coils of small intestine. It must be noted that the variations in the positions of the intestines that are met with in the pig are considerable. This especially applies to young animals and to the pregnant dam. The liver lies in the anterior part of the abdomen between the diaphragm and the stomach and duodenum. The pancreas lies up against the right kidney, and often touches the spleen and the left kidney. The spleen is situated under the last three ribs on the left side, and from here it passes downwards and forwards to the lower abdominal wall touching the left lobe of the liver.

Dog.—The abdomen of the dog is somewhat difficult to describe owing to the great differences that are met with in various breeds. In this respect it is only necessary to consider the shape of the body of the St. Bernard and compare it with that of the greyhound, to enable one to realise how incomplete an average description must be.

In a dog of the fox-terrier type the abdominal contents will be described as the nearest approach to an average that is possible. The stomach occupies a position which varies according to the amount of food it contains. On an average, it lies behind the liver and the left part of the diaphragm, in contact with the left lower part of the abdominal wall, as far back as the level of the 2nd or 3rd lumbar vertebra. Behind it on the left side is situated the spleen, and the coils of the small intestines lie on the right posterior aspect of this organ. The small intestines measure about 15 feet in length, and have a fairly definite position in the middle lower part of the abdomen. They terminate at the cæcum, which is situated against the middle of the upper part of the right flank. From the cæcum arises the colon, and travels for a short distance forwards and slightly upwards, where it is called the ascending colon. It soon turns across the body as the transverse colon, and, finally, slightly descends and runs backwards to end in the rectum. The liver lies close against the diaphragm, between that structure and the stomach, and mainly on the right side of the body. It is comparatively large. The pancreas occupies a position high up in the right part of the abdomen, lying against each of the kidneys. The kidneys do not occupy similar positions on each side of the body. The right organ is placed under the last rib and the first three lumbar transverse processes, and the left one lies under the 2nd to the 4th lumbar transverse process according to whether the stomach is full or empty. It is more loosely attached than the right. The situation of the spleen has been mentioned.

ABDOMEN, DISEASES OF. (*See under* STOMACH, DISEASES OF; INTESTINE, DISEASES OF; DIARRHŒA; LIVER, DISEASES OF; PANCREAS, DISEASES OF; KIDNEYS, DISEASES OF; BLADDER, DISEASES OF; PERITONITIS; TUMOURS; COLIC; DROPSY; HERNIA; etc.)

Symptoms.—PAIN.—Kicking at the belly and by gazing at the flanks by horses and cattle; pigs generally lie on one side or roll on the ground, and are sometimes seen sitting on their haunches in dog-fashion; they may grunt or groan in a distressed manner; dogs and cats usually object to being handled, keep the muscles of their abdominal walls tense and hard, may lie full length on a cold place, or may assume a characteristic crouching attitude with their backs arched. The commonest cause of abdominal pain in animals is digestive disturbance. (*See* COLIC; INTESTINE, DISEASES OF; STOMACH, DISEASES OF.) Straining, in an endeavour to pass fæces, either successfully or otherwise, generally indicates that there is some obstruction in the bowel. The assumption of the attitude for the passage of water by the horse points to an impaction of the large colon in the majority of cases of colic. Tenderness on pressure by the hand generally means that there is some inflammatory process going on in the organs below the painful area. (*See* PERITONITIS.)

VOMITING.—In animals that normally vomit, *i.e.* the pig, dog, and cat, this act may not be of a serious nature, for it is one of the provisions of Nature whereby objectionable material may be quickly eliminated from the system; but, on the other hand, it generally accompanies gastritis, enteritis, and kidney disease, as well as being present in the majority of cases of irritant poisoning. In the larger animals, vomiting is a very serious symptom of internal trouble, and, in the horse at least, frequently denotes either a ruptured stomach or a rupture of the diaphragm.

TUCKING UP OF THE ABDOMEN.—This symptom is seen in a variety of different troubles. In its most acute form it is generally indicative of serious starvation from some wasting disease, such as tuberculosis, infestation with parasitic worms, tumour formation, Johne's disease in cattle, chronic indigestion, etc.

In other cases it may be due to some

less serious condition. It is often seen as an accompanying symptom of pleurisy, when the term 'pleuritic line' is given to the groove that becomes very obvious between the edge of the rib-cage and the muscles of the flanks; in this condition the tucking up of the abdomen is due to an almost constant spasm of the abdominal muscles that are concerned in respiration, owing to the pain occasioned by full, deep breaths.

SWELLING OR DISTENSION of the abdomen is one of the signs of pregnancy, and it is also evident in dropsy or ascites, when large amounts of fluid collect in the peritoneal cavity, giving the animal a 'pot-bellied' appearance. The abdomen is often swollen in sheep affected with liver-rot, and in those that harbour various other parasitic worms. In other cases the distension is due to collections of gas in one or other of the abdominal organs, and in other cases yet it is due to collections of fæces that cannot be evacuated.

ABDOMEN, INJURIES OF.—These can be classed either as injuries to the abdominal walls, or as injuries to the contained organs. Owing to their mode of life, bruises, wounds, etc., affecting the muscles, subcutis, or skin of the walls of the abdomen, are common in the domesticated animals. They are frequently produced by kicks, blows, thrusts with horns, and by pressure against hard objects, such as the squeezing of many animals through a narrow gate entails. The nature of the injury depends upon the nature of the object which inflicts it. Severe blows and kicks may bruise the skin and cause tearing of the muscles below, so that a hernia is produced (*see* HERNIA). Sharp objects produce surface wounds when the injury is mild, and punctures of the walls of the abdominal cavity when severe. In less common cases both the muscles and the skin are torn or cut through and the contained organs escape from the cavity; in such cases there is generally injury to the internal structures and organs (for which see later). In the great majority of the injuries that are liable to be inflicted on the walls of the abdomen, there is a greater or less amount of bleeding into the tissues that are damaged. This in many instances produces large swellings, hard, sore, and painful at first, but soon becoming softer, fluctuating, and practically painless. These are collections of blood, or blood and serum, generally immediately under the skin, to which the name 'hæmatomata' is applied (*see* HÆMATOMA). They are particularly common among cattle that have been injured in transit by rail.

Injuries to the internal organs are not so common as might be expected, although they do occur. The reason is that the walls of the abdomen, in spite of being unprovided with a bony foundation, are of considerable thickness, enclosed by a tough skin with an appreciable amount of fat or connective tissue below, and are capable of being braced by the animal when it expects a blow or other injury, in a purely reflex manner. The arrangement provides a rubber-like cushion of from 1 to 2½ inches thickness over the organs, which, while yielding itself, is of sufficient substance to give great protection to the structures within. Extreme force must be exerted to overcome this protection, such as run-over accidents, falls from a height on to hard or irregular surfaces, severe crushes or trample, etc., or else the animal must be injured when not expecting the traumatic agent.

The commonest organ to suffer is the liver, especially in old or diseased animals. The intestines are less often damaged, since they contain fluids or air and recede from the impact, but the liver being a solid organ and fixed in a definite position has not the same chance of escaping. The kidneys are sometimes ruptured or bruised, particularly when the bones of the lumbar vertebræ are fractured; the urinary bladder is sometimes ruptured, especially if full at the time of injury; and the spleen has been found ruptured in some cases. When a sharp instrument has caused a large wound in the abdominal wall, the bowels may protrude through the opening, and if the incision be extensive, evisceration may take place. In the case of severe punctured wounds, such as are caused by a horned animal, by a stable fork, by gunshot at close range, or by some other penetrating body, actual damage is sustained by the internal organs. This is followed by the escape of their contents, and in some cases by hæmorrhage into the abdominal cavity. In any of these instances death may follow almost at once, either from shock or from internal hæmorrhage. When the abdominal wall only has been damaged little difficulty is experienced in securing healing, and the condition is not serious. With extensive bruises or wounds, cases are more serious and often fatal. If exposure of the abdominal contents has taken place, or if the organs have been themselves damaged, everything depends on the extent of the lesion and its nature. Some alarmingly serious abdominal injuries have made excellent recoveries when they are attended at once, and in a rational manner, especially when the vitality of the subject is great. It frequently happens, however, that the animal lives for a day or two, suffering intense pain, and gradually becomes weaker and weaker till it dies from absorption of the poisonous products that have escaped into the cavity. For this reason the injured animal should receive promptly the expert services of a veterinary surgeon or else be humanely destroyed. Simple wounds or bruises of the abdominal walls are treated in the same way as ordinary wounds (*see* WOUNDS).

ABDUCTION (*ab*, from; *ducere*, to lead) is a term meaning the movement of a limb in a sideway direction away from the central plane of the body. It is used to signify the action of certain muscles which are generally situated between the outside of the limb bones and some other part of the skeleton, and it is employed to describe a symptom of some forms of lameness where the limb is swung outwards in the stride, or is held out to one side as far away from the body as possible.

ABIOTROPHY.—A degenerative disorder not attributable to external causes, and occurring after birth—hereditary rather than congenital.

ABNORMALITIES, INHERITED (*see under* GENETICS, DEFORMITIES).

ABOMASUM is the name given to the 4th stomach of ruminating animals. It is also called the 'true' or 'rennet stomach', and the 'reed'. It is an elongated, pear-shaped sack lying on the floor of the abdomen, on the right-hand side, and roughly between the 7th and 12th ribs. It follows the 3rd stomach (or omasum), and it leads to the beginning of the small intestine. Above it lies the 3rd stomach, before it lies the 2nd stomach (or reticulum), and its deep face is in contact with the 1st stomach (or rumen).

Its walls are composed of three coats. On the outside it is provided with a peritoneal covering in common with practically all the abdominal organs, which reduces friction with surrounding structures to a minimum. Beneath this is the muscular layer which supplies the organ with its capacity for movement. Lining the muscular coat is the mucous membrane which carries the glands upon which digestion depends. These glands are of three kinds, known as *cardiac*, *fundus*, and *pyloric* respectively. They pour out a digestive fluid to which the collective name of gastric juice is applied. (For displacement of the abomasum, *see* STOMACH, DISEASES OF.)

ABORTION (*aborior*, I perish) means the premature expulsion of the fœtus, or of the contents of the pregnant uterus.

Cow.—Before the extensive use of Strain 19 vaccine, infection with *Brucella abortus* was the most frequent cause of abortion affecting the herd in Britain. (*See under* BRUCELLOSIS.) Other important causes are infection with *Trichomonas fœtus*, *Vibrio fœtus*, and *Salmonella dublin*; less commonly with a fungus, *e.g. Aspergillus fumigatus*. Listeriosis is another cause. In America, leptospirosis is important. (*See also Pasteurella pseudotuberculosis* under EWE below.) Tick-borne fever may be a cause, especially in Scotland. Mycoplasma may be responsible, and these organisms can withstand deep freezing of semen and the usual antibiotic buffers. (*See also* Q FEVER).

Abortion may also follow the death of the calf due to hereditary causes. For example, a recessive lethal gives rise to mummification of the fœtus, and this is commonly aborted at the eighth month. The neck is short, the legs are stiff, and joints prominent.

Hæmolytic disease may account for some cases of abortion in cattle.

Abortion may also occur during the course of parasitic bronchitis, or Husk; or as a result of fear. A terrified animal can be expected to abort, whereas this does not invariably occur in an animal seriously injured in an accident.

Other causes include: Malnutrition of the mother. Ill-treatment of the dam in the later stages of pregnancy, the unwanted attentions of the bull or the aggressive propensities of field-mates towards in-calf cows, are liable to cause abortion. Long journeys by road or rail, severe abdominal pain or purgation, ingestion of substances of a poisonous nature such as ergot of rye (*Claviceps purpurea*), pasture œstrogens, etc., are possible causal agents. Abortion has followed the feeding of silage contaminated by hormones. (*See* HORMONES.) (*See also under* RESORPTION, ALFALFA.)

Ewe.—Bacterial causes include infection with *Vibrio fœtus* and *Salmonella abortus ovis*. The latter is important in S.W. England. Other infections include Listeriosis and Toxoplasmosis. A virus disease, Enzootic Abortion of Ewes, occurs in the S.E. of Scotland and the N.E. of England. Tick-borne fever is another cause; occasionally Q Fever (*e.g.* in Yorkshire). *Pasteurella pseudotuberculosis* (from infected wild birds, hares, rabbits, or voles) has been found in some cases in the U.K.; also Brucellosis. (*See also* TURNIPS.)

The chasing of in-lamb ewes by dogs, careless handling, long journeys by road or rail, ergot and other poisons, malnutrition (especially the near-starvation of hill ewes in winter, and the feeding of cattle-cake containing a hexœstrol additive, are among other causes. In Australia clover œstrogens are important.

Mare.—*Salmonella abortus equi* is a cause of abortion; also the virus of Equine Rhinopneumonitis. (*See also* BRUCELLOSIS and under UTERINE INFECTIONS.) Working the pregnant mare in shafts, and other general causes mentioned in connection with the cow apply also. The presence in the uterus of twin foals very frequently results in abortion at 5 to 7 months or later. Failure to produce a sufficiency of the hormone *progesterone* may occasionally result in abortion in animals.

With reference to thoroughbreds, the Animal Health Trust has stated (1968) 'The vast majority of foals slipped early on in pregnancy from the 6th to the 20th week of gestation go completely unnoticed and the mare does not return to "season" immediately. One of the causes of this type of abortion may be an upset in the hormonal balance which is especially delicate from 6–14 weeks.'

Sow.—Overseas, *Brucella abortus suis* is an important cause of abortion. Investigations, reported in 1960, at Sutton Bonington into the causes of stillbirth and abortion showed that on eight farms swine erysipelas was responsible; on two abortion was probably the result of swine fever infection during pregnancy. Leptospirosis was the cause on four farms; and *E. coli* was isolated from all internal organs in five litters elsewhere. Forty-five sows had antibodies in their blood which indicated that they had encountered Toxoplasmosis infection, but the organism could not be found in the tissues. Faulty feeding and vitamin A deficiency accounted for other instances of stillbirth and abortion. (*See* Aujeszky's *also under* STILLBORN *and* INFERTILITY.)

A *Pasteurella multocida* infection has been reported in the U.K. as causing abortion. A *Bedsonia* infection may be responsible. Viruses causing breeding troubles in sows are widespread in the U.K. They include SMEDI viruses, enteroviruses, and the small hæmaglutinating virus. Before its eradication, swine fever virus was important in the U.K.

ABORTION, ENZOOTIC, OF EWES.—This disease occurs in lowland flocks in S.E. Scotland and N.E. England, as well as overseas.

Cause.—A virus, which multiplies only in the placenta where it causes necrosis of the cotyledons. It can, however, remain latent for long periods in non-pregnant sheep.

Symptoms.—Abortion occurs during the last 6 weeks, usually during the last 2 or 3 weeks of the normal period of gestation. Stillbirths and the birth of weak full-term lambs also occur. The aborted fœtus is dropsical. The ewes often remain ill for several weeks, but very few die. Infertility is temporary, since usually ewes lamb normally the following season.

Prevention.—This depends partly upon management, the avoidance of lambing-pens where the disease is known to exist. An effective vaccine is available for use in late summer, or early autumn. Re-vaccination is not necessary.

ABSCESS (*abscessus*) is a localised collection of pus or matter. A minute abscess is known as a pustule (*see* PUSTULE), and a diffused area that produces pus is spoken of as an area of cellulitis or erysipelas (*see* CELLULITIS). An abscess may be acute or chronic, and since these two forms possess little in common they are considered separately.

ABSCESS, ACUTE.—An acute abscess is one that forms rapidly and as rapidly comes to a head and bursts, or else becomes reabsorbed and disappears—a process that is called 'abortion'. Acute abscesses generally run their course in a week or ten days, and are, as a rule, accompanied by heat, pain, redness, and swelling, with often a slight fever.

Causes.—The direct cause of an acute abscess is either infection with bacteria, or the presence of an irritant in the tissues, either chemical or mechanical. Bacterial invasion is the more common cause, and even in many abscesses that are con-

ABSCESS, ACUTE

sidered to be of a mechanical nature, such as the presence of bullets or pieces of metal, thorns, splinters, etc., in the tissues, the production of pus is directly due to the germs that have been introduced.

The organisms that are most often associated with the formation of abscesses are *staphylococci* and *streptococci*, which are found in almost all conditions that are due to injury to the tissues from the outside, as well as in certain specific conditions, such as strangles and botriomycosis in the horse; *Clostridium pyogenes*; *Corynebacterium ovis*; *Actinomyces necrophorus*. *Shigella viscosa* may produce abscesses in the kidneys; *Escherichia coli*, or some allied germ, sometimes produces abscesses in connection with the

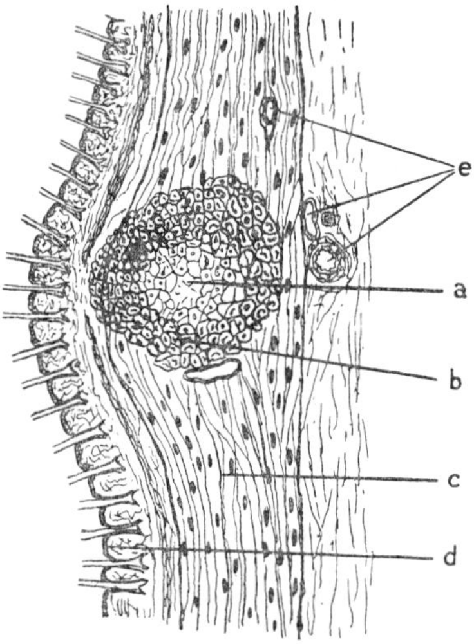

Diagram of a small abscess situated below the skin surface, and causing it to bulge. *a*, Centre of abscess undergoing a process of liquefaction; *b*, the surrounding ring of white blood-cells; *c*, subcutaneous tissues; *d*, the skin; *e*, blood-vessels in the vicinity of the abscess engorged with blood.

intestinal system, where this organism is normally found living in a harmless state; in addition to these, *Pfeifferella mallei*, *Mycobacterium tuberculosis*, and in rare cases *Clostridium tetani*, cause abscess formation.

Given the micro-organism in the tissues it is also essential that: (1) that the vitality of the tissues has been impaired, or that local or general disease or injury, bad health, unsuitable food, exposure, or some other condition has lowered the animal's powers of resistance; (2) that the germs shall be present in sufficient numbers; and (3) in certain instances the presence of a specific virus appears to be necessary before the organisms can produce abscesses.

Abscess-forming bacteria generally enter the body by a wound of the skin or mucous membrane, but they may also penetrate by the intestinal mucous membrane when this is in a weakened state through constipation, diarrhœa, inflammation, or from the effects of poisoning. They also invade the lining membranes of the nose, pharynx, throat, mouth, respiratory passages, or bladder, and in some cases they obtain access to the tissues by way of the minute sweat or sebaceous glands of the skin.

When bacteria have gained access they commence to multiply, and by the forma-

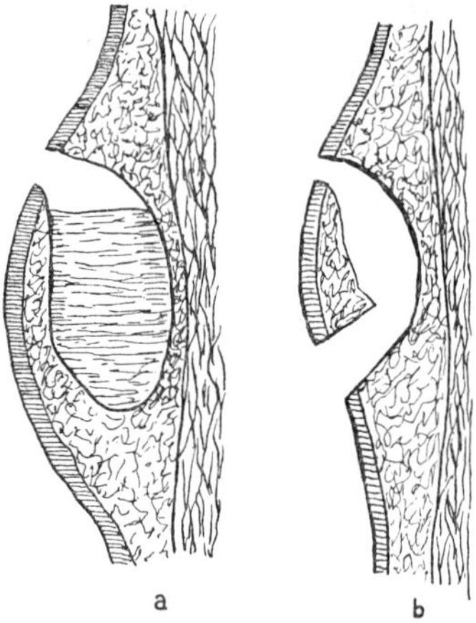

Diagram of section of an abscess which at *a* is not getting drainage for the pus, although the abscess has burst through the skin; *b* shows the effect of a counter-opening, or drainage wound, situated where the pus can escape by gravity.

tion of poisonous substances, among which are ammonia, trimethylamine, and certain 'toxins', they irritate the surrounding tissues, produce dilatation of the blood-vessels, slowing of the blood-stream, and a migration of white blood corpuscles towards themselves. These white blood corpuscles or leucocytes, collect around the invaded area, and there commence to devour, or destroy by the elaboration of fluids, as many of the bacteria as they are able. The white corpuscles themselves may be destroyed by the bacteria, or they may die from other causes. Ultimately the area of invasion becomes congested with dead or dying bacteria, dead or dying leucocytes, dead tissue cells which formerly occupied the site, débris, and a certain amount of fluid exuded from the gorged blood-vessels in the vicinity. This constitutes the pus or 'matter' of the abscess. Meanwhile the area has been cut off from communication with the rest of the body by the plugging of the blood-vessels and the lymph-ducts. The pressure inside the cavity rises as more and more leucocytes flock to the scene of action, and after a time it becomes essential that an outlet should be obtained. If the abscess has been developing near to the surface of the skin, the patch of that tissue lying immediately above the abscess cavity loses its blood-supply and consequently dies. Dead skin is easily dissolved by the contents of the abscess, and finally, when it gives way, the abscess has burst.

Symptoms.—In an abscess there are the classic symptoms of inflammation, *rubor, calor, tumor,* and *dolor, i.e.* redness, warmth, swelling, and pain; and besides these, when the abscess is of large size and is well developed, a considerable amount of fever, the temperature sometimes rising to 105° F., and an interference with the function of the part. 'Pointing' of an abscess means that it has reached that stage when the skin covering it is dead, thin, generally glazed, and bulging. This is only appreciable when the abscess is near to the surface. If it be deeply situated, the skin over the area becomes swollen, is painful, and 'pits' on pressure. The lymph glands in the vicinity become swollen and are tender, while it not infrequently happens that they become the seat of secondary abscess formation, either at the time or soon after. Immediately the abscess bursts, or when it is evacuated by lancing, the pain disappears, the swelling subsides, the temperature falls, and the tissues around regain their normal elasticity. If all the pus has been evacuated the cavity rapidly heals, and only a tiny pit remains. If, however, the abscess has burst into an internal cavity, such as the pleural or peritoneal sacs, into the bladder, or into a part of the bowel, death from a septic infection of the lining of the cavity (in the case of the pleura and peritoneum), or general ill-health for a considerable period, will result. When an abscess is deeply seated so as to be out of reach of diagnosis by manipulative measures, its presence can be confirmed both by blood tests and by a study of the temperature.

Treatment.—The introduction of penicillin and drugs of the sulphanilamide group have greatly facilitated the prevention and treatment of septic infection. These agents may be employed as the sole means of treating multiple or deep-seated abscesses, they may be injected into a cavity following aspiration of the pus, or they may be used in addition to the lancing of an abscess. This may be done as soon as there are sufficient grounds for forming a positive opinion as to the existence of the pus, as denoted by fluctuation, pitting on pressure, etc. Previous to this, the formation of pus in the area can be hastened by the application of a hot poultice, or better still (though not always convenient) by warm fomentations, which also relieve pain. Sometimes warm fomentation for long periods will cause the inflammation to subside without the formation of pus and an abscess; a process that is usually spoken of as 'aborting' the abscess.

When an abscess is to be opened the following points should be kept in mind:

(1) Important arteries, veins, and nerves in the vicinity should not be damaged. This is especially the case in those strangles abscesses that are very common in the throat region of the horse.

(2) The opening should be as far away from any new source of infection, such as the mouth, anus, or prepuce, as possible.

(3) The abscess cavity should always be opened by a large incision so that it will not heal over and imprison any pus which will often result in the formation of a second abscess at the same site.

(4) The opening should always be situated at the lowest part of the cavity so that its discharges will drain away by gravity. Failure to ensure this results in a collection of putrid fluid in the lower parts of the cavity, which will remain in place and form a sinus (*see* SINUS); for this reason it is sometimes necessary to make one or more 'counter-openings' by which the pus may escape. (*See* Diagram.)

After the abscess had been opened it is usually best to leave it uncovered, unless it is in such a position that the animal will bite or scratch it and reinfect the part. If it is necessary to cover the surface a wet pad of lint, or wool soaked in an antiseptic, should be first applied, and over this a piece of oiled silk or rubber-tissue, the whole kept in position by a loosely applied bandage. This dressing must be renewed at least every day if the discharge is copious. In abscesses where the cavity is larger it may be necessary to pack it with gauze, or with cotton-wool impregnated with an antiseptic, and in the most extensive cavities a drainage-tube of rubber is advisable.

Special varieties of acute abscess :

ABSCESS IN BONE (*see* BONE, DISEASES OF).

ABSCESS IN BRAIN.—The formation of an abscess in the brain is usually a secondary condition to some general disease.

ABSCESS IN THE LUNG may follow pneumonia or the intaking of some foreign body into the bronchial tubes, such as the awns of barley. During the course of tuberculosis, glanders, and strangles, abscesses sometimes develop in the lungs.

INTERDIGITAL ABSCESS IN THE DOG.

MAMMARY ABSCESSES may be caused by a piece of straw penetrating the teat-canal of the udder of the cow.

SHOULDER ABSCESSES (*see* SHOULDER TUMOURS).

ABSCESS, CHRONIC. — A chronic abscess is one which takes a long time to develop, seldom bursts, unless near to the surface of the body, and becomes surrounded by large amounts of fibrous tissue.

Causes.—Abscesses due to tuberculosis, actinomycosis, staphylococi, and caseous abscess formation in the lymph glands of sheep, are the most common types of cold or chronic abscesses. They may arise when an acute abscess, instead of bursting in the usual way, becomes surrounded by dense fibrous tissue which imprisons the offending germs, and remains more or less stationary. The tuberculous forms generally appear to be most common in the lymph glands and in certain of the bones, especially those of the neck in the horse. (*See* TUBERCULOSIS.)

Staphylococi cause the common 'shoulder tumour' or 'shoulder abscess', and abscesses following castration of horses and pigs. (*See* BOTRIOMYCOSIS.) (*See also* CASEOUS LYMPHADENITIS OF SHEEP.)

Symptoms.—Swelling may be noticeable on the surface of the body (as in actinomycosis or botriomycosis), or it may show no signs of its presence until the animal is slaughtered (as in the case of many tuberculous abscesses and in lymphadenitis of sheep). If it is present on the surface, it is found to be hard, cold, only very slightly painful, and does not rapidly increase in size. As a rule the health of the patient remains quite good, unless the swelling is in such a position that it will interfere with some of the vital functions of the body, such as swallowing or breathing.

Characters of the pus.—The contained fluid varies in its appearance and its consistence. It may be thin and watery, and contain some flocculi or little curdled masses, or it may be solid or semi-solid. To this latter type the name 'inspissated pus' is given, and the process is often spoken of as 'caseation'. In certain cases, especially in tuberculous abscesses that have been in existence for a long time, the contained material may show small centres of deposition of lime salts, and the name 'calcification' is applied to such a process. In the 'pus-centres' of actinomycosis and botriomycosis the fluid is similar to that found in an acute abscess, *i.e.* it is thick, white, and creamy, but there is generally only a very small amount present in each centre.

Treatment.—This absolutely depends upon the nature of the chronic abscess and its position in the body. Penicillin or the sulphonamide drugs may be employed. In the case of tuberculous abscesses it is not advisable to employ treatment. In nearly all cold abscesses the time taken to effect a cure is considerable, for there is almost always a great amount of fibrous tissue to become absorbed.

ACACIA POISONING has been recorded in cattle and goats. Different species of acacia contain different toxic principles.

ACANTHOSIS.—Increased thickness of the prickle cell layer of the skin.

ACAPNIA (ἀ, neg.; καπνός, smoke) means a condition of diminished carbon dioxide in the blood.

ACARUS (ἄκαρι, a mite) is the name given to a minute parasitic creature belonging to the natural order *Acarina*. This includes the mange mites, harvest mites, follicular mites, cheese mites, etc. (*See* PARASITES, p. 687.)

ACCIDENTS (*accidere*, to happen).—Injuries include almost every possible form of wounding of the skin, of muscles, tendons, blood-vessels, nerves, and internal organs, as well as many varieties of fractures, which are always serious in animals. Death is by no means an uncommon termination.

Horses.—If the horse falls while in harness, the first essential is to secure the head, either by kneeling upon the neck, or by seizing the bridle or the nose of the horse and forcibly pulling it round into such a position that the head and neck are well extended away from the chest, and held with the nose pointing to the sky. The animal will usually lie quiet in this position, when the harness may be loosened or removed, the cart or vehicle pulled back from the animal, and assistance given so that it may regain its feet. If it is unable to rise, expert advice should be sought as rapidly as possible, for the horse may have received some injury to the bones of the limbs, skull, or back which incapacitates it and renders destruction necessary. Meanwhile, it should be made as comfortable as circumstances will allow, by placing a sack or straw under its head, and prevented from doing itself further injury by restraining the head. In the event of the horse being able to rise, obvious injuries may be so slight as to warrant the continuance of the work, but it must be remembered that injuries do not always immediately manifest themselves, and if the horse appears lame or stiff it should be submitted to competent examination. If bleeding is profuse, endeavours should be made to check it by pads of cotton-wool. (*See* BLEEDING, ARREST OF.) Bruises and less severe lacerations call for no immediate attention, provided the horse can walk to its stable, but when extensive, these and sprains or strains should be subjected to hot and cold fomentations alternately (*see* FOMENTATION), and treated subsequently by suitable liniments. Fractures in most cases necessitate destruction, but some are not of such a serious nature.

Cattle, Sheep, Pigs.—These animals meet with accidents less often than horses and dogs, since they are not upon highways of traffic to any great extent. Injuries to cattle by others horning them, by kicks from horses, by falling timber—especially in woods—by bites, by breaking through fences, and by falling into ditches, etc., are among the most common accidents.

Dogs and Cats.—'Run-over accidents' and injuries from fights with other animals are the most usual casualties that befall these creatures, although in towns, cats sometimes fall from great heights on to pavements, etc., and the question of maliciousness must not be forgotten. Apart from fractures, the most frequent form of injury is a tear through skin and muscle; these are to be looked on as infected wounds. (*See* WOUNDS.) If fracture be suspected, no time should be lost in seeking skilled assistance, for diagnosis is incomparably easier and more accurate before the swelling of the injured part masks the physical signs; besides which, the speedy immobilisation of the parts spares the animal much suffering, and makes for more successful healing of the tissues involved.

ACCOMMODATION (*see* EYE).

ACCREDITED.—The Accredited Poultry Breeding Scheme is administered by the National Agriculture Advisory Service, 'to assist poultry keepers in obtaining healthy stock of good quality and to combat the spread of poultry disease, but gave way to the POULTRY HEALTH SCHEME (*which see*).

The Meat and Livestock Commission listed accredited herds of pigs, but this term was abolished in favour of nucleus and reserve nucleus herds, selected by an independent panel and accepted on condition that they joined the official PIG HEALTH SCHEME (*which see*).

For cattle, the Brucellosis (Accredited Herds) Scheme came into operation in 1967 but was replaced in 1970 by the Brucellosis Incentives Scheme as a further step towards eradication of the disease in the U.K. (*See also under* BRUCELLOSIS.)

A.C.E. MIXTURE.—One part alcohol, 2 parts chloroform, 3 parts ether. For use as an anæsthetic by inhalation. (*See* ANÆSTHETICS.)

ACERIN.—A substance obtained from the seeds of the Norway Maple, active *in vitro* against certain viruses.

ACETABULUM (*acetabulum*, a cup) is the cup-shaped depression on the pelvis with which the head of the femur forms the hip-joint. Dislocation of the hip-joint sometimes occurs as the result of 'run-over accidents', and fractures of the pelvis involving the acetabulum frequently result from the same cause. Owing to the extensive muscular coverings and to the important pelvic organs near by, which are liable to be damaged, both dislocations and fractures of this part are difficult to treat with any reasonable hope of complete success. (*See* Hip-Joint, Dislocation, Fracture.)

ACETIC ACID (*acetum*, vinegar), also called 'pyroligneous acid', is prepared in large quantities by the distillation of wood, and subsequent separation from tar. In the pure state it is solid, being then known as 'glacial acetic acid'. It is the active principle of vinegar. Weak acetic acid has all the actions of vinegar and is less expensive. Strong acetic acid is a caustic, and an irritant poison.

Acetic acid poisoning has caused the death of pigs fed a mash which had been allowed to stand. (After 24 hours in a warm place the acetic acid content of the mash reached 5 per cent.)

Acetic acid may also occur in silage and in fermenting hay.

ACETONE.—This is a substance found in small amounts in certain samples of normal urine, and present in greater quantities during the course of diabetes, pneumonia, cancer, starvation, and diseases of disturbed metabolism. Where there is an excessive intake of fats and a deficiency of carbohydrate, or incomplete oxidation of fats, acetone appears in blood (*acetonæmia*) and in urine (*acetonuria*).

ACETONÆMIA and **KETOSIS** are names given to a metabolic disturbance in cattle and sheep. It may be defined as the accumulation in the blood plasma, in significant amounts, of ketone bodies. It may occur at any time, but is commonest in winter in dairy cows kept indoors. Many cases are shown by cows up to about 3 weeks after calving, when receiving a full ration of concentrates. With these at least 6 lb. of hay should be fed daily. Heavy feeding with low-quality silage is stated to be a predisposing factor. It often follows hypomagnesæmia. It is very rare in heifers and seldom occurs before the 3rd calving.

Cause.—Whenever the glucose level in the blood plasma is low, as in starvation or on a low carbohydrate diet, or when glucose is not utilisable, as in diabetes, the concentration of free fatty acids in the plasma rises. This rise is roughly paralleled by an increase in the concentration of ketone bodies, which provide a third source of energy. In other words the moderate ketosis which occurs under a variety of circumstances is to be looked upon as a normal physiological process supplying the tissues with a readily utilisable fuel of respiration when glucose is scarce.

By contrast, the severe forms of ketosis met with in the lactating cow and the diabetic cow, and characterised by high concentrations of ketone bodies in the blood and urine, are obviously harmful pathological conditions where the quantities of ketone bodies formed grossly exceed possible needs. (*See also under* Ketone Bodies.)

Vigue (1963) found that there was a higher incidence of ketosis in cows which had been fed on low-quality roughage and low-protein concentrates (10 to 12 per cent), than in those which had been fed good roughage and high-protein concentrates (16 to 20 per cent).

Symptoms.—The cow ceases to feed normally, but may lick or chew the walls, chain, head-rope, or other objects. Depression is marked, but short periods of what would seem to be delirium may be shown, when the cow may become excited. Constipation and decrease in urine secretion occur, and rumination either ceases or is intermittent. Milk secretion is reduced. This may be the first symptom.

A peculiar sickly sweet odour (the odour of acetone) can be perceived from breath, urine, milk, and even from the skin in established cases. It is upon the presence of acetone in the body secretions, etc., that a diagnosis is based. To confirm the diagnosis a chemical test (Rothera's test) may be carried out.

Treatment.—The animal must be removed to a loose-box and made comfortable. Large quantities of glucose by injection are recommended (*Vet. Record* Feb. 5, 1966). Two or three tablespoonfuls of glycerine should be tried as a first-aid measure in sheep; half a pint for the cow, given with a little water in each case. Black treacle (half a pound in water) is the next best thing.

Resistant cases are met with which defy all treatment, the cow improves up to a point but does not feed properly and dies in 10 to 20 days.

Feeding should include adequate hay after recovery and exercise is important.

ACETONURIA means that acetone is present in the urine. It often accompanies acetonæmia.

ACETYLCHOLINE is a drug which in common with choline but in a more marked degree possesses the power to reduce arterial pressure and to stimulate peristalsis. It is given by injection and is of great use in a large number of abdominal disturbances in which gas formation, paralysis of intestinal movement, and 'abdominal shock' are in evidence. It is sometimes of great use in colic in horses.

Acetylcholine is produced in the areas of the nerve endings of the neuro-muscular system and is a link in the transmission of nerve impulse to the muscles controlled by each nerve. In cases of pain, shock, injury, etc., the normal supply may fail, so that nerve impulses cannot reach the muscle fibres and paralysis results. The administration of acetylcholine serves to correct this deficiency.

In health, acetylcholine is destroyed as soon as a nerve impulse has passed, by the enzyme cholesterinase. This, however, is itself destroyed by exposure to organic phosphorus insecticides; resulting in poisoning—convulsions and death. Excessive salivation is an important symptom in dogs so poisoned.

ACHONDROPLASIA (ἀ, neg.; χόνδρος, cartilage; πλάσσω, I form) is the name given to a form of dwarfing due to disease affecting the long bones of the limbs before birth. It is noticed in some calves of certain breeds of cattle such as the Dexter, and in some breeds of dogs.

ACHORION (ἄχωρ, dandruff) is a microscopic fungus causing favus or 'honeycomb ringworm'. (*See* RINGWORM.)

ACHROMYCIN is a chemically altered form of the antibiotic Aureomycin, over which it is claimed to have certain advantages.

ACHYLIA (ἀ neg.; χυλος, juice) means absence of chyle due to the absence or great diminution of the gastric ferments, so that in this condition the food is passed from the stomach in a state of incomplete digestion.

ACID-FAST ORGANISMS are those which, when once stained with carbolfuchsin dye, possess the power to retain their colour after immersion in strong acid solutions, which decolorise the non-acid-fast group. The method serves to differentiate between organisms belonging to the two classes. The more important of the acid-fast group are *Mycobacterium tuberculosis*, causing tuberculosis in man and animals; *M. paratuberculosis*, the cause of Johne's disease; and *M. lepros*æ, causing human leprosy. Many other non-pathogenic types are also encountered in sewage, dung, ear-wax, smegma, butter, and one, the *M. phlei*, occurs frequently on Timothy grass and may be mistaken for the *M. tuberculosis*.

ACIDOSIS.—A condition of reduced alkaline reserve of the blood and tissues, with or without an actual fall in pH. Sudden death may occur in cattle from acidosis after gorging on grain. (*See also* BARLEY POISONING.)

ACIDS.—These are substances which combine with alkalies to form salts. Most of them are oxygen compounds; they have a sour taste, and turn litmus red. They are divided into: (*a*) Inorganic, such as sulphuric, arsenious, phosphoric; and (*b*) Organic, such as acetic, citric, salicylic, and tannic acids.

ACIDS, POISONING BY.—It occasionally happens that animals are either accidentally or maliciously poisoned.

Symptoms.—Excessive salivation, great pain, and destruction of the mucous membrane lining the mouth (which causes the unfortunate animal to keep its mouth open and protrude its tongue), are seen. After a short time convulsive seizures and vomiting occur, and general collapse follows; while if a large amount of acid has been taken, death from shock rapidly supervenes. In those cases of poisoning by odorous acids the characteristic smell associated with the acid may be evident on examination of the mouth.

Treatment.—Alkaline demulcents should be given at once and in large quantities; bicarbonate of sodium or potassium, washing soda, chalk or slaked lime, given in gruels or barley-water or milk, are all quite useful. These neutralise the acids into harmless salts, and soothe the corroded and burnt tissues. They require to be given at once, since the greater the delay the greater the damage done, and the greater the amount of acid absorbed. Poisoning by particular acids which require special antidotes is treated under the respective headings of such acids. (*See* ACETIC ACID, ARSENIOUS ACID, CARBOLIC ACID, HYDROCYANIC ACID, OXALIC ACID, etc.)

ACINUS (*acinus*, a grape) is the name

applied to each of the minute sacs of which secreting glands are composed, and which usually cluster round the branches of the gland-duct like grapes on their stem.

ACNE.—An inflammation of sebaceous glands or hair follicles, with the formation of pustules.

ACNE, CONTAGIOUS.—The synonyms of this affection are many, but among the most common may be mentioned contagious pustular dermatitis, and Canadian horse-pox.

Contagious acne is a contagious affection of the skin of horses caused by the Preisz-Nocard bacillus (*Corynebacterium ovis*), and characterised by the formation of pustules; these, on bursting, liberate a quantity of thick sticky pus which rapidly dries and leaves a yellow crust. It appears to have been introduced into Great Britain by the importation of Canadian horses, and German authorities maintain that it was first brought to Germany by horses imported from England.

It is spread from one horse to another either by direct contact, or by means of the harness, grooming tools, clothing, etc., from an infected case being used upon a healthy animal. Those parts of the body in contact with the harness are most often affected, and parts that are irritated, wounded, bruised, or inflamed are more susceptible than the healthy skin. The period of incubation varies between 3 and 14 days, most cases occurring about one week after exposure to infection.

Symptoms.—Two forms are recognised—a *benign* and a *severe*. In both varieties the areas affected are: the skin of the back, the croup and shoulders, and more rarely the head, neck, and extremities.

In the *benign* form the involved skin presents a number of small round or oval prominences surrounded by hot and slightly painful areas. These prominences become covered with two or three vesicles in the case of the smaller types, while the larger raised areas may show as many as twenty. The vesicles develop into pustules, and these, after a variable time, burst and discharge a quantity of pus which on drying forms a yellowish-coloured crust, gluing together the hairs in the near vicinity. In about 7 or 8 days the crusts fall off, carrying with them the matted hairs, and leaving circular bare spots. No evidence of itchiness accompanies the formation of these lesions, and no general symptoms are shown.

In the rare *severe* form, the pustules, after they have developed, become confluent, and large areas of the surface of the body are affected. The virulence of the infection increases, and the skin tends to become thickened, with the production of large suppurating cavities, which, in some cases, extend into the underlying tissues.

Treatment.—The horse should at once be withdrawn from work and strictly isolated. Articles that are likely to be contaminated with the discharges, etc., as well as the litter, must be rendered safe by suitable disinfection or disposal. The skin lesions may be treated with astringent lotions if the attack be a mild one; but antibiotics are more effective.

Attendants should be warned that contagious acne is liable to affect man; washing of the hands in disinfectants after handling a case should not be neglected.

ACONITE (*Aconitum napellus*, commonly known as 'Monkshood', 'Wolfsbane', 'Blue-Rocket', etc.).—Aconite is an extremely poisonous plant found in all parts of the world, but especially in the cooler mountainous parts of both hemispheres. It is frequently cultivated in gardens in Great Britain for its decorative appearances. All parts of the plant are

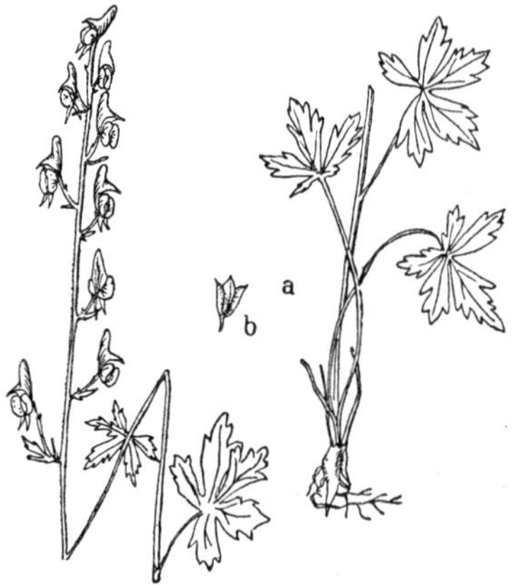

Aconite (*Aconitum napellus*). *a*, Root and stem with flowering top on left; *b*, seed capsule. The flowers are either blue or yellow, and are characterised by one of the petals assuming the shape of a helmet or hood, hence the name, Monkshood. All parts of the plant are poisonous.

poisonous, the parts above the ground being often eaten by stock (see later). Aconite owes its poisonous properties to an alkaloid (*Aconitine*), mainly found in the tuberous root, but present in smaller amounts in other parts of the plant.

Aconitine is irritant in large doses, but smaller doses have a sedative and paralysing effect on the sensory nerves.

Uses.—Locally applied, in virtue of its action on sensory nerves, it first produces irritation, tingling, and twitching, and later numbness and anæsthesia, while the muscular movements are slowed. In this manner it is sometimes employed as a liniment in painful swollen conditions. On account of the risks attending its administration, it should on no account be used indiscriminately by animal-owners.

ACONITE POISONING.—Poisoning by aconite generally occurs when herbivorous animals gain access to gardens in which the plant is cultivated for ornamental purposes and eat its upper parts. Pigs rooting in fields where it grows (especially on the continent of Europe) sometimes eat the horse-radish-like root with toxic results. Occasionally poisoning by an overdose of the strong tincture, given in mistake for the weaker, has occurred.

Symptoms.—The chief symptoms shown are general depression, loss of appetite, salivation, inflammation of the mucous membrane of the mouth and jaws, grinding of the teeth; pigs are nauseated and may vomit; and horses become restless and may be attacked with colic. Animals walk with an unsteady gait, and later become paralysed in their hind-limbs. The pulse becomes feeble or almost imperceptible, and unconsciousness is followed by convulsions and death.

Treatment.—Animals which have eaten aconite should be secured at once in a convenient building. An emetic must be given to the pig, dog, and cat to induce vomiting, and the stomach-tube should be passed in the large herbivorous animals that do not vomit. Stimulants, such as strong black tea or coffee, should be given by the mouth.

ACOPROSIS.—Absence or scantiness of fæcal matter in the intestines.

ACORN POISONING (*see under* OAK).

ACRIFLAVINE is the official name of the antiseptic flavine, a member of the acridine series. It is an orange or red crystalline powder; fluorescent in aqueous solution. Perhaps the most effective antiseptic against Gram-negative bacteria. Unlike most antiseptics it is quite harmless to the tissues, and being a potent germicide it need only be used in weak solution, one part dissolved in one thousand of boiled or distilled water making an excellent wound lotion, effective in the presence of pus. (*See* ANTISEPTICS.) Synergistic with the sulphonamides.

ACROPACHIA.—A condition in which new bone is laid down, first in the limbs and later in other parts of the skeleton. It may accompany tumours and tuberculosis in the dog.

A.C.T.H.—ADRENOCORTICOTROPHIN (*see* CORTICOTROPHIN).

ACTINOBACILLOSIS (ἀκτίς, a ray; *bacillus*, a little rod).—This is a disease of cattle similar in some respects to actinomycosis, and sometimes mistaken for it. (*See* ACTINOMYCOSIS.) It is widely distributed throughout temperate countries wherever cattle are kept under conditions of domestication, and while it does occur in cattle out at grass, it is not so common in them.

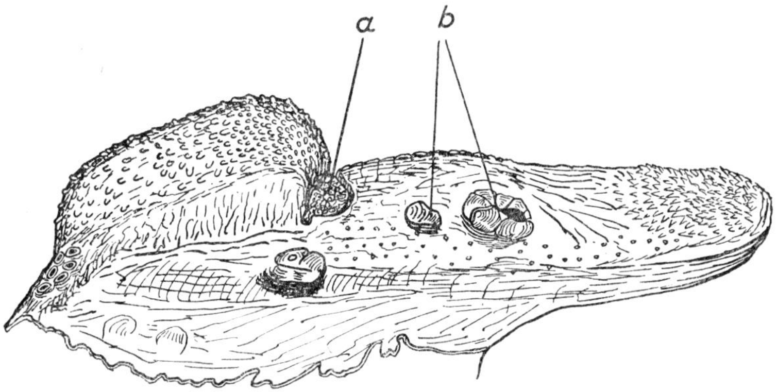

Actinobacillosis lesions on the tongue of ox. *a*, Lesion in the dorsal groove of the tongue; *b*, lesion on the surface.

Generally only one or two animals in a herd are affected at one time.

The disease occurs also in sheep, when the colloquial name 'Cruels' is sometimes applied to it. Swellings may be seen on the lips, cheeks, jaw, and at the base of the horn. Pneumonia, infection of the liver or alimentary canal may lead to death in untreated cases.

Cause.—Actinobacillosis is due to infection of the tissues with the organism *Actinobacillus lignièresi*. These are arranged at the centre of the lesions in a radiating manner. Infection occurs through injuries, abrasions, etc., of soft tissues, and when lymph glands are affected through invasion along the lymph vessels. Occasionally subcutaneous tissue may be involved without apparent lesions in the lymph glands. Abscesses form.

Lesions may involve the lungs, rumen, omasum, abomasum, and reticulum. A case of genital actinobacillosis in a bull was reported by the Milk Marketing Board in 1971. The semen at first appeared normal, but clots formed five minutes after collection. There were no lesions which could be felt.

Symptoms.—When lymph glands in the throat are affected, the swelling and pressure caused may make swallowing and breathing difficult; if the lesion is in the skin and superficial tissues only, it may attain to a great size without causing much trouble; when the tongue is affected the animal has difficulty in mastication and swallowing and there is usually a constant dribbling of saliva from the mouth. If this is examined there may be found in it small greyish or greyish-yellow flocculi, the so-called 'pus spots', in which the organism can be demonstrated by microscopic methods.

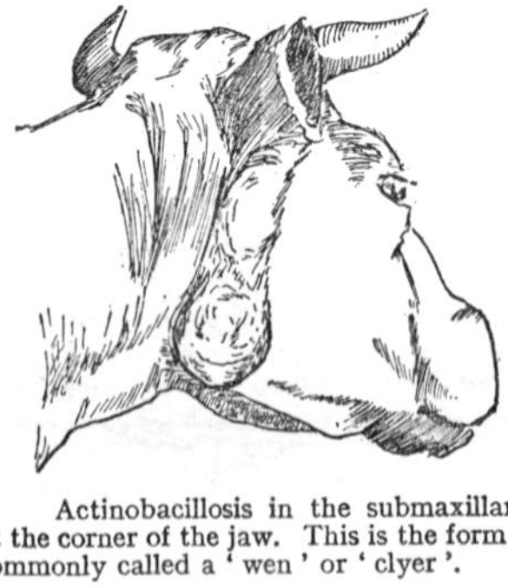

Actinobacillosis in the submaxillary gland at the corner of the jaw. This is the form which is commonly called a 'wen' or 'clyer'.

Later, the saliva may become thick, purulent, and foul smelling, and resemble pus from a wound. Saliva may show similar changes when the organisms are located in the mucous membrane of the cheeks, in the muscles of the soft palate or pharynx, or in the salivary glands.

When the swellings are near the surface, there is a copious discharge of thick creamy or greyish pus, after the abscesses have burst. This may gum the hairs together and pieces of straw, dust, chaff, etc., adhere to the surface. The skin may lose its hair and appear scalded and inflamed around the discharging sinus.

In those cases where feeding or breathing are hindered, animals, especially bullocks, rapidly lose flesh, and if neglected severe emaciation may occur, occasionally resulting in death. In cows, the yield of milk may be greatly reduced, especially where pain is severe, or feeding is difficult.

Treatment.—The intravenous injection of sodium iodide has made the treatment of this condition easier than formerly. There are many cases which show a complete recovery with only one or two injections. Antibiotics may also be tried.

The treatment of actinobacillosis is not always successful, and it is sometimes advisable to slaughter a fat bullock rather than to treat it.

Precautions.—The disease can be transmitted to man. Accordingly, care must be taken over washing the hands, etc., after handling an animal with actinobacillosis.

ACTINOMYCOSIS (ἀκτίς, a ray; μύκης, a fungus).—This disease has been known for many years, and before actinobacillosis was differentiated from it, a large number of cases of the latter were included as actinomycosis. It is called by many popular names, such as 'Lumpy jaw', and has been recorded in very many species of animals, including man, dogs, pigs, birds, and reptiles.

It is found, like actinobacillosis, in nearly all temperate countries.

One affected animal may occasionally infect others, but this is not usual, and in the absence of injury by which the pus or discharges from another animal can gain access, there is very little likelihood that in-contact animals will be affected.

The lesions produced bear a considerable resemblance to those of actinobacillosis, and are often indistinguishable from them, but typically actinomycosis affects the cheeks, pharynx and occasionally the nose, bone and periosteum of the

ACTINOMYCOSIS

jaws, and other bones of the skull, while actinobacillosis is more likely to attack soft tissues only. When bone and periosteum become affected by actinomycosis, the soft tissues adjacent usually become involved as the disease progresses, which may lead to a difficulty in diagnosis.

Cause is the so-called 'ray fungus'—*Actinomyces bovis*, an anærobic organism. It is present in the digestive system of cattle, and it is probable that it can only become pathogenic by invading the tissues through a wound. It is common during the ages when the permanent cheek teeth are cutting the gums and pushing out the milk teeth. It may then be carried into the tooth sockets by barley awns, pieces of straw, etc. The abdominal organs, especially the liver, are sometimes affected, while actinomycosis and actinobacillosis have both been found in lungs and bronchi.

Symptoms.—When the invading organism has gained entrance into the living tissues, a reaction of the cells of the part results, with the production of a small hard nodule around the foreign intruder. The fungus commences to increase in size, and, spreading deeper and wider from its original situation, causes a corresponding increase in the amount of body reaction, and consequently in the size of the swelling. The swelling in bone or other tissue is mainly composed of dense fibrous tissue and it may reach considerable dimensions causing interference with the function of the affected part, with resulting difficulty in mastication, in swallowing, or in breathing, depending on the situation of the lesion. In most cases when the mouth or throat is affected, there is a constant dribbling of saliva in varying amounts from the mouth. In the earlier stages this saliva is normal in its appearance, but later becomes offensive.

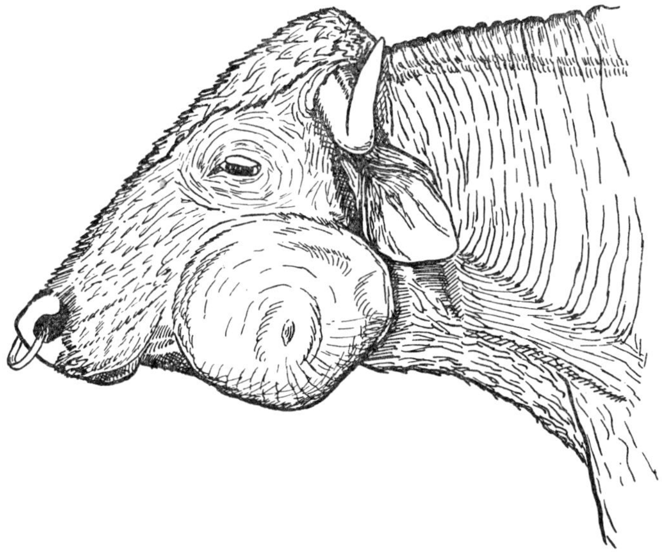

Actinomycosis affecting the left side of the face of the bull. The swelling involves the bones and muscles of the jaws, and makes chewing difficult.

The terms 'wens' and 'clyers' are generally reserved for swellings of the lymph glands at the corner of the jaw, or in the skin of that region. Many of these are actually actinobacillosis, and the terms are rather loosely used. The size varies from that of a walnut to that of a child's head in extreme cases. This form of the disease appears to be most commonly encountered in the Fen districts of England and in the north-western States of America.

Actinomycosis of the bone of the upper and lower jaws produces an increase in the size of the part and a rarefication of its bony structure, the spaces becoming filled with the proliferation of fibrous tissue which is characteristic of the disease.

When the udder is affected, hard fibrous nodules may be felt below the skin, varying in size from that of a pea to a walnut or larger, and firmly embedded in the structure of the gland itself. These swellings enclose soft centres of suppuration which, on occasions, may either burst through the covering skin, or else into an adjacent milk sinus or duct. The milk from such a cow should not be used for human consumption because of the danger of the consumer contracting the disease.

Treatment.—The use of penicillin or streptomycin. Sulpha drugs assist recovery. (*See also* ACTINOBACILLOSIS.) (*See* PRECAUTIONS *on* p. 18.)

ACTINORUBIN.—An antibiotic isolated from cultures of a strain (A.105) of *Actinomyces*. Active against certain micro-organisms, *e.g. Brucella abortus, B. anthracis, Salmonella enteritidis, Staphylococcus aureus*.

ACTIVE PRINCIPLES are the substances in a drug which are responsible for its effects. Many are alkaloids, others are glucosides or saponins. They are mostly able to be extracted from the crude drug, formed into salts (sulphates, hydrobromides, salicylates, etc.), and when dissolved in water are used as hypodermic injections. For example, the alkaloid morphine is the chief active principle of the crude drug opium. (*See* ALKALOIDS, GLUCOSIDES, SAPONINS.)

ACTUAL CAUTERY is the method of burning by a heated body, as distinct from 'potential cautery', which owes its action to chemical activity.

ACUARIA UNCINATA.—This roundworm has caused outbreaks of disease in geese, ducks, and poultry. The life-cycle of this parasite involves an intermediate host, *Daphnia pulex*, the water flea. On post-mortem examination of affected birds, worms may be found in nodules scattered over the mucous membrane of the œsophagus and proventriculus. Mortality may be high among geese and ducks.

ACUTE DISEASE.—A disease is called acute in contradistinction to 'chronic' when it appears rapidly, and either causes death quickly or leads to a speedy recovery. As examples of acute disease in the lower animals, anthrax and black-quarter (where the animal may be dead within 12 hours), acute pneumonia, and acute distemper, may be mentioned. Sometimes 'acute' is used as an indication of a very severe painful condition.

***AD LIB.* FEEDING** is a labour-saving system under which pigs or poultry help themselves to dry meal, etc., and eat as much as they wish. The self-feeding of silage to cattle might also come under this heading. (*See also* DRY-FEEDING.)

ADDITIVES.—Substances added to a compound or a protein concentrate in the course of manufacture for some specific purpose other than as a direct source of nutrient.

The current list of additives is a long one, and includes such diverse products as those for treating ringworm in cattle and horses without the necessity to handle the animals; vitamin, mineral and trace element additives; those containing urea; additives for planned moulting in laying hens; and those for the control of worm infestations, coccidiosis, and 'scours' in pigs, respectively. In 1971, following the recommendations of the Swann Committee, regulations made under the Therapeutic Substances Act 1956 came into force, making unlawful the retail sale or supply of feeds containing penicillin, chlortetracycline (Aureomycin), oxytetracycline (Terramycin) and tylosin 'unless on prescription or in accordance with a written authority of a veterinary surgeon'. In other words, these antibiotics will not be feed antibiotics, in terms of the Swann Committee Report, and are placed in the category of therapeutic antibiotics.

Under the same regulations other antibacterial agents are no longer obtainable as feed additives unless prescribed. They are: four nitrofurans (nitrofurazone, furazolidone, nitrofurantoin, and furaltadone) plus the sulphonamides. There are two relevant exceptions in the case of the sulphonamides in that, subject to certain conditions, sulphaquinoxaline and sulphanitran may be included in poultry feeds as coccidiostats.

Feed antibiotics, obtainable without prescription for adding to animal feeds as growth promotants, number three: Flavomycin, virginiamycin, and zinc bacitracin. The criteria for their inclusion in this category, as laid down by the Swann Committee, are that they must: (1) be of economic value in livestock production under UK farming conditions; (2) have little or no application as therapeutic agents in man or animals; and (3) must not impair the efficacy of a prescribed therapeutic antibiotic or antibiotics through the development of resistant strains of organisms. In addition to these freely available feed antibiotics, continuing use may be made of copper sulphate and of the three arsenicals listed in Table 2, plus a new quinoxaline additive, and Emtryl containing dimetridazole, newly introduced as a specific for the control of swine dysentery.

TABLE 1. ON PRESCRIPTION ONLY

THERAPEUTIC antibacterial agents

Antibiotics	Penicillin Chlortetracycline Oxytetracycline Tylosin
Nitrofurans	Nitrofurazone Furazolidone Nitrofurantoin Furaltadone

Sulphonamides—except that sulphanilamide may be used for wound dressings; sulphaquinoxaline and sulphanitran may be used as coccidiostats.

TABLE 2. FREELY AVAILABLE

FEED antibiotics

Zinc bacitracin (for poultry, pig, calf and lamb feeds)
Flavomycin (moenomycin) (for poultry and pig feeds)
Virginiamycin (for poultry feeds)

Other additives

Copper sulphate	Nifursol
Arsanilic acid/ sodium arsanilate	Nitrovin (Payzone)
	Carbasone
Quinoxaline-di-N-oxide (Grofas)	3 nitro-4-hydroxy-phenylarsonic acid
Dimetridazole (Emtryl)	

The object of these regulations is to ensure as far as possible that the benefits gained from the use of antibiotics in animal feeds are not offset by hazards to human and animal health. The benefits may include a faster growth rate, a more efficient use of food, and the possibility of successfully rearing unthrifty or runt pigs.

It has to be admitted that antibiotics have been widely used at low dosage, often in large quantities on a hit-or-miss basis—to mitigate the effects of stress.

Admittedly, not all stress can be avoided, *e.g.* that arising at weaning or resulting from the mixing of litters, castration, etc. At such times the veterinary surgeon will, if circumstances warrant it, prescribe a suitable drug *at full dosage for a brief period.* He may well do the same thing if convinced of the need for what has come to be called 'blanket coverage', where animals are in contact with others suffering from disease, or where exposure to infection is thought to have occurred, or is likely to arise in the immediate future. The danger of using therapeutic drugs at less than the full therapeutic dosage was emphasised by the Swann Committee in view of transferable drug resistance. This is very important from the public health angle, and concerns the farmer and his family as much as the urban consumer of his produce. For example, UK strains of *Salmonella typhimurium*, notorious as a cause of scouring in farm animals and of 'food poisoning' in man, are already resistant to several antibiotics and other antibacterial agents. This means that medical treatment may become difficult or impossible, and that a person's life could be endangered.

With regard to future development, it is likely that new products will be submitted for approval as feed additives. (*See also under* FEED ANTIBIOTICS.)

ADENITIS (ἀδήν, a gland) means inflammation of a gland. (*See* LYMPHADENITIS; PAROTID GLAND, DISEASES OF.)

ADENOMA (ἀδήν, a gland; *-oma* termination meaning a tumour).—An adenoma is a non-inflammatory new growth or tumour which presents the appearance of gland tissue when viewed under the microscope. Adenomata are commonly found in positions where gland tissue is not normally present. (*See* TUMOURS, CARCINOMATA.)

ADENOVIRUS.—This is a contraction of the original term 'adenoidal-pharyngeal conjunctival agents'. These cause canine virus hepatitis, warts, respiratory disease in cattle, scouring in pigs, etc.

ADHESIONS.—Adhesions occur by the uniting or growing together of structures or organs which are normally separate and freely movable. They are generally the result of acute or chronic inflammation, and in the earlier stages the uniting material is fibrin, which later becomes resolved into fibrous tissues.

Causes.—Inflammation of a serous membrane results in the pouring out of a fluid serum, or of semi-viscid flocculent material, which, in the case of a covering layer of membrane (visceral pleura or peritoneum), adheres to a similar deposit thrown out on the inside of the chest or abdominal wall by the lining layer of the membrane (parietal pleura or peritoneum).

Sometimes the deposit occurs between adjacent folds of the serous membrane covering two or more organs which touch each other, as when a foreign body penetrates from the stomach towards the liver or some part of the intestines, and the organs involved become coherent from the resulting adhesion. The surfaces involved become glued together during the course of the inflammation, limiting the normal movement, and in the majority of cases being attended with considerable pain. With recovery, a resolution of this fibrinous material should take place and almost complete absorption result, but when the causal inflammation was very acute, or when recovery was prolonged, the extravasated fibrin is not removed in its entirety, and adhesions result. In these latter cases the fibrinous material becomes organised or colonised by fibrous tissue cells, and ultimately a strong fibrous band binds the two previously freely movable surfaces to each other. In the case of pleurisy the outer surface of the affected lung adheres to the inside of the chest wall or to some other pleural surface; in peritonitis an abdominal organ may adhere to another organ or to the abdominal wall; in sprained tendons in the horse, the affected structures adhere to surrounding skin, to other tendons, to bones, or to ligaments, etc., with consequent interference with the normal functions of the parts affected.

Symptoms.—Shortness of breath after an attack of pleurisy, the recurrence of colic or indigestion following a laparotomy (the opening of the abdominal cavity by surgical means), continued lameness or stiffness of a limb subsequent to sprain of a tendon or ligament, or after some joint disease, unfruitful coition following a difficult parturition, are all suggestive of adhesions.

Treatment.—Surgical division of the obstructing bands is often necessary in the abdominal cavity and in adhesions of the walls of the vagina following injuries received at a previous parturition. (*See* PLEURISY, PERITONITIS, etc.)

ADIPOSE TISSUE, or FAT (*adeps*, fat)—This consists of a loose matrix or network of fibrous tissue in the spaces of which lie cell envelopes each distended with several small globules, or one large globule, of fat. Tissue of this structure replaces fibrous tissue under the skin, between muscles and muscle fibres, etc., when the amount of food taken is in excess of the needs of the healthy body. During periods of excessive muscular exercise, or when an insufficiency of food is taken, or during debilitating disease, this store is drawn upon and utilised by the body. In such cases each cell yields up its fat-content to the blood, thereby growing smaller and smaller until once more the tissue structure resembles ordinary fibrous tissue.

ADRENAL GLANDS (*ad*, prefix meaning to-; *ren*, kidney), also called SUPRARENAL GLAND, are two small organs situated at the anterior extremities of the kidneys, one on either side of the body. These organs belong to the class of ductless glands, or endocrine organs, which are remarkable in that their secretions are poured into the blood-stream direct, instead of gaining another part of the body by a duct. Their size varies in the different animals, and also at different stages in the life of the individual. In the horse they measure about 3½ inches long and ½ an inch thick, and weigh one to two ounces, while in other animals they are comparatively small.

Structure.—An adrenal gland consists of an outer capsule of fibrous tissue enclosing the gland substance proper. When cut through, it is seen to be formed of two very distinct parts: an outer, firm, red-brown, *cortical* layer, and an inner, soft, yellow, *medullary* centre. In the cortical substance the cells are arranged in long columns radiating outwards from the centre. If these are followed inwards the columnar appearance gives place to an irregular arrangement with numerous blood-vessels of considerable size, and in the middle of the gland is a central vein.

Function.—In common with the other ductless glands of the body, much yet remains to be learned concerning their function. Removal of the adrenals is rapidly followed by death, preceded by muscular prostration and a fall in blood-pressure. The adrenals produce more than one hormone, but the best known is *adrenalin.*

ADRENALIN is the name given to an extract of the adrenal glands of various animals, chiefly sheep, which is used in medicine and surgery. The active principle of this extract (one of the internal secretious or hormones) was first prepared in 1901. In the purified form it consists of a white crystalline substance, but for use it is dissolved in distilled water, and employed as a 1-in-1000 solution. Its chief property is that of raising the tone of all involuntary muscle fibres, stimulating the heart, constricting the walls of the smaller arteries, and producing a rise in the blood-pressure. It is used for checking capillary hæmorrhage in wounds, for warding off shock or collapse by raising the blood-pressure, and is frequently used as a constituent of local anæsthetic solutions, where it limits the area of insensibility. It gives good temporary results in acutely inflamed conditions, *e.g.* in conjunctivitis it is dropped into the pouch of the eyelid; in laminitis it is injected into the digital region of the horse's foot; in each case it reduces the inflammation by contracting the gorged and swollen arterioles and capillaries. The action of adrenalin is fleeting, however, and in from 2 to 4 hours the area to which it was applied is found to be as acutely inflamed as before; in fact, the inflammation may be even greater. Its use is consequently restricted to special cases.

Other substances of similar composition are suprarenin, adnephrin, vasoconstrictine, renaglandin, hemisine, etc. Many of these are now frequently prepared synthetically. (*See* ADRENAL GLANDS.)

ADRENOCORTICOTROPHIN. — Commonly abbreviated to A.C.T.H. It has been used in the treatment of acetonæmia in cattle, and is a naturally occurring hormone obtained from the anterior pituitary glands.

ADULTERATION OF FOOD-STUFFS.— At one time food-stuffs put on the market for animal consumption were very grossly adulterated, but since the passing of the Food-Stuffs and Fertilisers Act in Britain the practice has become much less frequent.

One of the commonest methods of adulterating, or 'faking', foods is to add to the bulk a small proportion of an inferior article, which may be damaged or musty. This addition may be actually harmless, or it may be extremely dangerous. In almost all cases the unscrupulous vendor aims at adding an adulterant which is difficult of detection, and which has a cheaper market value than the bulk of the food-stuffs. The chemical detection of adulterated foods is often very difficult if not impossible, but there is a method which, although tedious, is reasonably certain. This consists in the taking of a sample of the suspected food-stuff, separating the various particles by means of graded sieves, and examining the resultant pieces of similar size, by means of the naked eye and the microscope, either stained or unstained.

An example of an adulterated food would be bean meal, sold and invoiced as such, which is found to contain an admixture of mill sweepings, finely ground oat husks, coarse barley dust, or other mill refuse. It sometimes happens that a compound feeding meal has as an adulterant a small proportion of finely ground poisonous lupin seeds or extracted castor bean meal incorporated with it in such a cunning way that provided it is thoroughly mixed no harmful effects are likely to accrue from its use. There is always the risk, however, that some of the poisonous substance has not been properly mixed, or has gathered into a mass (called 'pocketing'), and one or two animals unlucky enough to eat this unmixed portion may become fatally ill. Detection in such cases is very much more difficult than ordinary.

Mixed horse-feed (commonly called 'chop') frequently contains inferior oats, or 'sport oats', obtained from the large milling establishments, and are so bruised and disguised that they pass for sound oats upon casual examination. Such oats, as well as barley and oat husks and lentil and bean shells, often command a price far above their actual nutritive value.

Among adulterants found from time to time in animals' feeding stuffs are the following: Sawdust in maize; French chalk in barley meal; castor seeds or castor seed husks in various oil-cakes; rape or mustard seeds in linseed cake; Lathyrus peas in pea meal; Java beans and Rangoon bean pickings in bean meal; ground-up oat husks and various offals from mills in bean and pea meals, or in calf meals; wheat and other cereal screenings in poultry foods and game-bird foods; etc. In the case of adulterants in poultry food it should be remembered that they often contain common weed seeds which are objectionable for two reasons: (1) some are poisonous, and (2) when grain is spread on cultivated land for poultry to pick up, many of the weed seeds germinate in the ground.

One other example of adulteration must be given, *i.e.* the mixing of herring or other offals with white-fish meals. Manufacturers of the better class of fish meals give a reliable guarantee that their product does not contain any deleterious offal, and prospective purchasers of this material are well advised to demand such a guarantee before buying. (*See also under* BONE-MEAL.)

ADYNAMIC (ἀ, neg, δυναμις, power) means a state of great depression of vital power occurring in disease. The animal lies in a weak, almost or quite unconscious state, the pulse may either be just perceptible, or cannot be felt at all, the respirations are shallow, irregular, or 'sighing', and the temperature is usually subnormal.

ÆROBE (ἀήρ, air ; βιόω, I live) is the name given to micro-organisms which require oxygen, and consequently air, before they can grow and multiply. Many such organisms are pathogenic, producing disease in animals or man, *e.g. B. anthracis*. (Cf. ANÆROBES.)

ÆROSOL.—A liquid agent or solution dispersed in air in the form of a fine mist for insecticidal and other purposes. If ærosols are used over a long period, *e.g.* by a continuous evaporator, thought must be given to the effect of the chemicals used (a) on the health of the livestock; (b) on organo-chlorine, DDT or other residues left in the carcase to the detriment of people eating the meat; (c) on the health of the stockmen.

ÆROSPORIN.—An antibiotic.

ÆROTROPISM.—The tendency of micro-organisms to group themselves about a bubble of air in culture media.

ÆTHER (*see* ETHER, ANÆSTHETICS).

ÆTIOLOGY (αἰτία, cause ; λόγος, a discourse).—That part of the subject of medicine in which the causes of disease are studied is called ætiology.

AFFERENT (*afferens*, carrying towards) is the name given to nerve fibres or tracts which carry impulses in towards the central nervous system to distinguish from efferent fibres which conduct impulses outwards to organs or tissues. Broadly speaking, afferent fibres have mainly sensory functions, while efferent fibres are concerned with activities of organs, such as movement, secretion, vascular changes, etc.

AFLATOXIN.—A toxin produced by the fungus *Aspergillus flavus* and the cause of poisoning in animals eating contaminated GROUNDNUT MEAL (which see). While not yet proven, evidence strongly supports the idea that aflatoxin is a carcinogen, giving rise to cancer of the liver. A 100 per cent incidence of this was found in young pigs which survived symptoms typical of groundnut poisoning in a 1945 outbreak in Morocco.

AFRICAN HORSE SICKNESS (*see* HORSE SICKNESS, AFRICAN).

AFRICAN SWINE FEVER (*see entry after* SWINE FEVER).

AFRIKANER.—A synonym for Brahman or Zebu cattle.

AFTERBIRTH, PLACENTA, 'CLEANSING', etc., are the names given to the fœtal membranes which serve as a connection between the dam and its offspring while the latter is retained in the womb, and which are expelled from the uterus either with or soon *after* the young animal, according to the species of the animal in question. The size, shape, and appearance of the afterbirth varies considerably in the domestic animals. Normally, the membranes should be discharged from the uterus with or soon after the young animal, but it is not uncommon to find their expulsion delayed for a

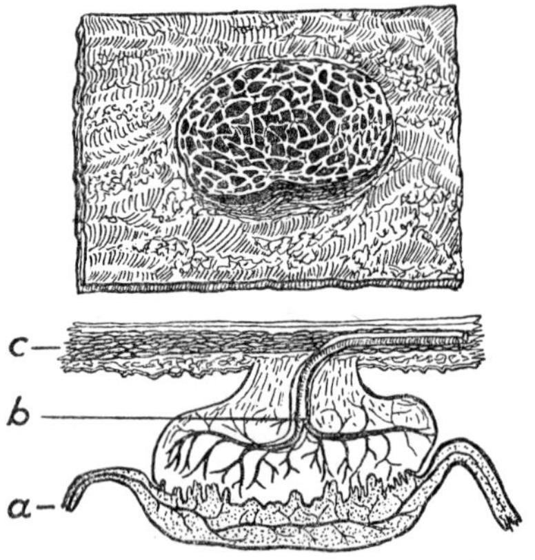

Cotyledon from the uterus of cow. Above—appearance when seen from the inner surface of the uterus. Below—diagram showing intimate attachment of placenta. *a*, Placenta; *b*, vessels of cotyledon; *c*, wall of uterus.

variable time, depending upon the species and the individual. Immediately after the birth of the young animal the uterus contracts to a size smaller than when pregnant with the result that the attachment between fœtal envelopes and maternal uterus is severed in greater or lesser extent. Afterpains follow, similar to those of normal labour, but less severe, with the object of expelling the membranes.

In the mare, with a scattered and slight attachment, the afterbirth separates rapidly and is soon expelled ; indeed, not infrequently the foal is born still enveloped in, or attached to, its membranes. These appear as a complicated mass of pinkish-grey tissue, plentifully supplied with blood, and often possessing little bladder-like pockets of amniotic or allantoic fluid. The weight and extent varies, but in an average-sized draught mare the afterbirth fills an ordinary stable-bucket more than half-full. If in six hours the placenta has not been discharged naturally, measures should be taken to effect its prompt removal, for the mare is very susceptible to metritis (inflammation of the uterus, often caused by decomposition of the afterbirth), and death frequently follows. (*See* RETENTION OF AFTERBIRTH.)

In the cow, where the attachment is cotyledonary, the fœtal membranes may be expelled at any time during the first six hours after calving, or not for one or two days, without any serious consequences. Retention occurs very frequently. (*See* RETENTION OF AFTERBIRTH, BRUCELLOSIS.)

In those animals which normally produce multiple offspring at a birth—ewe, sow, bitch, and cat—as each fœtus is born the corresponding membranous envelope either accompanies or else immediately follows it. The exception to this otherwise almost invariable rule is in the case of the last fœtus to be born, that fœtus which occupied the extremity of one or other horn of the uterus ; the envelopes of this, the youngest member of the family, are sometimes retained, and may occasion a mild or severe metritis, until such time as they are expelled.

The bitch, cat, sow, cow, and even the mare, will commence to devour the membranes after expulsion unless they are prevented. This is Nature's insurance that the enveloping folds of the afterbirth do not obstruct the free passage of air to and from the lungs of the young creature, and it is almost always the preliminary to the licking of the newly born, which ensures stimulating surface massage and comparative dryness in the hair-clothed animals. Although untoward results do not always follow this ingestion of large quantities of animal protein, even by the herbivora, there is some risk, for choking, indigestion, colic, superpurgation, and gastritis sometimes result from the practice. In dogs and cats, there is some evidence to show that the eating of the afterbirth supplies to the animal's system hormones which have accumulated in it. These in turn play a part in stimulating the flow of milk or involution of the uterus. (*See* PARTURITION.)

AFTERPAINS are rhythmic contractions of the uterus often assisted by the abdominal muscles (straining), very similar to, but less powerful than, those occurring during normal labour, commencing a variable time after the birth of the young animal, and resulting in the expulsion of the fœtal membranes. (*See* AFTERBIRTH.)

AGALACTIA.—The absence of milk in the udder, following parturition. (*See* SOW'S MILK, ABSENCE OF; COW'S MILK, ABSENCE OF.)

AGALACTIA, CONTAGIOUS (ἀ, neg.; γάλα, milk).—This is a contagious disease of goats particularly, and sheep less commonly, characterised by inflammatory lesions in the udder, eyes, and joints. It is chiefly met with in France, Switzerland, the Tyrol, Italy, the Pyrenees, North Africa, and India.

Causes.—*Mycoplasma agalactia*, one of the pleuro-pneumonia group of organisms. It often occurs in the spring and the summer, and disappears with the advent of the colder weather. There appears to be some relationship between the presence of certain flies and the incidence of the disease. The infection may be carried by the hands of the milkers and by the litter in a shed becoming contaminated, while the fœtus may be infected before birth.

Symptoms.—Two forms are recognised —an acute and a chronic.

Acute form.—In this, the animals show signs of high fever. The udder appears swollen, hot and painful, and may be the seat of abscesses. The milk secretion becomes less in quantity, and has a serous, clotted, dirty-yellowish appearance. The joints become affected after a variable time, especially those of the knee and hock, and the intense swelling and painfulness constrain the animal to lie almost continually. Abscesses form around the joint, burst, and discharge pus. When the eye is affected, it is found to be intensely inflamed, extremely painful, and a milky-white coloration appears over the anterior surface. About 15 per cent of the animals affected with the acute type of the disease die, and the others usually pass into the chronic form.

Chronic form.—In time the function of the udder is lost and the organ atrophies. The joints show changes somewhat similar to those of the acute type, but much milder and more prolonged. The eye becomes the seat of a chronic inflammation, ulcers appearing upon the cornea. Meanwhile the animal has been losing condition. Rams or he-goats show an inflammation of the testicle (orchitis), with or without abscess formation.

Treatment.—Isolation of the affected animals and strict segregation of the in-contacts should be carried out.

In most instances it is more economical to slaughter all but the most valuable animals and burn their carcases.

AGAR is a gelatinous substance prepared from Ceylon moss and various kinds of seaweed. It dissolves in boiling water, and, on cooling, solidifies into a gelatinous mass at a temperature slightly above that of the body. It is extensively used in preparing culture-media for use in bacteriological laboratories, and also in the treatment of chronic constipation in dog and cat, for which purpose it may be shredded and mixed with the food.

AGENE PROCESS.—The bleaching of flour with nitrogen trichloride. The use of such flour in dog foods may give rise to nervous symptoms. (*See* HYSTERIA.)

AGES OF ANIMALS.

The Horse.—By the time it has reached 17 years, which generally means about 14 years of work, a horse's powers are on the wane. Many at this age are still in possession of their full vigour, but these are generally of a class that is better looked after than the average, *e.g.* hunters, carriage-horses, or favourites. On an average, the feet of the horse are worn out first, not the arteries as in man, and consequently horses with good feet and legs are likely to outlast those inferior in this respect, other things being equal. After the feet come the teeth. In very many cases a horse's teeth wear out before their time. It often happens that the upper and the lower rows of teeth do not wear in the normal way; the angle of their grinding surfaces becomes more and more oblique, until the chewing of the food becomes less and less perfect, and the horse loses condition.

Instances are on record of horses attaining the age of 35, 45, 50, and one of a horse that was still working when 63 years old. These, however, are very exceptional. The average age at which a horse dies or is destroyed lies somewhere between 20 and 25 years. The following is a rough but fairly accurate comparison between the ages of the horse and man as computed by Blaine: A horse at 5 years is *comparatively* as old as a man at 20; at 10 he equals a man of 40; at 15 he is as a man of 50; at 20 a man of 60, and so on.

The Ox.—The great majority of bullocks are killed before they reach 4 years of age, and in countries where 'prime beef' is grown they are fattened and killed between 2½ and 3 years. In the majority of herds, few cows live to be more than 8 or 10 years of age. Pedigree bulls may reach 12 or 14 years of age before being discarded. Records are in existence of cows up to 39 years old, and it is claimed that one had 30 calves. Sixteen and 22 calves are claimed for other cows in Britain.

Sheep.—Here again the requirements of the butcher have modified the age of the animal at death. Wether lambs are killed at ages ranging from 4 to 9 months (Christmas lambs), and older fat sheep up to 2½ years. Ewes, on the average, breed until they are from 4 to 6 or 7 years, when they too are fattened and slaughtered for mutton. Exceptionally, they reach greater ages, but unless in the case of pure breeding animals, each year over six reduces their ultimate value as carcases. Rams are killed after they have been used for two or three successive seasons at stud, that is, when they are 3 or 4 years of age, as a rule.

Pigs.—In different districts the age at which pigs are killed varies to some extent, according to the requirements of local trade. Pigs for pork production are killed at about 3½ to 4 months; bacon pigs are killed between 6 and 7½ months, and only breeding sows and boars are kept longer. Ages up to 12 years have been recorded in the case of the sow.

Dogs and Cats.—These are the only domesticated animals which are generally allowed to die a natural death. The average age of the dog is about 12 years, and of the cat 9 to 12, but instances are not uncommon of dogs living to 18 or 20 years of age, and of cats similarly. (*See also* BREEDING OF LIVESTOCK, DENTITION OF ANIMALS.)

AGGLUTINATION (*agglutino*, I cause to adhere) is the adherence together of small bodies in a fluid. For instance, a quantity of normal healthy blood serum, when added to a uniform suspension of organisms in a test-tube, causes them to collect together into groups which may number from about 20 to over 100. Similarly, the blood serum of one animal will cause the red blood corpuscles of another to become grouped together or agglutinaed. The phenomenon is explained by the presence in the serum of an *agglutinin* which combines with an agglutinable substance, or *agglutinogen*, possessed by the organisms.

The principle is made use of in the Agglutination Test, which depends upon the principle that in the blood serum of an animal harbouring in its body disease-producing organisms (though it may show no symptoms) there is a far greater concentration of agglutinins than in a normal animal. Minute doses (*e.g.* dilutions of 1 part to 100 or even 1000) of such serum will cause agglutination, while serum from a normal animal will not cause agglutination when diluted more than 1 part in 10. Incubation of the mixture at body heat usually hastens the results and enables a rapid diagnosis to be made. The agglutination test is largely employed to detect so-called ' carriers ' of brucellosis of cattle and bacillary white diarrhœa in fowls.

AGGRESSINS (*aggressio*, aggression) are toxic products of bacteria found in body fluids of animals affected with certain bacterial diseases. They are used to produce immunity against attack by some specific organisms, such as *Clostridium* (*Bacillus*) *chauvœi*, which causes Black-quarter.

AIR.—Atmospheric air contains by volume 20·96 per cent of oxygen, 78·09 per cent of nitrogen, ·03 per cent of carbon dioxide, ·94 per cent of argon, and traces of a number of other elements the most important of which are helium, hydrogen, ozone, neon, zenon, and krypton, as well as variable quantities of water vapour. In addition to these normal constituents, impurities, such as soot, dust, particles of organic matter, etc., are present in larger or smaller amounts. (*See* SMOG.)

Air that has been expired from the lungs in a normal manner shows roughly a 4 per cent change in the amount of the oxygen and carbon dioxide, less of the former (16·96 per cent) and more of the latter (4·03 per cent). The nitrogen remains unaltered.

In enclosed spaces to which fresh air has not free access, it is obvious that if animals are housed for any length of time, the composition of the contained air must change ; the concentration of the oxygen becomes increasingly less, while that of the carbon dioxide and water vapour gradually rises. The body reacts to such conditions, greater volumes of blood are sent to the lungs to be exposed to the respired air, the heart-beats and the rate of respiration increase, and when the reduction of the oxygen content in the air inhaled is excessive, the blood becomes imperfectly supplied with that gas. Disease-producing organisms which may be present are enabled to survive longer and their numbers increase to a much greater extent than can occur in an atmosphere which is being constantly changed by the introduction of fresh air. It is under these circumstances that respiratory diseases, such as tuberculosis, influenza, bronchitis, pneumonia, etc., gain ground. The importance of a free supply of fresh air in stables, piggeries, and in cow-sheds especially, is immense, but unfortunately it is disregarded by many owners of animals. (*See* VENTILATION, RESPIRATION, SMOG, SLURRY.)

AIR PASSAGES.—These consist of the nasal cavity, pharynx, larynx, trachea, and bronchi. The nasal cavities, one on each side of the head, conduct the air to and from the pharynx or throat. Each is a more or less cylindrical passage into which two coiled bones project. These are known as the conchal or turbinated bones, and being covered by a very vascular mucous membrane during life, they ensure that air entering the lungs shall be warmed, moistened, and to some extent relieved of its grosser particles, before it has left the cavity. Opening from the nasal cavities there are air sinuses which act as air reservoirs and in some animals as resonating chambers. These are lined with mucous membrane continuous with that of the nostrils. (*See* SINUSES OF THE SKULL.) The horse, ox, sheep, and pig, do not habitually breathe in any other manner than by the nose, but they may, upon occasion, respire by the mouth, and the dog does this always when out of breath and panting. Air entering the lungs is therefore, in nearly all circumstances, compelled to pass through the nostrils and nasal passages, and any obstruction in these is more serious than in man, where mouth-breathing is easy.

The pharynx is a chamber at the back of the mouth cavity, situated where the respiratory and digestive passages cross each other. It has muscular walls which are used in swallowing, and from it opens the larynx or 'voice-box'. This latter organ guards the upper end of the trachea. It is composed of cartilages that give support to the vocal cords, and regulate the space by which the air enters or leaves. It is extremely sensitive, being well supplied with nerve-endings, irritation of which results in a cough, with the object of expelling any irritant body or material. From the larynx the trachea carries the air onwards towards the chest cavity. It is a cartilaginous flexible tube, composed of a number of incomplete rings, whose circumference is completed by a strip of muscle, and which are held to each other by a fibrous membrane, the whole being lined on the inside by a continuous mucous membrane. The trachea runs from the larynx down the middle of the lower part of the neck, enters the thorax, and ends by splitting into two or three bronchi, as the case may be (*i.e.* two in the horse and dog, and three in the ox, sheep, and pig). The bronchi, in their upper part, are of similar structure to the trachea, but they soon split up into bronchioles, which lose much of their cartilage as they divide and subdivide. They give off a large number of bronchial tubes which radiate through the whole of the lungs, becoming smaller and smaller till finally they open into the air alveoli of the lungs.

The whole of the air passages are lined by mucous membrane. In the nasal cavity this contains the organs of smell, and glands which elaborate the mucous secretion that carries the larger particles of foreign matter, extracted from the air, to the outside. In the larynx and trachea the mucous membrane is provided with epithelial cells that possess long whip-like processes which, by constant movement, drive small particles of dust, soot, etc., as well as mucous or bronchial secretion, towards the larynx, from where it may be coughed up. In addition to these ciliated epithelial cells, the bronchial mucous membrane contains numerous glands which keep its surface moist and soothed.

AIRSAC DISEASE (*see under* SINUSITIS, INFECTIOUS of turkeys).

ALBINISM (*albus*, white).—This is the absence of colouring matter in the skin, which may occur locally or may involve the whole of the superficial tissues of the body. Local albinism (white patches of hair) is very often met with in the faces and legs of horses, and in various parts of the body in certain breeds of cattle. The skin of such areas is usually pale pink in colour. Occasionally the iris of one or both eyes is devoid of the characteristic colouring matter in the horse, and the dark shining lens appears to be surrounded by a ring of white; the terms 'ring-eyed' and 'wall-eyed' are applied to this condition. In horses possessing this feature the face is very often a full 'blaze' (*i.e.* nearly all white). Albinism may affect the whole surface of the body as in 'white' (*i.e.* cream-coloured) horses, when the skin is always pink. Horses possessing white hair but brown or grey skins are not albinos; they are generally old and were definitely grey in their younger days; in such cases the whitening process is due to an absorption of the pigment (melanin) of the hairs themselves, and its subsequent deposition in the surface layers of the skin, in lymph glands, or in other parts of the body, especially where growth is occurring very rapidly, *e.g.* tumours. The mating of albinos with each other produces a family of albinos, while albinism in one of the parents only gives a coloured generation which, when interbred, yields a proportion of albino offspring in the ratio of one to three coloured; as a result of this feature albinism is scientifically considered to be a Mendelian recessive. (*See* COLOURS OF HORSES, GENETICS AND HEREDITY, MELANIN, MELANOTIC SARCOMA, etc.)

ALBUMINS (*albus*, white) are bodies closely resembling white of egg and composing in great part all the tissues of the body. Their characters are that they are soluble in pure water; can be dried into a light, flaky non-crystalline powder; are coagulated by heat; and are precipitated by such substances as nitric acid, tannin, alcohol, corrosive sublimate, etc.

Varieties. — Albumins are divided according to their source of origin as muscle-albumin, milk-albumin, blood- or serum-albumin, egg-albumin, vegetable-albumin, etc. These differ in their chemical and physiological actions; for example, although serum-albumin occurs in the blood-stream, egg-albumin, if injected direct, is highly poisonous.

Uses.—When taken into the stomach they are all converted into a soluble form by the process of digestion, and being in this state are absorbed into the blood to build up tissue gradually worn out by the general bodily activity. (*See* DIET, ALBUMINURIA.)

ALBUMINURIA.—The presence of albumen in the urine: one of the earliest signs of inflammation of the kidneys (a common condition in the dog). It may also indicate derangement of the urinary system below the kidneys, *e.g.* cystitis. Albuminuria, however, occurs also during fevers of several types. Detected by chemical tests, it is a useful aid to diagnosis.

ALCOHOL (an Arabic word).—There are two kinds of alcohol used in connection with the treatment of animals: ethyl alcohol and methyl alcohol. The latter is an active poison if given internally. Ethyl alcohol is produced by the action of yeasts on solutions of sugars, especially grape-sugar or glucose. Carbon dioxide is another product of the same action, but being a gas it escapes into the air. The alcohol in the resulting solution is secured by subsequent distillation.

Absolute alcohol is prepared by concentrating weaker mixtures until a solution consisting of 99 per cent of ethyl alcohol, with not more than 1 per cent of water, results. It is a mobile, colourless fluid, with a spirituous odour and an intensely burning, fiery taste.

Rectified spirit.—This contains 90 per cent of ethyl alcohol and 10 per cent of water, by volume. It is used in the preparation of many of the tinctures of the *British Pharmacopœia* and for the painting of the skin prior to operation.

Proof spirit is a solution of ethyl alcohol in water of the strength of 57·09 per cent.

Characters of alcohol.—Alcohol freezes at a very low temperature. It has considerable powers of solubility and is used to dissolve fats, oils, resins, balsams, and many alkaloids. When mixed with wood-naphtha or methyl alcohol it forms *methylated spirit*, a compound used in many external applications, liniments, etc., as well as for heating purposes. Owing to the presence of methyl alcohol, methylated spirit is a poisonous substance, most unsuited for internal administration.

Alcohol, taken internally, has a stimulating effect, which is later followed by depression. When applied to the surface of the skin or to a mucous membrane, alcohol withdraws water from the uppermost layer of cells, coagulates the protoplasm, and fixes and hardens the area, so that micro-organisms are imprisoned in these outer layers and prevented from contaminating any surgical wound in the near vicinity. It has, in addition, a solvent action upon any fatty material present on the skin, which often harbours and protects such organisms.

Varieties of alcoholic liquors.—The following list gives an average percentage by volume of alcohol in the preparations:

Whisky	44 to 50 per cent
Brandy should contain	43½ per cent, but is variable
Rum	57 to 62 per cent
Bitter ales	7 to 10 ,,
Beer	2 to 4 ,,

Uses.—A temporary stimulant, but one which gives rise to later depression and is greatly inferior to those drugs mentioned under STIMULANTS. Too much reliance must not be placed upon its so-called 'heating properties'; the primary effect is a dilatation of the surface blood-vessels resulting in a *sensation* of warmth of temporary duration. (*See also* SURGICAL SPIRIT.)

ALCOHOL POISONING.—Acute alcoholism is usually the result of too large doses given *bona fide*, but occasionally the larger herbivora and pigs eat fermenting windfalls in apple orchards; or are given, or obtain, fresh distillers' grains, or other refuse permeated with spirit, in such quantities that the animals become virtually *drunk*; or in more serious cases they may become comatosed, while fatal cases are sometimes recorded. The symptoms described are great excitement, prancing and striking out with the fore-feet, an unsteady gait, and a great tendency to fall to the ground, from which the animal only recovers itself with difficulty. Intermittent or almost continuous winking with one or both eyes is often seen. The head, feet, horns, and the ears become hot; the pulse-rate and respirations increase; the temperature may rise, and in serious cases unconsciousness or paralysis supervenes. Horses and dogs are more susceptible than ruminants, with pigs mid-way between. Dogs receiving large doses, *e.g.* from ½ to 1 ounce of whisky, on an empty stomach, may suddenly fall on their sides, become unconscious, and die very rapidly.

Antidotes are hot tea or coffee, cold douches to the head and spine.

ALDRIN.—An insecticide. It is a chlorinated naphthalene derivative used in agriculture against wireworms, etc. Misuse of it—as a dressing for orf affecting lambs' mouths—led to the death of 105 out of 107 lambs over a period of a week or so. Symptoms included: blindness, salivation, convulsions, rapid breathing. (*See* GAME BIRDS)

ALEUTIAN DISEASE.—First described in 1956 in the U.S.A., this disease of mink also occurs in the U.K., Denmark, and Sweden. The cause is believed to be a virus. Symptoms include: failure to put on weight or even loss of weight; thirst; the presence of undigested food in the fæces—which may be tarry. Bleeding from the mouth and anæmia may also be observed. Death usually follows within a month. Mink other than the dark-grey Aleutian ones may be affected.

ALEXIN.—A labile substance present in both normal and immune serum, possessing bactericidal and hæmolytic properties when combined with immune body.

ALFALFA, fed in large quantities, has in Israel given rise to infertility in cattle—owing, it is believed, to contained œstrogens.

ALGÆ POISONING.—Occurs in the mid-West, U.S.A., chiefly in the months of June to September, when a strong wind may blow a thick greenish scum of algæ from their normal habitat in the centre of a lake to the shore. In such cases an oily, paint-like layer several inches thick may accumulate, and decomposition of this liberates some toxic substance which has given rise to poisoning in all types of farm, and many laboratory, animals. The toxic substance is unstable, losing its potency within 24–48 hours. As soon as an offensive odour is noticeable, the danger is past.

Symptoms.—Stupor, collapse, narcosis, sometimes convulsions if touched, death in from half an hour to a few hours. In the guinea pig foamy-white tears are observed in addition to restlessness, sneezing, coughing, salivation, and weakness of the hindquarters.

ALIMENTARY CANAL.—The route taken by the food from the time that it enters the mouth until it is voided to the outside is through the alimentary canal. It is composed of the mouth, pharynx or throat, œsophagus or gullet, stomach or stomachs, small intestines and large intestines, which are arranged in this order. In this route or passage the food is broken down from complex into simpler compounds; it is subjected to the actions of the digestive juices and to bacterial activity; insoluble food substances are changed to soluble and therefore absorbable compounds; the useful constituents are absorbed by the blood- and lymph-streams, and such substances as are not required by the body are passed to the outside and eliminated.

ALKALI (Arabic word) is a substance which neutralises an acid to form a salt, and turns red litmus blue. Alkalies are generally the oxides, hydroxides, carbonates, or bicarbonates of metals.

Varieties.—Ammonium, lithium, potassium, and sodium salts are the principal alkalies, their carbonates being weak and their bicarbonates weaker. Calcium (lime), magnesium, barium, and strontium compounds are called the alkaline earths and act as alkalies, while certain substances which in the body are converted into alkalies are called indirect alkalies, the chief of these being acetates, citrates, and tartrates.

Uses.—In poisoning by acids, alkalies in dilute solution should be administered at once. (*See* ACIDS, POISONING BY.) Alkaline caustics (*i.e.* concentrated alkalies) are sometimes used to destroy or repress warts and surface tumours, where operation is inadvisable or impossible. Most stinging or biting insects produce their effects by the injection into the skin of irritating acid compounds; in such cases weak alkaline solutions, particularly ammonia, give relief from the subsequent inflammation. Alkalies are used in some forms of dyspepsia to counteract excessive secretion of acid in the stomach.

Alkalies, especially sodium hydroxide and sodium carbonate have a cleansing and solvent action upon grease and fatty substances. They are used in hot solution in water to cleanse premises, harness, clothing, various utensils such as milk pails, troughs, etc., prior to the disinfection of these by other compounds or steam. Some are themselves disinfectants, especially against viruses. (*See* DYSPEPSIA; STOMACH, DISEASES OF; ACIDITY; DISINFECTION; DETERGENTS.)

ALKALIES, POISONING BY.—Poisoning may occur as a result of the accidental administration of ammonia, caustic soda, or potash, but it is of rare occurrence.

When such a case does arise it is necessary to give weak solutions of the weaker acids —for instance, vinegar and water, diluted acetic and hydrochloric acids—and follow this with substances soothing to the mucous membranes such as gruel, thin flour paste, linseed tea, olive oil, beaten-up eggs and milk, etc.

ALKALOIDS.—A large number of the active principles of plants are classified under the name of alkaloids. They all possess a very powerful physiological action. Like alkalies, they combine with acids to form salts, and turn red litmus blue. Many of the active principles of the powerful drugs are alkaloids, and their names have an almost constant ending . . . *ine, e.g.* atropine, morphine, quinine, etc. Certain other active principles of some species of plants only differ from alkaloids in that their reactions are neutral; such often end in . . . *in, e.g.* digitin, santonin, etc. Most alkaloids are obtained pure from their plants by complicated chemical processes depending on the fact that they themselves are soluble in alcohol or ether, while their salts, formed by the addition of an acid, are soluble in water. For administration, alkaloid salts are usually dissolved in water and injected under the skin or into the muscles. (*See under* ANTIDOTES.)

Below is a list of the most common and important alkaloids and similar substances, with the parent plant from which they are derived:

Aconitine, *Aconine* } from Monk's-hood (*Aconitum napellus*).
Arecoline, from Areca nut (*Areca catechu*).
Atropine, from Belladonna, the juice of the Deadly Nightshade (*Atropa belladonna*).
Caffeine, from the Coffee Plant (*Coffea arabica*) and from the leaves of the Tea Plant (*Thea sinensis*), also found in the Kola nut, Guarana, and species of Holly, etc.
Cocaine, from Coca leaves (*Coca erythroxylon*).
Digitoxin *, *Digitalin* * } from Foxglove (*Digitalis purpurea*).
Ephedrine, from various species of *Ephedra*.
Ergotoxin *, *Ergotinin* *, *Ergometrine* } from the fungus Ergot of Rye (*Claviceps purpurea*).
Hyoscyamine, from Henbane (*Hyoscyamus niger*).
Hyoscine or Scopolamine } also from Henbane.
Morphine, *Codeine*, *Thebaine*, *Heroin* } from Opium, the juice of the Opium Poppy (*Papaver somniferans*)
Nicotine, from Tobacco leaves (*Nicotiana tobaccum*).
Physostigmine or *Eserine* } from Calabar Beans (*Physostigma venenosum*)
Pilocarpine, from Jaborandi (*Pilocarpus jaborandi*).
Quinine, from Cinchona or Peruvian Bark (*Cinchona*, and *Cinchona rubra*).
Santonin *, from Wormwood (*Artemesia pauciflora*).
Sparteine, from Lupins (*Lupulinus*, sp.) and from Broom (*Cytisus scoparius*).
Strophanthin *, a glucoside from an East African Creeper (*Strophanthus kombé*, or *S. hispidus*).
Strychnine, from Nux vomica seeds (*Strychnos nux vomica*).
Veratrine, from Green hellebore (*Veratrum viridi*).
Veratrine, from Cevadilla seeds (*Cevadilla officinale*, or *Schœnocaulon officinale*).

Those marked * are neutral principles.

ALLANTOIS (ἀλλᾶς, sausage; εἶδος, form) is one of the component parts of the fœtal membranes. It arises early in embryonic life as an outgrowth from the hind-gut, leaves the abdomen of the fœtus by the umbilicus, and insinuates itself between the chorion on the outside and the amnion on the inside. That part of it remaining inside the abdominal cavity of the fœtus forms the urinary bladder in after-life, and, until the time of birth, is in direct communication with the extra-fœtal portion by means of the urachus—that part passing through the umbilicus. Fluid secreted by the kidneys of the fœtus and passing to the urinary bladder gains exit to the allantoic cavity which is outside the fœtus until just before the time of birth, when the communication is occluded. (*See* AFTERBIRTH, PERVIOUS URACHUS, EMBRYOLOGY.)

ALLELOMORPHS are genes which influence a particular developmental process, processes, or character, in opposite ways. They occupy the same positions on the same chromosomes, and both allelomorphs cannot be present in the same animal. They result from a previous mutation, and the original gene and its mutated form are called an 'allelomorphic pair'. (*See also* GENETICS AND HEREDITY.)

ALLERGIC DERMATITIS ('Queensland Itch') is seen in horses in Australia, where it is a result of hypersensitivity to *e.g.* the bites of a sandfly; in Japan it follows bites of the stable-fly. It is a disease of the hot weather, and is intensely itchy in character. Treatment involves the use of antihistamines. (*See also* ECZEMA.)

ALLERGY means specific sensitivity to a plant or animal product, usually of a protein nature. The tuberculin reaction is an example. In the dog and cat sensitivity occurs most commonly to agents present in bedding, carpeting, rubber products, household cleaners, plants, and some skin dressings.

The three main symptoms are itching, self-inflicted damage as a result, and redness; sometimes œdema of the face, ears, vulva or extremities, or skin weals.

Many foodstuffs have caused allergy in the dog, *e.g.* cow's milk; horse, ox, pig, sheep and chicken meat; eggs.

Allergy may sometimes arise following flea-bites, and sometimes after bee or wasp stings. Pollens can produce skin changes; likewise avianised vaccines horse serum, antibiotics, and synthetic hormone preparations. (*See also* ANAPHYLAXIS; ANTIHISTAMINES; LIGHT SENSITISATION; LAMINITIS; ECZEMA.)

ALOES is the dried or inspissated juice of the leaves of various species of the aloe plant. There are three chief varieties: Socotrine aloes from *aloe perryi*, Cape aloes from *aloe ferox*, and Barbados or Curacoa aloes from *aloe vera*. The latter is the most suitable for animal use. It is a powerful purgative, being the chief constituent of the common 'physic ball' so much used and abused by many horsemen. If used without care or suitable preparation aloes balls are distinctly dangerous owing to their extremely violent and painful purging action on the bowel, particularly when that contains quantities of semi-dry food material.

Uses.—Purgatives in the horse must act chiefly upon the latter part of the alimentary canal to be satisfactory; and this aloes does. Aloes are much less used now than formerly and ALOIN (which see) may be preferred, or Dihydroxyanthraquinone.

It may be advisable here to remark upon some of the contra-indications when aloes should *not* be used; these are:

(1) When inflammatory processes exist in the alimentary or the urinary systems;
(2) During the course of fevers;
(3) In old, weak, or debilitated animals;
(4) In pregnant mares, when it is liable to induce abortion;
(5) In mares that are suckling their foals, for it is excreted in the milk and may harm the foal;
(6) In respiratory diseases if aloes are used at all a smaller dose is necessary, since in these cases there is an increased liability of superpurgation resulting.

Administration and precautions.—Owing to their nauseating and bitter taste aloes are usually given in ball form, coated either with paper or gelatine, and swallowed whole.

In the use of aloes balls it is necessary to observe some precautions. For 24 hours previously the horse should have been prepared by stopping the most of his feed of corn and hay, and substituting mashes of bran, bran and linseed, or bran and turnip. It is advisable to take care that the horse does not eat his bedding in an attempt to alleviate the hunger occasioned by the starving process. Water may be allowed freely up to the time of the giving of the ball, but should be restricted subsequently. He may receive the ball last thing at night. If the weather be at all cold it is wise to rug the horse and house him in a warm loose-box until the action of the purge has ceased.

In some horses the purging is over in from 2 to 4 hours after its inception, but in others it may last as long as 24 hours or more.

In certain cases, for some reason not well understood, an average dose of aloes fails to act. The dose should never be repeated in such cases until at least 48 hours have elapsed, as superpurgation is otherwise likely to follow. (*See* SUPERPURGATION.)

ALOIN is the name of the active principle of Barbados aloes. It is more reliable than the crude aloes and is often given to horses with calomel. (*See also* ALOES.)

ALOPECIA (ἀλώπηξ, a fox) is another name for baldness. (*See* BALDNESS.)

ALPHACHLORALOSE.—(*See* CHLORALOSE.)

ALUM or **ALUMEN** is the compound sulphate of aluminium and potassium, or, in the case of ammonia-alum, of aluminium and ammonia. Alum is slightly irritant, astringent, and antiseptic; it is mainly used as an external dry dressing for wounds on account of these actions. In solution, it is useful as a lotion for the eyelids when these are inflamed or the seat of suppurative processes, and is often given combined with zinc sulphate. It is sometimes prescribed as a mouth-wash, dissolved in glycerine, for injuries to the gums after the extraction of teeth, and in some cases of pyorrhœa. In acute laminitis in the horse, alum in doses of about one dram was once used, administered by the mouth, well diluted in warm water, to which a little treacle or syrup has been added. It was the chief constituent of powders given to cows to check the secretion of milk (*i.e.* to 'dry them off') about six weeks or two months before calving.

ALVEOLAR ABSCESS is the name given to those abscesses which develop in the root-cavity of a tooth. (*See* SINUSES OF THE SKULL, CARIES, TEETH.)

ALVEOLUS (*alveoli*) is a term applied to the sockets of the teeth in the jawbone. The term is also applied to the minute divisions of glands and to the air sacs of the lungs.

AMAUROSIS (ἀμαύρωσις), gutta serena, or 'glass eye', means a deprivation of sight.

AMBLYOPIA (ἀμβλυωπία) means a diminution in the power of vision.

AMBULANCE (*ambulo*, I move about). 'Cattle-floats' are often used for cattle, sheep, and pigs, and specially made ambulances for horses and the largest cattle. To be able to deal with cases that are unable to rise from the ground, horse-ambulances are usually provided with a low platform on rollers which can be removed from the bottom of the vehicle, and replaced by means of a windlass. The platform is removed, secured alongside the recumbent animal, which is then turned over on to the platform or lifted on to it, tied in position, and the whole wound up into the ambulance and fastened there.

AMERICAN QUARTER HORSE.—A breed derived mainly from dams of Spanish origin, for long bred by American Indians, and from Galloway sires brought by the early settlers. 'It was Barb blood spiced with a Celtic infusion and refined with a dash of Eastern blood that fashioned the present-day Quarter Horse.'—R. M. Denhardt.

AMINE.—An organic compound containing nitrogen.

AMINO-ACID, or **AMIDO-ACID**, is the name given to substances derived from the ultimate products of digestion of protein foods, from which the protein materials of the body are again built up.

There are 24 of these important substances, which constitute all the proteins in the animal and vegetable world. They can be compared to 24 different kinds of 'bricks': from them many different kinds of 'buildings' (*i.e.* the numerous proteins) can be made. Just as buildings can be broken down into bricks, so the proteins can be broken down into amino-acids, and in a similar way the amino-acids can be used again, perhaps in quite different numbers, proportions or arrangements, to form entirely different proteins. In the animal's body, the unwanted amino-acids are rendered harmless and discarded in urine or fæces.

The list of known amino-acids includes the following: *glycine, alanine,* and *cysteine,* which, with others, can be oxidised into glucose and are called **glucogenic**; *leucine, isoleucine, phenylalanine,* and *tyrosine,* which during oxidation may give rise to harmful ketones, and are known as **ketogenic**; *tryptophane, lysine, arginine, histidine, threonine,* and *methionine,* which with *cysteine* are known as the 'essential' amino-acids, because unless they are present in a diet it cannot sustain life. Other importan, amino-acids are *serine, glutamic acid, aspartic acid, iodogorgoic acid, valine*t *proline,* and *thyroxine.*

Two amino-acids contain sulphur and supply sulphur to the body as the raw material for all the sulphur-containing compounds used in the body—such as glutathione, taurine, the thiosulphates and the thiocyanates. These two are *cysteine* and *methionine*. Lysine is particularly important for growth and for milk secretion in all animals. Good milk-producing rations for dairy cows should contain proteins rich in lysine, such as those from grass, beans, peas, or those of animal origin (fish meal, blood meal, or meat and bone meal), if the best results are to be obtained. Tryptophane is very important for growth of all cells and normal development. It is used for all cell proliferation. Arginine and histidine play an important part in maintaining the blood-stream normal and healthy and have other complex functions.

The pig and rat require, for rapid growth: lysine, tryptophane, leucine, isoleucine, methionine, threonine, phenylalanine, valine, and histidine. The chick needs glycine in addition to these.

AMINONITROTHIAZOLE. — A drug

used in the treatment and prevention of Blackhead in turkeys.

AMMONIA is a pungent gas formed by heating a mixture of sal-ammoniac and quicklime. When dissolved in water it forms the well-known 'spirits of hartshorn' or liquor ammoniæ. Ammonium carbonate, itself extensively used as a stimulant, is the chief constituent of aromatic spirits of ammonia : sal-ammoniac is the chloride of ammonia : while the acetate of ammona is also used as a medicine.

Uses.—Externally, strong ammonia is an irritant blister. It is diluted by adding 1 part to 15 or 20 of water and used as an application to parts stung by wasps, clegs, or bees, etc. Strong ammonia and ammonium chloride are constituents of most embrocations. Internally, ammonia is extensively used as the carbonate.

Ammonia when given by the mouth is a rapid and diffusible stimulant acting on the heart, respiration, and on the bowel wall. It is often given in those colics which are due to an atonic condition of the intestinal wall resulting in overloading or stoppage, when its stimulating effect on the sluggish bowel movements is well marked. If ammonia has to be given by the mouth as a liquid preparation, great care in its administration is very necessary, especially in the case of the carbonate. It should always be given in *cold gruels* or in *cold oily or demulcent vehicles*, for when heated, the irritant volatile ammonia gas is given off and exercises a burning or blistering action upon any part of the mouth or throat with which it comes in contact.

An excess of ammonia in the rumen has been cited as a cause of hypomagnesæmia in spring following massive applications of nitrogenous fertiliser. (*See also* UREA.)

As an inhalation a few drops of ammonia on a piece of cotton-wool held a few inches from the nostrils has a good effect in reviving animals which have collapsed. (Inhalation of concentrated ammonia can prove fatal.) Ammonia fumes are helpful to cattle when the atmosphere becomes full of SMOG (which see). Ammonia fumes from litter may adversely affect poultry. (*See* DEEP LITTER.) (*See also* QUATERNARY AMMONIA COMPOUNDS.)

AMNION (ἀμνίον, a bowl for blood).—This is the innermost of the three fœtal envelopes. It is continuous with the skin at the umbilicus (navel), and completely encloses the fœtus but is separated from actual contact with it by the amniotic fluid, or the 'liquor of the amnion', which in the mare measures about 5 or 6 litres (*i.e.* 9 to 10½ pints).

This 'liquor amnii' forms a kind of hydrostatic bed in which the fœtus floats, and serves to protect it from injury, shocks, extremes of temperature, allows free though limited movements, and guards the uterus of the dam from the spasmodic fœtal convulsions which, late in pregnancy, are often vigorous and even violent.

At birth it helps to dilate the cervical canal of the uterus and the posterior genital passages, forms part of the 'water-bag', and, on bursting, lubricates the maternal passages. (*See* PARTURITION)

AMPOULE is a small glass container having one end drawn out into a point capable of being sealed so as to preserve its contents sterile. It is used to contain solutions of drugs for hypodermic injection, while many vaccines and other biological products are also distributed in ampoules.

AMPUTATION (*amputo*, I prune) means the severing of a limb or other appendage from the body. An amputation through a joint where no actual sawing of bone takes place is called a **Disarticulation.**

Objects of amputation.—In the great majority of cases the operation of amputation is undertaken where a limb or other member is damaged beyond all possible hope of recovery. This does not apply to the horns of cattle, tails of dogs, nor to the tails of lambs. (*See* DOCKING, DEHORNING OF CATTLE.)

AMYL NITRITE is a volatile, oily liquid, prepared by the action of nitrous and nitric acids upon amyl alcohol. It is used sprayed upon a piece of cotton-wool and held to an animal's nostrils so that the vapour may be inhaled. It is useful in cases of collapse from shock or under chloroform anæsthesia. It is unsafe in any but skilled hands.

AMYLASE.—A starch-splitting enzyme.

AMYLOPSIN or **AMYLASE** (ἄμυλον, starch ; ὄψις, appearance) is the name of a ferment secreted by the pancreas, which converts starch into maltose during the process of digestion. (*See* DIGESTION.)

ANABOLIC.—Relating to anabolism,

which means tissue building, and is the opposite of catabolism or tissue breakdown.

An **anabolic steroid** is one derived from testosterone in which the androgenic characteristics have been reduced and the protein-building (anabolic) properties increased in proportion. Examples are nandrolone, ethylestrenol. These are used in malnutrition, wasting diseases, virus diseases, and severe parasitism.

ANÆMIA (ἀ, neg.; αἷμα, blood).—This is a term meaning literally ' no blood ', but one which refers to a deficiency of red corpuscles or of hæmoglobin.

(*a*) *Primary anæmia* implies the failure of the body to produce sufficient red corpuscles or hæmoglobin. This failure may be due to lack of food or of certain food constituents, *e.g.* iron, cobalt, and copper. Disease of the bone marrow, bracken poisoning, ' Radiation Sickness ', and chronic sepsis are among other causes of aplastic anæmia.

(*b*) *Secondary anæmia* occurs: (1) after severe hæmorrhage, when it is called acute; (2) during the course of certain diseases such as strongylosis, piroplasmosis, trypanosomiasis, and when the animal is affected with malignant tumours, when the loss of blood is a chronic condition. It may occur during chronic salicylate poisoning (*see* SALICYLATES), and as a result of infestation by lice, ticks, and other external parasites. In sheep, pigs and cats, *Eperythrozoon* parasites in the blood-stream cause anæmia; in cattle it is associated with Redwater. Parasitic worms other than strongyles also cause secondary anæmia; *e.g.* liver flukes.

Symptoms.—In the acute cases following hæmorrhage the animal shows symptoms varying with the intensity of the hæmorrhage. Cold sweats, a staggering gait, pallid mucous membranes, a rapid, weak pulse becoming thready, cold extremities, and muscular quiverings, are encountered. The animal soon lies down and dies in convulsions if the hæmorrhage is not checked.

When the anæmia depends on the presence of some other disease in the body the symptoms develop gradually. The animal becomes dull, is easily tired when exercised or at work, the visible mucous membranes are paler than usual, and palpitation of the heart occurs when the beast is excited. The appetite is diminished, the coat stares, and in the later stages, or in extreme cases, emaciation is marked. Œdematous swellings may develop in the lower parts of the body, especially about the limbs and the undersurface of the abdomen and thorax. Unless checked, the animal may die from sheer exhaustion.

Treatment must be directed against the primary disease responsible for the anæmia, whenever such treatment is at all possible. Nutritious food, plenty of fresh air, well-regulated exercise along with suitable preparations of iron are indicated; and, in the smaller animals especially, vitamin B_{12} or liver extract is often a valuable method of treatment. Where cobalt or copper or iron are lacking, these must be supplied. Lice or ticks and fleas should be destroyed. (*See* PIGLET ANÆMIA, DEFICIENCY DISEASES, FELINE *and* EQUINE INFECTIOUS ANÆMIA.)

ANÆMIA, EQUINE INFECTIOUS (*see under* EQUINE INFECTIOUS ANÆMIA.)

ANÆROBE (ἀ, neg.; ἀήρ, air; βιόω, I live) is the term applied to bacteria having the power to live without oxygen. Such organisms are found growing freely, deep in the soil, as, for example, the tetanus bacillus.

ANÆSTHESIA (ἀναισθησία) means a temporary loss of the faculty of feeling. It is either applied to a loss of sensation over a limited area (such as is produced by injecting procaine solution), when it is called local anæsthesia, or to a total loss of sensation along with unconsciousness (as is produced by chloroform and ether), when it is known as general anæsthesia. Epidural anæsthesia is that induced by injecting a local anæsthetic into the sub-dural space of the spinal canal. Loss of sensation occurs posterior to the site of the injection. (*See* EPIDURAL, REGIONAL, *and* ENDOTRACHEAL ANÆSTHESIA.)

ANÆSTHETICS.—These are drugs and other measures used for the production of insensibility to external stimulation. The use of general anæsthetics for operations on animals dates back to 1847, when several veterinary surgeons used ether. Chloroform was also used in 1847. Ether is still much used to-day in conjunction with oxygen, but chloroform has very largely been abandoned, on account of its toxicity, for the horse, dog, and cat.

Chloral hydrate solution given intravenously is used in the larger animals, and barbiturates—given by the same route—in all species. (*See also* NITROUS OXIDE,

ETHYL CHLORIDE, CYCLOPROPANE, TRILENE, FLUOTHANE; *and under* CHLOROFORM, ETHER, *and* CHLORAL HYDRATE.)

'Anæsthetic drugs all act by limiting the oxygen uptake of tissues. The effect on an individual tissue is proportional to its normal oxygen requirement. Since the oxygen requirement of nervous tissues is disproportionately high, these tissues are the first to be affected by anæsthetic drugs. Unconsciousness, abolition of reflexes, muscular atony, and respiratory paralysis are due to depression of the cerebral cortices, the mid-brain, the spinal cord, and the medulla respectively.

'A constant action of any anæsthetic agent is its effect on the respiratory centre which is always depressed. This has the effect of lowering the sensitivity of the centre to its physiological stimulant—carbon dioxide.' (J. R. Campbell and D. D. Lawson.)

General anæsthesia in the Horse.—Professor J. G. Wright stated (1958):

The most satisfactory method we possess for inducing deep narcosis and light general anæsthesia in the horse is chloral hydrate administered by slow intravenous injection. The method has two main disadvantages; the first, great technical care is necessary during injection, and secondly, the recovery rate is relatively slow. Whenever possible the horse is cast and restrained before administration so that injection shall be precise and the degree of narcosis assessed as administration proceeds. An efficient casting team is essential.

For deepening the induction anæsthesia and its maintenance for prolonged interferences, an ultra-short- or short-acting barbiturate is preferred to inhalation anæsthetics. (*See* NEMBUTAL.)

General anæsthesia in the Ox.—Cattle take chloroform with very little trouble, and as a rule are good subjects. One feature in the administration of chloroform to cattle is the extraordinary rapidity with which they regain sensation, and the speed with which they get to their feet again when the mask is removed. Endotracheal intubation has, however, been recommended in order to preserve a free airway and prevent inhalation of regurgitated rumen contents. Methohexitone sodium and chloral hydrate are also used. (*See also* EPIDURAL ANÆSTHESIA.)

General anæsthesia in Pigs, Sheep, and Goats.—These may be given ether with a large-sized dog-muzzle generally, and take it quite well, provided a free supply of fresh air is allowed. Nembutal is far preferable. Epidural anæsthesia has been found convenient for castration of adult boars, and for operations for hernia, imperforate anus, prolapsed rectum, etc. The resulting paraplegia usually lasts 2 or 3 hours.

With methohexitone sodium, 'an estimated dose of 5 mg. per kg. bodyweight (approximately 1 ml. of 2·5 per cent solution per 10 lb. bodyweight) was injected into the ear vein through a 23 or 22 gauge needle. This dose provided satisfactory anæsthesia for foot inspecting and hoof trimming, detusking boars, catheterisation of a sow and inserting nose rings secured with screws.

'The repair of unilateral scrotal hernia, and castration, was carried out in two 8-week-old pigs. Anæsthesia was induced by an initial injection of methohexitone sodium (5 mg. per kg. bodyweight intravenously) and maintained by additional doses of 25 to 50 mg. administered intermittently as required to maintain surgical anæsthesia for a total of 12 to 17 minutes.

'Response to noise or disturbance during recovery from methohexitone sodium anæsthesia is more marked in pigs than in ruminants, but in only one sow did there appear to be a risk of self-inflicted injury as a result of incoordinate movements. The pig's propensity for violent headshaking, especially after injection into an ear vein, should be borne in mind', and animals anæsthetised by this means should not be left to recover on bare concrete. (Gerald A. Emberton.) (*See also* STUNNING *and* CARBON DIOXIDE ANÆSTHESIA.)

General anæsthesia in the dog and cat.—The agent in most common use for this purpose is pentobarbitone ('Nembutal'). Given slowly into a vein, it is rapid in action and obviates the struggling and excitement involved when chloroform, ether, etc., are administered. Ether is often used, sometimes in conjunction with oxygen, but it has certain disadvantages. (*See* ETHER.) The risks attending the use of chloroform in the dog and cat have diminished its application, except for purposes of euthanasia. Nitrous oxide, T.C.E., and ethyl chloride have been used to some extent. Electro-narcosis may prove of value in the future.

General anæsthesia in Monkeys.—Phenicyclidine, which can be given intramuscularly, has been found very suitable as a tranquillisation agent, which will prevent biting and render monkeys easy to handle. It is given by intra-muscular injection. For anæsthesia, pentobarbitone sodium ('Nembutal') may then be given intravenously. Halothane may be used as an alternative.

General anæsthesia in Birds.—Ether may be used, or a 25 to 40 per cent mixture of cyclopropane in oxygen. Nembutal, given subcutaneously, may be used—preferably for prenarcotisation. Post-anæsthetic excitement may be considerable and dangerous, and Mr. L. Arnall, B.V.Sc., recommends immobilising the bird with a cylinder of paper rolled round it and fixed with adhesive tape.

General anæsthesia in Fish.—'Propoxate'—dl-l- (l-phenyl - ethyl) - 5 - (propoxy-carbomyl)-imidazole HCl—is a safe and powerful anæsthetic for cold-blooded vertebrates, soluble in both fresh and salt water. (*See Vet. Record*, Aug. 7, 1971.)

Uses of general anæsthesia.—Anæsthetics are extensively used in veterinary surgery. Humanity apart, for all painful, delicate, or protracted operations, it is almost essential for success of the procedure that the animal shall be anæsthetised, and a general anæsthetic is given (*but see* CASTRATION). It is also customary to use a general anæsthetic for many minor operative procedures, where formerly the animal was secured and given a local anæsthetic. In severe cases of difficult parturition in all animals; in the reduction of strangulated herniæ; in the removal of foreign bodies from the mouth and throat; in the relief of choking in cattle; and to enable a diagnosis to be made in cases of extreme abdominal tenderness, or in fractures, when manipulation of the parts affected produces excruciating pain, anæsthesia of a general nature is employed. The powerful muscular surroundings of the shoulder and stifle make the use of a general anæsthetic necessary when these joints are to be reduced after dislocation. For the use of local anæsthetics, *see* ANALGESICS.

ANÆSTHETICS, LEGAL REQUIREMENTS.—The Protection of Animals (Anæsthetics) Act, 1964, amended a previous Act of 1954, especially in the matter of castration. It is now obligatory to use an anæsthetic when castrating dogs, cats, horses, asses, and mules of any age; goats and pigs over 2 months old; calves and lambs over 3 months. The use of rubber rings or similar devices for castrating bulls, pigs, goats, and sheep, or for docking lambs' tails, is forbidden unless applied during the first week of life. The Act also requires that an anæsthetic be used when de-horning cattle; and also for disbudding calves unless this be done by chemical cautery applied during the first week of life.

A requirement, still in force, of the 1954 Act is the use of an anæsthetic for any operation, performed with or without the use of instruments, which involves interference with the sensitive tissues or the bone structure of an animal.

Exceptions are the rendering in emergency of first-aid to save life or relieve pain; the docking of a dog's tail or amputation of its dew claws before its eyes are open; any minor operation performed by a veterinary surgeon or veterinary practitioner, being an operation which, by reason of its quickness or painlessness, is customarily so performed without the use of an anæsthetic; any minor operation, whether performed by a veterinary surgeon or veterinary practitioner or by some other person, being an operation which is not customarily performed only by such a surgeon or practitioner.

Any person guilty of an offence under this Act is liable to a penalty of up to £50, with or without three months' imprisonment.

ANÆSTHETICS, RESIDUES IN CARCASES.—Dogs and cats have shown severe symptoms of poisoning after being fed on meat from animals humanely slaughtered by means of an overdose of a barbiturate anæsthetic.

ANAL.—Relating to the anus.

ANAL GLANDS (*see under* ANUS).

ANALEPTICS.—Restoratives.

ANALGESIA (ἀ, neg.; ἄλγος, pain) means the loss of the power to feel pain without loss of consciousness or of the power of movement of the part although that may in some instances be interfered with. It is induced by the injection of certain drugs. (*See* ANALGESICS.)

ANALGESICS are drugs which cause a temporary loss of the sense of pain without a loss of consciousness. Some act upon the brain or the whole nervous system and are called ANODYNES (which see), while others act locally and are often called local anæsthetics, such as cocaine, procaine.

Uses.—For minor operations, local anæsthetics are generally employed to minimise the pain in preference to general anæsthetics. They are injected under the skin with a hypodermic syringe. For *regional anæsthesia* the local anæsthetic solution is injected into the connective tissue around a sensory nerve trunk. Analgesics are often prescribed as constituents of eye-lotions to allay the pain and prevent further damage by rubbing or scratching. Some analgesics, such as quinine and urea hydrochloride, have the power of rendering areas into which they are injected insensible for from two to four or more days according to the dose. For the diagnosis of occult forms of lameness it is customary to inject an analgesic over the sensory nerves of the limb at various levels until the lameness ultimately disappears. A knowledge of the parts of the limb supplied by the particular nerve trunk which has been 'blocked' in this way localises the seat of the painful condition causing the lameness in such part or parts. Regional anæsthesia is also used to relieve pain, *e.g.* in cases of laminitis. The process of freezing is but little used on account of the risks of sloughing of the skin in the vicinity which attends its application. Substances such as adrenalin are often combined with local anæsthetics.

The use of epidural anæsthesia in animals has greatly increased. For cattle in particular, the method enables many minor operations on the vagina, uterus, rectum, and parts of the hind-limbs to be carried out without pain. Examinations which may involve painful manipulation of these parts, difficult calvings, etc., are rendered easier. (*See* ETORPHINE, EPIDURAL ANÆSTHESIA.)

ANAMNESIS (ἀνάμνησις) is the term applied to the past history of some particular patient.

ANAPHRODISIA.—Impairment of sexual appetite.

ANAPHYLAXIS (ἀνά, against; φύλαξις, protection) is the state of unusual or exaggerated susceptibility to a foreign protein which sometimes follows a primary injection of such protein. It is frequently encountered on giving a second dose of a vaccine or of a serum in the process of immunising an animal against some disease, *e.g.* distemper. It may also occur if a warble is crushed while still in a cow's back. (*See* ANTIHISTAMINES.)

ANAPLASMOSIS (ἀνά, backwards; πλάσσειν, to form).—This is an infectious disease of cattle, characterised by anæmia. In the U.S.A., it causes a loss of between 35 and 50 million dollars annually through deaths and decreased yields of beef and milk. No completely effective treatment has been developed for the acute stages of the disease. A vaccine was produced in the U.S.A. in 1965, and gives protection for one year. Two injections at 6 weeks' interval are necessary. Where the disease is seasonal, vaccination should begin after the last cases appear and finish about 2 months before cases are expected to appear next season. Animals that have been vaccinated and re-exposed, or that have recovered, can remain as 'carriers' for life. (*See* '*Gall-sickness*', under PARASITES.)

ANASARCA (ἀνά, up; σάρξ, the flesh) is a condition of general dropsy, particularly of the tissues below the skin. It is occasionally met with in fœtuses of various species, especially calves and puppies, and sometimes renders parturition difficult.

ANASTOMOSIS (ἀναστόμωσις, an outlet) is a term describing the means by which the circulation is carried on when a large vessel is severed or its stream obstructed, and in anatomy the term is applied to a junction between two or more arteries or veins which communicate with each other. In the abdominal cavity, inthe limbs, and in the brain, branches from the larger arterial trunks unite with each other to an enormous extent. The result of this is an even pressure of blood all over the area, and after injury or the ligaturing of one of a set of anastomosing trunks, it ensures that the flow of blood to any part shall not be cut off. When even the very large femoral artery of the hind-limb is cut and tied the blood-supply is not much interfered with after the first few hours, for the branches which come off above the seat of the ligature dilate and carry an extra amount of blood, some of which finds its way to areas of the limb below the ligature. Some arteries in the animal body do not anastomose, and if they become damaged the blood-supply is cut off from the areas which they supply. Degeneration of such areas follows and their functions are lost.

They are known as 'infarcts', and are common in the kidneys and liver, less common in the valves of the heart, and sometimes found in the brain. (*See* ARTERY.)

ANATOXIN.—A toxin rendered harmless by heat or chemical means but capable of stimulating the formation of antibodies.

ANEURIN is the name given to vitamin B_1, the anti-neuritic vitamin.

ANEURISM or **ANEURYSM** (ἀνεύρυσμα), means a dilatation upon an arterial trunk due to the yielding of one or more of its coats with a resulting bulge or swelling at the affected parts.

Varieties.—(1) *True aneurism.*—In this the vessel wall is dilated but still remains intact. It may assume a variety of shapes such as *cylindrical, fusiform, circumscribed, saccular,* etc. (2) *False aneurism.*—When the wall of an artery is injured or ruptured the blood may become localised in the surrounding tissues and produce a swelling to which the name hæmatoma is applied. This must be distinguished from another variety of swelling also called a hæmatoma,

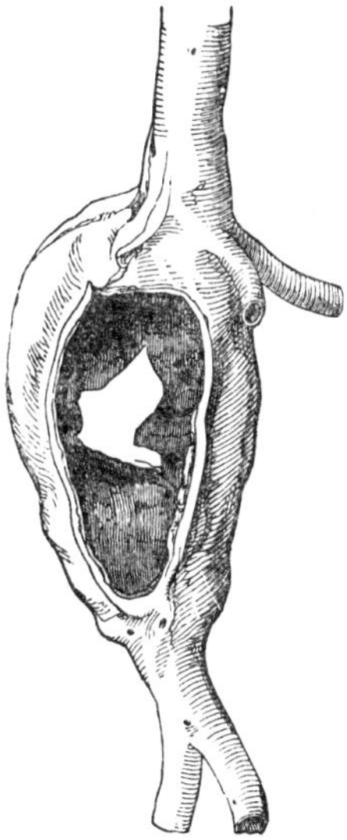

Aneurism of fusiform type, on the abdominal aorta. The aneurism has ruptured. (Miller's *Surgery*.)

but produced by the bruising and laceration of the capillaries of the part. A false aneurism is rare among animals, and generally pulsates at the rate of the heart-beat, while an ordinary hæmatoma is of common occurrence and does not pulsate, neither does it contain pure blood but rather blood-serum. (3) *Arterio-venous aneurism.*—This is produced when both an artery and a vein are injured in the same vicinity, as was frequently the case when the custom of bleeding was in vogue. A direct communication is established between the cavity of the artery and that of the vein, the blood passing by this route without any apparent discomfort to the animal. (4) *Verminous aneurism.*—The mesenteric artery of the abdomen is often the seat of immense numbers of a young stage of certain worms, which produce an aneurism and even a thrombosis of the main trunk or some of its branches. (*See* PARASITES, p. 658; THROMBOSIS.)

Causes.—Sudden and violent muscular efforts are regarded as the chief factors in the production of aneurisms; and as would be expected, the horse is more subject to this trouble than any of the other domesticated animals. The elastic arteries expand and contact with each successive heart-beat to provide the extra space required when a considerable amount of blood is forced into a system already full. The process of expansion begins at the base of the heart, where the aorta leaves to distribute the blood to the body by means of its multiple branches; it proceeds along the aorta and down each division until what was a definite perceptible stretching in the larger vessels (*i.e.* a pulse) finally becomes so slight that only by the microscope can it be recognised. In a condition of perfect health the elasticity of the arteries is quite equal to any strain that the heart may impose as the result of severe sudden or sustained muscular effort, and in such cases aneurism does not occur. It is only when the walls of the arteries are weakened by disease, atheroma (which see), or old age, that these bulbous swellings are liable to be produced as the result of some unusual strain. Direct injuries to the back have been blamed as the cause of aneurisms of the posterior part of the aorta, where they are most frequent, but in all probability there had been some pre-existing abnormality in this region in such cases. In the verminous variety, aneurism is the consequence of the obstruction to the free flow of the blood, by the presence in the artery or its branches of large numbers of the immature stage of *Strongylus vulgaris*, a parasitic worm. (*See* PARASITES, p. 658.)

Symptoms.—In the great majority of instances the presence of aneurism is never suspected until the animal suddenly falls dead from rupture and internal hæmorrhage, when the cause is discovered on post-mortem examination. In some cases, however, the affected animal shows a partial loss of power in its hind legs—what is often regarded by the layman as an injury to the spinal column; the muscles of the loins and croup degenerate later on, and control of the hind legs may be lost, or these may become lame after exercise. Such symptoms point to the possibility of an aneurism of the abdominal part of the aorta. In other cases when the lesion is situated in another part of the body the symptoms shown are dependent on circulatory disturbances of the area supplied by the involved artery, and vary with each case.

Treatment.—In animals it is seldom that treatment can be undertaken. Those that can be operated upon are either exposed, ligatured, and excised, or else are punctured with a special needle which lacerates the internal wall and induces a local clotting of the blood, so that when the clot is organised the wall may be strengthened and the risk of rupture minimised. Horses that are known to possess aneurisms must be treated with extra care.

ANDROGEN is the name given to those hormones which influence the growth and development of male sex organs and male characters. (*See* HORMONES.)

ANGIOMA (ἀγγεῖον, a blood-vessel) is a tumour composed of a large number of blood-vessels. They are common in the livers of cattle, when they are called hæmangiomata. (*See* TUMOURS, HÆMANGIOMA.)

ANGITIS, or **ANGIITIS** (ἀγγεῖον, a vessel), means inflammation of a vessel, such as a blood-vessel, lymph-vessel, or bile-duct.

ANHIDROSIS.—A failure of the sweat mechanism. This occurs in horses especially, but also in cattle, imported into tropical countries with humid climates.

At first, affected horses sweat excessively and their breathing is distressed after exercise. Later, sweating occurs only at the mane; the skin becomes scurfy; and breathing becomes more laboured. Heart failure may occur.

ANHYDRIDE.—An oxide which can combine with water to form an acid.

ANHYDROUS.—Containing no water.

ANILINE is a substance derived from indigo by distillation, from coal-tar by extraction, or manufactured from benzene. It is a colourless liquid with a peculiar aromatic smell and a burning taste. From it many vivid and beautiful dyes are made and extensively used, such as fuchsine or rosaniline, eosine, magenta, Congo red, methyl blue, Hoffmann's violet. Aniline itself is a narcotic poison, although most of its dyes are harmless.

ANIMAL BOARDING ESTABLISHMENTS ACT, 1963.—This requires that the owner of a boarding establishment shall obtain a licence from the Local Authority, and that this licence must be renewed annually. The applicant has to satisfy the licensing authority on certain personal points, and that the 'animals will at all times be kept in accommodation suitable as respects construction, size of quarters, number of occupants, exercising facilities, temperature, lighting, ventilation, and cleanliness'. The Act also requires that animals boarded 'will be adequately supplied with suitable food, drink, and bedding material, adequately exercised, and (so far as necessary) visited at suitable intervals'. Isolation facilities and fire precautions are covered by the Act, which empowers the Local Authority to inspect both the boarding establishment and the register which must be kept there.

ANIMALS, BREEDS OF (*see* BREEDS OF STOCK; also separate sections on HORSES, CATTLE, etc.).

ANIMAL FOOD (*see* DIET, RATIONS, PROTEINS, POISONING, ADULTERATION, ADDITIVES, TINNED FOODS; *also sections on* HORSES, CATTLE, SHEEP, *etc.*)

ANIMAL HEALTH SCHEMES.—(*See under* HEALTH SCHEMES.)

ANIMALS, HOUSING OF (*see* HOUSING OF ANIMALS and the various illustrations).

ANIMAL NURSING AUXILIARIES.—A Register of lay assistants who have passed the requisite examination is maintained by the Royal College of Veterinary Surgeons. Their qualification is designated by the letters R.A.N.A.

ANIMAL WELFARE CODES.—(*See under* WELFARE CODES FOR ANIMALS.)

ANISE, or **ANISEED.**—This is the dried fruit of *Pimpinella anisum* or of *Illicium anisatum*, a Chinese plant. Powdered aniseed is used as a constituent of cough powders, of electuary, and is incorporated in many of the compound feeding cakes for cattle. It has a soothing action on the throat, has a pleasant taste and acts as a spice increasing the appetite. An oil is extracted from it.

ANKYLOSIS (ἀγκύλος, crooked) is a term meaning the condition of a joint in which the movement is restricted by fibrous bands, by malformation, or by actual union of the bones. It is most common in the limb joints of horses, especially the coffin, pastern, knee and hock joints. (*See* JOINTS, DISEASES OF.)

ANKYLOSTOMA (ἀγκύλος, crooked; στόμα, mouth) is a parasitic worm affecting domesticated animals and man. (*See* PARASITES, p. 656.)

ANODYNES (ἀ, neg.; ὀδύνη, pain).—These are curative measures which soothe

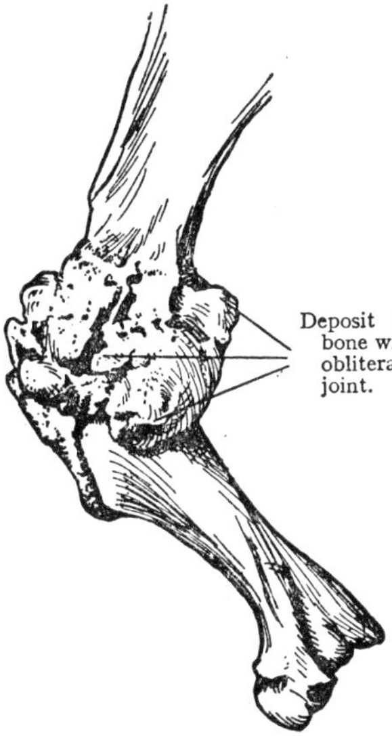
Deposit of new bone which has obliterated the joint.

Ankylosis of shoulder-joint (horse).

pain. They act either by removing the cause of the pain, by soothing the irritated nerves of the painful part, or by paralysing that part of the brain where the impressions of pain are received. Substances which destroy the power of feeling altogether are called 'anæsthetics'; those which only destroy the power to feel pain are 'analgesics'.

Varieties.—Alkaline applications are anodyne to the stings and bites of insects. Hot or cold applications to inflamed areas are anodyne when administered for considerable periods. Aconite, belladonna, cocaine, eucaine, camphor and menthol, and opium are local anodynes; while internally these drugs, as well as bromides, chloral, hyoscyamus, and aspirin, soothe pain in remote parts of the body.

(*See under* CHLORAL HYDRATE, ASPIRIN; etc.)

ANŒSTRUS is the state in the female when no œstrus or 'season' is exhibited. (*See* ŒSTRUS.)

ANOREXIA (ἀ, neg.; ὄρεξις, appetite) means loss of appetite. It is a symptom of many different diseases, especially of the stomach and intestines. (*See* APPETITE.)

ANOXIA.—Oxygen deficiency. Cerebral anoxia, or a failure in the oxygen supply to the brain, occurs during nitrite and prussic acid poisoning; in copper deficiency in cattle; and in the thoroughbred 'barker foal'.

ANTACIDS are medicines which correct acidity, whether general or stomachic. (*See* ALKALIES, DYSPEPSIA.)

ANTAGONISM.—When one drug with a certain physiological action is given simultaneously with or soon after another which has an opposite action, the result is *antagonism* in the animal subject. The action of the one substance diminishing that of the other and *vice versa*; thus if strychnine and morphine are given together in suitable doses the marked effects of neither are exhibited.

ANTE-NATAL INFECTION.—Examples of this may occur with the larvæ of the dog hookworm, *Ancylostoma caninum*, and with the larvæ of certain roundworms. (*See* TOXOCARA.) Toxoplasmosis is another example of an infection which may occur before birth.

ANTE-PARTUM PARALYSIS is a fairly common condition in the cow, has been seen in the sheep and goat, but is rare in the mare, in which the hind-quarters of the pregnant animal suddenly become paralysed. It appears from 6 to 25 days before parturition, and is liable to affect animals in almost any condition—those that are well kept as well as others.

Cause.—The actual cause cannot be established in all cases, but probably most are due to mechanical results produced by the compression of the nerves and vessels of the hind-limbs by the greatly enlarged and heavy uterus. Debility from an insufficiency of good food, lying for long periods in the same position, and accidental injuries received when lying or rising, are also accountable for some cases.

Symptoms.—The condition suddenly appears without any warning. The pregnant animal is found in the lying position, and is quite unable to regain her feet. The position of the body is natural: there is no interference with the pulse, breathing, or temperature, and the animal appears to be quite happy. The sensation in the hind-limbs and the quarters is generally retained, and movements are shown.

Treatment.—As a rule, the nearer to the day of parturition that the paralysis appears, the more favourable will be the result. Those cases that lie for two or more weeks are very unsatisfactory. The condition usually disappears after parturition has taken place, either almost at once or in two or three days. As a consequence, treatment should be mainly directed to ensuring that the animal is comfortable, provided with plenty of bedding, is turned over on to the opposite side three or four times a day, if she does not turn herself, and receives a laxative diet so that constipation may not occur. Mashes, green food, occasional doses of salts or oil, and a variety in the food-stuffs offered, are indicated. Tonics, such as strychnine, bitters, etc., and stimulating embrocations applied near to the spine, along with vigorous hand massage, are useful. If the cow does not rise by the end of a week after calving she should be destroyed, as she never will be an economic proposition subsequently. When the paralysis has occurred a considerable time before parturition is due, it is often necessary to produce artificial abortion of the fœtus and so relieve the uterus of its heavy encumbrance. All pregnant animals should be kept in as good hygienic surroundings as is possible, and should receive regular daily exercise.

ANTHELMINTICS (ἀντι, against; ἕλμινς, a worm).—These are substances which are given to expel parasitic worms. They include phenothiazine, thiabendazole, methyridine, piperazine compounds, tetramisole, hygromycin B, santonin, rafoxanide, haloxon, morantel tartrate, oxyclozanide, dichlorves, parbendazole. Niclosamide and bunamidine preparations are used against tapeworms in the dog.

Certain criteria apply to anthelmintics. For example, will the drug in question kill worm eggs? Is it effective against immature worms? Is it effective against adult worms of the economically important species? Does the drug discolour or taint milk? Can it be given to pregnant, or emaciated, animals?

Methods of administration include drenching; injection (in the case of tetramisole, for example); and in the feed.

ANTHISAN—An antihistamine.

ANTHRACOSIS (ἄνθραξ, coal) is that condition of the lungs and bronchial lymph glands which is due to the deposition of particles of carbon, soot, etc., from the inspired air.

ANTHRAX (ἄνθραξ, coal).—Synonyms: Splenic fever; splenic apoplexy; in human medicine, malignant pustule and woolsorter's disease; in India, loodianah disease and Manipur horse disease; in France, charbon and fièvre charboneuse; in Germany, Milzbrand; etc.

Anthrax is characterised by a high fever, an enlarged spleen, swellings of the throat in some animals, and by the presence of the casual organism in the blood-stream.

Animals attacked.—It may attack all the domesticated animals and man, while numerous of the wild animals are also liable to the disease, but it is commonest among the herbivora, and of these, cattle and sheep are the most frequently affected. The order of frequency among other animals is horse, pig, dog (including the fox), cat, rabbit (tame and wild), and the guinea-pig. Rats and mice may become affected by gaining access to the carcases of other animals that have died from the disease or to bone-meal, but birds possess a considerable degree of immunity.

Occurrence.—The disease is widespread, occurring in all parts of the world, particularly in tropical and sub-tropical areas where it kills thousands of cattle and sheep annually. In temperate countries cases only occur spasmodically, and in the majority of the outbreaks only a few cattle are affected.

Cause.—Anthrax is caused by the *Bacillus anthracis*. Under certain adverse circumstances each rod-shaped bacillus is able to form itself into a spore. The spores of anthrax are the hardest of all bacterial life to destroy. They resist drying for a period of at least two years, and very probably they can retain their vitality for a longer time than that if they are not exposed to sunlight. They are able to live in the soil for ten years or more and still be capable of infecting animals. The spores resist boiling for about half an hour, and are only killed with difficulty by the strongest disinfectants. Consequently pastures that have been infected by spilled blood from a case that has died are extremely difficult to render safe to stock on future occasions, and most particularly if these are at all wet or marshy. Cases have been known to occur on fields that were under grass ten years previously when an outbreak occurred, and which in the meantime had been cultivated every year in an effort to eradicate the organisms from the soil. It has been thought that the earthworm is to blame for cases that have broken out on fields in which on some previous occasion carcases dead from anthrax were buried. The contention is that the earth-worms carry the spores from deeper layers of the soil up to the surface. Spores have been found in bone manure, in blood fertilisers, in wool and hides from infected countries, and in feeding cakes imported from abroad. The fodder grown upon land that has been infected is liable to reproduce the disease, and streams of running water are a possible cause of the spread from one field to another, if they become contaminated. The bacillus itself is a comparatively delicate organism, and easily killed by the ordinary disinfectants.

Method of infection.—In cattle and the lower animals generally, it appears that infection nearly always occurs by way of the mouth and alimentary system. Either the living organisms or else the spores are taken in on the food or with the drinking water. The powerful gastric juice probably destroys most of the bacilli, but is unable to harm the spores. These latter under the influence of heat and moisture commence to vegetate, and, invading the walls of the intestines, reach the bloodstream, where they find conditions ideal for their subsequent very rapid growth. In certain cases it seems probable that both the house-fly (*Musca domestica*) and the horse-fly (*Stomoxys calcitrans*), by feeding upon the blood or upon the carcase itself and becoming contaminated, are factors in the spread of the disease, the latter, at least, causing infection by way of the skin. In man infection through the skin is the most frequent (for obvious reasons). Inhalation of the spores from dust, etc., although it occurs in man (woolsorters' disease), does not appear to be applicable to animals, but the disease has been caused through inoculation of vaccine contaminated by spores. Sheep should not be inoculated, therefore, in a dusty shed. Unsterilised bone meal is an important source of infection. (*See* BONE-MEAL.)

Symptoms.—Three forms of the disease are recognised: the *per-acute*, the *acute*, and the *sub-acute*.

In Cattle.—It is not often that any one connected with the animal has an opportunity to observe the symptoms, for in most cases the animal is found dead without having shown any noticeable symptoms beforehand. In those instances where the termination is not quite so sudden the animal may be noticed to be standing alone in a dazed, stupefied state, reeling and staggering if made to move, fighting for breath, perhaps bathed in perspiration, and showing all the signs of a high fever—a temperature of 106° or 107° F., a thin, rapid pulse, coldness of the ears, feet, and horns, and 'blood-shot' eyes and nostrils. After a few hours this picture is followed by one of prostration, unconsciousness, and death. In either of the above types there may have been considerable or small quantities of a blood-stained diarrhœa passed with some straining. In the so-called sub-acute form the affected animal may linger for as long as 48 hours, showing nothing more than a very high temperature, laboured respirations, and the symptoms that mark the onset of an attack of acute pneumonia. Such animals as these may get better or may die from an acute complication. Occasionally cattle may be infected through the skin, when a 'carbuncle' follows, similar to that seen in man. Diffuse, painless, doughy swellings are seen in other cases, especially about the neck and the lower part of the chest.

In Sheep and Goats.—Anthrax in these animals is almost always of the per-acute or apoplectic type. The animals are found dead without having shown any warning signs. The wool around the tail may be soiled by a blood-stained watery diarrhœa, and there is very rapid decomposition of the carcase, manifest by excessive and rapid formation of gas in the alimentary system, which dilates the abdominal walls.

In Horses.—There are two notable forms of anthrax in the horse; one in which there is a marked swelling of the throat, neck, and chest, and one in which there is exhibited an acute abdominal pain, not unlike that seen in acute inflammation of the bowels. In the first instance the signs are almost typical and characteristic. The swellings start at the throat and gradually form down the lower part of the neck until they reach the chest. Accompanying this there is all the evidence of an acute fever such as is seen in cattle. The swellings of the head and neck increase to such a size that the horse assumes the appearance of a hippopotamus. Movement becomes impossible, the head and neck being held forward in a stiff, wooden manner. The animal is unable to swallow, and a thin flow of saliva falls from the mouth, while respiration becomes more and more laboured until the horse finally expires in convulsions. In the other form of equine anthrax a fit of shivering ushers in the fever. The pulse-rate becomes increased, the horse lies and rises again with great frequency; he shows signs of slowly increasing abdominal pain by kicking at his belly, by gazing at his flanks, or by rolling on the ground. The bowels move frequently. Excitement gives way to a dull stupor, the gait is uncertain, until finally he dies in convulsions. From the beginning to the end of such a case in the horse, 3 to 7 or 8 hours only elapse.

In Pigs.—The disease may follow the feeding of slaughter-house refuse or the flesh of an animal that has died from an unknown disease, which has really been anthrax, or raw bone-meal intended as a fertiliser. There is sometimes swelling of the throat; or the intestine may be involved. In this abdominal form the symptoms may be very vague. Otherwise the pigs are dull, lie a good deal, show a gradually increasing difficulty in respiration, present in the early stages a swelling of the throat and head which later invades the lower parts of the neck, becoming more and more exaggerated, until finally the pig dies from choking. The disease takes from about 8 to 16 hours to run its course, death being quiet and unaccompanied by convulsions.

In Dogs, Cats, and Poultry.—These animals, although less frequently affected, usually present the acute or per-acute type. The symptoms shown are similar to those seen in cattle.

Prevention and Treatment.—In Great Britain, as in most civilised countries, anthrax is a disease which must be reported to the police or ministry responsible for the control of animal disease. In so far as its prevention is concerned the important points to remember are (1) the disposal of the carcase by efficient and safe means (*see* DISPOSAL OF CARCASES); (2) the careful observation of animals that have been in contact with the victim and their isolation from others if they show any rise in temperature; and (3) the strict supervision of the carcase until such time as it can be disposed of, with efficient methods of sterilisation of any blood or discharges that have been spilled. In this respect certain disinfectants are little better than useless if spores have had time to form. Bleaching powder in a hot 10 per cent solution kills both bacilli and the spores almost instantaneously.

The prompt use of anti-anthrax serum in large doses has been useful in a proportion of animals already showing symptoms, but it is essential that it is given at once. Penicillin may be used; also sulphathiozole. It is customary to use serum for the passive immunisation of animals which have been in contact with a case, and vaccination to give a longer immunity where outbreaks are common.

The milk from in-contact animals must be regarded as dangerous until such time as these are considered to be out of danger. It should be mixed with an equal amount of the chlorinated lime (bleaching-powder) solution, and after standing for ten minutes should be poured down a drain, or on to arable land which is some considerable distance from a water-course. Should the hands or clothes of a human being become contaminated with infective material, they should be washed in a suitable disinfectant as soon as possible, or in the case of clothing it should be destroyed, and the medical adviser informed. The law forbids any one who is not authorised to cut an anthrax carcase for any purpose whatsoever. Cases of death from this procedure are by no means unknown, and illness following the dressing of a carcase must always be considered suspicious of anthrax until the contrary has been established. The need for reporting illness to the medical authorities in all persons whose work brings them into contact with carcases of animals cannot be too strongly stressed.

ANTIBIOTICS.—Chemical compounds derived from or produced by living organisms which are capable, in small concentration, of inhibiting the life process of micro-organisms. To be useful in medicine an antibiotic must (1) have powerful action in the body against one or more types of bacteria; (2) have specific action; (3) have low toxicity for tissues; (4) be active in the presence of body fluids; (5) not be destroyed by tissue enzymes such as trypsin; (6) be stable; (7) be not too rapidly excreted; (8) preferably not give rise to resistant strains of organisms.

'Antibiotics can be divided, on a basis of their mode of action, into three groups: (1) those acting on the bacterial cell wall, such as the penicillins and bacitracin; (2) those affecting the cell membrane in a manner similar to that of detergents, and including polymixin, novobiocin, and nystatin; (3) this group appears to act by interfering with protein synthesis in bacteria and includes the tetracyclines, chloramphenicol, neomycin, streptomycin, and erythromycin.

'*The antibacterial activities of all antibiotics require the intervention of the cellular and humoral defence mechanisms of the body.* Evidence of this requirement is shown by the fact that in diseases such as agranulocytosisis, leucæmias, etc., the administration of even a competent antibiotic such as penicillin is useless, although the organism causing the infection is penicillin-sensitive.'—F. Alexander, D.SC., M.R.C.V.S.

Antibiotics are much used in veterinary medicine to overcome certain infections, and they have been of notable service, for instance, in the control of certain forms of mastitis in dairy cattle, in the avoidance of septicæmia following badly infected wounds, deep-seated abscesses, peritonitis, etc. Abdominal and other surgery has been rendered safer by the use of antibiotics. They must not, however, be used indiscriminately, be regarded as a panacea, or given in too low a dosage. It is unwise to use antibiotics of the tetracycline group in either pregnant or very young animals owing to the adverse effects upon bone and teeth which may result.

Selection of Antibiotic.—It is often necessary to begin antibiotic therapy before the results of bacteriological examinations are available, and therapy must depend on the clinical features. However, the taking of material for culture and carrying out sensitivity tests are most important procedures. Another factor in veterinary practice is the cost of the drug.

Only in a very few instances are mixtures of antibiotics superior to a single drug, and the use of fixed dose mixtures can be very misleading. In those cases in which more than one antibiotic is required, it is much better to use full doses of each of the individual antibiotics. Moreover, there is a degree of antagonism between penicillin and the tetracyclines. Combined antibiotic therapy does not improve the outlook in chronic urinary infections or, indeed, many chronic infections. Mixtures of antibiotics have been most successful when used in local applications or in infections of the alimentary canal. (*See* ADDITIVES, SIDE-EFFECTS, RESISTANT STRAINS, *and under* MILK.)

ANTIBIOTIC RESISTANCE.—Dr. F. Alexander stated (1966), 'There appear to be two types of antibiotic resistance. Acquired resistance, which is due usually to the organism being exposed to increasing concentrations of the antibiotic, and the second type, namely, selective survival. Organisms with the latter type of resistance survive exposure to antibiotics and are either naturally occurring resistant strains or mutants.

'The relatively new phenomenon of transferable resistance, first discovered by Watanabe and his colleagues (1963) must be mentioned. It has been shown that resistance to antibiotics can be transferred from one organism to another by so-called resistant factors or R factors. The R factor consists of R determinants which are genetic, and RT factors which are present in the cytoplasm, and it is these latter factors which are involved in the transference of the resistance from one strain of organism to another.'

Studies in the U.K. (Anderson, E. G., 1965) have shown that *Salmonella typhimurium* strains are commonly resistant to the following—streptomycin, tetracycline, sulphonamides; or chloramphenicol, streptomycin, tetracycline, sulphonamides; or streptomycin, tetracycline, neomycin, kanomycin, and sulphonamides. To these combinations of antibiotic resistance furazolidone resistance can now be added.

ANTIBIOTIC SUPPLEMENTS are subject to certain Government regulations in the U.K. (*See under* ADDITIVES.)

ANTIBODY.—A substance in the blood-serum or other body fluids formed to exert a specific restrictive or destructive action on bacteria, their toxins, or any foreign protein, *e.g.* an antitoxin.

Antibodies are not produced, like hormones, by a single organ, the blood then distributing them throughout the body. Antibody production has been shown to occur in lymph-nodes close to the site of introduction of an antigen, in the skin, fat, and voluntary muscle, and locally in infected tissues.

ANTICOAGULANTS.—Agents which inhibit clotting of the blood. They include dicoumarol and heparin. They have been used in the treatment of coronary thrombosis in humans, but not without a number of fatalities. (*See also* WARFARIN.)

ANTICOAGULINS.—These are substances secreted by hookworms in order to prevent clotting of the blood, which they suck.

ANTICONVULSANTS (*see* ANTISPASMODICS and PHENYTOIN SODIUM).

ANTIDOTES (ἀντί, against; δίδωμι, I give) are remedies which neutralise the effects of poisons either (*a*) by changing the poisons into harmless substances through some chemical action, or (*b*) by setting up an action in the body opposite to that of the poison.

Alkaloids.—Tannic acid, strong tea, or coffee.

Alkalies.—Vegetable acids; dilute acetic, citric, tartaric, vinegar and water; oils and demulcents.

Ammonia.—Acetic acid, vinegar, oils, and demulcents.

Antimony.—Tannin and purgatives, strong black boiled tea and linseed oil, oils and sedatives.

Arsenic.—Sodium thiosulphate in solution and lime-water.

Atropine and Belladonna.—Emetics, opium, stimulants, such as caffeine, hypodermically.

Barbiturates.—'NP13' (β-methyl-ethyl glutarimide) or Leptazol or Picrotoxin.

Cantharides or 'Fly Blister'.—*Internally*: Emetics, soothing or emollient drinks, opium; *avoid oils.* **Locally**: Wash with warm water containing potassium or sodium bicarbonate.

Carbolic acid.—White of egg, lime water, sulphate of soda (Glauber's salts), strong tea or coffee, and castor oil.

Carbon monoxide gas.—Fresh air, cold douches to the head and neck, diffusible stimulants, inhalations of ammonia, ether, etc.

Chlorinated lime or Bleaching powder.—Emetics, white of egg, milk, flour; *not acids.*

Chloroform.—Prussic acid, inhalations of ammonia or amyl nitrite, fresh air, artificial respiration, heart stimulants such as coramine or caffeine.

Copper salts.—Potassium ferrocyanide, soap, white of egg, metallic iron, oily purges, alkalies, and demulcent drinks.

Croton oil.—Emetics, starch-, barley-, or linseed-gruels, opium and astringents.

Cyanides and Prussic acid.—Inhalations of amyl nitrate, the intravenous injection of 3 per cent sodium nitrite and 25 per cent sodium thiosulphate solution. Artificial respiration.

Digitalis.—Emetics, tannin, empty the stomach and give stimulants, aconite hypodermically, and massage.

Hellebore, Hemlock, Henbane, Hyoscyamus.—Emetics, oil purges, strong black tea that has been boiled and allowed to stand, tannin, gallic acid or oak-bark infusion, atropine hypodermically.

Iodine.—Starch in solution, followed by barley-gruel.

Iron salts.—Carbonate of sodium ('washing soda'), magnesia, mucilages.

Lead salts.—Epsom and Glauber's salts, linseed oil, milk. If treatment can be given intravenously—calcium disodium versenate.

Mercury salts.—Eggs, wheat flour, starch milk, protochloride of tin, sulphuret of iron Epsom salts.

Mineral acids.—Alkalies; chalk, magnesium, the bicarbonates of soda and potash; demulcents; olive, whale, linseed, and rape oils, gruels, etc.

Morphia.—Strychnine (*see* Opium.)

Nembutal.—Picrotoxin or Leptazol or NP13.

Opium and Stramonium (Thorn Apple).—Emetics, animal charcoal, potassium permanganate with vinegar, oily purges, vigorous massage, exercise, inhalations of ammonia, cold douches; atropine, or caffeine hypodermically.

Oxalic acid.—Chalk or magnesia in water.

Phosphorus, as in rat-poisons.—Emetics, turpentine, gallicum, soothing drinks.

Organo-phosphorus compounds as in farm sprays—atropine sulphate by injection. (*See* ORGANO-PHOSPHORUS POISONING.)

Physostigmine or eserine.—Atropine hypodermically, chloral and stimulants.

Pilocarpine. — Atropine hypodermically, tincture of belladonna by the mouth.

Strychnine.—Emetics, chloral, chloroform, bromide of potassium, tobacco, nicotine, anodynes and sedatives.

Tobacco.—Emetics, tannin, strong black tea, purges, strychnine, external and internal stimulants.

Yew.—Operation of rumenotomy, active purges, mucilaginous drinks such as thick linseed- or barley-gruel, sedatives.

Zinc salts.—Milk, white of egg in cold water, tannin, copious draughts of warm water.

ANTIFEBRIN (*see* ANTIPYRINE).

ANTIGEN is a substance which causes the formation of antibodies.

ANTIHISTAMINES are drugs which neutralise the effects of histamine in excess in the tissues. They are useful in treating shock following burns and also allergic disorders, *e.g. some* cases of: laminitis, urticaria, azoturia, light sensitisation, bloat, acetonæmia, anaphylaxis, acne, etc. They include mepyramine maleate, promezathine hydrochloride, Anthisan, Benadryl, and Phenergan. They should not be used except under professional advice.

Recently, eosinophil cells have been found to be a rich source of an anti-histamine factor. (*See* EOSINOPHIL.)

ANTIHORMONES.—True antibodies formed consequent upon the injection of hormones.

ANTIKETOGENIC is the term applied to foods and remedies which prevent or decrease the formation of ketones.

ANTIMONY is a metallic element belonging to the class of heavy metals. Antimony salts are less used now in veterinary medicine than formerly, less toxic substitutes being preferable.

Uses.—Tartar-emetic, the double tartrate of antimony and potassium, used for intravenous injection against certain trypanosomes and other protozoon parasites. (*See* ANTIDOTES.)

ANTIPERISTALSIS is a term used to indicate a reverse action of the movements of the stomach or the intestines. The contraction starts in a part distant from the commencement of the alimentary system and carries the ingesta nearer to the mouth. It is opposite to PERISTALSIS. (*See also* POISONS, ANTIDOTES).

ANTIPHLOGISTICS (ἀντι, against; φλέγω, I burn) are remedies used in inflammation of tendons or muscles, in orchitis, and in parotiditis. They commonly consist of mixtures of kaolin and glycerine with some antiseptic added, or of cold packs applied to the part affected. Proprietary antiphlogistics are sold in containers which require warming before application; some of these are of great value, such as ' Antiphlogistine '.

ANTIPYRETICS (ἀντι, against; πυρετός a fever) are measures or drugs used to reduce temperature during fevers.

ANTIPYRINE, or **PHENAZONUM,** is one of the coal-tar derivatives which is of crystalline form, possesses the following properties: It dulls pain, reduces temperature, produces profuse perspiration, in the horse especially. The principal of these drugs, in addition to antipyrine, are acetanilide or antifebrin, and phenacetin.

Uses.—Antipyrine may be used for reducing temperature in equine influenza, and as a sedative for the central nervous system. Acetanilide is much more serviceable in the treatment of animals, having more powerful although also more poisonous characters. It is used in cases of hæmoglobinuria and for fevered conditions in horses, cattle, and dogs, when its lowering effect on the temperature is well marked. It has not such a sedative action on the nervous system, but large doses slow the heart-beat. Phenacetin lowers temperature, decreases pain, and slightly depresses the heart, being less powerful than the two aforementioned drugs. It is safer than acetanilide, but larger doses are needed to produce the same effects.

ANTISEPTICS (ἀντί, against, and σηπτός, putrid, from σήπω, I make rotten). —Strictly speaking, the term ' antiseptics ' should be reserved for agents which prevent fermentation, putrefaction, or disease by hindering or disallowing the growth of micro-organisms without necessarily killing them. Preparations designed to kill organisms are properly called ' disinfectants ' or ' germicides '. Many substances may be either antiseptic or disinfectant according to the strength used.

Very strong antiseptic or disinfectant solutions should not be used for wounds because of the destruction of cells they cause. The dead cells so formed may retard healing, and in some cases are later cast off as a slough.

The chief of the chemical antiseptics which are of service in animal medicine are as follows:

Acriflavine is one of the best antiseptics for a healing wound. It is potently lethal to organisms, yet, even in strong solution, it is practically non-irritant to the cells. It is used as a solution of 1 part in 1000.

Chlorine compounds in several different forms are used for cleansing wounds from the presence of organisms. During war they are extensively used for continuous irrigations of large septic shot-wounds and give good results. Among the class may be mentioned eusol, eupad, bleaching powder solution, 'T.C.P.', ' Fecto,' etc. They include sodium hypochlorite and chloramines, both also used as disinfectants.

Quaternary Ammonium compounds (see under this heading), are widely used in dairy hygiene. They include cetrimide (see under separate heading) and benzalkonium chloride.

'Dettol', Liquor Chloroxylenolis, B.P.—Powerful bactericides of low toxicity. Much used for skin cleansing, obstetrical work, and disinfecting premises. The bactericidal action is reduced in the presence of blood or serum.

Crystal Violet—A 1 per cent solution forms a useful antiseptic for infected wounds, burns, fungal skin diseases, and chronic ulcers. Similarly, **gentian violet**.

Common salt (a teaspoonful to a pint of boiled water) is useful as a wound lotion and is usually easily obtainable when other antiseptics may be lacking. It promotes a flow of serum and lymph from the cells of the part, stimulates granulating tissue, acts as a mechanical cleanser of the area, and although somewhat irritating in a wound is non-poisonous.

Sulphonamides have proved of great use in wounds infected with streptococci and certain other organisms. They are to be regarded as bacteriostatic, in this respect that below effective strength they may have very little beneficial action. When properly used, however, they have revolutionised wound treatment.

Iodoform is a powerful, poisonous but soothing antiseptic formerly often used for dusting on to wounds as a powder with boric acid.

Iodine in an alcoholic solution is more penetrating and irritant, especially to delicate skins. For use on the unbroken skin *only*.

Alcohol is a very powerful antiseptic chiefly used for removing grease and septic matter from the hands of the surgeon and the skin of the patient. (Ether is used in this way also).

ANTISERUM (*anti*, against).—A serum for use against a specific condition is produced by inoculating a susceptible animal with a sub-lethal dose of the causal agent or antigen and gradually increasing the dosage until very large amounts are administered. The animal develops in its blood serum an anti-substance which can be made use of to confer a temporary protection on other animals. Antisera may be either *antibacterial* or *antitoxic*. In the former, dead or attenuated cultures are used for injection; in the latter, a toxin of known strength produced by filtering a culture of the organism is employed. In either case, the tissues of the animal are able to mobilise a defensive mechanism by producing an antidote which circulates in the blood serum. The reaction bears a direct proportion to the amount of the antigen used.

The use of antiserum alone confers a temporary immunity, and in most cases this probably does not protect for longer than from 10 days to a maximum of about 21 days. Antisera are used in the treatment of existing disease, and also as a means of protecting animals exposed to infection.

ANTISIALICS.—Substances which reduce salivation; *e.g.* atropine.

ANTISPASMODICS (ἀντί, against; σπάσμα, a spasm) are remedies which diminish spasm or 'cramp'. They mostly act upon the muscular tissues, causing them to relax and making the vital contractions more regular, or soothing nerves which control the muscles involved.

Modern anti-convulsive drugs include LARGACTIL and MYSOLINE (*see under those headings*).

ANTITETANIC SERUM is a serum used against tetanus. Nowadays the antitoxin is preferred. (*See* TETANUS.)

ANTITOXINS, or **ANTITOXIC SERA** (ἀντί, against; τοξικόν, arrow poison) are substances calculated to neutralise the harmful effects of a toxin. (*See* SERUM THERAPY.)

ANTIVENINE is a substance produced by the injection of snake venom into animals in small but increasing doses. In course of time the animal becomes immune to the particular venom injected, and the antivenine prepared from its serum is highly effective in neutralising venom injected by the bite of a snake of the same species. To be of any use it must be administered within one hour of the snake bite.

ANTIVIRAL.—Used against viruses.

ANTIZYMOTIC.—An agent which inhibits fermentation.

ANTRYCIDE.—A synthetic drug used in the control of trypanosomiasis.

ANTS are of veterinary interest as intermediate hosts of the liver fluke *Dicrœlium dendriticum*. This fluke, which is smaller than *Fasciola hepatica*, the common fluke, is found in sheep, goats, cattle, deer, hares, rabbits, pigs, dogs, donkeys, and occasionally man. In the British Isles, the fluke occurs only (it is believed) in the islands off the Scottish mainland.

The fluke's eggs are swallowed by a land-snail of the genus *Helicella*. From the snail, cercariæ periodically escape and slimy clumps of them are eaten by ants (*Formica fusca* in the U.S.A.). Grazing animals, swallowing ants with the grass, then become infested.

Ants also act as the intermediate host of a tapeworm of the fowl, guinea-fowl and pigeon, *Raillietina tetragona.*

ANTU.—Alphanaphthylthiourea, used to kill rodents. One gram may prove fatal to a 20 to 25 lb. dog. The poison gives rise to œdema of the lungs. (*See also* THIOUREA.)

ANURIA is a condition in which little or no urine is excreted or voided for some time. (*See* URINE, KIDNEY.)

ANUS is the opening of the digestive tract to the outside, by means of which the unused and unusable portions of the food material are evacuated. In health it is kept closed by the *sphincter ani,* a ring of muscle fibres about one inch thick in the horse, which is kept in a state of constant contraction by certain special nerve fibres situated in the spinal cord. If this ring fails to relax, constipation may result, while in some forms of paralysis the muscle becomes unable to retain the fæces. In the dog there are two small anal glands situated one on either side of the opening and slightly to the inside of the actual ring. These secrete a musky material, and are considered to be scent-glands. Under certain circumstances the ducts by which they open become occluded and the secretion does not escape. The glands swell and become inflamed, while the pain is sufficient to prohibit the attempt of evacuation, and the dog gets constipated as a result. They require to be evacuated by squeezing, and some soothing ointment should be applied afterwards. On occasion they require surgical attention. (*See also* IMPERFORATE ANUS.)

AORTA is the principal artery of the body. It leaves the base of the left ventricle and curves upwards and backwards, giving off branches to the head and neck and fore-limbs. About the level of the 8th or 9th thoracic vertebra it reaches the lower surface of the spinal column, and from there it runs back into the abdominal cavity between the lungs, piercing the diaphragm. It ends about the 5th lumbar vertebra by dividing into the two internal iliacs and the middle sacral arteries. The internal iliacs supply the two hind-limbs and the muscles of the pelvis. At its commencement the aorta is about 1½ inches in diameter in the horse, and from there it gradually tapers as large branches leave it. It is customary to divide the aorta into *thoracic aorta* and *abdominal aorta.* (*See* ARTERIES, ANEURISM.)

AORTIC RUPTURE.—This follows degenerative changes in the aorta, and is a not uncommon cause of death of male turkeys aged between 5 and 22 weeks. It was first reported in the U.S.A. and Canada. In Britain most cases occur between July and October. No symptoms are observed ; the birds being found dead. ' In a flock of 500 turkeys, 30 or more may die from this disease over a period of 2 to 3 weeks ' (BOCM Poultry Advisory Service). The use of Reserpine has been recommended in order to lower blood pressure and so prevent further deaths in a flock.

APERIENTS (*aperio,* I open) are medicines which produce a natural movement of the bowels. (*See* CONSTIPATION, PURGATIVES.)

APEX (*apex,* summit) means the pointed extremity of an organ, such as the heart, lungs, or cæcum, which has a roughly conical general outline.

APHTHA, MALIGNANT.—This, and contagious aphtha, are other names for FOOT-AND-MOUTH DISEASE (which see).

APLASTIC.—Relating to aplasia, the congenital absence of an organ. In aplastic anæmia, there is defective development or a cessation of regeneration of the red corpuscles, etc.

APNŒA (ἀ, neg. ; πνέω, I breathe) means the stoppage of respiration which occurs when the blood is artificially supplied with too much oxygen ; for instance, when several deep breaths are taken in quick succession. (*See* ASPHYXIA.)

APOMORPHINE is a derivative of morphine which has a marked emetic action in the dog, and is used in that animal to induce vomiting when some poisonous or otherwise objectionable material has been taken into the stomach. It has a very rapid action, passes off quickly, and leaves no bad after-effects. It is given in doses of $\frac{1}{25}$th to $\frac{1}{10}$th of a grain by hypodermic injection, or double these amounts by the mouth.

APONEUROSIS is the name for a sheet of tendinous tissue providing an insertion or attachment for muscles, which is sometimes itself attached to a bone, and sometimes is merely a method of attaching one muscle to another.

APOPLEXY (ἀποπληξία)—an extravasation of blood into some one or other organ, but usually the brain, and resulting in a sudden insensibility.

Causes.—Cerebral apoplexy may occur as a complication during the course of certain specific diseases, such as anthrax, and it is also seen in animals that are suffering from such conditions as heart disease, kidney disease, or chronic inflammation of the liver. Severe excitement, violent coughing fits, or excessive muscular exertion when the animal is in a weakened state, may bring on an attack, and it is seen in some cases of tumour formation. In each of these conditions some of the smaller blood-vessels that supply the brain become burst and allow the blood to escape into the brain substance or on to its surface. This collects and presses on the vital nerve tissue, producing the symptoms of the condition.

Symptoms. — The symptoms vary according to the extent of the hæmorrhage. In the mildest cases only the slightest amount of staggering, sweating, or excitability is exhibited. In more serious instances the animal becomes unsteady in its gait, stumbles, falls to the ground, and lies in an unconscious state. In the most acute conditions when the hæmorrhage is extensive the beast falls as if shot, performs a few convulsive movement, stiffens, and is soon dead. The breathing is generally much troubled and even stertorous, while occasionally it is hardly perceptible. In nearly all cases there is no complete recovery. The animal may live for a considerable time, but remains weak and uncertain in its movements. It may receive a total or partial paralysis of one or a group of muscles ; its eyesight is sometimes destroyed ; or it becomes affected with a permanent lameness.

Treatment.—In most instances the only course is destruction of the animal. If treatment is to be attempted the first essential is to lower the blood-pressure as rapidly as possible. Perfect quietness is essential, and the animal should be taken to a dark loose-box and soothed if it be excited.

APOTHECARIES' WEIGHT is the measure by which medicines used to be dispensed.

The apothecaries' table is as follows:

20 grains (gr.) . .	1 scruple (℈)
3 scruples . .	1 drachm (ʒ)
8 drachms . .	1 ounce (℥)
12 ounces . . .	1 pound troy (lb.)

Further, 437·5 grains make one ounce, and 7000 grains are 1 lb. avoirdupois. A fluid ounce is the bulk of one ounce by weight of water, and the minim and fluid drachm are the corresponding bulks of the weights of one grain and one drachm, which are $\frac{1}{480}$th and $\frac{1}{8}$th of an ounce respectively. A minim of water is about one drop. There are 20 fluid ounces in one imperial pint, and 8 pints in a gallon. One grain is equal to ·0648 of a gramme, and there are 15·432 grains in a gramme. (*See* EQUIVALENTS, TABLES OF.)

APPALOOSA.—The Appaloosa Horse Society of America and the British Spotted Horse Society are concerned with the breeding of this horse, which has some Arab blood and is characterised by a silky white coat with black (or chocolate-coloured) spots which can be felt with the finger.

APPETITE is a desire to take food. When the word is applied to the sexual activities it is used to indicate a desire for satisfying reproductive impulses.

' Depraved ' appetite. — Sometimes an animal will eat rubbish such as cinders, coal, stones, soil, plaster, wire, old clothes, fæces, etc., the reason in some cases being a mineral or vitamin deficiency. In some diseased conditions, especially rabies, hysteria, and dyspepsia, and during pregnancy, the tendency to ingest foreign bodies is so great as to be an important feature of the conditions. Another cause of ' depraved ' appetite or pica is infestation with parasitic worms, and this may cause the victims (dogs, cats, and carrion birds) to eat moles poisoned by strychnine or birds poisoned by dieldrin, etc., and so themselves become poisoned. (*See* COPROPHAGY, BARK, *and* MORTAR EATING.)

Excessive appetite may be a sign of dyspepsia or diabetes, of internal parasites, of tuberculosis, listeriosis, or of the early stages of malignant tumour formation.

Diminished appetite is common to very many diseases which result in a weakening of the system, as the activity of the stomach and the gastric juice are among the first body functions to become impaired. Anorexia, or a diminished appetite, is present in the later stages of tuberculosis, cancer, especially of the stomach, in most forms of dyspepsia, in gastritis and enteritis, in many fevers, and in abnormal conditions of the throat and the mouth, when the act of swallowing is difficult or painful. In other cases the appetite is in abeyance for no apparent reason, and after a course of tonics and stomach stimulants it returns and becomes normal. During disease, when the appetite is capricious or uncertain, endeavours should always be made to keep the animal's interest in its food by giving as great a variety of suitable food-stuffs, and as small quantities at a time as possible for it is important to maintain the animal's strength. (*See* NURSING OF SICK ANIMALS, MINERALS, VITAMINS.)

APPLES.—Windfalls beginning to ferment occasionally give rise to mild alcohol poisoning (which see) in horses, cattle, and pigs in orchards.

APYREXIA (ἀ, neg. ; πυρέσσω, I am fevered) means that stage in certain diseases in which the temperature falls or there is no fever.

ARACHIS OIL (*see* BLOAT.)

ARACHNIDS (ἀράχνη, a spider) is the name of the class of Arthropoda to which belong the mange mites, ticks, and spiders. (*See* PARASITES, p. 681.)

ARACHNOID MEMBRANE (ἀράχνη, a spider ; εἶδος, form) is one of the membranes covering the brain and spinal cord. (*See* BRAIN.) Arachnoiditis is inflammation of this membrane.

ARBOVIRUSES.—This is an abbreviation for arthropod-borne viruses. They are responsible for infectious diseases (such as louping-ill, blue-tongue) transmitted by ticks, insects, etc.

ARECA-NUT is the seed of *Areca catechu*, the betel-nut tree. The freshly ground powdered nuts were formerly used for the expulsion of tapeworms from the intestines of the dog, but have largely been superseded by more efficacious preparations, such as arecoline-acetarsol (' Tenoban '), ' Dicestal ', etc.

Arecoline is the chief alkaloid found in areca-nut, and as the hydrobromide it is used when a rapid stimulation of peristalsis, an evacuation of the fæces, and an increase in the secretions of the intestinal glands is desired, such as in certain forms of colic. Its use requires great care ; for if the heart be at all weak it may cause collapse, and if there is acute obstruction of the bowel it is liable to give rise to rupture of the intestines. It is given to the horse in doses of from ½ to 1½ or even 2 grains by hypodermic injection. About twenty minutes after its injection the horse commences to salivate profusely, sometimes to an alarming extent, but this passes off in 30 to 40 minutes, and leaves no bad after-effects. It may also cause a temporary sweating. The use of arecoline in cattle practice is not always satisfactory. It should never be given to a pregnant animal.

AREOLA means a small space, and is the term applied to the red or dusky-brown coloured ring around the nipple in the human female and in the dog, or to an inflamed ring. In some breeds of toy dogs it is possible to distinguish a darkening of the areolæ of the nipples in early pregnancy, but this feature is not so marked nor so reliable as it is in the human subject.

ARGENTUM is the Latin word for silver.

ARIZONA INFECTION in turkeys was reported for the first time in the U.K. in 1968. The infection is caused by the Arizona group of the enterobacteriaceæ—closely related to the salmonellæ and the coliform group. Young birds can be infected by contact or through the egg. Nervous symptoms and eye lesions are characteristic in birds surviving the initial illness.

ARNICA is a medical preparation derived from the root of *Arnica montana*, a plant of the Western States of America and of Europe. The tincture of arnica is used as a lotion for application to sprains and bruises, relieving the pain.

AROMATICS include most of the essential oils of plants, such as anise, cloves, turpentine, camphor, thymol, as well as benzene, phenol or carbolic acid, aniline, etc. All these have a distinct aroma or smell, and most are strong antiseptics.

ARRHYTHMIA is a word used to signify that the heart-beat is not occurring regularly, or that a beat is being periodically missed. It may be only a temporary manifestation to which little or no importance should be attached, or on the other hand it may be a symptom of some form of cardiac disease. It requires a very careful examination before an opinion can be pronounced as to its harmlessness or otherwise.

ARSANILIC ACID.—One of the organic compounds of arsenic used as a growth supplement for pigs and poultry, and for the control of swine dysentery.

It should not be given within ten days of slaughter, nor should the recommended dosage rate be exceeded, as residues—especially in the liver—may prove harmful if consumed. The permitted maximum of arsenic in liver is 1 part per million. In a random survey (1969), 4 of 93 pig livers contained from 1·2 to 3·5 p.p.m. of arsenic.

Blindness, a staggering gait, twisting of the neck, progressive weakness and paralysis are symptoms of chronic poisoning with arsanilic acid in the pig.

ARSENIC is a metal, but by the word as commonly used is meant the oxide, or arsenious acid. It is contained in a great variety of substances, among the most common of which are: Scheele's green and emerald green—the two arsenites of copper; Orpiment or King's yellow, and Realgar—sulphides of arsenic; Fowler's solution—the liquor arsenicalis of the *British Pharmacopœia*, which contains arsenic trioxide; older varieties of sheep-dip, especially those sold as a powder; weed-killers, haulm destroyers, rat-poisons, fly-papers, wall-papers; and in lead shot as a hardening agent.

Uses.—Externally, arsenic is still used as a component, with derris, of some sheep dips, though arsenic has largely been replaced by BHC, etc. Internally, it was formerly employed for many different purposes, the chief being: (1) to expel worms in the horse, with action also as a digestive tonic by stimulating the muscles of the alimentary canal; (2) as a nerve tonic in asthma, chorea, and epilepsy; (3) as a tonic with a special action on the skin in eczema and grease; (4) in combination with salts of iron in anæmia and general debility; and (5) as an intravenous injection in cases of trypanosomiasis and infection with sclerostome worms in horses. Arsenic is sometimes given to horses in the hope that it will improve their condition; but if left to the unskilled to administer, too large doses are generally given, sometimes with fatal results. Arsenic is incorporated in some compound animal feeding-stuffs in order to improve growth rate. The disposal of dung containing arsenic residues from poultry-houses, etc., may accordingly be fraught with danger. (*See also* ARSANILIC ACID, ADDITIVES.)

Administered in small doses over a long period, arsenic may give rise to cancer.

ARSENIC, POISONING BY.—Arsenic is an irritant poison producing in all animals gastro-enteritis, no matter whether given by the mouth or otherwise. The rapidity of its action depends on the amount that is taken, on the solubility of the compound, on the presence or otherwise of food in the digestive system, and on the susceptibility of the animal.

Horse.—The symptoms shown are violent purging, severe colic, straining, a staggering gait, coldness of the extremities of the body, unconsciousness, convulsions, and death in a variable time, when a large amount has been taken. When the poisoning is the result of the taking of small doses for a considerable period, cumulative symptoms are observed. These consist of an unthrifty condition of the body generally, swelling of the joints, indigestion, constant or intermittent diarrhœa, often with a fœtid odour resembling decomposing flesh, great thirst, emaciation, and distressed breathing and heart action on moderate exercise.

Ox.—Cattle show symptoms somewhat similar to those seen in horses, but larger doses are needed to produce toxicity, and owing to the peculiarities of the alimentary canal the arsenic takes longer to act. Profuse watery diarrhœa is a common feature of chronic poisoning.

Cattle have died after straying into a field of potatoes sprayed with arsenites to destroy the haulm. Others have died following the application to their backs of an arsenical dressing, and of the use of arsenic-contaminated, old bins for feeding purposes.

Sheep.—Probably most cases of arsenic poisoning in sheep occurred from the use of arsenical dips before BHC was introduced. The source of this poisoning is in many cases the herbage of the pastures which becomes contaminated either from the drippings from the wool of the sheep, or from the washing of the dip out of the fleece by a shower of rain on the second or third day after the dipping. Absorption through wounds or laceration of the skin may result in arsenic poisoning, and when dips are made up too strong absorption into the system may also occur. The signs of poisoning are dullness, frothing at the mouth, colicky pains, and rapid respirations. Death takes place quickly. The obvious precautions, apart from care in the actual dipping, are to ensure that the sheep are kept in the draining pens long enough to ensure that their fleeces are reasonably dry (some 15 to 20 minutes) and subsequently are not allowed to remain for long thickly concentrated in small fields or paddocks. Where double dipping is carried out, the second immersion in an arsenic dip must be at half-strength.

Dog and Cat.—These animals are particularly susceptible to poisoning by arsenic, especially the dog. The symptoms are nausea, vomiting, abdominal pain, dark fluid evacuations, and death preceded by convulsions.

Antidotes.—Sodium thiosulphate is a better antidote than ferric hydroxide, and a solution can be given intravenously. (*See* DIPPING, TONICS, etc.)

ARTERIES (ἀήρ, air ; τηρέω, I keep) are the vessels which carry the blood away from the heart to the tissues and organs of the body. With the exception of the pulmonary artery, which carries venous blood to the lungs, the arteries carry oxygenated blood ; that is, blood which has recently been circulating in the lungs, has absorbed oxygen from the inspired air, and has become scarlet in colour. The pulmonary artery carries blood of a purple colour which has been circulating in the body and has been returned to the heart, to be sent to the lungs for oxygenation.

The arterial system begins at the left ventricle of the heart with the aorta (*see* AORTA). This is the largest artery of the body. It divides and subdivides until the final branches—so small that they are invisible—end in the capillaries which ramify throughout the whole of the body tissues except cornea, hair, horn, and teeth. The larger of these branches are called *arteries*,, the smaller ones are *arterioles*, and these end in the *capillaries*. The capillaries pervade the tissues like the pores of a sponge, and bathe the cells of the body in arterial blood. The blood is collected by the venous system and carried back to the heart.

The chief arteries of the horse are : (1) two *coronary arteries*, which supply the heart-muscle with blood ; (2) two *common carotids*, each of which runs up the neck and gives off branches to its muscles on the same side, and ends by dividing into an *internal* and an *external carotid* and an *occipital artery*. These terminal branches supply the brain and the head and face generally ; (3) two *subclavians*, which supply the fore-limbs. Each runs to the level of the first rib on either side ; from there to the shoulder-joint they are called the *axillary arteries* ; after passing this joint they become the *brachials* till the elbow-joint is reached where they are called *medians*, and *common digitals* at the carpus ; (4) *intercostal arteries* arise opposite each space between two adjacent ribs, either from the aorta or from some other large artery in the vicinity. These supply the muscles, etc., between the ribs and the spinal column and its associated structures ; (5) *phrenic arteries* to supply the diaphragm arise just as the aorta leaves the thoracic and enters the abdominal cavity ; (6) *cœliac artery*, which divides into *gastric*, mainly to the stomach, *hepatic*, chiefly to the liver, and *splenic*, to the spleen ; (7) *cranial mesenteric* supplies branches to the small intestines, the cæcum, and the colon ; (8) *renal arteries* to the right and left kidneys ; (9) *caudal mesenteric*, which supplies the colon and rectum ; (10) *internal spermatic arteries* or *utero-ovarian arteries*, according to whether the animal is a male or female, nourish the genital organs ; (11) *lumbar arteries*, which are arranged similarly to the intercostals ; and after these the aorta ends by dividing into two *common iliac trunks* and a *middle sacral artery*. Each common iliac gives off branches to the pelvic structures and then divides into an *internal* and an *external iliac artery*. The internal iliac or *hypogastric* is distributed to the inner aspect of the pelvis and to its contents, and the external iliac runs past the brim of the pubis out of the pelvic and becomes the *femoral*, which is the chief trunk of the hind-limb. The femoral artery runs down the inside of the thigh to the back of the stifle-joint, where it becomes the *popliteal* ; this, after a short course, divides into a small *posterior tibial* and a large *anterior tibial*. This latter runs down the anterior surface of the tibia to the hock, where it becomes the *dorsal pedal*, and is continued onwards as the *common digital* below the hock.

Each of these larger branches gives off numerous smaller branches to supply muscles, bones, skin, or parts of organs in the vicinity of its course.

Structure.—The arteries are highly elastic tubes which are capable of great dilatation with each pulsation of the heart—a dilatation which is of considerable importance in the circulation of the blood. (*See* CIRCULATION.) Their walls are composed of three coats : (*a*) *adventitious coat*, consisting of ordinary strong fibrous tissue on the outside ; (*b*) *middle coat*, composed of muscle fibres and elastic fibres, in separate layers in the great arteries; (*c*) ***inner coat*** or ***intima***, consisting of a layer of yellow elastic tissue on whose innermost surface rests a single continuous layer of smooth, plate-like ***endothelial cells***, within which flows the blood-stream. The walls of the larger arteries have the muscles of their middle coat replaced to a great extent by elastic fibres so that they are capable of much distension. When an artery is cut across, its muscular coat instantly shrinks, drawing the cut end within the fibrous sheath which surrounds all arteries, and bunching it up so that only a comparatively small hole is left for the escape of blood. This in a normal case soon becomes filled up with the blood-clot which is Nature's method of checking hæmorrhage. (*See* HAEMORRHAGE; BLEEDING, ARREST OF.)

ARTERIES, DISEASES OF.—These include:

1. **Arteritis** occurs during specific virus diseases such as African Swine Fever, Equine Viral Arteritis, Rubarth's disease, etc.

2. **Chronic inflammation,** or **Arterio-sclerosis,** is a process of thickening of the arterial wall and subsequent degenerative changes, resulting in an abnormal rigidity of the tube and hindrance to the circulation.

3. **Degenerative changes** also occur in the arteries of pigs, especially, during the course of several diseases. Examples are hæmorrhagic gastritis and Herztod disease. Rupture of the aorta is not uncommon in young male turkeys.

Generalised arterio-sclerosis must be rare among animals, but when present gives rise to a very high blood-pressure, a tendency to fainting fits, and an ever-present risk of sudden death from rupture of the right side of the heart, or of the aorta, when the animal exerts itself.

4. **Thrombosis.**
5. **Embolism.**
6. **Aneurism.**

ARTHRITIS (ἄρθρον, a joint) means inflammation of a joint or joints. The chief forms are traumatic, rheumatic, or specific, such as the arthritis that is met with during the course of certain of the febrile diseases, *e.g.* swine erysipelas and tuberculosis. A mineral deficiency may also be responsible. (*See* JOINTS, DISEASES OF; BRUCELLOSIS; RINGBONES; SPAVIN; CORSTIONE.)

ARTICULAR RHEUMATISM is a manifestation of rheumatic conditions in one or more of the joints, where the lesion produced is known as rheumatic arthritis. (*See* RHEUMATISM.)

ARTIFACT.—An apparent lesion in a histological or pathological specimen, not existing during life, but made accidentally in preparing the specimen.

ARTIFICIAL ABORTION means the removal by means of hormone preparations or manipulative interference of the fœtus and its membranes at some time previous to parturition. It may be necessary to effect premature birth in some cases of dropsical disease of the uterus or its contents, when eversion of the vagina, accompanied by persistent straining, occurs, when a monstrosity is present in the uterus, and when a severe accident has caused the death of the fœtus but not its expulsion. The manual methods are of an intricate nature and demand the greatest care lest infection results. (*See* STILBŒSTROL, MALUCIDIN.)

ARTIFICIAL BONES.—In racing greyhounds, badly fractured scaphoids have been removed and replaced with plastic replicas. (Hare Spy won a race on January 16, 1958, after such an operation.)

ARTIFICIAL HIBERNATION.—A fall in the rate of metabolism and of body temperature, such as may be produced by 'Largactil' (a phenothiazine derivative) in conjunction with an anæsthetic. A French technique for combating shock in human beings.

ARTIFICIAL INSEMINATION. — The introduction of male germ cells (*spermatozoa*) into the female without actual service.

The practice is a very old one. In the fourteenth century Arab horse-breeders were getting mares in foal by using semen-impregnated sponges. In Italy bitches were artificially inseminated as long ago as 1780, and at the close of the nineteenth century the practice was applied, to a very limited extent, to mares in Britain.

It was the Russian scientist Ivanoff who saw in A.I. the possibilities of disease control, and in 1909 a laboratory was established in Russia for the development and improvement of existing techniques. 'By 1938 well over a million cattle and 15 million sheep had been inseminated in the U.S.S.R., where all the basic work was done.' Denmark began to take a practical interest in A.I. in 1936 (and within eleven years had a hundred co-operative breeding stations inseminating half a million head of cattle annually); the U.S.A. in 1937. The United Kingdom began to practise A.I. on a commercial basis in 1942, and by the end of 1950 had close on a hundred centres and sub-centres in operation, serving over 60,000 farms. From the Milking Marketing Board's A.I. centres more than 1,784,000 cows were inseminated during 1970–71.

Uses.—The use of A.I. in commercial cattle breeding is dependent upon the fact that, in normal mating, a bull produces between 50 and 100 times as much semen as is required to enable one cow to conceive. By collecting the semen, diluting it and, if necessary, storing it in a refrigerator, the insemination of many cows from one ejaculate becomes possible.

A.I. reduces the spread of venereal disease, and hence greatly reduces the incidence of the latter. Farmers in a small way of business are able to dispense with the services of a communal bull—an animal seldom well bred and often infected with some transmissible disease. At the same time, the farmer has the advantage of the use of a healthy, pedigree bull without the considerable expense of buying, feeding, and looking after it. Owners of what are sometimes called commercial herds are enabled to grade these up to pedigree standard, with an increase in quality and milk yield. In many of the ranching areas overseas, where stock-raising is carried out on an *extensive*, rather than an *intensive*, scale, to achieve satisfactory production of animals for trade and commercial purposes, sires have to be imported at regular intervals from the essentially sire-producing countries—of which Britain is the chief. The method of artificially inseminating a large number of females from an imported sire enables bigger generations of progeny to be raised and consequently more rapid improvement to be achieved.

Methods.—Various methods are employed. Those which give best results involve the use of an artificial vagina in which to collect the semen from an ejaculation. This is used outside the female's body, being so arranged that the penis of the male enters it instead of entering the vagina. The full ejaculation is received without contamination from the female.

After the ejaculate has been collected it is either divided into fractions, each being injected by a special syringe into the cervix or uterus of another female in season, or—in commercial practice—it is diluted 20 times or more with a specially prepared 'sperm diluent', such as egg-yolk citrate buffer. Dilution rates of up to 1 in 100 have been successful, but it appears desirable to inseminate 12 or 13 million sperms into each cow.

The method requires skill to carry out successfully, and necessitates the employment of strict cleanliness throughout. (*See* CONCEPTION RATES.)

With the object of making A.I. more practicable in sheep, a technique for the control of the breeding cycle has been developed at the University of Sydney. A plastic sponge impregnated with the hormone progesterone or an equivalent substance to suppress heat is inserted into the vagina. When the sponge is removed—with the aid of an attached drawstring—normal ovulation occurs 2 to 4 days later.

Artificial insemination has also been carried out in pigs (*see* FARROWING RATES), goats, dogs, turkeys and other birds, bees, etc.

Storage of Semen.—Diluted semen may be stored at A.I. centres for a few days if kept at a temperature of 5° C. In practice, a good deal is wasted because its fertilising power has diminished before it is all required for use. Research work, carried out at Cambridge, has made it possible, however, to store semen for months and even years. In this technique, glycerol is added to the sperm diluent, and it is this addition which enables the spermatozoa to withstand a temperature of −79 degrees Centigrade (110 degrees below zero, Fahrenheit) without losing their power to fertilise when thawed. In practice the diluted semen was stored in special cabinets containing solid CO_2. Nowadays it is stored and transported at −196 degrees Centigrade, using liquid nitrogen.

The advantages of this method are many. There is less wastage of semen, more can be stored, and the semen of any particular bull can be made available on any day. It is possible for several thousand cows to be got in calf by a given bull. In fact, a Hereford bull owned by the Milk Marketing Board, had by 1960 sired 50,000 calves. The disadvantages of using a given bull or bulls too widely must be borne in mind, but that is a matter of policy and not of technique.

The deep freezing of boar semen did not lead to conception until it was introduced directly into the sow's oviducts. By this method it is possible to inseminate a thousand sows with one ejaculate of a boar. A simple surgical operation is at present necessary but Agricultural Research Council work is continuing to find a surgery-free technique.

ARTIFICIAL LACTATION (*see* p. 490).

ARTIFICIAL REARING OF PIGLETS.—Cows' colostrum makes a satisfactory substitute for sows' colostrum, and may be frozen and later thawed when required. Pigs' serum as an addition enhances the value of cows' colostrum.

ARTIFICIAL RESPIRATION.—This is resorted to in: (1) Cessation of respiration while under general anæsthesia; (2) cases of drowning when the animal has been rescued from the water—chiefly applicable to the smaller animals; (3) poisoning by narcotics or paralysants, such as morphia and prussic acid; (4) cases of asphyxia from fumes, smoke, gases, etc.

Horses and Cattle.—If indoors, open all poors, windows, etc., of the building so as to ensure thorough circulation of air. Release from all restraint except a loose halter or head-collar, extend the head and neck to allow a straight passage of the air into the lungs, open the mouth, and pull the tongue well out. If any fluid—blood, saliva, or water—is suspected in the throat it is advisable to raise the neck to a higher level than the head by placing under it a sackful of straw, a bale of hay, or a rolled-up overcoat, so that the fluid may escape by the mouth. Should the ground slope the horse must be placed with his head downhill. While such adjustments are being carried out one or two assistants should have been engaged in compressing the elastic posterior ribs by alternately leaning the whole weight of the body on the hands pressed on the ribs, and then releasing the pressure about once every 4 or 5 seconds, in an endeavour to stimulate the normal movements of breathing. As an alternative in a larger animal a heavy person may sit himself with some vigour astride the ribs for about the same time, rise for a similar period, and then re-seat himself. If no response occurs, these measures should be carried out more rapidly.

It is advisable to extend the uppermost fore-limb (by means of a rope round the pastern) as far forwards as possible, and at the same time as the release of the pressure on the thorax.

The inhalation of strong solution of ammonia upon a piece of cotton-wool and held about a foot from the upper nostril often assists in inducing a gasp which is the first sign of the return of respiration, but care is needed not to allow the ammonia to come into contact with the skin or burning will occur. After 2 or 3 minutes' work the animal should be turned on to the opposite side to prevent stasis of the blood. Sometimes the mere act of turning will induce the premonitory gasp. So long as the heart continues to beat, no matter how feebly, the attempts at resuscitation should be pursued.

Pigs and Sheep.—The outlines of procedure given for the larger animals are equally applicable here. In addition, if the size of the animal will allow, an assistant should grasp the two fore-limbs and raise the fore-quarters off the ground as high as possible for a second; then, as he lowers the fore-end a second person raises the hind-quarters in a similar manner. The two people should face each other.

Dogs and Cat.— In these smaller animals the methods of artificial respiration more nearly resemble those that are employed in human work. A reliable method, that is, a modification of the Schafer system, is to lay the dog on its side with the head at a lower level than the rest of the body, place one hand flat over the upper side of the abdomen and the other on the rib-cage, lean heavily on the hands, and in a second or two release the pressure. Another method is to lay the dog on its back, and standing behind the head grasp the fore-limbs above the wrists or carpus and forcibly extend the legs upwards and outwards, bringing them to the side of the head. Now return them to the thorax and, still holding the legs, compress the dog's thorax between the hands. An assistant should hold the hind-limbs to steady the body.

The motions of artificial respiration should in all cases be a little faster than those of normal respiration, but a slight pause should always be observed before each rhythmic movement.

A respiratory stimulant may be given by injection. (*See* CORAMINE.) A carbon dioxide 'Resuscitator' may be used.

ARTIFICIAL SOMATIC MUTATIONS in birds have, it is claimed by French scientists, been obtained by their use of Desoxyribonucleic acid (DNA). This was prepared from the nuclei of testicular tissue and from erythrocytes of donor Khaki Campbell ducks, and injected intraperitoneally into Pekin ducks and drakes starting when the animals were 8 days old. Nine ducks were used and they were injected with DNA weekly for 19 weeks. The 3 drakes used were given 5 injections over one month.

About 9 months afterwards 8 of the ducks and one drake showed marked deviation from the Pekin type having developed characteristics much more like the donor Khaki Campbell breed. Changes in beak colour, feathering, conformation of the head, and size of the body were apparent. The artificial 'hybrids' differ greatly from the normally produced cross between Khaki Campbell and Pekin, which reverts to the primitive Rouen type.

The mutations produced by DNA behave quite normally, the ducks laying eggs regularly and the drake showing normal sexual activity.

ASCARIDÆ is the name of a class of worms belonging to the round variety, or *Nemathelminthes*, which are found parasitic in the intestines of horses, pigs, dogs, and cats particularly, although they may affect other animals. They attain a size of 15 or 18 inches in the horse, but are smaller in other animals. (*See* PARASITES, p. 657).

ASCITES (ἀσκός, a wine skin) means dropsical swelling of the abdomen; a very common complication of abdominal tuberculosis, of liver, kidney, or heart disease, as well as of some parasitic infestations. (*See* DROPSY.)

ASCORBIC ACID.—Synthetic vitamin C.

ASEPSIS (ἀ, neg.; σήπω, I make putrid) is a term used in surgery, and means that principle employed during the conduct of an operation where, instead of the use of strong germicides, sterilised water, boiled dressings and instruments, and rubber gloves are utilised. The object aimed at is to cleanse thoroughly everything which is to come into contact with the wound, as well as the skin covering the part, and to maintain that scrupulous cleanliness until the wounds are healed. Aseptic surgery is the ideal, but among animals it may be difficult to attain if carried out under farm conditions. Moreover, it is an exceptionally difficult matter to prevent accidental infection in a surgical wound after the operation, for the animal cannot be put to bed; and it may object to the dressings and do all in its power to remove them. (*See* ANTISEPTICS, SULPHONAMIDES, PENICILLIN.)

ASH POISONING has been reported in cattle. Symptoms include: drowsiness, dropsical swellings over ribs and flanks, purple discoloration of perineum.

ASPERGILLOSIS, or **PNEUMOMYCOSIS,** is the name given to a disease of animals and birds produced by the growth of the fungus *Aspergillus* in the tissues of the body. The various parts of the respiratory system are the most commonly affected, but the disease is also met with in the ears, liver, and sometimes in the mouth and throat. It runs a slow chronic course which in some ways resembles that of tuberculosis and in fact, is occasionally mistaken for it. (For poisoning by the toxin produced by *Aspergillus flavus*, *see under* GROUNDNUT MEAL.)

Cause.—The disesae is produced by the presence of the fungus in the tissues of the body, where it causes a necrosis or death of the cells and the formation of small abscesses in its vicinity. The spores are abundantly present in hay, fodder, and grain, and gain access to the body by inhalation. Once within the body they grow out *hyphæ*, which in turn produce more spores and these spread the infection further. It is very rare in sheep and cattle that live wholly in the open air.

Symptoms.—The air passages become filled with a cheesy material in which the fungus develops, and breathing gets progressively worse. The bird gapes with its beak, gasps for breath, exhibits frequent sneezing and coughing, and there is a constant rattle in the throat. A discharge with a repulsive odour trickles from the mouth and nostrils, or is expelled with each cough or sneeze. The sick birds isolate themselves from the rest of the flock, and gradually waste in condition. In some cases there is a marked diarrhœa, while in others the joints swell and become painful, with resulting lameness. Eggs from sick birds show an opaque, nonmotile, dense spot in the enlarged airchamber, which, if th ‹ egg be carefully broken, is found to be composed of the greenish mould or fungus.

In young turkey poults, involvement of the brain has been reported; the symptoms being: unsteady gait, walking backwards, and turning of the neck to one side.

In the Ox the disease somewhat resembles contagious pleuro-pneumonia and tuberculosis, although the symptoms are not very characteristic. The animal does not thrive, but appears dull and weak; the appetite is poor. The breathing is laboured and often accompanied by a hard, dry cough, or a moan or grunt on expiration. When there are areas of fungus growth in the lung the sides of the beast 'lift', and there are evidences of obstruction of the bronchi if the ear be placed over the sides of the animal. The temperature is rarely above normal. There often is some nasal discharge in which the fungus or its spores may be found.

In the Horse the disease resembles a sore throat, bronchitis, pneumonia, anthrax, or anæmis according to the seat of the fungus. It is not by any means common.

In the Dog, which may contract the infection from poultry, the disease runs a rapid course, often accompanied by epileptiform convulsions, or symptoms that are not unlike those of rabies. There is always a considerable amount of scratching or rubbing of the muzzle and the nose, as if the dog was trying to rid itself of some irritating object. A discharge runs from the nostrils or is sneezed from them; it is usually blood-stained.

Treatment is very unsatisfactory and should only be attempted in the more valuable animals. They should be given the best of food, and whenever possible turned outside into the open air.

ASPHYXIA (ἀ, neg.; σφύξις, pulse) means literally an absence of pulse, but is applied to the whole series of symptoms which follow stoppage of breathing and the cessation of the heart's action.

Causes.—Asphyxia may occur during the administration of anæsthetics by inhalation, during the outbreak of fires in animal houses, where the fumes and the smoke present are responsible for œdema, and in cases of poisoning. In isolated cases asphyxia may be caused by the presence of large abscesses or tumours in the respiratory passages, either in the throat or nose. These, if of a chronic nature, cause little distress until some occasion arise when the respiratory system is overtaxed and an insufficiency of air enters the chest, with consequent unconsciousness.

In Africa, cattle have been deliberately strangled—a cause of asphyxia seldom encountered elsewhere in domestic animals.

Symptoms.—The direct cause of death from asphyxia is an insufficiency of oxygen supplied to the tissues by the blood. The first signs are a rapid and full pulse, and a quickening of the respirations. The breathing soon changes to a series of gasps, and the blood-pressure rises, causing the visible membranes to become intensely injected and later blue in colour. Greater struggles for breath occur, and soon general convulsions supervene. The convulsions are followed by quietness, when the heart-beat may be almost imperceptible and respiratory movements practically cease. The actual time of death is unnoticed as a rule, since death takes place very quietly.

During the stage of convulsions, when the amount of carbon dioxide circulating in the blood is increased, the smaller arteries vigorously contract and cause an increase in the blood-pressure. This high blood-pressure produces an engorgement of the right side of the heart, which cannot totally expel its contents with each beat, and becomes more and more dilated until such time as the pressure in the ventricles overcomes the strength of the muscle fibres of the heart and the organ ceases to beat. During this stage immediate relief follows bleeding from a large vein.

Treatment.—The first essential in all cases of asphyxia is to remove the cause by opening all ventilating openings, or by carrying the animal into the open air and adjusting the head and neck so that no pressure is placed on the air passages. So long as the heart is beating, recovery may be hoped for with vigorous measures. If the breathing is shallow and the membranes livid, artificial respiration (which see) should be begun. Inhalations of ammonia upon a piece of cotton-wool held to the nostrils are useful. Where the cause is situated in the larynx, the immediate use of a tracheotomy tube may save the animal's life.

ASPIRATION (*aspiro*, I breathe) means the withdrawal of fluid from the natural cavities of the body or from cavities produced by disease. It may be performed for either curative purposes, when a large quantity is usually removed, or for diagnostic purposes, when only a small amount is removed with a hypodermic syringe.

Uses.—*Dropsy* of the chest or abdominal cavity is the commonest condition requiring aspiration. It is generally relieved by a small metal tube or canula which is provided with a sharp-pointed stilette or trocar. The trocar fits into the canula and the two are inserted into the cavity to be drained, the trocar is withdrawn and the hollow canula left in position for the fluid to escape into an air-tight bottle by rubber tubes. There is usually required some suction to withdraw the fluid, and this is supplied by a hand vacuum pump. *Pleurisy*, when there has been a throwing out of fluid, is another condition that benefits from the operation of aspiration. *Pericarditis* may be treated by aspiration when there is a collection of fluid present. *Inflammations of joints and bursæ*, particularly of the limbs of horses, are often aspirated.

Before the operation the skin is very carefully cleansed, and the instruments are previously boiled ; scrupulous care is necessary to prevent any infection of the cavities opened.

ASPIRIN is a preparation of acetylsalicylic acid. It is sedative to nerves, antiseptic, anti-rheumatic. Owing to its expense it is seldom given to the larger and less valuable animals. It has been given in influenza, pneumonia, distemper, rheumatism, and pachymeningitis, etc., but 5 gr. daily is said to prove fatal to cats within 12 days. (*See Vet. Record* November 11, 1963.) A dose of 22½ gr. over 2½ days proved fatal to one cat. Symptoms of aspirin poisoning in the cat include loss of weight, salivation, vomiting, unsteady gait. Aspirin can also prove harmful in the dog, injuring the mucous membrane of the stomach, and should *not* be given in cases of gastro-enteritis. (*See* SALICYLATE POISONING.)

ASTHENIA (ἀ, neg. ; σθένος, strength) is another name for debility. *Asthenic* is applied to the exhausted state that precedes death during some fevers.

ASTHMA (ἆσθμα, a gasping ; ἀσθμαίνω, I gasp for breath) is a term somewhat loosely applied. Strictly speaking, the term should be reserved for those conditions where a true spasmodic expulsion of breath occurs without the effort of a cough. Broken wind in the horse is a condition difficult or impossible to distinguish from asthma upon certain occasions, as the two diseases have some common features. (*See* BROKEN WIND.) The so-called ' asthma ' of birds is due in nearly every case to aspergillosis. (*See* ASPERGILLOSIS.)

Causes.—These are obscure, but it is generally held that true spasmodic asthma is of nervous origin, and due to a sudden distressful contraction of the muscle fibres which lie around the smaller bronchioles. In some cases asthma may be an allergic phenomenon. In other cases a chronic inflammation of the lining mucous membrane of the small tubes is the cause.

Botanical and clinical studies have shown that the spores of fungi (*e.g.* cladosporium, botrytis, and alternaria) are potent allergens, and can account for many cases of asthma, especially recurrent summer asthma, in man. There are, however, a number of patients with seasonal (summer or autumn) asthma who are not sensitive to spores of any of the above nor to pollen.

Symptoms.—The horse is suddenly seized with a painful and distressing difficulty in breathing, frequently when at rest in the stable. The inspiratory actions are abrupt and sudden, while expiration is drawn out and jerky. In some cases a shallow cough accompanies the expiratory effort, but it is not constant. The animal stands with the fore-limbs apart, the elbows turned outwards, and the head and neck extended. The face has an anxious, worried expression, and the nostrils are dilated. Movement causes an increase in the severity of the attack, and the horse prefers to stand in one position. After a period normal respiration becomes restored and the horse commences to feed as if nothing had happened. It may remain quite normal for a few hours or even a month, but is liable at any time to a recurrence. Nasal discharge often appears later in the course of the disease, but it is absent at first. The pulse-rate is increased and there may be some cardiac disturbance, as shown by a purplish hue of the visible mucous membranes—eyes, nose, and mouth.

Treatment.—Administration of various antispasmodic drugs has been recommended ; also antihistamines.

Asthma in the Dog.—Many cases that are really chronic bronchitis are spoken of as ' bronchial asthma ' owing to their similarity to asthma in man, with which many owners of animals are familiar. In true asthma the attacks of dyspnœa (*i.e.* distressed respiration) occur at irregular intervals, and there are periods between them when the dog is to all appearances quite normal. The attacks occur suddenly, are very distressing to witness, last for from ten minutes to half an hour, and then suddenly cease. The dog gasps for breath, makes violent inspiratory efforts without much success, exhibits a frightened, disturbed expression, and stands till the attack passes off.

The condition appears to be hereditary in some breeds, especially the Maltese terrier. Cardiac dysfunction also gives rise to ' asthma '.

Treatment.—Inhalations of amyl nitrite often serve to cut short an attack; internally antispasmodics. Antihistamines or heart tonics may be of service. Regulation of exercise and diet is necessary.

ASTIGMATISM (ἀ, neg.; στίγμα, a point) is a defect of vision due to irregularities in the curvatures of the cornea (*i.e.* the clear anterior membrane of the eye), in which the curve is longer in one axis than in the other. The eyes of the horse and the ox are very frequently astigmatic, but it appears that there is some compensating nervous provision by which the animal is able to appreciate objects in the usual way although its eyes possess defect. In human beings similarly affected round objects appear to be elliptical and square figures are oblong.

ASTRAGALUS, or **TALUS**, is the name of one of the bones of the tarsus (hock), with which the tibia forms the main joint. The articulation between these two bones is sometimes referred to as the 'true hock joint', the others being more or less secondary and less freely movable joints. (*See* BONES.)

ASTRINGENTS (*astringo*, I bind) are substances that cause contraction of mucous surfaces, blood-vessels, or tissues, or which stop secretions.

Examples.—Dilute acids; acetate or sugar of lead, sulphate of copper (bluestone), sulphate of zinc, alum, tannic acid, witch-hazel.

ASUNTOL.—An anti-tick organo-phosphorus compound.

ASYSTOLE (ἀ, neg.; συστολή, a contraction) means a failure of the heart to contract, generally due to the walls having become so weak that they are unable to contract and expel the blood, with the result that the organ becomes distended —a feature found after death.

ATAVISM (*atavus*, a grandfather) means the inheritance of disease or bodily characters from grandparents or remote ancestors, the immediate parents not having been so affected. (*See* HEREDITY.)

ATAXIA (ἀ, neg.; τάξις, order) means the loss of the power of governing movements, although the necessary power for these movements is still present. A staggering gait results.

ATELECTASIS (ἀτελής, imperfect; ἔκτασις, expansion) is applied to that condition of the lung either at birth or in the adult state, when the air cells become obliterated and fail to expand with each

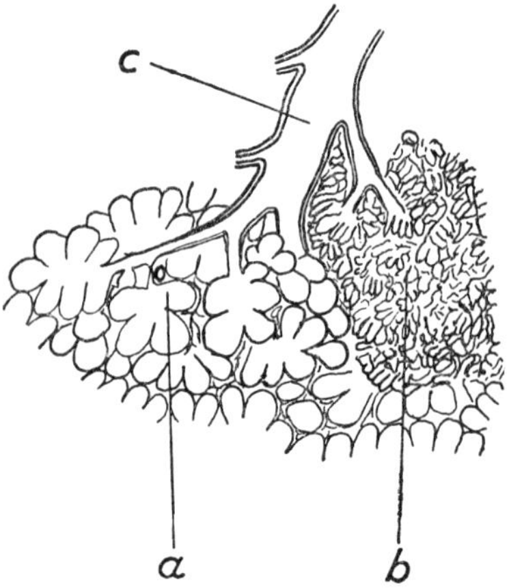

Atelectasis of the lung. *a*, Area of normal lung *b*, area of atelectasis; *c*, a small bronchiole.

respiratory movement. An area thus affected is collapsed, solid to the touch after death, and gives a dull note on percussion of the chest-wall.

ATHEROMA (ἀθήρη, porridge) is a degenerative change in the inner and middle coats of the arteries. (*See* ARTERIES, DISEASES OF.)

ATLAS is the name given to the first of the cervical vertebræ, which forms a double pivot joint with the occipital bone of the base of the skull on the one hand, and forms a single gliding pivot joint with the epistropheus—the second cervical vertebra—on the other hand. The freedom of movement of the head is due almost solely to these two joints. The large space between the bony surfaces of the upper aspect of the first of these joints is sometimes made use of in humane destruction of animals—a knife blade being inserted in the space to divide the spinal column.

ATOMIC EXPLOSIONS (*see under* HYDROGEN BOMB).

ATONY (ἀ, neg.; τόνος, strength) means want of tone or vigour in muscles or other organs. (*See* TONICS.)

ATOPIC DISEASE.—A hypersensitivity to pollens and other inhaled protein particles. (*See* ALLERGY.) Hay-fever-like symptoms may be produced in the dog; also intense itching affecting the feet, abdomen, and face.

ATOXYL, or SODIUM ARSANILATE, is a white powder constituting an organic preparation of arsenic. It is used by intramuscular and intravenous injection for treatment of certain diseases due to the presence of trypanosomes in the blood.

ATRESIA (ἀ, neg.; τίτρημι, I pierce) means the absence of a natural opening, or its obliteration by membrane. Atresia of the bowel is found in newly born pigs, lambs, calves, and foals. Atresia is sometimes met with in the vaginæ of heifers, when it constitutes what is known as 'white heifer disease'. (*See* WHITE HEIFER DISEASE.)

ATRIAL.—Relating to the atrium or AURICLE (which see) of the heart.

ATROPHIC MYOSITIS (*see under* MUSCLES, DISEASES OF).

ATROPHIC RHINITIS.—A disease of pigs. (*See under* RHINITIS.)

ATROPHY (ἀ, neg.; τρέφω, I nourish) is a wasting of the tissues. Atrophy may be local or general according to whether only an area or particular tissue or the whole of the body be affected. General atrophy is seen in most of the severe diseases, sooner or later; in old age, following starvation, when it is often called *emaciation*; and in certain conditions where defective nutrition of the fœtus in its dam's uterus has taken place. Localised atrophy is much the more common, and is in many cases important, since it may be the only indication of disease that can be recognised from the outside. A wasting away of the muscles of a limb owing to disuse—what is called the 'atrophy of inaction'—is a very common symptom of old-standing lameness in the horse. After a 'slipped shoulder' or a 'slipped stifle' (*i.e.* a dislocation of these joints), the mass of muscular tissue that is normally found around these joints becomes less. If only one side of the body is affected, as is the most usual, the right and left sides of the animal are no longer symmetrical, the affected side showing a smaller mass of muscle over the particular joint. Following paralysis of a motor nerve, when the muscles supplied by it are no longer able to contract, atrophy of the area takes place. This is seen in paralysis of the radial nerve in the horse, which often results from a fracture of the first rib and consequent pinching of the nerve between the broken ends. Here the large mass of muscle immediately above the elbow (triceps muscle) and those on the anterior aspect of the fore-arm (extensors) become flabby and decrease in size. In long-standing cases they almost disappear, and leave well-marked hollows. Atrophy may also result from the cutting off of the blood-stream, as by the ligaturing of an artery. Again, delicate tissues that are subjected to great or continuous pressure become atrophied; for instance, the sheep's brain is atrophied when the cyst stage of the tapeworm *Cœnurus cerebralis* has been in existence for some time. (*See* PARASITES.) Organs in the vicinity of rapidly growing tumours and pressed upon by them atrophy. (Cf. HYPERTROPHY.)

ATROPINE is the alkaloid contained in the leaves and root of the deadly nightshade (*Atropa belladonna*). Preparations of belladonna owe their actions to the presence of atropine, and are active in such proportions as the percentage of the alkaloid varies. It depresses sensory nerve-endings and thus relieves pain and spasm in parts to which it is applied. It checks secretion in all the glands of the body when given internally; and whether given by the mouth or rubbed on the skin it causes a dilatation of the pupil of the eye and paralysis of accommodation. In large doses it induces a general stimulation of the nervous system, but this action is rapidly followed by depression, and the primary effect is not noticed in the administration of ordinary doses. The action on the heart is one of stimulation, since the inhibition fibres are paralysed, while the accelerator nerves are not interfered with, except when large doses are given and paralysis of all motor fibres occurs.

Uses.—Externally, the chief use of

belladonna preparations is for the relief of pain in delicate structures such as the udders of all animals, the testes, and the eyes. It is also used to dilate the pupil for the examination of the eye in daylight. Internally, it is given in conditions where there is great pain in the abdominal organs. In painful and inflamed conditions of the respiratory passages, such as bronchitis, pharyngitis, laryngitis, and in inflammation of the mouth, salivary glands, and tongue, it is used to check the secretions from the glands and allay the pain. Finally, it is the antidote to morphine poisoning, when it is given as the sulphate of atropine by hypodermic injection, and also to some of the organo-phosphorus compounds used as farm sprays.

ATROPINE POISONING may occur as the result of the unintentional administration of too large amounts of the alkaloid or of the drug belladonna in one form or another, or it may be induced by feeding on the plant growing wild in Nature, and it may happen that after the application of a belladonna liniment or plaster the drug is absorbed into the circulation, or the animal may lick the area, and toxic symptoms result.

The signs of poisoning shown are restlessness, delirium, dryness of the mouth, a rapid and weak pulse, quick, short respirations, an increase in temperature, and dilatation of the pupil. In addition there is sometimes seen a loss of power in the hind-limbs, but apart from this no signs of paralysis have been noticed. In the dog, convulsions usually precede death.

Antidotes.—To those animals that vomit, an emetic should be given at once. if the poison has been taken by the mouth. Horses and cattle should have their stomachs emptied by the passage of the stomach-tube, in so far as that is possible. Stimulants such as ammonia should be given, and pilocarpine, by hypodermic injection, is the physiological antidote. Artificial respiration, hot and cold douches to the head and neck, and the emptying of the bladder, are indicated.

ATTENUATED (*see under* VACCINE).

AUDITORY NERVE, or **ACOUSTIC NERVE,** is the 8th of the cranial nerves, and is concerned with the special sense of hearing. It arises from the base of the hind-brain just behind and at the side of the pons. It is distributed to the middle and internal ears, and in addition to its acoustic function it is also concerned with the balance of the body. (*See* EAR.)

AUJESZKY'S DISEASE.—Also known as Pseudo-rabies and Infectious Bulbar Paralysis, occurs in cattle, pigs, dogs, cats, and rats, and is caused by a virus. The disease has a very short incubation period, and is characterised by intense itching. It was first described in Hungary by Aujeszky in 1902, is not very common in the United Kingdom; and has been encountered in several parts of the U.S.A., South America, Australia, the continent of Europe, etc.

Symptoms.—Cattle.—The first symptom to be observed is usually a persistent licking, rubbing or scratching of part of the hindquarters (or sometimes of the face) in an attempt to relieve the intense itching. The affected part soon becomes denuded of hair, and may be bitten or rubbed until it bleeds. Bellowing, salivation, and stamping with the hind-feet may be observed. Within 24 hours the animal is usually recumbent and unable to rise on account of paralysis. Death, preceded by convulsions, usually occurs within 36 to 48 hours of the onset of symptoms.

Pigs.—In these animals the disease may run a milder course, with a mortality of 5 per cent or less. Symptoms may include, besides some evidence of pruritus, loss of appetite, vomiting, diarrhœa, convulsions, drooling of saliva, paralysis of the throat. Mummification of the fœtuses may occur in pregnant sows affected with Aujesky's disease. Such sows may show loss of appetite and constipation, or stiffness and muscular inco-ordination without itching at all.

Dogs and Cats.—Restlessness, loss of appetite, vomiting, salivation, signs of intense irritation (leading to biting or scratching) about the face or some other part, and occasionally moaning, groaning, or high-pitched screams are among the symptoms observed.

The disease often occurs in the animals named above following an outbreak among rats, and may be spread by rat-bites. Cattle are often infected by pigs. Dogs have died after eating meat from carcases of cattle dead from Aujeszky's disease. Recent work has suggested that the rat may be an incidental rather than a reservoir host of the virus, and less important in the spread of the disease than was previously thought.

AURAL.—Relating to the ear.

AURAL CARTILAGES are the supporting structures of the ears. There are three chief cartilages in most animals, viz. the *conchal*, which gathers the sound waves and transmits them downwards into the cavity of the ear and gives the ear its characteristic shape; the *annular*, a cartilaginous ring below the former which is continuous internally with the bony acoustic canal; the *scutiform*, a small quadrilateral plate which lies in front of the others and serves for the attachment of muscles which move the ear.

Accidents and diseases of the cartilages of the ear are not common in animals, with the exception of two conditions. Ulceration of the cartilages, chiefly the annular, occurs as a complication of ear inflammation in the dog. Laceration of the conchal cartilage is seen as the result of the application of a twitch to the ear in the horse. In severe cases the cartilage may be actually split, and owing to the poor blood supply, healing is very slow,

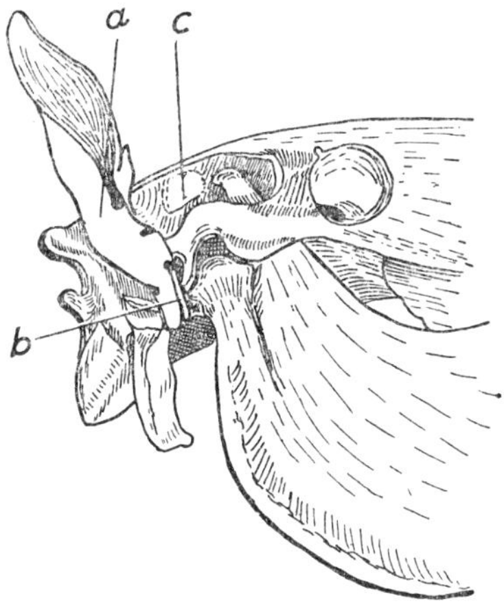

Aural cartilages of horse. *a*, Conchal; *b*, annular; *c*, scutiform.

and malformation often results. If the damage is considerable, amputation may be necessary. The tips of the flaps of the ears of dogs sometimes become lacerated, and prove resistant to treatment. As soon as healing begins, the dog further irritates the wound by continually shaking its head, and the damaged area does not get an opportunity of healing. In such cases the hair should be clipped from the ear-flap, the surface cleaned with alcohol (*e.g.* methylated spirits), the wounded part covered with a small amount of pure iodoform, and a broad piece, or several narrow strips, of adhesive tape should be stuck on to the inner surface of the ear, carried over the edge, and then stuck on to the outer surface. It should be firmly pressed on to the surface of the skin, and left in position for a week. At the end of that time it is removed, and may be reapplied if necessary. Occasionally it is necessary to remove the piece of damaged cartilage by a surgical operation.

AUREOMYCIN.—An antibiotic obtained from a mould *Streptomyces aureofasciens*. (*See* ANTIBIOTICS; *also* ANIMAL PROTEIN FACTOR.) In cattle it has been used in cases of streptococcal and staphylococcal mastitis. In horses it is used in the treatment of strangles, and infected wounds. In dogs it is effective against leptospirosis and coccidiosis. It has a low toxicity, though side-effects have been reported; occasionally shock at the first injection.

Aureomycin is the brand name for CHLORTETRACYCLINE. In the U.K. it is now classed as a therapeutic antibiotic and is no longer used as a feed additive for growth promotion. (*See under* ADDITIVES; *also* SIDE EFFECTS.)

AURICLE, or ATRIUM.—The auricles, right and left, are the chambers at the base of the heart which receive the blood from the body generally, and from the lungs respectively. Opening into the right auricle are the cranial and caudal vena cavæ, which carry the venous blood that has been circulating in the head and neck and the abdomen and thorax. This blood is pumped into the right ventricle through the tricuspid valve. Opening into the left auricle are the pulmonary veins which bring the arterial blood that has been purified in the lungs; when this auricle contracts the blood is driven into the left ventricle through the mitral valve. (*See* HEART, CIRCULATION.)

AUSCULTATION (*ausculto*, I listen) is a method of diagnosis used in medicine by which the condition of some of the internal organs is determined by listening to the sounds they produce. Auscultation is practised either by placing the ear over the part concerned or by means of the stethoscope (στῆθος, the chest, and σκοπέω, I examine).

The stethoscope consists of a small chest-piece connected by rubber tubing to ear-pieces made of metal. The phonendoscope is an instrument in which the chest-piece is replaced by a vulcanite and metal drum, with devices for the modification or intensification of the sounds heard. The application of electricity, by means of microphones and amplification of the sound waves may become of greater use in future.

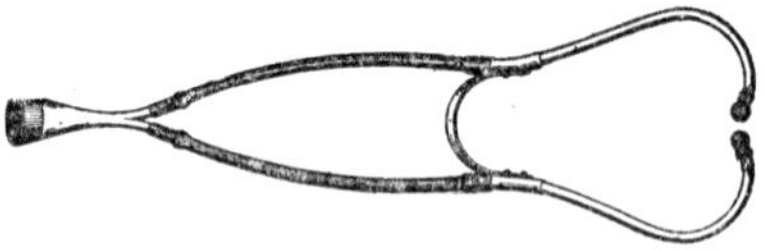

Binaural stethoscope.

The stethoscope is a most valuable aid to the accurate diagnosis of heart and chest affections in all animals. Some difficulty is always encountered in horses and cattle that are very fat or that have thick chest walls, and in those that are of a nervous or irritable disposition. The chief diseases that affect the lungs, pleura, and heart are fairly easily recognisable by the method of auscultation, and a number of other conditions are able to be better interpreted by its use than otherwise; chief among these are crepitation in deeply seated fractures, the heart sounds of the intra-uterine fœtus, and the grating sound that accompanies certain joint affections when ulceration of the articular cartilages has taken place.

AUTOCLAVE (αὐτός, self; *clavis* a key, or *clavus*, a nail) is a strong closed vessel, generally of metal covered with felt, which is used to sterilise utensils, instruments, or dressings before they are used for bacteriological or surgical measures.

AUTOGENOUS (αὐτογενής, self-produced) means self-generated, and is the term applied to products which arise within the body. It is applied especially to bacterial vaccines manufactured from the organisms found in discharges from the body and used for the treatment of the particular individual from whom the bacteria were derived.

AUTO-INFECTION (αὐτός, self; *inficio*, I taint) is a term used to indicate the infection of one part of the body, hitherto healthy, from another part that already is suffering from the disease. Thus, sheep suffering from 'orf' on their feet may bite the painful areas and convey the organisms to their mouth, where the disease becomes established.

AUTO-INTOXICATION (αὐτός, self; τοξικόν, poison) is any condition of poisoning brought about by substances formed in or by the body. During the process of digestion harmful materials are produced which, if not removed, will become absorbed into the general circulation and result in intoxication or poisoning. Auto-intoxication is particularly well marked in diseases of the liver when that organ, instead of eliminating the unwanted products of digestion, is unable to cope with them, and allows them to increase in the circulation until they induce collapse, or even death.

AUTOLYSIS.—Self-digestion.

AUTONOMIC NERVOUS SYSTEM is that part of the nervous system which governs the automatic or non-voluntary processes, such as the beating of the heart, movements of the intestines, secretions from various glands, etc. It is usually regarded as composed of two distinct

Organ.	Stimulation by chemical or other means of	
	Parasympathetic.	Sympathetic.
Pupil	Contracts	Dilates.
Heart	Slows	Accelerates.
Salivary glands	Thin watery secretion	Thick glairy secretion.
Stomach and Intestines	Causes movement	Inhibits movement.
Pyloric, anal, and ileocæcal sphincters	No act on	Causes constriction.
Bladder	Contracts	Relaxes.
Bronchial muscles	Causes contraction	Causes relaxation.
Gastro-intestinal and bronchial glands	Produces secretion	No action.
Sweat glands	No action	Causes secretion.

but complementary portions: the *parasympathetic* and the *sympathetic* systems.

The parasympathetic system is composed of a central portion comprising certain fibres present in the following cranial nerves: Oculomotor, Facial and Glossopharyngeal; and the whole of the outgoing (efferent) nerves in the important Vagus nerve. There is also a sacral set of autonomic nerve fibres present in the ventral roots of some of the sacral nerves.

The sympathetic system is composed of nerve fibres present in the ventral roots of the spinal nerves lying between the cervical and lumbar regions.

The two systems are mutually antagonistic in that stimulation of each produces opposite effects. These effects are shown in the form of the now classic table above.

Under normal circumstances there is a harmony preserved between the working of the two systems, which are flexible enough to provide for the ordinary exigencies of life, but this harmony or balance may readily be disturbed under the action of various toxic products (elaborated in diseased conditions) when these gain access to the circulation, or by certain drugs and the hormones of some endocrine glands.

AUTOSOMES are the chromosomes present in the nuclei of cells other than the sex-chromosomes. They are of the same type in both sexes in each species of animal, whereas the sex-chromosomes of the female are different from those of the male. (*See* GENETICS AND HEREDITY.)

AUXINS.—Plant hormones. These include œstrogens in pasture plants.

AVERTIN.—An anæsthetic now little used in veterinary practice, but at one time much used for cats. It is given *per rectum*, and is a solution of tribromæthanol. It must be freshly prepared and tested for acidity before use.

AVIAN ENCEPHALO-MYELITIS.—A disease of chicks under 6 weeks old caused by a virus. One form of 'Crazy Chick Disease'. Leg weakness is seen, and this is followed by partial or complete paralysis of the legs. The chicks struggle to balance with the help of their wings.

Trembling of the head and neck are also seen in a varying proportion of birds, or may be felt.

A mortality rate of 40 per cent is by no means unusual. When the disease first appeared in Britain in about 1954, the disease was less serious. Diagnosis depends upon laboratory methods. Drugs are ineffective but vaccination has proved very successful.

AVIAN CONTAGIOUS EPITHELIOMA (*see under* FOWL-POX).

AVIAN LEUCOSIS COMPLEX.—This includes Marek's disease and avian leucosis (*see* LEUCOSIS COMPLEX).

AVIAN LISTERIOSIS.—An infectious disease of poultry, occuring as an epidemic among young stock (often as an accompaniment of other diseases) or sporadically among adults.

Cause.—*Listerella monocytogenes*, a Gram-positive motile rod-shaped organism.

Symptoms.—In the epidemic type wasting occurs over a period of days or even weeks. For 48 hours before death birds refuse all food.

The sporadic type is characterised by sudden death without much loss of condition.

Diagnosis.—Depends upon bacteriological methods. (*See also* LISTERIOSIS.)

AVIAN MONOCYTOSIS (*see* 'PULLET DISEASE').

AVIAN PLAGUE, or **FOWL PLAGUE** also known as BIRD PEST, INFECTIOUS PERITONITIS OF FOWLS, and BRUNSWICK BIRD PLAGUE, attacks domesticated fowl chiefly, but turkeys, geese, ducks, and most of the common wild birds, are sometimes affected. It is not known to affect the pigeon. The disease is chiefly found in India and Middle East countries, and to a less extent in parts of the continent of Europe, and is always liable to be introduced to countries hitherto free from its scourges by the migrations of wild birds. An outbreak occurred among turkeys in Norfolk in 1963. This was the first recorded outbreak in Britain since 1929. Mortality is usually 100 per cent of the infected birds.

This disease is embraced by the term Fowl Pest which, however, usually refers to Newcastle Disease.

Cause.—A virus.

Method of spread.—The natural discharges from infected birds contaminating the food or water, forms the chief method by which the infection spreads to other fowls. In certain cases it is seen in the domesticated birds of an establishment first, and wild birds are not noted ill until later, but in other cases the disease is seen in the commoner varieties of wild birds before it attacks the poultry. Rats and mice, although not themselves affected, are capable of carrying the virus from one place to another by contamination of their feet. It appears probable that external parasites of the bird, such as flea and louse, may spread the infection.

Symptoms.—The disease is generally seen at its worst in the early spring, declines in virulence during summer, and lies dormant in winter. In an outbreak not all the birds are affected, nor do those that are suffer to the same degree. In some cases the number attacked is small, while on the same premises the next year 80 or 90 per cent of the total inhabitants of the runs die. The affected birds often die quite suddenly. They may be discovered dead on their nests, or are found curled into a ball with their heads under their wings, although normal a short time previously. In other instances the sick birds isolate themselves from the rest of the flock, preferring some dark out-of-the-way corner where they will be undisturbed. They are dull, disinclined to move, the tail and wings droop, the eyes are kept closed, and there may be a discharge from eyes and nose; the bird may squat on its breast with its head tucked under a wing or in amongst the shoulder feathers; food is refused, but thirst is often shown; the respirations are fast and laboured but not impeded by mucus; the temperature is very high at the commencement (110° to 112°), but falls shortly before death to below normal. (The normal temperature of birds is 106·5° F.) The comb and wattles are at first purple or blue, but become brownish and covered with yellowish grey deposits after a day or so. The illness seldom lasts more than 24 to 36 hours, and often not more than 6.

The symptoms in general resemble those shown in fowl cholera and the peracute form of Newcastle Disease, and may lead to confusion.

As general preventative measures, vermin should always be kept down in poultry-runs, food-houses, etc.; newly purchased birds should not be mixed with other stock until two weeks have elapsed; hampers, cages, crates, etc., that have been used at shows, sales, etc., should be disinfected before being again used; and the birds that return from such shows, etc., should be isolated as if they were newly bought.

Control in Britain.—(*See under* NEWCASTLE DISEASE.)

AVIAN TUBERCULOSIS.—This disease is known to the poultry-keeper as 'Going light', rheumatism, liver disease, spotted liver, etc. It is due to the *Mycobacterium tuberculosis* (avian). The disease has a wide distribution, but is particularly prevalent on general farms where birds are kept for many years, and less prevalent on the modern poultry farm where birds are rarely kept for more than two years. Occasionally, however, cases are met with in birds from good premises, and less than a year old. Fowls, turkeys, guinea-fowl, and pea-fowl are readily affected; ducks and geese less commonly, although cases are met with where ducks and fowls run together. Wild birds, such as pheasants and swans, which may feed occasionally in poultry-runs are sometimes found affected. In zoological gardens almost all species of wild bird, from the eagle downwards, have been found affected with tuberculosis. Pigs are readily susceptible, and a large percentage of porcine tuberculosis is traceable to an avian origin. In cattle avian tuberculosis rarely causes progressive disease, but quite commonly one or two lymphatic glands become infected, and this will affect the interpretation of the tuberculin test. (*See* the COMPARATIVE TEST.) Cases have occurred in man.

Symptoms.—Infection occurs following ingestion of food and water contaminated by the droppings of affected birds. Young birds are susceptible, but the disease is slow in progression, and deaths do not occur till a later period. Several birds of the flock appear unthrifty, and an occasional death is recorded. The comb and wattles become pale, and flesh is lost rapidly, the sternal muscles in some cases almost disappearing. Lameness is sometimes noticed. Inappetence may be seen, but other birds feed well till near the end, many being affected with diarrhœa. In a few cases no loss of condition is noticed, the birds dying suddenly without symptoms of illness.

Post-mortem.—Emaciation is usually well marked, and whitish yellow nodules are present in the liver and spleen. These nodules are easily shelled out from the substance of the organ and vary in size from a millet seed up to a pea, or larger. Nodules of varying sizes are found associated with the intestines. These nodules vary in size from a pea to a pigeon's egg and may be few in number, or many. They open into the lumen of the intestine, and large numbers of organisms may be shed from such lesions. The lungs are rarely affected in avian tuberculosis. In birds which have died suddenly death is often found to be due to rupture of the liver, which when affected with tuberculosis is often enlarged and friable. The above findings must be confirmed by making a film from the lesion, staining by Ziehl Nielsen, and demonstrating the acid-alcohol-fast *Mycobacterium tuberculosis*.

It is very important that even apparently healthy birds be destroyed, as these may be in the early stages of the disease, and if retained may be the cause of a fresh outbreak. The houses should be thoroughly disinfected. With valuable pedigree birds the intradermal tuberculin test may be employed, but before applying this test all birds should be examined and all thin birds destroyed, since those in the advanced stages of the disease may fail to react. Birds which pass the test should be put in clean houses on fresh ground.

As a general preventive measure newly purchased birds should be kept in quarantine for a period of 4 to 5 weeks and expensive breeding fowls should only be purchased subject to passing the tuberculin test.

(*See* DISPOSAL OF CARCASES.)

AVITAMINOSIS is a term used to describe the diseased conditions produced by a deficiency or lack of a vitamin in the food. Thus 'avitaminosis A' means a deficiency of vitamin A. (*See* VITAMINS.)

AXILLA is the anatomical name for the region between the humerus and the chest wall, which corresponds to the armpit in the human being. Although the area is protected to a great extent by the powerful muscles and the bone of the foreleg, penetrating injuries are not uncommon both in the horse and in the dog. Such injuries are liable to be very serious, since the axilla contains the large blood-vessels of the fore-limb and the important brachial plexus of nerves. Wounds in the posterior part are less dangerous than those occurring in the anterior and upper regions. Accidents in the hunting field, often from a stake in a hedge, etc., are the commonest origin of wounds in this part in the horse. Rupture of blood-vessels, tearing or laceration of the nerves, as well as extensive muscular rending, are the usual results. (*See* WOUNDS.)

AZOTURIA, or more correctly **MYOHÆMOGLOBINURIA,** is a disease of the horse and sometimes of the ox. It is seldom seen in horses under four years old, and practically never in those that are out at pasture. It is reputed to be commoner among mares than in the entire or castrated male, although these latter are by no means immune.

Cause.—The direct cause of the disease is as yet unknown, but breakdown of the myohæmoglobin of the skeletal muscles occurs. Certain conditions predispose to an attack, and are looked upon as being indirect causes. When horses that have been in continuous work are suddenly rested for a few days, fed very well meanwhile, and then returned to work or exercise, a certain proportion become affected, particularly those that are in good bodily condition. Cases are most commonly met with after spells of frost, and always occur after the horse has left the stable and has been put to work. (For a suggestion that azoturia and laminitis have the same cause, see *Vet. Record*, 4 Feb. 1967.)

It has been suggested that the cause is an accumulation of glycogen in muscle, liberating excessive amounts of lactic acid during exercise.

Symptoms.—The hind-limbs suddenly become stiff and weak or staggering, and there is a tendency to 'knuckle-over' at the fetlocks. The muscles of the hindquarters become tense, hard, and often painful. They feel like wood to the hand. Colicky symptoms are observed in some cases, but they pass off after a short time.

If the horse is pulled up at this stage and taken to a stable near by and treated, the symptoms soon pass off in most cases, but if the work be continued and the horse forced to move, they become rapidly worse, the hind-quarters collapse, the horse goes down, and is quite unable to rise again. When the horse falls to the ground he will often struggle very violently, and may do himself considerable damage if measures are not taken to quieten him. In some cases only one of the hind-legs is affected, and this appears to be oftener the case in light than in heavy horses. In such cases the horse is unable to sustain weight with the affected leg, although he makes efforts to do so. At some stage during the attack the horse will generally pass quantities of urine which varies in colour from a light Burgundy wine colour to a dark coffee-like black or brown. In some cases the urine is retained, and it is necessary to relieve the bladder by the passage of the catheter. This urine almost always contains quantities of albumin and often sugar as well, besides blood-pigment. The temperature is generally elevated in severe cases, but seldom reaches more than 104° F. The muscular areas of the hind-quarters show a hardening, and often a swelling, which results from tonic contraction occurring without relief. Occasionally, the muscles of the fore-quarters are similarly affected. The hind-limbs are not incapable of movement, although quite unable to sustain the body weight in a severe case.

Treatment.—Generally speaking, those cases that are taken from work and housed in the nearest stable at once, after the first noticeable symptoms, recover without leaving any bad after-effects, and in the course of two or three days. Horses that are worked on after the disease has appeared—the driver often mistaking the conditions for a colic—are much more serious and often end fatally. It is advisable therefore that the horse should be taken from work at once when the slightest stiffness or rigidity is noticed. It should be placed in a loose-box for preference with plenty of bedding, and if the weather is at all cold one or two rugs should be applied. The urine is drawn off with a catheter if it tends to be retained, and the horse made generally comfortable. A number of medicinal agents have been employed from time to time, but no specific cure has so far been discovered, though antihistamines may help. General measures: evacuation of the bowels and the application of hot packs, etc., to the loins and over the hard muscles, along with massage or grooming of the other parts of the body that are not affected, to promote a vigorous circulation. If the horse is unable to stand on his feet, he will require to be turned over on to the other side at least four times during the day, and if possible he should be lifted with a set of slings for some minutes each day until he regains control of his affected limbs, and is able to stand without assistance.

Prevention.—When horses are out of work they should be given some amount of exercise, and have their concentrated diet restricted. A good system of rationing consists in the giving of a bran mash with a handful of Epsom or Glauber's salts whenever the horses are expected to be idle for a few days. Since cold is at least a predisposing cause of the disease, it is wise to provide those animals that have been affected before with a warm rug when they leave the stable after a holiday, and the work should not be too strenuous to begin with. Horses of a naturally lively disposition should be restrained until they have warmed up to their work, for it is often the sudden exertion when they are very fresh that brings on an attack.

B

B. COLI.—*Bacillus coli.* This is now more usually known as *Escherichia coli* or *E. coli* (which see).

B. VIRUS.—This is a virus of the Herpes type, which gives rise in Man to a rare disease with an almost 100 per cent mortality. It may be transmitted to Man from monkeys—especially newly imported Rhesus and Cynomolgus monkeys. Lesions on the face and lips of monkeys should arouse suspicion of this condition.

It is believed that B. virus, Herpes virus, and Aujeszky's disease virus have a common origin.

BABESIA (*see* p. 636).

'BABY PIG DISEASE'.—The provisional name for a condition associated with a fall in the level of blood sugar within 48 hours of birth. The piglets cease suckling and appear dull. Temperature is subnormal. Artificial rearing is indicated. Otherwise, piglets will die from the condition itself or as a result of overlaying by the sow.

The causes are now considered to be: (*a*) failure of sow's milk supply; (*b*) failure—due to hæmolytic disease or to one of several infections—of the piglet to suck.

BACILLARY NECROSIS (*see* NECROSIS, BACILLARY).

BACILLARY WHITE DIARRHŒA (*see* PULLORUM DISEASE).

BACILLUS (*bacillus*, a little rod) is a micro-organism which has a rod-like appearance when seen under the microscope. (*See* BACTERIOLOGY.)

BACITRACIN.—A feed antibiotic. (*See under* ADDITIVES.)

BACK-CROSS is the progeny resulting from mating a heterozygote offspring with either of its parental homozygotes. Characters in the back-crosses generally show a 1 : 1 ratio. Thus if a pure black bull is mated with pure red cows (all homozygous), black calves (heterozygotes) are produced. If the heifer calves are 'back-crossed' to their black father, their progeny will give one pure black to every one impure black. If a black heterozygous son of the original mating is mated to his red mother, the progeny will be one red to one black.

Back-crossing can be employed as a means of test-mating, or test-crossing to determine whether a stock of animals is homozygous, when it will never throw individuals of different type, or whether it is heterozygous, when it will give the two allelomorphic types. (*See* GENETICS AND HEREDITY.)

BACK-FENCE (*see* STRIP-GRAZING).

'BACON-WEIGHT'.—This is between 200 and 230 lb. (liveweight), attained at an age of 26 to 28 weeks. (Cf. 'Heavy Hog Weight'—260 lb.).

BACTERIA (βακτήριον, a rod) is a term which used to be reserved for micro-organisms which had the form of rods, but the term is now applied to organisms as a whole quite irrespective of their shape. It is synonymous with such words as 'germs', 'microbes', 'organisms', and 'micro-organisms'. Rod-shaped varieties are now called 'bacilli'.

BACTERIOLOGY (βακτήριον, a rod; λόγος, study) is the name given to the science which deals with the study of bacteria. Veterinary bacteriology deals in particular with those forms of bacteria which are responsible for the production of disease in domesticated animals. Bacteria, however, are not the only microscopic forms which cause disease; just as bacteria are the lowest form of vegetable life, so protozoa are the lowest forms of animal life, and in this latter group are classified the causal organisms of such diseases as red water in cattle, coccidiosis, nagana, surra, and dourine. Other diseases, *e.g.* swine fever, foot-and-mouth disease, and rinderpest or cattle plague, are due to exceedingly minute forms of life, the viruses and rickettsiæ, most of them invisible under the highest powers of the ordinary microscope, and so small that they are able to pass through the pores of a porcelain filter.

(*a*) **Moulds** may be found growing on any damp surface which offers a sufficient degree of nutriment. Many of these, such as the cheese mould, are not associated with disease, but on the other hand some types flourish in the animal body, giving rise to disease, *e.g.* ringworm, mycotic pneumonia, sporotrichosis, moniliasis.

(*b*) **Yeasts** may sometimes be the cause of disease, *e.g.* scouring in pigs.

Types of bacteria.—According to peculiarities in shape and in group formation, certain names are applied : thus a single spherical bacterium is known as ' coccus ' ; organisms in pairs and of the same shape (*i.e.* spherical) are called ' diplococci ' ; when in the form of a chain they are known as ' streptococci ' ; when they are bunched together like a bunch of grapes the name ' staphylococcus ' is applied. Bacteria in the form of long slender rods are known as ' bacilli ', wavy or curved forms are called ' spirilla ', ' vibrio '.

Reproduction.—The mode of multiplication of some bacteria is exceedingly simple, consisting of a splitting into two of a single bacterium. Since the new forms may similarly divide within half an hour, multiplication is rapid and may result in the formation of millions of organisms from a single type in 24 hours. In order to multiply, bacteria must be kept in a suitable medium of heat and moisture, but some bacteria have the power of protecting themselves from unfavourable conditions by changing their form to that of a more resistant body known as a ' spore '. One bacillus gives rise to one spore. The anthrax bacillus is of this type, and so resistant is the spore that the bacillus may by this means resist boiling for several minutes, or retain its vitality under ordinary conditions for a period of eighteen years, after which, if suitable conditions present themselves, each spore gives rise to a bacillus.

Size.—Even the largest forms of bacteria are much too small to be visible by the naked eye ; and when it is considered that some may only measure $\frac{1}{25000}$th of an inch, it will be obvious that a drop of water may contain many hundreds of organisms.

Mobility.—All bacteria do not possess the power of movement, but if a drop of fluid containing certain forms of organism which are called ' motile ' be examined microscopically, it will be observed that they move actively in a definite direction. This is accomplished, in the motile organisms, by means of delicate whip-like processes which thrash backwards and forwards in the fluid and propel the body onwards. These processes are called ' flagella ', and the movement is spoken of as ' flagellate movement '.

The methods of diagnosis are :

(1) **Microscopical.**—In order satisfactorily to examine bacteria microscopically a drop of the fluid containing the organisms is spread out in a thin film on a glass slide. The organisms are killed by heating the slide, and the details of their characteristics are made obvious by suitable staining with appropriate dyes. Since bacteria of a certain size, shape, or group formation are known to cause diseases of a certain variety, a consideration of the form presented enables a diagnosis to be made. Further, it is known that certain bacteria will not stain by certain dyes ; thus the tubercle bacillus will not stain by methylene blue, and organisms can be differentiated by special staining methods. (*See* ELECTRON MICROSCOPE.)

(2) **Cultural characters.**—By copying the conditions under which a particular bacterium grows naturally, it can be induced to grow artificially, and for this purpose various nutrient substances known as ' media ' are used. The commoner media that are employed are broth, gelatin, agar, potato, blood-serum, and milk, according to the special requirements of particular organisms. A convenient amount of the medium is placed in a glass culture-tube and the tube is plugged with a piece of cotton-wool to make entrance or exit by further germs impossible. At this stage the tube will already contain many micro-organisms, and before it is ready for use these must be destroyed. For this purpose steam is the most efficient agent, and it is best employed by one or other of the modifications of Koch's steam steriliser. The period of exposure is about 30 minutes on each of three successive days. On the first day the bacteria themselves are killed. On the second day any spores which may have survived the first sterilisation are destroyed, and on the third day any life which has withstood the previous steamings is rendered incapable of existence. The medium in the tube is

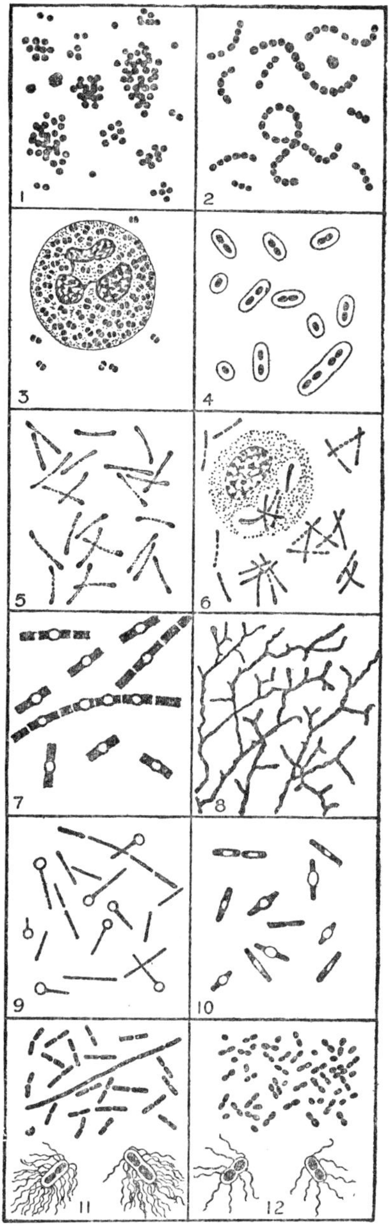

Various types of bacteria which cause disease: 1, staphylococcus; 2, streptococcus; 3, diplococcus; 4, pneumococcus with capsule; 5, diphtheria bacillus; 6, tubercule bacillus; 7, anthrax bacillus; 8, streptothrix of actinomycosis; 9, tetanus bacillus; 10, bacillus of gas gangrene; 11, typhoid bacillus; 12, bacillus coli. (Drawn by R. Muir.)

now inoculated with the material under examination, which contains the bacteria, by means of a sterile platinum needle, the plug being removed before and replaced afterwards. The tube and its contents are placed in an incubator at a constant temperature of 37° C. At the end of 2 or 3 days, or perhaps sooner, examination will show that the bacteria deposited by the needle have grown, forming masses or colonies, which are now visible to the naked eye. This growth is known as a 'culture'. If material, such as the discharge from a wound, be inoculated, it is probable that various different types of growth will be observed at the end of the incubation period, as the discharge may contain several types of germs, each having a characteristic colony appearance, and the colonies may be so mixed that

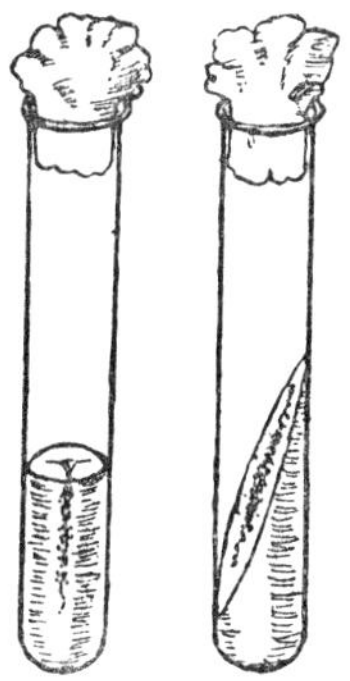

Culture-tubes for bacteria. The tube on the left shows a 'stab culture' in gelatine, that on the right a 'stroke culture' on agar.

careful scrutiny of any one is difficult or impossible. It is necessary to separate the colonies by sub-cultivation, or it may be advisable to treat the discharge previous to inoculation on to the medium. Sub-cultivation consists in picking up any one particular colony on the sterile platinum needle and introducing it into a separate culture-tube and cultivating it still further. After a time a pure culture of the special organism can be thus obtained. Mixtures of various organisms can be separated by other methods. (*a*) Heating to such a temperature as can be comfortably borne by spores, *e.g.* about 80° C., will kill all those organisms which have not the power to sporulate, and yet leave the spores of other germs intact. Inoculation of some of the heated material will result in a growth of the sporulating organisms only. (*b*) Dilution of the discharge or other material under examination with quanti-

Modern Name.	Synonyms.	Associated or Specific Diseased Conditions caused.
Actinobacillus lignièresi	—	Actinobacillosis and actinomycosis.
A. bovis	*Streptothrix bovis*	Actinomycosis.
A. mallei	*Pfeifferella mallei*	Glanders in equines and man.
A. whitmori	*Pfeifferella whitmori*	Melioidosis in rats and man; occasionally in dogs and cats.
Bacillus anthracis	—	Anthrax in all susceptible animals.
B. Calmette-Guérin	B.C.G.—an avirulent strain of *Mycobacterium tuberculosis*, specially grown for many years	
Bacterium viscosum equi	*Shigella equirulis*	Causes 'sleepy foal disease', septicæmia, nephritis, and arthritis.
Bordetella bronchiseptica	*Bacillus bronchisepticus*	Complicates distemper in the dog.
Borrelia anserina	*Spirochæta gallinarum*	Spirochætosis in geese and fowls.
Brucella abortus	*Bacillus abortus*; Bang's bacillus	Contagious abortion in cattle; undulant fever.
Brucella melitensis	—	Contagious abortion of goats; undulant fever in man (in part).
Clostridium botulinum (three types—A B and C)	*Bacillus botulinus*	Botulism in man and animals.
Cl. chauvœi	*Bacillus chauvœi*	'Black-quarter' in cattle and partly in sheep.
Cl. œdematiens	*Bacillus œdematiens*	'Black-quarter' in cattle and pigs in part; 'black disease' in sheep; septicæmia in horses and pigs (wound infection).
Cl. septique	*Vibrion septique; Cl. œdematis-maligni*; bacillus of malignant œdema; gas-gangrene bacillus	Gas gangrene in man; black-quarter in in-door cattle and pigs; braxy in sheep; 'grass ill' in lambs; putrefaction in moribund animals.
Cl. tetani	*Bacillus tetani*	Tetanus in man and animals.
Cl. welchii	*Bacillus ærogenes capsulatus; B. phlegmonis emphysematosæ; B. perfringens; B. enteritidis sporogenes*	Lamb dysentery; present in many cases of gas gangrene.
Corynebacterium ovis	Preisz-Nocard bacillus; *Bacillus pseudo-tuberculosis; Corynebacterium pseudo-tuberculosis*	Caseous lymphademitis in sheep; some cases of ulcerative lymphangitis and acne in horses.
C. pyogenes	*Bacillus pyogenes*	Abscesses in liver, kidneys, lungs, or skin in sheep, cattle, and pigs especially; present as a secondary organism in many suppurative conditions, such as mastitis in ewes and cattle.
C. equi	—	A cause of pneumonia in the horse and of tuberculosis-like lesions in the pig.
Escherichia coli (sub types are many)	*Bacillus coli communis; B. coli*	Always present in alimentary canal as commonest organism; becomes pathogenic at times, partly causing enteritis, dysentery (lambs), scour (calves), cystitis, abortion, mastitis, joint-ill, etc. Associated with other conditions also.
Fusiformis necrophorus	*Actinomyces necrophorus*	Necrosis of the liver in the ox-calf diphtheria; quitter, poll evil, and fistulous withers in horses; necrosis of the skin in dogs, pigs, and rabbits; navel ill in calves and lambs; various other conditions in bowel and skin associated with necrosis of tissue.
Klebsiella pneumoniæ	*Friedlander's bacillus*	Metritis in mares; acute suppurative pneumonia in dogs, etc.
Leptospira ictero-hæmorrhagiæ	—	Leptospiral jaundice, or enzoötic jaundice of dogs; Weil's disease in man.
Lept. canicola	—	Canicola fever in man, and nephritis in dogs.
Mycobacterium paratuberculosis	*Bacillus paratuberculosis*	Johne's disease of cattle.
Myc. phlei	*Bacillus phlei*; Timothy-grass bacillus	Non-pathogenic, but may be present in milk or butter; is impossible to distinguish from *M. tuberculosis* when stained.
Myc. tuberculosis (bovine, human, and avian types)	*Bacillus tuberculosis*; Koch's *bacillus; tubercule bacillus*	Tuberculosis in man and animals.
Mycoplasma	P.P.L.O. organisms	Pleuro-pneumonia, etc.
Pasteurella multocida	—	Fowl cholera, Pasteurellosis in cattle.
P. pestis	*Bacillus pestis*	Plague in man and rats.
P. tularensis	—	Tularæmia in rodents.
Salmonella abortus equi	—	Contagious abortion of mares naturally, but capable of causing abortion in pregnant ewes, cows, and sows experimentally.
S. abortus ovis	—	Contagious abortion of ewes occurring naturally.

Modern Name.	Synonyms.	Associated or Specific Diseased Conditions caused.
S. anatum	—	'Keel' disease of young ducks in Britain and America.
S. enteritidis	*Bacillus enteritidis* Gaërtner's bacillus	Enteritis in cattle, sheep, pigs and rats; causes 'food poisoning' in man.
S. gallinarum	—	Klein's disease or fowl typhoid.
S. pullorum	*Bacillus pullorum*; bacillus of white diarrhœa of chicks	Bacillary white disease; pullorum disease.
S. choleræ suis	*Bacillus suipestifer*	Ulcerations and diphtheritic lesions in bowel of pigs during swine fever (virus infection).
Staphylocossus albus	—	Botriomycotic abscesses in horses; joint-ill in lambs; suppurative and purulent conditions in animals and man, especially wound infections where other pus-producing organisms are also present. Present in various types of abscess, and in pyæmic and septicæmic conditions. Cause about 5 per cent of mastitis in cows. 'Bumble-foot' in fowls. *Sta. aureus* is the most, and *Sta. citreus* the least, virulent.
Sta. aureus	—	
Sta. citreus	—	
Sta. pyogenes	—	Often associated with the other staphylococci in above conditions; causes so-called 'actinomycosis' of the udder in cows and sometimes in sows.
Str. equi	—	Strangles in horses, secondary to a filterable virus; partly responsible for joint-ill in foals, and sterility in mares.
Str. agalactia	—	Mastitis in cows.
Str. pyogenes	—	Many suppurative conditions, wound infections, abscesses, etc.; joint-ill in foals. [In the above conditions various other streptococci are also frequently present.]
Vibrio fœtus	—	Abortion in ewes, and infertility in cattle.
V. jejuni	—	Winter dysentery in cattle.

ties of sterile water and the inoculation of a drop of the mixture will result in a thinning of the bacilli over the surface of the culture, and the colonies that grow will be fewer and farther between.

(3) **Inoculation of animals.**—In the case of slow-growing organisms the separation from fast-growing organisms is very difficult, for the rapidly growing germs soon swarm over the whole surface of the medium and mask or obliterate those which do not grow so fast. In such cases inoculation into certain animals is resorted to. The mixture of germs is introduced into the body of a laboratory animal, and when disease develops the animal is killed and tubes of media are inoculated from the various organs which show the characteristic appearances of a particular disease.

BACTERIOPHAGES are viruses which multiply in and destroy bacteria. Some bacteriophages have a 'tail' resembling a hypodermic syringe with which they attach themselves to bacteria and through which they 'inject' nucleic acid. 'Phages' have been photographed with the aid of the electron microscope.

BACTERIOSTATIC.—An agent which inhibits the growth of micro-organisms, as opposed to killing them.

BALANITIS.—Inflammation of the termination of the penis which is covered by the prepuce. It is common in the dog, when it is usually only a fleeting trouble in all but tropical countries. (*See* VENEREAL TUMOURS.) Enzootic Balanoposthitis ('Pizzle Rot'; 'Sheath Rot') is a disease mainly of Merino sheep in Australia. The cause is not known. Some deaths may follow, especially after complications from blow-flies.

BALANTIDIUM.—A protozoan parasite which can cause scouring in pigs.

BALDNESS, or LOSS OF HAIR.—In the great majority of cases where the hair becomes thinner and thinner in patches, accompanied by greater or less itchiness in the skin, the actual cause is one or other of the parasitic skin diseases—mange, lice, ringworm, etc.—or it is due to eczema. (See these sections.) Alopecia or baldness may be due to malnutrition, hormone deficiency, or to selenium poisoning.

Female animals of all species that have recently given birth to young sometimes become bald in large patches, especially in the posterior parts of their bodies—a condition which is called 'parturient alopecia'. In these, there is no irritation of the skin, and new hair rapidly grows in the denuded areas without any treatment.

Foals and calves sucking their mothers are sometimes attacked with baldness during the first few weeks of their life. They may lose practically all their hair in a very short time, but, as in the case of parturient alopecia, new hair soon grows over the body.

Old animals, particularly dogs, are sometimes affected with baldness similar to that seen in human beings, except that parts of the back and sides are rendered devoid of hair. In the male dog, there is a form of alopecia which responds to castration. The animal is usually five years old or more, and commonly seen to be attractive to other male dogs. The skin feels soft, and often there is hardly any hair on the body. There is no response to treatment with thyroid extract, but a new coat can be expected to grow within three months of castration. In the bitch, a form of alopecia with a harsh coat and bare patches mainly under the throat and on the flanks and at the back of the thighs is seen. Often she is dull and lacking in energy. Thyroid extract, with or without massage and ultra-violet rays, may prove effective.

There is a form of alopecia or baldness which affects young animals at birth. In at least some cases this appears to be due to a failure of the secretion of the thyroid owing to lack of iodine in the food of the dam.

Baldness in spayed cats has been treated successfully with implants of testosterone propionate.

Baldness is sometimes associated with diabetes.

BALING WIRE.—Discarded pieces of this are often eaten by cattle and give rise to traumatic pericarditis. (*See under* HEART DISEASES.)

BALLING.—The administration of medicines to the larger animals is known as 'balling' when the drugs are compounded into a 'bolus' or 'ball'. Balls are generally made use of when it is desired to give drugs in a solid state, when the ingredients are irritant or bitter, when drenching must be avoided owing to inability to swallow easily, or when an accurate dose of a particular drug must be received by the patient—a condition which is not fulfilled by drenching, or by giving medicines in power form in the food.

Of the drugs which are often given in this manner the following are the commonest: aloes, chloral hydrate, ammonia salts, quinine, nux vomica, camphor, iron salts, and phenothiazine. The exact dose of the drug required is reduced to a fine powder, and worked into a stiff paste with some excipient such as treacle, syrup, glycerine, honey, or soft soap. The 'mass', as the paste is called, is then moulded into a short cylinder, from 1½ to 3 inches in length, and up to about ½ inch in diameter, and wrapped in thin white paper or filled into a gelatine capsule. In this form it keeps quite well for a time provided it is kept dry and that no volatile drugs, such as ammonia, are used.

Administration.—The horse or ox is held by a halter; the assistant, standing on the near side of the animal, holding the halter-shank in his right hand, places the left hand on the animal's nose to prevent it raising the head too high. The ball is taken in one's right hand and held by the first three fingers arranged as a cone, while the animal's tongue is securely gripped by the left hand. The tongue is turned in between the upper and lower jaws so as to keep them apart, and the right hand is boldly and quickly thrust back over the root of the tongue to the entrance to the throat. The ball is released, the hand is withdrawn, and the tongue freed. As the animal withdraws its tongue the ball is carried farther back and a swallowing movement begins which passes the ball down the gullet, where it can be seen as a small swelling travelling down the left side of the neck. The chief precautions are to draw the tongue as far forwards as possible, to keep the back of the right hand against the palate, to drop the ball as far back as possible, and to withdraw the hand as quickly as may be. The animal should never be frightened by undue noise or commotion, but the man should work quickly, quietly, and firmly. Sometimes a horse that has been previously balled has learned to bring the ball back by lowering his head and opening his mouth. To prevent this his head should be kept well up, and if he still refuses to swallow, a few mouthfuls of water will wash the ball down. In difficult or refractory animals a balling gun may be necessary, but this must be used with care.

BALSAMS (βάλσαμον) are substances which contain resins and benzoic acid; balsam of Peru, balsam of Tolu, and Friar's balsam are the chief. They are given internally to promote expectoration during colds and bronchitis in all animals, especially when these are accompanied by a hard, dry cough. Externally Friar's balsam is useful to check hæmorrhage from the smaller vessels.

BANDAGES and BANDAGING.—The protection of wounds when healing is of considerable importance. Not only is it necessary to protect them from further injury, but it is also essential to prevent infective agents gaining access from the outside, to keep flies away from wounds, to give support to the healing tissues by lessening tension of the skin, and to supply an absorbent covering which will soak up any discharges and render them harmless. The application of bandages to veterinary patients is much more difficult than in human practice, because not only must the bandage remain in position during the movement of the patient, but it must also be comfortable, or it will be removed by the teeth or feet, and it must be so adjusted that it will not become contaminated by either the urine or the fæces. Generally speaking, bandages are most useful and most often used after surgical operations where the wound is aseptic, and where it is advisable that it shall remain so until healed. For accidental wounds, unless these are first rendered as free from organisms as possible, it is often better to allow them to remain open to the action of air and sunlight than to cover them with bandages.

The best materials for covering wounds are medicated gauzes, medicated cotton-wool, lint, compresses of linen, cotton, flannel, wool, and, in some cases of surface abrasions, collodion and a thin film of cotton-wool. These are held in position by bandages or by adhesive tapes. Bandages are generally made of calico, tarlatan, cotton, or knitted wool. They should be soft enough to adapt themselves to irregularities of the surfaces to which they are applied, and they must be of sufficient substance to give support and to remain in position. When they are intended to immobilise a limb, such as those applied to fractures or dislocations, they are saturated with dextrin, pitch, plaster of Paris, or some other substance which will set hard and firm. Various compounds incorporated in cotton or other bandaging material are on the market. These are soaked with water

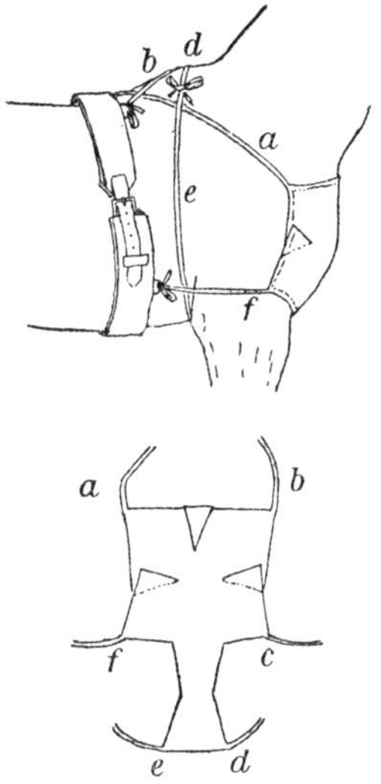

Bandage for point of shoulder of horse

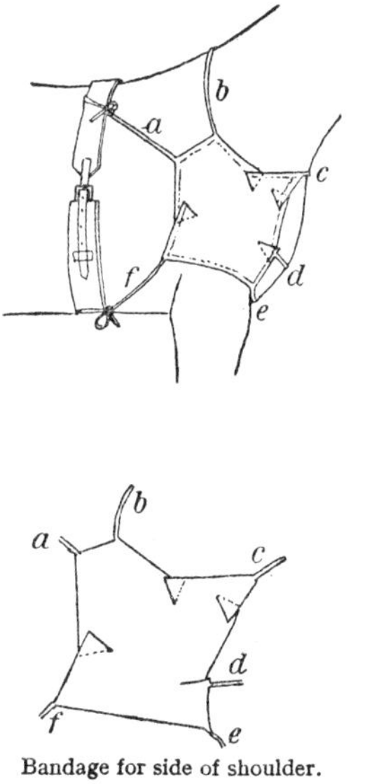

Bandage for side of shoulder.

during application and set firm subsequently. Such substances as 'elastoplast' or 'cellona' are of this type. Those used to give support to sprained tendons, etc., are made of elastic rubber or of Newmarket stockinette, and are applied tightly.

BANDAGES AND BANDAGING

Bandages are made in the form of either single or double roller, or 'many-

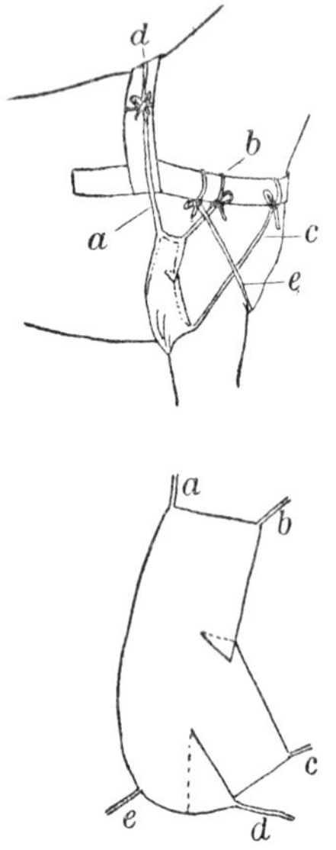

Bandage for elbow.

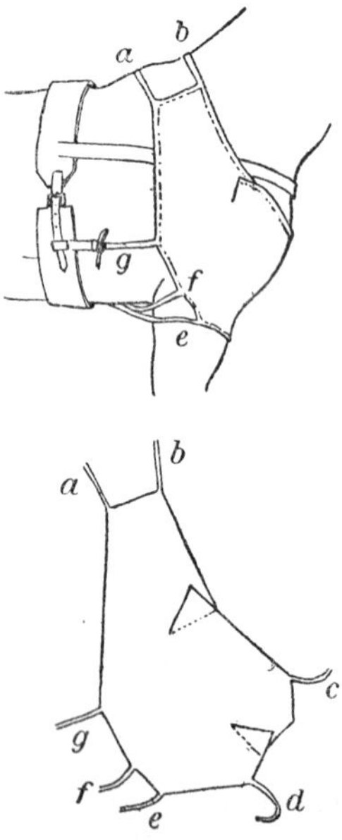

Bandage for a large wound on the front and side of shoulder.

tailed'. A single bandage is a long strip of fabric rolled up from one end only; a double bandage is rolled from each end and the middle of the strip is applied first; and a 'many-tailed' is a broad piece of material with a number of ends that fasten round the part and are tied together. There are various methods of

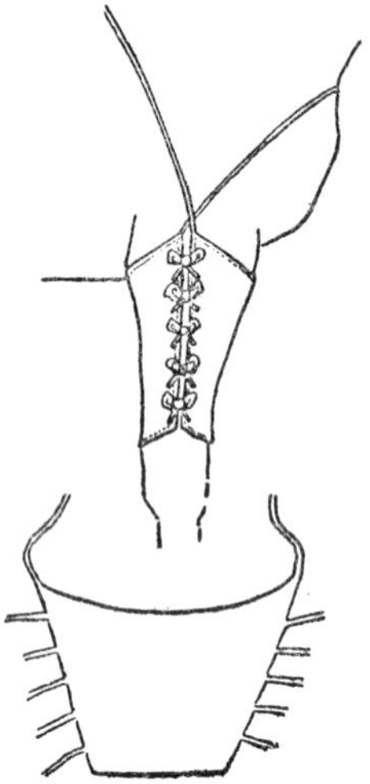

Bandage for fore-arm.

applying the single bandage: viz. the spiral, the circular, the spiral-reversed, and the spica or figure-of-eight methods, The spiral and the circular are usually

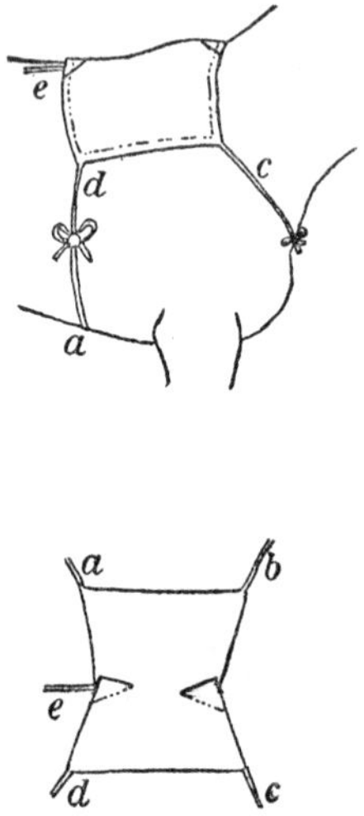

Bandage for withers.

used together for parts that are of the same circumference all the way up, such as the cannons of horses and the lower parts of the limbs of other animals. The bandage commences as a circular turn round the part, and each succeeding turn overlaps that before it until the area is covered, when one or two circular turns

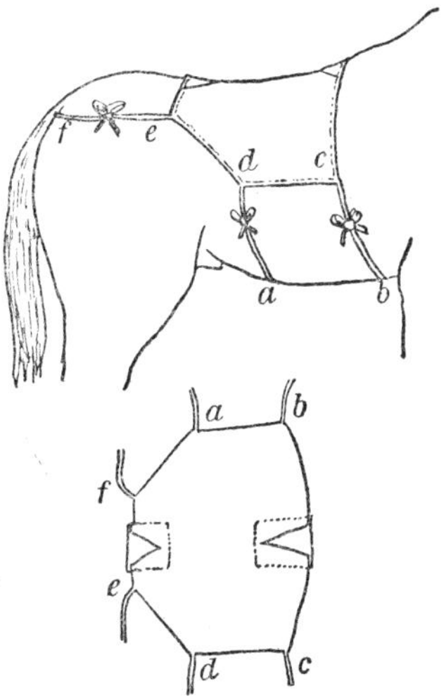

Bandage for back or loins.

are taken to finish off. In the spiral-reversed, which is used for parts that are conical, such as the fore-arms, thighs, and the tail, each turn is doubled sharply

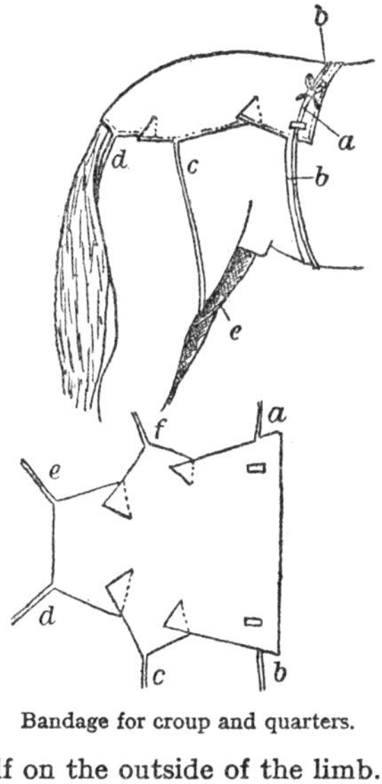

Bandage for croup and quarters.

on itself on the outside of the limb. This allows the bandage to come into immediate contact with the changing shape of the limb for its whole length. The spica or figure-of-eight is used for covering joints

BANDAGES AND BANDAGING

where movement must be provided for, and where the surface to be covered is greater on one aspect than on the opposite. It is generally begun by taking

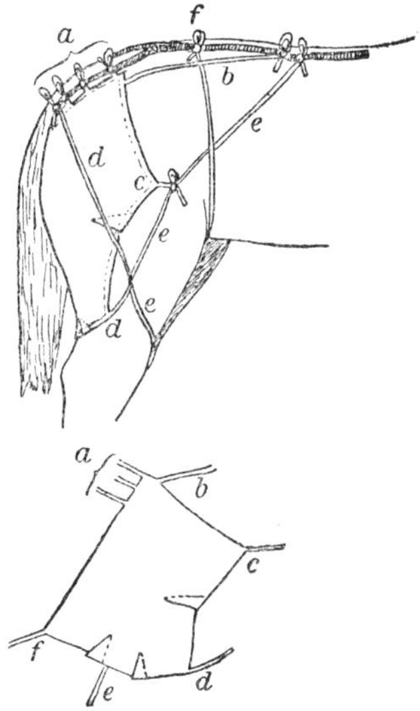

Bandage for wound over buttock, thigh, or hip-joint.

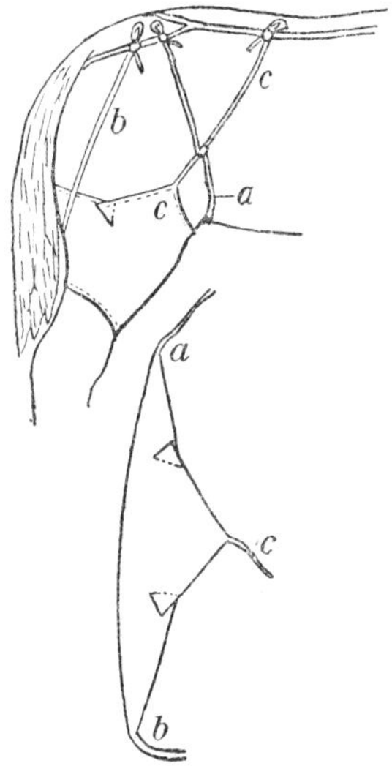

Bandage for gaskin.

a few circular turns around the limb below or above the joint to fix the bandage in position. For covering the abdomen and the thorax of the smaller animals the 'many-tailed' bandage is used. It is made by taking a piece of material large enough to encircle the trunk and leave a few inches to spare, and wide enough to cover the area. Along the two sides an equal number of slits are made towards the centre for a short distance, each one being opposite to that on the other side. The bandage is wrapped round the body, and the ends, or tails, are tied to each other along the back of the animal. As a modification of this, two holes may be cut out at one end and the fore-limbs passed through them; this gives the bandage greater stability and lessens the risk of its coming off.

For the bodies of the larger animals it is not customary to use roller bandages

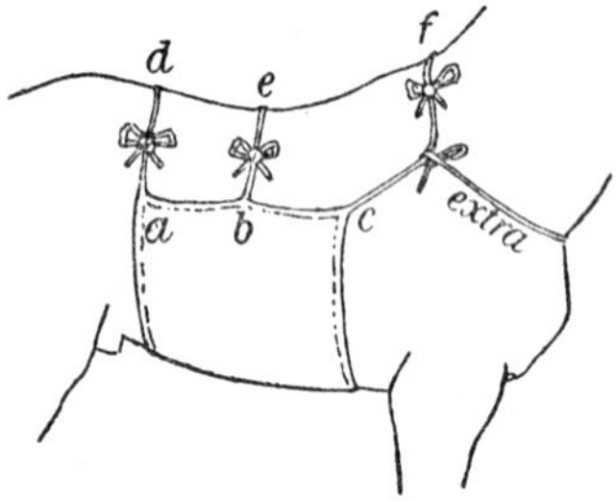

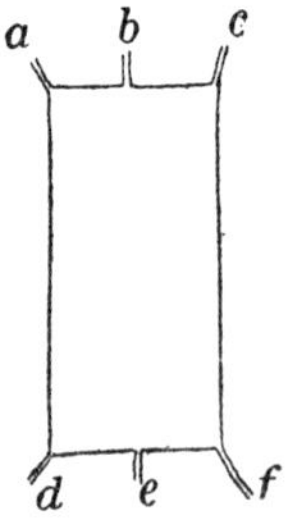

Bandage for abdomen, or, if extended further, for sides.

owing to the difficulty of keeping them in position, and 'many-tailed' bandages require too much material; pieces of towelling, or other suitable material, are employed instead. These are cut to the shape of the part to be covered, have tucks or hems sewn at various places, and are provided with tapes that tie to a surcingle, or around some convenient part of the body, such as the tail, neck, or to a limb. (*See* Diagrams.)

Stable and exercising bandages.—It is sometimes necessary to bandage the limbs of horses when these are travelling by rail, when their limbs are wet, or when they are likely to be exposed to extremes of cold. For these purposes the stable bandage, made of thick woollen fabric, is used. It is applied from the upper part of the fore or hind cannon right down to the coronet and back again, and is tied, either to the outside or to the inside of the limb, by tapes sewn on to one end. Exercising bandages are used for horses that are in training, to give some support to the

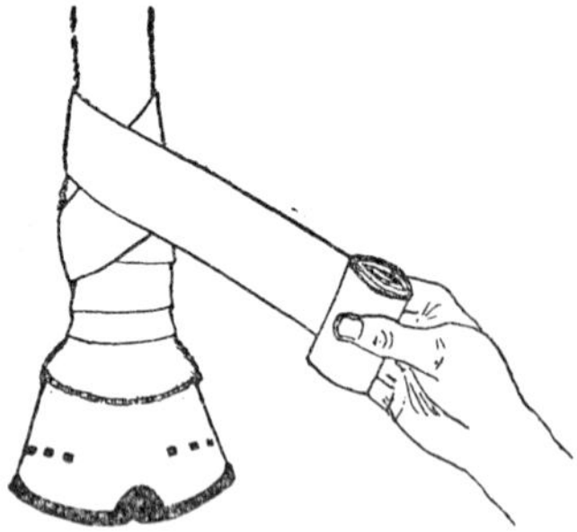

'Figure-of-eight' bandage (roller) for fetlock, also known as a 'spica'.

tendons, and are often applied to hunters and steeplechasers to protect their shins should they strike their jumps. It is usual to cover the limbs from below the knees and hocks down to the fetlocks with a layer of cotton-wool or teased tow, and to apply the bandage above this part fairly tightly. An exercising bandage should never interfere with free flexion and extension of the fetlock joint. They are made of cotton, mixtures of cotton and wool, or of Newmarket stockinette, which, being flexible and elastic, will remain in

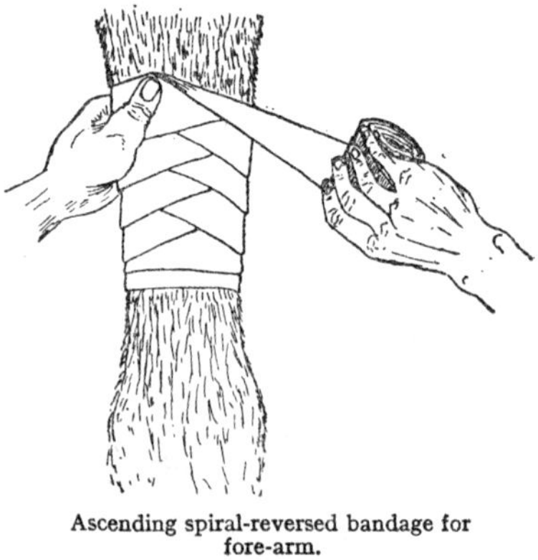

Ascending spiral-reversed bandage for fore-arm.

position and not loosen as the others are liable to do.

BANG'S BACILLUS is the old name for *Brucella abortus*, which causes 'contagious abortion' of cattle, and was first discovered by Professor Bang of Denmark.

BARBITURATES are derivatives of barbituric acid (malonyl-urea). They include a wide range of very valuable sedative, hypnotic or anæsthetic agents. Several are used in veterinary practice, including Nembutal (pentobarbitone) and Luminal (phenobarbitone).

In case of barbiturate poisoning, use a stomach tube, keep the animal warm, give picrotoxin, or leptazol, or strong coffee, strychnine.

NP13 has been described as very promising in human medicine.

BARBONE is the name given to hæmorrhagic septicæmia of the buffalo. (*See* PASTEURELLOSIS.)

BARIUM POISONING sometimes takes place through the ingestion of rat-poison, which is frequently prepared with the chloride of barium as its active toxic agent.

The symptoms are excessive salivation, sweating (except in the dog), muscular convulsions, violent straining, palpitation of the heart, and finally general paralysis.

Treatment.—As soon as the cause is established the stomach contents should be evacuated, either by inducing vomiting, or by means of the stomach-pump.

Doses of Epsom salts given by the mouth in a watery solution act as antidotes by converting the chloride into the insoluble sulphate of barium, and the administration of demulcent fluids, such as milk, barley-water, white of egg, etc., should follow. Anæsthesia may be needed.

BARIUM SULPHATE being opaque to X-rays, is given by the mouth prior to a radiographic examination for diagnostic purposes. (*See* X-RAYS.)

BARIUM SULPHIDE is sometimes used as a depilatory for the site of surgical operations.

BARLEY POISONING.—As with wheat (and to a much less extent, oats) an excess of barley can kill cattle and sheep not gradually accustomed to it.

During the severe weather of early 1963 trouble of this kind was experienced in several Pembrokeshire flocks fed in various ways, *e.g.* crushed barley 80 per cent, oats 20 per cent, with cake and hay; whole barley and hay; crushed barley and turnips. Owing to the continued hard frost there was no access to grass. In the first 2 types of feed, deaths occurred about the 10th day after commencement of the diet. In the third, deaths were seen on the 4th day. It was noted that the greedy feeders were the first to be affected. Symptoms comprised staggering and blindness, with subnormal or normal temperatures. This was followed in 24 to 48 hours by recumbency, and finally coma and death. A profuse yellowish diarrhoea was present. Milder cases recovered when the barley ration was discontinued. The flock mortality varied from 5 per cent to 20 per cent.

Similar symptoms, with dullness and loss of appetite have been seen in young cattle the day after *ad lib.* feeding of an 85 per cent barley ration began, with deaths following in about 18 per cent of those affected.

The sudden introduction of cereal feeding is known to give rise to acidity in the rumen, and to acetonæmia. It has been suggested also that very acid conditions in the rumen may damage the lining mucous membrane, allowing bacteria to enter the bloodstream and reach the liver, injuring this.

Recent observations made at the Rowett Research Institute suggest that the penetration of swallowed hairs into the epithelium of the rumen may be an important cause of rumenitis in cattle fed on barley. It is possible that a proportion of the liver abscesses mentioned above may result from inoculation with bacteria of the rumen walls by the entry of contaminated hairs, including the sharp, hollow ones from barley grain. (VR 30.12 67)

It is important that barley should not be fed in a fine, powdery form. To do so is to invite severe digestive upsets, which may lead to death. Especially if ventilation is poor, dusty food also contributes to coughing and may increase the risk of pneumonia.

(*See also under* BEEF FROM BARLEY.)

BARLEY-WATER is a demulcent drink prepared by allowing about two ounces to the quart of barley-meal or pearl barley to simmer in water for two hours, and straining while hot. It is useful for animals suffering from sore throats when solid food is not taken, for soothing the mouth and gullet when irritant substances have been accidentally ingested, and for correcting simple diarrhœa in dogs, foals, and calves. When the temperature is high and during the course of kidney disorders, barley-water is of assistance in maintaining the animal's appetite and quenching thirst.

BAR-PAD is a leather sole for a horse's foot which carries a rubber or leather pad across the whole of its posterior portion, and is fitted along with a short shoe. The pad covers the whole of the frog, and extends across to each heel over the bars of the foot. It acts as an anti-slipping device, it prevents concussion on hard surfaces, and is useful for giving protection to the heels in cases of 'corns', chronic laminitis, bruises of the sole, etc.

BARRENNESS (*see* INFERTILITY).

BARRIER CREAM.—A protective dressing for the hands and arms of veterinarians engaged in obstetrical work or rectal examinations.

BARROW.—A castrated male pig.

BAR SHOE is a shoe that has a strap of iron running across from one heel to the other. This is the 'bar', and it acts by making the frog take a share in the support of the weight of the horse. It is applied for the correction of atrophy of the frog, when this condition has not progressed too far, for easing the heels, when there is some painful condition situated in them, and for giving attachment for a steel plate when the sole of the foot has to be packed with dressings.

BARK EATING by cattle should be regarded as a symptom of a mineral deficiency, *e.g.* manganese and phosphorus. The remedy is use of an appropriate mineral supplement.

'BARKERS', THE 'BARKING' FOAL.—In thoroughbred studs in Britain the word 'barkers' is applied by stud grooms to new-born foals which, during the cause of an obscure illness, make a sound like a yapping terrier. Normal at birth, the foal may be seen soon afterwards jerking its head up and down, and moving its legs aimlessly without attempting to get to its feet. A foal already on its feet may wander aimlessly around, colliding with the walls, or stagger and fall. In other instances, the groom may return at the sound of 'barking' to find the foal in convulsions. These may continue intermittently for a matter of hours or days. Mortality is sometimes as much as 50 per cent. Treatment involves the use of mysoline. The trouble is believed to be associated with human interference with the navel cord, leading to a loss of blood.

BARS OF FOOT.—At each of the heels of the horse's foot the wall turns inwards and forwards instead of ending abruptly.

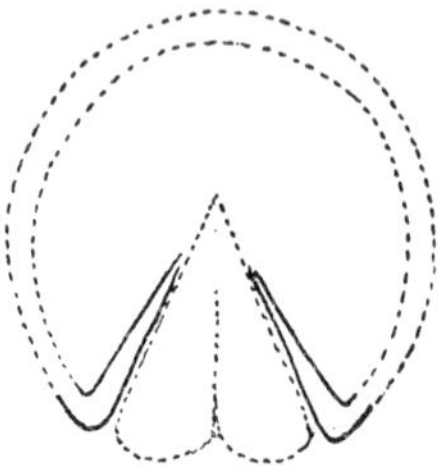

Diagram of the position of the bars of the horse's foot. The dotted line shows the outline of the wall and frog.

These 'reflected' portions are called the bars of the foot. They serve to strengthen the heels; they provide a gradual rather than an abrupt finish to the important wall; and they take a share in the formation of the bearing surface, on which rests the shoe.

The bars are sometimes cut away by smiths or others, who hold the erroneous idea that by so doing they allow the heels of the foot to expand; what actually happens in such instances is that the union between the component parts of the foot is destroyed, and the resistance to contraction which they afford is lost. They should therefore be allowed to grow and maintain their natural prominence.

BARTONELLOSIS. — Infection with *Bartonella* organisms, which occasionally occurs in dogs and cattle but is of most importance in laboratory rats. Symptoms are mainly those of anæmia.

Treatment.—Neoarsphenamine has been used.

BASEDOW'S DISEASE (*see* GRAVE'S).

BASIC SLAG has caused poisoning in lambs, which should not be allowed access to treated fields until the slag has been well washed in to the soil. Adult sheep have also been poisoned in this way, scouring badly, and so have cattle. In these animals the symptoms include: dullness, reluctance to move, inappetence, grinding of the teeth, and profuse watery black fæces.

BATHS.—Among animals bathing may be undertaken for the sake of cleanliness, for the cure of a parasitic skin disease, for the reduction of the temperature or of high blood-pressure in small animals, or it may be intended to exert a tonic effect upon the body generally.

Horses.—When it is desired to wash a horse's coat it is customary to employ bucketfuls of water, hard soap, and a soft brush, and to wash the skin and coat by hand. The legs and the feet are more often washed, especially for shows or sales, and in the heavier breeds when 'feather' is abundant. In all cases the subsequent drying is of great importance. The body of the horse is rinsed with cold clean water when the actual washing is complete, the surplus water is scraped out of the coat with a sweat-scraper, the whole body is well wisped with either hay or straw, and often rubbed with a rough towel, and an armful of clean wheat straw is laid cross-wide over the horse's back, withers, and quarters, and a warm rug is applied over the whole. This is left in position for about an hour. It allows a free circulation of air around the body without any risk of a draught, and prevents too rapid evaporation of the moisture which remains. In many cases the horse is given a hot mash while his coat is drying, and a small feed of hay; when he has finished this he is given ten minutes' vigorous exercise in the open air, and rugged with a warm, dry rug. The legs are rinsed with clean water in the same way, the surplus water is squeezed out by hand, and dry, clean pine sawdust of fine texture is thoroughly rubbed into the hair; this absorbs the remaining moisture, scours the locks of hair, and when brushed out afterwards leaves the feather dry and silky-looking.

Actual immersion in water is sometimes carried out for the cure of mange. Gammexane or lime-sulphur preparations may be used. After coming out of the bath the animals stand in a dripping-pen for a few minutes so that they may shake a good deal of the solution out of their coats, and are then led away and dried. The bathing is repeated as often as the condition renders necessary.

Sulphur dioxide and steam baths have also been used for the cure of mange.

Sand baths exercise a tonic and stimulating effect on the surface of the body, and have some slight scouring action of the skin and hair. The horse is allowed into a small enclosure bedded with fine silver sand (which has been collected from a fresh-water stream and does not contain any salt which he may lick), and is allowed to roll for a few minutes. Young horses coming in from work hot and sweating soon learn to roll and cool themselves if they are allowed out after their harness has been removed and before they are groomed.

Cattle, Sheep (*see* DIPS AND DIPPING).

Dogs.—These animals are bathed much more frequently than any of the other domesticated creatures; sometimes more frequently than is necessary, but at the same time it is essential that they should be kept as clean as possible on account of their close relationship with man. Excessive washing is apt to irritate the skin and predispose to attacks of eczema, and unless some care is exercised afterwards the dog may contract a chill as the result of being improperly dried.

With foxhounds, beagles, otter hounds, etc., which are kept together in numbers, the whole pack should be washed on the same day if possible, all the old litter being burnt and the kennels cleansed with hot water and disinfectant.

For ordinary purposes the dog is bathed in warm water to which a pinch of soda has been added (about a dessert-spoonful to two gallons) contained in a tin or wooden bath. It is bad practice to bath the dog in a human bath or in a sink, for obvious reasons. It is necessary to add derris, or a proprietary preparation containing BHC, to the water to ensure the destruction of fleas, lice, etc. The dog is firstly thoroughly soaked in the water (which should be about blood-heat) and then lathered with hard toilet soap. (Soft soap contains a certain amount of free alkali, and is apt to blister the more delicate parts of the skin.)

When the skin has been cleansed the soapy water should be rinsed out with cool, clean water poured over the back. The surplus water is then wrung out of the coat by the hand, and the dog is dried with a rough towel. An electric drier, as used by barbers, which gives a hot, a warm, and a cold blast of air, is excellent. The dog should be allowed to exercise himself in the house, or out of doors if the weather permits, for a few minutes, and is finally well brushed or rubbed to stimulate the skin circulation. In the most delicate breeds, the animal may be allowed to lie beside a fire until it is dry, but should be protected from draughts for two hours afterwards.

Upon certain occasions a hot bath will lower the temperature of a dog suffering from some fevered condition more rapidly than any other means. The dog is plunged into a bath of water of a temperature of about 110° to 115° F. for about ten minutes. Is is then taken out, rapidly dried before a fire, and wrapped up in a woollen blanket or cotton-wool, and provided with two or more hot-water bottles.

BATS (*see* RABIES, VAMPIRE BATS).

BATTERY SYSTEM.—A method of keeping pullets in cages; one, two, or even three birds per cage. Feeding and watering may be on the 'cafeteria' system, with food containers moving on an endless belt, electrically driven. Advantages: ease of culling, since it is easy to see which birds are laying well; labour-saving; disadvantages: high capital cost, an unnatural system which is not much used for breeding stock.

The practice of keeping two or three birds in one cage, where they can hardly move, has been deplored by the B.V.A. 'If cannibalism occurs, the victim cannot escape.'

'Cage Layer Fatigue', a form of leg paralysis, is sometimes encountered in battery birds. Birds let out of their cages on to a solid floor usually recover. A bone-meal supplement may help. (*See* INTENSIVE LIVESTOCK PRODUCTION, EGG YIELD.)

B.C.G. VACCINE is the name given to a vaccine of the so-called *Bacillus Calmette-Guérin*. This was originally a strain of the *Mycobacterium tuberculosis* repeatedly cultivated upon a potato medium with glycerin and bile, so that the organisms lost their power to produce the disease. Such organisms are *avirulent* in consequence.

Upon injection of a suitable dosage of these living but avirulent germs into calves soon after birth, a resistance against virulent organisms is developed. The protection so obtained lasts for at least one year, when re-inoculation may become necessary.

B.C.G. vaccine is used in human preventive medicine (*see Brit. Med. Journal*, June 6, 1959), but in veterinary medicine the emphasis on tuberculosis control is by means of testing with tuberculin and eradication of reactors. B.C.G. was found disappointing as regards cattle. B.C.G. may be used for dogs and cats in Britain in households where the owner has tuberculosis. (*See* TUBERCULOSIS.)

BEAK (*see* DE-BEAKING, 'SHOVEL BEAK').

BEDDING and BEDDING MATERIALS.—Whenever animals are housed in buildings it is both necessary and economical to provide them with some form of bedding material. The reasons are as follows:

(1) All animals are able to rest more adequately in the recumbent position, and the temptation to lie is materially increased by the provision of some soft bedding upon which they may more comfortably repose than on the uncovered floor. Indeed, there are some which, in the event of the bedding being inadequate, or when it becomes scraped away, will not lie down at all.

(2) The extra comfort provided by bedding ensures more beneficial rest.

(3) The provision of a sufficiency of some non-conductor of heat (which is one of the essentials of a good bedding) minimises the risk of chills.

(4) The protection afforded to prominent bony surfaces—such as the point of the hip, the points of the elbow and hock, the stifles and knees, etc.—is important, and if neglected leads to bruises and injuries of these parts.

(5) From the point of view of cleanliness, both of the shed or loose-box and of the animal's skin, the advantages of a plentiful supply of bedding are obvious.

(6) In the case of sick animals, the supply and management of the bedding in the sick-box makes all the difference between a rapid recovery or a protraction of the sickness which may terminate in death. (*See also* SLATTED FLOORS.)

Horses: Wheat straw.—Wheat straw undoubtedly makes the best litter for either stall or loose-box, but on board ship it has certain disadvantages, the chief of which are: (*a*) its inflammability; (*b*) its bulkiness; and (*c*) the difficulty of its disposal.

Wheat straw should be supplied loose or in hand-tied bundles for preference. Trussed or baled straw has been pressed and has lost some of its resilience or elasticity in the process. The individual straws should be long and unbroken, and the natural resistive varnish-like coating should be still preserved in a sample. The colour should be yellowish or a golden white; it should be clean-looking and free from dustiness. Straw should be free from thistles and other weeds, and should be crisp and firm to the touch.

Wheat straw has a particular advantage in that horses will not eat it unless kept very short of hay ; it is neither sweet when chewed, nor is it easily masticated. It is firm and yet soft enough for bedding purposes, and if the bed is made with the individual straws crossing each other as much as possible, when the horse lies down any urine which may have been voided previously is able to trickle through the bedding and escape without much of it being absorbed and held to soil the skin.

Oat straw.—This straw is also very good for bedding purposes, but it possesses one or two disadvantages when compared with wheat straw. The individual straws are not so long as wheat, since the plant is not so tall, and the stubble is often left longer so as to protect the clover or rye-grass that is often sown with the oats. The straw is considerably softer, more easily broken and compressible than wheat, and being sweet to the taste, horses are often induced to eat it.

Barley straw is inferior to either of the two preceding for these reasons : it is only about half the length ; it is very soft and easily compressed and therefore does not last so long as oat or wheat ; more of it is required to bed the same-sized stall ; and it possesses numbers of awns or avels. The awns of barley are sharp and brittle and are provided with a series of backwardly directed barbs, which enable the broken pieces to travel in one direction when they gain entrance into a part where there is any movement.

Awns irritate the softer parts of the skin, cause scratches, and sometimes penetrate the soft tissues of the udder, lips, nose, or the region about the tail. In fine-skinned horses they sometimes set up a diffuse itchy condition of the skin which is not unlike the appearance of mange.

Rye straw.—It has the same advantages as wheat straw, but it is a little harder and rougher.

Peat-moss litter, also called **Moss litter, Peat moss,** and **Peat litter,** is quite a useful litter for horses that are in a healthy condition and in an ordinary stalled stable. It is specially recommended for town stables and for use on board ship, or in other circumstances where the economic storage of straw is a difficulty, or where the supply of straw is inadequate. A good sample should not be powdery, but should consist of a matrix of fibres in which are entangled small lumps of pressed dry moss. It is of a brownish peaty colour, and therefore never looks clean, and it is very absorbent—taking up six or eight times its own weight of water. Peat-moss litter is specially recommended for use on board ship and in railway loose-boxes, since it affords a good foothold even when wet, is practically non-inflammable, and can be conveniently stored in bales of from ½ to 1 cwt. In the stable it has the disadvantage of clogging up horses' feet ; and if there are covered drains in the building it works into the gratings over the traps and blocks them also. When it is used the drains should be of the open or 'surface' variety, or covered drains should be covered with old sacks, etc.

It should never be used in a sick-box in which there is an animal suffering from any respiratory disease, for on account of its dusty nature it pollutes the atmosphere whenever a fresh supply is given or when it is otherwise disturbed. Peat-moss litter is very effective for bedding those horses that eat their litter, since no horse, however hungry, will eat the dry, dusty peat moss. About 20 to 25 lb. are required per horse per day in an ordinary stall.

Sawdust is good when of suitable quality and when it can be obtained in regular and sufficient amounts. It should not contain any chips of wood or nails, etc.

If used as a bedding it must be renewed frequently and the stall thoroughly cleansed once a week, for the dung and urine cause it to ferment and the atmosphere of the stable becomes fouled. Pine sawdust possesses a characteristic odour, and while this is to be desired in a stable, the pine smell is apt to mask the smell of any decomposition that may be taking place in the deeper layers, and a sense of false security is induced. It is especially sweet and cool in the summer time, and so long as it is fresh itself it keeps the hoofs hard and sound. It is clean-looking, and the soiled portions can be easily removed. It is not likely to be eaten by horses that habitually eat their litter, and it is more easily removed from the skin than peat-moss litter or sand. In some parts of the country it is usual to bed stallions and very valuable mares as well as blood-stock upon sawdust during the summer months, and in the winter a layer of wheat straw is laid over the sawdust. It has the disadvantage of blocking drains if these are open. About 1 to 2 cwts. per week are required for a stall, and more than this in a loose-box, for every horse.

Sand makes a fairly good bed when the sample does not contain any stones, shells, or other large particles. It is clean-looking, has a certain amount of scouring action on the coat, is cool in the summer, and comparatively easily managed. Sand should be obtained from a sand pit or the bed of a running stream; not from the sea-shore, because the latter is impregnated with salt, and likely to be licked by horses when they discover the salty taste, of which they are very fond. If this habit is acquired the particles of sand that are eaten collect in the colon or cæcum of the horse and may set up a condition known as 'sand colic', which is often difficult to alleviate. For this reason, sand is not suitable for those animals that are used to eating their hay from the ground; here again quantities of sand are taken in with the hay and the same untoward results follow.

Ferns and bracken make a soft bed and are easily managed, but they always look dirty and untidy, do not last as long as straws, and are rather absorbent when stamped down. In connection with bracken it must be remembered that with horses that eat their bedding there is a slight risk of bracken poisoning. This is not great, however, for it is known that poisoning only occurs when the green shoots of the plant are eaten, and that drying and storing cause a deterioration of the poisonous principles.

Shavings, where abundantly procurable, make a fairly satisfactory litter if obtained from hand planes in a joiner's shop. Machine planes make the shavings harsh and rough. Unfortunately they often contain chips of wood from the joiner's shop, and as these are difficult to remove they should generally be avoided. Like sawdust, they have little manurial value for the land afterwards.

Management of the bedding.—Whatever material is used it is essential that it shall be kept as clean as the circumstances allow. All dung and soiled bedding must be removed in the morning and carried to the dung-pit. The cleaner portions of the bedding should be gathered and carried out into the sun to dry and become aerated whenever possible. It is often laid out in rows across the direction of the prevailing winds, and turned once or twice during the day. On wet days, or when the wind is very strong, it is usually left in the passage behind the horses, and the windows and doors are kept open. This is not possible in many stables, and alternative methods consist in piling the litter to either side of the stall, or up into a heap below the manger. In all cases it is better to remove the bedding from the floor so that this latter may get a chance of drying before it is again soiled with urine at night. It is important that the bedding, if left behind in the stable during the day, shall be as dry as possible, for otherwise it undergoes decomposition, and when the horses return at night they enter a close, damp atmosphere instead of a clean, dry, and sweet one.

The floor of the stable should be well swept down at least once during the day, and ought to be hosed once a week. A little disinfectant added to the water will be of use in keeping the building as germ-free as may be.

If horses have to stand in all day, they should stand on the bare floor in the forenoon and may be bedded about 2 P.M., when they can lie and rest if they so desire.

In the evening, either just before the horses return to the stable, or soon after, they should be bedded down for the night. The new material should be placed chiefly under the old, so that the latter may receive the dung and be removed next day. It is usual to bed as far forward as the manger, or to within about one foot of it, and back about the same distance past the heel-posts. The urine channel should always be left free, however. The bedding is slightly piled up at the sides of the stall, to protect the horse from the partition when it lies down, and is left thinner in the middle. The straws should cross each other as much as possible, thereby ensuring as elastic a bed as can be. Horses that habitually scrape their beds away from the front of the stall may be given an extra amount at this part, or the front of the stall may be bedded with peat moss or some other such substance. Those that eat their bedding may be muzzled after they have done feeding, or provided with some unpalatable material (see previously).

Bedding for cattle.—Wheat straw is the most satisfactory. Oat straw is used in parts where little or no wheat is grown. Barley straw is open to objection as a litter for cows on account of its awns, which may irritate the soft skin of the perineal regions and of the udder. Sawdust has been found very convenient in cow cubicles. (*See* CUBICLES.) Sand has been used on slippery floors below straw bedding, when it affords a good foothold for the cows and prevents accidents. (*See also* DEEP LITTER.)

In milk-fed calves, the ingestion of peat or wood shavings may induce hypomagnesæmia. (*See Veterinary Journal,* October, 1970, **126** 10).

Bedding for pigs.—Many materials are used for the pig, but probably none possesses advantages over wheat straw, unless in the case of farrowing or suckling sows. These should be littered with some very short bedding which will not become entangled round the feet of the little pigs, and will not irritate the udder of the mother. For this purpose chaff, shavings, oak leaves, and even hay, may be used according to circumstances. An insufficiency of litter along with a cold, damp floor is the chief cause of 'cold anæmia' of young pigs and of 'cramp'. (*See* Sow's Milk, Absence of.)

Piglets bedded on red African hardwood shavings have died, as explained under Bedding for dogs.

Slurry systems need not necessarily mean the total abandonment of bedding for pigs. Where vacuum tankers, as opposed to pipelines, are used for distributing the slurry on the land, moderate quantities of sawdust and shavings are not ruled out as bedding materials. Certainly, straw might well be thought of as the pig's best friend—and an ally of the farmer, too, despite its high handling costs.

For straw can make up for deficiencies in management and buildings as nothing else can. It serves the pig as a comfortable bed, as a blanket to burrow under, a plaything to avert boredom, and a source of roughage in meal-fed pigs which can help obviate digestive upsets and at least some of the scouring which reduces farmers' profits. Straw can mitigate the effects of poor floor insulation, of draughts, and of cold; and in buildings without straw ventilation, to quote Dr. David Sainsbury, 'becomes a much more critical factor'.

Bedding for dogs and cats.—Clean, long, soft oat straw is best for the larger breeds of dogs, although wheat straw is almost as good. It can be easily and quickly cleaned out, burns well, thereby destroying fleas, lice, mange mites, etc. It is warm enough in winter, but rather too warm in summer. When the weather is hot it is often replaced by clean sawdust in the larger sporting kennels. In the case of the long-haired breeds of toy dogs, and for cats (especially Persians), meadow hay is the most satisfactory litter. Sawdust is not advisable, because it is likely to get into the coat and is difficult to remove.

Dogs have died as a result of the use for bedding of shavings of the red African hardwood (*Mansonia altissima*), which affects nose, mouth, and the feet, as well as the heart.

The whole of the bedding should be removed and burnt at least once a week, especially where male cats are kept. The cages should be thoroughly scrubbed out with boiling water and a disinfectant once every three weeks or month, and allowed to remain vacant for the day, so that they will be quite dry before the animals sleep in them.

BEDDING, INSUFFICIENCY OF.—The provision of an inadequate amount of bedding for the domesticated animals is liable to occasion bruises and injuries of the prominent parts of the body which are not covered with masses of muscle, such as the elbow, the knee, fetlock, scapular region, hip, stifle, hock, etc. The tissues covering these parts are never very thick, and in many cases consist of the skin and a little fibrous tissue only. If they are subjected to long-continued or severe pressure against a hard object, such as the bare floor of a stable, the circulation is disturbed or cut off and the nutrition of the skin is impaired. This leads to bed-sores. Capped elbow, capped knee, and capped hock, are three similar conditions. (*See* Foot-rot in Pigs, Capped Elbow, Capped Hock, Hygroma.)

Other conditions that may result directly or indirectly from an insufficiency of bedding are tail-biting, chills, in young store pigs; sometimes broken legs from falling; eye injuries; 'bed-sores'; occasionally tetanus (lockjaw) from bruises and subsequent infection, etc. In addition to these serious conditions, there is a loss of time, money, and working capacity which results from the animals requiring longer to groom and failing to get comfortable and refreshing rest, taking longer to fatten, losing litters from cold and exhaustion, and so on. No good animal husbandman will neglect the bedding of his animals. (*See* Bedding Materials, Bed-sores, Slatted Floors, Tail Sores, and under the other sections mentioned.)

BEDSONIA.—Psittacosis type agents. (*See under* Calf Pneumonia.)

BED-SORES are areas of inflamed or ulcerated skin which appear upon certain parts of the body and limbs of animals which, owing to injury or disease, are forced to remain lying for long periods at a time. Thus cows affected with ante-partum paralysis are likely to develop bed-sores upon the skin over stifles, point of the hip, on the side of the shoulder, on the elbows and hocks, and sometimes on the side of the head if this cannot be held off the ground. Horses are sometimes affected, but generally only in the old or debilitated animal, since horses do not survive long periods of recumbency. Lack of bedding produces lesions which are of the same nature if the ground is hard or uneven. Old dogs, which spend a good deal of time lying, sometimes develop bed-sores on the elbows and hocks. The skin at first appears to be inflamed and sore to the touch, and later on begins to ulcerate and will eventually slough off, leaving a raw and painful sore which has little tendency to heal. The causes are pressure on the skin interfering with the blood-supply and infection occurring subsequently.

Prevention.—Animals that are unable to stand should be provided with an adequate supply of soft bedding and turned over on to the opposite side two or three times a day or more. If the skin becomes inflamed it should be bathed with warm solution of salt and water, dried, and painted with methylated spirit to harden the surface. If the sores have already developed when they are first noticed they should be thoroughly washed and afterwards dusted with an antiseptic dusting powder, and if possible they should be protected by bandages and cotton-wool. Poulticing will hasten the removal of a persistent slough.

BEEF-BREEDS and CROSSES.—The British beef-breeds are the Aberdeen-Angus, Scotch Shorthorn, Hereford, Devon, Sussex, Galloway, Belted Galloway, Highland, and Lincoln Red.

Very little of the beef eaten in Britain is, however, from purebred animals of these breeds—except meat in the luxury class. Most of the beef comes from crossbred animals, an increasing proportion from crossbred Friesian steers, or purebred Friesian steers.

Professor M. M. Cooper has commented: 'The better prospect for someone contemplating store production is one based on the purchase of week-old Friesian calves which are born in the autumn. One would like to advocate Hereford or Angus-cross Friesians, but these calves, according to locality, carry a premium that their subsequent performance does not warrant.'

Mr. P. I. Bichan has commented: Of the many breeds of cattle in this country, it is only really worth while considering those which make a significant contribution to meat production. Without doubt the dairy breeds are the most important source of supply, and of those the Friesian, Ayrshire and Shorthorn are the most numerous. The Friesian has shown itself beyond all doubt to possess the attributes required, and when fattened at 18 to 20 months of age it is satisfactory to both butcher and consumer.'

'Unless the buyer is gifted with the ability to select calves of the required conformation, the only really safe type to purchase is the white-faced calf with a black coat. This can only be either a Hereford × Friesian, Hereford × Welsh Black, or a Hereford × Aberdeen-Angus, all of which are good beef types. Of course, the progeny of Aberdeen-Angus crosses on the Friesian and Dairy Shorthorn are all black—and very useful types—but they are not easily recognisable as such.'

'Certainly the only really good cross on the Ayrshire seems to be the Scotch Beef Shorthorn, and, indeed, the ability of this breed to put flesh on the progeny of the Ayrshire may be even more marked when it is crossed with other dairy breeds.'

Since the above was written, the Charolais has become the third most important beef-breed as judged by A.I. figures. (*See under* CATTLE.)

Beef which is acceptable to the butcher can be produced economically by crossing the Charolais bull with Guernsey and Jersey cows. In a trial conducted by Spillers Limited, Charolais × Guernsey steers reached 850 lb. liveweight in 342 days—a performance equal to that of pure Friesian steers on a similar system. Daily liveweight gain was 2·24 lb. (*See* CHAROLAIS, LUING, *and* BEEVBILDE.)

BEEF CATTLE HUSBANDRY.—In Britain today there are four main systems of management for beef production: (1) Fattening of suckled calves; (2) intensive cereal beef; (3) semi-intensive grass/cereal beef; and (4) intensive grass/cereal beef.

What follows is not a series of dogmatic statements but a summary of what farmers have been practising in beef herds recorded by the MLC.*

Suckler herds.—Twenty per cent of our beef now comes from suckler herds, and this proportion is likely to rise. Under the traditional system, the average suckler cow produced a calf gaining less than 1½ lb. per day, and took three acres to do it. The new concept calls for a cow with plenty of milk; able to over-winter on arable by-products such as potatoes, pea-haulm silage, sugar-beet tops, straw and supplement; able to produce a calf gaining at least 2·5 lb. per day; and needing only one acre to do it.

Autumn-calving herds have usually proved the most profitable. All-the-year calving tends to suffer from the disadvantage that it does not allow either: (1) cheap over-wintering of spring-calving cows; (2) a heavier weaned calf at the summer sale by autumn calving.

It is recommended that bulls should be selected with weight-for-age records above average, and dams should be chosen on the basis of the weaning weights of their progeny.

With autumn-calving herds, the most efficient producers are those who are generous with creep feed.

Intensive cereal beef.—At the present time some 8 per cent of home-produced beef comes under the heading of 'barley beef'; though the MLC* prefers to speak of intensive cereal enterprises and defines them as those where roughage does not account for more than 2 lb. per head of the dry matter intake of the animal.

Dr. H. K. Baker has described it as 'the best documented, the most straightforward system of beef production; yet in a survey of many hundreds of groups of cattle we find that in the last three months before they're finished, live-weight performance ranges from 1·6 to 2·8 lb. a day'. In recorded units, steers are finished on average at 860 lb., when 11 months old.

Friesian steers remain the first choice for this form of beef production. 'The number of Charolais crosses being recorded is still relatively low in comparison with Hereford and, to a lesser extent, Aberdeen-Angus crosses.'

Charolais make Channel Island crosses suitable for intensive cereal beef. Aberdeen-Angus × Friesians will, in many cases, be calves out of heifers, and this may bias the results for that particular cross downwards.

Semi-intensive grass/cereal beef.—The winter fattening of semi-intensive grass/cereal beef appears to be uneconomic in many instances. Of 22 groups of light cattle, weighing 400–599 lb., nine groups were putting on weight at a financial loss to their owners. 'Any profit in most cases will be a reflection of "dealing" ability.' Poor-quality feed is usually to blame for the poor results.

* Meat and Livestock Commission.

BEEF CATTLE HUSBANDRY

The Friesian steer quite often loses much of its advantage when it comes to winter feeding. It takes longer, or requires more feed, to reach the required weight or finish as compared with a crossbred Friesian.

Hereford × Friesian cross steers gain on average 0·25 lb. per day more than Friesian steers at grass on the same farm.

Intensive grass/cereal beef.—Carried out, with modifications, from Devon to Aberdeenshire, this system involves the use of autumn-born dairy calves. These are reared indoors during their first winter and turned out to grass in spring at a liveweight of about 400 lb. Paddock grazing is an essential feature of the system, and the aim is to attain high production by a combination of stocking rate and performance per animal. The calves are brought into yards in the autumn at about 750 lb. liveweight and fed high-quality conserved fodders and a limited amount of cereals. The cattle are slaughtered when 14 to 19 months old, at weights ranging from 850 to 1,150 lb.

During the fattening period it is possible to replace some of the silage by arable by-products, but the amount of concentrates will then have to be increased. For example, the two following rations both gave similar animal performance when fed to Friesian and Hereford × Friesian steers at an EHF: (a) 25 lb. silage, 8 lb. concentrates, plus straw *ad lib*; (b) silage *ad lib* (average 50 lb. per day), plus 3 lb. concentrates. On ration (b) the steers took only 12 days longer to achieve the slaughter weight of 8¾ cwt. than those on ration (a). 'Pea-haulm and other arable silages are difficult to make well enough to support high performance (1¾ lb. per day) in beef cattle given less than 6–8 lb. cereal mix per day. Even good-quality arable silage will not compare with silage made from grass of 65 per cent digestibility, and the cost of the total ration will be higher owing to this greater reliance on concentrates' is the MLC conclusion.

Supplementary feeding at grass, states a 1969 MLC report improved daily gains of both semi-intensive beef and suckler calves, resulting in heavier yarding weights. Cattle used to concentrate feeding before yarding receive less of a check in growth when brought into yards.

Among yarded cattle, over 1,800 Friesian steers gained an average of 1·74 lb. per day. This figure was inferior to that achieved by all the beef breed × Friesian steers except A-A crosses. Among beef breed × Friesian steers, the highest gains were achieved by (1) South Devon, (2) Charolais, and (3) Devon crosses, in that order.

Systems of beef production

Type	Age at slaughter	Weight at slaughter*
Intensive beef	10 to 14 months	700 to 900 lb.
Semi-intensive	15 to 20 months	850 to 1150 lb.
Extensive	24 to 29 months	900 to 1300 lb.

* The wide range depends upon whether the cattle are of late, early, or medium maturing breeds (MLC figures)

BEEF FROM BARLEY-FED CATTLE.—Sudden and unexpected deaths among calves being fattened on barley have been reported from several parts of the country. Two entirely different causes account for many of these deaths. One is a failure on the part of the owner of the animals to make a gradual change from their previous diet to one mainly of barley. This brings about ill-effects in the rumen and is referred to under BARLEY POISONING.

The other health problem is the coughing which persists in some intensively reared cattle from a month or two after they are housed right through until they are slaughtered. For a few days, the calves may appear feverish and off their food, but then they usually rally and thrive reasonably well. From time to time, however—and this is the experience of several veterinary surgeons—complications occur with alarming suddenness, and there are deaths from what is technically known as Cuffing Pneumonia.

Such deaths have occurred under 'seemingly ideal conditions' to quote one report; but usually a predisposing cause is inadequate ventilation, and when this is improved health is found to improve, too. In one building, in an effort to increase warmth, sacks had been placed over wire netting above the calves, which became acutely ill—with constant coughing and distressed breathing—within 4 days; 3 dying after a further 2 days.

BEET TOPS (*see* FODDER POISONING, p. 736).

BEEVBILDE CATTLE.—There is now a Breed Society for these. Beevbilde breeding is based on 54 per cent polled Lincoln Red blood, 40 per cent polled Beef Shorthorn, and 6 per cent Aberdeen-Angus.

BELLADONNA is the common name for the deadly nightshade flower (*Atropa belladonna*) from which are prepared several compounds used in medicine. Externally, belladonna is useful for the larger animals for relief of painful conditions. Internally, it is often an ingredient of electuaries to relieve coughs. (*See* ATROPINE.)

BENADRYL is the proprietary name of beta-dimethylamino-ethylbenz-hydryl ether hydrochloride, which is of use as an antihistamine (which see) in treating certain allergic conditions.

BENZALKONIUM CHLORIDE.—One of the quaternary ammonia compounds. (*See under* QUATERNARY.)

BENZAMINE LACTATE is another name for eucaine, one of an important group of compounds used as local anæsthetics. It is particularly useful for operations on the eye.

BENZENE HEXACHLORIDE. — The gamma isomer of this is a highly effective and persistent parasiticide, of great value in destroying flies, lice, and fleas, ticks, and mange mites. It has a low toxicity for man and the domestic animals, and is the main ingredient of several well-known proprietary preparations, designed for use as dusting powder, spray, dip, smoke-generator, etc.

BHC is the common abbreviation for the gamma isomer. (*See* BHC POISONING.)

BENZOCAINE is a white powder, with soothing properties, used as a sedative for inflamed and painful surfaces. It is antagonistic to the sulphonamides.

BENZOIC ACID is an antiseptic substance used for inflammatory conditions of the urinary system. It is excreted as hippuric acid, and renders the urine acid. It is used in the treatment of ringworm, and as a food preservative.

BENZOIC ACID POISONING.—Suspected cases of this have been reported in the cat, giving rise to extreme aggressiveness, salivation, convulsions, and death.

BENZYL BENZOATE is a useful drug for treating mange in dogs and horses. It is usually employed as an emulsion. It is prepared from balsam of Peru. It should not be used over the whole body surface at once.

BEPHENIUM EMBONATE.—A drug which is used in sheep to kill nematodirus worms.

'BERENIL' is the proprietary name of a diamidinophenyl compound used in treating babesiosis and trypanosomiasis in the dog. Poisoning from overdosage gives rise to tremors, jerky eye movements, unsteady gait, opisthotonos, and death.

BHC (*see* BENZENE HEXACHLORIDE).

BHC POISONING.—This may arise, especially in kittens and puppies, from a single dose (*e.g.* licking of dusting powder). Symptoms include: twitching, muscular inco-ordination, anxiety, convulsions.

A farmer's wife became ill (she had a convulsion) after helping to dip calves, but recovered after treatment. Two of the calves died. This shows that even BHC must be regarded with respect, and precautions taken to avoid the use of too strong a dip or dressing, or of not washing all of the residue off one's own skin. (*See also* GAME-BIRDS.)

BHC is highly poisonous for fish.

B.H.S.—Beta hæmolytic streptococcus.

BICARBONATE OF SODA, or baking soda, is one of the most useful of the less strong alkalies both for internal and external application. (*See* ALKALIES.)

'BIG HEAD.'—A condition associated with Black Disease in rams which have slightly injured their heads as a result of fighting.

BILE is a thick, bitter, golden-brown or greenish-yellow fluid secreted by the liver, and stored in the gall-bladder when that organ is present. The *Equidæ* possess no gall-bladder, but it is present in the other domesticated animals and birds. Bile is composed of water, mucus, brown or green pigments, and salts of taurocholic and glycocholic acids. It is partly the result of the neutralisation of harmful products of digestion which are absorbed into the blood-stream, carried to the liver, changed into harmless compounds, and discharged to the intestines again. It is partly an elaborated secretion, and it has digestive functions which assist the saponification of the fat contents of the food. It has in addition some laxative action, stimulating peristalsis, and it prevents undue putrefaction of the ingested food. It is formed by the liver cells and passed into the smaller bile-ducts; these unite with each other to form the radicles of the main bile-duct, which either empties its contents into the gall-bladder or opens into the first part of the small intestine, *i.e.* the duodenum, about a foot from the termination of the stomach. In those animals which possess a gall-bladder another bile-duct leads to the duodenum, the bladder acting as a reservoir only.

Jaundice, a symptom rather than a disease, may be caused when the flow of the bile is obstructed and does not reach the intestines, but remains circulating in the blood. As a result the pigments are deposited in the tissues and discolour them, while the visible mucous membranes show a yellowishness or even a brown coloration in bad cases. In addition, the appearance of the urine changes, due to some of the bile salts being excreted by the kidneys.

Vomiting of bile usually occurs when the normal passage through the intestines is obstructed, and during the course of certain digestive disorders.

(*See also* GALL-STONES.)

BILHARZIOSIS is a disease produced

by bilharziæ or Schistosomes; these are parasites of about ¼ to 1 centimetre in length which are sometimes found in the blood-stream of cattle and sheep in Europe, and of horses, camels, cattle, sheep, and donkeys in India, Japan, and the northern seaboard countries of Africa. (*See* PARASITES, p. 648.)

BILIARY FEVER, or **CANINE PIROPLASMOSIS,** which is also called tick fever, malignant jaundice, and infectious icterus, is a disease of the dog occurring in South Africa, India, many countries in the Far East, Italy, and France. It is due to a blood parasite, *Babesia canis*, which is carried from an infected dog to a healthy one by means of a tick. (*See* PARASITES, p. 640.)

Cause.—The disease is caused by the presence of the piroplasm (pear-shaped) in the blood-stream. This results in a breakdown of the red blood corpuscles of the dog and anæmia, toxic symptoms and severe disturbances result. Ticks feeding on an infected dog and upon a recovered dog whose blood may still contain the piroplasms, take these organisms into their stomachs. From there they migrate to the reproductive organs of the tick and reach the eggs in due course. The new generation of nymph ticks are not themselves able to transmit the disease to dogs on which they feed until they attain the adult stage, in the majority of cases. Infection gains the body of the new host by being ejected along with the tick's saliva into the wound in the dog's skin.

Symptoms.—Between ten and twenty days after the introduction of the pear-shaped piroplasm the dog becomes fevered, its temperature rises to 103° or 105° F., respirations are rapid, and the pulse is fast. In the acute cases the dog rapidly becomes weak, the membranes are pale, and often tinged with yellow. Wasting of the flesh is very marked; the spleen is enlarged, and blood is passed with the urine. In the chronic forms the animals show the same symptoms, but these are less acute, and death may be delayed for several weeks. The mortality varies according to whether the animal has been imported from an absolutely clean locality or not.

Treatment.—Trypanblue has been replaced by the more specific diamidino-diphenyl ether compounds, *e.g.* Acapron, Phenamidine. In addition, it is necessary to attend to the nursing of the dog.

BINOVULAR TWINS are twins which result from the fertilisation of two ova, as distinct from 'monovular twins' which arise from a single ovum.

'BIO-ACTIVE' RATIONS contain selected animal substances: bovine liver, spleen and placenta; hæmoglobin; pig's stomach; and embryonic calf. These are reduced to powder by controlled heat in vacuum. The process has Ministry of Agriculture approval.

BIOPSY is a diagnostic method in which a small portion of living tissue is removed from the animal and examined by special means in the laboratory so that a diagnosis may be made.

BIOTIN.—Factor H of the B_2 complex; formerly known as vitamin H.

BIRD LOUSE is a parasitic insect belonging to the order *Mallophaga*, which attacks most domesticated and many wild birds. The lice eat feathers and the shed cells from the surface of the skin, but they do not suck blood. Dusting with BHC or other parasiticide powder is an efficient remedy. (*See* PARASITES, p. 681.)

BIRD MALARIA.—A tropical disease of fowls and turkeys caused by *Plasmodium gallinaceum* and *P. durae*, respectively.

It may run a rapidly fatal course, or a chronic one with anæmia and greenish diarrhœa.

BIRD REPELLENTS.—Thiram and anthraquinone are examples. In the U.K. birds have avoided contact with the chemical by picking out the cotyledons after germination of the treated seed.

BIRDS (*see* CAGE BIRDS, DUCK VIRUS HEPATITIS, FALCONS, GAME BIRDS, TURKEYS, and POULTRY. *See also* DESTRUCTION OF BIRDS).

BIRDSVILLE DISEASE occurs in parts of Australia, is due to a poisonous plant *Indigofera enneaphylla*, and has to be differentiated from Kimberley Horse Disease. Symptoms: sleepiness and abnormal gait with front legs lifted high. Chronic cases drag the hind limbs.

BIRTH (*see* PARTURITION).

When an animal gives birth to offspring which is alive at the time of birth but which never breathes, it is said to produce a *stillborn foal*, or *calf*, etc. Many of these could have been saved if there had been someone at hand to render assistance to the dam or to remove the membranes from the mouth and nostrils of the young animal. When such measures fail there is still hope of reviving the young creature by the adoption of more vigorous methods. It should be slapped about the head with a wet towel, turned over on to the opposite side, held by the hind-legs, and even hung up by them so as to allow the blood a chance of flowing from the heart to the head. Artificial respiration should be attempted and persisted in for so long as any movement at all can be detected on the part of the heart. (*See* ARTIFICIAL RESPIRATION.)

Abortion or *miscarriage* means the birth of a dead fœtus before the normal period of pregnancy has passed. *Premature birth* occurs before the appointed time, but the young animal lives, and although perhaps undersized develops quite normally.

BISMUTH is one of the heavy metals whose carbonate, oxide, subnitrate, salicylate, and oxychloride are much used in medicine.

Uses.—The carbonate, subnitrate, and the salicylate are used in irritable and painful conditions of the stomach and intestines to relieve diarrhœa and vomiting. The salts of bismuth are reputed to form a protective covering over any ulcerated areas used in these conditions. As astringents they are sometimes used for weeping sores on the surface of the skin, when they are often mixed with starch and oxide of zinc; for this purpose the oxide of bismuth is favoured.

The oxychloride and the subnitrate are used as bismuth meals prior to taking X-ray photographs of the abdominal organs for purposes of diagnosis. The massed bismuth salt forms a barrier to the passage of the rays; and the outline of the opaque bowel appears in the print. Barium sulphate has to some extent replaced the bismuth salts, being more readily taken in milk by dogs and cats. Bismuth compounds, when given in excess, tinge the motions a dark smoky-black colour, which is rather alarming to the uninitiated.

BITES, STINGS, and POISONED WOUNDS.—The bites of animals, whether domesticated or otherwise, are always to be looked upon as infected wounds, for, no matter how clean the mouth of an animal appears to be, it is always the seat of myriads of organisms, many of which are of a harmful nature, and if neglected may give rise to sepsis, toxæmia, and even death. (*See* WOUNDS.) In countries abroad where rabies is indigenous the spread of this disease is generally by means of a bite. (*See* RABIES.)

Cat-bites are usually followed by some degree of suppuration. (*See also* RABIES, CAT-SCRATCH FEVER.)

Dog-bites are usually inflicted upon other dogs, defenceless sheep or goats, and sometimes pigs; cattle may be bitten by the herd's dog and serious wounds result. The bite is generally a punctured wound, or large tear, depending upon the part that is bitten. Where an animal is bitten in numerous places, even though no individual bite is large, there is always a considerable degree of danger. The wounds should be dressed with some suitable antiseptic, the hair or wool being first clipped from the area; and left open. (*See* WOUNDS, RABIES.)

Snake bites. (*See* separate entry under this heading.)

Harvest-bugs, fleas, lice, ticks, mosquitoes, etc., are dealt with under section on PARASITES.

Bees, wasps, and hornets cause great irritation by the stings with which the females are provided. Death has been reported in pigs eating windfall apples in which wasps were feeding. The wasps stung the mucous membrane of the throat, causing great swelling and death from suffocation some hours later. So far as the actual sting is concerned a few drops of ammonia and the removal of the stinging apparatus that if often left in the wound are sufficient to allay the pain.

BITTERS are substances that are added to tonic powders for both cattle and horses, to increase appetite and promote a flow of the digestive juices of the stomach and the intestines. The chief are gentian, ginger, calumba, and cubebs.

BITTERSWEET POISONING. — The common 'bittersweet'—*Solanum dulcamara*—is a frequent denizen of hedgerows and waste lands, and, although not likely to be eaten to a great extent by domesticated animals, cases of poisoning due to its ingestion have been recorded. All parts of the plant—stem, leaves, and berries—contain the toxic principle, which is an alkaloid similar to *Solanine* found in the potato, but it appears that in different seasons and in diverse parts of the country the toxicity varies. In addition to solanine the stems contain a glucoside called *Dulcamarin*, which imparts a bitter taste when chewed.

Symptoms.—In cattle and sheep the symptoms are giddiness, quickening of the

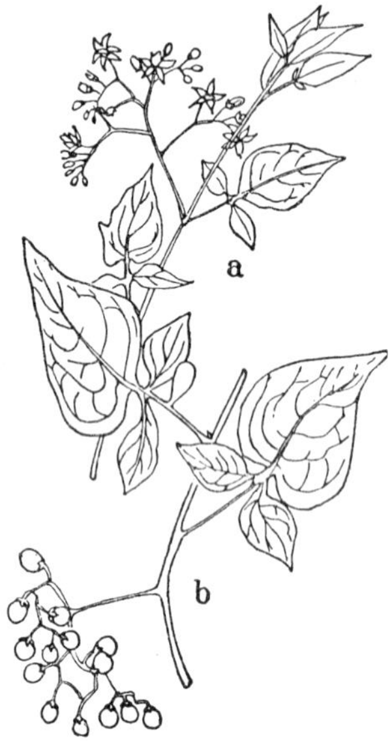

Bittersweet (*Solanum dulcamara*): *a*, flowering part; *b*, ripening berries. The flowers are purple with bright yellow anthers, and the berries are first green, then yellow, and finally change to a brilliant red, hanging loosely to the stem from which the leaves have usually fallen. All parts of the plant are poisonous—the berries especially so.

respiration, staggering gait, dilated pupil, greenish diarrhœa, and when the animal is closely examined the temperature is found to be raised, and the pulse is small and irregular.

Treatment.—Purgatives and stimulants.

BLACK DIARRHŒA occurs when blood from the stomach or earlier part of the intestinal canal becomes mixed with the fæces. There are many conditions in which this may occur, the following being important: gastro-enteritis of irritant origin, heavy intestinal parasitism in lambs, coccidiosis in calves, and a dark-coloured diarrhœa may be seen in the dog suffering from deficiency of the B vitamin complex.

The fæces become dark or black after administration of large doses of bismuth or iron salts, but this is a normal occurrence.

BLACK DISEASE is the name given to infectious necrotic hepatitis of sheep and occasionally of cattle in Australia, New Zealand, Scotland, Wales, and N.W. England. It is typically caused by a combined attack of immature liver flukes and bacteria: a strain of *Clostridium œdematiens*, which is one of the so-called 'gas gangrene' group, and is capable of forming resistant spores.

In black disease these spores are apparently present in the liver in an inactive state until, with the migration of (perhaps) large numbers of young immature flukes (*Fasciola hepatica*) from the intestine, the liver substance becomes injured and the spores become active. The liver becomes necrotic and there is a rapid toxæmia set up.

Symptoms.—The sheep are usually found dead in the early morning, death in some instances being so exceedingly rapid that the animal has food between the lips or teeth, indicating that death took place during feeding. Where affected sheep have been noticed ill, they are first seen to lag behind the others, then to lie down in the usual position on the sternum. Breathing becomes rapid and shallow and pulse-rate is greatly increased. The animal may yawn or gasp occasionally, and a little later respiration becomes distressed, stertorous, and death occurs quietly. The duration of illness in observed cases varies between a few minutes and 48 hours, most cases terminating within 20 to 30 minutes of having first been noticed ill. Gathering a flock by dogs, chasing sheep during dipping or clipping operations, and other circumstances which cause violent muscular exercise will precipitate attacks.

On *post-mortem* examination the most striking feature is the rapidity with which sheep dead from this disease have undergone decomposition. Within only a few hours the carcase has decomposed so much that characteristic lesions are masked. In carcases of sheep recently dead or killed in the later stages, the skin is a dark bluish-black colour, and the underlying tissues are congested and œdematous. In the liver, where the most constant lesions are found, there are one or more necrotic areas about 1 inch in diameter, roughly circular in outline and yellowish-white in colour. In some cases they may be seen to be associated with a 'fluke burrow', in others young flukes may actually be found. Exudation of fluid into the pericardium is typical, and usually the peritoneal and thoracic cavities contain inflammatory exudate.

A characteristic, unpleasant—but not repulsive or putrefactive—smell is perceptible from the carcase, and in particular from the affected liver.

Prevention. — An antiserum and a vaccine are available. Eradication of flukes and the avoidance of fluke-infected land for grazing sheep serve to some extent to prevent loss. Carcases of dead sheep should be burned or buried so that infection in them may not spread.

BLACKHEAD OF TURKEYS is a very common and fatal disease of young turkeys (from three weeks to four months old), which is caused by a small protozoön parasite, *Histomonas meleagridis*, which belongs to the class *Mastigophora*. It passes part of its life in the body of a worm (*Heterakis gallinæ*), which acts as an intermediate host. The histomonas is found in adult worms and eggs, ingestion of the latter is the chief means of spread.

Though turkeys are chiefly affected, the disease has been seen in chickens, partridges, pheasants, grouse, quail and pea-fowl.

Symptoms.—The birds become dull, droop their wings, head, and tail, lose condition, mope, and develop an appetite for unnatural substances. Weakness and emaciation are marked. The droppings are usually liquid and greenish in colour, and the featherless parts of the head become a dull bluish-black or black colour, from which the name is derived. Death, in 5 to 8 days, may occur in 70 to 90 per cent of young turkeys, in which the disease is very acute and most prevalent in summer and autumn. In adults, mortality is lower, and the disease may persist in winter. An acute form of the disease may be seen in which death occurs without any previous symptoms of illness.

Prevention. — This can be largely achieved by hygiene and (*a*) good management; (*b*) the use of certain preparations given regularly in the food.

With regard to (*a*) it is important to ensure when buying new stock that the birds are healthy and from disease-free premises. This may necessitate a microscopical examination of the motions before a clean bill of health can be given. Newly purchased birds should on all occasions be isolated from the rest of the flock for a month. Artificial rearing by means of incubators and foster-mothers, and preventing any contact between the young turkeys and adult birds is useful where it can be adopted. Clean land which has never been used for turkeys is essential when the chicks are old enough to leave the foster-mothers. If this cannot be ensured, the young turkeys may be successfully reared in intensive houses, fitted with 'sun-parlours' on wooden or wire-netting floors, so that the birds never come into contact with the infected soil.

Treatment.—This is always less hopeful than prevention.

'Entramin', a nitrothiazole compound, given in the food is very effective; likewise Furazolidone is also used. It is necessary to feed from hoppers that are not readily fouled by fæces, and to keep the drinking water free from pollution.

Disinfection.—Suspected coops, cages, baskets, crates, pens, runs, incubators, foster-mothers, rearers, brooders, and poultry houses should be periodically scrubbed out with boiling water and soda, and disinfected.

'BLACK-LEG' (*see* BLACK-QUARTER).

BLACK MOTIONS are passed when either iron or bismuth salts are given to dogs and pigs, or when there is constipation in these animals. Pigs may show this feature if they have access to heaps of coal and are allowed to eat to excess, but in such cases the coal can be recognised as small particles of a shiny blackness. The most serious cause of black motions is hæmorrhage into the early part of the digestive system, the blood mixing with the ingesta and becoming changed into a dark colour. Such conditions often result from ulceration of the stomach and hæmorrhage, or from injury by a foreign body that has been eaten and passed into the stomach, or from a hæmorrhagic inflammation in some part of the intestines.

BLACK-QUARTER, also called BLACK-LEG, QUARTER-ILL, SYMPTOMATIC ANTHRAX, EMPHYSEMATOUS ANTHRAX, FELON, etc., is an acute specific infectious disease of cattle, sometimes of sheep, and likewise of pigs, characterised by the presence of rapidly increasing swellings containing gas, and occurring in the region of the shoulder, neck, thigh, quarter, and sometimes on the trunk. Certain farms or districts—'black-leg lands'—are notoriously infected and well known locally. Most are either moorlands of poor quality or liable to become flooded at some period of the year. Young cattle between the ages of three months and two years are most susceptible, although animals outside these limits are occasionally attacked. In South Africa animals appear to be attacked at and age, from calfhood to senility. Sheep, theoretically more susceptible than cattle, are less often affected, probably on account of the greater protection afforded to their skins by the fleece (see later). The disease has been seen in the reindeer, camel, and the buffalo.

Causes.—*Clostridium chauvœi*, which lives in the soil until such time as it gains entry into the animal body either along with the food or else by abrasions of the skin (*see* TATTOOING). It remains at the seat of its lesions and does not invade the blood-stream. On exposure to the air—as, for instance, if the lesion bursts, and when the exudation falls on to suitable places—the organisms form spores which are resistant to extreme cold, or even exposure to 100 degrees Centigrade of dry heat. The incubative period is from a few hours to 5 days.

Symptoms.—Often all that is seen is that one or more of the young stock in a field is found dead without previous history of having been ill. At other times the affected animals are noticed to be very lame in one or more limbs, and on examination the corresponding quarter is swollen and very painful. If seen in the early stages, the swelling is hot and pits on pressure, but, increasing rapidly, it becomes puffed up with gas (emphysematous), and if pressed it crackles as if filled with screwed-up tissue-paper, while on tapping it gives out a hollow sound. These symptoms are accompanied or followed by the shrivelling and drying of the skin over the swellings, which assumes the appearance of leather, becomes cold and insensible, and is liable to crack. When it is incised, or if it becomes accidentally opened, a dark frothy fluid escapes, with a smell not unlike that of rancid butter. At some period of the disease there is a rise in temperature, but the incidence of this is not constant, and the temperature may be subnormal when taken. As the disease progresses the animal becomes duller and duller, lies down and refuses to move, becomes unconscious, and dies usually within 24 hours from the commencement of the symptoms. *Sheep* show somewhat similar symptoms, but they may be attacked at almost any age. There are often blood-stained discharges from both the nostrils and the rectum. The wool over the affected areas is raised above the level of that on the surrounding skin in the Down breeds especially; naturally, this feature is not so obvious in the long-woolled breeds.

Prevention.—Marshy ground that has been responsible for the loss of numerous animals in the past has often been rendered safe by the draining of the land, by heavy liming, and by intensive cultivation. Young animals should not be grazed on land that is suspected of harbouring organisms. Animals that are already badly affected should be isolated and killed, and their carcase buried in quicklime or burned, while the few square yards around an area where an animal has died should be treated with a top-dressing of lime and hurdled off for a few months to keep other members of the herd from eating the probably infected herbage.

Vaccine.—Immunity may be conferred by the use of serum, and a 'Black-quarter Aggressin' gives good results when used early in the season. A formalised vaccine also gives very good results.

Curative.—There is generally no opportunity to treat cases, since death occurs after only a few hours' illness; but, where the opportunity offers, success has been obtained with penicillin and antiserum.

'BLACK TONGUE.'—The counterpart of human pellagra. It is shown in the dog fed a diet deficient in nicotinic acid, and, experimentally, on jowar (*Sorghum vulgare*), a cereal containing nicotinic acid but also high levels of leucine. (*See also* SHEEPDOGS and 'BROWN MOUTH'.)

Symptoms.—Discoloration of the tongue, a foul odour from the mouth, ulceration, loss of appetite, and sometimes blood-stained saliva and fæces. Death will occur in the absence of treatment.

BLACK VOMIT is due to the presence of blood in the stomach. The appearance of the vomit may be either that of black masses of clotted blood, or it may resemble coffee-grounds.

BLACK-WATER FEVER is a popular name for Texas fever, which is caused by a piroplasmal parasite, and is of the same nature as British Redwater. The name 'black-water' is sometimes also applied to British red-water fever. In both diseases the urine becomes dark, even coffee-coloured, due to the excretion of blood pigment by the kidneys. (*See* PROTOZOÖN PARASITES, p. 637.)

BLADDER.—A bladder is a sac formed of muscular and fibrous tissue and lined by a mucous membrane whose surface is covered by smooth cells. The connection between the mucous membrane and the muscular and fibrous wall is loose, so that the cavity of the bladder will be capable of considerable distension. Bladders are designed to act as reservoirs for fluids produced by the body until such time as it shall be required, or until circumstances are convenient for its evacuation to the outside. They usually communicate with the exterior by a narrow tube-like passage, access to which is permitted or prohibited by a ring of muscular tissue called a *sphincter*. There are two important bladders in most animals—the *gall-bladder* and the *urinary bladder*—but the members of the horse tribe only possess one; the gall-bladder is absent.

Gall-bladder.—This is situated in a shallow depression in the abdominal aspect of the liver. Its function is to store gall, or bile, produced by the liver until such time as this product is required in the process of digestion. (*See under* LIVER.)

Urinary bladder.—In some animals the urinary bladder is situated in the pelvis, but in the dog and cat it is placed farther forward in the abdomen, while in the pig and ox it may be almost entirely abdominal when distended. The size of the organ varies with the breed and sex of the animal, and its capacity depends upon the individual. Two small tubes—called *ureters*—lead into the bladder, one from each kidney, and the larger, thicker *urethra* conveys urine from it to the exterior. The constricted portion from which the urethra takes origin is called the *neck* of the bladder, and is guarded by a ring of muscular tissue—the *sphincter*.

Structure.—The wall of the bladder is somewhat similar to that of the intestine, and consists of a mucous lining on the inside, possessing flat, pavement-like epithelial cells, a loose sub-mucous layer of fibrous tissue very rich in blood-vessels, a strong complicated muscular coat in which the fibres are arranged in many directions, and on the surface an incomplete peritoneal coat covers the organ. In places this peritoneal covering is folded across to parts of the abdominal or pelvic wall in the form of ligaments which retain the bladder in its position.

In young animals the bladder is elongated and narrow and reaches much farther forward than it does in the adult. In the unborn fœtus its forward extremity communicates with the outside of the body until just before birth, when the passage becomes closed at the umbilicus, or navel, and the bladder shrinks backwards.

BLADDER, DISEASES OF.—For disease of the gall-bladder *see under* GALL-BLADDER. The herbivorous animals, from the nature of their food, usually possess alkaline urine; in carnivorous and omnivorous animals the urine is generally either neutral or acid in reaction.

CYSTITIS.—Inflammation of the bladder is always caused by irritants or bacteria or both. Irritation may follow overdoses of such substances as turpentine, cantharides, croton oil, etc., which are excreted in the urine in such concentration that they cause inflammation of the walls of the bladder. The inflammation set up interferes with the natural resistance of the mucous membrane to bacteria in the urine, and bacillary invasion of the wall follows. In other cases the bacteria gain entrance from either the kidneys, by the ureters, or from the genital passages, by the urethra. Inflammation of the bladder may occur during the course of specific diseases, chills and colds. In these latter conditions the cystitis that occurs is fleeting and does not prove serious. In the specific diseases, however, it depends upon the nature and the extent of the infection. The presence of large or irregular calculi in the bladder sometimes causes inflammation of its walls, and the introduction of an unclean catheter for diagnostic or other purposes may bring about the same condition. In newly foaled mares and in newly calved cows the bladder sometimes becomes the seat of inflammation as the result of injury and the passage of organisms from the female genital canal down the urethra.

In pigs an infectious cystitis and pyelonephritis is caused by *Corynebacterium suis*. and gives rise to the presence of blood in the urine.

In dogs, cystitis may occasionally be caused by the bladder worm *Capillaria plica*.

Symptoms.—In acute cystitis, the urine is passed frequently and pain is shown at each effort. The amount voided is small, and it issues in a small stream accompanied by much straining (a condition called 'strangury'). Blood or pus may sometimes be seen if the urine—which is usually turbid, contains albumen, and smells strongly of ammonia—is collected and allowed to stand. The animal shows pain when the region of the bladder is palpated whether from the outside in the small animals, or from the rectum in the larger animals.

The larger animals may walk with their hind-legs apart and their backs hunched. In the dog and cat constipation often occurs. The symptoms of chronic cystitis are similar but less severe. A tendency towards retention of the urine generally appears after a time, and the animal suffers great discomfort.

Treatment.—When the cause has been irritant medicines these must be stopped and copious drinks of water, barley-water, given. Belladonna and hyoscyamus may be given to relieve pain, together with urinary antiseptics. (*See under* this heading.) Enemata may be necessary, and the application of hot packs to the abdomen and perineum is useful.

URINARY CALCULI.—The stone (or stones) varies from the size of a grain of sand up to a man's fist. It may be smooth, corrugated, or it may possess definite points. Sometimes there is only one stone and at other times they are multiple; in the latter case each possesses facets or smooth surfaces formed by friction with its neighbours. They are usually composed of a mixture of phosphates, urates, oxalates, and lime salts, in varying proportions.

Too many mangels may cause calculi in young rams and bulls, excessive amounts of fish are associated with calculi in dogs and especially cats of either sex. Large amounts of peas or beans are considered to induce calculi in stallions.

Symptoms.—Until the calculus has become of a large size it seldom causes trouble, unless there are numbers of small stones present, when by partially blocking the urethral opening they cause obstruction to the flow of urine, much pain, the passage of drops of blood. The animal may be suddenly interrupted while passing its urine, and may be convulsed by a severe pain. In a short while this passes off and nothing further may be noticed until urine is again passed. The horse or ox may kick at its belly immediately after urinating; sometimes a colicky pain arises which induces the animal to roll for a minute or two; and in the smaller animals a sharp scream or squeal may be heard. A dribbling of the urine is often seen, and in the male the penis may be protruded and swollen. The back is occasionally kept arched in the dog and cat, and palpation of the posterior part of the abdomen reveals the presence of a hard mass in the bladder which is painful on pressure. In the larger animals the stone can be felt through the wall of the rectum when the hand is inserted a few inches.

Treatment.—The diet should be corrected as far as possible, and copious allowances of water provided. A daily supply of common salt given either as rock-salt licks or mixed with the food, will stimulate thirst and induce the animal to drink more frequently than otherwise. The presence of stones, 'gravel', or concretions calls for surgical interference. The stone is taken out whole if it is not too large, either through the urethra or by opening the bladder through the abdominal wall in the smaller animals.

In the cat the bladder is not uncommonly found to be distended beyond its normal size by an accumulation of urine which is unable to escape—except a few drops at a time now and then—owing to blocking of the urethra with sand-like calculi which have passed down the bladder. Pain is intense, and unless relief is promptly obtained the animal will die. Where a catheter cannot be passed, skilled manipulation may free the sand-like material; in other cases the bladder must be emptied surgically. The above also applies, less commonly, to the dog. Hyaluronidase helps.

TUMOURS.—Cancer of the bladder may cause difficulty in the act of micturition. Sometimes irregular cauliflower-like tumours are found affecting only the mucous membrane of the bladder, and possessing a stalk which enables them to be removed quite easily.

RUPTURE of the bladder sometimes takes place through a violent fall, a run-over accident, or through some severe obstruction which results in the filling of the organ beyond its maximum capacity. The condition is invariably fatal.

BLASTODERM is the name given to a very early stage in the development of the fœtus, in which the mass of cells resulting from the fertilisation of the ovum, which is to become the new animal, assumes a hollow, spherical at first and then ellipsoidal, bladder-like form, in the centre of which there is a clear limpid fluid. The blastoderm stage is preceded by the **morula stage,** and is followed by the **differentiation stage,** when the *epi-*, *meso-*, and *hypoblast* are formed. (*See* EMBRYOLOGY).

BLASTOMYCOSIS OF DOGS.—A rare case of infection with *Blastomyces dermatitidis*, involving the liver and kidneys, was reported in the *Veterinary Record* of April 5, 1958. The animal suddenly lost appetite and showed persistent vomiting. Rubarth's disease was at first suspected.

The disease is fairly common in both man and dogs in North America. Diagnosis depends upon a laboratory demonstration of the parasite.

BLASTOMYCOSIS OF GEESE.—This is a condition of the livers of geese that have been crammed specially for fattening purposes, in which colonies of the yeast-like fungus called *Blastomyces* (*Cryptococcus*) *anseria* are found along the borders of the organ. The fungus colonies are enclosed in capsules that vary in size from a pea to a filbert, and are connected to each other by narrow channels. The centres of these capsules contain the fungus, and as the parasite is closely allied to that which causes thrush in the mouths of infants, affected livers should not be used for human consumption.

'BLEEDERS' (*see* HÆMOPHILIA).

BLEEDING, or **HÆMORRHAGE,** means an escape of blood from the vessels which naturally contain it. It may occur from wounding of the skin, in which case it escapes to the outside of the body; it may occur from an injury to internal organs which are very vascular—liver, spleen, lungs—in which case the blood is poured out into one of the body cavities; and when tissues are bruised through the skin the blood may escape into the spaces between the cells of the part. In each instance the blood is of no further use to the body, being outside the circulatory system. Bleeding may be classified according to the vessel or vessels from which it escapes: *e.g.* (*a*) *arterial*, in which the blood is of a bright scarlet colour and issues in jets or spurts corresponding in rate and rhythm to the heart-beats; (*b*) *venous* when it comes from veins, is of a dark colour, and wells up from the depths of a wound in a steady stream; and (*c*) *capillary*, when it gradually oozes from a slight injury to the network of capillaries of an area. (*See also under* INTERNAL HÆMORRHAGE.)

Natural arrest.—When an artery with a small calibre is cut, the muscular fibres in its middle coat shrink, and the cut end is slightly retracted within the stiffer fibrous covering. This results in a diminution in the size of the cut end and in a lessened capacity for output of blood. In the space between the end of the muscular coat and the end of the fibrous coat a tiny clot commences to form, which, later, is continued into the lumen of the vessel. This is added to by further coagulation of blood, until the whole of the open end of the vessel and of the cavity of the wound is sealed by a clot. A fall in blood-pressure, due to shock, and loss of blood, contributes to the natural arrest of bleeding. (*See* COAGULATION *and* PROTHROMBIN.)

BLEEDING, THE ARREST OF.—Arterial hæmorrhage is always serious, and where a large artery is severed, such as the femoral, brachial, or carotid, the beast may die in such a short time that remedial measures cannot be taken to control the flow. Venous bleeding is generally easily checked by pressure upon the side of the wound farthest away from the heart; and as the valves in the veins prevent any back flow this form of hæmorrhage is seldom serious except when some of the largest veins are damaged and when the bleeding is all internal. Capillary bleeding is of very little consequence, as the flow is never strong enough to wash away the clot which soon forms over the oozing area.

(1) **Control of the patient.**—It is essential to secure the animal in such a manner that the wounded area is easily accessible and that the animal may not injure itself or the persons around. In all cases it should be remembered that the more an animal is allowed to struggle, and the more excited it becomes, the more severe is the bleeding and the greater the difficulty in controlling it. (*See* RESTRAINT.)

In certain cases where severe wounds have been inflicted and where the pain is very great, it becomes necessary to submit the patient to general anæsthesia before the hæmorrhage can be stopped, since owing to the violence of the struggles it is impossible to locate and deal with damaged arteries.

(2) **Pressure.** — This may be either direct or indirect. When a definite bleeding point is seen in a wounded part, the cleansed finger or thumb should be applied to it until more permanent measures can be taken, but preferably interpose a clean

BLEEDING, THE ARREST OF

handkerchief or sterile dressing. If the blood is so great as to make it impossible to determine from what part of the wound the blood is flowing, a swab of cotton-wool soaked in either clean water, or preferably a solution of salt and water, should be pressed well into the depths of the wound, held there for a few seconds, considerable pressure being maintained, and then removed. If this is done once or twice the wound is cleansed and the bleeding point may be seen. In some cases a swab of dry cotton-wool introduced into a wound provides such a rough and complicated surface that the blood is induced to clot more rapidly and the bleeding is checked. If clean, this wool may be left in position, for, if it be carelessly removed, the clot is disturbed and the bleeding proceeds. Of measures that check hæmorrhage by indirect pressure, the tourniquet is the most effective. This can be improvised from a piece of soft rope, a length of bandage, a rolled-up handkerchief, piece of rubber tubing, etc. etc., formed into a loop around the limb above the wound, and twisted up tight enough to stop the circulation. It must never be left on for longer than twenty minutes, and when removed must be loosened very gradually. Bleeding from small arteries can be stopped by applying a pad and bandaging tightly. Another form of pressure is employed during surgical operations through the medium of specially constructed forceps called 'artery forceps'. These are used to grasp

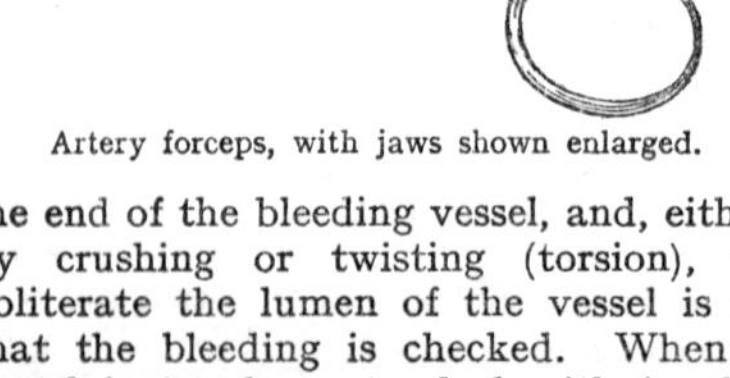

Artery forceps, with jaws shown enlarged.

the end of the bleeding vessel, and, either by crushing or twisting (torsion), to obliterate the lumen of the vessel is so that the bleeding is checked. When a vessel is too large to deal with in this way it is necessary to ligate its cut end. It is held as before with the artery forceps, and a loop of silk, catgut, or thread is slipped over the handles of the forceps; the end of the vessel is slightly pulled out from the surrounding tissues, the loop is placed round it and pulled tight; for this purpose the 'surgeon's knot' is used, a it does not tend to loosen with the elasticity of the vessel wall. A second knot is

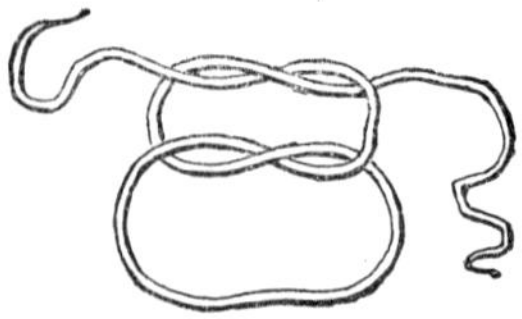

Surgeon's knot, or reef knot, used for ligaturing cut vessels.

subsequently applied and the cut end of the vessel released after the ends of the ligature have been cut short.

(3) **Styptics.**—The application of either cold or hot water to a bleeding wound will check the hæmorrhage from the smaller vessels and the capillaries. Lukewarm water tends to make the bleeding more profuse than before. Actual cautery is an excellent styptic, but it has the disadvantage that it destroys much tissue and it is attended with a great deal of pain unless a general or local anæsthetic has been administered. It is chiefly useful when the hæmorrhage is from surfaces where the artery or vein is imbedded in or surrounded by harder tissue such as bone, cartilage, or horn.

Of the substances of a chemical nature that are useful as styptics the following may be mentioned: a 10 per cent solution of alum, adrenalin, Friar's balsam, tincture of iron parchloride, medicinal oil of turpentine. Russell's viper venom and Thrombin Topical are also used professionally.

(4) **Packing and suturing.**—It sometimes happens that the actual point or points of bleeding cannot be located, especially when the wound is deep or ragged, and the blood issues in a more or less continuous stream showing no tendency to clot. In such cases it is necessary to resort to packing the wound with GELATIN SPONGE (which see).

BLEEDING FROM SPECIAL PARTS.—(1) **The nose.**—Within each of the nasal passages there are two coiled scroll-like bones, each of which is covered with mucous membrane very profusely supplied with blood-vessels. Blows or severe injuries to the faces of animals may result in fracture of these bones and damage to the vascular covering membranes. In the most of such cases the bleeding is capillary in nature and issues in a steady stream or trickle from one or both nostrils. It generally will cease of its own accord, but occasionally it proves troublesome. It may be checked by gently syringing a styptic solution into the affected nostril, taking care that the head is maintained in such a position that the solution will not flow back into the throat. Cold packs to the region of the face may also assist in checking the bleeding. The nostrils must obviously *not* be blocked with cotton-wool or tow since the breathing is thereby obstructed. When the horns of cattle are fractured but not separated the hæmorrhage (which is sometimes very copious) appears at the nostril on the side corresponding to the fracture.

(2) **The horns.**—The horns of cattle are sometimes broken by falls or blows, and severe bleeding follows. If the horn is broken completely off, the hæmorrhage is to the outside from the stump, but it often happens that while the bony horn-core is fractured the horn itself holds the broken end in position and the escaping blood finds its way down into the frontal sinus and out by the nostril. Hæmorrhage from a stump may be controlled by the application of a pad and bandage and the temporary use of a tourniquet round the base of the horn.

(3) **Legs and feet.**—The tourniquet described earlier in this article may be applied, to the lower side of the injury if the bleeding is venous, and above it if it be arterial. When the upper parts of the limbs are injured and the hæmorrhage is considerable, one of the methods of pressure is adopted. If the attendant has a knowledge of the arteries that supply the bleeding part, and when these are near enough to the surface to be compressible, he may press his two thumbs firmly over the artery above the wound until more permanent measures can be taken.

(4) **Stomach.**—The vomiting of blood by dogs, cats, and pigs in considerable amounts is a very serious symptom of severe injury or disease in the stomach, but in small amounts it is generally negligible, since it is often then due to rupture of very small vessels in the walls of the stomach under the influence of the muscular action accompanying vomiting.

Measures calculated to check it consist of giving of drinks or drenches of cold water in small amounts, of salt and water, of strong cold coffee or tea, diluted vinegar and water, or of forcing small lumps of ice down the throat. The animal should be kept as still as possible, and veterinary assistance obtained. Alcohol is not advisable, as it causes a dilatation of the vessels of the stomach wall and tends to promote the bleeding.

(6) **Intestines.**—Blood mixed up with the fæces but not changed in colour, indicates that the bleeding part is about midway along the alimentary canal. If the blood has become dark in appearance and of a tarry consistence, the hæmorrhage is from a part of the bowel high up, while if the blood is red or scarlet and only visible on the outside of the motions, some part of the rectum or colon has been injured. Injections of adrenalin into the bloodstream, or of normal saline solution are useful.

(7) **Uterus and vagina.**—After parturition in all animals there is a certain risk of hæmorrhage, especially in those which have a diffuse placenta, such as the mare and ass, and when the fœtal membranes have been forcibly removed. If it is copious, it may prove fatal; and if it is only slight it leaves a surface into which infective germs may more easily enter and cause inflammation of the uterus, so that it is a serious condition at all times and should be treated by a veterinary surgeon. The first essential in treatment is quietness of the patient, which should be ensured by suitable means. Next, it is absolutely imperative that all appliances to be used shall be *surgically clean*—*i.e.* free from germs. In emergency, in places overseas where prompt professional aid is not available, proceed as follows. First, wash the posterior part of the external genital region with some safe disinfectant, such as Dettol. The arm of the operator should be most thoroughly scrubbed in a similar solution, the finger-nails cut short, and the arm anointed with an antiseptic lubricant.

Meanwhile a sheet or large towel should be placed in a clean pail of water and the whole boiled for ten minutes. This kills germs present in the inside of the pail and in the interstices of the fabric. The pail should be lifted by a stick or iron rod (which is also previously boiled for a few minutes); immediately covered over with a second clean towel, allowed to cool down, either by standing in the open air, or by lowering it into a tank of cold water, and taken to the operator, who alone may handle the contents. He takes the towel, wrings the surplus solution from it, and gently inserts it into the genital passage When the towel is in the vagina and uterus it should be opened out so that it may lie against the bleeding surface, and it is left in position. At the same time cold packs to the loins and along the back should be applied, and the animal may receive draughts of cold water, or salt and water. The injection of adrenalin or pituitrin is also indicated. The towel is left in position for 8 or 10 hours or more, and is then carefully removed so that the clots that will have formed in the mouths of the bleeding vessels may not be disturbed. For the smaller animals the same principles should be applied, but swabs of cotton-wool, boiled in the same way, should be used instead of towels or sheets. (*See also under* WOUNDS *and* INTERNAL HÆMORRHAGE.)

BLENDING INHERITANCE. — When several pairs of additive factors are concerned in a character, a cross between an individual which possesses all the dominants, and one which possesses all the recessives, results in an offspring which is intermediate between the two parents for these characters. Interbreeding of individuals showing this blending of extremes of parental type results in a graduation of type stages from the homozygote for all the dominants to the homozygote for all the recessives.

In livestock breeding, the character of roaning in crosses between red and white, and the ' blue-grey ' (cross between black and white), can be regarded as examples of blended inheritance. (*See* GENETICS *and* HEREDITY.)

BLEPHARITIS means inflammation of the eyelids. It is usually associated with conjunctivitis.

BLEPHAROSPASM is a spasm of the eyelids.

BLINDNESS (*see* EYE, DISEASES OF; VISION).

BLISTERS are medicinal substances used for the purpose of counter-irritation : that is, to produce a superficial congestion of the skin and its underlying tissues which may relieve inflammation or congestion in some deeper-seated organ or tissue. The action is due partly to the friction by rubbing, partly to the irritant properties of the drugs used—cantharides, biniodide of mercury, ammonia preparations, etc., and partly to the effect which these substances have upon the nerves that control the size of the calibre of the smaller blood-vessels.

Varieties.—In animal practice cantharides or some of its preparations, biniodide of mercury, and compounds of ammonia used as liniments, are the chief blistering agents. These are divided into *rubefacients*, which cause a reddening of the skin and later peeling, such as mustard, turpentine, *vesicants*, which produce little blebs or blisters under the outside layer of the skin, such as cantharides or Spanish fly, pure ammonia and pure acetic acid, biniodide of mercury, and chloroform in delicate skins.

Uses.—Liniments are used in cases of inflammation of the throat, trachea, and in bronchitis in old animals, in acute congestion of the lungs and pleurisy, and in muscular rheumatism. Active counter-irritants are not used so much now as formerly, since other and better methods are available ; *e.g.* short-wave irradiation or inducto-therm treatment.

Application of a blister.—The hair is first clipped from the part which it is proposed to blister, and the surface of the skin is given a good rubbing with a brush to remove the débris and to quicken the circulation. The blister, either in ointment or in fluid form, is now rubbed thoroughly into the skin with the hand for about 10 minutes. Afterwards the horse should be taken into the stable, tied up so that he cannot reach the part with his teeth, and given a feed. (*See* RESTRAINT.)

Precautions.—Not more than two legs of a horse should be blistered at the same time. At least three weeks should elapse before repetition of a blister in any animal, either to parts already treated or to others. Always rub vaseline into the flexures of joints near the area. Blisters should not be applied during very hot weather, or when flies are very numerous. Cantharides blisters should not be used when there is any disease of the kidneys, bladder, or urethra, or when any acute inflammation exists in the part to be treated. If the blistered part is within reach of the tail, this latter should be secured to prevent it carrying portions to other parts of the body near. If the blister proves too severe it should be washed off with warm water in which some potassium or sodium carbonate has been dissolved.

BLONDE d'AQUITAINE.—A French breed of cattle, for which an English breed society has already been formed.

BLOAT is a condition of tympanites occurring in cattle, sheep, and goats.

With the increased use of lucerne and clovers, bloat has become of more common occurrence among cattle and is now a matter of serious economic importance. The rumen becomes distended with gas, and pressure is exerted upon the diaphragm; the animal eventually dying either from asphyxia or shock.

The precise cause of bloat, and the way in which it is brought about, are still something of a mystery. It appears that there is not so much an excess of gas produced in the rumen, as that this gas cannot escape by eructation. To account for this many theories have been postulated. For example, it has been suggested that an absence of roughage leads to atony of the rumen and affects the reflex of belching. Again, it has been suggested that hydrocyanic acid gas is liberated as the digestion of plants containing cyanogenetic glucosides proceeds, and that this is the cause. Allergy may be responsible, an animal sensitised to some particular plant protein experiencing shock which affects the œsophageal opening of the rumen. The finding, in many cases of bloat, that when the rumen is punctured there is no immediate rush of gas to the exterior, but merely a slow exudation of foam, has suggested that saponins in plants may be at least partly responsible —the gas being unable to escape owing to being intimately intermingled with the rumen contents. More recently, work at Wisconsin has suggested that an enzyme—pectin methyl esterase—is responsible for bloat. Released during rumination, this enzyme is said to react with the natural pectin in herbage, producing pectic acid and alcohol. Calcium salts may then lead to the production of a gelatinous honeycombed mass which traps gas in the rumen. Bloat, often of this frothy type, is common after grazing kale, perhaps especially so during wet weather.

Symptoms.—The left side of the body, between the last rib and the hip bone, is seen to be swollen; the whole abdomen gradually becoming tense and drum-like. There is obvious distress on the part of the animal which appears restless. Breathing is rapid.

Treatment.—As a first-aid measure, cattle may be given an ounce of oil of (medicinal) turpentine in a pint of linseed oil. This is not very effective against the frothy type of bloat, however, and New Zealand authorities recommended for first-aid purposes 12 fluid ounces of cream; or 4 ounces of arachis (pea-nut) oil shaken up in a pint of warm water. In emergency, if a veterinary surgeon is not available and death seems imminent, relief can be given by plunging a sharp, pointed knife into the left side. In the frothy type of bloat, however, a small puncture may do more harm than good, weakening the distended organ and perhaps causing it to split with leakage of some of the solid contents inside the abdomen. Normal therapeutic measures include the use of adrenalin, carbachol, antihistamines, and oil of turpentine; with the foamy type of bloat, good results have been obtained in the U.S.A. from polymerised methyl silicone, or in the U.K. from 'Avlinox'—an ethylene oxide derivative of ricinoleic acid.

Preventive measures.—Hungry cows should not be allowed access to lucerne or clover-rich leys where the sward is prolific. The feeding of fibrous hay (10 to 15 lbs. per head) prior to such grazing will greatly diminish the risk of bloat, or oat straw may be put in the field. Night grazing of old pasture is also recommended. In 1955 New Zealand authorities provisionally recommended spraying the total area to be grazed in 24 hours with a purchased emulsion of arachis oil at the rate of 3 fluid ounces per cow.

Strip grazing prevents selective grazing, and ensures that leaf and stem are eaten at the same time.

BLOOD is a red, slightly alkaline fluid which has the special functions of nourishing nearly all of the tissues of the body, aiding in their growth and repair, acting as a carrier of oxygen, carbon dioxide, water vapour, internal secretions, and various waste products of the body activity. The blood is circulated through the

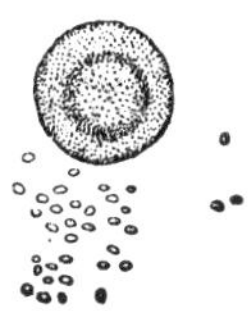

One red blood corpuscle with blood platelets below. Magnified × 1000.

body by a system of arteries, capillaries, and veins, and it receives its propulsion by pulsations of the heart. Its specific gravity varies in the different animals; it is about 1060 in the horse, ox, and pig,

1050 to 1058 in the sheep, 1050 in the dog.

Composition.—Blood consists of a fluid portion, or plasma, in which blood-cells, or corpuscles, are suspended. They are of three chief varieties: red blood corpuscles, white blood cells, and platelets.

Plasma forms about 66 per cent of the total amount of the blood and consists of three important proteins—*Fibrinogen, serum-globulin,* and *serum-albumin.* Serum-albumin is a substance allied to egg-albumin, and probably consists of more than one substance. Serum-globulin is also a mixture of proteins; its source is partly from the absorbed proteins of the food-stuffs and partly from broken-down white blood-cells. Fibrinogen is of great interest and importance, owing to its rôle in the coagulation of the blood. Its source is unknown, but is supposed to be formed in the liver, and in the destruction of the red blood-cells. It coagulates at a lower temperature than either serum-globulin or serum-albumin, and blood with the fibrinogen coagulated is incapable of further clotting.

Pure plasma is found in the pericardial, pleural, and peritoneal cavities in very small amounts normally. In some diseased conditions this plasma is thrown out in large quantities, becomes coagulated into fibrin, and forms the adhesions found after inflammations in these cavities, especially in the chest. While the blood is circulating the fluid portion is true plasma, but upon coagulation, when shed, it separates into two parts: a liquid,

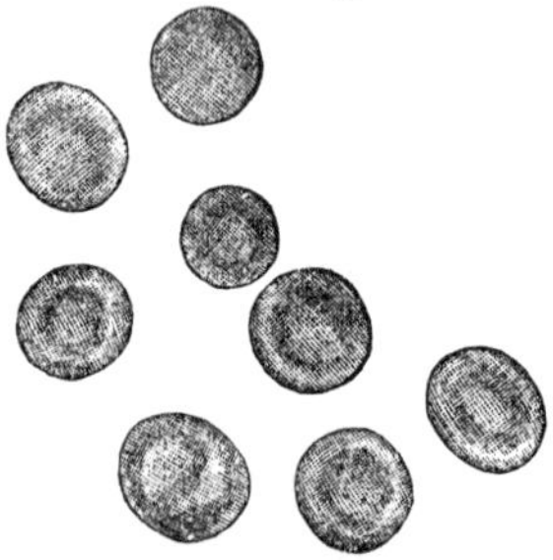

Red blood corpuscles. Magnified × 800.

which is called *serum,* and a solid, which is the fibrin clot. Blood serum is therefore plasma which has lost its fibrinogen, the latter having gone to form the fibrin of the clot; but it contains two newly formed proteins—*fibrino-globulin* and *nucleo-protein.* These are derivatives of fibrinogen which are split off from the fibrinogen when it forms the fibrin clot.

Corpuscles.—When examined by the microscope, blood is seen to consist of huge numbers of cells floating in the plasma. These are mainly of two kinds—red blood corpuscles and white blood-cells, with a very few blood platelets. *Red blood corpuscles* constitute about 32 per cent of the total amount of the blood. Seen under the microscope they appear as biconcave discs, circular in shape, and they possess no nucleus. (*Note.*—The red blood-cells of birds, fish, and reptiles possess a nucleus, while those of the camel are oval in outline and biconvex.) Red cells are soft, flexible, elastic envelopes or capsules containing the red blood-pigment known as *hæmoglobin,* which is held in position by a spongy lace-work of threads called *stroma.* They are present in large numbers in the blood. In the horse they number about 7 to 9 million per cubic millimetre, and about 6 million in the ox, on an average.

Blood platelets, or thrombocytes, are believed to originate in bone marrow, are oval discs of protoplasm which take many shapes when seen in smears. Their main function seems to be to reduce loss of blood from injured vessels by the formation of a white clot.

Hæmoglobin—a complex substance—has the power of absorbing oxygen in the u ngs, parting with it to the tissues, receiving carbon dioxide in exchange, and finally, of yielding up this carbon dioxide in the lungs. When hæmoglobin carries oxygen it is temporarily changed into a substance called *oxyhæmoglobin,* and when it is carrying carbon dioxide it is known as *carboxy-hæmoglobin.* The process of oxidation and reduction proceeds with every respiratory cycle. The red blood-cells are destroyed after 3 or 4 months in the circulation. The red blood-cells are formed in the red marrow of the bones, and appear first of all as nucleated red cells, called *erythroblasts.*

'Hæmolysis' is a process by which the hæmoglobin of the red blood-cells becomes dissolved and liberated from the cell-envelope. Anything which kills the cell or destroys the envelope can accomplish this phenomenon, such as alternate freezing and thawing of the blood, the passage of electric shocks through it, the addition of chloroform, ether, bile salts, tannic and boric fluids, etc. Most of the factors which induce hæmolysis act as protoplasmic poisons, and most of the poisonous principles elaborated by animals for killing their prey, or for purposes of self-defence, act in this way; thus, snake-venom and the materials produced by spiders, bees, wasps, scorpions, etc., are hæmolytic agents. Moreover, the natural serum of one animal can act as a hæmolytic agent when injected into the body of another animal of a different species. The serum from a dog is hæmolytic to the red blood-cells of a rabbit, but if this serum be heated to 135° F. it loses its hæmolytic powers. The heat has destroyed the agent which caused the hæmolysis.

'Agglutination' is the process by which the red cells of the blood are collected together into clumps, under the action of an agent in the blood called an 'agglutinin'. It sometimes precedes hæmolysis.

White blood-cells can be seen as colourless bodies in among the red cells when blood is examined by the microscope. They are larger and fewer than the red cells, are nucleated, and possess the power

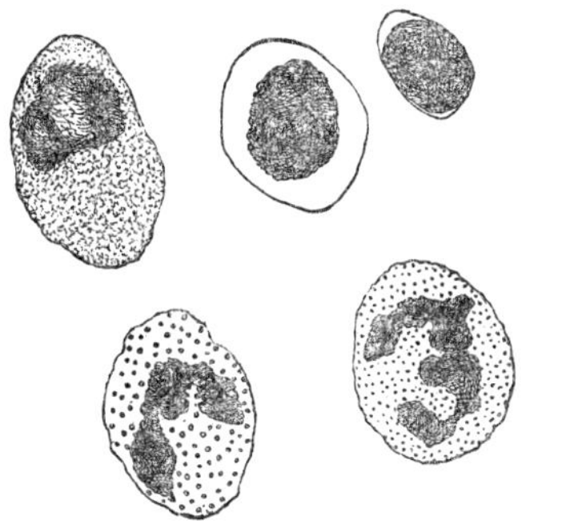

White blood-cells. Mononuclear leucocyte at top left; large and small lymphocytes, top right; eosinophile leucocyte, bottom left; and on the bottom right is a polymorphonuclear leucocyte. Magnified × 1000.

of spontaneous (*i.e.* 'amœboid') movement. They are collectively called white blood-cells, but are divided into certain classes. They exist in a varying proportion to the red cells, from 1 to 300, to as few as 1 to 700, and their numbers are liable to great fluctuation in the same animal at different times.

White blood-cells or *leucocytes* comprise the following:

Neutrophils, in which the cytoplasm contains granules which—with stains containing eosin and methylene blue—are not coloured markedly red or blue. The nuclei are of many shapes, and the term *polymorphonuclear leucocyte* is applied to neutrophils. They can migrate from the blood-vessels into the tissues and engulf bacteria (phagocytosis), are found in pus and are very important in defence against infection.

Eosinophils have red-staining granules, contain histamine, and have been observed to increase in numbers during the course of certain chronic diseases.

Basophils have blue-staining granules, and their function is unknown.

Monocytes have very few granules, engulf bacteria, and are important in less acute infections than those dealt with by neutrophils. When they migrate from blood-vessels into surrounding tissues, they increase in size and are called *macrophages*.

Lymphocytes also have few granules and are likewise formed in lymphoid tissue, *e.g.* lymph nodes, spleen, tonsils. They are possibly concerned with antibody formation and form barriers against local disease.

Coagulation. (*see under* CLOTTING).

Temperature.—The temperature of the blood is not uniform throughout the body. It is coolest near the surface, and hottest in the hepatic veins. It varies from 100° to 105° F.

Quantity.—It is impossible to estimate the total amount of the blood by measuring the quantity that can be obtained by direct bleeding, for a proportion is always left in the blood-vessels of the body. Roughly speaking, the amounts that have been calculated for the domesticated animals are as follows:

Horse .	1/15 or 6·6 per cent of the body weight.
Ox .	1/13 „ 7·71 „ „ „
Sheep .	1/12 „ 8·01 „ „ „
Pig .	1/22 „ 4·6 „ „ „
Dog .	1/11 to 1/18, or 9·1 per cent to 5·5 per cent of the body weight.

In an average-sized horse this is roughly about 50 pints.

Functions.—Briefly speaking, the functions of the blood can be enumerated as follows:

(*a*) The transport of oxygen and carbon dioxide to and from the tissues and lungs; (*b*) the destruction of harmful germs or other particles of foreign material; (*c*) the distribution of nutritive substances throughout the body; (*d*) the removal of waste products from the tissues; and (*e*) it acts as a medium for the distribution of the internal secretions to parts remote from the glands which produce them.

BLOOD, DISEASES OF.—These include: **Anæmia.** (*See* ANÆMIA; EQUINE PERNICIOUS ANÆMIA.) **Leukæmia, Pseudoleukæmia.** (*See also* PROTOzoön Parasites; Arteries, Diseases of; Hæmophilia; etc.)

BLOOD GROUP.—There is apt to be confusion over this term, since it is sometimes applied to single blood factors or agglutinogens, but usually to combinations of blood factors. It is preferable to speak of blood group systems, and the factors within these.

character on which the grouping is based, is inherited, examination of blood samples from within a breed might eventually prove a very useful means of selection. It might also indicate what matings could be expected to result in infertility.

BLOOD SPOTS IN EGGS.—Various foreign bodies are occasionally found in eggs and, while not harmful to the con-

Group Systems	Group Factors													
A	A_1,	A_2,	D,	H,	Z'									
B	B,	G,	K,	I_1,	I_2,	O_1,	O_2,	O_3,	P,	Q,	T_1,	T_2,	Y_1,	Y_2,
	A'_1,	A'_2,	B',	D',	E'_1,	E'_2,	E'_3,	I',	J',		K',	O',	P',	Y'
C	C_1,	C_2,	E,	R_1,	R_2,	W,	X_1,	X_2,	X_3,	L'				
FV	F_1,	F_2,	V_1,	V_2										
J	J													
L	L													
M	M_1,	M_2												
SU	S_1,	S_2,	U_1,	U_2,	U'									
Z	Z_1,	Z_2												
$R'S'$	R',	S'												

The blood group systems of cattle, and the factors within each system, are as shown in the table, reproduced here by courtesy of Dr. J. Moustgaard, Royal Veterinary and Agricultural College, of Copenhagen.

In dogs, seven major groups have been recognised in the U.S.A., and they are referred to as A to G.

The blood serum method of grouping is referred to under Electrophoresis, and shows that there are 6 types of pattern in British breeds of cattle.

BLOOD-POISONING is a popular name for 'septicæmia' or 'pyæmia'. (See these headings.)

BLOOD SERUM PROTEIN.—Examination of blood samples obtained from a large number of cattle have shown that the latter can be classified into six clearly defined groups. An investigation is proceeding in order to ascertain whether it is possible to correlate an important economic factor, such as high butterfat content of the milk, with a particular group. All five groups are found among Shorthorns and Friesians, but among Jerseys, Guernseys and South Devons, two groups have not been encountered. It is not yet known what the significance of this is.

Since the particular blood serum protein

sumer, are unpleasant. The commonest extraneous material is a 'blood spot'. In this condition, with the rupture of the follicle and the release of the yolk into the oviduct, there is often in the congested ovary an oozing of a little blood which accompanies the yolk down the oviduct and is incorporated into the egg. On cooking, the clot closely resembles a piece of meat, and is unsightly. Fæcal material, and occasionally a round worm, are also sometimes found in eggs, these having reached the oviduct from the cloaca. The only method of preventing such eggs reaching the consumer is to 'candle' all eggs before sale. This consists of examining them in front of a beam of light which shows up foreign materials as shadows in an otherwise translucent medium.

BLOOD TRANSFUSION is used in veterinary practice in cases of hæmorrhage and shock, and to a lesser extent as part of the treatment of certain infectious diseases. In cattle, donor and recipient are usually in the same herd, a fact which lessens the risk of introducing infection. Blood is collected from the jugular or other vein (after the skin has been cleaned and all precautions taken to achieve asepsis) by means of a suitable needle (*e.g.* 13 B.W.G.) and syringe, and is allowed to flow into a sterilised bottle containing sodium citrate solution (10 grains of sodium citrate in a little sterile water for every 100 c.c. of blood collected). The bottle must be shaken during collection. The donor's blood, 400 c.c. or more, thus collected, is transferred to the recipient's vein by the Simplex Apparatus.

Normal antibodies against the blood group factor J are sometimes found in cattle. Thus, if the donor's blood is J-positive, and the recipient's blood contains the normal antibody anti-J, so-called transfusion reactions might be expected immediately following blood transfusion, in the form of dyspnœa, muscular twitching, increased salivation, and circulatory disturbances (hypotension). In a very few cases, weak reactions of this kind do occur. If, however, an animal has been exposed to repeated blood transfusions, a different situation arises. The animal will now have formed antibodies against the blood group antigens it does not have itself. It is therefore by no means unlikely that the blood of donor and recipient are incompatible. If this is so, the blood transfusion will set off strong transfusion reactions. Such reactions can occur on the second or on subsequent blood transfusions, even though there are no serologically demonstrable amounts of antibody in the recipient's blood. (Dr. J. Moustgaard.)

In dogs, if not in cattle, it is desirable to inject a little local anæsthetic at the site where the needle is to be introduced, after clipping the hair and cleaning the skin. The jugular, radial, or external saphena vein will serve. A 19 B.W.G. needle is useful. Sodium citrate is used, as mentioned above. The blood is transferred to the recipient from the collecting bottle by the Simplex Apparatus or by means of a syringe.

In the new-born foal suffering from hæmolytic disease, exchange transfusion has been the means of saving life. Up to 5500 ml. of the foal's blood are removed, being replaced by up to 7000 ml. of compatible donor's blood. This process takes some three hours and is only practicable with special apparatus. (*See also* BLOOD GROUPS, PLASMA SUBSTITUTES.)

BLOOD TYPING.—In Canada extensive use is made of blood typing in respect of cattle, and results of a blood test have been accepted as evidence in court in a case where a man was convicted of falsifying a pedigree. The basis of this evidence was that to prove parentage of an animal all the factors found in the blood of a calf must be present in the blood of either the sire or the dam. If certain factors found in the blood of the calf could not be found in the blood of either the sire or the dam, then that calf could not have been of that particular mating—as was proved in this case.

Blood typing is also used in the diagnosis of freemartins. In one series 228 freemartins were found out of 242 sets of twins.

Blood-typing has been used to decide the paternity issue in a heifer calf born to a cow inseminated twice in the same heat period with semen from two different bulls; to reveal discrepancies in pedigrees; and to allay or confirm suspicion on the part of a Breed Society asked to register a calf born following a very short or a very long gestation period.

The preparation of test sera containing antibodies, or blood group reagents, is based on the injection of blood corpuscles from one animal into another of the same species, or into one of a different species. The first procedure is called iso-immunisation, the second heteroimmunisation. As a result of both procedures, the recipient animal produces antibodies to the antigenic factors associated with the donor blood corpuscles, provided that these factors are not already present in the recipient animal. (No animal can produce both an antigen and its antibody.) Figure 45 demonstrates the principle of iso-immunisation in cattle.

It shows that the donor possesses blood group factors A, B, and C while the recipient has only blood group factor A. On immunisation, the recipient will therefore form antibodies to blood group factors B and C. The antiobdies thus formed are called anti-B and anti-C. A serum containing several blood group antibodies is known as a crude serum. This serum will react with red corpuscles not only from the donor, but also from all cattle with the blood group factor B or C.

To obtain a blood group reagent which reacts with only one blood group factor, for example B, the anti-C antibody must be removed. To do this, the prepared crude serum is mixed with blood corpuscles which are C-positive but B-negative. The anti-C is then bound to the blood corpuscles and can be removed by centrifuging, as illustrated in Figure 45. This procedure is called antibody absorp-

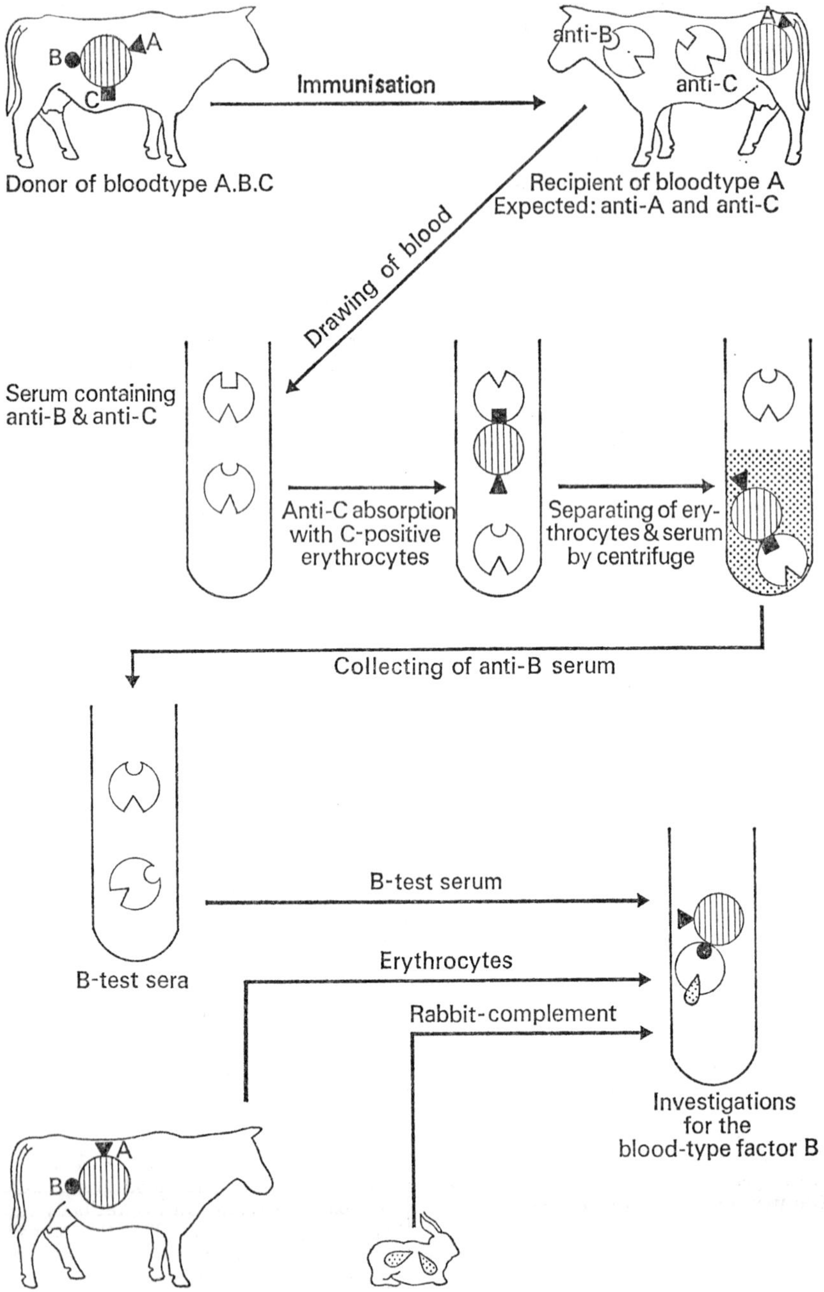

The principles of producing a test serum and its use in blood grouping
(*with acknowledgements to Dr. J. Moustgaard, Royal Veterinary and Agricultural College, Copenhagen*).

tion. As the figure indicates, a specific B-reagent prepared in this way can be used to decide whether the blood group factor B is or is not present in a cow or bull, provided that rabbit complement is also present.

To obtain sufficiently high concentration of antibodies, donor blood corpuscles are injected into the recipient once a week for 4 to 6 weeks. The antibody concentration of the recipient's blood serum, or its titre, is estimated by determining the power of the serum to react with donor blood corpuscles, or with blood corpuscles possessing a similar antigenic structure. In some cases, one single period of immunisation is inadequate to achieve a satisfactorily high antibody concentration in the recipient's blood. This can often be achieved, however, by repeating the immunisation a few months later (re-immunisation). (Dr. J. Moustgaard.) (*See also* BLOOD SERUM PROTEIN, ELECTROPHORESIS, **BLOOD GROUP.**)

BLOUWILDEBEESOOG.—A disease of sheep, cattle and horses, characterised by enlargement of the eyes leading to blindness. It occurs in Africa, and is apparently spread by blue-wildebeest. Cause: unknown.

BLOW-FLIES (*See* p. 672, *and also under* 'STRIKE'.

'BLOWS.'—Distention of the cæcum in the rabbit as a result of excessive gas formation. The rabbit assumes a huddled posture.

BLUEBOTTLE is the name of a dipterous fly, whose maggots live in decomposing flesh as a rule, but are sometimes found upon living sheep. (*See* p. 672.)

BLUE COMB (*see* PULLET DISEASE).

BLUE-GREY.—The offspring of a Galloway crossed with a Beef Shorthorn bull.

BLUE NOSE DISEASE.—This is apparently a form of Light Sensitisation occurring in the horse, following the eating of some particular meadow plant. The name arises from the blue discolouration observed in some cases on the muzzle (but not, for example, on the same animal's white socks). Sloughing of the non-pigmented skin occurs, and there is often intense excitement amounting to frenzy—during which the horse may do itself a fatal injury. (*See* LIGHT SENSITISATION, ANTIHISTAMINES.)

BLUE-TONGUE, or **BLAUTONG,** or **BLAWTONG,** also called 'malarial catarrhal fever', or sheep fever, is a disease formerly confined mainly to Africa but, of recent years, reported also in America, Portugal, Spain, and Cyprus, Israel, etc. In 1958 the Australian Government imposed a ban upon imports of cattle as well as of sheep on account of the risk of introducing this disease. Quarantine is not an effective safeguard in the case of cattle, since if infected they rarely become ill with the disease.* No reliable blood-test is at present available. It is characterised by fever and inflammation of the mucous membrane of mouth, nose, and alimentary canal. The feet are sometimes affected, when the hoofs may be shed. Wool may be shed after recovery. It is worst during wet, moist seasons, and certain localities are more seriously affected than others. Outbreaks always appear between December and April, *i.e.* in the summer and autumn, and the disease is never seen after the first frosts. Infection is carried by some biting insect, probably the mosquito, and consequently outbreaks are commonest near the breeding haunts of such insects—damp, marshy regions.

Cause.—The cause is a virus which is present in blood plasma, and is very resistant to drying and putrefaction. It is probable that 'virus reservoirs' occur in Nature in the form of some wild animal.

Symptoms.—A rise in temperature up to 107°, and after a week or ten days eruptions on the tongue, lips, and dental pad with a swelling and blueness of these parts, mark the typical appearance of an attack. Both the mouth and nose show a discharge, and there is an accompanying smacking of the lips. In spite of the soreness of the mouth the sheep are inclined to feed, but loss of fleshis very rapid, particularly when diarrhœa sets in. Thirst is usually great during the fevered stage. In from 3 to 5 days, the mouth lesions begin to heal, and the disease is seen in the feet. These

* At least one strain of virus (identical with a Californian strain) is stated to have caused an outbreak involving cattle in 1959–60. An interesting feature is that 10 per cent of the cattle died but that sheep were not affected at all. Death was mostly a result of thirst and starvation due to the difficulty of swallowing. Similar effects have been recorded in South Africa.

become sore ; sheep are stiff in their movements, and feed from the kneeling or recumbent positions. In bad cases the hoofs may be shed, but this is not always the history. The mortality is variable : in some outbreaks 5 per cent, in others 10, 20, or even 90 per cent of those attacked die. The loss from wasting and from the shedding of the wool is often more serious than the actual deaths.

Treatment.—Isolation of the affected into shady paddocks, sheds, or orchards, where they are immune from disturbance, antiseptic mouth washes, good feeding of a soft, succulent quality, the provision of a clean water-supply and salt-licks, milk or gruel for the very badly affected, and trimming of the feet. Vaccination is useful. It must be remembered that if the sheep can be kraaled at night, so that they have a roof over their heads, the number affected will be greatly reduced, or even, in many cases, the disease will never appear. Dipping has given good results.

Prevention.—A quadrivalent vaccine is available.

BOARDING KENNELS (*see* ANIMAL BOARDING ESTABLISHMENTS ACT).

BOBBY CALF.—A farmer's term for an unborn or very young calf of a quality not good enough for veal but only for the processed meat trade. Bobby veal is that of inferior quality from calves 1 to 3 weeks old.

BOAR LICENSING.—In Britain this was abolished in 1971.

BOG ASPHODEL.—A plant suspected of causing light sensitisation in sheep.

BOG SPAVIN is the name of a distension of the capsule of the true hock-joint. It appears as a puffy or ' boggy ' swelling on the front of the hock, one-third the way down and towards the inside. It may attain a considerable size and by its presence impede the free flexion of the joint, but in the greater number of cases it does not become larger than a bantam's egg and does not hinder movement. In some instances the inflammation in the capsule is acute and painful, and the horse is lame, but this is rare.

Causes.—Bog spavin is seen most commonly in horses that have straight or upright hocks, in which there is a considerable risk of spraining the structures at the front of the joint from over-extension. It may appear in young horses that are being broken-in to work, from slipping backwards with the hind-legs. In the heavy draught breeds a common contributory cause is heavy feeding on protein-rich foods with inadequate exercise or work. It is often seen in conjunction with thorough-pin, and the two conditions are taken to be an indication of weakness in the hock-joints. In the majority of cases, however, it does not make its appearance until comparative old age, and then it comes on so slowly that it is not noticed until it has reached a considerable size.

Treatment.—Bog spavin is not a serious condition except in those cases where the enlargement is acutely inflamed. In such, the inflammation should be reduced by cold applications to the joint, absolute rest until the pain has disappeared, and massage and stimulating liniments subsequently. For this purpose embrocations or strong liniments are useful. In chronic cases, where the tissue around the joint is thickened, treatment is not necessary. It should be remembered that young horses with very straight hocks need more careful handling when being broken-in than others, and should bog spavin develop it may often be checked by giving a complete rest and shoeing the hind-feet with moderate calkins on the heels of the shoes. Tincture of iodine painted on to the swelling once or twice daily will sometimes reduce a bog spavin of recent occurrence, but it is useless for one of considerable standing.

BOLLINGER BODIES.—Inclusion Bodies seen in cases of fowl-pox.

BOLTING OF HORSES.—Horses that have a tendency to bolt or run away when in harness may do so either from fright or from habit, and only occasionally from viciousness. Those that bolt as the result of fright should receive especial care when on the roads, and whenever the opportunity occurs they should be led up to the object which has frightened them, and allowed to smell it or touch it with their noses. A horse will not always trust his sight, but there are few that do not gain confidence from being allowed to acquaint themselves with strange objects in the manner mentioned. Vicious animals or those of a mischievous temperament sometimes run away for no apparent cause. The fact that some abnormality in the eye may account for the misbehaviour must not be forgotten. (*See* NIGROID BODIES, IRIS, *and* EYE.)

BONE forms the framework upon which the rest of the body is built. The collection of bones in the body is generally referred to as the 'skeleton', but this term also includes the cartilages which join the ribs to the breast-bone or sternum, form the larynx, etc.

Structure of bone.—Bone is composed partly of fibrous tissue, partly of bone-earth (phosphate and carbonate of lime), intimately mixed together. Since the bones of a young animal are composed of about 60 per cent fibrous tissue, and those of an old animal of more than 60 per cent of lime salts, one readily understands the toughness of the former and the brittleness of the latter. Two kinds of bone are considered: *dense bone*, such as forms the shafts of the long bones of the limbs, and *cancellous* or *spongy bone*, such as is found in the short bones and at the ends of the long bones. Dense bone is found in a tube-like form, with a central cavity in which normally *yellow marrow* is found, composed mainly of fatty substances; the walls of the tube are stout and strong, and the outer surface is covered by 'bone membrane' or *periosteum*. Cancellous bone has a more open framework, is irregular in shape, and, instead of possessing a cavity, its centre is divided into innumerable tiny spaces by a fine network of bony threads, which support the important *red marrow*. This red marrow is the tissue of the body that is engaged in the formation of red blood-cells. Periosteum also covers the outer surfaces of the short ones. All bone is penetrated by a series of very fine canals (Haversian canals), in which run blood-vessels, nerves, lymph-vessels, etc., for the growth, maintenance, and repair of the bone. Around these Haversian canals the bone is arranged in circular plates or scales which are called 'lamellæ', the lamellæ being separated from each other by spaces or 'lacunæ', each of which contains a single bone-cell. Even the lamellæ are tunnelled by fine tubes known as 'canaliculi' carrying processes of the bone-cells. Each lamella is composed of very fine interlacing fibres.

Growth of bone.—Bones grow in thickness from the periosteum surrounding them, the inner surface of which is being constantly transformed into hard bone; while the long bones grow in length from a plate of cartilage (epiphyseal cartilage) which runs across the bone at a short distance from each of its ends, and which on one surface is also constantly forming bone until the growth of the animal ceases. The existence of this cartilage is important to remember, because should it be injured in the young animal, the growth of the particular bone is interfered with and a deformity may result.

Repair of bone is effected by cells of microscopic size; some, called osteoblasts, elaborating the materials brought by the blood, and laying down strands of fibrous tissue, between which bone-earth is deposited later; while other cells, called osteoclasts, dissolve and break up the damaged or dead bone. When a fracture has taken place and the broken ends have been brought into contact and as accurate apposition as is possible, the ends are first surrounded by blood that has escaped from damaged vessels. This mass is partly absorbed and partly 'organised' by these cells, at first into fibrous tissue, and later into bone which seals the two divided ends firmly together. The irregularity of the bone thus produced would be inconvenient to the animal should it persist, so that after the bones have united a gradual process of reduction occurs on the surface of the mass, known as the 'callus', until in the course of several months the thickening has been reduced and the shaft of the bone is but little thicker than it was formerly. This is important, because it often happens that an animal will be lame for a long time after it has had a fractured leg, and the owner may despair of it ever becoming sound again. If the bone has been 'set' so that the ends are in as near a position to the normal as possible, there is little danger of the callus not becoming finally absorbed. It does, however, sometimes happen that the ends cannot be brought into accurate adjustment at the time of the fracture and a 'persistent callus' remains. Should this interfere with the action of an important muscle, tendon, or nerve, or should it interfere with the flexion of a joint, there is little hope of the animal ever becoming sound without surgical interference.

Varieties of bone.—Apart from their structural classification, bones are arranged according to their external shape into: (*a*) *long bones*, like those of the limbs; (*b*) *short bones*, such as those of the 'knee' and hock; (*c*) *flat bones*, such as those of the skull and the shoulder-blade; (*d*) *irregular bones*, such as those of the vertebral column; and (*e*) the so-called '*sponge-bones*' of the feet of horses and cattle and the claws of other animals. This latter type of bone is really extraordinarily dense in structure, but multitudes of both large and small blood-vessels penetrate into its depths from the outside and give it the appearance of being soft and spongy.

The skeleton is composed of a varying number of bones in the different animals, and the number varies even among individuals of the same species and breed. These variations are due to age in some cases—the younger animals having certain bones separate that fuse together later; sex may alter the number—the male dog has a bone in its penis that the female does not possess; while in the tails of all animals the number of bones is likely to differ according to the varying length of that structure in animals of the same breed and size. The skeleton is divided into: (1) an **axial** part, consisting of the skull, the vertebræ, the ribs with their cartilages, and the sternum or breastbone; and (2) an **appendicular** portion, consisting of the four limbs. In addition to these divisions, certain parts of the skeleton are embedded in the substance of organs, and are described as the **visceral** skeleton, *e.g.* the bones in the tongue, that in the heart of the ox, the snout of the pig, the penis of the dog, etc.

Skeleton of the horse.—1. **Axial part.**—*The skull* is divided into the cranium, which encloses the brain and its membranes, and the face, which includes the other bones of the head. The cranium is made up of one occipital, sphenoid, ethmoid, and interparietal, and two parietals, frontals, and temporals. The face has 20 bones as follows: Single bones: vomer and mandible; paired: maxilla, incisive, palatine, pterygoid, nasal, lacrimal, zygomatic, superior and inferior turbinals. (For further details *see* SKULL.) *The vertebral column* consists of 7 bones in the neck—the cervical vertebræ; 18 in the thoracic or dorsal region, called thoracic or dorsal vertebræ; 6 lumbar vertebræ in the loin region; 5 sacral vertebræ fused together to form a secure foundation for

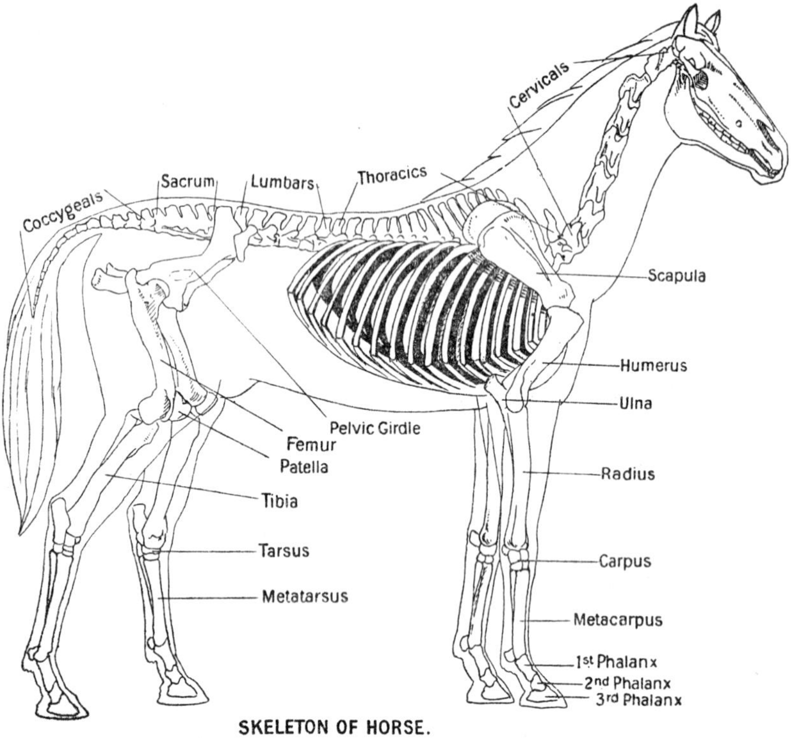

SKELETON OF HORSE.

the pelvis which has to carry the bones of the two hind-limbs; and a varying number of coccygeal vertebræ in the tail, usually from 18 to 20. Each vertebra has a solid part, the body, which lies lowermost in the living animal, and above this a ring through which passes the spinal cord. An *articular disc* of cartilage lies between each of the bodies and enables a more free movement to take place than would otherwise be the case. The first 12 thoracic

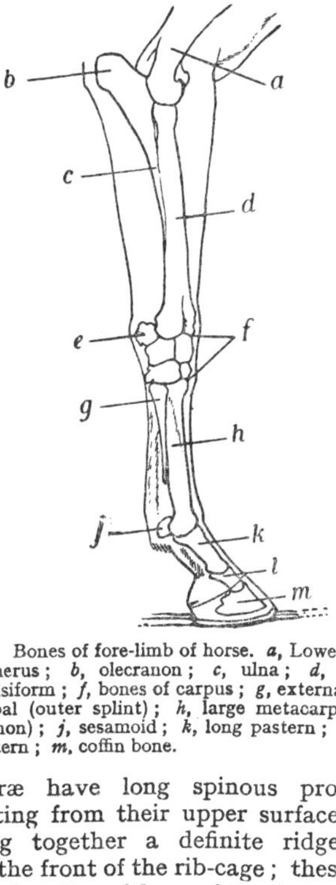

Bones of fore-limb of horse. *a*, Lower end of humerus; *b*, olecranon; *c*, ulna; *d*, radius; *e*, pisiform; *f*, bones of carpus; *g*, external metacarpal (outer splint); *h*, large metacarpal (fore cannon); *j*, sesamoid; *k*, long pastern; *l*, short pastern; *m*, coffin bone.

vertebræ have long spinous processes projecting from their upper surfaces and forming together a definite ridge just above the front of the rib-cage; these processes give the withers of the horse their characteristic shape. *The ribs*, 18 in number on each side of the body, are attached to the thoracic vertebræ above, and the first eight are continued to the breast-bone by their cartilages, thus forming a complete cage; the last ten have their cartilages joined to each other to form an arch, called the costal arch. It sometimes happens that a horse has a 19th rib on one or both sides of its body, and when such is the case the rib cartilage is usually free, and the rib is called a 'floating rib'. *The sternum*, or breast-bone, is shaped somewhat like a canoe in the horse, and except in old age it is formed mainly of cartilage with bony segments in its middle line.

2. **Appendicular part.**—*The fore-limb* comprises the shoulder-blade, or scapula, and five sections: the arm, the fore-arm, the 'knee' or carpus, the cannon or metacarpus, and the foot. The scapula is a triangular plate of bone which allows of a large area for attachment of the muscles that bind it to the body, and for those that control and attach the rest of the limb. It lies on the outer, upper, and anterior part of the rib-cage, but is not attached by any

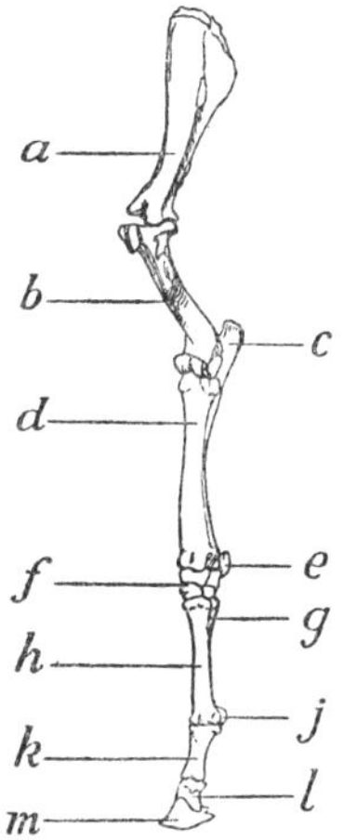

Bones of fore-limb of horse. *a*, Scapula; *b*, humerus; *c*, olecranon of ulna; *d*, radius; *e*, pisiform; *f*, carpus; *g*, small metacarpal; *h*, large metacarpal; *j*, sesamoid; *k*, 1st phalanx; *l*, 2nd phalanx; *m*, 3rd phalanx.

bony union to the rest of the axial skeleton. At its lower end it possesses a cup-like depression into which the head of the humerus fits to form the shoulder-joint. The humerus is the first bone of the fore-limb proper. It is a strong, powerfully made bone, which has a number of roughnesses for the attachment of muscles. Its upper extremity carries the head, which is received into the cavity of the scapula, to form the shoulder-joint. Its lower end is shaped somewhat like a broad pulley, and with the radius and ulna composes the elbow-joint. The humerus is covered with powerful muscles in the living animal, and it is seldom that it is injured by a direct blow, except perhaps at its upper end, where some of its projections lie near to the surface of the skin. The radius and ulna are the bones of the fore-arm. In animals with a number of digits, the two bones are distinct and complete, but in the horse the shaft of the radius has become over-developed at the expense of the shaft of the ulna. All that is now left of the latter bone is the upper part, which forms the 'point of the elbow', and which is called the 'olecranon process'. The shaft tapers away to end in fusion with the shaft of the radius. The radius bears the weight of the region, lies immediately under the skin for a great part of its length on the inner aspect of the fore-arm, and is consequently exposed to injury from blows, kicks, etc. At its upper end it forms the elbow-joint along with the humerus and the olecranon of the ulna, and at its lower end it comes into contact with the upper row of the bones of the carpus. The carpus, or 'knee', of the horse is a complex joint formed by the radius, two rows of small, roughly cuboid bones, and the heads of the metacarpal bones. The upper row is composed of 3 main bones (sometimes 4), and the lower row is similar. At the back and to the outside is an accessory bone which usually causes a quite noticeable prominence under the skin. An arrangement such as this allows of free flexion of the joint without sacrificing strength or efficiency. The metacarpus, or cannon region, possesses three bones, the central of which is much larger than the other two: these smaller bones, called the 'splint bones', are in process of disappearance, their uppermost ends only serving any useful purpose by helping to form part of the carpal or knee-joint. Their shafts taper away to end in little 'buttons' of bone about $\frac{2}{3}$ down the shaft of the central metacarpal. The large central metacarpal bone runs down to the fetlock and there forms a hinge joint with the long pastern bone or first phalanx. At the back of the fetlock joint are two small bones, each about half the size of a walnut, which are developed in the course of the flexor tendons to enable these structures to pass over the bend of the joint without exposing themselves to an undue amount of friction. These are called the sesamoids of the first phalanx, but they do not actually come into contact with the first phalanx. The first phalanx, or the long pastern bone, runs between the fetlock and the pastern joints. It is wider at its upper end than at its lower, and each end forms part of a hinge joint with adjacent bones. It is set at a slope of about 45° to the ground in the living animal. The second phalanx, or the short pastern—which is also called the 'os corona'—lies below the previous bones with which it forms the pastern joint. It, lower end is received into the joint surface of the third phalanx, both of which, along with the sesamoid of the third phalanx, form the 'coffin-joint'. The lower half of the second phalanx is below the level of the coronet, and consequently is embedded within the hoof. It is around the joint at the upper end of the second phalanx, *i.e.* the pastern joint, that high ring-bone forms, and low ring-bone is found around the lower, or coffin joint. The third phalanx, or coffin bone, has approximately the form of the external hoof, within which it is totally embedded. It is composed of extremely strong bone, but has the appearance of being soft and spongy by reason of the large number of foramina or holes which pierce its outer surface. These admit blood-vessels into the central parts of the bone. At its two posterior extremities (called angles) are attached plates of cartilage, one on either side. Under certain conditions these ossify and give rise to that disease known as 'side-bones'. The sesamoid of the third phalanx runs across the back of the coffin-joint, and like all sesamoids it is developed where a tendon would otherwise have to pass around the angle of a joint.

The pelvic girdle, although in adult animals it appears to be only one bone, is really composed of six bones, three on each side. These are: (1) ilium, (2) pubis, (3) ischium, but for convenience it is better to describe the wholeas a single bone. It lies in the region of the quarters and hips of the horse, forms the 'points of the haunch' and the 'points of the buttocks', and it assists in forming the 'point of the croup' in the middle line, as well as the hip-joints on either side. In outline it is roughly the shape of a bottomless basin with the side cut through and the ends bent towards each other, while that part of the basin opposite the cut ends has been pressed outwards. The part of the girdle attached to the fused sacral vertebræ is flattened and more or less triangular; the outer angle forms the point of the haunch, and the inner forms the one side of the point of the croup. Between these angles lies the large mass of gluteal muscles which gives the quarters their contour and symmetry. The third angle runs downwards and backwards to the cup-shaped depression (called the 'acetabulum'), which receives the head of the femur to form the hip-joint. This anterior flattened part of the pelvis is formed by the ilium. Immediately below, behind, and inside the third angle is a large hole through the bone (the obturator foramen), which is circumscribed by the two arms of the L-shaped pubis and the edge of the ischium. Just in front of and running between these two obturator foramina (one on either side) is the 'brim of the pelvis', which is so important in parturition cases. The third bone, the ischium,

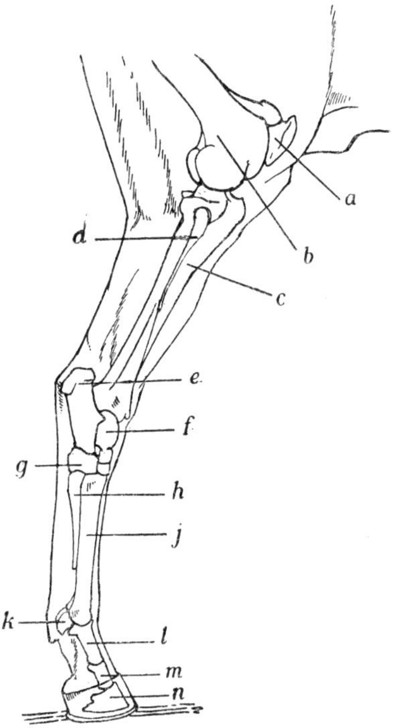

Bones of hind-limb of horse. *a*, Patella; *b*, head of femur; *c*, tibia; *d*, fibula; *e*, calcaneus; *f*, talus; *g*, cuboid; *h*, external metatarsal (outer splint); *j*, large metatarsal (hind cannon); *k*, sesamoids; *l*, *m*, *n*, 1st, 2nd, and 3rd phalanges.

is in the form of a more or less quadrilateral plate lying behind the obturator foramen, and helping to bound it posteriorly. A roughened and often very irregular protuberance stretches backwards from the plate of the ischium and forms the attachment for the muscles of the buttock, and is known as the 'point of the buttock' in the living animal. The two ischii and the two pubes lie alongside each other in the middle line of the body. In the young animal the bones of one side are separate from those of the other; but as age proceeds the layer of cartilage, which hitherto kept them apart, becomes ossified into bone, and the two halves of the pelvis fuse at what is called the 'symphysis of the pelvis'. The dimensions of the pelvis vary according to sex. In the mare the inlet of the pelvis measures about $9\frac{1}{2} \times 9$ inches, and in the stallion about $7\frac{1}{2} \times 8$ inches: the first of these being the vertical or conjugate dimension, and the second the transverse, in each instance.

The hind-limb possesses five sections, as does the fore-limb; these are: femur, tibia and fibula, tarsus, metatarsus, and the bones of the foot. The last two sections are similar to the corresponding regions of the fore-limb, and merit no

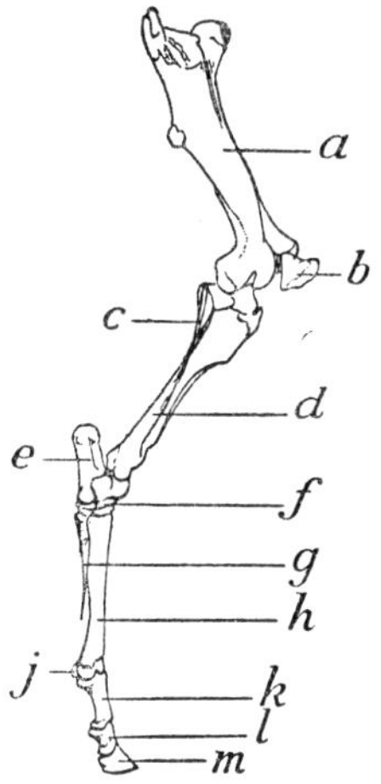

Bones of hind-limb of horse. *a*, Femur; *b*, patella; *c*, fibula; *d*, tibia; *e*, calcaneus *f*, tarsus; *g*, small metatarsal; *h*, large metatarsal; *j*, sesamoid; *k*, 1st phalanx; *l*, 2nd phalanx; *m*, 3rd phalanx.

further description here. The femur, or thigh-bone, is the largest and most massive single bone of the body. It has a shaft and two extremities, the uppermost of which carries the head, which is received into the acetabulum of the pelvis to form the hip-joint. Lying behind the head is a large irregular prominence called the 'great trochanter', which gives a basis of attachment to the powerful middle gluteal muscle —a very important agent in the acts of kicking, rearing, and in the propulsion of loads. At the lower end of the anterior aspect of the femur is a grooved surface along which slides the patella or 'knee-cap'—a sesamoid bone. Below this surface for the patella are two tubers or condyles which enter into the formation of the 'stifle joint'. These do not come into direct contact with the tibia, which lies below, but they rest upon two discs of cartilage that are found in the stifle. The shaft possesses several roughnesses to which muscles are attached. The tibia and fibula simulate the radius and ulna in that one has become more greatly developed than the other ; in this case it is the tibia that is the larger. At the upper end, its head lies below the cartilaginous discs of the stifle, and towards the inside of the leg. It gradually tapers down to the hock, where it forms the main hock-joint with one of the component bones. The fibula is unimportant. The hock is composed of six bones in most cases, but seven are found at times. The most posterior of these forms the 'point of the hock' to which the large Achilles tendon is inserted. The joint as a whole is somewhat intricate, but no more description is here necessary. The bones of the hind-limb from the hock downwards are similar to those of the fore-limb below the carpus, with only very minor differences.

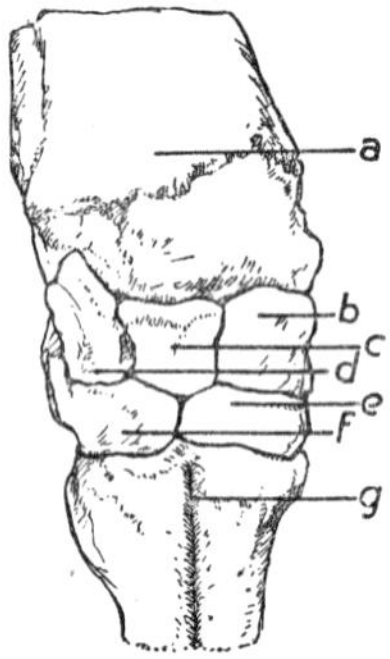

Bones of right carpus ('knee') of ox (anterior view). *a*, Radius ; *b*, scaphoid ; *c*, lunar ; *d*, cuneiform ; *e*, magnum and trapezoid (fused) ; *f*, unciform ; *g*, groove between the two metacarpals.

Skeleton of the Ox.—Only the most marked differences will be mentioned both as regards the ox and for the other animals that follow. *The skull* is remarkable from the fact that in the horned breeds the frontal bone carries variously shaped horn cores, and also because upper incisor teeth are absent from the incisive bone. (For other details *see under* SKULL.) *The vertebral column* differs from that of the horse in that (1) the bones of the neck are shorter and smaller ; (2) the thoracic vertebræ are larger but fewer, there being only 12 ; (3) the lumbar vertebræ are much longer, but number the same, *i.e.* 6 ; (4) the sacrum possesses the same number of bones, but they are longer and more completely fused ; and (5) the coccygeal vertebræ are longer and better developed and number from 16 to 21. *The ribs* are 13 in number ; each is broader, longer, less curved, and less regular than in the horse. The first 8 are sternal and the last 5 non-sternal. *The sternum* is longer than in the horse and does not possess any 'keel', being rather punt-shaped than canoe-shaped. *The fore-limb* presents a number of small and comparatively unimportant differences in the scapular and humeral regions, but it is not until the fore-arm that any striking variations are found. In this part the shaft of the ulna is much more developed than in the horse. It is still, however, almost completely fused to the shaft of the radius except for two small areas where fusion does not occur. The carpus consists of 6 bones, 4 in the upper row and 2 in the lower. The metacarpal region differs in that there are two large metacarpals completely fused together except at their lower ends, and a small metacarpal lying on the outside of the limb and only about 1½ inches in length. The lower extremity of the fused metacarpal is split into two parts, each of which meets the phalanx corresponding to it at the fetlock joint. Four small sesamoids are present at the back of the joint ; two to each joint surface. They meet the metacarpal and the phalanx in each case, while each member of each pair meets its fellow-bone. There are 4 digits present in the ox, but only the two central ones are at all well developed, the outer ones being very rudimentary and not attached to the rest of the skeleton. Each of the large digits has 3 phalanges which form the skeleton of the 'toes' of the ox. The third or lowermost in each case closely corresponds in shape to the outline of the claw. *The pelvic girdle* presents a number of minor

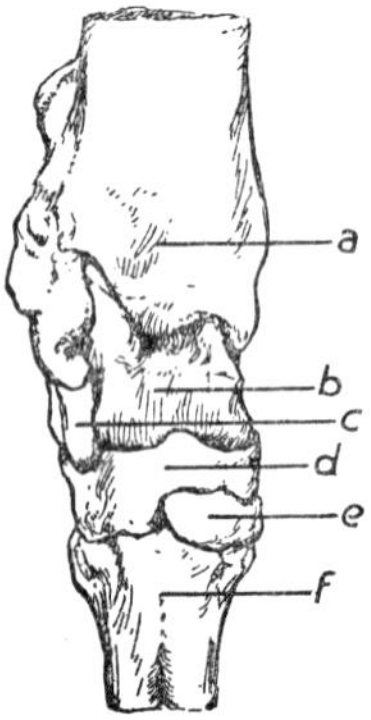

Bones of right tarsus ('hock') of ox (anterior view). *a*, Lower end of tibia ; *b*, talus ; *c*, lower extremity of calcaneous ; *d*, fused scaphoid and cuboid ; *e*, fused small and large cuneiforms ; *f*, upper extremity of cannon bone.

BONE

variations, but they are not important. The pelvis as a whole is comparatively larger and rougher than in the horse. The inlet is more elliptical, its dimensions being about 9½ inches by 7 inches in an average-sized cow. The femur has a small shaft and a smaller head than the horse's, and it does not possess so many muscular irregularities. The tibia and fibula are somewhat like the same bones in the horse. The shaft of the fibula is not developed in bone, but it can usually be distinguished as a fibrous or cartilaginous cord running between the two extremities, which are laid down in bone. The bones of the tarsus or hock number 5, fusion having taken place between two pairs. Below the hock the hind-limb is similar to the fore-limb.

Skeleton of the sheep.—For all practical purposes the skeleton of the sheep is the same as that of the ox in miniature, and no further description is needed.

Skeleton of the pig.—At first sight the skeleton of the pig seems much too small for the external size of the animal. This is partly due to the methods of artificial feeding of the present day, which result in a greater deposit of fat than occurs in the wild, and partly to the fact that all the bones of the pig are more dense and close in structure than in other common domesticated animals, and consequently stronger in proportion to their size. *The skull* is an irregular pyramid in outline and remarkable for the great size and strength of the frontal bones, as well as for the presence of very large canine teeth in the adult, and a small bone situated in the snout. (*See* SKULL.) *The vertebral column* is made up of 7 cervical bones, 14 to 15 thoracics, 6 to 7 lumbars, 4 sacrals, and 20 to 23 coccygeals. The cervical vertebræ are very short and wide, as would be expected from the shortness of the neck of the pig. The thoracic and lumbar vertebræ are unusual in that their numbers are not constant ; the smaller numbers are present as often as the larger in each case. The sacrum is made up of 4 bones which are fused later and less completely than in the other animals. The coccygeals are small and, with the exception of the first 5 or 6, which possess articular projections, are not specially remarkable. *The ribs* number 14 or 15 pairs according to whether there are 14 or 15 thoracic vertebræ. They are markedly curved in the improved domestic breeds but straighter in wild pigs. Seven are sternal and the last 7 or 8 asternal. *The sternum* resembles that of the ox in general, being broad and flat. *The fore-limb* is characteristically pig-like in that all the bones are comparatively shorter than in the other animals. The scapula is wide and short, and carries a wide spine. The humerus is bent somewhat like the italic *f* without the cross-bar. The radius is small, short, and narrow, with a thick shaft. The ulna is larger than the radius and the shafts of the two bones are less completely fused than in the horse or ox. The carpus consists of 8 bones ; 4 in each row. Four separate and distinct metacarpals are present, the two centrals being larger than those on the outsides. These laterally placed metacarpals form the skeleton of the two posteriorly situated small digits, which do not reach the ground normally. Each of the digits possesses three phalanges and three sesamoids, and those of the large digits resemble the bones of the digits of the ox. *The pelvic girdle* of the pig is flatter and wider, and not by any means so deep as in other animals. The inlet of the pelvis is elliptical and oblique, and in an average-sized sow measures from 5 to 6 inches vertically and about 3½ to 4 inches transversely. *The hind-limb* shows a femur with no great variation, a distinct tibia and fibula whose shafts are separated by a wide space, and a tarsus of 7 bones. Otherwise there is nothing of note to be mentioned.

Skeleton of the dog.—It is difficult to describe a typical dog's skeleton on account of the great divergencies that are seen in different breeds. It is only necessary to indicate such divergent types as the pekinese and the fox-terrier, or the bull-dog and the staghound, or the chow and the Great Dane, to emphasise this fact. It is usual to take a dog such as the fox-terrier, which has not been so bred that it is now deformed, for descriptive purposes, and the foowing remarks apply to a dog of the proportions and form of the fox-terrier. *The skull* of the dog shows a greater proportion of brain cavity to face than in the animals mentioned previously. This would be expected, for the high state of intelligence of the dog is proverbial. The skull generally is that of a carnivorous animal as judged by the teeth, which are adapted for piercing and tearing rather than for grinding, as in the herbivora or omnivora. The bony orbit is incomplete, there being no distinct bony socket for the eye. This is like the pig, but unlike the other animals. (*See* SKULL.) *The vertebral column* consists of 7 cervical, 13 thoracic, 7 (sometimes 6) lumbar, 3 sacral, and 20 to 23 coccygeal vertebræ.

The cervical vertebræ are somewhat like those of the horse. They are fairly long, more or less quadrilateral, and possess divided processes on their lower aspects, while the last three carry spinous processes. The thoracics and lumbars are not unusual in any important feature. The sacrum is short, wide, and triangular, and the fusion between the component parts is more complete than in pig or horse. The coccygeals are relatively long in the adult unmutilated tail. *The sternum* is long and laterally compressed, and *the ribs* are narrow, well curved, and long ; the last rib is usually floating. The first 9 are sternal and the last 4 asternal. *The fore-limb* of the dog possesses a small, badly developed clavicle, which is a small bone running from the shoulder to the middle of the breast ; it is often present only as a plate of cartilage, but in the cat the bone may reach a length of 1 inch. The scapula is long and narrow, and carries a definite and large spine. The humerus is very long but rather slender ; like the pig's humerus it has a shape somewhat like the italic letter *f*. There is often a foramen pierced through the bone at its lower end, just above the elbow-joint. The radius and ulna are long and unfused. A certain amount of movement is possible between them as in man. The carpus contains 7 bones : 3 in the upper row and 4 in the lower. Five metacarpals and five digits are usually present, although the first or innermost is absent in some individuals and only rudimentary in most. The first digit is called the 'dew claw', and never reaches to the ground. In sporting breeds it is often removed so that it may not interfere with the speed of the dog by becoming entangled in herbage, etc., which frequently happens when it is present. The four large functional metacarpals are plain shafts of bone with a joint surface at each end, the lowermost of which carries two sesamoids in each case. There is generally only one sesamoid in connection with the dew claw. The phalanges are simple, the two central digits being the longest. The last phalanx in each toe is shaped like the claw. *The pelvic girdle* is long and deep and narrow from side to side. Its angles are less distinct than in other animals, and fusion of its separate bones takes place later. *The hind-limb* has all of its sections lengthened in comparison with other animals. The femur is long and slender, and has a cylindrical shaft. Just above each of its condyles is an extra small sesamoid which carries the tendon of the gastrocnemius muscle over the back of the joint. The tibia is about the same length as the femur and larger than the fibula, which has a slender but quite distinct shaft. The tarsus is composed of 7 bones. The metacarpals are similar to those of the fore-limb, except that the dew claw is absent altogether in many cases, and is double in some. (*See* ARTIFICIAL BONES.)

BONE, DISEASES OF.—Since bones are deeply seated and not richly supplied with blood-vessels diseases of bone are apt to be overlooked for a much longer time than in the cases of other tissues similarly affected.

ACUTE INFLAMMATION of bone is divided into acute *periostitis*, or inflammation of the surface of the bone and its covering membrane, the periosteum ; acute *osteitis* or *ostitis*, inflammation of the bone substance itself ; and acute *osteomyelitis*, inflammation in the bone and the central marrow cavity. These three conditions are grades in severity ; the deeper the inflammation extends the more serious is the condition. It is seldom that the three can be separated from each other with a nice distinction, except after death.

Causes.—Acute inflammation of the bone almost always results from external violence. The most severe forms are due to bacterial activity, the germs gaining access either through the blood- or lymph-streams, or through the broken tissues resulting from a deep wound. The mildest types are often due to an inflammation in a ligament or tendon spreading to the periosteum in the near vicinity and causing it to become inflamed as a consequence. Some forms may be caused by rheumatism.

Symptoms.—These vary according to the bones affected. In all cases there are seen signs of pain when the affected part is handled, and if it be a limb bone, as is often the case, there is lameness. In very severe instances, where the bone tissue has become infected, there is fever ; dullness and a disinclination for movement ; the arteries of the affected part can sometimes be felt full and throbbing, and there are signs of severe general disturbance. If the bone is near the surface, such as in the case of 'sore shins', a condition that affects the cannon bones of young thorough-breds when their training has been too severe or when the ground is very hard, the bone seems to be swollen and hot to the touch during the first few days; and later, when the acuteness of the symptoms gets less, the bone is found to be still more swollen, but the pain and heat are less. This thickening of the bone often remains for long periods and in some animals never wholly disappears.

Treatment.—Success depends upon the state to which the inflammation has progressed when treatment commences. Complete rest from work is essential: in fact work, or even walking, is often impossible. Hot fomentations, soothing and cooling liniments or applications, are usually sufficient to cut short mild attacks. For this purpose 'Antiphlogistine', a preparation of glycerine and kaolin with other agents, is very useful. The severer cases, in which infection has reached the bone, call in the first place for penicillin or the sulphonamides, or immediate opening up of the area and the elimination of any pus that has collected. After that, any pieces of dead bone that are present are removed, and the wound treated as an infected open wound. This is not always practicable in animal patients, but the alternative is often septicæmia and death.

CHRONIC INFLAMMATION includes several diverse conditions, such as tuberculosis, actinomycosis, etc.

Symptoms.—Generally speaking, when a chronic suppurative inflammation affects a bone, sooner or later the pus and débris of a liquid nature will burrow through the surrounding tissues and burst on to the surface of the skin. A discharging sinus results which proves intractable to treatment. At the bottom of this sinus lies the dead piece of bone, and until it has been removed or absorbed the leakage of purulent material will continue in spite of antiseptic injections and other surface treatment. It often happens that the pus in its burrowing to the exterior does not take a direct course. In such cases the damage sustained by the tissues may be very considerable, may interfere with the functions of the part, and continual lameness or other debility may persist.

Treatment.—The offending dead portion of bone must be removed in the first instance, and the whole sinus tract must be laid open. This is not always an easy matter, and much depends upon the situation of the 'sequestrum', as well as on the mouth of the sinus. The area afterwards is treated as an open wound, and if all the necrotic parts have been removed, recovery generally takes place.

EXOSTOSIS is an outgrowth of rarefied bone tissue upon the surface of a bone, which may be produced by a long-continued irritation, *e.g.* the bony growths that appear upon the outsides of the hocks of horses that work in pairs on a pole, and often strike their hocks when turning; or it may be due to a slight but frequent sprain of a ligament, which tugs up the periosteum to which it is attached; and it is often due to concussion in some form or other in horses. Among the commonest forms of exostoses are the following: certain forms of splints, ring-bones, bone spavins, some side-bones, 'cab-horse disease', curb-chain galls that appear in horses that have hard mouths, and the hard bony swellings that often are found on the cannons of both light and heavy horses. (*See also* ACROPACHIA.)

TUMOURS OF BONE are sometimes met with. The commonest of these is the osteo-sarcoma of the limb-bones of dogs. The bony tissue is invaded by the cells that are characteristic of the tumour, and the size enlarges until, in extreme cases, the bone affected may be as much as four times its normal thickness. In such a condition it is liable to bend under the action of the muscles, and is easily broken. The only thing that can be done to prolong the life of the animal is immediate amputation. Chondromata, small tumours of bone and cartilage, are sometimes met with in the larynx of the horse after operation.

RICKETS is a disease of young animals in which the bones of the limbs are affected, and often small pea-like swellings are found at the junction of each of the ribs with its cartilage. (*See* RICKETS.)

OSTEOMALACIA, or OSTEOPOROSIS, is a disease of bones that is confined to adults, causing diminished resistance, hypertrophy of the animal matter, and an increase in size. (*See* OSTEOMALACIA.)

OSTEODYSTROPHIC diseases are a group of diseases which are due to errors in feeding in which the minerals—calcium, phosphorus, magnesium, and sometimes manganese—and vitamin D have been inadequate in amount in the food eaten for some considerable time. (*e.g. see* OSTEOFIBROSIS).

PORPHYRIA is a rare disease, hereditary in origin, occurring in man, cattle, and pigs. It is characterised by brown or pinkish discoloration of the bones and teeth, and by changes in the urine. In cattle a hairless, scabby condition of the skin is also a symptom. (*See also under* HEXACHLOROBENZENE.)

BONE-MEAL is made from green or dry bones by grinding or crushing. It may be coarse (meal) or fine (bone-flour). It is useful for all young growing animals, for breeding dams and poultry owing to the calcium, phosphorus, and magnesium it contains. It should be sterilised before use. Unsterilised bone-meal intended as a fertiliser should not be fed to livestock owing to the danger of anthrax.

In bone meal produced by the low-temperature method much of the proteins in the red marrow and periosteum, and of the fat present in the bone, are preserved in the final product, which has a consequent added value in feeding to animals. (*See also* SALMONELLOSIS).

BONE PINNING.—A method of treating fractures. In medullary pinning, a pointed stainless steel 'pin' is driven down the marrow cavity of the bone concerned; in ordinary pinning transverse 'pins' are used, driven through the bone at right angles to its length, and the pins held in position by a special adjustable metal splint.

These methods obviate the use of cumbersome plaster casts, and they also enable cases of serious and multiple fracture (*e.g.* as caused in a dog or cat knocked down by a car) to be successfully treated—a result often impossible of achievement by older methods. These techniques require a high degree of specialised professional skill and strict asepsis and, of course, the use of a general anæsthetic. (*See* PLATE 5.)

BONE SPAVIN, also called 'spavin', 'spaved hock', and having a variety known as 'occult spavin', is a disease of the hock or tarsus of the horse in which changes take place in the small bones on the inner lower aspect of the joint, usually resulting in a deposition of new bone which interferes with freedom of movement, or actually produces lameness. There are many different types of spavin, and it is often very difficult to diagnose the exact nature of the condition affecting a particular horse. It is important to remember that while a horse may suffer from a 'spavin' serious enough to cause lameness and to necessitate rest from work, bony enlargements do not invariably accompany the condition, so that a horse's hock may appear and feel normal to the touch, and yet be affected with the condition: such cases are referred to as 'occult spavins', occult meaning hidden.

Causes.—There is still a good deal of controversy but certain factors are definitely associated, and are at least pre-

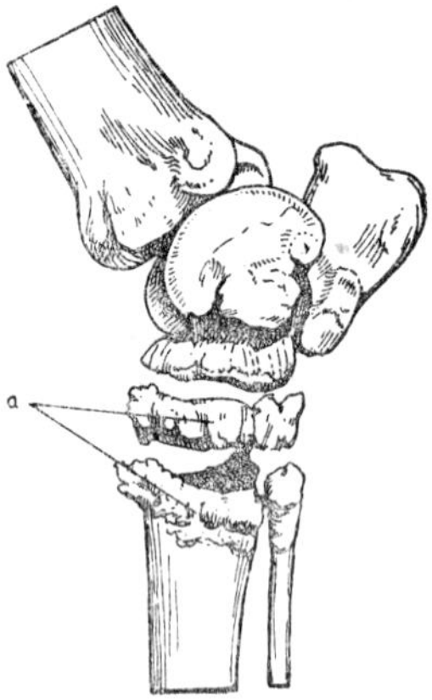

Bones of horse's hock, showing the preliminary stage of inflammation of the surfaces of the small bones of the hock at *a*, which leads to the formation of bone spavin later.

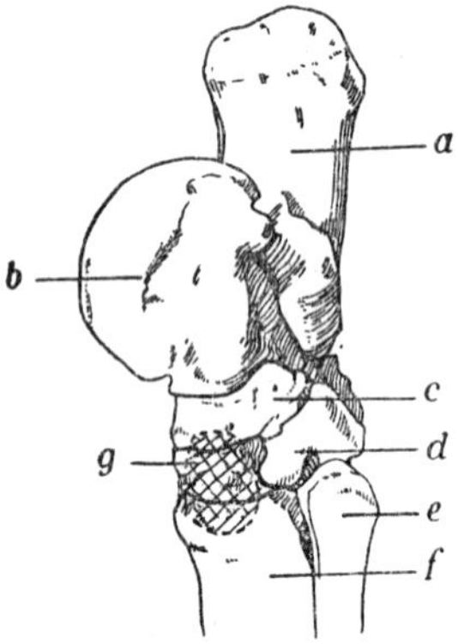

Diagram of bones of hock of horse viewed from the inner aspect: *a*, Calcaneus; *b*, talus; *c*, scaphoid; *d*, small cuneiform; *e*, upper extremity of small metatarsal; *f*, upper extremity of large metatarsal; *g*, the area usually involved by bone spavin.

disposing causes. (1) *Heredity*; (2) *Inflammation* of some of the soft structures in the region of the hock, spreading to the membrane covering the bone (periosteum) and inducing in it a deposition of lime salts and fibrous material, is to blame; (3) *Concussion*, whether due to bad conformation, faulty shoeing, to working young horses too severely, or to working horses of any age upon very hard surfaces before they become accustomed to them, is looked on by many as a cause of the condition ; and (4) *Rotation* of the lower section of the limb, from the hock downwards, whenever the weight of the body is

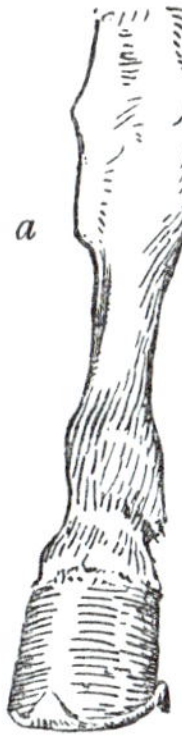

Spavin, at *a*.

taken by a hind-limb, is regarded as straining the ligaments of the small bones and inducing spavin. These causes are certainly blameworthy in some cases ; but it is a fact that many perfectly shaped hocks, in horses that have been well looked after, rationally worked, born from healthy parents, and in which none of the above conditions have obtained, do frequently develop spavins quite as severe as those found in untoward conditions. On the other hand, the reverse holds good, and horses are encountered that have hocks so badly formed that one would expect spavins to be present, horses that are badly shod, and have been subjected to much rough usage, and yet their hocks remain normal. We can only conclude that there is some factor connected with the cause of the disease that has not yet been brought to light.

Spavin affects all classes of horses whatsoever, and is not more prevalent in one breed or class than another. It may occur in a two-year-old, or it may not make its appearance until extreme old age. It has been seen in wild horses and zebras, it affects the ass, but is uncommon in the mule.

Symptoms.—Lameness may be noticed before there is any bony enlargement. In occult spavin the latter doesnot occur, the lesion being solely confined to the joint surfaces between two or more of the bones, but lameness is very marked. In a typical case it is noticed that the animal starts off in the mornings definitely lame, but that after a time the gait improves and it may become sound. In occult cases, however, owing to the damage that has been done to the joint surfaces the lameness persists continually. If an ordinary case be followed it is found to become gradually worse with the lapse of time and provided the horse is kept at his work, until when the horse comes out in the mornings it may drag the toe along the ground for a few steps. The toe of the shoe begins to wear faster than the heel. The affected hock is not flexed so fully as the other, but is moved forwards as if the leg were made in one piece, and the affected quarter is dropped at each forward stride. Later on the muscles of the hip and quarter on the same side as the spavin begin to atrophy, especially if the horse is kept at work. The tendons at the back of the cannon shorten and the fetlock 'knuckles over'. In such a case as this it is probable that the owner would have noticed the lameness in the early stage, would have rested the horse, and the condition would have been relieved ; but owing to the fact that the horse 'worked his lameness off' there is always the temptation for an owner to take a less serious view of the case than the condition actually demands. Generally speaking, after the lameness has persisted for a time an enlargement of bone occurs and the horse recovers so far as to be able to work sound at slow paces at least. The larger the deposit of new bone that is thrown out the less chance there is that a relapse will occur, but in young horses spavin is always more serious than in the older animals. At the same time some horses never recover their capacity for work, and unless they are of value for breeding purposes, their utility is at an end. Cases of occult spavin are always most serious. The joint surface is affected, and there is but little likelihood of the horse ever becoming sound for more than a short period.

Treatment.—In all cases rest is essential, so that the granulating areas of the bone may be allowed to unite. When the joints between the small bones of the hock, and between the lower row of small bones and the head of the cannon, become fused together the pain and lameness disappear, and it is the attainment of this that is aimed at in treatment. So long as the horse is kept at work the desired union seldom or never occurs. It may be 12 weeks before the horse is fit for work. Where counter-irritants fail, the operation of 'cunean tenotomy' has often been performed with about 80 per cent successes. Shoeing with raised heels to the shoes of the hind-feet gives relief to the tendons at the back of the cannon and tends to prevent the knuckling over that otherwise is often seen.

In all cases of spavins it will be found of the greatest ultimate benefit if the horse is given a fortnight to a month at grass, where he will get gentle exercise, *after he is apparently sound, and before he is put to work.*

BONE-SPAVIN TEST consists in the holding of the suspected limb with the fetlock as near to the stifle as possible, so that all the joints of the limb are fully flexed for about half a minute, and then releasing the limb and making the horse walk a few steps. It used to be considered that a distinct increase in the amount of the lameness was a sure sign of the presence of a spavin, but this is not necessarily the case. Any painful condition of any of the joints involved will be exaggerated by the enforced flexion of the limb.

BONES thrown to pigs, or given raw to dogs and carried by them to ground to which pigs have access, have caused outbreaks of foot-and-mouth disease in pigs; the bones having come from imported beef carcases infected with the virus.

For troubles caused in dogs by unsuitable bones, see under CHOKING and INTESTINES, DISEASES OF.

BOOTS.—The varieties used for the horse, and upon occasion for valuable cattle travelling to shows or sales by rail, are as follows: Yorkshire boot, buffing or brushing boot, speedy-cutting boot, sausage boot, hock boot, and tail boot.

Yorkshire boot is simply a piece of felt or blanketing about 8 to 10 inches square which has a piece of tape sewn across it parallel to and not far from one edge. It is wrapped round a horse's fetlock and the tapes tied above the joint, the longer portion being left upwards, and finally pulled down over the tapes. It is used for protecting the fetlock from injuries by the shoe of the opposite foot.

Buffing or brushing boot is usually made of leather lined with felt, sometimes strengthened with a steel plate inside, and provided with a strap which can be buckled round the fetlock to hold the boot in position. There is a long and a short variety, the long giving some amount of protection from speedy-cutting as well as preventing damage by brushing, and being used mainly for the fore-limbs. The short boot is simply a disc of leather which protects the fetlock from brushing injury, and is used chiefly for the hind-limbs. Long boots have from three to six straps.

Speedy-cutting boot is similar to a long brushing boot, but it reaches right up to the lower part of the knee, and protects the whole of the inside of the cannon from injury.

Sausage boot is a leather sausage-like bag which is strapped round the hollow of the pastern. It is filled with stuffing of tow or wool, and projects beyond the calkins or heels of the shoe. It is used at night to prevent the heels of the shoe from coming into contact with the elbows of the fore-limbs of the horse and causing 'capped elbow'.

Hock boot is used somewhat similarly to a knee-cap but applied to the hocks. It consists of felt inside and leather facings outside, and is made to cover the whole of the hock. It is strapped on to the hock by two straps, one above and one below, the latter of which must not be fastened too tightly lest the flexion of the joint be hindered. Hock boots are used to protect the hocks from injury when travelling in railway boxes, and are applicable to cattle as well as horses.

Tail boots, also called 'tail-savers', are flat pieces of leather which are rolled round the tail and provided with a number of straps. They generally have a long strap reaching forward to the surcingle or roller to prevent them from slipping off. They protect the tail from abrasions, etc., while horses are travelling by rail.

Boots for dogs, made of leather, and provided with holes for lacing, are sometimes used when a dog is suffering from injuries or diseases of the feet, such as blistered or tender pads. They reach about half-way to the knees or hocks, and are often lined with felt or other fabric.

Boots for sheep have been introduced as an aid in the treatment of foot-rot. They are made of rubber and are fastened by metal snaps or by laces.

BORACIC, or BORIC, ACID, is found in volcanic districts, or is prepared from borax.

Uses.—Boracic acid is a popular but inefficient antiseptic. In solution, it was widely used as an eye-lotion. In human medicine, babies have died as a result of topical applications of boracic acid. In poultry boric acid poisoning gives rise to loss of appetite, diarrhœa, depression, and progressive weakness, coma, and death.

BORAN.—An East African type of Zebu cattle.

BORAX has many of the properties of boric acid except that it is not acid in reaction.

BORBORYGMUS (βορβορύζω, I rumble) means flatulence in the bowels.

'BORDER DISEASE' OF SHEEP.—A disease occurring on the English-Welsh border, and first described in 1959. The cause is a transmissible agent, which can be acquired congenitally. The birth-coat is altered; the amount of hair in the fleece being increased. Lambs are smaller than normal, and grow more slowly. The shape of the head is slightly abnormal—likewise the gait which, however, shows only a slight swaying motion. Mortality is very high; most lambs dying during their first few weeks.

The disease has been recognised in New Zealand, the U.S.A., Switzerland.

BORDETELLA (*see under* BACTERIOLOGY).—*B. bronchiseptica* is a secondary invader complicating cases of canine distemper, and is associated with some cases of 'fading' in puppies. The organism may be associated with chronic respiratory infections of many species of animal.

BOREDOM.—Among housed stock, this can undoubtedly have a serious effect upon health and consequently upon the farmer's profits. Boredom is regarded by many people as one cause of TAIL-BITING (which see) in intensively reared pigs. In laying batteries, it is one cause of egg-eating. In horses, it is a cause of weaving, windsucking, and crib-biting.

BORNA DISEASE, also called BORNA SICKNESS, CRAZY DISEASE, and ENZOÖTIC CEREBRO-SPINAL MENINGITIS of horses, is a disease caused by a virus, and occurs in Germany. It is similar to Equine Encephalomyelitis.

Symptoms.—The temperature rises to 104° F., or even more; there is violent trembling, an unsteady gait with a tendency to fall, inability to swallow, with strings of saliva hanging from the mouth, and areas of extreme painfulness in various parts of the body, in some cases. In others a dumb type is seen, where the horse stands quiet; has no interest in external surroundings; refuses to feed; and appears to be in a deep stupor. In yet other cases, delirium is the chief symptom; the horse becomes violent, may persist in turning round and round in one direction without ceasing until he becomes dizzy, or he may stand with his head firmly pressed against a convenient wall. Most serious cases end by the horse falling, failing to regain his feet, and dying in convulsions. Less severe affections get better after from 8 to 14 days' illness, but these often leave some permanent injury behind them which may render the horse quite useless for any other purpose than as a carcasefor food.

Treatment.—In many instances the most economic and humane course is immediate destruction, especially if the horse is affected with the raging form. Continental workers claim good results from the use of hexamethyltetramine by intravenous injection. Mild cases should be placed in a darkened loose-box and kept quiet. If they will eat they should be given a bran-mash containing a full dose of purgative medicine. Cold packs to the head and neck, or where available ice-bags to these regions and the spine are indicated.

BOROGLUCONATE.—The salt of calcium used in solution for intravenous or subcutaneous injection in cases of hypocalcæmia ('Milk Fever').

BOROTANNIC COMPLEX.—An antifungal preparation of use in the treatment of ringworm, and said to produce a local acidity, to coagulate the proteins of the fungus, and to 'tan' the skin.

BOSS COWS (*see* BUNT ORDER).

BOT-FLIES belong to the Œstrus family, and their maggot forms are parasitic upon various of the domestic animals, chiefly the horse, sheep, and deer. (*See* PARASITOLOGY, p. 675.)

BOTHRIOCEPHALUS (βοθρίον, a pit; κεφαλή, the head) is one of the parasitic tape worms.

BOTRIOMYCOSIS (βοθρίον, a pit; μύκης, a fungus) is the name formerly given to

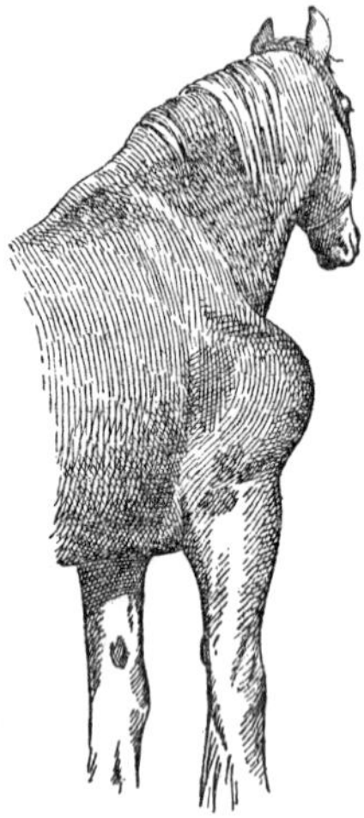

A large shoulder abscess, formerly cited as an example of 'botriomycosis.'

very large chronic staphylococcal abscesses especially in horses after castration.

BOTULISM is infection with the organism *Clostridium botulinus*. In man, the organism is responsible for some cases of food poisoning, when the very powerful toxin it produces is present in improperly preserved foods. It is the cause of illness and death in animals kept under conditions where they receive inadequate amounts of phosphorous, and are constrained to remedy this deficiency by eating the bones of dead animals, as in parts of the veldt country of South Africa.

An outbreak of botulism among broiler chickens has been reported in the U.K., and also outbreaks among waterfowl. (*See* LAMZIEKTE, MINK.)

BOUGIES are solid instruments which are inserted into the natural passages of the body either for purposes of dilatation or for the conveyance of medications, with which they are provided. There are urethral bougies, teat bougies, uterine bougies (or tents), etc. They are usually made of steel, rubber, vulcanite, or gum-elastic.

BOULIMIA (βουλιμία) means exaggerated appetite. (*See* APPETITE.)

BOVINE ENCEPHALOMYELITIS, SPORADIC (*see* BUSS DISEASE).

BOVINE HERPES MAMMILLITIS.—An ulcerative disease of the cow's teats and udder, caused by a herpes virus. (*See* VIRUS INFECTIONS OF COWS' TEATS.)

BOVINE INFECTIOUS PETECHIAL FEVER.—Also known as Ondiri disease, this affects cattle in Kenya, and is characterised by hæmorrhages of the visible mucous membranes, fever, and diarrhoea. There may be severe conjunctivitis and protrusion of the eyeball. Death within 1 to 3 days is not uncommon, though some animals survive for longer, a few recovering. The cause is a rickettsia, believed to be spread by a biting insect.

BOVINE PAPULAR STOMATITIS.—This disease was first described in Germany and during recent years has been reported in the United Kingdom, Australia, East Africa, etc. The disease is not accompanied by fever or systemic upset. Slightly excessive salivation may occur.

Characteristically, early lesions are rounded areas of intensive congestion up to 1·5 cm. in diameter, which in pigmented mucous membrane are visible as roughened areas with greyish discoloration. The centre of such areas becomes necrotic and in a later stage shows a depressed centre. Removal of the caseous material leaves a raw granulating ulcer but normally epithelial regeneration occurs in three to four days. A feature of the disease is the occurrence of concentric rings of necrosis and congestion.

BOWEL, ŒDEMA OF THE.—This disease affects mainly piglets of 8 to 14 weeks old, though occasionally it is seen in the newborn and in pigs of up to 5 months. In most cases a gelatinous fluid is found in the thickness of the stomach wall and other parts. The disease can be experimentally transmitted by inoculation of this fluid.

Cause.—*E. coli.*

Symptoms.—The finding of a dead pig—often the best in the litter—is usually the first indication. Puffy eyelids, from which there may be a discharge, and puffiness of snout and throat may be observed; together with leg weakness and convulsions.

Treatment.—This is seldom practicable; laxatives have been tried in affected herds.

BOWELS (*see* INTESTINE).

'BOWIE'.—A disease of unweaned lambs, resembling rickets, in New Zealand. A supplement of phosphates appears to be effective.

BOW-LEGS obtain normally in some breeds of dogs, such as the pug and bulldog, but in other breeds they are usually the sign of rickets. The shafts of the long bones become softened and bend outwards under the weight of the body, so that the fore-limbs especially become curved outwards. (*See* RICKETS.)

BOXWOOD POISONING may sometimes occur through farm animals gaining access to gardens where the plant grows, or by eating the trimmings from box hedges along with other green food taken from the garden. The plant, known botanically as *Buxus sempervirens*, contains several toxic alkaloids, the chief of which is *buxine*. In animals that are able to vomit, small amounts induce this action, and the harmful material is expelled with little further trouble. When larger quantities have been taken, or if the beast is not able to vomit, nervous symptoms, lameness, muscular twitching, dizziness, diarrhœa, and acute abdominal pains are seen. In very severe cases there is the passage of blood-stained motions, great straining, convulsions, delirium, unconsciousness, and death. Pigs are the most susceptible of the farm animals.

Treatment.—Animals that vomit, if they have not already done so, should be given an emetic to clear the stomach. Draughts of strong tea or coffee should be given in order to neutralise the alkaloid as soon as possible after it is known that boxwood has been eaten. An oleaginous purgative such as linseed or castor oil may be given.

BRACHIAL is a word meaning 'belonging to the upper arm'. There is a brachial artery, a brachial vein, and a brachial plexus of nerves. This latter, situated immediately within and slightly above and behind the point of the shoulder, is an important and complicated network of nerves, most of which supply the fore-limb. It is the place where the arrangement and distribution of the nerve-fibres takes place, and from whence the large motor and sensory nerves have their origin, before travelling on to the respective parts of the limb. It is liable to be injured in accidents to the shoulders.

BRACHYCEPHALIC SKULL means a short skull, and is applied to the skulls of such dogs as the bulldog, toy spaniel, or pug. In such the forehead is high, the skull broad, and the face foreshortened.

BRACKEN POISONING.—The eating of bracken (*Pteris aquilina*) by horses, cattle or sheep may lead to serious illness and death; symptoms appearing a month or two after the first meal of the plant. The cause is some substance within the plant which has yet to be identified. It is *not*, as was at first thought, the enzyme thiaminase. There are complex changes in the blood and bone-marrow. Poisoning is more prevalent in dry seasons than in wet weather, and young store stock are more often affected than adult cattle. The rhizomes are said to be five times as poisonous as the fronds—a fact of importance where the plough is being used for reclamation.

Symptoms.—In the horse these take the form of a general loss of condition and an unsteady gait; with later on loss of appetite, nervous spasms, and death. There is no fever; the animal's temperature remaining normal. Affected cattle, on the other hand, run a high temperature. They segregate themselves from the rest of the herd and cease grazing. The visible mucous membranes are pale in colour, and numerous small red spots (petechial hæmorrhages) are found scattered over the lining of the nose, eyes, and vagina. Diarrhœa, passed without straining, is usually bloodstained. The temperature is elevated to about 105° or 107° F., the pulse cannot be felt, respirations are accelerated, and on the slightest exertion the animals fall and have some difficulty in rising. In many cases a knuckling of the fetlocks, especially of the hind-limbs, is noticeable. In some cases the throat becomes swollen, so that there is difficulty in breathing. The illness last from 1 to 6 days, and death occurs quietly in the majority of instances. In other cases, death may occur much sooner, and be accompanied by bleeding from nose and anus, when the carcases have some similarity to deaths from anthrax. Pigs may be affected.

Treatment.—DL-Batyl alcohol injections have been recommended for cattle in the early stages of bracken poisoning.

Vitamins of the B group are often ineffective.

Prevention.—Avoid the use of green bracken as bedding, and avoid the situation in which animals turn to bracken out of sheer hunger or thirst—semi-starvation of live-stock is ever a false economy. Especially where the grazing is poor, it is essential to move animals to bracken-free land every three weeks. (*See also* BRIGHT DISEASE of sheep.)

BRADSOT, or BRADSHOT (*see* BRAXY).

BRADYCARDIA (βραδύς, slow; καρδία, the heart) means slowness in the beating of the heart, with corresponding slowness of the pulse-rate. (*See* HEART, PULSE.)

BRAFORD.—A breed of cattle formed by crossing the Brahman and the Hereford.

BRAHMAN.—Cattle of this name in the south of the U.S.A. are Indian in origin, but may have some European cattle blood.

BRAILING.—A means of temporarily preventing flight in pheasant poults, etc., by means of leather straps.

BRAIN.—The brain and the spinal cord together form what is called the *central nervous system.* The twelve pairs of cranial nerves and the many pairs that leave the spinal column, together with the complicated network of nerve-fibres originating from or associated with the ganglia in the chest and abdomen, form the *peripheral nervous system.* This latter is composed of two kinds of nerves: (a) *cranial and spinal,* and (b) *sympathetic nerves.* These are all closely connected with each other, but their functions differ. The cranial and spinal nerves are concerned in the transmission of messages to and from the brain, generally either messages of sensation (by sensory nerves), or orders of movement to the muscular system (motor nerves). Sympathetic nerves govern the activities of the abdominal and thoracic organs chiefly. (*See* NERVES.)

Divisions.—The brain in its simplest form in lowly vertebrate animals is a thickened part at the front end of the spinal cord, developed to govern the organs of special sense, viz. smell, hearing, and taste, lodged close at hand. Higher in the scale, in fishes for example, there are marked bulgings of nervous matter forming the *fore-*, *mid-*, and *hind-brain,* and that part connected with nerves of sight seems to be the most highly developed. In the animals of a more highly complicated standard still, the fore-brain is the most specialised, and not only does it form the bulk of the brain, but it controls the activities of the rest. This fore-brain is in the form of two hemispheres, connected with each other by a white, fairly dense mass, called the 'corpus callosum', and connected with the rest of the brain

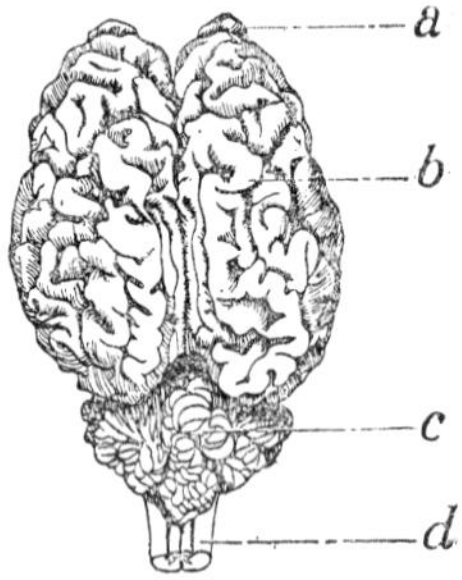

Upper aspect of brain of horse. *a*, Olfactory bulb; *b*, cerebral hemisphere; *c*, cerebellum; *d*, medulla, which is continued into spinal cord.

by the 'cerebral peduncles', elongations of the mid-brain. The hemispheres of the fore-brain are known as the 'cerebral hemispheres'; the mid-brain is formed by the peduncles chiefly; and the hind-brain is composed of the 'cerebellum', 'pons', and 'medulla'.

(1) **Cerebrum,** or cerebral hemispheres, occupies the anterior part of the bony brain cavity. The two hemispheres are separated from each other by a deep cleft, the 'median longitudinal fissure', which has in its deeper part the corpus callosum, and are divided from the posterior part of the brain (*i.e.* the cerebellum) by the 'transverse fissure'. Other 'fissures', nearly all of which have names, and vary in the different animals, make deep grooves or impressions over the surface of the hemispheres. A number of shallower depressions lying between raised portions that are called 'convolutions', cross and recross the surface and are known as 'furrows', or 'sulci'. In the dog, sheep, monkey, and man, it has been found that the centres for the perception of certain impressions, and the origin of some of the body movements, lie on or near the surface of the cerebrum, and these fissures and sulci serve to locate these centres. They are not of such great importance in animals as in man, however, and they have not been as fully investigated. Lying at the front end of each of the hemispheres

is a little lobe which receives numerous small nerves from the organs of smell in the nose; it is the 'olfactory lobe'. The corpus callosum passes between the two parts, and immediately below it are the two 'lateral ventricles', spaces in the brain, and the remains of the primitive tube around which the whole edifice of the brain has been built.

Beside the lateral ventricles and around them lie important parts of the 'basal' part of the brain, called the 'basal ganglia'. These are the centres of the senses already referred to. Lower than these, lying in a little depression in the bone in the middle line, is the 'pituitary body'.

(2) The **mid-brain** is a short stalk that connects the fore and hind parts. It is composed of the peduncles and four rounded eminences called 'corpora quadrigemina', that lie above them.

(3) The **hind-brain** is formed by the 'cerebellar hemispheres', which lie in the most posterior and upper part of the bony cavity; the 'pons', a bridge of fibres which connects the various parts of the brain with each other; and the 'medulla'. The medulla is the direct continuation forwards of the spinal cord, and is similar to it in appearance, though larger. In it are the centres that govern the heart, respiration, circulation, and the action of the digestive system from the mouth to the large intestine. In addition to this it is the highway for all the tracts of nerves that are leaving or entering the brain, and it gives rise to all the cranial nerves except those of smell, sight, and the muscles of the eyeball.

Structure.—The brain is composed of white and grey matter. In the cerebrum and cerebellum the grey matter is arranged mainly as a layer on the surface, though both have grey areas imbedded in the white matter. In other parts the grey matter is found in definite masses called 'nuclei', from which the nerves spring. The grey matter consists of cells, in which all the activities of the brain commence, and variously arranged nerve-fibres. The cells vary in size and shape in different parts of the brain, but all of them give off a number of processes, some of which form nerve-fibres. The cells on the surface of the cerebral hemispheres, for instance, are numerous, and arranged in layers of five or six deep; they are roughly pyramidal in shape, and each one gives off numbers of nerve-cell projections, called 'dendrites', from one end, and a single long process, called an 'axon', from the other. The white matter is made up of a large number of nerve-fibres, each of which is connected to a cell in the grey matter, arranged in various 'paths'. The chief of these paths are either *efferent, afferent*, or *associative*.

Efferent paths are the arrangements of fibres that are outgoing to some part of the muscular system, either directly or else indirectly, after having been changed in some other part of the brain, *e.g.* the cerebellum, or in the spinal cord. The afferent paths convey sensations of heat, cold, touch, pain, vision, smell, taste, and hearing, in towards the brain from the outlying parts of the body. They nearly all converge to one point, called the 'optic thalamus', where a change takes place before the sensations are transmitted to the grey matter on the surface. The association paths simply connect one part of the brain with another, or the right side with the left. The fibres in this latter case in the cerebral hemispheres pass through the corpus callosum, which has been already mentioned. In both the grey and the white matter there is a framework of fibrous tissue cells, extremely fine and delicate, which acts as a supportive structure for the fibres and nerve cells, to which the name 'neuroglia' is applied. Permeating the grey matter is a complex system of blood-vessels, and in the white matter there are also vessels but to a less extent.

Size.—The brain varies very much in different animals and in different breeds, but the following table gives the average relation of the weight of the brain to the weight of the body:

Cat	1 to 99
Dog	1 ,, 235
Sheep	1 ,, 317
Pig	1 ,, 369
Horse	1 ,, 593
Ox	1 ,, 682

From this it will be seen that the cat has proportionately to the size of its body the largest brain; but while the weight of the brain in relation to the body weight has been suggested as a measure of intelligence, it must not be thought that the cat is the most intelligent of the animals given. Intelligence depends not only on the weight of the brain, but rather on the proportion of grey and white matter, especially in the case of the cerebrum, and on the complexity of the arrangements of nerve processes of the large pyramidal cells of the cerebrum.

Functions.—*The Cerebrum.*—In the first place the cerebrum is non-sensitive: it can be handled, cut, or injured without any signs of pain in the subject.

A dog which had both its cerebral hemispheres removed was kept alive by Goltz for as long as 18 months.

The cerebrum is concerned with the higher senses, such as memory, initiative, volition, intelligence, and, as well as these, that it is the receiving station of the impulses that originate from the organs of the special senses, viz. those of sight, smell, taste, hearing, and touch. In addition to this the movements of the skeletal muscles that are not purely reflex are controlled in various areas of the surface of the cerebral hemispheres.

The Cerebellum—Accurate knowledge of the functions of the cerebellum is almost as meagre as in the case of the cerebrum. Main functions of this part are to co-ordinate muscular movement, to preserve the body balance, and, by assistance from the visual centres, to govern direction. Each half of the cerebellum controls the muscular system of its own side of the body, and is in communication with the opposite side of the cerebrum. It closely communicates with the nerves, internal ear, and with certain nerves of muscle-sense that bear messages dealing with the state of contraction that is in process in any particular skeletal muscle.

The Medulla, etc.—The functions of those parts that lie below the cerebellum and behind the cerebral hemispheres are very complex. In the first place, it is through the medulla that communication between the brain and the rest of the body takes place. There are areas composed of outgoing fibres, and other areas composed of incoming fibres. It is the central controlling station of such vital functions as heart action, respiration, circulation, the action of the whole digestive system; it gives rise to all the cranial nerves except three, viz. those of smell, vision, and of the muscles of the eyeball; and it possesses the centres that control mastication, swallowing, sucking, vomiting, voice-production, coughing, the calibre of the arteries, movements of the iris, the secretion of saliva and sweat, the amount of sugar in the urine, and the act of shivering. It is remarkable that such a large number of important centres should be situated in a matter of only a few inches of nerve tissue.

Membranes.— The brain proper is covered over by a thin membrane called the 'pia mater', the bones of the cranium are lined by a thick membrane called the 'dura mater', and between these is an irregular network called 'the arachnoid'. Between the arachnoid and the pia mater is a small amount of fluid, which serves as kind of water-bed in which the brain floats.

Nerves.—The nerves which leave the surface of the brain are twelve in number in the domesticated animals:

1. Olfactory, to the nose (smell).
2. Optic, to the eye (sight).
3. Oculomotor } to the muscles of the eyes.
4. Trochlear } to the muscles of the eyes.
5. Abducent } to the muscles of the eyes.
6. Trigeminal, to the skin of the face, etc.
7. Facial, to the muscles of the face.
8. Auditory, to the ear (hearing).
9. Glossopharyngeal, to the tongue (taste).
10. Vagus, to heart, larynx, lungs, and stomach.
11. Spinal accessory, to muscles in the neck.
12. Hypoglossal, to the muscles of the tongue.

Blood-vessels.—The brain obtains its blood-supply from four main sources: two internal carotids and two occipital arteries. These branch and unite to form an irregular circle under the brain within the skull, called the 'circle of Willis'. From this numerous smaller branches leave to supply the whole of the brain substance. By such an arrangement any possibility of deficiency of blood is obviated, for should one of the main branches become cut or occluded, the others enlarge and the same amount of blood is still supplied. The blood leaves the organ by means of large venous sinuses situated in the membranes covering the brain, and finally finds its way into the jugular veins of the neck.

BRAIN AND ITS MEMBRANES: INJURIES AND DISEASES OF.—ABSCESS OF THE BRAIN, or Cerebral Abscess, is a condition in which pus-forming organisms gain entrance to the cranium and cause suppuration. The organisms may enter through an injury to the bone, through the medium of the ear (especially in the pig and dog), or may arrive by the blood-stream. Sometimes a foreign body, such as a needle that has become lodged in the throat, may pass upwards into the brain and set up an abscess. The condition may be produced during the course of glanders, strangles, pneumonia, metritis, endocarditis, etc., when the causal germs invade the blood-stream and get carried to the brain among other tissues.

Symptoms.— There is often a primary stage of excitement and frenzy, but this

BRAIN AND ITS MEMBRANES

is soon followed by a period of dullness or unconsciousness. The temperature is high, but does not remain constant. The head is carried low down, sometimes to one side, and there may be blindness. Convulsions of a violent nature often take place, and during these the animal does itself serious damage. Finally coma sets in, and the animal generally dies after having been ill for less than a week.

Treatment.—Antibiotics may be tried.

CONCUSSION.—The reception of heavy blows on the surface of the head, such as those received when horses run away, fall, are kicked, or injured by falling obstacles, when dogs are run over, etc., results in an interference with the normal functions of the brain, even although the skull itself is not always fractured.

Symptoms.—Generally, immediately after the accident, the animal becomes unconscious, with all its muscles relaxed. It lies stunned for a variable period, and then rises and may walk as if nothing were the matter. In more severe cases it attempts to rise, but fails, and lies, conscious but without the power of co-ordinated movement. These symptoms may slowly pass off, and in a few days the brain gains its customary control of the body and the animal quite recovers. In the most serious cases the animal may never regain consciousness (where the brain has been deeply injured), or consciousness may return and then a stage of convulsive seizures takes place, generally ending in permanent paralysis of some set or sets of muscles. During any of these stages, or varieties, vomiting may occur in those animals that vomit, and the fæces and urine may be voided in all animals.

Treatment.—Absolute quiet and rest are essential, and a stimulant, preferably given hypodermically, should be administered.

CONGESTION.—An excessive amount of blood in the brain may be either active or passive.

(1) *Active congestion* is produced sometimes by poisons, bacterial, chemical, or alkaloidal; by changes in the wall of the blood-vessels of the brain; by heat-rays, as in sunstroke; and by parasites in the blood-stream.

Symptoms.—Excitability, which shows itself either in the form of actual convulsions, or in milder cases as a 'frenzy' or 'mad staggers'. Animals plunge about without any regard for objects around them; they show fear of men, often howling and screaming when touched; the pupil is generally dilated, the pulse is fast and full, the breathing is laboured and rapid, and the head of the creature feels hotter than normal. The symptoms may last for only a few seconds and then pass off, or they may continue for hours at a time. Those cases in which the 'fits' are of short duration are usually the least severe, and those that continue often pass into inflammation of the brain substance, known as 'encephalitis'.

Treatment.—Endeavours should be made to lessen the amount of blood in the head by the application of cold packs of ice or water to the poll. The animal should be kept as quiet as possible, and must be watched to ensure that it does not do itself damage against surrounding obstacles.

(2) *Passive congestion* is brought about by anything that obstructs the free return of blood from the head to the heart, such as tightly fitting collars, tumours, disease in the heart valves, and by the action of bacteria themselves in the blood, when free circulation is interfered with.

Symptoms.—Contrary to what is seen in active congestion, the animal affected with passive congestion is dull and depressed. It may show one or two spasmodic and violent plunging movements, after which it often falls or lies down and becomes quiet, often making a few half-hearted movements without any real attempt to rise. The pulse is weak and slow, the breathing is blowing, and there is often a bluish tinge seen in the mucous membrane of the eye and mouth.

Treatment.—Should the animal be on the ground the head should be raised on a sack of straw, etc., and any pressure on the veins of the neck relieved. Cold water splashed over the head and into the ears will often revive a case; but when these measures fail, the congestion of the brain should be relieved by the withdrawal of blood and the administration of stimulants to the heart, such as camphor, strychnine.

HÆMORRHAGE (*see* APOPLEXY).

INFLAMMATION (*see* ENCEPHALITIS; MENINGITIS).

PARASITES IN BRAIN (*see* GID).

TUBERCULOSIS OF BRAIN (*see* TUBERCULOSIS).

TUMOURS OF BRAIN are sometimes met with in the horse and dog. They often cause erratic movements, a tendency to stagger and even fall, circular motion, and sometimes violent attacks of frenzy.

ŒDEMA, or dropsy, of the brain is

seen in salt poisoning in pigs, and in Polioencephalomalacia. Blindness and convulsions are produced.

(*See also* sections on 'DAFT LAMBS', HEAT-STROKE, LIGHTNING STROKE, HYDROCEPHALUS, SWAYBACK, EPILEPSY, ECLAMPSIA, CHOREA, etc.)

BRAMBELL COMMITTEE REPORT.—This was published in Britain in 1965 by H.M.S.O. (price 6s. 6d.) under the full title *Report of the Technical Committee to inquire into the Welfare of Animals Kept Under Intensive Livestock Husbandry Systems*, under the chairmanship of Professor F. W. R. Brambell, a distinguished zoologist.

The British Veterinary Association presented evidence to the Committee, and made the following principal recommendations :

1. Salmonellosis in cattle should be made a notifiable disease.
2. In veal calf production, total darkness and close confinement in boxes are both undesirable and unnecessary.
3. Declaration of the addition of non-nutritional additives to feeding-stuffs should be made compulsory.
4. Close confinement in two- or three-bird battery cages is deplored.
5. Birds should be effectively stunned before slaughter.

The Brambell Committee had in mind mandatory rules, but the Government decided instead upon non-mandatory codes for the welfare of cattle, pigs, domestic fowls and turkeys. The codes contain many departures from Brambell Committee recommendations, but several points not covered by their report. Details will be found in Section 3 (1) of the Agriculture (Miscellaneous Provisions) Act, 1968.

BRAN (*see* OSTEOFIBROSIS).

BRAN MASH (*see* p. 602.)

BRANDING can be achieved with the minimum of pain by the technique of freeze-branding developed in the U.S.A. by Dr. R. K. Farrell, a veterinarian.

When the branded area thaws the hair falls out. The new hair which grows in 2 or 3 weeks is white, and therefore shows up well on a darkish animal. For a white animal, the brand has to be left on longer to kill the hair roots. The brand-mark then resembles a hot-iron brand, but the hide damage may be less. (Early claims that 'there is no damage to the hide' have been disproved.)

A copper branding 'iron', cooled to −70° C. with dry ice and alcohol, is applied to a clipped or shaved area for about 27 seconds ; this is not a final recommendation.

Laser beams have been used for branding cattle in the U.S.A. It is claimed that 'with the 5,000° C. temperature of the branding beam, the speed of branding is faster than the pain reflex of an animal'.

BRANDY (*see* ALCOHOL).

BRASSICÆ SPECIES.—Illness may occur in cattle fed excessive amounts of kale, cabbage, Brussels sprouts, and rape, especially if other foods are not available or if the kale is frosted. Anæmia, hæmoglobinuria, and death may result. (*See under* KALE.)

BRAXY.—Synonyms : Bradshot, Bradsot, Red-water of sheep, White-water, Sheep-sickness, etc. This is a disease of sheep characterised by a very short period of illness, by a seasonal and regional incidence, and, in the natural state, by a high mortality. It occurs in various parts of Scotland, Ireland, the north of England, Scandinavia, etc., chiefly on hilly land. It attacks young sheep under the age of two years, weaned lambs being very susceptible ; the best members of the flock are more liable to become attacked than poorly nourished sheep, and it is most frequently seen during a spell of cold, severe weather with hoar frosts at night.

Causes.—*Clostridium septique.* It affects the mucous membrane of the 4th stomach of sheep and from there invades the tissues. It gains entrance to the alimentary canal by way of the mouth along with the grass from a 'braxy pasture'. There is no proof of infection spreading from one infected sheep to another. Weather seems to have a considerable influence on the disease, for cases occur between the months of October and March inclusive. The first and any subsequent severe frost appears to lower the natural vitality of the sheep and render it liable to an attack.

Symptoms.—It is seldom that the signs of the disease are seen, unless by shepherds or continual attendants, for the length of the visible illness rarely exceeds 5 or 6 hours, and the sheep is often found dead when nothing unusual was seen previously. The affected animal shows a loss of

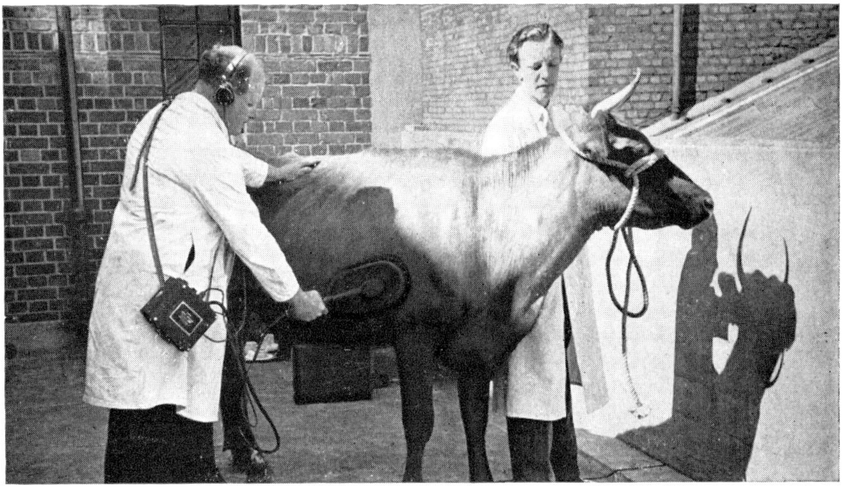

Cattle frequently ingest metal objects, often without ill effects. Sharp-pointed objects such as nails, however, may perforate the wall of the reticulum and then the pericardium. When this is suspected, a metal-detector may prove helpful in confirming a professional diagnosis.

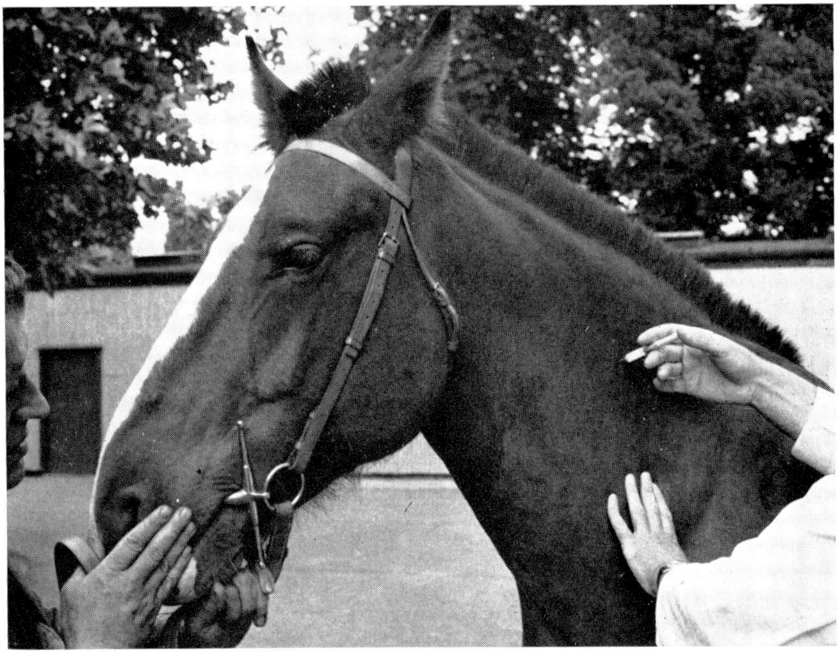

A tetanus vaccine introduced in 1971 by Burroughs Wellcome is claimed to overcome the disadvantage experienced hithero in active immunisation of horses against this disease – it does not give rise to a painful swelling at the site of inoculation.

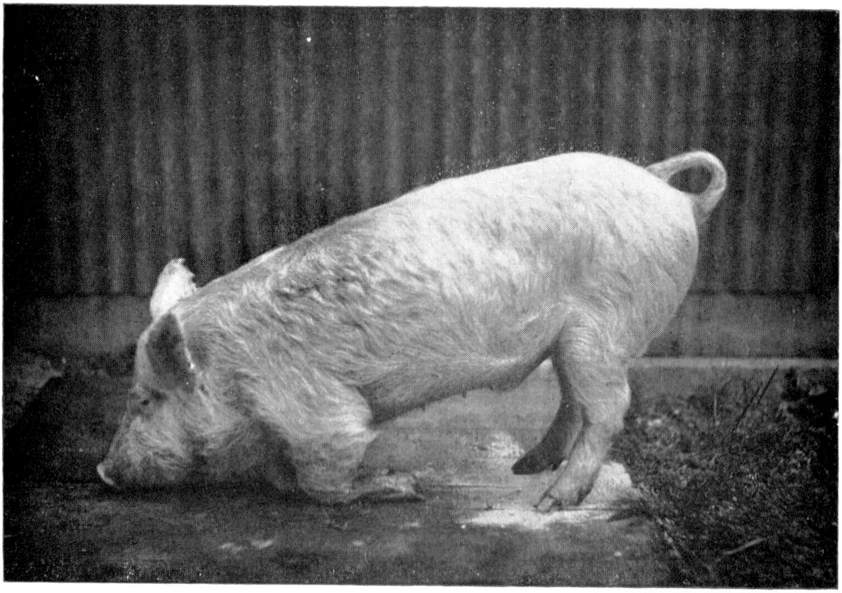

A pig suffering from rickets as the result of an excess of yeast being included in its diet. For explanation see under Yeast and Vitamins.

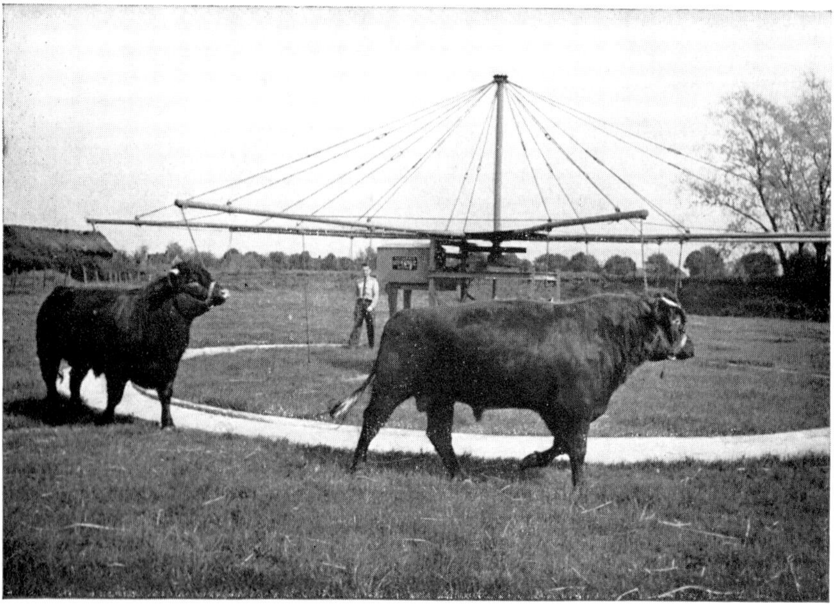

This mechanical bull-exerciser, installed by a Cambridge breeder, is a reminder that bulls need exercise and sunlight if they are to have maximum health and fertility.

See EXERCISE *and* INFERTILITY.

appetite, dullness, abdominal pain, and usually diarrhœa. It may walk in short, jerky movements, and fall in a dazed manner. The temperature is raised to 107° F., breathing is laboured, and the pulse absent or very weak. Just before the onset of death a characteristic odour is perceptible from the breath and body fluids. Decomposition is very rapid. The lesions are those of a gastritis in the 4th stomach (abomasum). The mucous membrane is intensely congested with black or purple blood, and in some cases parts are stripped off. The peritoneal membrane is also similarly congested.

Prevention.—Vaccination at the beginning of September, so that the animals have time to establish an immunity before the frosts begin, has given good results. On farms where the losses have been very heavy a second vaccination 14 days later may be needed. (*See* VACCINATION.)

BREASTS (*see* MAMMARY GLAND).

BREATH, BAD.—May be associated with dyspepsia, some forms of pneumonia, bronchitis, and decay or caries of the teeth in all animals. Decay of the delicate bones inside the nostrils, and actinomycosis affecting the throat or mouth may give rise to it.

BREATHING (*see under* RESPIRATION).

BREATHLESSNESS may be due to any condition that hinders the thorough oxygenation of the blood.

Causes.—Anæmia is one of the commonest causes of difficulty in breathing or an increase in the rate of respiration. In such a case the lessened amount of red blood corpuscles is not able to carry a sufficient supply of oxygen to the tissues, and in order that these be not starved more air has to be introduced into the lungs during a given time.

Many diseased conditions of the lungs give rise to breathlessness, since the area available for the exchange of gases is considerably reduced, *e.g.* in bronchitis, emphysema, pneumonia, solidification of the lung, tuberculosis, 'husk', lymphosarcoma in the cat, pleurisy with effusion.

Anything that results in a narrowing of the passages of respiration gives rise to breathlessness, for obvious reasons. Nearly all affections of the heart result in an interference with breathing, especially if the animal is subjected to any special exertion.

Many general diseases and all fevers, or conditions when the metabolism of the body is hastened, are accompanied by an increase in the rate of respiration.

BREEDING OF LIVESTOCK.—Information about animals coming 'on heat' or being 'in season' is given under ŒSTRUS. Other information is given under PREGNANCY and PARTURITION.

Number of females per male varies according to the age of the male and to the conditions under which the breeding animals are kept. The more carefully the males are looked after the more sexual vigour do they possess. The stallion when he is four years old and upwards and in good condition will serve from 80 to 120 mares during a season. A three-year-old can take up to about 50 or 60, and from 15 to 20 are enough for a two-year-old. From 60 to 80 cows are sufficient for an average adult bull, but he should not serve more than 35 or 40 between 1 and 2 years of age. Twenty to 30 ewes are as many as the ram lamb will successfully serve, but shearlings may have as many as 40 to 50. Adult rams may successfully impregnate 80 ewes or more. The year-old boar should not be allowed more than 20 sows during a season, but when he is older he may have up to 30 or 35. In this connection it must be remembered that when a large number of females are served by a male, those served at the later stages are not so likely to prove fruitful as those served earlier.

In Old Age.—There is little reliable data, but mares have bred foals when over 30 years, cattle and sheep up to 20 years, and cats till 14 years old. These, however, were all animals that had bred regularly in their younger days. It is difficult to breed from an aged female that has not previously been used for stud purposes. (*See also under* REPRODUCTION, ARTIFICIAL INSEMINATION, ARTIFICIAL SOMATIC MUTATIONS.)

BREEDS OF STOCK.—The British breeds of livestock are not only of local interest, since they have been exported to many parts of the world. A list of the breeds is given under the headings HORSES, CATTLE, BEEF BREEDS, SHEEP, etc.

BREWERS' GRAINS are used both in the wet state and dry. They are a by-product of brewing, and consist of the malted barley after it has been exhausted. In both forms they are used for feeding cattle and pigs, while dry grains are sometimes fed to folded sheep. If stored in the wet state for any length of time they become mouldy and fermented unless packed tightly so as to exclude air. In the dry they can be kept for a considerable length of time without harm. They are rich in proteins and carbohydrates, but if fed to excess they are liable to cause a mild form of intoxication, and if continued for long they are said to cause chronic inflammation of the liver, or cirrhosis.

BRIDLE INJURIES are usually not severe unless they are allowed to go unnoticed for any length of time. They take the form of: 1, injuries to the poll; 2,

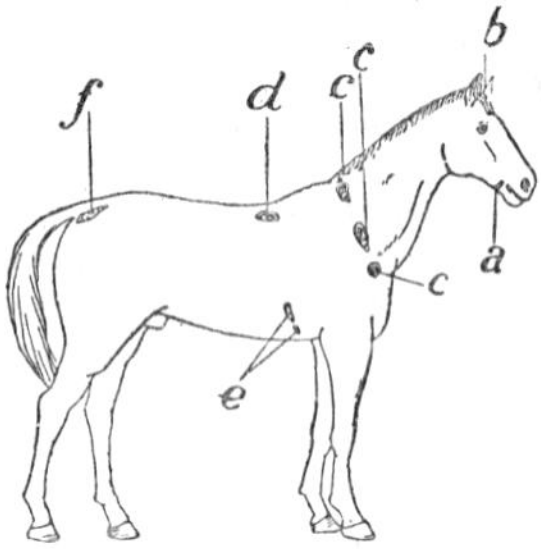

Injuries from harness. *a*, Curb-gall; *b*, poll injury; *c*, chafed shoulders from collar, high, medium (over spine of the scapula) and low (at point of shoulder); *d*, sore back from saddle; *e*, girth-galls; *f*, crupper-gall saddle.

injuries to the chin, caused by the curb-chain; and 3, injuries of the mouth from the bit. Injuries to the poll are produced by outside agencies generally, and are aggravated by the poll-strap rubbing or chafing the skin. The damage is generally only superficial, but in a few cases pus forms and may burrow down into the ligamentous tissue of the poll and produce ' poll evil '. (*See* POLL EVIL.) In ordinary cases it suffices to protect the damaged skin by winding a piece of sheep-skin round the strap that is causing the injury, and dressing the abraded areas with weak tincture of iodine each night. Those injuries to the chin that are caused by the curb-chain are usually only slight, and mainly affect young horses when they are being broken in. When they learn to answer the reins and acquire what is called a ' soft mouth ', the chafed skin is allowed to heal and the condition passes off. In older horses that have ' hard mouths ' and that constantly require the use of the curb-chain, the skin becomes thickened and calloused, and the surface of the bone may become irritated with a resulting deposition of new bone in the groove of the chin. Rarely this new bone grows to a large size and becomes unsightly, but in ordinary cases it is not apparent except to the touch. The injury may be obviated by using a leather curb for young horses that have very tender skins, and by changing the bit for older animals. A leather or webbing curb is sometimes used for older horses that pull, but it often happens that such is not sufficiently severe. Care in the driving of the horse, avoiding all sudden or severe pulls on the reins, will often do more to ' soften ' a horse's mouth than the use of more drastic measures. Bit injuries consist of the abrasion of the mucous membrane of the lower jaw, just opposite the corners of the lips, where the bit crosses. Sometimes the membrane becomes actually ulcerated and a foul-smelling discharge escapes, but in the majority of cases the injuries are slight and heal in a few days. In rare instances the ulcerating process reaches as deep as the surface of the bone, and attacks the covering membrane. Such a case requires a cessation from work, the daily use of mouth washes.

BRIGHT BLINDNESS.—This, a prevalent condition in Yorkshire hill sheep, was first described in 1965, and is characterised by progressive degeneration of the retina. The disease is of considerable economic importance in some flocks. The cause is not yet known, but there appears to be an association between this form of blindness and the grazing of bracken. Sheep are known to be partial to bracken wilting as the result of a fungus infection, and perhaps this is of significance.

Bright blindness has been found in several breeds of sheep, in Scotland and Wales as well as in Northern England. In some flocks the incidence may be 5–8 per cent among the ewes, with a peak incidence in those two to four years old. The blindness is permanent.

In ewes moved to bracken-free grazing before the disease is well advanced the condition will not progress further.

BRIGHT'S DISEASE is a term applied by many people to any disease of the kidneys. It is used very little in veterinary work, but may be taken to mean either acute or chronic nephritis. (*See* KIDNEY, DISEASES OF.)

BRISKET DISEASE (*see* MOUNTAIN SICKNESS).

BRITISH DANE.—A breed established by the Red Poll Cattle Society in the U.K. following the import of Danish Red cattle.

BRITISH VETERINARY ASSOCIATION.—Its principal objects are the advancement of veterinary science in all its branches, the publication of scientific and clinical material, and the promotion of the welfare of the profession. It is intimately concerned with all matters of professional policy, and maintains contact with many outside bodies and Government Departments. (*See* B.V.A.)

BROILERS.—Good quality table chicken of either sex, about 10 or 12 weeks old, and weighing $2\frac{1}{2}$ to 4 lbs. (liveweight).

Mortality.—If the chicks and their management are good, the total mortality for a broiler crop should be less than 5 per cent, frequently only 3 per cent. Most of these deaths will take place during the first fortnight. In fact, a $1\frac{1}{2}$ per cent mortality is normal and to be expected during the early period.

For commercial reasons there is often the temptation to overcrowd broilers in their houses, and this practice will inevitably increase stress and hence the liability to disease—the effects of which may be the more severe. (*See also under* NEWCASTLE DISEASE; POULTRY, DISEASES OF.)

'BROKEN HOCK'.—In greyhound racing circles this means a fractured scaphoid.

'BROKEN MOUTH' is the name given to the mouths of old sheep that have lost some of their teeth. Loss of incisor teeth is not uncommon in hill sheep and is of economic importance because a ewe needs her incisors if she is to support herself and a lamb on the hill.

Loosening of the teeth, followed by their falling out, is a form of disease comparable to pyorrhœa in man. A predisposing factor is the way in which the incisor teeth meet the pad. Lambs with a 'sow mouth', in which the incisors bite *behind* the pad, should never be kept for breeding; nor those in which the incisors bite on to the *front* of the pad or—being placed too far forward—do not meet it at all. The lambs with incisors which meet the pad 'squarely' are those to breed from, if broken mouth is to be avoided in future.

The feeding of turnips in winter is said to result in the incisor teeth falling out if they are placed too far forward; *i.e.* only just meeting the front of the pad. Mineral deficiencies may, perhaps, aggravate the trouble.

Symptoms.—Difficulty in feeding, drop ping some of the food back into the trough, and 'quidding'.

'BROKEN WIND', also called 'HEAVES' and CHRONIC ALVEOLAR EMPHYSEMA, is a condition affecting the respiration of the horse which may be due either to a breakdown of the walls of the air-cells in the lungs, resulting in the formation of large cavities in the lung structure with a resulting reduction of the area through which the normal exchange of gases takes place, or it may be due to an asthmatical condition. Broken wind often follows pneumonia, acute bronchitis, or a chronic cough. It may follow chronic bronchitis.

Infestation with *Dictyocaulus arnfieldi* (p. 658) may, it has been suggested, be a cause of some cases of emphysema. Another suggestion is that a fungal toxin may be responsible, the fungi gaining entrance to the body in inhaled dust from straw or hay, and sometimes if not always producing an allergy; but the precise nature and cause of broken wind remain obscure.

Symptoms.—In most cases the symptoms develop very gradually. A cough attacks the animal in paroxysms, especially on leaving the stable in cold weather. This persists, and may be accompanied by a nasal discharge. On violent exercise, a rapidity and a difficulty in breathing are seen which are quite in excess of the amount of exercise undertaken. When the horse is resting nothing unusual may be seen in the early stages, but later the nearly typical 'broken-winded breathing' commences. This may be described as a cough, generally single, short, shallow, feeble, and jerky, and not followed by a 'sneeze'. A series of these short coughs may occur after or during exercise, but at rest only one of these hollow (sometimes called 'graveyard') coughs is heard. Accompanying the above symptoms there gradually develops a change in the respiration. It becomes irregular, faster than normal, and while the inspiratory movement is not very much altered, the expiratory effort is first of all prolonged and then doubled, so that two definite columns of breath can be seen at each expiration on a frosty day. A groove between the posterior edge of the rib-cage and the muscles of the flank is almost characteristic of the condition, but it does not develop until the disease is advanced.

Treatment.—When the air-cells are broken down nothing can be done to alleviate the condition.

BROMIDES are the salts of bromine. They have a sedative action on the nervous system, lessen the capacity for feeling the stimuli of pain, and were used in overcoming excitement or a tendency to hysteria. The dose for a dog is about 10 to 20 grains. (*See also* TRANQUILLISERS which have to some extent replaced them.)

BROMISM is the name given to a group of symptoms that are associated with the excessive use of bromides. In animals it has occurred when small dogs were given sleeping powders composed of bromides and where the nightly dose of the salt had been too large. The chief signs are cerebral depression, feebleness, an unsteady gait, anæmia, and in some cases the appearance of a rash.

BRONCHIAL TUBES are the smaller divisions of the air passages which arise from the bronchi—the two (or three) main divisions of the trachea or windpipe. They carry the inspired air into the lungs and discharge the expired air into the trachea, from whence it passes by the throat and nasal passages to the outside. Bronchial tubes are composed of a basis of incomplete cartilaginous rings joined to each other by fibrous tissues, and lined on the inside by respiratory mucous membrane. A small band of muscle completes the cartilage and allows of a certain amount of alteration in the size of the lumen of the tube. (*See* AIR PASSAGES, LUNGS.)

BRONCHIECTASIS (*βρόγχος*, windpipe; *ἔκτασις*, lengthening) means dilatation of the walls of the bronchial tubes due to weakening through excessive coughing. The condition is often met with in chronic bronchitis, and the cavities produced are often filled with pus.

BRONCHIOLITIS is a name sometimes applied to bronchitis affecting the finest bronchial tubes (bronchioles), also known as capillary bronchitis.

BRONCHITIS (*βρόγχος*, windpipe) means inflammation of the lining mucous membrane of the bronchial tubes. It is a very common complaint of all animals in temperate or cold climates. An acute and a chronic type are recognised.

(*a*) **Acute Bronchitis : Horse.**—This usually follows an attack of nasal catarrh, laryngitis, influenza, a common cold when the animal is still kept at work or exposed to a chill, or mechanical irritation, *e.g.* caused by smoke from burning buildings, drenches. And it may occur during the course of specific fevers such as strangles and glanders.

Symptoms.—A rise in temperature, accompanied by faster respiration, loss of appetite, a cough, and nasal discharge, are seen. The cough is at first hard and dry, but becomes softer and easier in the later stages. The breathing may often be heard to be wheezing and bubbling in the later stages.

Treatment.—Attention to hygienic conditions is of first importance. The horse should be removed to a loose-box, provided with a plentiful supply of bedding, rugged if the weather demands, given plenty of clean water to drink, and fed on soft foods. It must on no account be drenched, for there is nearly always difficulty in swallowing, and a great risk of some of the medicine entering the trachea and complicating an already serious case. Medicines—such as belladonna, camphor, ammonium carbonate, liquorice—are best mixed with treacle and given as an electuary. Penicillin and the Sulpha drugs are indicated. (*See* NURSING OF SICK ANIMALS.)

Cattle.—Acute bronchitis is not so often met with in the ox as it is in the horse, if we except the parasitic form commonly called ' hoose ' or ' busk '.

Dog.—Acute bronchitis may occur as the result of exposure to chills, wettings, imperfect drying after a bath, and it is often present in cases of distemper and pneumonia. It is generally regarded as being of an infectious nature, and isolation is practised as a routine.

Treatment.—The animal should be placed in comfortable quarters and kept quiet. A flannel jacket is advisable. Penicillin may be given. Inhalations of medicated steam are useful in the dry stages of the disease. Good nursing, along with the administration of halibut-liver oil.

(*b*) **Chronic Bronchitis : Horse.**—This may follow the acute form ; it may be a complication of valvular disease of the heart ; it is sometimes seen along with broken wind, and it may arise as a primary condition. The smaller capillary bronchial tubes are affected and not the larger passages.

Symptoms.—A loud, hard cough, often appearing in spasms, respiratory distress on the least exertion, an intermittent, white, clotted, or pus-containing nasal discharge, which is most in evidence after coughing or exercise, and a gradual loss of condition, characterises this form of bronchitis. The chronic, although not so alarming as the acute, type of bronchitis is to be considered a serious illness, for it very often leaves behind it that permanent injury which is commonly called 'broken wind'. (*See* BROKEN WIND.)

Treatment.—Antibiotics. The animal should not be drenched; its diet should be the best of food, linseed meal or mash, minced roots, green food, and the restriction of the hay constituent, are advisable. Nursing should be along the lines indicated under ACUTE BRONCHITIS.

Cattle.—Chronic bronchitis is often associated with some other disease, *e.g.* tuberculosis.

Dog and cat.—Aged and obese domesticated carnivora are very prone to suffer from the chronic form of bronchitis. It is often associated with disease of the heart. It may be mistaken for asthma.

Treatment.—Skilled attention is advisable, since if treated early by modern methods there is good hope of recovery.

(*c*) **Bronchitis in the Sheep.**—There are two kinds met with, one of which is benign and soon clears up with treatment, and the other is a contagious type mostly seen in pedigree rams that are being kept and fed for shows or sales.

Causes.—Worm larvæ or the adult 'lung worm', chills, exposure to wet, inclement weather, going from a warm sheep-pen into the open air in cold, windy weather, shearing and dipping in bad weather. (*See* HUSK.)

(*d*) **Bronchitis in the Pig.**—This is often the result of cold, damp surroundings, or associated with pneumonia, etc. Parasitic worms are often the cause of outbreaks of bronchitis that affect store pigs. (*See* PARASITES)

Treatment.—Drenching is a proverbially dangerous process in the healthy pig, and it is much more so in those that are affected with bronchitis, since there is often an associated laryngitis, and swallowing is difficult. They should be housed by themselves in a warm, dry, well-bedded sty, given the best and most easily swallowed foods, and clothed with a jacket made from a piece of old blanket (with two holes cut out for the fore-limbs), which is tied, stitched, or fastened with safety-pins along the back. They should be disturbed as little as possible, and when apparently recovered should not be placed with the other healthy pigs for at least a week, as relapses are common and often lead to a chronic form that persists for a considerable time. (*See under* Ascaris lumbricoides, PARASITOLOGY; *also* NURSING OF SICK ANIMALS.)

(*e*) **Bronchitis in Chickens.**—(*See under* INFECTIOUS BRONCHITIS.)

BRONCHO-PNEUMONIA (*see* PNEUMONIA).

BRONCHUS (βρόνχος, windpipe), or bronchial tube, is the name applied to tubes into which the windpipe divides, one going to either lung. The name is also applied to the later divisions of these tubes distributed throughout the lungs.

BROOM POISONING is not so common as would be expected, considering the plentifulness of the plant, *Cytisus scoparius*. It is when animals, sheep especially, are extremely hungry that it is cropped. It contains an active volatile alkaloid called *sparteine*, and another called *cytisine*, and it appears that the former is mainly concerned in the production of the symptoms of poisoning.

Symptoms. — When taken in large amounts the plant causes at first a temporary stimulation of all the body functions. This is very soon followed by drowsiness, general weakness, and later complete narcosis and paralysis. Sheep are most frequently affected, and the mortality is comparatively low.

First-aid.—The administration of tannic acid or strong tea.

'BROWN MOUTH'.—A syndrome characterised mainly by gum necrosis and dysentery, occurring as a complication of virus diseases in the dog. It appears to be infectious and yields to penicillin.

'BROWN NOSE'.—A form of light sensitisation (which see) in cattle.

BRUCELLOSIS is an infection with organisms of the *Brucella* group. The commonest is the disease due to *B. abortus*, which causes abortion in cattle. Malta fever in goats and human beings, due to *B. melitensis*, is another form of brucellosis. In man, brucellosis often takes the form of 'undulant fever', with characteristic undulating fluctuations of the temperature. Human infection with *B. abortus* may follow the drinking of raw milk or the handling of infected fœtal membranes. Accidental self-inoculation with S19 vaccine is another cause. Infected uterine discharge drying on the cow's skin may be inhaled.

Overseas, abortion in pigs is caused by *B. abortus suis*, and commonly hares have been found to harbour this organism, which caused orchitis in them. The American strain of *B. suis* is pathogenic for man, causing undulant fever and arthritis. What was formerly referred to as *Br. melitensis* in the U.S.A. is now known as biotype 3 of *Br. suis*.

In horses, *B. abortus* may cause fistulous withers and lameness due to infection of other ligaments. In the mare, abortion may (rarely) occur (see *Vet. Record*, Feb. 4, 1967); in dogs: arthritis, abortion.

B. canis has been recognised as a separate species in the U.S.A., where it has caused outbreaks of severe illness in beagles. *B. canis* also caused illness in man.

It is now recognised that what was thought to be *B. melitensis* infection in cattle in Britain was infection with the biotype 5 of *B. abortus*. *B. melitensis* var. *ovis* gives rise (in Australasia, U.S.A., and Europe) to infertility and scrotal dropsy in rams. Abortion may occur in infected ewes.

In Britain, brucellosis is not a serious problem in goats, and does not occur in pigs.

In parts of Africa *Brucella* agglutinins have been recorded in wild animals, and *B. abortus* has been isolated from a waterbuck, and from rodents.

In Argentina foxes are commonly infected with *Br. abortus*.

Brucellosis is not an important disease in sheep in Britain. The infection can exist in rams, and ewes have been known to carry it for up to three successive lambing seasons. Four outbreaks of abortion due to *Brucella abortus* were reported in 1969. On one Cumberland farm 12 in-wintered ewes (vaccinated against enzootic abortion) aborted. The findings suggested a low and sporadic incidence of brucellosis with little lateral spread within the flocks. They also pointed to a possible connection between the infection in cattle and sheep on the farms. There is no evidence that deer, infected with *Br. abortus*, have infected cattle grazing the same pasture.

(*See* CHEESE, FISTULOUS WITHERS, BUMBLE-FOOT.)

BRUCELLOSIS IN CATTLE ('Contagious Abortion') is a specific contagious disease due to the *Brucella abortus*. Since the infection may exist and persist in the genital system of the bull, *Brucellosis* is to be preferred as a name for the disease. In females it is characterised by a chronic inflammation of the uterus (especially of the mucous membrane); usually, but not invariably, followed by abortion between the fifth and eighth months of pregnancy.

It is important to note that not all infected animals abort. Indeed, in over half of them pregnancy runs to full term. 'Any animal that has aborted once may be almost as dangerous at its next and subsequent calvings—which are generally at full term—as on the occasion it aborted.' (Mr. A. C. L. Brown, M.R.C.V.S.)

Infection may occur by the mouth or through the vagina during service, when a bull which has served an infected cow is called upon to serve a clean one afterwards, or when the bull is a 'carrier'. Contamination of litter with discharges from a previous case is an important factor in the spread of the disease in a herd. The hand and arm of the man who handles an aborted foetus may also transmit infection.

In the pregnant cow a low-grade chronic inflammatory reaction is set up in the uterus with the result that an exudate accumulates between the fœtal membranes and the uterine mucous membranes, especially around the cotyledons. The cotyledons may appear necrotic, owing to the presence of fibrinous adherent masses upon their surfaces, and the fœtal membranes may show similar areas after they have been expelled. Quite commonly in cattle the membranes are thickened and tough. The fœtus may be normal or may show a dropsical condition of the muscles and the subcutaneous tissues, and there may be fluid present in the cavities of chest, abdomen, and cranium. In some cases the fœtus undergoes a process of mummification, and when it is discharged it is almost unrecognisable as a fœtus.

Cows at pasture may become infected by older 'carrier' cows (which are liable to harbour the organisms in their udders) or by wild animals (*e.g.* foxes), dogs or birds, which have eaten or been in contact with infected membranes or discharges upon other farms near by where the disease already exists. (*See also* BUMBLE-FOOT.)

Symptoms.—Very often there are no well-defined symptoms. There may be a slight discharge of a catarrhal nature from the vulva, and the lips of the latter may become congested and swollen. The discharge increases in quantity, sometimes becomes blood-stained or purulent, and abortion occurs shortly afterward. In other cases abortion may occur without any preliminary symptoms, and except that the calf is not a full-term one, may be practically the same as normal calving. Most cows which have aborted once will carry their next calf to full term, or to practically full term; while only very few cows will abort a calf three times.

As a rule, if abortion occurs early in pregnancy the fœtal membranes are expelled along with the fœtus, but if towards the end of the period there is almost always retention of these. A continuous reddish-brown or brownish-grey discharge follows, and persists for about 10 to 20 days (often for about 2 weeks). In some instances it slowly collects in the cavity of the uterus, little or nothing being seen at the vulva, and then it is discharged periodically, often in large amounts at a time.

In the bull symptoms of infection may be very slight or absent, and laboratory methods are usually necessary to establish a diagnosis.

Brucellosis is not the only cause of abortion in cattle due to an infective agent, and in arriving at a diagnosis it must be differentiated from infections listed under ABORTION.

Immunity.—Infected animals gradually produce an immunity in themselves against further abortions. The organisms may persist in the system for long periods, and a cow which does not herself subsequently abort may spread infection to other cows in the herd. This natural immunity, however, is wasteful, both in the matter of calves and milk supply, so that methods have been adopted in which an effort is made to provide animals with an artificial immunity.

Agglutination Test.—This consists of taking a sample of blood from a cow suspected of being or having been infected, allowing it to coagulate so that the blood serum is expressed. The serum is diluted 1 in 10, 1 in 20, 1 in 40 and so on, and is mixed with a suspension of the organisms (the antigen). After 24 or 48 hours, agglutination of the organisms occurs in positive cases where the antibody content of the serum is high. This indicates that at some time previously the cow has acquired infection, though it does not mean that she will necessarily abort if she subsequently becomes pregnant. The test is not a test of infection or infectiveness to other cattle, but it indicates that the antibodies are still present in the cow's blood-stream. (*See* MILK RING-TEST, ROSE BENGAL TEST.)

Treatment.—There is no curative or preventive treatment for pregnant cows. Antiseptic irrigations of the uterus after abortion, and the use of pessaries, may do a certain amount of good by preventing the discharge of such large numbers of germs, but the results from their usage have been indifferent. In the bull treatment is usually impracticable. 'Carrier' animals should be no longer used for service but slaughtered.

Prevention.—There is no doubt that prevention by a regular system of vaccination of all heifer calves with S.19 vaccine offers the best protection against the disease so far available. It has already reduced losses to minor proportions in countries where it is used. An immunity is developed sufficient to protect against natural infection and consequent abortion for at least five pregnancies and probably for the normal milking life of the cow.

Calves so vaccinated generally pass the Agglutination Test successfully from 6 to 12 months afterwards, and nearly always before they calve their first calf.

There are two main objections to adult vaccination. One is that it interferes with the interpretation of the agglutination tests by causing 'false positives', so that it becomes difficult or impossible to distinguish between the effects of the last dose of vaccine and the effects of a natural infection. In adults vaccinated only as calves there is no such difficulty—it is easy to determine natural infection from the effects of the vaccination.

The second objection to adult vaccination is that, to quote a former president of the B.V.A., 'vaccination of adult cattle can lead to the excretion of apparently virulent strains of *Brucella abortus* in the milk'.

Strain 19 vaccine had been of excellent service in preventing actual abortions, but it does not get rid of the disease, and there have been abortion 'storms' despite it in recent years.

Public Health.—While the abortion rate is now 5 per cent, and the majority of

BRUCELLOSIS IN CATTLE

abortions not nowadays associated with *Br. abortus* at all, the occurrence of this organism in the nation's milk supply is still high—as many as 10 per cent of samples in some areas contain it. This contamination of the milk supply is frequently associated with the presence of cows which have a localised infection in the udders.

Legislation.—In Great Britain the law provides against the exposure for sale of aborted cows until at least two months have elapsed since they aborted.

Towards eradication.—A free calf vaccination service was introduced by the Ministry of Agriculture in 1962.

In order to obtain an estimate of what would be involved if a policy of eradication was decided upon, a serological survey was made by the Animal Health Division in 1964. 'This revealed that about 14 per cent of breeding cattle (representing between ½ and ¾ million cattle) would react to the diagnostic tests. Clearly many of these animals would be reacting as a result of vaccination and the radical slaughter of this vast number of cattle and the replacement created by depletion on this scale would not be possible.'

Mr. F. V. John, past president, B.V.A., commented in 1969: 'Unfortunately about this time came evidence of an increasing incidence, particularly in herds changing from the traditional cowshed to yard-and-parlour systems. This change in husbandry was often accompanied by an expansion in herd size—usually by the purchase of cattle of unknown brucella status. It soon became evident that S 19 vaccination was quite unable to give adequate protection under the new conditions . . . the immunising value of S 19 itself had fallen.'

The Brucellosis (Accredited Herds) Scheme was brought into operation in April, 1967. 'The primary aim of this voluntary Scheme is to identify and register those herds already free of brucellosis and to maintain a standard of periodic testing and management designed to maintain that state. This will enable a nucleus of stock to be formed from which replacements can be safely obtained by those who are eradicating the disease from their herds by elimination of reactors,' stated a senior Ministry official.

Dairy herds first become Supervised after passing three Milk Ring tests.

Since April, 1967, two further steps have been taken with a view to later eradication. The first was to limit the use of Strain 19 in the Free Calf Vaccination Service to calves not more than 180 days old. The second (Nov. 1967) limited the use of Strain 19 to herds within the Free Calf Vaccination Service. 'This, together with the previous reduction in the upper age limit, had the effect of preventing the use of Strain 19 in any animal over 180 days. It is generally recognised that vaccination over this age may be beneficial in certain circumstances, and Strain 45/20 dead vaccine can be used for this purpose. The circumstances when such vaccination is considered to be of possible benefit are:

'1. Where a herd is uninfected and unprotected but there is a heavy infection in adjoining herds.

'2. Where a herd may be infected and it is necessary to introduce animals which may not have been vaccinated or it is thought necessary to protect animals within the herd which may not yet have been infected.

'It is hoped that the use of this vaccine rather than the strongly agglutinogenic Strain 19 will create less of a problem for diagnosis by blood tests. Its indiscriminate use can only cause further confusion at blood tests and it should only be used in carefully selected circumstances.'

The use of 45/20 dead vaccine, while it does not have as lasting an effect on the serum agglutination test as Strain 19, tends to interfere to a greater extent with the complement fixation test used to distinguish between inconclusive and positive serum agglutination tests. Therefore herds in which 45/20 has been used will not be accepted for testing under the Scheme until at least 12 months after the last vaccination.

Mr. F. V. John commented (1969): 'Most (veterinary) practices are now encountering abortion storms which we all hoped were things of the past . . . It is doubtful if more than 10 per cent of herds will, under the present regulations, seek enrolment—a percentage far too small to allow progress towards an eradication programme . . . Unless we can move very quickly to some form of area eradication, the effort and expense involved will be disproportionate to the results achieved.'

Both Mr. John and many others advocated the compulsory slaughter of reactors. Failure to prohibit the circulation of infected animals from farm to farm was (1969), of course, one of the greatest weaknesses of the Scheme; which as a whole, however, the B.V.A. supported.

In 1970 the (voluntary) Brucellosis Incentives Scheme was introduced to replace the former Scheme, and to facilitate a programme of area eradication, with compulsory slaughter of reactors.

The map shows the three initial eradication areas announced in 1971; N.W. England, between the rivers Esk and Lune; western Scottish seaboard: Argyll and Bute; and south Wales: a coast-to-coast corridor of Cardigan and Carmarthen; plus the Isle of Wight, the Shetland Isles, and the Uists. Extension zones for 1972–73 are also shown, together with potential eradication zones in S.E. England, East Anglia, Devon, and north and west Scotland, which will be selected 'in the light of the industry's response to voluntary eradication'.

With herds still qualifying or accredited under the earlier scheme, over 31,000 herds were engaged in voluntary accreditation, and over 13,000 of them had already gained registration by March 31, 1971.

November 1, 1971 saw the beginning of what the Ministry terms the 'voluntary year' in the initial eradication areas, and during this period herd-owners will have the option of joining the incentives scheme or of applying for eradication terms on a voluntary contractual basis. It will mean that owners will have at least 18 months' notice before compulsory slaughter begins.

The programme was due to open with compulsory blood testing of all herds not already in the voluntary schemes.

Movement restrictions are likely to be applied, for all cattle other than steers, on the following lines. Movement into and within an eradication area will be confined to accredited animals under normal licence; once tested animals subject to isolation and a check test as in the incentives scheme; and calves under 14 days into isolation for test within 7 days and again after 60 days. All other cattle may be moved into and within the area only if consigned direct for immediate slaughter. Movement through the area will be permitted without licence provided that there is no de-trucking. Movement out of the area will be unrestricted except for reactors, which must be consigned for slaughter under approved arrangements. Scheme animals will require the usual permits. Restrictions may also be applied on the movement of skim milk, slurry, and other 'risk' products.

The use of 45/20 vaccine will be prohibited, except under licence, in initial eradication areas and extension zones. **As this vaccine (especially after calfhood vaccination with S.19) can affect test results for at least a year and sometimes for up to 18 months, it is important for the veterinary authorities to know in which herds and individual animals it has been used.**

The use of S.19 vaccine in calves up to six months old is encouraged in that the owner who uses the free calf vaccination service continuously from July 1 (or takes equivalent precautions if he does not rear calves) will be paid a higher replacement grant for any reactors in his herd.

Eradication in other countries.—Brucellosis has been successfully eradicated from many overseas countries, including Denmark, Sweden, Norway, Finland, Czechoslovakia, and Eire. Farmers' co-operation and discipline played an important part.

Precautions.—The greatest care must be taken in handling and disposing of an aborted fœtus, fœtal membranes, discharges, etc., both in the interests of human health and in order to prevent the spread of the disease among cattle. It is worth having a veterinary surgeon examine the cause of *any* abortion. There can be danger from the infected cow that has carried a calf to full term. Avoid buying in replacements from non-Accredited herds.

BRUISED SOLE is a condition of bruising of the sensitive sole of the foot, due to a badly fitting shoe, or the result of the horse having stood upon a projection, such as a stone, etc. Its characters and its treatment do not differ from what is given under 'CORNS', except that while the corn has a more or less definite position in the foot, bruising of the sole may occur anywhere. (*See* CORNS.)

BRUISES, or **CONTUSIONS,** are more or less extensive injuries of the deeper parts of the skin and the underlying tissues, generally accompanied by an outpouring of blood from the damaged vessels, but unattended by corresponding open wounds.

The simplest type of bruise is one in which the deeper layers of the skin only are damaged, and which is visible only on those parts of the animal body that are not covered by hair, such as below the arm and inside the thighs of dogs, sheep, and cattle, the udders of those breeds where the skin covering it is white, etc. A slight

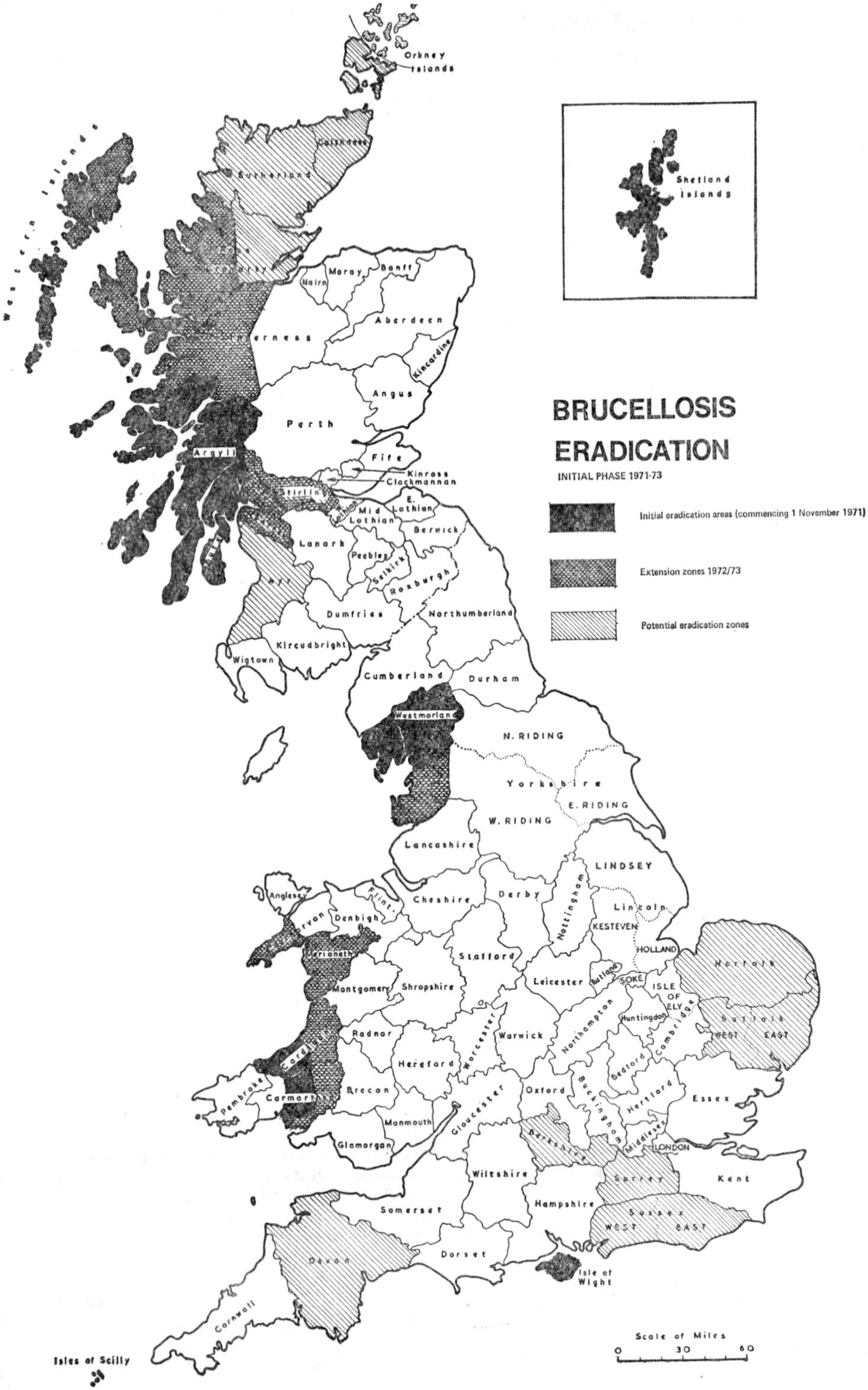
BRUCELLOSIS
ERADICATION
INITIAL PHASE 1971-73
Initial eradication areas (commencing 1 November 1971)
Extension zones 1972/73
Potential eradication zones
Shetland Islands
Orkney Islands
Western Islands
Caithness
Sutherland
Nairn
Moray
Banff
Aberdeen
Inverness
Kincardine
Angus
Perth
Argyll
Fife
Kinross
Clackmannan
Stirling
E. Lothian
Mid Lothian
Berwick
Lanark
Peebles
Selkirk
Roxburgh
Ayr
Dumfries
Northumberland
Kircudbright
Wigtown
Cumberland
Durham
Westmorland
N. RIDING
Yorkshire
E. RIDING
W. RIDING
Lancashire
LINDSEY
Lincoln
KESTEVEN
HOLLAND
Anglesey
Flint.
Denbigh
Cheshire
Derby
Nottingham
Merioneth
Stafford
Norfolk
Leicester
Rutland
SOKE
ISLE OF ELY
Montgomery
Shropshire
Northampton
Huntingdon
Cambridge
Suffolk
WEST
EAST
Radnor
Warwick
Worcester
Hereford
Bedford
Cardigan
Pembroke
Carmarthen
Brecon
Oxford
Buckingham
Hertford
Essex
Gloucester
Monmouth
Glamorgan
Berkshire
Middlesex
LONDON
Wiltshire
Surrey
Kent
Somerset
Hampshire
Sussex
WEST
EAST
Devon
Dorset
Isle of Wight
Cornwall
Isles of Scilly
Scale of Miles
0
30
60

bluish mark is seen, which is caused by the tearing of minute vessels and the escape of the blood into the cell spaces of the region. When the injury is the result of a severe blow, the muscles may be bruised and torn without any wound in the skin, and the resulting effusion of blood may cause a large swelling, in which, after the first day or so, fluid may be detected. If the injury is inflicted on a part that lies immediately above a bone, the damage done is often serious, for, owing to the bruising of the vessels of the periosteum and the consequent effusion of fluid, along with the reparative processes that are set up in that tissue, a permanent thickening of the bone (or *exostosis*) results, which may interfere with the free movement of a joint, tendon, or ligament in the vicinity. Moreover, when the bruise is near a joint and blood effuses into the cavity and complete absorption does not occur, adhesions will be set up and the joint may be permanently stiffened. Yet again, it sometimes happens, in cases where a severe blow has been received on a bone that is only slightly protected with overlying tissues, that an actual fracture of the bone occurs, although there is no separation of the fractured ends, and only very little evidence of injury on the skin above it. Such cases, called *stellate* or *star fractures*, are liable to remain undetected until later when, after a false step or an abnormal strain, the cracked bone separates. Blows on bones near the skin surface must always be regarded as potentially serious.

The appearance of a bruise in an animal varies. Often little or nothing can be seen during life, but on post-mortem examination an appalling amount of blood is found to have escaped from the vessels into the tissues, and the animal has died literally from internal hæmorrhage or from shock following that. The parts of the body that are most commonly bruised in the horse are those bony prominences that come into contact with the ground when the horse has a fall; these are the skin over the orbit above and below the eye, the side of the face, the lips, the side of the shoulder, the knees, elbows, and fetlocks, the point of the hip, the stifle, hock, and sometimes the point of the buttocks in old or very thin animals. These parts should be carefully examined after a fall, and any particles of grit removed.

Treatment.—In slight cases cold applications should be carried out as soon after the injury as possible, so that the blood-vessels of the part may be induced to constrict and the effusion of blood checked. For this purpose there is nothing to beat the hose-pipe gently applied. Ice is useful if it can be obtained. Failing either of these, a pad of cotton-wool or a clean cloth should be soaked in cold water and applied. After the first day much benefit will be derived from hot fomentations. Gentle exercise and hand massage may be given when the acute pain has gone from the part, which will usually be about the third or fourth day after the accident. When there is much grit, etc., in the surface layers of the skin, it is advisable, after clipping away the hair, to use an antiseptic. (*See* WOUNDS.)

BRUIT and **MURMUR** are words used to describe several abnormal sounds heard in connection with the heart, arteries, and veins on auscultation.

BRUSHING and CUTTING.—By these terms is meant an injury to the inside of a fetlock joint or coronet occasioned by the inside of the opposite foot striking this part during the walk, trot, or canter. At a natural pace the unbroken horse does not show this fault; it is almost always found in either young animals shod for the first time, in old or weak animals that are overworked, at the beginning of the training season when the horses are out of condition, or at the end of a long journey when the horse is tired out. A few cases do result from bad shoeing, especially the fitting of too wide a heel on the inside, and from some disease of the joints, but these are not numerous. (*See* SPEEDY-CUT.)

The injury inflicted varies from a mere scratch of the skin to a deep torn wound that involves the fibrous tissue surrounding the joint. Hind-legs are more often affected than are the fore-limbs, but the condition is much more serious in the front feet. When a horse brushes himself in front he is very apt to stumble, and may easily fall. If he brushes behind he can usually recover himself without coming down.

Treatment.—Ill-conditioned horses should be given lighter work and better feeding until they have regained their condition; young animals, especially those shod for the first time, should be allowed to become accustomed to their shoes before being put to fast or severe work; horses that have become tired at their work should be driven more slowly and carefully.

If, in spite of the observance of these measures, the horse still continues to injure himself, his shoes should receive attention. If calkins have been fitted they should be removed and plain shoes worn. Failing this a 'knocked-up' shoe is applied. This has the innermost branch narrowed from side to side, and left plain, without any nail-holes except at the toe, A calkin may be worn on the outside heel, and to make the height equal, the inner branch is made deeper. The shoe is fitted close on the inside of the foot, or even within the wall, which is then allowed to project beyond it. Some smiths fit the outer heel lower or higher than the inner, but unless the conformation of the limbs is abnormal, there is nothing to be gained from this procedure. It is always better to keep the horse's heels at the same height and alter the shoe accordingly. Three-quarter shoes—those with the inner branch cut short by 1½ to 3 inches—are useful in some cases which prove intractable to other methods.

BRUSSELS SPROUTS.—Cattle strip-grazing these for 6 weeks, without other food, became ill with anæmia and hæmoglobinuria. The illness caused by members of the *Bassicæ* species is said to be always more serious near to the time of calving.

BUCCOSTOMY.—An operation for the creation of buccal fistulæ in order to prevent wind-sucking.

BUCHU (*see* URINARY ANTISEPTICS).

BUDGERIGARS (*see* CAGE BIRDS).

BUFFALO FLY.—This is *Lyperosia exigua*, a parasite of importance in Australia and in India and Malaya. It causes great irritation and even anæmia. (*See* p. 674, Horn-fly, for life history.)

BUFFALO GNAT.—Swarms of these, which breed in running water, attack cattle, often causing them to stampede, and producing serious bites which may lead to death. Man is also attacked. They are also known as Black Flies (*Simulium* species).

BUFFER.—A substance which, when added to a solution, causes resistance to any change of hydrogen-ion concentration when either acid or alkali is added.

BUFFING is a term applied to the striking of the inside of one hoof at the quarter with some part of the opposite one. It is due to the same causes as BRUSHING (which see), but it occurs in horses that do not lift their feet very high. Less damage is done than in brushing, and it is not so likely to cause stumbling or lameness. It is corrected by the adoption of the same measures as those given under BRUSHING.

BUFOTALIN.—The principal poisonous substance present in the skin and saliva of the common European toad, *Bufo vulgaris*. Very small quantities will cause vomiting in dogs and cats, and ·00917 mg. per kg. bodyweight has caused death from heart-failure in the cat. (*See* TOADS.)

BUIATRICS.—The study of cattle and their diseases.

BUILDINGS (*see* HOUSING OF ANIMALS).

BULBAR PARALYSIS, INFECTIOUS (*see* AUJESZKY'S DISEASE). The term 'bulbar' relates to the *medulla oblongata* or the prolongation of the spinal cord into the brain.

BULL BEEF.—This is beef from the entire animal as opposed to the castrate. (*See under* CASTRATION.)

'BULL-DOGS'.—A small metal appliance used temporarily for the restraint of cattle. They are applied to the inside of the nose for holding an animal steady.

BULL-DOG CALVES.—In Dexter cattle commonly, and in other breeds occasionally, a hereditary condition, which is scientifically known as *achondroplasia*, occurs. Calves are born in a deformed condition in which the short limbs, dropsical swollen abdominal and thoracic cavities, and a marked foreshortening of the upper and lower jaws give the calf an appearance resembling a bull-dog. Such calves are usually dead when born.

The condition is governed by a semi-dominant gene.

BULL HOUSING.—Ministry of Agriculture advice is as follows: The best system of housing is where a bull is kept loose and has constant access to an uncovered exercising yard or pen. The house may be a loose-box, at least 12 feet × 10 feet; the door which leads into the pen should be kept open during the day. An open fronted shelter, from 12 feet to 15 feet deep, across one end of the pen, and with a short baffle wall to shelter the sleeping area, is satisfactory also.

The yard or pen should be up to 30 feet long, if sufficient space is available, and at least 12 feet wide. The walls of the pen or exercising yard should be built to a height of $3\frac{1}{2}$ feet and thereafter continued to a height of 6 feet with stout tubular steel rails. This allows the bull a good view of his surroundings and helps to prevent boredom, which can be one cause of viciousness in an animal. There should be a fodder rack and feeding trough, at the end away from the shelter, provided with just sufficient cover to give protection to the fodder and concentrates during rain and snow, and also to the animal whilst feeding. This arrangement encourages the bull to stay out in the open rather than in the box or shelter and is considered beneficial. The entrance to the pen should be convenient to the feeding area.

The feeding trough should be about 2 feet above ground level and should be fitted with a tubular tying arrangement which can be closed on the bull's neck when he puts his head through to the trough, if it is required to catch him. This equipment is very desirable as an added safety measure, as it permits the bull to be securely held before the attendant enters the pen. It is stocked by merchants specialising in cowshed fittings.

An arrangement which is very useful for dealing with vicious bulls is the provision of a strong overhead wire cable running from inside the house or shelter to the opposite end of the pen. This cable is threaded through a strong ring, about $2\frac{1}{2}$ inches in diameter. This ring, which slides along the cable, is attached to a chain which passes up through the bull's nose ring, then around the back of the horns and is hooked to the upright chain in front of the forehead. In this way, the weight of the chain is carried by the head instead of by the nose ring and considerable discomfort to the animal thereby avoided. The chain should be just sufficiently long to allow the animal to lie down comfortably. The advantage of this arrangement is that a cow can be brought into the pen for service without the necessity of having to release the bull from his tying.

Another safety device which should be provided, where possible, in the walls or railings surrounding the pen, is escape slits. These are upright openings about 15 inches to 18 inches wide, sufficient to allow the attendant to pass through in case of emergency, but through which a bull could not pass. If, due to the location of the pen, it is not possible to provide these escape slits, the blind corners of the pen should be fenced off by means of sturdy upright steel rails set 15 inches to 18 inches apart, behind which an attendant could seek refuge.

BULL LICENSING.—In Britain, all bulls must be licensed by the Ministry of Agriculture when 10 months old. (Application being made at least 28 days in advance.) In 1963 arrangements were made for up to 500 bulls to be kept on, unlicensed, for beef production trials. In 1969 some 3,000 bulls were reared for beef. (*See under* CASTRATION.) General class licences for bulls of the Ayrshire, British Friesian, British-Canadian, Holstein-Friesian, Red and White Friesian, Guernsey and Jersey breeds will not be issued unless the bulls reach the standards laid down for a Dairy Bull licence. In 1971 the licensing of cross-bred bulls was introduced.

BULL MANAGEMENT includes good feeding so that a youngster may be well grown and fit for service when 10 to 11 months old; exercise to keep him healthy, active, and with good hoofs; grooming to keep the skin clean and to keep him used to handling; service according to his age—not more than 1 per week or 3 in two weeks until 15 to 16 months old—and firm treatment always without either petting or teasing. Bulls should not be turned loose in a field with a herd of cows; the defects of this practice are that accurate records of dates of service cannot be kept, the fecundity of the bull may be impaired by unnecessary service, and there is a risk of breaking out of the field, especially if cows and heifers are in adjacent fields. Owners should realise that the bull is 'half the herd' and take care that in selection and management this 'half' is in no way neglected. Bulls should never be kept shut up in dark quarters—a cause of infertility. (*See* BULL HOUSING, *also* PROGENY TESTING *and* BULL LICENSING.)

'BULLETS.'—These are administered to cattle and sheep by means of a special dosing 'gun', and are used as a means of supplying the animal with a long-lasting supply of *e.g.* magnesium or cobalt, in order to prevent hypomagnesæmia or cobalt deficiency. Bullets are somewhat costly and not always retained.

BULLING (*see under* Œstrus, *in the paragraph headed Cow*).

BUMBLE-FOOT is a condition of the feet of poultry in which an abscess forms in the softer parts of the foot between the toes. It is caused by the penetration of some sharp object, such as a piece of glass, thorn, stone, etc., or by bruising of the tender tissues below the hard cuticle. An abscess slowly forms, accompanied by distinct lameness, and generally bursts by a small opening to the outside. Since pus in domestic fowls is always of a dry cheesy nature, the small hole formed does not afford an exit, and the lameness continues.

Treatment.—It is necessary to open thoroughly the pus-containing cavity and evacuate every small piece of the cheese-like contents. The inside is dressed with tincture of iodine, and a protective pad of cotton-wool is applied by bandaging afterwards. A second dressing may be necessary at the end of four days.

Brucella abortus has been isolated from a case of bumble-foot in Germany. Experimentally infected fowls excreted this organism. There is, however, no evidence that poultry act as a reservoir of brucellosis infection for cattle, though the possibility cannot be lightly dismissed.

BUNT ORDER.—Equivalent to the 'peck order' among poultry, this is the order of precedence established by cattle and pigs. With a newly mixed group of these animals there will be aggressiveness or actual fighting, until the dominant ones (usually the largest) establish their position in the social order. Once this is established, fighting will cease and the group will settle down, with the top animal being accorded precedence without having to fight for it. The second animal will be submissive to the first, but will take precedence over the rest; and so on down through the herd, with the bottom animal submissive to all. Occasionally two animals will be of equal rank, or there may be a somewhat complicated relationship between a small group as in the 'dominance circle'.

The bunt order can be important from a health point of view, and it can affect the farmer's profits. If, in large units, the batching of animals to ease management means frequent mixing or additions to established groups, stress will arise, and productive performance will decline. Stress will be *reduced* in the system whereby pigs occupy the same pen from birth to slaughter time. The health factor—as well as daily liveweight gains and feed conversion ratios—will be involved when there is, for example, insufficient trough space, and those animals at the bottom of the social scale may go hungry or thirsty. Similarly, the dominant animals will be able to choose more sheltered, less draughty places, while their inferiors may be cold and wet, and may suffer less from internal parasites because they can eat clean food. (*See* Stress.)

BURDIZZO EMASCULATOR (*see under* Castration, Cattle).

BURNS and SCALDS are injuries caused by heat, and though the former is caused by dry heat and the latter by moist heat their lesions and the treatment of these are similar.

Burns are often classified according to their depth and penetration as follows:

1st degree—affect hair and skin but do not destroy the skin;

2nd degree—destroy the skin superficially;

3rd degree—destroy the whole of the skin but not the underlying fascia and muscles;

4th degree—destroy skin, fascia, and muscles or other soft tissues;

5th degree—penetrate down to and involve bone or cartilage.

In animals a burn is usually easily recognised by singeing of the hair, or its destruction, but with a scald there may be little to be seen for several hours or even days. Moreover, a scalded area may remain concealed by a scab.

Burns and scalds are extremely painful, and will give rise to shock unless they are slight. After a few hours the absorption of poisonous break-down products from the damaged tissues may give rise to toxæmia; while destruction of skin affords means of entry for pathogenic bacteria, against which the burned tissues can offer little or no resistance. Death is a frequent sequel to extensive burns—the result of shock, toxæmia, or secondary infection.

Treatment.—Where the burn or scald is at all extensive, no time should be lost in calling in the veterinary surgeon, who may have to administer a narcotic or anæsthetic before local treatment can be attempted (and in order to relieve pain, and hence lessen shock).

In an emergency occurring where no first-aid kit is available, a *clean* handkerchief (or piece of linen) either dry or soaked in strong tea may be applied as a first-aid dressing. The part should be covered, the animal kept warm and offered water to drink.

The object of treatment, besides reducing pain, is to form rapidly a coagulum of protein on the surface of the burned area and diminish absorption of those altered proteins, from the damaged tissue, which give rise to toxæmia ; and also to prevent infection—to which the damaged tissue is so susceptible. Tannic acid (the useful constituent of the strong tea mentioned above) forms the desired coagulum. A tube or two of tannic acid jelly should be included in every first-aid kit for dealing with small burns. It should not be applied over large areas.

In remote areas overseas, where the animal-owner cannot obtain professional assistance, subsequent treatment must aim at avoiding sepsis ; the damaged tissues being very prone to infection. Sulphathiozole or sulphanilamide powder may be dusted lightly on to the area before a first or second application of tannic acid jelly. Subsequent irrigation of the part may be carried out with a hypochlorite solution, *e.g.* ' T.C.P.'.

For burns caused by caustic alkalis use vinegar or dilute acids ; for phenol and cresol burns, swab with cotton-wool soaked in alcohol and then smear with vaseline, oil, or fat.

Blood transfusion and the use of normal saline may be indicated in all serious burns.

BURNT SOLE is a condition which results from the fitting of a hot shoe to the horse's foot when the horn has been reduced to too great an extent, or when the hot shoe has been held to the foot for too long a time. It is most likely to occur when the horn is naturally thin, and when the sole is flat or convex. The heat penetrates through the thickness of the horn, and burns or blisters the sensitive structures below. It causes great pain and lameness, and may result in the production of a piece of dead sensitive tissue, with resultant separation of the horn and the production of pus. Professional advice should be sought.

BURSÆ are natural small cavities interposed between soft parts of the structure of the body where unusual pressure is likely to occur. They are found between a tendon or muscle, and some underlying harder structure, often a bony prominence, between fascia and harder tissue, and some are interposed between the skin and the underlying fascia. They are lined by smooth cells which secrete a small quantity of lubricating fluid, and they answer the purpose of allowing free movement without straining or tearing or undue friction of the parts.

BURSATI, or BURSATEE, is a diseased condition of the skin and underlying tissues of the horse, which is characterised by the formation of fibrous tumours and the ulceration of the covering skin. It occurs chiefly in India during the rainy season—June to October.

BURSITIS means inflammation within a bursa. **Acute bursitis** is generally due to external violence. It commonly occurs after runaway accidents, falls, continued slipping when driven at fast paces, and after kicks in the shoulder, where the bursa of the biceps tendon is involved. The cartilage over the groove through which the tendon of this muscle plays (called the intertubercular groove), may become inflamed. Lameness becomes gradually more and more marked and the horse becomes useless. Acute inflammation may attack the so-called ' bursa of the knee ', which is really a tendon sheath, as the result of punctured wounds at the back of the knee, the horse getting his foot

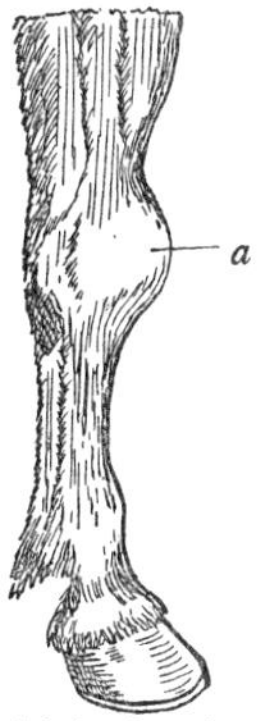

Example of bursitis in a horse's carpus (knee).
a, The swelling caused by the inflamed bursa.

into the manger and struggling to get free, and from bruises in this region. The acute form often leads to the chronic in this situation, with the production of ' knee thoroughpin ', a fluctuating swelling above and below the joint and to the inside. The bursa over the point of the elbow in the horse may become the seat of an acute inflammation as the result of the animal lying on a hard or rough floor with an insufficiency of bedding, or from injuries made by the calkin of the shoe when the horse lies. This is not so common as the chronic form, which in this situation leads to 'capped elbow'.

Chronic bursitis is much the commoner type of the disease among animals. It is due to an overuse of a bursa, or to a more or less continuous but mild irritation or pressure over the structure involved. The blemishes resulting are very commonly seen in all the domestic and many wild animals. The walls of the bursa increase in thickness, more fluid than usual is poured out, leading to a soft, almost painless swelling in which fluid can be detected. Later this fluid coagulates, the swelling becomes hard, and fibrous tissue invades the clotted material. In extreme cases the skin over the part becomes definitely horny in character, and the increase in size is very marked. 'Capped elbow' and 'capped hock' in the horse are instances of the condition due to lying on hard floors for a long period, or in the case of the elbow to the calkins of the shoe; 'lumpy withers' are of the same nature, due to the pressure of a badly fitting saddle, and often lead to fistulous withers; hygromata or 'big knees' in cattle result either from a shortage of bedding at the front of the stance, or from the animals continually striking their knees on a too high feeding-trough when rising; in dogs the same conditions are often seen both on the knees, hocks, sternum, and stifles, particularly in old and very lean individuals which lie a lot; monkeys, both in captivity and in a free state, develop similar lumps on the points of their buttocks.

Treatment.—In the early stages of bursitis, rest, cold applications alternated with hot fomentations, stimulating and absorbent liniments, painting with tincture of iodine or other mild counter-irritants, and massage will reduce the inflammation in most instances. When the condition is perverse or after it becomes chronic there is little hope of effecting a cure, but considerable benefit may be effected by surgical means. Sometimes when the swelling is large and organised (filled with fibrous tissue cells), complete amputation of the whole mass is practised with good results (*See* KNEE THOROUGHPIN, CAPPED ELBOW, CAPPED HOCK, LUMPY WITHERS, FISTULOUS WITHERS, HYGROMA, etc.)

'BUSH FOOT'.—This is a term applied to a severe lesion associated with foot-rot in pigs in New Zealand, Australia, the U.K., etc. The infection involves *Fusiformis necrophorus* and spirochætes in the U.K. (*See Vet. Record* September 18, 1965.) (*See* FOOT-ROT IN PIGS.)

BUSH SICKNESS.—A cobalt deficiency disease occurring in certain sheep-rearing districts of North Island, New Zealand. It is characterised by inability to thrive, emaciation, anæmia, and ultimate prostration, and affects probably all herbivorous animals, although sheep and cattle suffer most. One of the greatest sources of loss is the difficulty experienced in getting females to breed in a bush sick area.

The type of soil is usually blown coarse sand, coarse-textured gravelly sand, or 'sandy silt', and the disease is always worst on land that has been recently cleared and burnt. With time, especially if cultivation is undertaken, the severity of the condition decreases, and it may entirely disappear.

The cause is a deficiency in the soil, and consequently in the herbage, of the small amounts of cobalt, which is the trace element needed to enable the body to utilize iron needed for the formation of the hæmoglobin of the red blood cells. In this respect, bush sickness is very similar to conditions which are called by other names in various parts of the world, such as 'Pining', 'Vanquish' or 'Vinquish' in Scotland; 'Nakuruitis' in Kenya; 'Coast disease' in Tasmania; and 'Salt sickness' in Florida.

Earlier, it was shown in New Zealand that the oxide of iron deposit known as 'limonite' may be used on bush sick holdings as a lick, and will prevent or cure the disease very effectively. It contains very small amounts of copper and cobalt as impurities. Various medicinal compounds may be administered to ailing animals by hand. A mineral lick in which small amounts of the essential trace elements are incorporated is used for preventing illness in deficient areas; also cobalt pellets which disintegrate slowly in the (usually 4th) stomach, giving protection for 9 months or so.

BUSS DISEASE.—This occurs among cattle in the U.S.A., Australia, and Japan. It is also called Sporadic Bovine Encephalomyelitis. The cause is a virus.

Affected calves become dull and may show a drooling of saliva and a discharge from the nose. Laboured breathing, a cough, diarrhœa, and a staggering gait are other symptoms. Control of the disease is difficult.

'BUTCHER'S JELLY' (*see* LICKED BEEF).

BUTTERCUP POISONING.—The common buttercups of meadowlands may be divided into two classes: (1) those that are dangerous when eaten by cattle, and (2) those less poisonous. Of the former class *Ranunculus scleratus*, the celery-leaved buttercup; *R. acris*, the acrid buttercup or the tall crowfoot; *R. flammula*, the lesser spearwort; *R. bulbosus*, the bulbous buttercup, are the most common; while *R. ficaria*, the lesser celandine, and *R. lingua* may be mentioned among the latter class. In addition to these there are certain varieties which appear to be practically harmless except when eaten in large amounts, such as *R. ripens* and *R. aquatilis*. Notwithstanding these facts there is no doubt that at certain times of the year almost any of the plants enumerated above may be eaten by stock with impunity, while at other times the plants are all dangerous to a greater or lesser degree. The toxicity of buttercups varies in different localities and probably on different soils in the same locality. (*See under* WEEDKILLERS.)

The growing flower-heads are the most dangerous, then the leaves, and the stem contains least of the poison. The fruits or seeds of the plant seem to be practically harmless. Drying in the sun destroys the toxic principles, and consequently buttercups in dried hay are harmless.

Symptoms.—Buttercups are acrid, burning, and narcotic. They cause irritation and inflammation of the intestinal mucous membranes, gastro-enteritis, colic, and black, foul-smelling liquid motions are passed. Loss of condition appears, and the milk yield of cows falls off. The milk may have a smoky-red appearance and a bitter taste. In cattle that have eaten large amounts of buttercups the pulse is small and irregular, the breathing is stertorous (snoring), the pupil is dilated, there is difficulty in mastication, and the eye-lids, lips, and ears show quivering movements. Convulsions and death follow.

Treatment.—Cathartics or purgatives should be given hypodermically if possible.

When sucking lambs are affected with purging and indigestion on a pasture where buttercups are numerous, they should be moved onto a field of young grass (seed hay), or to a cultivated green crop.

BUTTERFAT (*see under* FIBRE *on* p. 257, *and also* MILK).

BUTYL CHLORIDE.—An anthelmintic.

B.V.A.—The British Veterinary Association, of 7 Mansfield Street, Portlan Place, London, W.1.

B.W.D. (*see under* BACILLARY WHITE DIARRHŒA).

C

CAB-HORSE DISEASE is met with in the limbs of old horses. An exostosis or new growth of bone occurs on the inner and posterior surface of the long pastern bone (first phalanx) of the fore-leg. Generally, it is nothing more than a blemish, since it is not situated near to either of the joints. It may cause lameness when it is developing, but this subsides when the swelling becomes established. Cab-horse disease is often associated with RINGBONE (which see).

CABBAGE contains a goitrogenic factor and may cause goitre if it forms too large a proportion of the diet over a period.

Excessive quantities of cabbage fed to cattle may lead to anæmia, hæmoglobinuria and death.

CACHEXIA (κακός, bad; ἕξις, condition) is the feeble state produced by serious disease, especially cancer or tuberculosis.

CADERAS, MAL DE (*see* PARASITES).

CADMIUM ANTHRANILATE is used in America against ascarid worms in the pig, the dose being given mixed in the food. The Food and Drug Administration there, however, insists that it must be used only once during a store pig's lifetime, owing to the danger to human consumers. Acute cadmium poisoning results in vomiting. In the rat, chronic poisoning is characterised by bleaching of the incisor teeth, anæmia, hypertrophy of the heart, and hyperplasia of the bone-marrow.

CADZOW IMPROVER RAM.—A hybrid developed from the Dorset Horn and the Finnish Landrace breeds, with the object of crossing with a British native hill ewe to give vigorous progeny. The ewe of the cross is likely to have a lambing percentage of 200 plus, it is claimed.

CÆCUM (*caecus*, blind) is the blind end of the large intestine, into which opens the termination of the small intestine. Its shape varies in the domesticated animals; it is largest in the horse, smaller and less important in the ox, sheep, and pig, and quite small in the dog. (*See* INTESTINES.)

CÆSAREAN SECTION means the removal of the unborn young from the dam by surgical incision into the walls of the abdomen and the uterus, which are afterwards sutured. It is so called because it is believed that Julius Cæsar made his entry into the world in this way. This delicate and somewhat intricate operation is chiefly performed in bitches, sows, cows, and ewes; occasionally in the mare.

The operation is performed when the pelvic passage is for some reason unable to accommodate and discharge the fœtus; when the fœtus has become jammed in such a position that it cannot pass through the pelvis, and its delivery cannot be effected; when the value of the progeny is greater than the value of the dam; and when the dam is *in extremis* and it is believed that the young is or are still alive. (In this latter case the dam is usually killed and the abdomen and uterus are opened at once. There is a possibility of saving the fœtus in the mare and the cow by this method, provided that not more than two minutes elapse between the time when the dam ceases to breathe and when the young animal commences. The foal or calf will die from lack of oxygen if this period be exceeded.)

Other indications for Cæsarean section are: cases of physical immaturity of the dam, failure of the cervix to dilate, torsion of the uterus, the presence of a monster and, perhaps, pregnancy toxæmia.

CAFFEINE is a white crystalline substance obtained from the coffee plant, of which it is the active principle. It is almost identical with *theine*, the alkaloid of tea, and similar to *kreatine*, which gives beef-tea its stimulating properties. Caffeine is used as a heart stimulant for cases of collapse, or when it would not be wise to administer strychnine. It can be given either hypodermically or by the mouth.

CAGE BIRDS, DISEASES OF.—Budgerigars, canaries, parrots, and other birds commonly kept in cages are subject to a wide range of diseased conditions, and the veterinary reader is referred to the article by L. Arnall, B.V.Sc. (*Vet. Rec.*, 73, 173, 237). Diseases include: rickets (common in young budgerigars and to be suspected if the wings are powerless and the legs stunted), osteomalacia and ostetodystrophy, 'feather cysts' (hard, yellow swellings under the skin of back and wings in the canary), fatty tumours and malignant growths.

The crop may be impacted, and if medicinal liquid paraffin has no effect, it may have to be opened surgically. A torn crop is a common condition, and requires sutures. Persistent vomiting may indicate 'sour crop'; for which 0·1 per cent gentian violet solution, given by eye-dropper into the mouth, may be tried, and the diet varied. Prolapse of the rectum may be due to, or simulated by, a tumour. Rupture of the abdomen may follow fatty degeneration of the abdominal muscles. An ill bird with a soft swelling of the abdomen may have a ruptured oviduct and peritonitis. Prolapse of the oviduct may occur.

Laboured breathing, associated with rhythmical dipping of the tail, and closing of the eyes while on the perch, suggests heart disease and dropsy of the lungs. Gape-worms, mucus, or aspirated food material may block the upper air passages. Air-sacs may be punctured by the claws of cats, and if infected, or filled with blood or exudate, pneumonia is to be expected as a sequel.

Faulty diet, infestation by mites, and injury are among the causes of beak abnormalities, which need correcting at an early stage with scissors. In the female budgerigar especially, the nostrils may become blocked by sebaceous or other material. Horn-like excrescences near the eyes may be associated with mite infestation.

Dry gangrene of the feet may follow a fracture of the limb or the presence of ergot in the seed. Fractures of the legs result from their being caught in the wires of the cage. Dislocation of the hip is not rare. Overgrown and twisted claws are common. (*See also* PSITTACOSIS, TUBERCULOSIS.)

For more about budgerigars, the veterinary reader is referred to the *Journal of Small Animal Practice* for February 1965.

The over-heating of 'non-stick' frying pans in kitchens gives rise to vapour which was shown in 1969 to kill budgerigars and other small birds within half an hour. The substance involved is polytetrafluoroethylene.

'CAGE LAYER FATIGUE.'—A form of leg paralysis in poultry attributed to insufficient exercise during the rearing period. (*See* BATTERY SYSTEM.) Most birds recover wit hina week if removed from the cage or if a piece of cardboard is placed over the floor of the cage.

The long bones are found to be very fragile. The precise cause is obscure. A bone-meal supplement may prove helpful.

CAKE POISONING (*see also* GOSSYPOL POISONING).—Under suitable conditions of warmth and moisture, linseed cake is capable of producing small amounts of prussic acid, owing to the interaction of an enzyme, *linase*, with a glucoside, *linamarin*, both of which are normally present in linseed. The amount of prussic acid formed may be sufficient to produce symptoms of poisoning in calves and lambs. Linseed cake should consequently be fed in a dry form, and soaking in warm water, making pastes, and so on should be avoided. Gruels made with linseed or linseed cake meal should be boiled for 10 to 15 minutes to render them safe by destroying the enzyme. Prussic acid is very volatile, and is given off into the atmosphere almost as soon as it is formed; when formed in the body it is very rapidly absorbed and eliminated, so that cumulation of the poison in the system does not occur. It is not advisable to feed linseed cake to young animals along with mashes, yeast, or malt products, or with large quantities of succulent green food, because these foods materially assist in the formation of the acid.

Linseed cake, and certain compound cakes which include linseed that has been grown in India particularly, sometimes contain proportions of rape and mustard seeds; the latter, when it exceeds about 3 per cent of the bulk of the original sample (*i.e.* before manufacture of the cake), is liable to produce symptoms of mustard poisoning. Young store cattle and sheep are attacked with violent diarrhœa and straining a few days after the cake is first fed. If the cake is stopped immediately the symptoms disappear, but if more of it is fed the diarrhœa increases in severity and death occurs. The treatment consists in administering a mild saline purge to eliminate any dangerous material from the bowels, and thereafter giving demulcent drinks, such as milk, gruels, and lime-water. The contaminated cake should, of course, be fed no longer.

CALABAR BEANS are the ripe seeds of *Physostigma venenosum*, from which the alkaloid *eserine* or *physostigmine* is obtained. (*See* PHYSOSTIGMINE.)

CALAMINE, or CARBONATE OF ZINC, is a mild astringent used to protect and soothe the irritated skin in cases of wet or weeping eczema, and is used in the form of calamine lotion.

CALCIFEROL is a crystalline substance extracted from irradiated ergosterol. (*See* VITAMIN D.)

CALCIFICATION is a term used in pathology to indicate that condition of a tissue in which there is a deposit of calcium carbonate laid down as a sequel to an inflammatory reaction. In animals, the commonest instances are those met with in old-standing tuberculous abscesses in cows, where the body cells have formed a fibrous ring round the seat of the tubercle bacilli, and a deposit of calcium salts has occurred inside this barrier. Areas of calcification have been described as Nature's gravestones erected over the bodies of the dead invaders.

For calcification in the lungs of puppies, leading to death at 10 to 20 days old, see the *Vet. Record* for September 4, 1965.

CALCINED MAGNESITE.—This contains 87 to 90 per cent magnesium oxide, and being cheaper than pure magnesium oxide is used for top-dressing pastures (10 cwt. per acre), and for supplementary feeding of cattle, in the prevention of hypomagnesæmia. In the powder form, much is apt to get wasted, but if the granular kind is well mixed with damp sugar-beet pulp or cake, the manger is usually licked clean.

CALCIUM is a metallic element which combines with bases to form salts. The commonest of these are: **Calcium oxide,** or *quicklime, calx,* or *lime*; **Calcium hydrate,** or *slaked lime*; **Calcium carbonate,** or *chalk,* from which is formed the *prepared chalk* used in medicine; **Calcium sulphate,** or *plaster of Paris*; **Calcium chloride**; **Calcium hypochlorite,** also called *chlorinated lime* or *bleaching powder.* **Calcium borogluconate** is a compound of calcium, boric acid, and glucose, which is used to replace lowered blood calcium in milk fever and other diseases. In addition to these, the phosphate, the hypophosphate, and the sulphurate are used in medicine.

Actions and Uses.—Quicklime is a caustic and irritant much used for the destruction of carcases of animals that have died from an infectious disease, when it is buried in the grave in which the animal is interred. (*See under* QUICKLIME.) Purified quicklime slaked with distilled water forms lime-water, an agent used as a sedative, antacid, and astringent. Saccharated lime-water contains refined sugar in solution and is about five times richer in lime content than the plain lime-water. Prepared chalk has similar actions to lime-water, but it is less rapidly absorbed and is able to act as an astringent on the walls of the intestines. It is useful in diarrhœa when the bowel walls are in an irritable state. It is an antidote to poisoning by the mineral acids and by oxalic acid. Plaster of Paris is mixed up with water, spread on to bandages, and used to immobilise the broken ends of the bones in fractures. It sets hard when dry. Bleaching powder is a compound which, when fresh, is rich in chlorine, and is used as a disinfecting, deodorising, and cleansing agent for the walls and floors of byres, stables, etc. (*See also* CAT FOODS, HYPOCALCÆMIA.)

CALCIUM SUPPLEMENTS.—These may consist of bone meal, bone flour, ground limestone, or chalk.

Such supplements must be used with care, for an excess of calcium in the diet may interfere with the body's absorption or employment of other elements. A high calcium to phosphorous ratio will depress the growth-rate in heifers. Dr. Ruth Allcroft has also pointed out that: ' This effect of excess dietary calcium on absorption of magnesium and on growth rate make it pertinent to consider that many modern rations for cattle and sheep supply very high intakes of calcium. For example, the majority of proprietary pelleted rations for cows, calves, and sheep contain from 1 to 4 per cent of a mineral supplement consisting of limestone, bone flour and salt. These concentrate rations are frequently fed as well as grass, hay, and silage. Legume hays, and to some extent, grass-clover hays are very high in calcium. In addition most stock are offered *ad lib.* compound mineral mixtures which may contain a high percentage of calcium as limestone, bone flour or dicalcium phosphate and often contain limestone as well as either of the other calcium-phosphorus compounds. Thus, the heavily yielding dairy cow, or the calf which is being 'done extra well', may be ingesting excessive amounts of calcium in relation to magnesium and other essential minerals, thereby causing conditioned deficiencies.

'For many years now there have been indications that too much calcium is a contributory cause of goitre.

'The inter-relationship of zinc and calcium in the development of parakeratosis in pigs is well known', and a calcium carbonate supplement in excess can increase the risk of Piglet Anæmia. Calcium without phosphorus will not prevent rickets; both minerals being required for healthy bone.

CALCULI (*calculus*, a pebble).—Stones or concretions containing salts of calcium that are found in various parts of the body, such as the bowels, kidneys, bladder, gall-bladder, urethra, bile and pancreatic ducts, etc. They are either the result of the ingestion of a piece of foreign material such as a small piece of metal or a stone (in the case of the bowels), or they originate through some one or other of the body secretions being too rich in salts of potash, calcium, sodium, or magnesium.

Urinary calculi, found in the pelvis of the kidney, in the ureters, urinary bladder, and often in the male urethra, are collections of urates, oxalates, carbonates, or phosphates, of calcium and magnesium. Urates are common in the dog and cat; carbonates in the horse and ox; and ammonium-magnesium phosphate is often found in stones from the sheep and pig. They weigh almost anything up to 8 ounces, and may be few and large, or many and small. (*See also* p. 96.) The nucleus of the calculus is a mucoprotein. Secretion of this and the occurrence of urinary calculi are linked, though the cause is not fully understood.

Urinary calculi associated with high grain rations, and the use of œstrogen implants, produce heavy losses among fattening cattle and sheep in the feedlots of the United States and Canada. 'However, this condition does not seem to present the same problem in the barley beef units in this country, although outbreaks do occur in sheep fed high grain rations. Udall found that the inclusion of 4 per cent NaCl in the diet decreased the incidence of urinary calculi.' —H. C. Wilson.

Intestinal calculi (enteroliths) are found in the large intestines of horses particularly, especially when fed upon large amounts of bran. They are usually formed of phosphates and may reach enormous sizes, weighing as much as 22 lb. in some instances. In many cases they are formed around a nucleus of metal or stone which has been accidentally taken in with the food, and in other instances they are deposited upon the surfaces of already existing oat-hair balls, dung-balls, etc. (*See* Wool Balls.)

Salivary calculi, found in the duct of the parotid gland (Stenson's duct), along the side of the face of the horse. A hard swelling can usually be both seen and felt, and the horse resents handling of this part. They are rarely seen in the ox and dog.

Billiary calculi are found either in the bile-ducts of the liver or in the gall-bladder. (*Note*.—There is no gall-bladder in animals of the horse tribe.) They may result either from bile which has undergone concentration and 'inspissation', or they may be salts deposited from it in the same way as with urine. They are combinations of carbonates, calcium, and phosphates, along with the bile pigments, and have, accordingly, many colours; they may be yellow, brown, red, green, or chalk-white in colour.

Pancreatic calculi in the ducts of the pancreas have been observed, but are rare.

Lacteal calculi, either in the milk sinus of the cow's udder or in the teat canal, are formed from calcium phosphate from the milk deposited around a piece of shed epithelial tissue. They may give rise to obstruction in milking.

Treatment.—In many cases the only method of dealing with themis surgical excision, whenever they are in a position and of such a nature as to allow of this being performed. Recent reports claim success with Hyaluronidase in treating urinary calculi.

CALF DIPHTHERIA is a disease of calves generally under 6 weeks of age, in which greyish patches appear on the mucous membrane of the mouth and throat, and less often on the nose, caused by the *Actinomyces necrophorus*. Generally speaking, it can be regarded as most frequently associated with bad housing, feeding, and management.

Symptoms.—Affected calves lose their

spirits, cease to suck or feed, salivate profusely, have difficulty in swallowing, become fevered, and may be affected with diarrhœa. The mouth is painful, the tongue swollen, and grey patches of a variable size are seen on the surface of the mucous membrane of the cheeks, gums, tongue, and throat. On removal of one of these thickish, easily detached, membranous deposits, the underlying tissues are seen reddened and inflamed, and are very painful to the touch. The bone or muscle below the patch may be the seat of necrosis, and the tissues in the vicinity are then much swollen. In the course of 3 or 4 days the weaker or more seriously affected calves die, but the majority live for 2 or 3 weeks, develop complications in the form of pneumonia or diarrhœa with enteritis, and die from intoxication and exhaustion. A few cases do recover.

Treatment.—Since the disease can be transmitted by indirect means as well as by immediate contact, by the feeding-pails, attendants, etc., it is necessary to remove the healthy calves from the diseased ones as soon as calf diphtheria makes its appearance, and to ensure rigorous isolation. Internally, the use of penicillin under strict supervision gives good results when used early in an outbreak.

CALF MORTALITY (*see* CALVES, DISEASES OF, GROUNDNUT MEAL).

CALF PNEUMONIA.—Virus pneumonia of calves occurs in Britain, the rest of Europe, and North America. It is a disease of housing, and the practice of good hygiene and the avoidance of damp, dark, cold surroundings will go a long way towards preventing it. Scours are often associated, probably the result of secondary bacterial infections.

In 1962, Mr. A. B. Paterson, Ministry of Agriculture, referred to 5 transmissible pneumonias of calves: Calf Influenzal Pneumonia, Enzootic Pneumonia, Calf Pneumonia—Enteritis, Cuffing Pneumonia, and Inclusion Body Pheumonia. All these are caused by viruses of which at least eight have been incriminated, namely :—

Parainfluenza 3	—a myxovirus
Bovine adenovirus 1	—an adenovirus
Bovine adenovirus 2	—an adenovirus
Bovine adenovirus 3	—an adenovirus
Infectious bovine rhinotracheitis—	—a herpes virus
Mucosal disease virus	—a pseudo-myxovirus
Bovine reovirus(es)	—reovirus
Bedsonia organisms	—psittacosis-type agents

CALF PENS.—Housing for calves must be warm but not stuffy (well ventilated), dry, well lit by windows, and easy to clean and disinfect. Individual pens prevent navel-sucking.

CALF-REARING.—*In dairy herds*, as a rule, only bull calves being kept for breeding are ever allowed to suckle for the normal period or are pail-fed with whole milk throughout.

Otherwise, calves are either removed at birth, or are allowed to suckle the dam for 3 or 4 days before being removed ; in the latter case, they receive the colostrum at the normal temperature. (*See* COLOSTRUM.)

After colostrum, the calves receive ordinary whole milk (which should be fed warm three or four times a day for the first three weeks) ; or sometimes they are given a proprietary milk substitute. For an average calf, three quarts of milk per day will be enough for the first couple of days. This quantity may be increased gradually to four quarts at the end of the first week and to six quarts in the third week. At a fortnight old, a gruel (often incorporating a special 'calf-starter' mixture) may replace whole milk. Another method is to give whole milk until the fourth week, and then gradually change to a 'follow-on' concentrate mixture—upon which the calf will be subsisting at 8 weeks. Yet another method consists in offering whole milk and an 'early weaning' concentrate mixture from 4 days or a week old onwards ; entirely replacing the milk between the third and fifth weeks. (*See* EARLY WEANING, *and below*.)

Clean water should be offered *ad lib.* from 3 weeks of age. The use of skim milk or whey may, where convenient, be introduced as variants of the systems given above.

In beef herds, single suckling is the rule in typical beef-producing areas where only beef animals are bred ; but multiple suckling on nurse cows is common practice in beef-rearing herds where calves are bought in for the purpose. Under this system a cow suckles two or more calves at a time for at least 9 to 10 weeks and these are then weaned and replaced by another two which suckle for a similar period. Another two calves, or perhaps only one, may follow these and then, as a rule, one more calf is suckled. Thus, one cow, according to her milk-yielding capacity, may suckle from 3 to 10 calves in the course of the lactation. (*See* NURSE COWS.)

Professor M. M. Cooper has commented : ' Except where it is a means of utilising an otherwise idle cow, multiple suckling is not advocated. It is expensive in terms of milk usage, it is a " messy job ", and it results in uneven lots of cattle which are not easily bunched. Quite the best approach is the new method of early weaning, using a high-quality dry food. Provided the calf has had colostrum, it can go on to a reputable proprietary milk substitute until about a month old. Meanwhile, it has been offered, and will be eating the palatable dry food which need not be expensive proprietary pencils. At Cockle Park we have reared many calves very successfully on the following type of home mix :

45 parts of flaked maize.
25 ,, ,, rolled oats.
10 ,, ,, dried skim milk.
10 ,, ,, molassine meal.
10 ,, ,, soya bean or linseed meal.
Plus vitamins and minerals.

' This is fed, along with good hay *ad lib.*, up to a maximum of 5 lb. daily, till the calves are 10 weeks old, when they are switched to a cheaper mix, such as the following :

35 parts of rolled oats.
30 ,, ,, crushed barley.
20 ,, ,, flaked maize.
15 ,, ,, soya bean meal.

' This is fed at 3–4 lb. per day along with hay and silage to appetite.

' The system is an economical one, in terms of both food and labour ; and once calves are weaned from milk, which is best done abruptly, there is a virtual absence of scouring. By the time the calves are four months old they will have attained their normal weight for age.'

(*See also* BEEF-BREEDS AND CROSSES.)

The bought-in calf often arrives, from market or dealer, suffering from exposure, exhausted by a long journey, or nearing starvation. Often the calf has been exposed to infection on the way ; and it should be remembered that antibodies received from its dam in the colostrum protect only against infections current in its original environment—not necessarily against infections present on another farm. Liquid feeding for the first day may consist of three feeds of two pints warm water into which has been dissolved two tablespoons of glucose. An early-weaning concentrate should be on offer *ad lib.*

CALF SCOUR (*see* WHITE SCOURS).

CALF VACCINATION SERVICE.—In 1963 the Ministry of Agriculture in Britain introduced a free service for vaccinating heifer calves against Brucellosis. (Which see.)

CALIFORNIA MASTITIS TEST (C.M.T.).—Using Teepol as a reagent, this test may be carried out in the cowshed for the detection of cows with subclinical mastitis. The test can also be used as a rough screening test of bulk milk in order to determine the approximate extent of mastitis in a herd.

CALKINS are the portions of the heels of horses' shoes which are turned down so as to form projections on the ground surface of the shoe, which will obtain a grip upon the surface of the roadway. They are most common in Scotland and the North of England, but they are met with in countries abroad as well. Where there are small spaces left between the stones of pavements or causewayed surfaces, calkins may assist a horse to keep its feet better than when shod with a flat shoe ; but upon smooth surfaces, and on the land, they serve no useful purpose. If they are too high they lead to atrophy of the frog and induce contracted heels unless the shoe possesses a bar.

In winter when the roads are slippery the calkins are sometimes ' roughed ', *i.e.* they are sharpened so that they will cut into the ice and give a better grip.

CALLOSITY (*callositas*, hardness of skin) means thickening of the skin, usually accompanied by loss of hair and a dulling of sensation. Callosities are generally found on those parts of the bodies of old animals that are exposed to continued contact with the ground, such as the elbows, hocks, stifles, and the knees of cattle and dogs. (*See* HARNESS GALLS, HYGROMA.)

CALLUS (*callus*, hard skin) is the lump of new bone that is laid down during the first 2 or 3 weeks after fracture, around the broken ends of the bone, and which holds these in position. Three stages can be recognised: (1) the formation of the soft callus; (2) formation of the hard callus; (3) absorption of the hard callus. (*See* FRACTURES.)

CALOMEL, or **MERCURIC SUBCHLORIDE,** should not be confounded with the much more active and poisonous *perchloride*, which is used as an external antiseptic and disinfectant. Calomel is a useful purgative having a special action on the bile-mechanism of the liver. (*See* MERCURY.)

CALORIE, or **CALORY,** is the name applied to a unit of energy. Two units are called by this name—the small calorie, *gram calorie*, or standard calorie, is the amount of heat required to raise 1 gram of water 1 degree centigrade in temperature; the large calorie, or *kilocalorie*, which is used in the study of dietetics and physiological processes, is the amount of heat required to raise 1 kilogram of water 1 degree centigrade.

CALVES, DISEASES OF.—These include WHITE SCOUR, JOINT-ILL, CALF DIPHTHERIA, TUBERCULOSIS, JOHNE'S DISEASE, HUSK, PARASITIC GASTRO-ENTERITIS, PNEUMONIA, RINGWORM, MUSCULAR DYSTROPHY. PARATYPHOID, GASTRIC ULCERS, RICKETS, SALMONELLOSIS.

CALVING (*see* PARTURITION and TEMPERATURE).

CALVING INDEX, INTERVAL.—In England and Wales in 1968 the average calving interval was about 13 months, but farmers' profits could be higher if it was 12 months.

In order to achieve a calving index of 365 days, it is necessary to get the cows in calf between the 8th and 12th week after calving. This entails regarding the period up to 7 or 8 weeks after calving as a 'preparation period', during which all heat periods, and expected subsequent heat periods, should be recorded on a wall chart or breeding calendar.

Cows that do not come into season regularly generally have cysts or other infertility disorders which, when spotted at an early stage, can be treated by the veterinary surgeon so that they are cycling regularly again before they have been calved more than eight weeks, thus improving their chances of holding to the first service to calve within the year.

Sometimes, however, these irregularities do not become apparent until they have been calved longer than eight weeks so, as a further precaution, it is advisable, as a routine measure, to have each cow inspected three weeks after calving to see whether she has returned to normal again. If she has not, this allows additional time for treatment during this limited preparation period.

CAMBOROUGH.—A hybrid female developed from Large White and Landrace pigs. Litter size consistently averages 10 or more.

CAMPHOR is a solid oily substance distilled from the wood of a species of laurel—*Cinnamomum camphora*. Camphor possesses sedative, carminative, expectorant, and antiseptic actions. Externally it is primarily stimulating to nerve endings in the skin, and later sedative, and is employed in many liniments to allay superficial inflammation.

Internally, camphor was used as a heart stimulant, as an expectorant, and as an intestinal antiseptic in some cases of diarrhœa.

CANADIAN HORSE-POX (*see* ACNE. CONTAGIOUS).

CANALICULUS means a small channel, and is applied to the minute passage leading from the lacrimal pore on each eyelid to the lacrimal sac in the nostril.

CANCELLOUS is a term applied to loose bony tissues as found in the ends of the long bones.

CANCER is a group of diseases and not a single disease entity. (*See under* CARCINOMATA AND SARCOMATA for possible causes, research, and treatment; *also under* LEUKÆMIA, MELANOTIC, TUMOURS.) Cancer is not uncommon in domestic animals and farm-livestock.

CANDIDA ALBICANS.—A fungus which gives rise to the disease MONILIASIS or CANDIDASIS, both in humans and in farm livestock.

CANICOLA FEVER.—The disease in man caused by the parasite *Leptospira canicola*, which is excreted in the urine of infected dogs. Paresis may occur and some few cases of this disease may resemble poliomyelitis. 'Mild conjunctivitis and nephritis accompanying symptoms of meningitis are suggestive of

Canicola fever'. The parasite may be harboured by pigs and the disease has been recorded among workers on pig farms. (*See* LEPTOSPIROSIS.)

CANINE DISTEMPER (*see* DISTEMPER)

CANINE HERPESVIRUS.—A virus isolated from vesicles affecting the genital system of the dog and associated with infertility, abortion, and stillbirths. It is abbreviated for convenience to CHV.

CANINE RICKETTSIOSIS.—A tick-borne fever caused by *Rickettsia canis* and occurring in Africa, the Mediterranean region, and India. Symptoms include a high temperature (up to 107 degrees Fahrenheit), thirst, loss of appetite, a staring coat, a brown discolouration of mouth and teeth with an unpleasant odour. A discharge from eyes and nose, and a Distemper-like rash may be seen. Death may occur within days or weeks. Dogs which recover may become 'carriers'. Antibiotics are said to be effective in treatment.

CANINE TEETH are the so-called 'eye-teeth', which are such prominent features of the mouths of carnivorous animals. In different animals they are known by different names, *e.g.* 'tusks' in the pig, dog, and cat, and 'tushes' in the horse and ass. (*See* DENTITION, TEETH.)

CANINE TRANSMISSIBLE VENEREAL TUMOUR.—A few cases of this have been seen in the U.K. and Eire, and it may cause infertility.

CANINE VIRUS HEPATITIS.—This is also known as Rubarth's disease or *Hepatitis contagiosa canis*, or C.V.H.

Dogs of all ages may be affected—even puppies a few days old—but perhaps the disease occurs most frequently in young dogs of 3–9 months.

Cause.—A virus.

Symptoms.—Infection may exist without symptoms, and in such cases it can be recognised only by means of laboratory methods. In the very acute form of the disease a dog, apparently well the night before, may be found dead in the morning. In less acute cases the dog may behave strangely and have convulsions. A high temperature, wasting, anæmia, lethargy, and coma are other symptoms observed in some cases. A thin, thready pulse is characteristic.

Vomiting, diarrhœa, and dullness may persist for 5 or 6 days, and be followed by jaundice.

Such cases may be thought to be leptospiral jaundice.

Puppies may show symptoms of severe internal hæmorrhage, and have blood or blood-stained fluid in the peritoneal cavity, with petechial hæmorrhages from several organs. Hæmorrhages, including subcutaneous ones, may also occur in older dogs.

More commonly, there is fever, dullness, some vomiting, tenderness of the abdomen. Of those that survive 5 days or so, many recover.

Keratitis ('blue eye') occurs a week or two after the beginning of the illness in some cases.

In older dogs, restlessness, convulsions, and coma are common.

Antiserum is useful in treatment. Glucose and vitamin K are also recommended.

Canine Virus Hepatitis may occur simultaneously with Distemper (which see).

Dogs which have recovered may continue to harbour the virus and act as 'carriers', spreading the disease to other dogs via the urine. (*See also under* GLOBULIN.)

Diagnosis.—A gel diffusion test is useful at *post-mortem* examination, especially where decomposition of the animal's body has involved cell disintegration.

'CANKER OF' THE EAR (*see* EAR, DISEASES OF).

CANKER OF THE FOOT is a chronic, hypertrophic condition of the horny sole, frog, and walls of the horse's foot; moist softening in which considerable production of soft cheesy material and overgrowth of the sensitive tissues occur. Since the horn is a modified form of skin, the condition is similar to wet eczema in other parts. This disease was at one time one of the most common of the troubles of the feet of draught horses in the heavy clay districts of England. It is pre-eminently a disease of the foul, badly drained, damp stable, where the horses are called upon to stand for long periods upon layers of decomposing dung soaked with urine, and especially when they get their feet wet several times a day through wading in muddy or stagnant ponds. The continual wetting of the hoof softens it and causes it to swell, and later decomposition occurs, whereby organisms gain entrance below the horn, set up irritation and slow inflammation, producing an abnormally soft growth. The hind-feet are more often affected than the fore. One, two, three or all four feet may be affected at the same time, or it may appear in one foot first, and at a later stage it may develop in one of the others. Animals of the heavy draught type are the most often affected, especially Shires, Clydesdales, and Suffolks, but the lighter breeds are also liable to be attacked. It is extremely rare in the mountain breeds of ponies, in Arabs and thoroughbreds; and hackneys are only seldom affected. It is seen in horses of all ages above 3 years, and is as common in young adults as in the aged. It is rare in the mule and never seen in the donkey.

Many different organisms have been isolated from cases, but those most frequently found are spirochætes, species of necrophorus bacilli, and staphylococci. None of these are capable of attacking healthy horn, but all may do so when the horn is already soft and spongy.

Symptoms.—The appearance of and the odour from a typical case of canker are familiar to owners of horses who have had experience, and they are so characteristic that they can be very easily recognised. Two forms are common. In the first there is a moist, soft condition of the horn at the back of the heel-bulbs, which is generally covered with a foul-smelling discharge, and which, when pressed, breaks away in a manner resembling wet cheese. The skin immediately above the area is red, devoid of hair, and eczematous in appearance. From the original site the condition gradually progresses around the coronet and under the thin horn of the heel. In the second type, canker commences under the hard outer crust of horn, usually in association with the central cleft of the frog, or in one of the side clefts. Its progress is slow at first, and it may remain in existence for a long time without causing any inconvenience to the horse. Sooner or later it spreads over part of the bulbs of the frog or underneath the sole, and is eventually exposed when the horn is being pared down preparatory to shoeing. In such cases there is usually but little moisture until the canker has progressed to the surface. In well-established cases the lower surface of the foot has an appearance as if it had been soaked in oil, and the normally hard, tough horn is soft, friable, whitish, and cheese-like, while in some parts the sensitive structures may be exposed, and the whole area is sodden and 'rotten-looking'. The amount of pain varies; in some apparently very bad cases the horse is not lame except when it stands upon a stone or some other projection which presses upon the sensitive tissues. In other cases, what appears to be a very slight attack is accompanied by severe lameness. Usually the lameness is not marked unless the wall is under-run.

Treatment.—Often the owner of a horse is tempted to persevere with treatment himself, encouraged by the absence of lameness and apparent progress, until what was a simple case has developed into an incurable one through failure to check the spread of the canker at the margins of the affected areas. In all cases of this condition, no matter how simple, the horse-owner is well advised to seek competent veterinary advice as early as possible. All but the very extensively affected cases are curable, provided attention is given to the dressings and after-treatment. Usually the surgeon removes all obviously affected tissue and a margin of the healthy horn for a distance of about half to three-quarters of an inch around the lesions. A special form of shoe, which will retain dressings in position is usually applied. Some cases take 8 to 10 months' treatment before they are cured, but the majority are fit for work in from 3 weeks to 2 months. Some success is claimed following intravenous injection of sulphonamide compounds in early cases, but canker in the horse does not yield to this treatment so satisfactorily as does the somewhat similar condition in cattle, 'foul in the foot'.

The prevention of canker consists in keeping the horses upon a dry stable surface, laying down a concrete floor where necessary, and providing troughs, instead of allowing horses to wade into muddy water. The feet should be periodically inspected, and all adherent mud and dung should be scraped out daily.

CANNIBALISM.—**In poultry,** this may follow feather-picking—especially if blood is drawn—or a case of prolapse. The crowding together of housed birds is a common cause; and boredom (no scratching for insects as out-of-doors) is a factor, too. Occasionally a nutritional deficiency may be involved. In broiler plants, debeaking or subdued red lighting is resorted to. (*See also* SPECTACLES.)

In pigs, tail-biting is a serious vice. (*See under* TAIL SORES. These can lead to death.) Cannibalism, where sows eat piglets mainly at birth or shortly afterwards, has been seen increasingly among farrowing sows kept on free range, chiefly on arable farms. The cannibal sow does not eat her own litter but guards it fiercely against other predatory sows. Thus this vice is entirely different from the occasional savaging of a litter by an hysterical sow or (more commonly) gilt in intensively kept pig herds.

CANNULA is the tube through which a trocar is inserted, when puncture of the rumen to relieve tympany in the ox is necessary. After puncture the trocar is withdrawn and the cannula remains in position to allow escape of gas.

CANTHARIDES is a powder made from the dried bodies and wings of the Spanish fly *Cantharis vesicatoria*, or *Lytta vesicatoria*, and in some cases the Chinese blister fly *Mylabris phalerata*, although this latter is generally used as an adulterant.

Cantharadin poisoning has been reported in a horse and a mule, which died after eating hay contaminated by beetles (*Epicanta vittata*) which contain cantharadin.

Actions.—When made into an ointment with some oily or fatty material and rubbed into the skin, cantharides causes smarting, pain, and the formation of vesicles in the surface layers of the skin. Primarily it acts only on the surface of the skin, but when applied more copiously it similarly affects the deeper structures and is absorbed into the body. When a sufficient amount has been absorbed, the drug has an irritant action on the genital and urinary organs by which it is eliminated from the body. Cantharides was sometimes employed to stimulate the sexual appetite, but the risk of setting up acute inflammation of kidneys or bladder —leading to very serious illness or death —is very great. (*See* BLISTERS, APPLICATION OF.)

CANTHUS (κανθός) is the name applied to the angle at either end of the aperture between the eyelids.

CAPILLARIASIS.—Infestation with Capillaria worms. *Capillaria obsignata* has been increasingly recognised as of economic importance in intensely reared poultry in Britain. Haloxon, given in the drinking water, has been recommended as treatment.

CAPILLARIES are the very minute vessels that join the ultimate arteries (or arterioles) to the commencement of the veins. Their walls consist of a single layer of fine, flat, transparent cells, joined together at their edges, and the vessels form an intricate mesh-work throughout

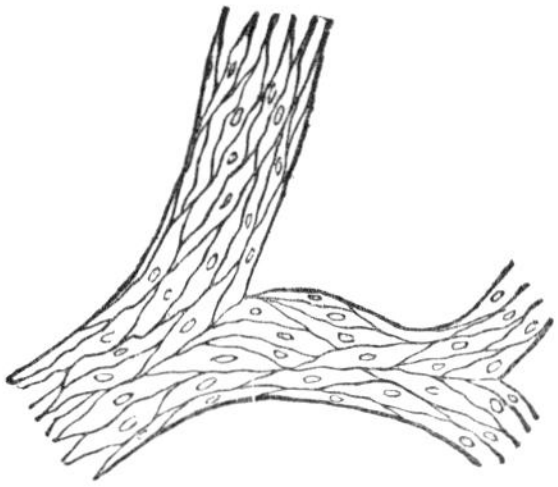

The endothelial walls of capillaries from the retina. Magnified × 300. (Turner's *Anatomy*.)

the tissues of the body, bathing them in blood, with only the thin walls interposed, and allowing free exchange of gases and fluids. These vessels are less than $\frac{1}{1000}$th of an inch in diameter. (*See* BLOOD, CIRCULATION.)

CAPONISATION.—The castration of cockerels, carried out in order to provide a more tender carcase, and also to obviate crowing and fighting. Surgical caponisation has now been largely superseded by chemical methods—the implantation of pellets of stilbœstrol or hexœstrol. This is done under the skin high up the neck, about 4 to 6 weeks before killing at 12 to 16 weeks of age. Older birds may need 2 injections, one 6 and one 12 weeks before killing.

It is important that offals or residues from chemically caponised birds should not be fed to mink or to pet animals, as sterility or abortion may result.

CAPPED ELBOW, which is also called 'hygroma of the elbow', and 'shoe-boil', is due to a distension of the false bursa between the skin and the olecranon bone at the point of the elbow, and is produced by constant irritation either from lying upon hard surfaces, from injury by the calkin or heel of the shoe in the horse, or from some other cause of a similar nature. It is seen in horses especially, but it also sometimes occurs in the heavier breeds of dogs during old age. It may arise from acute irritation, *e.g.* after a blow, when it appears quickly and is usually accompanied by lameness, but it generally follows chronic irritation, *e.g.* such as occurs from the elbow continually coming into contact with the heels of the shoe, or with the hard floors in badly bedded stables, etc., when the horse lies down.

Symptoms.—These differ with age and the type of the lesions produced. The *acute* type appears suddenly as an œdematous painful swelling with a diffuse base, and is in most cases accompanied by lameness. The acute symptoms usually subside in a few days, leaving the swelling more circumscribed, and this swelling may disappear altogether. In other cases the swelling recurs and becomes chronic. The *chronic* type appears slowly, but unless the cause be removed it becomes steadily larger. The walls thicken and become hypertrophied, the skin hardens and gets more and more insensitive, and finally the weight of the newly formed tissue leads to its displacement, causing it to drag out a stalk for itself from the skin around the elbow.

Treatment.—*Acute* cases associated with inflammation, are treated on the general lines for an inflammation. They are fomented with hot water alone, or may be fomented with hot and cold water alternatively; and after drying are rubbed with a soothing and astringent absorbent liniment, such as the soap liniment of the *British Pharmacopœia.* The horse meantime is prevented from doing itself further damage by being kept standing for a few days; in bad cases, which will take some time to resolve, it may be necessary to put it into slings, but it is usually sufficient to tie it up in a stall so that it cannot lie down. When the acute swelling has subsided, it is necessary to prevent a recurrence of the condition by providing plenty of bedding, by keeping the heels of the fore-shoes as short as possible, and, if necessary, by using a 'sausage-boot', or by fastening a thick pad of straw rope round the fetlock so that when the horse lies the straw will protect the elbow point. Alternatively, a thick straw rope may be fastened round the fore-arm, just above the knee, or a fore-arm boot, made of stuffed leather, may be used in the same place. In *chronic* types the sooner the swelling is noticed and preventive measures are applied the less the permanent blemish. The use of sausage- or straw-boots as indicated above will prevent further irritation, and the tumour will very often disappear without any further treatment. In other cases, although the tumour persists, and may be quite hard and of considerable size, it does not interfere with the utility of the horse nor cause pain. Sometimes, surgery is necessary.

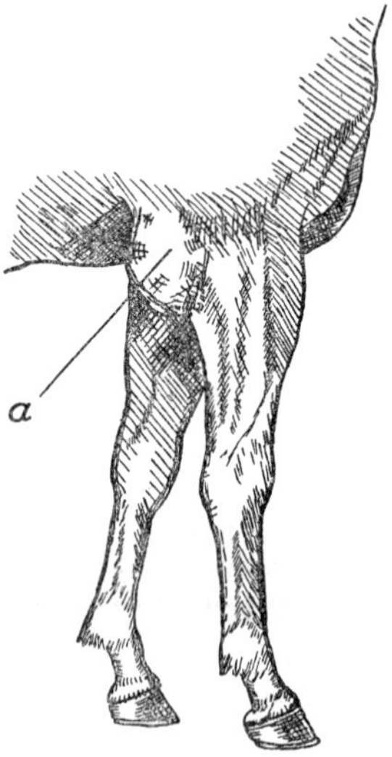

Capped elbow in the horse; the swelling is seen at *a*. This is a comparatively early stage and will become progressively worse unless treated.

CAPPED HOCK is a term loosely applied to any swelling over the point of the

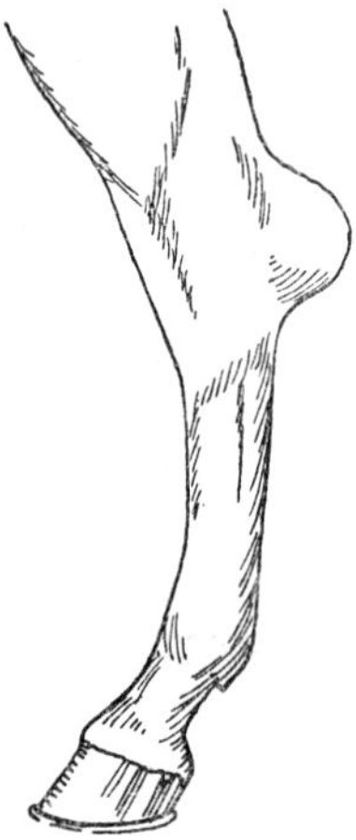

Capped hock.

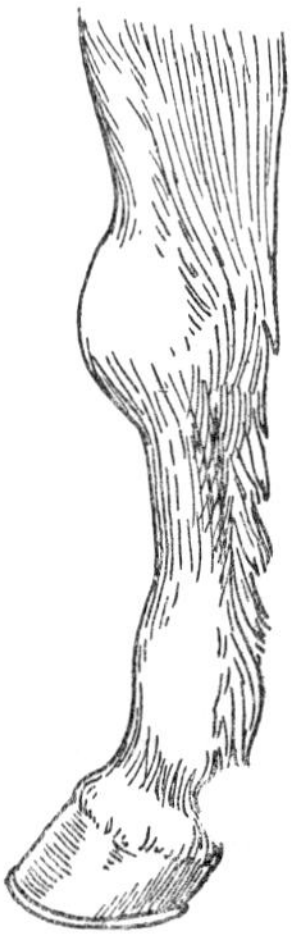

Capped knee, a condition essentially the same as capped hock.

hock. At this point there are two bursæ: the first, a false bursa, distention of which constitutes true 'capped hock', lies between the skin and the tendon which plays over the bone, and the second, the true bursa, separates the tendon from the bone.

As in capped elbow, the condition arises as the result of irritation, and it may be acute or chronic according to the nature of the irritation. The lesion is virtually identical with that of capped elbow except as to its position, and the course, symptoms, and treatment are practically the same. Fluid occupying the centre of the tumour is more often met with than in capped elbow, and it is possible to reduce materially the swelling by aspirating the fluid.

Since the condition may be brought about in the mare by continual kicking at the heel posts of the stall (*e.g.* in cases of nymphomania), it is necessary to pad the heel posts with sacks of straw or chaff, or to house the horse in a loose-box.

'CAPPIE,' a disease of sheep. (*See under* 'DOUBLE SCALP'.)

CAPSULE (*capsula*, a little box) is a term used in several senses. The term is applied to a soluble case, either of gelatine which dissolves in the stomach, or keratin which only dissolves in the small intestine, for enclosing small doses of medicine. The term is also applied to the fibrous or membranous envelope of various organs, as of the spleen, liver, or kidney. It is also applied to the ligamentous bag surrounding various joints, and attached by its edge to the bones on either side, when it is called a 'joint capsule'. Capsules of fibrous tissue may also be laid down around an area of disease, such as an abscess.

CAR EXHAUST FUMES.—These are used for the humane destruction of mink, and have been used to destroy—on public health grounds—a large flock of turkeys. (*See under* DESTRUCTION OF ANIMALS.)

CAR SICKNESS (*see under* TRAVEL SICKNESS).

CARBACHOL, or **CARBAMYLCHOLINE CHLORIDE,** is a drug which has the action of stimulating the parasympathetic nervous system. It is a synthetic ester of choline, and like acetyl choline is a powerful stimulant to glands which are under parasympathic control—lachrymal, salivary, gastric, and the intestinal glands. It slows the heart-rate, lowers blood-pressure, and stimulates the plain muscle fibres of many organs to contract, in particular that of the bowels and stomach. It is of use in treating cases of bowel atony, especially in certain forms of colic in the horse. It is useful in constipation and tympany of abdominal organs in horses and cattle but is dangerous in all forms of obstruction of the bowels, since the powerful contractions it induces may cause rupture at the obstruction. In the dog, it can be used to induce vomiting, and it has been of assistance in dystokia due to uterine inertia.

It should not be used in pneumonia, late pregnancy, and if severe debility exists. Its action is neutralised by atropine which can be regarded as an antidote.

CARBOHYDRATE is a term used to include organic compounds containing carbon, hydrogen, and oxygen, the two latter being in the same proportions as they are present in water, viz., two parts of hydrogen to every one part of oxygen. The simplest carbohydrates are the monosaccharid sugars (*e.g.* glucose), then come disaccharid sugars (*e.g.* cane sugar), and the various higher compounds. The complex carbohydrates, *e.g.* such as the starches, celluloses, and lignified compounds in hay, must be broken down into simpler sugars by both bacterial and protozoa action and by the processes of digestion before they can be absorbed and made use of in the system.

CARBOLIC ACID, or **PHENOL,** is a coal-tar antiseptic.

Actions.—Carbolic acid first paralyses and then destroys all forms of life, particularly the lower kinds of plant life, such as bacteria. When applied to the skin in strong solution it causes death of those cells on the surface and paralyses the superficial sensory nerves. It has a very penetrating action, being more powerful in this respect than either alcohol or the mercury compounds. Used to excess on the surface of the skin it produces an almost painless slough, becomes absorbed into the tissues, and may cause carbolic acid poisoning. As carbolic oil it was erroneously employed as a wound dressing. In combination with oil much of its antiseptic property and penetrating qualities are destroyed, and it is not now used.

Uses.—Externally, carbolic acid is

sometimes used to cauterise ulcers, but for cleansing the skin or dressing wounds more modern antiseptics of less toxicity and greater efficiency are to be preferred.

Carbolic acid should only be used with the greatest of care for the dog, since this animal (and the cat) is extremely liable to suffer from poisoning. (*See* DISINFECTANTS, CARBOLIC ACID POISONING.)

CARBOLIC ACID POISONING may occur from the application of too strong dressings to the skin; from the internal administration of the drug by mistake; and cases have been recorded from the use of strong carbolic disinfecting powders sprinkled on to the floors of animal buildings.

Symptoms.—When taken by the mouth there are signs of burning about the tongue throat, and pharynx. The animal shows profuse salivation, and a whitened, hard appearance of the mucous membrane where the acid has come into contact with the living tissues; and there is the characteristic odour of the drug perceptible from the breath. Later, muscular tremors, a staggering gait, accelerated respirations, coldness of the extremities, convulsions, paralysis, and ultimately unconsciousness, follow each other in rapid succession. In those animals that are able to vomit, this act is frequent in the early stages, but is not seen after the case becomes serious. If the drug has been taken by the mouth in any quantity, perforation of the walls of the stomach may occur with consequent escape of the acid into the peritoneal cavity, and death from shock takes place.

Treatment.—In all animals chemical antidotes are two: Epsom, and Glauber's salts, given in as large doses as possible; 1 to 2 ounces for the dog; 2 to 4 ounces for the sheep and pig; and from 1 to 2 lb. for the larger animals. The insoluble sulphocarbolate is formed in each case. When the carbolic acid has been absorbed from the skin, the area should be washed with pure glycerine, after removing any excess acid by warm-water swabs.

CARBONATES OF SODA, POTASH, etc. (*see* ALKALIES).

CARBON DIOXIDE is formed by the tissues, taken up by the blood, exchanged for oxygen in the lungs, and expired from them with each breath. In a building, the ventilation must be such as will get rid of it rapidly so that it does not accumulate in the atmosphere. (*See* VENTILATION.) It is poisonous in quantity, inducing a condition of deep sleep, stupor, and asphyxia. It is present in the atmospheric air to the extent of about 0·03 per cent by volume, although this amount varies. CO_2 is used as a respiratory stimulant by anæsthetists.

CARBON DIOXIDE ANÆSTHESIA.—CO_2, derived from dry ice, has been successfully used in America for anæsthetising pigs prior to slaughter. The pigs are driven in single file through a tunnel and inhale the CO_2 for less than a minute, after which a very brief period of unconsciousness follows—long enough, however, for shackling and 'sticking' to be accomplished without causing pain. There is no adverse effect upon the carcase.

CARBON DIOXIDE SNOW is formed when CO_2 is first compressed in a cylinder to a liquid and then released through a small nozzle. The temperature falls to about —70° C and the CO_2 solidifies as a snow. This is then compressed into solid blocks, which are used for a variety of purposes where a low temperature is required for a considerable time, such as to cool meat, milk, or fish in transit by rail, to preserve tissues, bacteria, or foods, so that normal enzyme action is arrested, and sometimes to produce local anæsthesia by freezing or to cauterise a surface growth on the skin.

A piece of 'dry ice' or carbon dioxide 'snow' placed on the floor of an infested building will act as a bait for ticks which will gather round it and can then be collected and destroyed.

CARBON MONOXIDE (*see* COAL-GAS POISONING; CAR EXHAUST FUMES).

CARBON TETRACHLORIDE is a powerful agent for use against liver flukes and round worms in animals, **but it is not safe for use in cattle.** It is lethal not only to the adult worms, but also to some immature forms, and in a few cases even to the eggs. It can be given in capsules of gelatin which are dissolved in the stomach. It is not necessary that the animal should be starved, although it is better that the alimentary canal be not full, and it is not necessary to give a purgative dose before or after administration. When its vapour is inhaled it may bring about general anæsthesia for a few moments.

The doses are: horse, 1 to 2 ounces; pigs, 1 to 6 drams; sheep, ¼ to 1 dram (1 to 4 c.c.); dogs, ½ to 2 drams, according to size.

The introduction of a carbon tetrachloride preparation which can be given by injection has not much reduced the risk of poisoning so often associated with carbon tetrachloride given by mouth. It is still advisable to treat a trial pen of sheep first, and fasting them for 18 hours before injection has been recommended. If he takes the former precaution, the farmer can expect to lose fewer ewes.

CARCINOGENS are substances which give rise to cancer.

CARCINOMATA and SARCOMATA are two divisions of the class of tumours called 'cancers'. Although a carcinoma is very distinct from a sarcoma upon microscopic examination, to the naked eye, and from a clinical point of view, they frequently much resemble each other. They can be defined, in common with other *malignant tumours*, as non-inflammatory, non-encapsulated new growths, parasitic in a measure upon the body cells from which they derive nourishment and which they gradually supplant, not conforming to the usual body laws, and having a tendency to reproduce themselves in other parts of the body remote from the seat of the original lesion. They tend to simulate the cells of the normal tissues in which they are found, and in many cases it is difficult to determine the extent of the tumour and the margin dividing it from the surrounding normal tissue. Carcinomata and sarcomata are the most malignant and dreaded members of the tumour class, and are characterised by a rapid unencapsulated growth destroying the normal tissue at the site of the habitat, and infiltrating the deeper structures so that, when fully established, removal by the surgeon becomes difficult or impossible; they tend to reproduce themselves in other parts of the body by spreading along the lymph-vessels (or perhaps blood-vessels) to new organs or tissues, forming *metastatic*, or secondary, tumours there, and very often causing rapidly fatal changes in important organs like lungs, liver, stomach, etc.

Causes.—Many theories have been advanced to account for the origin and development of these growths.

Virchow's theory that malignant tumours originate from repeated irritation of a part, is one of the oldest theories and is in some ways substantiated by the production of tumours experimentally. It gains enhanced credence from the fact that in certain 'occupational conditions' where repeated irritation occurs, tumours tend to appear spontaneously; *e.g.* cancer of the scrotum in chimney-sweeps, cancer of the horn cores in yoke-oxen, cancer of X-ray operators, and cancer of the lips of men addicted to clay-pipe smoking. Repeated irritation of a healing wound may result in the formation of sarcomata from the granulation tissue; repeated stimulation or irritation of mucous membranes, such as may occur in the stomach from unsuitable or irritant foods, may cause cancer; parasites in the bowels of the fowl may result in the formation of proliferations from the epithelium which burrow into the adjacent tissues and form tumours, and somewhat similar growths are sometimes seen in the bile-ducts of the rabbit's liver affected with coccidiosis.

Based on this irritation theory interesting results have been obtained. It has been found that in rats fed with the eggs of a tape-worm of the cat (*Tænia crassicollis*) an infiltrating tumour growth appears at the margins of the cysts which form in the rat's liver. Japanese workers showed that by repeatedly painting the skin of the mouse with tar or paraffin oil, or, better, with the actual chemical carcinogenic compound in them, a cancer may be produced in a great majority of cases. In addition to these facts it has been found that tumours of the mammary gland of the mouse can be successfully transmitted through successive generations of mice by aseptic transplantation of minute portions of the original tumour to another animal.

There is a chemical relationship between one of the carcinogenic agents in tar, dibenzanthracene, and the hormone œstrin. This has suggested that hormones may be concerned in the production of tumours.

Successful transplantations have been made in the case of Rous sarcomata of fowls. This type of tumour has been shown to be associated with a virus.

The virus theory: cancer is due to a virus which is universal, *i.e.* the virus causing cancer in man is the same as that causing cancer in the dog and other animals; with the virus is associated a 'specific factor', which varies with different animals. This hypothesis clears up a difficulty which had previously been insurmountable. It had been noted that while it was possible to transplant tumour cells from mouse to mouse, it was not possible to transmit them to another animal, even of a closely allied species; but the union of mouse specific factor with tumour tissue from rat or other animal will produce tumour in the mouse. On the other hand, the union of non-specific mouse factor with tumour tissue from the mouse will not reproduce tumour in the mouse. This obscure specific tumour cell factor is, then, absolutely necessary before cancer can be produced in an animal. Pieces of perfectly fresh infective sarcomata from fowls when engrafted on healthy fowls *infallibly* reproduce the tumour in the latter; when treated so as to remove from the tumour cells the specific fowl factor, however, no tumour results. The specific factor may be likened to the chemical catalyst which introduces and unites two chemical substances without in any way actually entering into the constitution of the new compound resulting.

Further information on this subject can be obtained from the annual report for 1965 of the Imperial Cancer Research Fund. This mentions that both a virus and a mycoplasma may be involved in leukæmia, and that 13 viruses have been isolated from 10 cases of Burkitt's lymphoma. The part played by hormones is also referred to. (*See also under* Treatment at the end of this section.)

By 1971 it was accepted that 'a wide variety of animal tumours are caused by viruses. Several oncogenic RNA viruses have been isolated: the Rous chicken sarcoma virus, the Bittner mouse mammary carcinoma virus, the Gosse mouse leukæmia virus and, more recently, the Jarrett cat lympho-sarcoma virus and possibly the Northern European bovine leukosis complex. Of the DNA viruses, several oncogenic viruses have been isolated, but of special importance are the herpes viruses causing Marek's disease in chickens and, recently, a fatal lymphoreticular tumour in monkeys.'

'Several of the malignant conditions outlined above also occur in man, and the evidence, although inferential and circumstantial, must point towards a viral aetiology. Direct proof of a viral cause of malignancy in humans may be impossible but long-term development of an experimental vaccine to a suspected causative virus may show a subsequent decrease of neoplasia in the vaccinated group.' (*Lancet*, June 26, 1971.)

Immunology of Cancer.—Some light has been thrown on this by studying the development of immunity towards further tumour implants in experimental animals. H. Rinderknecht, Los Angeles, has reported in *The Lancet*:

'In 93 per cent of the mice bearing Ehrlich's adenocarcinoma, when treated with mycetin from the culture medium of *S. felis*, complete regression of the tumour was observed and the animals became resistant to further implants of this tumour. Transplanted lymphomas in mice, treated with colchicine, permanently regressed, and immunity towards this tumour developed. Complete regression of lymphosarcoma transplants was observed in mice receiving a combination treatment consisting of riboflavine deficiency and cortisone. 70 per cent of rats bearing Flexner-Jobling carcinoma when treated with triethyleneimino-s-triazine responded with complete destruction of the tumour and development of resistance to further implants of the same tumour. When chickens with metastasising lymphomatosis were infected with Russian summer and spring encephalitis, louping-ill, and Japanese encephalitis, the tumour quickly regressed and immunity developed. Ligation of methylcholanthrene-induced tumours in mice produced regression and immunity to further implants. Spontaneous tumours, however, when destroyed by ligation, did not produce immunity to later implants of the same tumour. When tumour tissue mixed with adrenaline was implanted, the implants were resorbed and resistance to the same type of tumour developed. Complete regression of leukæmia in mice under treatment with polycarbonyl compounds was accompanied by immunity fo further implants.'

In 1971 it was reported that the growth of Walker sarcoma was entirely suppressed or greatly enhanced in *Nippostrongylus brasiliensis* infected rats depending on the timing of the tumour-cell inoculum in relation to the parasitic infection. Early in the immune response to the parasite, the tumour did not grow, but, once the immune response had developed, tumour growth was enhanced. The enhancing effect could be transferred with antiserum from animals immune to the parasite only, suggesting that the tumour and parasite share antigens. (Keller, R.; Ogilvie, B. M. and Simpson, E., *Lancet*, April 3, 1971.)

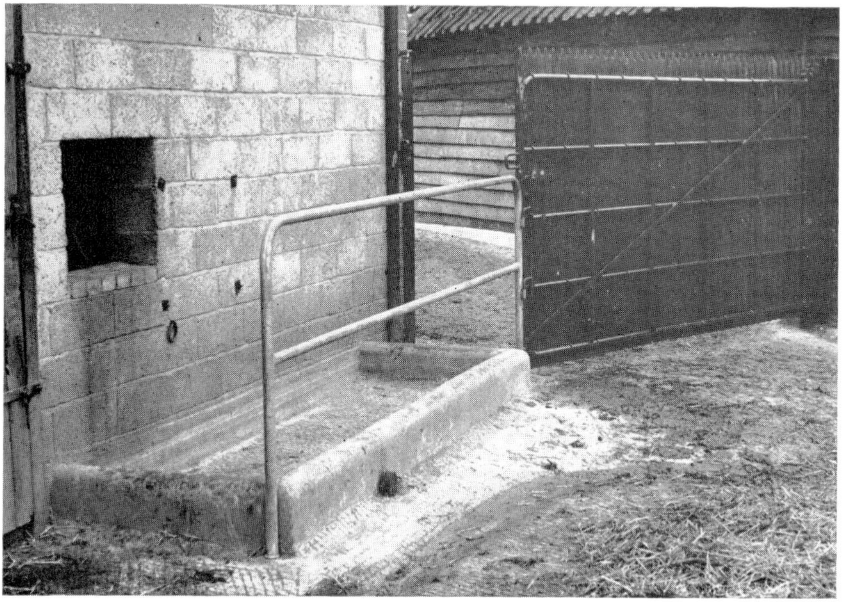

A foot-bath for cattle and two-way gate useful on farms where there is a high incidence of Foul-in-the-foot.

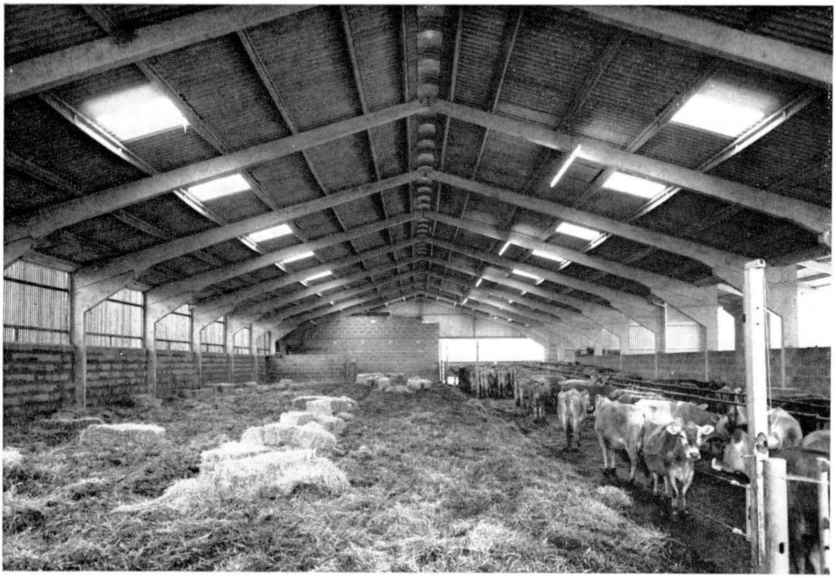

A modern dairy unit, with lying area, parlour, and dairy under one roof. Note the Yorkshire boarding to the left of the picture – a good means of ensuring good ventilation and an absence of condensation.

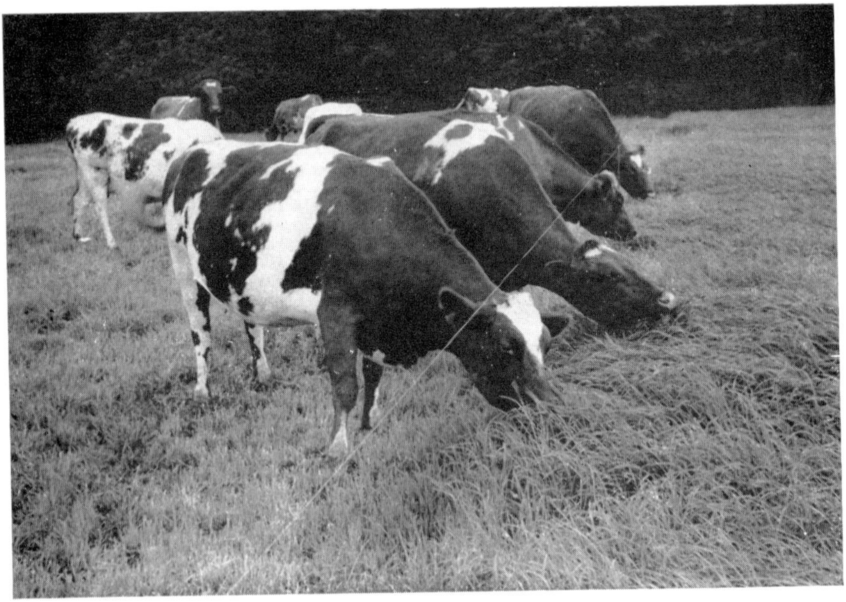

Controlled grazing, showing use of an electric fence.

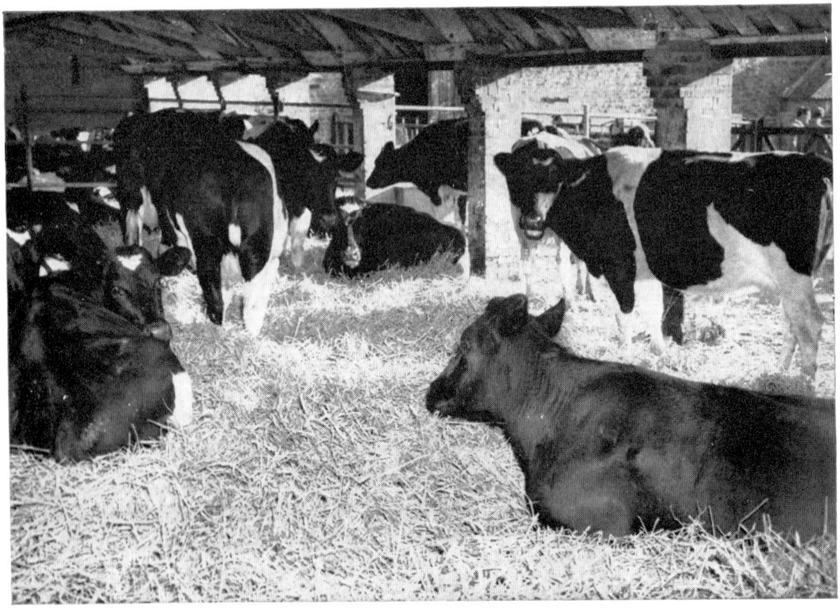

Warm and dry: cattle on deep litter in a covered yard.

SARCOMATA.—These tumours develop from tissue which is formed from the mesoblast of the embryo, *i.e.* connective tissues, bones, cartilage, muscle, etc., and when present as primary growths are usually found in sites where connective tissue is abundant, such as under the skin, in among the muscles, and in connection with bones or cartilages. They may occur in the scaffolding tissue of organs like the kidney, liver, parotid gland, etc. These primary tumours may be as soft as brain, or as hard as a lymph gland, but they are generally fleshy in appearance. Sarcomata are amongst the most malignant of all tumours, and the malignancy varies according to the type of the sarcoma. The main types found are as follows: (*a*) small round-celled; (*b*) large round-celled; (*c*) spindle-celled; (*d*) myeloid, or giant-celled; (*e*) lympho-sarcoma; (*f*) melanotic sarcoma; (*g*) fibro-sarcoma; and (*h*) osteo-sarcoma. All of these types are malignant, destructive, infiltrating, unencapsulated growths. When incised the cut surface is greyish-white with numerous red spots (the cut ends of blood-vessels). Upon microscopic examination the whole tumour is found to be composed of cells without any scaffolding tissue; the cells resemble the round lymphocytes of the blood-stream, having a large nucleus and a small amount of cellular material (protoplasm). The blood-vessels are primitive in the extreme, and it is owing to this fact that sarcomata are so prone to bleed upon the slightest provocation, and that there is a great tendency for small collections of tumour cells to be carried away by the blood-stream, and to set up new centres of tumour growths in parts of the body remote from the seat of the original growth. These secondary tumour growths are spoken of as *metastases*, and the principle of spread is known as *metastatic spread*. Secondary metastases are common in the lungs, kidneys, liver, spleen, heart, and other tissues where the vessels are naturally very small. In spindle-celled sarcomata the cells are spindle-shaped instead of round, the secondary growth are often rounded in outline, but they are never encapsulated, and the spindle-celled variety is never exceedingly malignant. Myeloid or giant-celled sarcomata are not very common; they usually arise from bone or periosteum and often contain spicules of bone. They are commonest in domesticated fowls. They owe their name to the presence in them of a certain number of large nucleated cells, which are called 'giant cells'. They are not so malignant as other forms, and metastases are not so frequent. Lymphosarcomata are found in lymph glands, especially in those superficially situated in the dog, where they have a tendency to ulcerate through the skin. They are very malignant and tend to recur after surgical excision. In the horse they may cause superficial swellings which can be easily seen. They remain more or less discrete without destruction of the surrounding tissues, and metastases do not usually occur. Melanotic sarcomata are commonest in man, where they often affect the eye; this form of tumour being probably the most malignant known. They are also found in subcutaneous situations in the dog, but in animals melanotic sarcomata are not so malignant as they are in man. They are dark or even black in appearance, owing to the presence of melanin, which is deposited around and in the cells. These tumours must not be confounded with the subcutaneous melanomata which are commonly found in grey horses and roan cattle, round the anus, tail, head, neck, hip, and shoulder, when the coat colour becomes lighter with advancing age. They are particularly common in old grey horses, and consist of fibrous tumours the cells of which are heavily laden with melanin, due to the depigmentation of the skin and coat. The process may be so acute in some cases that the melanin may be passed in the urine on account of its excess in the body tissues. Their chief interest lies in that they spread by the blood-vessels and lymphatics, forming metastases in the lungs, liver, spleen, kidneys, etc., exactly like malignant tumours elsewhere.

The so-called 'infective sarcomata' are found in fowls and dogs. Sarcomata are the commonest tumours of the fowl, except for lymphomata and the swellings of lymphatic leukæmia, conditions which hardly come under this heading. They, sarcomata, are subcutaneous in position, tend to be less malignant, and have been transplanted to healthy fowls; they may also be transmitted by the inoculation of filtered cell-free tumour extract into healthy fowls, but they are not infective in the sense that an affected bird may spread sarcomata by running with healthy birds. (*See* LEUKÆMIA.)

CARCINOMATA, or EPITHELIOMATA.—These are tumours composed of modified epithelial tissue, derived from and arising

CARCINOMATA AND SARCOMATA

in epithelium or epithelial structures. They are chiefly tumours associated with advancing age, and for that reason are chiefly found in the dog and the horse, since the food animals do not usually reach old age, although they are liable to form in any animal. Primary carcinomata occur in the skin, muco-cutaneous junction of lips, eye, and anus, in the stomach, intestines, and testicles in the dog; and in the eye, lips, blind sac and

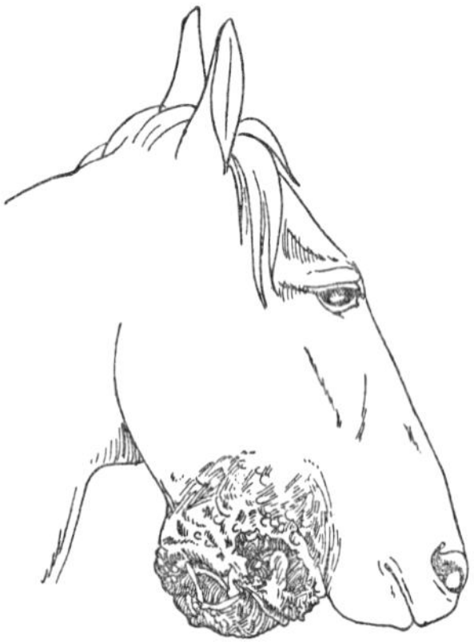

Cancer of the lower jaw. The muscles of the cheek, and the right half of the mandible are affected.

other parts of the stomach, air sinuses, and the penis (where they are very common), in the horse. Carcinoma of the mammary gland, which is so common in the human subject, is not often met with in the domesticated animals, but it may occur in the bitch, where it is not very malignant.

Carcinomata are divided into: (*a*) epitheliomata; (*b*) adenomata; and (*c*) carcinomata proper. *Epitheliomata* arise from skin, especially where there is a junction between skin and mucous membrane, and from the edges of old-standing unhealed ulcers. They are also met with in the proliferating edges of warts. To the naked eye the growths are irregular, warty, or cauliflower-like, often with ulcerations upon their surfaces, and frequently discharging a foul-smelling purulent material. On microscopic examination the normal skin papillæ appear to be abnormally clothed with epithelium, particularly well seen at the edges of an ulcer. The papillæ, however, instead of growing outwards in the normal way, have become inverted and are growing *inwards*, into the substance of the skin, and even through it into the subcutaneous tissue. The papillæ branch and re-branch, so that the area of the carcinomatous growth becomes very congested with cells; and if the part is a sensitive one the nerves are subjected to pressure, and great pain is felt. In the centre of each mass there is seen a concentric area of homogeneous keratinised cells—the so-called 'bird's nest bodies of cancer'. *Adenomata* almost always imitate the structure of a gland, and arise from mucous membranes whose surfaces are lined by secreting glands. The female genital organs are the commonest seat of this tumour in the human being; while in the horse adenomata are found in the stomach and intestines, the thyroid gland, kidney, and rarely in the liver. In the sheep the liver is affected in some cases, and the kidneys or pancreas in others. In the dog, the gastro-intestinal tract, the region of the anus, and occasionally the mammary gland and the uterus, are the common sites, while the thyroid gland and the kidney are also affected. In structure an adenoma resembles a gland. The epithelium may be primitive, probably representing developing gland tissue, or resting gland tissue, in which there is a single layer of cells upon a basement membrane, which does not enclose a secreting space, and in which no secretion is produced. Fibrous tissue supports the epithelial cells, well-developed blood-vessels are present, but there is no encapsulation. Such a tumour is seen in the anal adenoma of the dog. In a second type the epithelium is more fully developed: secreting spaces (acini) are present, a secretion is produced, sometimes in such large amounts that it fills the acinus and distends it, forming a 'cystic adenoma', but no ducts are present. Such forms are seen in the mammary gland, in the thyroid kidney, and ovary. Columnar-celled epitheliomata (or adenomata) are specialised adenomata found in the gastro-intestinal tract. In them long processes are sent out which burrow in the submucous tissues of the bowel until large areas are invaded by the tumour. To the naked eye these growths appear somewhat 'succulent', eroded, and often show a tendency to ulcerate.

Carcinoma proper (or *carcinoma simplex*) is the simplest type of the group, but it is the most malignant. It is commonly found in the heart of man, and in the domesticated animals it may arise in the skin and gastro-intestinal system, especially in the œsophagus and rectum; it is

CARCINOMATA AND SARCOMATA

also found in the vagina, uterus, ovary, kidney, and air sinuses of the horse, and sometimes in the testes of dogs, and in the liver of the ox, associated with fluke infestations. It is not at all common. The tumour is essentially one in which fully developed fibrous tissue supports cancer cells arranged in an orderly or irregular manner. It may be hard (scirrhous) or soft (encephaloid) in consistency. Blood-vessels are well developed, but in the softer kinds hæmorrhages may be present. In some cases the arrangement of the cells appears as though the fibrous tissue enclosed spaces around the walls of which the cancer cells were grouped; the formation resembling adenomata, and being known as an adenocarcinoma. This is one of the types often found in the ox's liver. The softer types contain a greater proportion of cells to fibrous tissue, and are accordingly more malignant. A special type of carcinoma, known as a 'rodent ulcer', derived from the deeper layers of the skin, is sometimes found on the face, head, and occasionally on the fore-limbs of animals, more particularly in old age, and therefore commoner in the horse and dog than in others. This form is relatively benign in that it does not form metastases, but it tends to spread and destroys much of the surface tissue. It is called 'rodent ulcer', because of its unsightly appearance, which suggests that rats or other rodents were in the habit of coming there to feed.

In the earlier stages carcinomata spread by the lymph-stream to other parts of the body, and at later stages by the blood-stream. The softer types, on account of the ease with which blood-vessels are damaged, may spread by the blood-stream from the start, with especial liability to involvement of liver, heart, and circulatory organs. Where lymph-stream spread occurs the first site of the new growth is the nearest lymph gland, and the nature of the spread is of importance, because when surgical removal of a tumour becomes advisable it is very often necessary to remove the adjacent lymph glands as well.

Effects produced.—Symptoms produced vary with the seat of the growth.

In some cases the tumour undergoes degeneration. It may become necrotic and soft, in which case metastatic spread is encouraged; it may be crushed or bruised when in a necrotic state and a fatal hæmorrhage occur; it may become infected with inflammatory organisms, and fever follows; or it may ulcerate on to the skin, or into the lumen of a hollow organ.

Treatment.—The best results are to be looked for from surgical excision undertaken as early as possible. There is some difference of opinion as to whether surgical removal of *primary growths* is always advisable, for it frequently happens that following the removal of a primary growth from the surface of the body *secondary metastases* in some deeper part are stimulated to grow with increased speed, and cause serious changes in internal organs, which might not have been so rapid if the primary growth had been untouched. Unless surgical removal of the growth is prompt and complete a recurrence of the tumour in its original seat is much more to be feared, but in the domesticated animals, as a general rule, early and extensive operation is strongly advisable. The great difficulty in removing an old-standing tumour is that much infiltration of the surrounding tissues is almost sure to have occurred, and complete removal is not possible. There is no line of demarcation between the tumour and normal tissue to guide the surgeon, such as is present in typically benign growths. It is important to remember that excessive handling of soft growths is very likely to induce some amount of breaking down of the tumour and favour metastatic spread to other parts. Treatment by X-rays directed on to the growth in such a way that the new tissue is soaked in the rays but that healthy tissue is protected as much as possible, has given beneficial results in some cases, but it is by no means always successful. The insertion of radium tubes into the growth or near to it has also been satisfactory in a number of cases, but the economic question is very often insuperable. Progress in human cancer control has been achieved in certain cases by the use of stilbœstral or hexœstral, especially for cancer of the prostate gland. Some success has also attended its use in old dogs.

A search for antigenic materials in tumours undergoing autolysis, and their evaluation in the production of specific anti-tumour hyperimmune sera, seems to hold much promise.

There is also the possibility of 'reforming' cancer cells by means of some chemical substance, such as ribonucleic acid (RNA), which stimulates normal development.

It has been suggested that there may be a place for thalidomide in the treatment of cancer.

CARDIA (καρδια, the heart) is a term applied to the upper opening of the stomach at which the œsophagus terminates. It lies close behind the heart.

CARDIAC DISEASE (*see* Heart Diseases).

CARDIOGRAPHY is the name given to the process by which graphic records can be made of the heart's action. Thus, auricular and ventricular pressures can be recorded, the sounds of the heart-beat can be converted into waves of movement and recorded on paper, and the changes in electric potential that occur can be similarly recorded by the use of an electrocardiograph. (*See* Electrocardiograph.)

CARDIOLOGY is the name given to a study of the heart and heart diseases.

CARDIOSPASM means a spasmodic contraction of the muscle fibres of the cardia of the stomach. It occurs in horses in particular when fed upon dry foods such as large amounts of chaff or dried sugar beet pulp. It interferes with the normal passage of food from the œsophagus into the stomach and may be very serious unless relieved.

CARIES (*caries*, decay) is a process of gradual decay of bone, teeth, or cartilage, which is sometimes analogous to ulceration of soft tissues. The word is usually restricted in application in veterinary literature to decay of the teeth, the process in bone and cartilage being more often spoken of as 'necrosis'. (*See also* under Teeth, Diseases of.)

CARMINATIVES are substances which produce a healthy action of the muscular walls of the stomach and intestines, and assist in the expulsion of gases. They lessen pain and spasm and promote a more regular peristaltic action. Almost all the aromatic oils are carminatives.

CAROTENE is a pigment, present in carrots among many other foodstuffs, which is a precursor of vitamin A and can be converted into this vitamin in the liver and stored there. (*See* Vitamins.)

CARPUS is the name given to the bones of the wrist in man, or the 'knee' of the fore-limbs of animals.

'CARRIER', A.—An animal recovered from a disease, or not showing symptoms, but capable of passing on the infection to another animal. For example, a bull may be a carrier of brucellosis; dogs may be carriers of *leptospiræ*; a cow may be a carrier of *Salmonella dublin.*

CARRION CROWS often cause injury to ewes and lambs, sometimes death, and in addition they may transmit vibrionic abortion. Crows may also kill piglets or injure older pigs.

CARTILAGE is a hard but pliant tissue forming parts of the skeleton, *e.g.* the rib cartilages, the cartilages of the larynx and ears, and the lateral cartilages of the foot, as well as the cartilages of the trachea or windpipe. Microscopically it consists of cells arranged in pairs or in rows, embedded in a clear homogeneous tissue devoid of blood-vessels and nerves. The surfaces of the bones that form a joint are covered with *articular cartilages,* which provide smooth surfaces of contact and minimise shock and friction. In some parts of the body there are discs of cartilage interposed between bones forming a joint, *e.g.* between the femur and tibia and fibula there are the cartilages of the stifle joint, and between most of the adjacent vertebræ there are similar discs. When a bone is still growing, there are layers of cartilage interposed between the shaft and its extremities; these are called *epiphyseal cartilages,* and it is by addition to the surfaces of this type of cartilage that bones increase their length. These epiphyseal cartilages disappear when the animal stops growing, and no further growth in a longitudinal direction can take place after that.

Diseases of cartilage.—Two chief diseases affect cartilages in animals, although there are several affections that may rarely be encountered.

Necrosis, or death of the cells of the cartilage, results from accident, injury, or in some cases from pressure. These factors, which would only produce a temporary inflammation in the case of softer tissues of the body, are serious in cartilage because of its normally poor blood-supply, which does not allow of rapid recovery. This disease is commonest in the lateral cartilages of the horse's foot, when it produces the disease called 'quittor' (which see). It may affect the rib-cartilages from accident or injury, and it is sometimes met with affecting the cartilages of the larynx and ears. The treatment is wholly surgical, and consists in the removal of the dead piece or pieces and the provision of drainage for discharges.

Ossification.—Many of the cartilaginous structures of the body become ossified into bone in the normal course, especially in old age; but as the result of a single mild or many slight injuries to a cartilage the formation of bone may take place prematurely, and interference with function results. This is seen in the case of the lateral cartilages of the foot, from continued concussion, tramps, sprains of ligaments, etc., when the condition resulting is called 'side-bones' (which see). After operation on the larynx, ossification of the cartilage sometimes occurs as a sequel, but is not important so long as the openings through which the air passes remain patent.

CARUNCLE.—A small fleshy protuberance, which may be a normal anatomical part.

CASCARA SAGRADA is the dried bark of *Ramnus purshianus*. It acts as a tonic laxative, producing gentle purgative effects, and is useful for chronic constipation in the dog.

CASEATION (*caseus*, cheese) is a process which takes place in the tissues in tuberculosis and some other chronic diseases. The central part of a diseased area, instead of forming into pus and so producing an abscess, changes into a firm, cheese-like mass, which may either be absorbed and result in healing with the production of a scar, or, more often, becomes the seat of numbers of crystals of calcium salts, when the process is called calcification. (*See* CALCIFICATION.)

CASEIN.—A protein of milk and an important constituent of 'Solids-not-fat'.

CASEOUS LYMPHADENTITIS.—**Definition.**—A chronic disease of the sheep and goat, characterised by the formation of nodules containing a cheesy pus ('matter') occurring in the lymphatic glands, lungs, skin, or other organs; exhibiting a tendency to produce a chronic pneumonia or pleurisy.

Distribution.—The condition is widely spread amongst flocks in most countries. Amongst the domesticated animals it only occurs in the sheep and the goat, but can be produced in the rabbit, the guinea-pig, and the rat by artificial means.

Cause.—The *Corynebacterium ovis*, or previously known as the bacillus of Preisz-Nocard. The 'droppings' of affected sheep contain the organisms and so aid in spreading the disease. Wound infection is a common source.

Treatment.—This is difficult as the lesions become encapsulated and so inaccessible to antibiotics. Veterinary advice should be sought.

CASTOR OIL is the oil expressed from the seeds of the castor oil plant *Ricinus communis*, or it may be extracted from the crushed seeds by using a solvent such as petroleum or benzene. The solvent is subsequently removed by steam.

Actions.—On the external surface of the skin castor oil lessens irritation and acts as a protective. It is useful as an application to the eyes to relieve the irritation subsequent to the removal of foreign bodies from that organ. Internally it is a simple purgative, mild in action and free from any griping effects. It acts upon the small intestine in all animals, but if the stomach is in an inflamed or irritable condition it is apt to be vomited before it reaches the intestines.

Uses.—Castor oil is a common purgative for dogs, cats, foals, and calves. It is not suitable for the adult horse. It is most eminently suited for those cases in the smaller animals where a single dose of purgative medicine is indicated, for after the primary effect there is a slight tendency to constipation. For chronic constipation it is unsuited.

CASTOR SEED POISONING is not uncommon through animals being accidentally fed either with the castor seeds themselves or with some residue from them. The seeds of the castor plant (*Ricinus communis*) contain an oil which is used not only as a medicinal agent, but also for lubricating. Processing leaves behind in the press-cakes the great majority of the poisonous toxin, called *ricine*, and so renders these 'castor-cakes' unsuitable as a food-stuff for all live-stock. Overseas, however, unscrupulous cattle cake merchants sometimes sell them for feeding cattle after treating the residual press-cakes to the action of steam, with the result that the ricine is not all destroyed and poisoning may occur.

The toxic principle, ricine, bears a great resemblance to snake venom, both in its action and its composition. It acts like a bacterial toxin, to some extent, and animals can be immunised against its toxic effects by repeated small sub-lethal doses given either by the mouth or by hypodermic injection. After immunisation they can withstand doses from four hundred to eight hundred times the ordinary toxic dose without ill effects.

Symptoms.—These consist of dullness, loss of appetite, elevation of the temperature, severe abdominal pain, and usually constipation. The heart's action is tumultuous, the surface of the body is cold; there may be a watery cold sweat, and the respiration is distressed. Purgation occurs in some instances. In cattle there is often a blood-stained diarrhœa, especially if comparatively small amounts have been taken. Where large amounts have been eaten the fæces are usually hard, dry, and brown in colour. Upon *post-mortem* examination there is an intense inflammation of the stomach and intestines, with 'false membrane' formation in the small bowel particularly.

Treatment.—Give milk or oatmeal gruel pending veterinary advice.

CASTRATION consists of the removal of the essential sex organs—testes and ovaries—from either male or female. In the latter case, *i.e.* the removal of the essential female gonads, as they are called, it is more often referred to as 'ovariotomy', 'spaying', or oöphorectomy. (*See also* SPAYING.)

In Britain, it is illegal to castrate horse, ass, mule, dog, or cat without the use of an anæsthetic. For other animals, an age limit is in force. (See ANÆSTHETICS, LEGAL REQUIREMENTS.)

Reasons for Castration.—To the humanitarian who has not an extensive acquaintance with animals the necessity for this operation may not be obvious, and it is advisable at the outset that the reasons for castration should be given.

Bullocks are able to be housed along with heifers without the disturbance which would otherwise occur during the œstral periods of the female, and they live together without fighting, and without becoming dangerous to man, in a way that is not possible with bulls. The uncertainty of the temper of an entire male animal, especially of the larger species, and the risk of injury to attendants, are well known The same remarks apply to horses, asses and mules.

Another reason for castration of domesticated animals living under artificial conditions is that breeds and strains can be more easily kept pure, desirable types can be encouraged and retained and undesirable types eliminated.

It used to be held that meat from uncastrated animals was greatly inferior to that from castrated ones. In fact, apart from such considerations as obtaining docility and avoiding promiscuous breeding, meat-quality was the main reason advanced for doing the operation. Nowadays that phrase 'greatly inferior' has tended to become 'slightly inferior'.

Some Disadvantages of Castration.—The growing practice of early slaughter of meat-producing animals, so that the majority never fully mature, has posed the question: is castration still necessary or, for efficient meat production, even advisable?

In all species, the entire male grows more quickly and produces a leaner carcase than that of the castrate. Since rapid and economic production of lean flesh is essential in modern meat production, the principle of male castration may seem to be becoming out of date.

The problem differs from one species of farm animal to another. Veal calves are not castrated. They have a better food conversion ratio than castrated calves. In 1963 a trial with up to 500 'beef bulls' was authorised by the Ministry of Agriculture. But experts favour castration of lambs; and while beef from the entire is used fairly extensively in the south of France and in Italy (beasts being killed at 14 to 16 months), it does not find favour in Britain. With pigs, a change may come. At the 6th B.O.C.M. Boar Performance Test, the average boar took only 151 days to reach bacon weight (200 lb.), and had a food conversion ratio of 2·87 between 70 and 200 lb. liveweight. If the animals in the test had been castrated they would each have required about ¾ cwt. more food to reach 200 lb. liveweight. (*See also under* STRESS, BULL BEEF.)

Methods.—Briefly speaking, the operation consists of opening the scrotum and coverings of the testicle by a linear incision, separating the organ itself from these structures, and dividing the spermatic cord well above the epididymis which lies on the testicle, in such a way that hæmorrhage from the spermatic artery does not occur. In very many cases the larger animals are operated upon in the standing position, but lambs and young pigs are usually held by an assistant. There are also the 'bloodless' methods of the emasculator and rubber rings. After the operation the animal is allowed to go free, but care should be taken that it is not subjected to exertion for some hours, so that the risks of post-operative hæmorrhage are decreased.

The Russian method, advocated by Dr. Baiburtejan, aims at leaving the hormonal functions of the testes unimpaired, but eliminating the parenchyma, seminiferous tubules, and associated structures. The epididymis and the tunica albuginea are left. (The technique was described by W. C. Miller, *Veterinary Journal*, December 1963.)

Horse.—Entire colts are usually castrated when one year old, *i.e.* in early spring of the year following their birth, but they may preferably be castrated as foals, at an age of 5 months or younger. The colt may be caught with a long neck rope, have a canvas anæsthetic mask applied. When the foal can no longer stand as a result of the anæsthetic, a hind-leg is pulled forward to expose the operation site, and castration performed with the foal lying on its side. By this method,* 6 colts can be castrated in an hour ; less assistance is required ; the gelding is not frightened when handled later, as occurs when the 2-year-olds are castrated. Owners have been well pleased with the results of this early castration, which is more humane.

The operation should be performed when the weather is mild, extremes of temperatures and rainy days being avoided if possible. It should not be delayed until the hot weather of summer, for then there is some danger of irritation and even of septic infection of the wounds from flies. A number of colts are castrated every year about September and October—particularly such as were late foals, or those of a backward nature whose testes had not descended into the scrotum earlier in the year—and a number of colts are left until they are 2 years old—especially those pedigreed animals which give early promise of turning into good breeding types, but which later do not fulfil that promise. The colts are shut up the day before operation, and fasted for from 12 to 24 hours, so that their internal organs may not be overloaded with ingesta.

The animal may be operated upon in the standing position, or it may be cast in the corner of a good grass field or in a clean yard. Each operator has his own particular preference. Probably the majority of surgeons use an écraseur. This is an instrument which carries a strong adjustable chain, a loop of which passes through a loop at the end of a hollow metal rod, the chain being actuated by a long screw or by a ratchet. The chain is passed round the spermatic cord and gradually tightened by winding the screw until it severs the cord, crushing the artery so that it does not bleed. In another type of instrument, known as an 'emasculator', the cord is crushed between two grooved jaws, and cut off clean below the level of the crushed part. In a few cases it becomes necessary to ligature the spermatic artery, after which the testicle is cut away below the ligature, but it is usually only in castration for the relief of some disease that this is necessary.

After castration the colt is either turned out into a well-strawed yard or put into a roomy loose-box and given a feed ; or, if climatic conditions are favourable, it may be turned out to grass again. It is always advisable to see the colt at intervals during the 24 hours after castration, to ensure that there is no bleeding, that hernia has not developed, or that no other untoward accident has happened. It is hardly necessary to state here that castration of colts should be carried out by a veterinary surgeon. Cryptorchid castration is briefly mentioned under the heading RIG.

Cattle.—Bull calves are usually castrated between the ages of 2 and 8 months, but in some districts it is quite usual to leave them until they are somewhat older than this. A number of male calves are also left in the expectation that they will materialise into animals which may be fit for breeding purposes, but some of these must be castrated later on when they are between 12 and 15 months old. Aged bulls the breeding days of which are over are often castrated before being shut up to fatten for the butcher. The operation may either be performed standing, or the animal may be thrown on to one side, and the uppermost hind-leg drawn forward by a rope and held by an assistant. The steps of the actual castration are essentially the same as those in the horse, but a smaller type of instrument is usually used. In very young calves—*i.e.* those between a month and six weeks old—castration is very often carried out by merely opening the scrotum

* Recommended in the *Veterinary Record* of March 3, 1960.

and scraping the spermatic cord through with the edge of the knife. Bleeding resulting in such cases is but slight and negligible. The quickest, easiest, and cleanest method of castrating cattle is to use a 'Burdizzo emasculator'. This is made in the form of a pair of very powerful blunt pincers with heavy, non-elastic jaws, and an arrangement of levers in the handles by which the force applied to the handles is very considerably multiplied when it is transmitted to the jaws. The instrument is arranged with the jaws over the neck of the scrotum in such a way that when closed they will crush the spermatic cord through the skin of the scrotum. An assistant presses the handles together while the operator holds the cord from moving away from the closing jaws. The skin of the scrotum is not severed, there is no hæmorrhage and very little danger of septic infection, and the method is expeditious and clean. The disadvantages of the Burdizzo emasculator are that the cord is liable to slip away from between the jaws of the instrument and so escape crushing, and that, even when the cord is properly crushed in the larger young bulls, the blood-supply of the testicle may not be completely cut off, and a certain amount of its function remains. To avoid these disadvantages as much as possible, the majority of practitioners make a point of crushing each cord separately in two places about an inch apart, the second crush being below the first, and therefore painless. In satisfactory cases after use of the Burdizzo emasculator the testicle swells up for a day or two, and there is also some swelling of the scrotum, but the animal is not greatly inconvenienced, does not go off its food, and in a few days the swelling has disappeared. The testicle gradually shrinks and atrophies, until in a month's time it is but little larger than a walnut.

The rubber-ring method (*see* 'ELASTRATOR') has of recent years come into use. It is not, as might be supposed, a painless method. Pain is caused immediately after the application of the ring; and also, in a proportion of cases, after two or three weeks when ulceration occurs.

Sheep.—The most convenient age at which lambs are castrated is when they are between a week and a month old, the operation usually being carried out at the same time as docking. The point of the scrotum is cut off transversely and each testicle exposed by the one incision. They are then seized alternately by a pair of rubber-jawed forceps, turned round and round so as to twist the cord, and then pulled off, or the cord may be scraped through with a knife. Various patterns of forceps are used, but they are all essentially the same in principle. Special small emasculators, similar to those used for cattle and horses, are also employed.

The rubber-ring method (*see* 'ELASTRATOR') is also used, and the Department of Agriculture, New Zealand, has stated that there was no significant difference in the fat quality of lambs castrated at three weeks of age by (*a*) rubber ring, (*b*) knife, and (*c*) emasculator. Lambs castrated at birth by the rubber-ring method were lighter and smaller.

This method is not ideal. Pain immediately following application may be severe, and subsequent ulceration of the skin may also be painful and conducive to tetanus infection.

For the castration of adult rams the Burdizzo emasculator is probably the best instrument. Any method of castration of adult rams which involves opening the scrotum is usually attended by a high percentage of deaths, no matter with how much care and asepsis the operation is performed.

Pigs.—Young male pigs are usually castrated at the time they are weaned or a little before it, *i.e.* between 7 and 9 weeks old, although a number are operated upon when only about 5 weeks old. Many people consider that the earlier period is not to be recommended because it entails placing the newly castrated pigs back with the sow; with a fractious gilt, or with an irritable old sow, the small amount of bleeding which may occur is apt to induce the mother to attack and perhaps kill her unfortunate little ones. At the same time many other owners prefer to have the pigs castrated before they are weaned, so that the check to their growth which always follows weaning does not coincide with the check they receive from the operation. Probably the best arrangement is to leave the little pigs with the sow until they are about 8 weeks old, and then to castrate them and wean them at the same time, giving extra good feeding for a short while afterwards. Young pigs should always be starved for 12 hours before castration, as bleeding is always less if the pigs are hungry and are fed immediately after the operation—a procedure which diverts the greater proportion of the blood in the body to the digestive organs away from the more distant parts of the body. The little pigs are held by the hind-legs by a man who grasps them above the hocks, the animal's belly being turned towards his knees. The process of castration is practically the same as for lambs, except that the scrotum is opened by two incisions, and the cords are usually scraped through with the knife instead of being broken.

In the United States it is becoming common practice for piglets to be castrated when they are between 4 and 7 days old. Instead of the conventional incising of the scrotum, small incisions are made at different sites and, by means of a surgical hook, the spermatic cords are withdrawn and severed. The testicles may be left in position. It is claimed that this method reduces the danger of subsequent wound infection.

Dog and Cat.—It is customary to castrate the male cat when it is to become a household pet, for by so doing the very pungent and penetrating smell from the prostatic secretion, which mingles with the urine, is abolished, and, moreover, the tendency to stray away at night-time in response to the powerful call of sex never exhibits itself in the castrated animal. Male dogs are usually only castrated when they become troublesome in the house, or on account of disease. In each of these animals in Great Britain a general anæsthetic is necessary if they are over the age of 6 months (under the Animals Anæsthetics Act). The operation is a simple one, and is performed in a manner similar to the castration of other animals. Castration of kittens is best done at 3 to 4 months of age.

Accidents following castration.—*Hæmorrhage* may occur either immediately following the operation or at any time afterwards up to the sixth or seventh day (usually within the first 24 hours). As a rule the small amount of hæmorrhage which nearly always occurs immediately after the operation can be disregarded, since it comes from the vessels in the skin of the scrotum. When bleeding is alarming it is necessary to pack the scrotum with sterilised cotton-wool or gauze or to throw the animal, search for the cut end of the cord, and apply a ligature. This is a task for a veterinary surgeon. (*See* BLEEDING, ARREST OF.)

Hernia of bowel or of omentum may occur where there is a very wide inguinal ring. The replacement or amputation of any tissue that has been protruded from the abdomen demands the services of a skilled practitioner. All that the owner should do until he arrives is to secure the animal, pass underneath its abdomen a clean sheet that has been soaked in a weak solution of an antiseptic, such as potassium permanganate solution the colour of port wine, and fix this sheet over the loins in such a way that it will support the protruded portions and prevent further prolapse. A good way is to tie the ends roughly over the loins, insert a stick, and twist the sheet tightly in the manner used to tighten a tourniquet.

Peritonitis, which is almost always fatal in the horse, may follow the use of unclean instruments, or may be contracted through contamination from the bedding, or by attack by flies subsequent to the operation. The symptoms are usually serious enough not to escape notice. The animal is dull dis inclined to move or eat ; temperature is high ; pulse is fast and thready, and there is a distinct pause between inspiration and expiration. The fæces are usually coated with mucus, and passed with considerable straining. The expression is haggard and anxious, and the case rapidly gets worse and usually dies in from 24 to 60 hours after the operation.

Tetanus may arise as a complication following castration in horses and lambs particularly. Sometimes there is a considerable loss among lambs from this cause. (*See* TETANUS.) In districts where tetanus is common, colts should be given a dose of tetanus anti-toxin before castration, which will protect them until the wounds have healed.

CASTS of hollow organs, or of parts of them, are found in certain diseases. During bronchitis membranous casts are sometimes coughed up from the lungs ; they consist of exudate and catarrhal material which filled up one or more of the larger bronchial tubes, and which were dislodged by the coughing. Casts of the microscopic tubules of the kidneys are passed in the urine in nephritis, and form an important diagnostic feature of this condition.

CAT, DISEASES OF (*see* FELINE ENTERITIS, FELINE INFLUENZA, FELINE INFECTIOUS ANÆMIA, FELINE INFECTIOUS PERITONITIS, FELINE JUVENILE OSTEODYSTROPHY, FELINE INFECTIOUS RHINOTRACHEITIS, RABIES, TOXOPLASMOSIS, and under diseases of the ear, bladder ; also diabetes, eczema, pleurisy, ringworm, thrombosis, tuberculosis, dropsy, steatitis, leukæmia, pasteurellosis of cats, Benzoic acid poisoning, etc.). (*See also under* CAT FOODS and succeeding paragraphs.)

CAT FOODS.—A diet of heart is injurious and if fed exclusively can lead to paralysis within a matter of weeks.

An all-liver diet is also dangerous since it gives rise to an excess of vitamin A, which in turn can lead to ankylosis of the cervical vertebrae. The 'angry cat' position may be observed by the veterinary surgeon called in to examine the animal. An exclusive diet of minced beef can also cause deformity of the skeleton. (*See* FELINE JUVENILE OSTEODYSTROPHY.) (*See also* TINNED FOODS, STEATITIS.)

CAT LEPROSY.—A disease resembling human and rat leprosy, and associated with acid-fast bacilli indistinguishable from *Mycobacterium lepræmurium.* These are found in granulomata affecting the skin and subcutaneous tissue, and in lymph nodes. The disease is transmissible to rats.

CAT LUNGWORM—*Aleurostrongylus abstrusus* can give rise to symptoms such as coughing, sneezing, and a discharge from the nostrils.

Recent research has disclosed a relationship between infestation with this lungworm and abnormality (hypertrophy and hypoplasia) of the pulmonary arteries. This condition may persist for two years—or even a lifetime.

CAT, WORMS IN.—In a survey of 110 cats autopsied in the University of Sheffield, *Toxocara cati* were found in 35·4 per cent, the tapeworm *Dipylidium caninum* in 44·5 per cent, *Tænia tæniæformis* in 4·5 per cent. (*See also* 'LIZARD POISONING'.)

CAT-SCRATCH FEVER.—A disease of man caused, it is believed, by a virus. The main symptom is a painless swelling of the glands nearest the scratch; sometimes fever, and a rash.

CATAPHORESIS (*καταφορέω*, I carry down) is a method of treatment by introduction of medicine through the unbroken skin by means of electric current.

CATAPLASM (*κατάπλασμα*) is another name for a poultice.

CATARACT (*cataracta*, a waterfall or portcullis) is an opacity of the crystalline lens of the eye. (*See under* EYE, DISEASES OF.)

CATARRH (*κατά*, down; *ῥέω*, I flow).—Inflammation of mucous membranes, particularly those of the air passages, associated with a copious secretion of mucus. This complaint, very prevalent among horses and dogs in cold weather, usually begins as a nasal catarrh or coryza, accompanied in the early stages by sneezing fits and the discharge of large quantities of watery material from the nose and eyes. There is generally some irritation in the throat which leads to a cough and perhaps difficulty in swallowing. Laryngeal and bronchial catarrh may accompany the above manifestations, and in severe cases bronchitis may result. Generally, however, the discharges assume a whiter and thicker character, and in the course of a few days the trouble clears up. There is always some temporary discomfort, and symptoms of fever may be seen.

Catarrhal inflammation may attack any of the mucous membranes of the body (*see* DYSENTERY, DIARRHŒA, *and* DISEASES OF INTESTINES) and of the genital organs (*see* METRITIS, BALANITIS, VAGINITIS, etc.).

CATECHU is an extract of the leaves and young shoots of *Uncaria gambier*, or, in the case of black catechu, from the wood of *Acacia catechu.* Catechu is a powerful astringent in caes of persistent diarrhœa and in dysentery in horses and cattle.

CATGUT is used in surgery for tying arteries, and for suturing wounds. It was originally made from the fibrous coats of the intestines of cats, although those from sheep are now almost exclusively used and serve equally well. It requires careful purification and preparation, and, being animal tissue, it has the advantage that it may be left in position until it is finally absorbed.

The catgut must be treated so as to render it sterile, and is sometimes further treated so that its absorption is delayed. (*See also* NYLON.)

CATHARTICS (*καθαρτικόν*) are substances which produce an evacuation of the bowels. (*See* PURGATIVES.)

CATHETERS (*καθετήρ*) are tubes used for passing along the urethra, the narrow passage which connects the bladder with the exterior, in order to draw off urine when for some reason or other natural voidance is impossible or difficult. They differ in shape and size according to whether they are intended for male or female use, and according to the breed of animal. For females they are generally rigid, made of metal which does not rust with the action of the urine, *e.g.* silver or electro-plated steel. For male use they are often constructed of gum-elastic or rubber, when they are flexible and less likely to damage or irritate the tortuous passage in the male. Their use requires considerable knowledge of the anatomy of the parts, and as fatal damage may very easily be inflicted by unskilled persons, they should only be employed by surgeons.

CATTLE : Names given according to Age, Sex, etc.—Different localities have their own names for particular cattle at particular ages, periods of life, etc., and these names vary somewhat. The following is a list of the most usual names :

Bobby or **Slink Calves :** immature or unborn calves used for human food, and often removed from the uteri of cows when the latter are killed. The flesh of slink calves is often called **Slink Veal.**

Freemartin : a cow calf born as a twin with a bull calf, and often barren.

Calf : a young ox from birth to 6 or 9 months old ; if a male, a *bull calf* ; if a female, a *cow* or *heifer calf.*

Stag : a male castrated late in life.

Steer or **Stot :** a young male ox, usually castrated, and between the ages of 6 and 24 months.

Stirk : a young female of 6 to 12 months old, sometimes a male of the same age, especially in Scotland.

Bullock : a two-year-old (or more) castrated ox.

Heifer or **Quey :** a year-old female up to the first calving.

Maiden Heifer : an adult female that has not been allowed to breed.

Cow-heifer is a female that has calved once only.

Bull : an uncastrated male.

Cow : a female having had more than one calf.

CATTLE, BREEDS OF.—**Beef Breeds :**

Shorthorn (Beef type).	Aberdeen-Angus.
Devon „	Galloway.
Sussex.	Belted Galloway.
Hereford.	Highland.

Lincoln Red (*and see* CHAROLAIS, LUING, LIMOUSIN, MEUSE–RHINE–IJSSEL).

Dual-Purpose Breeds :

Shorthorn (Dairy type).	Welsh Black.
South Devon.	Dexter.

Red Poll. (*and see* SIMMENTAL).

Dairy Breeds :

Ayrshire.	Jersey.
British Friesian.	Guernsey.
Kerry.	British Dane.

The Milk Marketing Board reported that during 1959–60, over 1,600,000 cows were artificially inseminated, and that of the bulls used, 48 per cent were Friesians ; 7 per cent Ayrshires ; 6 per cent Dairy Shorthorns ; 4 per cent Guernseys ; 3 per cent Jerseys ; 10 per cent Aberdeen-Angus ; 15 per cent Herefords.

Comparable figures for 1965–66, covering the Board's 23 A.I. centres in England and Wales, were : total cows bred, 1,705,000 approximately. Of the bulls used, 52 per cent were Friesians ; 3·8 per cent Ayrshires ; 1·1 per cent Dairy Shorthorns ; 4 per cent Guernseys ; 3·2 per cent Jerseys ; 7·8 per cent Aberdeen-Angus ; 21·2 per cent Herefords ; 3·2 per cent Charolais (now the third most important beef breed, with over 54,000 first inseminations).

BEEF CATTLE.—Beef cattle differ from dairy and dual-purpose cattle in that they are primarily intended for the production of meat. Their milk yield is of secondary importance ; indeed for many purposes they are satisfactory when they produce just sufficient milk to raise their own calves. There are parts of the world —*e.g.* the La Plata river basin of South America and the western ranges of U.S.A. —where animals of the extreme beef type are pre-eminent. This is because their capacity for converting bulky and coarse forage, corn, etc., into human food has made them the most profitable outlet for farming enterprise. Beef cattle are well adapted to rough land and sparse grazing ; they are suitable for unimproved and arid areas. In arable belts it is sometimes difficult and costly to market corn, and cattle may be kept to convert it into beef ; in other cases they are kept to consume by-products such as straw.

Quality must necessarily depend upon the purpose for which the animal is required, and is best considered from the view-points of (1) the farmer, (2) the butcher, and (3) the consumer.

The farmer requires an animal that will make rapid gains of weight on a minimum of food : docility and high digestion capacity are associated with this quality. The animal should put on fat while it is still growing, so that, in order to obtain the high prices offered in normal times for small animals in prime condition, it may be marketed before it has reached maturity. The beast should have the conformation and finish which enable it to command the highest price per unit of weight. (*See* BEEF BREEDS AND CROSSES, BEEF CATTLE HUSBANDRY.)

The rapidity with which an animal will make gains is nothing to the butcher. He wants a bullock which carries a high proportion of the most expensive cuts, and the score card is a fairly true reflection of his requirements. He wants the animal to 'kill well', *i.e.* he wants a carcase with a minimum of offal. A well-finished bullock will dress about 58 per cent of its live weight; very highly finished show specimens may produce even more than 70 per cent of carcase to live weight. Cattle bought on the farm where they are in a rested condition probably lose 40 to 100 lb. by the time they reach the abattoir.

A well-finished animal has a 'marbled' appearance owing to the deposition of fat between the bundles of muscle fibres, and when cooked it has fine flavour and juiciness. A joint from an animal of a dairy breed or an animal fattened after it has grown to maturity has not the same quality, because the fat is put on externally and internally without developing the requisite marbling of the flesh.

BRITISH BEEF BREEDS.—The following are the British breeds of beef cattle (*but see* BEEF BREEDS AND CROSSES. Most of our beef in Britain comes from dairy herds):

The Beef Shorthorn.—*Origin and history.*—The beef and dairy Shorthorns have a common origin in the short-horned cattle of Durham, Yorkshire, and Northumberland. Before the middle of the eighteenth century these had been improved by importations from the Continent of animals of good milking quality. The earliest of the famous improvers were the brothers Colling, who farmed near Darlington. By close in-breeding on the lines that had been adopted by Bakewell, the pioneer stock improver, they soon produced cattle far above the standard of their district. The Collings' herds were sold in 1810 and 1820. Thomas Booth and Thomas Bates, using Collings' stock, continued the improvement and spread the fame of the breed, the former developing a beef and the latter a stylish dual-purpose strain.

Amos Cruickshank (1808–1895) of Aberdeenshire developed the type of beef Shorthorn which is now so highly favoured at home and abroad. Cruickshank did not follow the craze of fashion, but added to his herd animals of any strain provided that they conformed to the type he had in mind. His aim was to develop a phlegmatic, easily fed, short-legged, compact and thickly fleshed butcher's beast. For long he gathered together selections from far and near, and he acquired an enviable assortment of vigorous cattle; but his type was not fixed. Then, and unexpectedly, he bred a calf which he named Champion of England. This bull so nearly approached what had long been his ideal that he used him and his progeny for judicious in-breeding. Thus the type ultimately became fixed and the Scotch Shorthorn acquired its vigorous prepotency.

Beef Shorthorns are registered along with Dairy Shorthorns in Coates's *Herd Book*, started in 1822. The book is 'open' to females that have four top pedigree crosses; *i.e.* non-pedigree stock can be 'graded up' to eligibility for entry in the herd book by using pedigree bulls on four successive generations of females.

Appearance.—The Shorthorn is one of our large-sized breeds. In general it closely adheres to the beef type, but it has a characteristic squareness of conformation. The short horns are preferably waxy throughout, being curved more in the cow than in the bull. A dark muzzle is objectionable. The shoulders are sometimes too prominent and bare. The body is extremely broad and deep; the lines are straight. The hind-quarters are as a rule extremely well fleshed, and in this respect the breed surpasses all others; older animals tend to develop patches of subcutaneous fat about the root of the tail. The colour may be red, red-and-white, white, or roan. Yellowish reds and red-and-whites are not popular.

Characteristics and usefulness. — The breed stands in the first class as a beef producer; a large proportion of commercial beef cattle have Shorthorn blood predominating. However, the dressing percentage is barely as good as in the case of the Aberdeen-Angus, to which breed the Shorthorn usually stands second at fatstock shows. Owing to the outstanding prepotency of the breed, nothing has done so much to improve the beef cattle of the world as the use of Shorthorn bulls on grade cows. For this purpose the Argentine has been the chief market for British pedigree stock. The milking capacity of the beef Shorthorn is poor, and in many pedigree herds nurse cows of other strains are required to assist in feeding calves for shows and sales.

The Hereford. — *Origin and history.* — The breed originated in the county whose name it bears. The ancestry is undoubtedly mixed and is somewhat obscure, but the characteristic white faces are believed to have been acquired from cattle imported from Holland. Early records show that Herefords were generally employed for draught purposes, and the earliest selections were probably made with a view to size, strength, and vigour. The colours of the early cattle were variable, and the present red-and-white markings were fixed only about 110 years ago. The most famous of the early improvers was Benjamin Tomkins the younger (1745–1815). He boldly adopted the system of 'in-and-in' breeding, and he effected a marked advance in early maturity, refinement, and general beef character.

The *Herd Book* was started privately in 1846, and it was not until thirty years later that the Hereford Herd Book Society was formed to continue its publication. In 1883 the book was closed except to the progeny of stock already entered.

Appearance.—The size of the Hereford is large, being about the same as that of the Shorthorn. Its colour is deep red with a white head, chest, and underline; the eyes may be surrounded by a red mark. The horns are waxy, of medium length, and drooping; black points are objectionable. The shoulder is beautifully laid and covered with flesh; the quality of the fore-quarters is noteworthy, and is seldom reached in other breeds. On the other hand, the hind-quarters are sometimes deficient in depth and thickness. The back is good, and the depth of chest indicates a sound constitution. The skin approaches that of the Galloway in thickness and mellowness, and in being covered with a dense, fine coat of hair.

Characteristics and usefulness. — The Hereford surpasses all other breeds in combining hardiness with early maturity and fattening qualities, and this makes it the pre-eminent breed for grass beef production. In its own district the animals are kept on grass the whole year round, and the cows have only to raise their own calves. At home, pure-bred herds are found mainly in the west of England but cross-bred Herefords are now widely distributed. The progeny of Hereford bulls always show the characteristic white face of the breed and this colour-marking prepotency is valued as it shows that the progeny are at least half of beef breeding and that the females are not suitable for dairy herds. The use of Hereford bulls at A.I. centres since 1949 has led to an ncrease in the number of cross-bred He eford stock suitable for beef production. It is overseas that the characteristics of the Hereford find their greatest usefulness, and there is hardly a pastoral district throughout the world where the breed is not firmly established. Nowhere has it been more successful than in North America, where it is found from Texas to Alberta, and surpasses all other breeds for the utilisation of the sparse herbage of the ranges.

The milking capacity of the cows is generally only sufficient to raise their own calves well; but the breed is probably better than the beef Shorthorn in this respect. The quality of the meat is good.

Aberdeen-Angus.—*Origin and history.* The origin is speculative, but the oldest records show that polled and horned cattle, variable in colour, were common in parts of Aberdeenshire and Angus. Apparently the early breeders selected for hornlessness, and this character was fixed before that of colour. Some Shorthorn blood may have been used by early improvers.

Hugh Watson (1789–1865) of Keillor, Angus, was the first great improver of the breed. He took black cattle to Keillor, and, having learned something of the methods used in developing the Shorthorn, set about improving his stock by 'in-and-in' breeding. His results were extremely satisfactory, particularly in promoting early maturity and in developing fineness of bone and thickness of flesh. Watson laid the foundations of those qualities which make the Angus such an admirable butcher's beast. Another name associated with the development of the Angus is that of William McCombie of Tillyfour. He was not only a very successful improver, but he attracted international attention by winning the grand championship against all breeds at the Paris International Exposition in 1878.

The *Herd Book* was established in 1862; it is open only to the progeny of registered stock.

Appearance.—The Aberdeen-Angus is smaller than the Shorthorn but weighs exceptionally heavy for its size. The conformation is more cylindrical or rounded than the Shorthorn; it has not the same square lines. The Angus is hornless and the head is unusually fine and free from coarseness; its poll is more Pointed than that of the Galloway. It is fine in the bone, short in the leg, round in the thigh, and smoothly fleshed all over. These points, and the way in which the hocks are well covered and laid in, all tend to give the breed its characteristic appearance.

Characteristics and usefulness. — The breed surpasses all others in quality from the butcher's point of view, and it has a unique record in carcase competitions. Its percentage of carcase to live weight is the highest; moreover, the fat is perfectly distributed and free from patchiness. The Angus is very early maturing, and is admirably suited for intensive feeding such as is given in the production of baby beef. No cattle are more satisfactory for court or byre feeding. However, the breed does not have the hardiness of the Hereford and is not suited for poor grazing conditions; nor has it the usefulness of the Shorthorn in grading up unimproved native stocks. The Angus is found in all parts of the world, but nowhere can it be said to form the national breed of cattle. The cows are better milkers than the beef Shorthorns, and it is probable that quite good milking strains could be obtained by selection. Cross Angus cattle make excellent feeders; the best known is the 'blue-grey', which is by a white Shorthorn. Aberdeen-Angus bulls almost invariably beget progeny which are black and hornless and this prepotency has led to the mating of Angus bulls with inferior milking cows in dairy herds either by natural service or artificial insemination.

The Devon.—*Origin and history.*—The Devon breed of cattle has been developed from the native cattle of the county. Old records show that the Devon was a hardy draught animal that made a good feeder and the breed came gradually to be valued primarily for beef purposes, giving meat of the finest quality with small weight of bone. Improvement was brought about by selection within the breed and not by crossing, and credit is due to Francis Quartly and Col. L. T. Davy for their early efforts in this direction. Col. Davy published eight herd books of the Devon breed between 1851 and 1881 and his pioneer work led to the foundation of the Devon Cattle Breeders' Society in 1884. The breed has been developed mainly in the hilly, rough country of north Devon and the cattle are considerably smaller than the Shorthorn. Herds that have been bred for a considerable time on good lowland pasture tend to produce bigger animals of somewhat poorer quality. Typical North Devons are strikingly refined in appearance and their shapely build and smoothness of flesh are very marked. In respect of quality of carcase, the breed may be said to occupy among English cattle the position that the Aberdeen-Angus holds among Scottish breeds. A criticism that is sometimes made is that the Devon does not mature very rapidly. Abroad, the breed has done well wherever animals are wanted to withstand conditions of great heat. There were always possibilities of selecting useful dairy strains in herds of Devons and in the south-east of the county and adjacent districts a dual-purpose type was once popular (*see under* DUAL-PURPOSE BREEDS).

Characteristics and size.—The Devons are a uniform dark red in colour, sometimes with a slightly curly coat; the horns are larger and longer than in Shorthorns, growing forward and slightly upward and of a creamy colour, with the tips showing a darker shade. The nose should be flesh coloured. The body is of compact shape and supplies medium-sized, high-grade, nicely marbled joints; it is said to be difficult to judge their weight in comparison with other breeds; this is no doubt due to the density of their flesh and the proportion of lean meat to fat. The average live weight may be given as 11 cwt.

Adaptability.—The great majority of pedigree Devon herds are found in the four south-western counties of England but recently additional herds have been established in other counties. Large numbers of commercial Devons have always been found in the grazing and fattening districts in the midlands and a feature of the last seven years has been the consignment of large numbers of calves and yearlings to be fattened in the eastern counties. There has also been a considerable export trade to South Africa, Australia, and South America.

The Sussex.—*Origin and history.*—The similarity between the Sussex and the Devon shows a common ancestry, which is believed to be the old Celtic cattle of Britain. As far as records go, the Sussex was originally developed as a draught animal in the Weald of Sussex and Kent. Doubtless the earliest selections were made with a view to obtaining size and strength. The animals were then long of leg, far from refined, and slow to mature; many, when mature, could be fed to weights exceeding a ton. When oxen were no longer wanted for draught purposes, the breed was developed along beef lines. The *Herd Book* was founded in 1874; in order to include good non-pedigree stock it was re-opened in 1902 for animals that passed an inspection.

Appearance.—The size is as large as that of the Shorthorn. The colour is a whole dark red, being of a deeper shade than in the Devon. The horns are large, and black or brown tipped. Although the breed has been greatly improved in recent years there is still a slight coarseness and largeness of frame inherited from the draught stock. The fore-quarters are particularly well developed, and the back is good. The loin is but medium, and in depth and thickness of flesh the rump and thighs do not equal the quality of our most improved breeds. Formerly somewhat 'leggy', the breed has been greatly improved in this respect.

Characteristics and usefulness. — The breed is extremely hardy and can subsist on very poor fare. Sussex cattle are good grazers and are noted for their ability to clean up rough, coarse herbage. They are not now slow to mature and will fatten while young, but are chiefly noted for producing well-finished carcases as three-year-olds. The cows are poor milkers and unsatisfactory except for raising their own calves. The breed has done well in South America and in South Africa.

The Galloway.—*Origin and history.*—The Galloway has been developed in the wet and hilly south-west of Scotland, but its origin is unknown. The breed has no outstanding improver; it is exceptional in that in-breeding has never been used to fix its type and so there has been no risk of losing its robustness. The breed has long been noted for producing beef of first-rate quality and towards the end of the eighteenth century many thousands of Galloway store cattle were travelled annually to Norfolk and Suffolk to be fattened for the London market. Galloways were first registered with Aberdeen-Angus cattle in the *Polled Herd Book*, but the Galloway Cattle Society started a book of its own in 1877.

Appearance.—The Galloway is about the size of the Aberdeen-Angus, which it resembles in being whole black in colour and hornless. The coat is very characteristic, and is made up of long wavy hairs forming an outer protection, and a soft mossy inner coat. The head is very short and broad; the poll is less pointed than in the Aberdeen-Angus. The ear is broad, low set, and covered with long hair. The body is rather long and is narrower than in most other beef breeds; the back tends to be slack. The hind-quarters are well developed, but the shoulder is sometimes not so good.

Characteristics and usefulness. — The Galloway produces beef of superlative quality and flavour, but its percentage of carcase to live weight barely reaches that of the most improved beef breeds. The breed has been kept in the open throughout the year in a severe climate. It is superior abroad in some extremely cold climates, because the horns of Highland cattle are affected by frost-bite. Like the Highland breed, its greatest usefulness is in converting into beef the herbage of wild and rough grazings where other cattle would fail to find subsistence. It is too slow to mature and fatten to be satisfactory for intensive court feeding. The cows are quite good milkers. Galloway bulls, when crossed with horned breeds, beget hornless calves.

When Galloway cows are crossed with a white Shorthorn bull the highly esteemed Galloway 'blue-grey' is produced which is well known as a superior fattener. A useful hardy dual-purpose animal can be got by crossing with the Ayrshire. The breed has extended into the North of England and has done well in North America.

The Belted Galloway.—This is a variety of Galloway cattle that is probably as old as any other. The colour may be black or dun, with a white belt extending from the shoulders to the haunch. In addition to beef qualities it is claimed that the belted strains are such good milkers that they might be included in the dual-purpose group.

The Lincoln Red.—This branch of the great Shorthorn breed has been developed from the Lincolnshire cattle of the 18th century, chiefly by the introduction of Shorthorn bulls from Durham; in fact, three bulls were purchased for Lincolnshire herds at Charles Colling's sale in 1810, and the most famous of the early herds of 'Lincoln Reds' was that of Thomas Turnell, which originally came from the neighbourhood of Darlington. Lincolnshire breeders, however, adhered to the popular red colour, and registered Shorthorn bulls introduced to give greater and quicker maturity were always red in colour. In 1895 the Lincolnshire Red

Shorthorn Association was formed to promote the interests of the breed and its owners, and since that date a separate herd book has been published. Many herds have been bred entirely on beef lines, but in others milk production has been developed, and during recent years many excellent specimens of this dual-purpose breed have been exhibited at the chief shows throughout England.

Characteristics and size. — The predominant colour is a whole cherry red, with occasionally a little white on the udder and in the switch of the tail. The horns and colour of the muzzle should conform to the recognised Shorthorn type. In size the Lincoln Reds are very similar to the Shorthorns, but on good soil they may be somewhat larger; the average weight is 12 cwt.

Milking properties. — Similar to the Dairy Shorthorn.

(*See also* CHAROLAIS and LUING. These two breed societies were scheduled as approved beef cattle breeding societies in 1969.)

DESCRIPTION OF THE DUAL-PURPOSE BREEDS.—**The Dairy Shorthorn.**—*Origin and history.* — The Shorthorn breed of cattle originated in the county of Durham, chiefly in the valley of the Tees. For many years it was known as the Teeswater breed, and in parts of America the breed is still known as the Durham.

Characteristics and size. — Shorthorns may be red, red-and-white, roan, or white in colour, but light red is not popular, though occasionally associated with high milk production; the most popular colours are dark red and dark roan. The horns should be of medium size; flat creamy yellow in colour and curving gracefully forward; they should not be coarse at the base, not waxy white in colour, nor should they grow upwards from the head (cock-horned). The muzzle should be flesh-coloured and without a stain of black, and the nostrils wide and expansive. As regards size the Shorthorn may be taken as setting the standard of size for the larger breeds, the average live weight of mature cows being 11 to 12 cwt.

Milking properties.—The average yield of milk-recorded Dairy Shorthorn cows in some 3285 herds is fully 809 gallons at 3·84 per cent butter-fat. Many Shorthorn cows have given over 10,000 lb. per annum, and several have given over 20,000 lb. in 365 days. The world's record for butter-fat production is held by an Australian-bred Dairy Shorthorn—Melba of Darbalara—which gave 32,522 lb. milk containing 1614 lb. fat in a lactation period of 365 days.

Danish Red semen has been used as part of a breed improvement plan. (*See also* MEUSE–RHINE–IJSSEL.)

Crossing qualities.—The bulls as a rule cross well with other breeds. The first cross from Ayrshire cows with a Shorthorn bull and from Shorthorn cows with a British Friesian bull is usually highly thought of as a dual-purpose animal.

The Northern Dairy Shorthorn.—This type of Dairy Shorthorn is found in the hilly parts of the counties of Northumberland, Cumberland, Westmorland, Durham, and north-west Yorkshire. Cattle of Dairy Shorthorn type have been maintained in the dales of this area for probably 200 years and are noted for their healthiness, hardiness, and good milk production under exposed conditions. When in 1940–1941 it was found necessary to stimulate milk production throughout the country, in order to obtain more milk for direct human use, many farmers in the above counties changed over from butter-making and rearing store stock on the farm to the sale of milk. This led to the introduction of bulls of the pure dairy breeds and there appeared a danger that the characteristic type of the cattle of the area would be lost through cross-breeding. To counteract this tendency the owners of many herds of non-registered but typical Dairy Shorthorns formed the Northern Dairy Shorthorn Breeders' Society in 1944 and opened a herd book to which bulls and cows were admitted by inspection. A very large proportion of the cattle accepted for entry would also have been eligible for the grading register of the Shorthorn Society of Great Britain and Ireland, but, as pedigree status and entry in Coates' *Herd Book* could, through this register, only be attained after four generations, it was apparently considered more advantageous to begin a new herd book. Considerable progress has been made and several volumes of the herd book have now been issued. The Northern Dairy Shorthorn has not yet been recognised as a separate breed for milk-recording purposes and the records made in the herds are included in the annual reports under Dairy Shorthorns.

The Devon.—*Origin* (*see under* BEEF BREEDS).

Characteristics and size.—The dairy type of Devon is somewhat larger and is coarser in bone than the beef type. In

1918 the publication of milk records in the herd book was begun.

Milking qualities.—The breed is not noted for high yields but produces milk of good quality. The average yield of the recorded cows in 24 herds is 570 gallons and that of heifers is 450 gallons. Butter-fat tests are made for some 10 per cent of the recorded cows and the average fat percentage is 4·10.

The South Devon (sometimes called the South Hams). — *Origin and history.* — It is probable that this breed is an offshoot from the Devon breed and has acquired its distinctive colour by the introduction of Guernsey blood in the first half of the 19th century. The South Devon Herd Book Society was formed in 1891.

Characteristics and size.—The colour is described as a rich medium red by breeders, but to owners of other red breeds South Devons appear light or yellowish red. The horns are white or yellow, wide at the base, and fairly long, and the nose is creamy. This is the largest English breed of cattle, being appreciably larger than Shorthorns ; the average live weight of a mature cow is 14 cwt. or more.

Milking qualities.—The average milk yield of recorded South Devon cows is about 660 gallons and that of heifers in their first lactation is approximately 520 gallons. Half the number of cows and heifers which are milk-recorded are also tested for butter-fat and the average percentage for the breed is approximately 4·25 per cent. The milk is well suited for butter-making and for the manufacture of clotted (Devonshire) cream.

The Red Poll.—*Origin and history.*— The Red Polls of the present day are descended from the native breeds of Norfolk and Suffolk, which were respectively red and horned, and dun and polled. It may be also that other breeds such as the Galloway have been used to bring in occasional crosses. The present types have been recognised as one breed since 1846, and since the first issue of a herd book in 1874, followed by the formation of the Red Poll Cattle Society some years later, great progress has been made towards uniformity in type and colour by careful selection and breeding. The breed is now popular and widely distributed in Britain, and is well known for its dual-purpose qualities in other English-speaking countries.

Characteristics and size. The outstanding features are the lack of horns and the uniform deep red colour ; the poll should be distinct, and there should be no sign of ' scurs ' or abortive horns. The tip of the tail and the udder are occasionally white, and the nose should also be white without any sign of a darker coloration. In size the Red Polls are slightly smaller than Shorthorns, the average live weight of mature cows being 10 cwt.

Milking qualities.—The Red Polls are as good milkers on the average as Shorthorns. Since the development of milk-recording in England the high yields obtained in the Norfolk Society have often attracted attention. The average milk-yield in some 500 herds is fully 740 gallons. (1956 figures.) About three-quarters of the recorded cows and heifers are tested for butter-fat and the average for the breed is 3·6 per cent. The milk is well suited for direct consumption and cheese-making.

Crossing qualities.—The Red Poll is not much used for crossing, but it is valuable where polled stock are desired, because the progeny are almost entirely polled.

The Society is now known as the British Dane and Red Poll Cattle Breeders' Society, and is concerned with the breeding of: (1) Red Polls, (2) Red Polls × Danish Reds, (3) British Danes. The change was officially approved in 1969.

For the **British Dane** the following qualifying yield is prescribed for any lactation: minimum milk yield 1,000 gallons ; minimum percentage of butterfat content 3·8.

The Welsh Black.—*Origin and history.* —Early writers on the live-stock of Wales usually referred to several varieties of Welsh cattle, all of which appear to have had a common origin. At the beginning of this century there were two herd books in use—one prepared by breeders in North Wales, and the other by breeders in South Wales, but fortunately in 1904 the two societies amalgamated, and the Welsh Black Cattle Society now represents the interests of all breeders of Welsh cattle. The breed has long had a good reputation for beef purposes, and annually large numbers of Welsh steers are fattened on the pastures of the English midlands. The milking qualities have received more attention in recent years, and the yields of milk obtained have substantiated the claims of breeders that the Welsh Black is worthy of inclusion amongst the dual-purpose breeds.

Characteristics and size. — The only recognised colour is black, with occasionally a little white on the udder ; the horns are long, growing forward and upwards, and are creamy in colour with black tips. The frame is sometimes rather coarse-boned and lacking in symmetry, but breeders are gradually lessening these defects. In size the Welsh Black is slightly less than the Shorthorn, the average live weight of mature cows being 10½ cwt.

Milking qualities.—Average yield of cows in fully 100 Welsh Black herds is 540 gallons and that of heifers in their first lactation is about 450 gallons. About half the recorded cows and heifers are tested for butter-fat and the average percentage is about 4·10 per cent.

The Dexter.—*Origin and history.*—The Dexter breed originated in the West of Ireland, but the mode of origin is uncertain. It is most probable that it originated from the other native Irish breed—the Kerry—either by mating together Kerries of a low, thick-set type or by mating short-legged Kerry cows with bulls of other breeds, especially the Devon. It is known that Devon bulls were imported into the South of Ireland early in the 19th century. In recent years the breed has fallen out of favour.

Characteristics and size.—Its small size is its chief characteristic; it is the smallest of British breeds, mature cows averaging only 6 to 6½ cwt. live weight. The colour is either black or red, with occasionally a little white on the udder, and the horns are of moderate size. The body is very compact and the legs are short, and the Dexter has a definite value for beef purposes where small joints of high quality are required.

Milking qualities.—Often surprisingly large yields have been obtained from Dexter cows, the daily yield reaching 3 gallons or more, and many cows have given 6000 to 7000 lb. in a normal lactation period. The average yield for 19 milk-recorded herds is 496 gallons for the cows and heifers, taken together. Fully 80 per cent of the cows and heifers in recorded herds are tested for butter-fat and the average percentage is approximately 4·20 per cent.

DAIRY BREEDS. — **The Ayrshire.** — *Origin and history.* — This noted breed takes its name from the county of its origin. The native cattle of the country were improved by the introduction of Dutch or Teeswater stock in the latter half of the 18th century, and later Highland crosses were used in a number of herds. During the 19th century improvement was brought about by selection within the breed. A hardy, heavy milking breed, Ayrshires are now found throughout the Commonwealth, and in the United States, Sweden, Finland, Japan, China, and many other countries. In recent years also the Ayrshire has gained popularity in England by reason of the reliable milking qualities it possesses.

Characteristics and size.—The Ayrshire is noted for her large symmetrical udder, roomy, wedge-shaped frame, short legs, and horns with a characteristic forward and upward curve. The colour is red and white in varying proportions and clearly marked—sometimes flecked but never roan—and occasionally black-and-white. In size the breed is smaller than the Shorthorn, mature cows averaging 9 to 9½ cwt. live weight, but many of those bred and reared in good dairy districts in England attain larger weights.

Milking qualities.—From the point of view of quantity of milk the present-day Ayrshire stands next to the British Friesian. The average yield of the recorded cows in some 4148 herds in England and Wales is approximately 873 gallons at 3·84 per cent butter-fat. Many cows have given over 2000 gallons in 365 days and several have achieved 3000 gallons in the same period.

Crossing qualities.—The first cross Ayrshire usually inherits the shapely udder and good milking qualities of the Ayrshire parent, and is a useful type of dairy cow.

The British Friesian. — *Origin and history.*—This breed is descended from animals of the famous Dutch dairy breed imported into England prior to 1892, since which year importation of cattle for breeding purposes has only been possible under Government licence. The British Friesian Cattle Society was constituted in 1909 and importations of Friesians have been made from time to time since then. There have been three importations from Holland, one from South Africa and one from Canada. These importations were permitted for the purpose of introducing new blood and assisting in improving the type and milk-yielding qualities of British Friesians. In other dairying countries throughout the world the Friesian is one of the most popular breeds, and the British herds have greatly increased during the last forty years, spreading from Cornwall in the south to Inverness-shire in the north.

Characteristics and size.—The colour is black and white in varying proportions and clearly defined, with white below the knees and hocks; dun and dun-and-white are undesirable colo urs. The horn resemble the Shorthorn's in size, but have black tips. Friesians are as large as Shorthorns, and mature cows average 11 to 12 cwt. live weight.

Milking qualities.—The Friesian is the heaviest yielding of all dairy breeds, and the British Friesian maintains this position in Britain. The average yield for some 8900 herds of recorded cows in England and Wales is 1000 gallons at 3·53 per cent butter-fat. Large numbers of cows in Britain have given over 20,000 lb. in 365 days and upwards of 100 have given over 30,000 lb. The British Friesian Cattle Society has spared no effort to improve the fat content and their efforts have been highly successful.

Crossing qualities.—Much beef in Britain comes from this breed.

There is also the British Canadian Holstein Friesian Society.

The Jersey.—*Origin and history.*—This breed is native to the island of Jersey, where it is said to have been bred without any addition of foreign blood for over 500 years. Since 1789 importation of other cattle into the island has been forbidden except for slaughter. Jerseys were introduced into Britain early in the 19th century.

Characteristics and size. — Jerseys are small to medium in size, the average live weight of mature cows being 7 cwt. They are very fine-boned and carry very little flesh, but have excellent udders. The colour is fawn of various shades, grey, and some with dark brown colouring ; a few have small white patches. The horns are fine and incurving, and the muzzle is black. The skin is noticeably yellow inside the ears, and on the udder.

Milking qualities.—Jerseys milk very well for their size and produce the richest milk of all breeds in Great Britain. The average yield for the milk-recorded cows in 1924 herds is about 742 gallons at 5·01 per cent butter-fat. Numerous cows have given over 1000 gallons per annum. Jersey milk has a characteristic creamy yellow colour ; it is very suitable for a butter-making or cream trade, or where a higher price can be obtained for a richer milk. The quality and colour of the milk often lead to a few Jerseys being kept in a herd of cows in order to improve the bulked milk from the herd. The cream layer in bottled milk is made more apparent.

Crossing qualities.—Cross-bred cows of Jersey blood often give high yields of rich milk, but cross-bred bull calves are of very little use.

The Guernsey.—*Origin.*—The breed has been bred on pure lines for several hundred years, and no cattle allowed to be imported except for slaughter. They were imported into England many years ago, and became very popular in Cornwall, where they are now the commercial farmer's breed, particularly in the extreme west of the county. The breed has become more popular and more widely distributed throughout England in recent years, and the English Guernsey Cattle Society does much useful work in encouraging breeders to have accurate milk and butter-fat records taken. The breed is also widely distributed in the Commonwealth and the United States.

Characteristics and size. — In general conformation the Guernsey resembles the Jersey, but is larger in size, the average weight of mature cows being about 9 cwt. live weight. It is coarser in bone, and lacks the refined appearance of the Jersey. The colour is fawn or yellowish-red with distinct patches of white ; horns are incurving, and the nose should be creamy, though occasionally black-nosed animal sare found in pure-bred herds. The yellow coloration of the skin is even more marked in the Guernsey than in the Jersey.

Milking qualities.—The breed is noted for the rich colour of the milk, and good yields are obtained. The average yield of milk-recorded cows in 2170 herds is 765 gallons at 4·55 per cent butter-fat. The milk is most suitable for butter- or cream-making, or where rich milk of good colour is specially desired ; it is also helpful where milk is sold in bottles, because the cream layer is then deepened and more easily seen.

Crossing qualities.—Not much used for crossing purposes, and cross-bred progeny have the same advantages and defects as Jersey crosses.

The Kerry.—*Origin and history.* This breed is native to Eire, but is now found primarily in the south-west of that country, having been gradually replaced by the larger English breeds on the better soils and pastures of the midlands.

Characteristics and size.—The Kerry is black in colour, sometimes with a little white about the udder ; the horns are creamy with black tips, and in cows often turn upwards. In size the Kerry resembles the Jersey, the average weight of mature cows being about 8 cwt. live weight.

Milking qualities. — Good, especially when the size of the animal is considered and the short time during which systematic improvement has been carried on. The average yield in 9 Kerry herds is 729 gallons. Butter-fat averages about 3·9 per cent. Individual cows have yielded over 10,000 lb. per annum. The milk is of all-round value for direct use, butter- or cheese-making.

OTHER BREEDS.—In addition to the above-mentioned breeds, all of which are well known and have classes provided for them at the larger agricultural shows, there are in England still a few herds of Longhorns and British White (Park Cattle).

(*See also* COWS, BULL MANAGEMENT, BULL LICENSING, BEEF-BREEDS AND CROSSES, CALF-REARING, HOUSING OF ANIMALS.)

CATTLE, DISEASES OF.—Surgical conditions include displaced abomasum, bloat, gastric ulcers, traumatic pericarditis, foul-in-the-foot. Other diseases include: ACTINOBACILLOSIS, ACTINOMYCOSIS, ANTHRAX, BLACKQUARTER, BLOUWILDEBEESOOG, BLUETONGUE, BUSS, BOVINE ENCEPHALOMYELITIS, BRUCELLOSIS (including CONTAGIOUS ABORTION), CATTLE PLAGUE, CEREBROCORTICAL NECROSIS, CLOSTRIDIAL ENTERITIS, COCCIDIOSIS, CONTAGIOUS PLEURO-PNEUMONIA, ENTEQUE SECO, FOOT-AND-MOUTH DISEASE, HUSK, HYPOCUPRÆMIA, HYPOMAGNESÆMIA, INFECTIOUS OPHTHALMIA, JOHNE'S DISEASE, LEPTOSPIROSIS, MALIGNANT CATARRH, MASTITIS, MILK FEVER, MUCOSAL DISEASE, MUCORMYCOSIS, PARASITIC GASTROENTERITIS, PASTEURELLOSIS, POLIOENCEPHALOMALACIA, POST-PARTURIENT HÆMOGLOBINURIA, PYELONEPHRITIS, RABIES, RED-WATER, RHINOSPORIDIOSIS, RHINOTRACHEITIS, SALMONELLOSIS, 'SKIN TUBERCULOSIS', TICK-BORNE FEVER, TRICHOMONIASIS, TUBERCULOSIS, VIBRIO FŒTUS INFECTION, VIRUS INFECTIONS OF COWS' TEATS, VULVO-VAGINITIS. (*See also* CALVES, DISEASES OF.)

CATTLE PLAGUE, which is also known as RINDERPEST, BOVINE TYPHUS, CONTAGIOUS TYPHUS OF THE OX, is an acute, specific, inoculable, and febrile disease of cattle, characterised by an ulcerative inflammation of mucous membranes, especially those of the alimentary tract. This disease ravaged Europe intermittently for fifteen centuries. In the United Kingdom the 1865–66 outbreak alone involved over 324,000 cattle, but the disease was finally eradicated in 1877. Vast areas of Asia and Africa are still subject to cattle plague, which remains one of the most serious threats to world food-supplies, and which—like foot-and-mouth disease—is caused by a virus, but one far more deadly. Indeed, when cattle plague strikes a herd, nine out of ten animals may die—a catastrophe which is not infrequently followed by famine—and the total loss of food and draught animals (cattle and buffaloes) from this cause runs into two million a year.

Susceptibility.—Cattle are by far the most susceptible animals. Eland and bush pig are known to contract rinderpest, and ailing wild game may carry infection to healthy cattle. Sheep and goats occasionally become infected; pigs also. The majority of infected pigs show only a mild, febrile response, with some depression and anorexia; they could, therefore, act as a very dangerous means of transfer of virus from contaminated meat to cattle. There is evidence that Asiatic pigs are more susceptible than those of European origin to infection with rinderpest virus, and they have long been known to be affected naturally in Indo-China. Horses are immune. Meat, skins, offal, manure, food, water, grooming tools, rugs, and so on, may carry in-

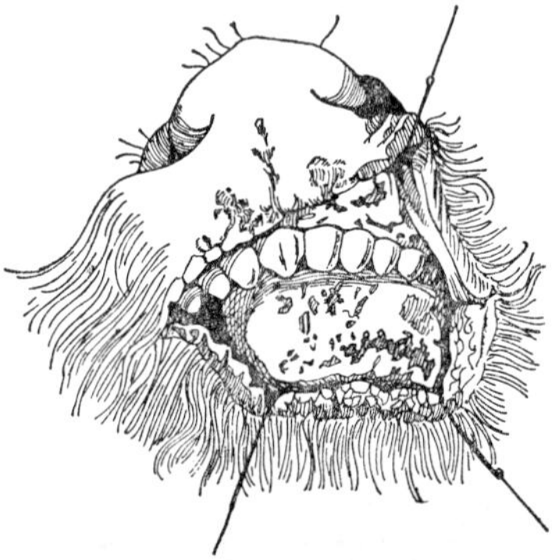

Diagram to show the appearance of the lesions in the mouth of an ox affected with cattle plague. Each of the pitted areas appears bright red in the living animal.

fection. Thus, cattle-markets, pens railway trucks, boats, or any places where diseased cattle have been, are a source of contamination and spread. The virus is fairly easily destroyed by ordinary disinfectants. Infection may lurk about cow-sheds or farm premises for considerable periods, although direct exposure to sunlight rapidly kills the virus. If an animal contracts the disease and recovers, it retains a strong and probably lifelong resistance to infection. Instances have occurred of an animal suffering from a second attack, though of a mild nature; but for all practical purposes this risk may be ignored.

Incubative period.—3 to 9 days.

Symptoms.—The first sign of illness is a rise of temperature, which may reach 104° to 105° F. This, which may escape observation, is quickly followed by dullness and depression. The animal, if free, stands away from the rest of the herd with drooping head, ears hanging down, and back arched. Many animals may eat fairly well for a couple of days after the initial temperature rise, but in other cases the appetite falls off sooner. Rumination is suspended ; the animal grinds its teeth, stands uneasily, and there may be slight constipation and some straining on defæcation. On the second day the changes on the mucous membranes commence ; the eyes appear red, and a slight discharge of tears occurs which soon mats the hair down the cheeks.

The muffle seems dry and has lost its normal dew ; the nasal mucosa becomes red and gives off a watery discharge which soon becomes mucoid. The mouth is found to be pasty and inflamed, and around the incisor teeth there is an angry red appearance. In some outbreaks there is a slight vesicular eruption of the skin over the neck, shoulders, vertebral column, and on the udder or scrotum. This causes slight matting of the hair and scar formation, but in many countries this symptom is absent or so slight as to escape notice.

As the disease progresses the symptoms become aggravated. The eyes are sunken and discharge a dirty mucoid matter ; the conjunctivæ are scarlet or livid in hue ; the muffle is dry and of a cracked or chapped appearance. The nose discharges a sticky mucus (not nearly so 'ropy' as in foot-and-mouth disease), and on the inflamed areas of the mouth ulcers may appear, which may be the size of a 6d. or 1s. piece. These occur in front of the incisor teeth, on the gums, inside the cheeks, on the borders of the tongue, and in front of the dental pad. The epithelium comes off in bran-like scales, leaving a ragged surface. This feature of the ulcers is important as one of the distinguishing characters from the ulcers found in foot-and-mouth disease.

The fever, with its usual accompaniments, last for 5 or 6 days or even more. On recovery the temperature falls gradually, but a sudden drop to normal or sub-normal usually portends approaching death. From the 3rd to the 4th day the constipation gives place to diarrhœa of a fœtid nature, and much straining takes place. The diarrhœa is followed by dysentery, dark clots of blood being evacuated with the diarrhœic discharges. In other cases almost pure blood may be passed. The anus becomes dilated and the mucous membrane of the rectum is exposed, appearing dark, or purple.

In milking cows the milk gradually falls off with the increase of the symptoms, and what milk is given is of a yellowish or watery consistency. Pregnant cows usually abort about the height of the disease.

The affected animal becomes very weak and emaciated. In a few cases a peculiar emphysematous condition of the skin appears, as though the subcutaneous tissues had been blown up with air. This is chiefly noticeable on the upper part of the neck, over the withers, and may extend along the spine as far as the lumbar region. It is a bad sign, only occurring as a rule in fatal cases.

Course and duration.—The disease is usually acute, lasting 4 to 10 days. Outbreaks of a more chronic type do occur in some countries. These last much longer, and produce a greater number of recoveries. In new outbreaks of cattle plague death may claim up to 90 per cent of the victims, while at other times the death-rate may be as low as 20 per cent.

Diagnosis.—In countries where the disease is known it is usually fairly easy to diagnose, provided that several animals in different stages of its course are seen. Nevertheless, diagnosis may prove more difficult in new outbreaks. Cattle plague most not be confounded with—

1. *Foot-and-mouth disease.*—In this disease the onset is more sudden, the ulcers in the mouth are larger, and the mucous membrane of the ulcers comes away more in one piece. The nose and eyes are not affected to the same extent nor so painfully as in cattle plague, and the lesions in the feet and consequent

lameness are distinguishing factors. Foot-and-mouth usually spreads more quickly through a herd, and if left unchecked its death-rate is very low.

2. '*Red scour*' or *Coccidiosis.* — In some cases this may simulate plague, but is confined to the digestive tract and is not infectious in the same sense.

Examination of scrapings from the rectal mucosa reveals the presence of coccidia.

3. '*Tick fever.*'—Some form of this, or piroplasmosis, as it is termed, may in certain countries be mistaken for cattle plague in the early stages, but a trained veterinarian can rapidly distinguish the diseases by blood examination, if not from the clinical symptoms.

Other conditions that might lead a layman to suspect cattle plague are hæmorrhagic septicæmia of the ox, malignant catarrhal fever, and even acute mineral poisoning.

Post-mortem appearances.—In no civilised country is it permissible for a layman to open a cattle plague carcase. The lesions are mostly confined to the eyes, nose, and alimentary tract, and are usually very characteristic and easily determined by a veterinary surgeon. The true digestive or 4th stomach (abomasum) usually shows the most characteristic appearance.

Treatment.—In the United Kingdom no form of treatment is permitted, but in countries where they do not follow the slaughter policy, careful nursing and attention to the animal's comfort may make all the difference to a case on the border-line between death and recovery. No drugs are of any use, and a severe case will die, no matter what is done for it.

Prevention. — In 'clean' countries this can be most readily achieved by stringent quarantine laws governing the importation of susceptible animals, but should an outbreak occur immediate notification is essential. Once the disease gets a hold in a country, enormous loss is occasioned before it is possible to stamp it out. The immediate slaughter of all infected or in-contact cattle, sheep, goats, or other ruminants, must be carried out, and all movement of stock prohibited in a given area. This, along with compulsory notification, is provided for in 'The Diseases of Animals Acts' and in the special Cattle Plague Order of 1895. This order also lays down the methods for the destruction of carcases, disinfection, and so on.

With regard to methods of immunisation used overseas, great progress was made in Kenya, especially, by improving a method of attenuating the virus first carried out by Edwards in India. In this the virus is passaged through more than 100 goats. At about the 130th passage the virus is found to be so attenuated that it fails to reproduce the disease in cattle, though still retaining its powers to stimulate the production of an immunity. The virus can be dried and stored, and is now commonly known as the 'K.A.G. virus', meaning Kabéte Attenuated Goat virus. Later, virus was passed through rabbits as well as goats. Then, during the 1939 war it was feared that the enemy might use cattle plague virus as a biological weapon and spread it in Canada and the United States. Since existing methods of vaccine production would have been far too slow and costly to protect all the herds of North America, intensive experimental work was carried out, as a result of which it was found possible to produce the vaccine—in bulk and cheaply—by growing the virus in hens' eggs. It is this method which the Food and Agriculture Organisation of the United Nations Organisation is using to-day.

Cross-immunity.—Infection of dogs with the rinderpest virus apparently confers immunity against distemper.

CAUDA EQUINA, meaning 'tail of a horse', is the name given to the termination

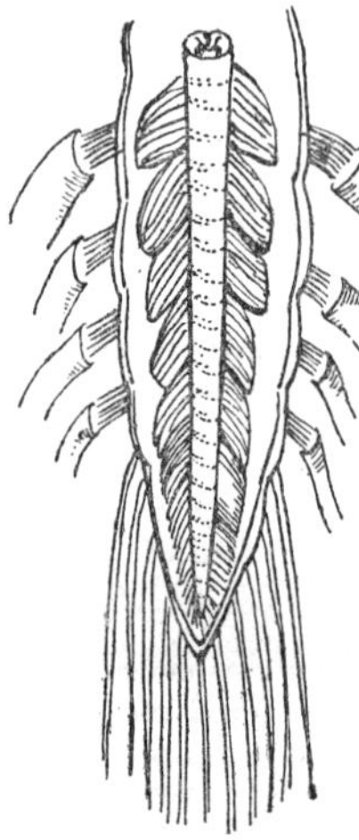

The 'Cauda Equina', or termination of the spinal cord. The membranes have been slit and laid back. The last four coccygeal branches are shown.

of the spinal cord in the sacral and coccygeal regions where it splits up into a large number of nerve fibres giving the appearance of a 'horse's tail', whence the name.

CAUSTICS and CAUTERIES (*καίω*, I burn) are bodies used to burn diseased or healthy tissues, the former acting by chemical energy, and the latter by their high temperature.

Varieties.—The chief chemical caustics in veterinary use are pure acetic, carbolic acids, caustic potash and soda, silver nitrate, copper sulphate, zinc chloride, and caustic collodion. The usual cauteries are the hot iron or firing-iron, and the electric cautery—a platinum point or blade heated by a current of electricity.

Uses.—Caustics are used to destroy small warts or tumours on the surface of the skin, etc. The cautery is used for the checking of arterial hæmorrhage, and for the removal of certain superficial new-growths. Cautery is sometimes used for operation upon vascular organs, such as the liver, in human surgery. (*See* SPRAINS, and DISHORNING, etc.)

CAVITY.—There are three main cavities in the animal body: those of the head, thorax or chest, and abdomen. That of the head, often called the cranium, is lined by a smooth membrane or meninge, which allows slight movement of the contained organ. That of the chest is lined by three similar membranes which prevent friction between the heart, right and left lung respectively, and the chest walls; while the abdomen is lined by the very complicated peritoneum, which serves the same purpose, and enables the body to store fat in such a position that it may cause no interference with vital structures. Cavities are produced in certain diseases of a destructive type. (*See* CONTAGIOUS BOVINE PLEURO-PNEUMONIA, TUBERCULOSIS, ABSCESS.)

C.C.K.—Contagious conjunctivo-keratitis. (*See* CONTAGIOUS OPHTHALMIA, p. 325.)

C.C.N.—Cerebro-cortical necrosis.

CELANDINE, GREATER and LESSER *see* BUTTERCUP POISONING).

CELLS (*cella*, a cell in a honeycomb) are the microscopic units of which all the tissues of the animal and plant kingdoms are composed.

Every cell consists essentially of a cell-body of protein material called 'protoplasm', in which lies a small kernel or 'nucleus' which controls the activities of the cell. Within the nucleus may be seen the 'nucleolus', a minute body which seems to control the process of cell-division or 'mitosis'; and there may or may not be a 'cell-envelope' surrounding all. In some cells various other structures can be seen, such as cilia, mitochondria, and Golgi bodies.

Cells vary very much in size, the smallest being about $\frac{1}{10000}$th of an inch in diameter, and the largest being the egg of a bird, which is still a simple cell, although much distended with food.

All animals and plants consist at first of a single cell (the egg-cell or *ovum*) which begins to develop after fertilisation by a male germ-cell or *spermatozoön*, derived from the opposite sex. Development commences by a division of the fused male and female cells into two new cells; these give rise to four after further division, and the process continues until a large mass results. In this mass differentiation into the various structures of the body gradually takes place, the ultimate result being the fœtus and its membranes, which are discharged by the act of parturition, after which the process of cell division still goes on until death occurs.

At first little difference can be discerned between the individual cells of the embryo, but slowly certain cells become differentiated, and give rise to the various tissues of the body: thus, cells of the nervous system send out long processes which develop into the nerves; cells of the muscular system assume a longitudinal shape and become muscle fibres; fat cells become filled with fatty globules; some deposit lime salts and form bone; others form cartilage, tendon, or ligament; and others again retain many of their primary characteristics and form liver-cells and white blood corpuscles.

From these differentiated cells others of a similar type are produced, and gradually all the tissues of the body are built up, and as they become worn out they are replaced or added to, according as the exigencies of the life of the animal demand.

Certain tumour growths are formed of cells that have a resemblance to other cells of the body, but they occur in parts where such cells are not normally found, or else in superabundance to what is usual. (*See* FŒTUS, TUMOURS, EMBRYOLOGY.)

'CELLULAR TISSUE' is the old name for the areolar or fibrous tissue found between the skin and the muscles of the body, between muscles, and around the various organs of the body. It is in this tissue that fat is stored by the body.

CELLULITIS means an inflammation taking place in the 'cellular tissues' of the body. (*See* ULCERATIVE LYMPHANGITIS.)

CENTRIFUGE—a hand- or electrically-driven machine used in the laboratory to separate cells, organisms, worm eggs, or other particles from a fluid suspension.

CERCARIA is the name given to an intermediate stage in the life-history of the liver fluke, viz., the tadpole-like form, which is produced in the body of the fresh-water snail *Limnœa truncatula*, bores its way out of the snail, and attaches itself to a suitable blade of grass to wait for the arrival of a sheep which will eat it. In the sheep's stomach and intestines further development takes place. (*See* PARASITES, p. 646).

CEREAL (*cerealis*) is the name given to plants belonging to the great class of grasses (Graminea), which produce edible seeds, such as wheat, barley, oats, rye, maize, millets, rice, and so on. They are all rich in starch and comparatively poor in proteins and minerals, and the seeds are mostly poor in calcium but richer in phosphorus. (*See* BARLEY POISONING.)

CEREBELLUM and CEREBRUM (*see* BRAIN).

CEREBROCORTICAL NECROSIS.—A condition first reported in ewes and calves in Britain in 1959. The cause may be connected with a thiamine deficiency. Symptoms include: circling movements, a staggering gait, excitement, and convulsions. Only a few animals in a flock or group become affected; but nearly all of those die. (*See also* POLIOENCEPHALOMALACIA.)

CERVICAL (*cervicalis*) means anything pertaining to the neck.

CERVICITIS means inflammation of the *cervix uteri* or neck of the womb.

CETAVLON (*see* CETRIMIDE).

CETRIMIDE.—An antiseptic of value in wound treatment and for cleaning cows' udders and teats; a 0·1 per cent solution being effective against *Streptococcus agalactiœ*, a cause of mastitis. A 1 per cent solution acts as a detergent.

CHAFING OF THE SKIN occurs almost solely among horses and animals that wear harness, and is caused by the improper fitting or adjustment either of the part of the harness that actually causes the injury, or else of some remote part throwing the rest out of place. The commonest parts of the body that are injured are the backs of horses, from badly fitting saddles or pads; the region of the chest behind the elbow, from the girths; the withers, from collars, breast-harness, or the pommel of a riding saddle; the poll, from the poll-piece of the bridle; the sides of the root of the tail, from the crupper; the points of the shoulders, from the collar being too wide usually; the buttocks, from the breeching-web during much backing of loads; and the most prominent parts of the sides of in-foal mares, from the rubbing of the plough-chains, or from the traces. Those parts of the bodies of working cattle or dogs that are in contact with harness are liable to become chafed in hot weather or if the adjustment of the harness is bad.

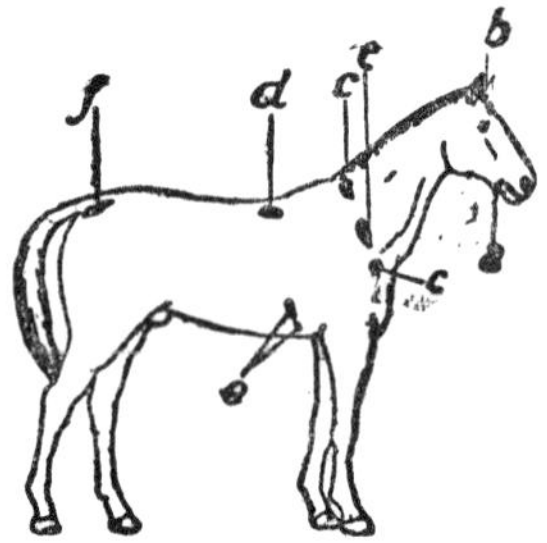

Injuries from harness. *a*, Curb-gall; *b*, poll-injury; *c*, chafed shoulders from collar, high, medium (over spine of the scapula) and low (at point of shoulder); *d*, sore back from saddle; *e*, girth-galls; *f*, crupper-gall.

Treatment.—Primarily it is necessary to prevent chafes occurring by ensuring that the harness is of a good fit, that it is kept clean, that it is not put on so loosely as to allow it to move over the surface of the horse's body during walking, etc., and that there are no projections to injure the skin. With pregnant mares, whippletrees should be wide enough to enable the chains, etc., to clear the sides, and such animals should not be worked in shafts when they are heavy in foal. Should a chafe occur, the part of the harness responsible must be eased from the sore place and arranged so that no further damage will result, or if serious, the work must be stopped altogether. Binding a piece of sheepskin with the wool outside over the chain or other part of the harness causing the chafe, is an excellent way of preventing further damage. The area should be cleansed with warm water and a suitable antiseptic, and the sore dressed with dry dusting powder. After healing, swabbing with methylated spirit will harden the skin.

Young horses that have fine or thin skins should have their shoulders, etc., bathed with a strong solution of salt and water, 3 ounces to the pint, before going to work and after the harness is removed. This, or painting with methylated spirit, hardens the skin and prevents the surface from being abraded.

CHAGAS' DISEASE.—This is an infection with *Trypanosoma cruzi*, mainly occurring in wild mammals (such as oppossums, armadillos, and wood rats) of Central and South America, and occasionally infecting man, dogs, cats, and pigs. The disease occurs mainly in children and young animals, and is characterised by fever, anæmia, emaciation, and dropsy, with death from heart failure following myocarditis. Blood-sucking bugs transmit the disease.

CHALAZA is the spiral band of albumen joining either end of the yolk to the shell of a bird's egg.

CHALAZION is a small swelling of the eyelid caused by a distended Meibomian gland. It is commonly seen in dogs.

CHALK (*see* LIME and CALCIUM).

CHAMPIGNON is the name given to a form of suppurative inflammation of the cut end of the spermatic cord in the horse. It is often due to botriomycosis (q.v.).

CHARLIER SHOE is a special type of shoe which is sometimes used for applying to horses' feet when they are to be turned out to grass. It is narrow and light and possesses no toe-clip which may injure the sole of the foot if the shoe becomes loose. It is fitted by taking a groove of horn out of the lower margin of the wall, into which the shoe is nailed. Charlier shoeing demands considerable skill on the part of the shoeing-smith lest burning of the sensitive tissues of the foot occur.

CHARLOCK POISONING.—The common charlock plant *Brassica sinapistrum* is only dangerous to live-stock after the seeds have formed in the pods, and then only when eaten in large amounts. The seeds contain small amounts of the volatile *oil of mustard*, as well as of the alkaloid *sinapine* and the alkaloidal glucoside *sinalbin*. The symptoms recorded are loss of appetite, colic, diarrhœa; inflammation of the kidneys, shown by tenesmus, excessive or blood-stained urine; great exhaustion, nervousness, and the emission of a large amount of yellowish frothy liquid from the nostrils, causing grave interference with respiration. The treatment should consist of large drenches of milk containing tannic acid in the form of strong black tea or coffee. Hypodermic injection or morphine or atropine may be necessary. Poisoning by charlock is fortunately rare.

CHAROLAIS.—This is the second (numerically) largest breed of cattle in France, and they have been exported throughout Europe and the U.S.A. The Charolais, white, is an excellent beef animal, a most efficient grazer, with a rapid growth-rate and a quiet disposition. The loin and thigh muscles are exceptionally well developed. The bulls are colour-marking and highly prized for crossing purposes. U.K. trials of this breed for crossing purposes were approved in 1961, and it is now the third most important beef breed.

'CHASTEK PARALYSIS'—A condition of secondary vitamin B_1 deficiency, seen in foxes and mink on fur farms as a result of feeding raw fish. An enzyme in the latter has the property of destroying the vitamin, probably in much the same way as occurs in 'bracken poisoning'. Administration of vitamin B_1 is curative in the early stages.

CHECK LIGAMENT.—This is joined to the Perforans tendon, and acts as a check on the movement of the pastern joint. The check ligaments are often strained in the racehorse.

CHEESE.—A high proportion of all cheese is made from raw milk. *Brucella* organisms may live in such cheese for two years. (*See* BRUCELLOSIS.)

CHELATING AGENTS are substances which have the property of binding divalent metal ions to form stable, soluble complexes which are non-ionised and so virtually lacking in the toxicity of the metal concerned. Derivatives of ethylene-diamine-tetra-acetic acid (E.D.T.A.) afford examples. E.D.T.A. itself is poisonous, as it removes calcium; but the calcium-E.D.T.A. complex has been recommended in the treatment of acute lead poisoning, being given repeatedly for several days. It would possibly be of service in mercury, copper, and iron poisoning.

CHEMOSIS (χήμη, a hole) means swelling of the conjunctival membrane that covers the white of the eye, leaving the cornea depressed.

CHEMOTAXIS, or **CHEMIOTAXIS** (χημεία, chemistry; τάξις, arrangement) means the property possessed by certain cells of attracting or repelling other cells, possibly by the pouring out of a secretion into the vicinity. It is in this way that white blood-cells are induced to leave the smaller arteries or capillaries when there are foreign particles present in the tissues. (*See* ABSCESS.)

CHEMOTHERAPY means the treatment of disease by chemical substances. Modern chemotherapeutics generally denotes the use of the newer anti-bacterial chemicals such as sulphanilamide, sulphapyridine, sulphathiazole, sulphaguanidin, and so on. Among others are penicillin, gramicidin, the range of stilboestral compounds, and the aromatic diamidines which are so useful in the trypanosome diseases.

CHENOPODIUM, OIL OF.—This is a volatile oil distilled from the Jerusalem oak — *Chenopodium anthelminticum* — which consists of a mixture of terpene substances. It is used as a vermifuge against round worms in the horse and the dog. It is, however, somewhat toxic for cats. In the horse, thiabendazole is now preferred.

The drug requires to be given along with a mild, oily purgative, such as linseed oil for horses or castor oil for dogs, and animals, especially horses, require to be fasted before administration. Its action is materially assisted if, some hours prior, horses and dogs are given a dose of salts to remove mucus and as much intestinal matter as possible; this allows the drug to exert its anthelmintic action more directly upon the worms.

Oil of chenopodium must not be given to pregnant or old or very debilitated animals. Symptoms of poisoning including vomiting, diarrhœa, and great prostration. (*See also* ANTHELMINTICS.)

CHEST, or **THORAX**, is the more anteriorly situated of the two large cavities of the body, occupying the space bounded by the anterior ribs, the sternum, the thoracic or dorsal vetrebræ, and the diaphragm. It is a conical cavity, with the apex directed forwards and continued into the root of the neck for a short distance. The base is formed by the diaphragm, while the sides are formed by the ribs, sternum, and vertebræ. Lying between adjacent ribs on the same side there are two layers of intercostal muscles, those on the outside running almost at right angles to those on the inside. The intercostal muscles fill up the spaces between the ribs and their cartilages, and are active agents in moving the ribs during respiration. The outsides of the chest walls are covered with the masses of the shoulder muscles, and the shoulder-blades or scapula lie one on either side, anteriorly over the rib-cage, but not attached to it by bony connections.

Contents.—The chest contains the two lungs, one on either side, with the termination of the trachea and the bronchial tubes. Occupying the middle of the space between the lungs, but projecting towards the left more than to the right, lies the heart and its associated vessels. The œsophagus or gullet, which carries food down from the mouth to the stomach, runs through the chest, passing for the greater distance between the upper parts of the lungs, and enters the abdomen through an opening in the diaphragm. The thoracic duct, which carries lymph from the abdomen, runs forwards immediately below the bodies of the vertebræ and ends by opening into one of the large veins in the apex of the cavity. Various important nerves, such as the two vagi which control the abdominal organs, the phrenics, which supply the muscles of the diaphragm, and sympathetics, etc., pass through the chest in particular situations. In the young animal the thymus gland lies in the anterior portion of the chest, but as time goes on and growth, which this gland has to do with, ceases, the gland atrophies and its place is occupied by lung and other organs. Lining each of the two divisions of the chest cavity is the pleura, a fold of which also covers the surface of the lung, and the heart is enclosed in a special sac or pericardium. (*See* HEART, LUNGS, PLEURA, PERICARDIUM.)

CHEST DISEASES (*see* LUNGS, DISEASES OF; HEART DISEASES, BROKEN WIND, BRONCHITIS, PLEURISY, PNEUMONIA, TUBERCULOSIS, GLANDERS, CONTAGIOUS BOVINE PLEURO-PNEUMONIA, VERMINOUS BRONCHITIS; THORACOTOMY).

CHESTNUTS (*see under* POINTS OF THE HORSE).

CHEYLETIELLA PARASITOVORAX.—A mite which infests dogs, cats, birds, rabbits, squirrels, etc. It gives rise to itching and scurfiness of the skin. In man Cheyletiella species (including *C. yusguri*) may cause urticarial weals of trunk and arms, together with intense itching.

CHEYNE-STOKES' RESPIRATION is an abnormal form of breathing in which the respirations become gradually less and less until they almost die away; after remaining almost imperceptible for a short time they as gradually increase in depth and volume until they are exaggerated; after attaining a maximum they again decrease until nearly imperceptible. This alternation proceeds with considerable regularity.

Cheyne-Stokes' breathing is always a very serious condition, which is generally associated with severe nervous disturbance, shock, and collapse, or with heart or kidney disease. It is most obvious in the dog and horse after they have sustained very severe injury but without internal hæmorrhage (which induces what is generally known as ' sobbing respiration ').

CHICK ŒDEMA (*see* ' TOXIC FAT SYNDROME ').

CHICKEN-POX (*see* AVIAN CONTAGIOUS EPITHELIOMA).

CHICKS require no food for the first 36 hours. The hover temperature should be 90° F., and the room temperature must be kept above 60° F. during the first 5 weeks or so of life. Chilling is one of the commonest causes of pullet chick mortality. Chicks require artificial heat for 3 to 8 weeks, depending upon the type of house, weather, etc.

CHILLING (*see under* CHICKS and CHILLS).

CHILLS and COLDS, although in themselves frequently very trivial ailments, are important because of the danger of serious complications, such as pneumonia, bronchitis, pleurisy, roaring, broken wind, etc., following them.

Causes.—A cold usually follows prolonged chilling of the surface of the body, such as exposure to a draught of cold air, living in a foggy atmosphere, prolonged wetting by rain or snow and subsequent standing in the open air, sudden immersion in cold water, railway journeys in open trucks in cold weather, standing in a cold, wet, draughty saleyard or showyard for long periods with insufficient food and under great nervous excitement. In many instances the introduction of an animal suffering from a cold among healthy young animals of the same species results in an outbreak. A virus is regarded as the cause though various organisms are also associated with the secondary symptoms.

Symptoms.—Everyone is familiar with a ' cold in the head ' among human beings, and in animals the condition is similar. As a rule, in simple cases there is only a slight elevation in temperature. When the cough becomes troublesome, laryngitis or bronchitis may be suspected. When there is persistent refusal of food, difficulty in drinking, and the return of certain amounts of either food or water through the nostrils, pharyngitis may be suspected, especially if the outside of the throat is swollen and painful on pressure. When great difficulty and rapidity in breathing are shown, congestion of the lungs, pleurisy, or even pneumonia, may be presumed. In addition to these not infrequent complications, others less common may be exhibited; the animal may become attacked with diarrhœa, indicating that the catarrhal condition has spread to the stomach and intestines; scantiness of urine and pain and stiffness in the lumbar regions point to inflammation of the kidneys; reddening and discharge of tears from the eyes mean that the conjunctiva have become infected, and if high fever is also present, ' pink eye ' or strangles may be suspected in the horse or distemper in the dog or cat.

Treatment.—Isolate and house in a warm, airy, well-ventilated place, provide with clothing if necessary, give easily digested food to eat and clean water to drink, and rest for a few days. In the large majority of cases prompt measures such as these will cut short an attack, and if the animal is otherwise healthy, complications will not occur.

Since it is well known that animals living continually out of doors, such as hill sheep, wintered-out colts and store cattle, ranch cattle, etc., seldom or never take colds or chills, so long as they are not housed indoors at night-time, it is very rightly considered that *fresh air* is a most potent preventative of chills and colds. (*See also under* BRONCHITIS; PLEURISY, PNEUMONIA, STRANGLES; LARYNX, DISEASES OF; VENTILATION; EQUINE VIRAL RHINOPNEUMONITIS etc.).

CHINCHILLA.—In domestication the average litter-size is two: in the wild state it is believed to be four. In their natural surroundings, chinchillas live at 10,000 feet above sea-level in the Andes. Those at lower levels are said to have poorer coats. There are two species.

The period of gestation is about 111 days. The life span may be over 7 years. Composition of the urine and fæces is such as to make this an odourless animal. A favourite diet in captivity is dried bread and hay.

CHINCHILLA, DISEASES OF.—Enteritis sufficiently severe to cause death is common in chinchillas, judging by the sparse literature on the subject. Out of a series of 1000 post-mortem examinations made in the U.S.A., 'epidemic gastro-enteritis' was found in 23 per cent of the chinchillas, as against 25 per cent with pneumonia, and 12 per cent with impaction (blockage of the intestine). In a further series of 1000 examinations, the figures were: impaction, 20 per cent; pneumonia, 22 per cent; and enteritis, 24 per cent.

Lying on one side and stretching the legs are said to be symptoms of impaction. The feeding of too many pellets with too little roughage is believed to be a cause, and clearly the means of prevention lies largely in the breeder's hands.

Intussusception is not uncommon and sometimes follows enteritis.

Fur-chewing—that bane of the North American chinchilla industry—has been attributed to 'environmental stress'—the frustration and depression associated with captivity. Of course, the wrong diet may enter into it, too; so a little more freedom, combined with some fresh greenstuff, is always worth an immediate trial—with a little apple and a raisin or two now and then for good measure.

CHLAMYDIA.—An alternative name for Bedsonia.

CHLORAL HYDRATE, usually called 'CHLORAL', is a substance produced by prolonged action between alcohol and chlorine gas. It is a clear, crystalline substance with a sweetish taste, dissolves rapidly in water, forming a solution which, when concentrated, has the property of blistering mucous membranes.

Actions.—Internally, chloral acts as a hypnotic, or a depressant to the central nervous system, according to the quantity administered. It diminishes the sense of pain, causes a fall in the blood-pressure, and interferes with co-ordination of movement. Extremely nervous or very vicious horses are quietened by the drug.

Uses.—It is given when animals require to be calmed before shoeing, clipping, travelling by railway; before service by the male in nervous or vicious females; to control bulls that are liable to 'run amok'; and before giving a general anæsthetic for some operations, and as the principal anæsthetic for others. It is used in some forms of colic, when the bowels are in an irritable condition; and as it is not supposed to interfere with peristalsis, it is probably the best sedative for this purpose. It should not be used in all colic cases, however, as in those that are due to impaction it serves to mask the real symptoms and may leap to a false sense of security concerning the case. In the cow it is used in many diseases when an agent which has both sedative and antiseptic actions is required internally. In the dog, in company with an equal part of bromide of potassium, it was much used. (*See also under* ANÆSTHETICS, TRANQUILLISERS.)

CHLORAL HYDRATE POISONING.—In the horse large doses of chloral produce a relaxation of the muscles, staggering, lowering of the temperature, and finally a deep stupor. The respirations gradually become weaker and weaker, until they are imperceptible, and death results from respiratory failure. In the dog the general signs are similar, but a fleeting stage of excitement is often noticed first.

Antidotes.—Artificial respiration, strong coffee, or hypodermic injections of cocaine, caffeine or strychnine, massage to the surface of the body by wisping or hand-rubbing, and the maintenance of the body-heat by hot-water bottles for the smaller animals and rugs for the horse and ox, are the chief measures to be employed.

CHLORALOSE.—A narcotic which has been used experimentally in wood-pigeon baits and also for the destruction of mice, and has led to unintentional poisoning in dogs and cats. Treatment with methylamphetamine has been recommended.

CHLORAMINES are widely used as a disinfectant. Their activity depends upon the amount of available chlorine.

CHLORAMPHENICOL.—An antibiotic effective against rickettsiæ, certain viruses, bacilli, staphylococci, streptococci, brucella, and certain salmonella organisms. It has been used in the treatment of keratitis of rickettsial origin, secondary infections in virus diseases of dogs, and infectious feline enteritis, and in cases of contagious foot-rot in sheep, and of diarrhœa in foals and calves.

In human medicine poisoning by chloramphenicol has led to aplastic anæmia, skin eruptions, and moniliasis. It is a synthetic product, formerly obtained from a soil-living organism, *Streptomyces venezuela*.

Intramuscular injections of chloramphenicol are painful, in the dog at least. The toxicity and high cost of this antibiotic limited its use and its use in veterinary medicine in the U.K. has been greatly restricted following the recommendations of the Swann Committee.

CHLORDANE.—A highly toxic insecticide of the chlorinated hydrocarbon group. It is volatile and poisoning through inhalation may occur.

CHLORETONE, or **CHLORBUTOL,** is a white powder with an odour like camphor. Internally it acts as a hypnotic. It is chiefly used as a remedy for sustained vomiting and travel sickness in dogs and cats.

CHLORIDE OF ZINC is the main constituent of Burnett's disinfectant. In the form of sticks, the chloride is used to repress exuberant granulations (proud flesh) in healing wounds, and to cauterise the surfaces of small tumours and ulcers.

CHLORINATED HYDROCARBONS.—The newer insecticides are mostly either organo-phosphorus compounds or chlorinated hydrocarbons. These include : DDT, DDD, methoxychlor, benzene hexachloride, toxaphene, aldrin, dieldrin, isodrin, and endrin plus a range of others less well known. Ingested at toxic levels, or absorbed through the skin, they act primarily on the central nervous system causing increased irritability at the outset followed by muscular tremors leading to convulsions in acute cases. Species capable of vomiting do so. Loss of appetite with marked loss of body weight is usual in subacute poisoning.

Most compounds—methoxychlor is an exception—can be stored in the body fat and excreted in the milk and so may constitute a public health problem. It is interesting to note in passing that out of 901 samples of market milk collected throughout the U.S.A. in the autumn of 1955, 62 per cent contained residues of chlorinated organic parasiticides, some samples containing up to 1·5 parts per million.—(P. J. Barden and H. Paver, *Vet. Record*, Oct. 14th, 1961.)

CHLORODYNE is very similar in composition to the compound tincture of chloroform and morphia. It is a sedative and hypnotic, and is useful for the purpose of controlling simple diarrhœa in dogs, horses, and cattle.

CHLOROFORM is a colourless, mobile, non-inflammable liquid, half as heavy again as water. It is prepared by distilling alcohol with a mixture of slaked lime and chloride of lime. It is used as a solvent for sulphur, phosphorus, fats, resins, and most substances rich in carbon, and consequently is much used for cleansing purposes. It was first applied to medicine by Sir J. Y. Simpson, who used it as an anæsthetic in place of ether, which had been introduced just previous to 1847 by an American—Morton. (*See* ANÆSTHESIA.)

Uses.—Internally, when given by the mouth, it acts as a carminative, antispasmodic, and anodyne. It should be given well diluted in gruel, or irritation of the gastric and intestinal mucous membrane results. Inhaled by the nostrils it induces general anæsthesia in all animals.

Four stages are recognised :

(1) *The stage of excitement* begins immediately the drug is administered. Vigorous animals struggle violently, and when in the standing position may rear or strike out with their fore-feet and shake their heads in an endeavour to dislodge the mask. In the recumbent position there is in nearly all horses an attempt to

get their heads doubled down towards their fore-feet; a position which should be prevented in all cases, for there is a risk that in such positions the spinal column will be fractured. (*See* CASTING.) Deep breaths are taken often in a gasping manner, and in from 3 to 6 or 7 minutes the second stage follows.

(2) *The stage of depression* follows the stimulation stage, and is marked by a quieting of the movements of the voluntary muscles, by a lessening of the force and volume of the pulse, and by slower and deeper breathing. Pain is still felt, and if inflicted induces reflex movements.

(3) *The stage of anæsthesia* produces complete muscular relaxation, unconsciousness, and insensibility. This is the safe or operating stage; all the centres of the brain are subdued except those that govern respiration and heart action. The animal may be kept in this stage for 2 hours or more by the administration of small amounts of the anæsthetic, viz. ¼ to ½ ounce every 7 to 12 minutes or so, depending on the individual.

(4) *The stage of paralysis* occurs when the anæsthetic is pushed beyond the safe stage. The centres of respiration and heart action, in common with all the other nervous centres, become paralysed. It consists of two phases: firstly, the cessation of the respiration; and secondly, the cessation of the heart-beat. The heart stops beating about two minutes after respiration ceases, and it is owing to this fact that any attempts at artificial respiration must be prompt. (*See* ARTIFICIAL RESPIRATION.)

CHLOROMYCETIN is an antibiotic (*see* CHLORAMPHENICOL).

CHLOROPHYL (χλωρός, green; φύλλον, leaf) is the name of the green colouring matter of plants. It is responsible for the greenish tinge of the bile, and consequently of the fæces in grazing animals. Though it is not of much food value itself, its presence is to some extent an index of the presence of the carotene compounds (which are yellowish orange) and from which vitamin A is formed in the liver. (*See* VITAMINS.) Chlorophyl preparations are used in the treatment of wounds and indolent ulcers, and as an internal deodorant in the dog.

CHLORPROMAZINE hydrochloride (Largactil) has been used with success in the dog, and in cattle, for pre-anæsthetic medication, and also as a tranquilliser, but Professor J. G. Wright stated (1958): 'Its place in equine surgery is not established. Its use can be associated with danger to the animals.' A dilute (0·5 per cent) solution is preferable, as chlorpromazine is irritant and stronger solutions may make the injection painful. The dose is ½ mg. per lb. body-weight, given intramuscularly 1½ hours before induction of anæsthesia. The drug has been used in human medicine to control the convulsions of tetanus. (*See also* ARTIFICIAL HIBERNATION.)

CHLORTETRACYCLINE.—(*See under* TERRAMYCIN.)

CHOKING means an obstruction to respiration, but through long usage it has come to have a particular significance when applied to animals, meaning an obstruction to the passage of food through the pharynx and œsophagus, either partial or complete. (*See also* OBSTRUCTION TO RESPIRATION.)

The domesticated animals, especially the ox and dog, are very prone to attempt to swallow either foreign bodies or masses of food material too large to pass down the œsophagus (gullet), with the result that they often become arrested in the throat or in some part of the gullet, perhaps in the neck, or perhaps in the thorax. These substances hinder the free passage of solid or fluid food, give rise to pain and discomfort, and are very often attended by serious and even fatal consequences. The agents which cause choking are very varied indeed; among them may be mentioned the handle of a whip, a small lamp chimney, a domestic fork, large bent wire nails, pieces of tin cans, hens' eggs, potatoes, apples, small turnips, pieces of larger turnips, swedes, mangolds, kohl-rabi or other roots, and even small grass snakes, in cattle; nests of field mice, dry chaff and collections of hay or straw, in horses; needles, pins, stones, bones, golf or other balls, buttons, corks, pieces of wood, and other such objects, in cats and dogs. The ox has a peculiar habit of attempting to eat the most unusual objects. It is a well-known fact that it is unsafe to leave small articles of clothing about a yard where cattle are kept, or in a field to which they have access. It is even reported that a man has lost a waistcoat containing a gold watch in this way! Speaking generally, it may be said that choking in the ox, dog, and cat is usually due to a hard, large, sharp-pointed, or irregularly shaped object; while in the horse it is most often due to a mass of dry impacted food material, or to a portion of a mangold or turnip.

CHOKING IN CATTLE.—In the ox, choking is of comparatively common occurrence, particularly in districts where roots are fed whole to the animals, and where there is a quantity of rubbish scattered about the pastures, such as in the vicinity of thickly populated cities. Cattle are somewhat careless in masticating their food, and have a habit of elevating their heads while feeding. It is not uncommon to see a cow shaking its head upwards and downwards so as to enable the larger particles of roots or other objects to find their way back between the molar teeth. In some cases the object, instead of being arrested in the mouth by the dorsum of the tongue, slips over into the pharynx (throat). A swallowing movement occurs either at once or shortly afterwards, and the large object sticks in the throat or becomes arrested farther down in the gullet.

Symptoms.—The animal immediately stops feeding, and becomes uneasy. It coughs and gasps, and may lower the head and attempt to vomit. In a few minutes there is a profuse flow of saliva from the mouth, particularly when the object is lodged in the pharynx or high up in the œsophagus. A remarkable feature of nearly all cases of choking in cattle is the rapidity with which gas formation occurs in the rumen (a condition known as 'tympany'), and the left side of the abdomen, especially the hollow immediately in front of the angle of the 'haunch-bone', swells up. This sudden production of gas is due to two chief causes: (1) where the obstruction is complete the normal regurgitation of stomach gases up through the mouth is prevented; and (2) the pain and discomfort resulting from the presence of the 'choke' cause an almost immediate cessation of the normal churning movements of the rumen, and the gas given off by the fermenting food, instead of being dispelled, rapidly accumulates. The accumulation of this gas rapidly leads to great distress to the animal, difficulty in breathing, grunting and groaning; and unless the pressure is relieved it may cause death from suffocation. The distended stomach and abdominal organs press forwards against the diaphragm, embarrassing its action and causing it to bulge forward and press upon the lungs.

In other cases, especially in lean animals and where the obstruction is low down in the neck or chest, there may be but little distress; the animal may even drink water—which is, however, presently discharged by way of the mouth and nostrils without apparent discomfort.

When the object is lodged in the pharynx or upper part of the œsophagus, it usually causes a swelling which can be seen or felt from the outside, but if it is situated in the part of the gullet which passes through the chest its presence can only be suspected from a consideration of the symptoms—salivation, discomfort, retching, ejection of fluids swallowed previously, and distension of the left side of the abdomen with gas. The careful passage of the probang down the œsophagus will, of course, definitely establish the presence or absence of an obstruction.

In a number of cases of choking relief occurs quite spontaneously after the lapse of from ½ to 2 or 3 hours from the origin of the symptoms. This is because the muscles of the gullet, which have been tightly gripping the obstruction, gradually become fatigued and relax, thereby allowing the object to pass down into the stomach. Naturally, such a satisfactory termination cannot occur wherever there is a sharp projecting point on the object causing the obstruction, but it frequently happens with eggs, apples, potatoes, and other smooth bodies. Otherwise, if the object is allowed to remain, one of two things may happen—either the œsophagus becomes inflamed and septic and the animal dies from sepsis, or it succumbs from suffocation brought about by the presence of the gas in the stomach. Occasionally the wall of the gullet ruptures during the struggling of the animal, or from other causes, and if the obstruction is located in the thoracic part of the œsophagus septic pleurisy kills the animal. Rupture is most often brought about by the interference of an unskilled person who violently thrusts a long object down the throat and endeavours to force the body into the stomach by brute strength.

Treatment.—In all cases of choking, no matter how simple they appear to be, the owner should seek skilled assistance as soon as possible, and confine his 'first-aid treatment' to the use of a trocar and cannula only—in the event of asphyxia appearing imminent—rather than to amateurish endeavours to remove the offending object. It should be emphasised here that in all cases of choking, when tympany of the stomach occurs, where the degree of distension is great and the animal becoming distressed, it is advisable to puncture the rumen and a low escape of the contained gas. Very often the object will at once move onwards into the stomach when the pressure of gas is relieved, and in any case the immediate danger of death from asphyxia is removed. (*See under* TYMPANY; TROCAR AND CANNULA.) The cannula should be left in position until the choking has been relieved.

In remote places overseas where veterinary assistance is unobtainable by the owner, an attempt must be made to remove the obstruction. In the first place, the animal must be well secured. With a man on either side of the head, steadying it and holding it out in as straight a line as possible, a search should be made to locate the object from the outside of the neck. It will be recognised as a hard, often painful swelling, situated towards the left of the middle line above the windpipe, manipulation of which usually causes the animal to make swallowing movements or to flinch with pain. It may lie at almost any level in the neck, or it may be found at the back of the throat. If it can be easily moved about it may be worked gently upwards into the mouth and removed, but if it is difficult to move it should not be forced. If external palpation fails to reveal the obstruction the cavity of the mouth should be examined. A gag should be fixed between the teeth, and the right hand should be passed along the roof of the mouth and back into the throat. In many cases the object can be discovered in the pharynx just at the entrance to the œsophagus, where it is firmly fixed. If it can be easily reached from the mouth the fingers should be gently forced past it, and it can then be dislodged and removed. In some cases pressing upwards from the outside of the neck will assist removal, and the use of a little butter or linseed oil on the fingers to smear around the walls of the throat greatly facilitates the process. Where the obstruction is situated lower down in the neck, or in the thorax, a little butter or oil should be poured down the throat (taking great care that the animal is not made to swallow too rapidly), so that a certain amount of lubrication between the walls of the gullet and the object may occur. After this, time should be allowed for the object to pass onwards if it will do so of its own accord. The head should be lowered, and a drink of water may be offered. If it still persists, the next procedure should be the passage of a probang or stomach-tube, should the owner possess one. It is most unwise to improvise a probang from a rigid whip-handle or other similar object, for with such an instrument great damage can be inflicted, and the procedure is fraught with danger to the life of the animal.

The passage of the probang is not a difficult matter, even for an unskilled person, provided time is taken and no force is used. The animal's head is secured by two men as before, and a gag with a hole through its middle is inserted between the jaws and held on either side by the two men. The shank of the probang (which is made in the form of a spiral steel spring covered over with smooth leather) is lubricated with oil or grease, and its blunt end is passed through the hole in the gag. At first it meets with a slight obstruction from the dorsum of the tongue, and it may be necessary to have a man hold the tongue well out of the mouth until the end has passed into the pharynx. The probang should be kept well down outside the mouth, so that its point is directed rather upwards, to avoid entering the trachea. As the blunt end passes into the throat the animal usually makes a swallowing movement, and the end can be felt as if it were suddenly gripped. From this point onwards a slight hindrance to the passage of the instrument is encountered, and the pressure should be gentle but sustained. As soon as the obstruction is encountered the progress should be slow. If it gradually gives with slight pressure, it may often be pushed right down into the stomach, and the animal will be immediately relieved. If it fails to move after a minute or two the probang should be removed. In cases where the obstruction is firmly fixed, the veterinary surgeon must either administer some drug which will relieve the spasm of the muscles, or else to perform an operation for removal of the foreign body.

CHOKING IN HORSES—Fortunately, the horse is less often choked than the ox, but owing to the long and narrow equine œsophagus, the accident is more serious.

Symptoms.—Essentially the same as those seen in the choked ox.

Treatment.—Avoid raising the head or giving drenches, lubricating or otherwise. It is imperative to secure professional assistance at once.

CHOKING IN DOGS AND CATS.—
Symptoms.—At first there is usually a

sudden pain, which causes the animal to cry out or scream. If it has been feeding it immediately ceases, and becomes very restless, perhaps running backwards and forwards holding the head and neck rigid, or standing with the head and neck outstretched. It may paw at its mouth with the fore-feet, and sometimes injures the lips or gums with its claws. Any attempt at control by the owner is resented, and a dog which has been otherwise quiet may be liable to bite at a person who handles it. Attempts at vomiting alternated with endeavours to swallow the foreign object are noticed, and each swallowing movement generally causes the animal to cry out with the pain. Salivation is nearly always very profuse, even when the obstruction occurs low down in the neck or in the thoracic portion of the gullet. When a threaded needle has become fixed in the throat or below it, the end of the thread may often be seen.

Treatment.—As in the case of the horse, unskilled manipulation is inadvisable and the owner is strongly advised to seek skilled assistance before irremediable damage has been inflicted.

CHOLAGOGUES (χολή, bile ; ἄγω, I move) are drugs that act on the liver, increasing the secretion of the bile. The only true cholagogues are bile and bile salts or preparations made from them. Drugs which have a beneficial action in promoting a flow of bile already formed include some mercury salts, and certain saline sulphates.

CHOLECYSTITIS (χολή, bile ; κύστις, a bladder) means inflammation of the gall-bladder.

CHOLECYSTOGRAPHY is the term used for X-ray examination of the gall-bladder after its contents have been rendered opaque by administration of lipiodol or pheniodol compounds.

CHOLERA, FOWL (*see* FOWL CHOLERA).

CHOLESTERIN (χολή, bile ; στερεός, solid) is a substance which can be derived from many of the tissues of the body, from many tumours, and from certain secretions, such as the bile. It can be obtained pure by extraction of nervous tissue with alcohol or ether, and is then found to be chemically a complex alcohol which crystallises in rhombic plates. Its practical interest lies in the fact that many gall-stones consist almost wholly of masses of cholesterin mixed with bile pigment and shed epithelial cells.

CHOLINE is found in egg-yolk, liver, and muscle, and is a member of the vitamin B complex. Acetyl choline is an essential part of the transmission of an impulse from nerve to muscle and choline chloride is used as a drug in veterinary medicine for certain cases of acetonæmia.

CHOLINE-ESTERASE is an enzyme necessary for the proper action of the stomach's nervous system. It is inactivated by a substance isolated from white clover S.100.

CHONDROMA (χόνδρος, cartilage ; *-oma*, termination meaning tumour) is a tumour composed of cells which very closely resemble those found in normal cartilage.

CHOREA (χορεία,, a dance), which is also called 'St. Vitus's Dance', is characterised by a succession of involuntary spasmodic contractions (clonic spasms) affecting one or more of the voluntary muscles. The spasm is of a rhythmic nature, occurring at fairly regular intervals, and between the individual contractions relaxation of the affected muscle takes place.

The condition affects dogs almost exclusively, although muscular spasms of a similar nature have been seen in horses, cattle, and pigs. In lambs, congenital chorea is described under BORDER DISEASE. (*See* TREMBLING.)

Causes.—The cause is as yet unknown, although the condition is associated with intoxication of the central nervous system by substances resulting from infection with a virus or bacterial agent. Chorea generally follows an attack of distemper. It may appear within a few days after apparent recovery, or its appearance may be delayed. Many very mild cases are followed by chorea, while after some of the most severe attacks chorea does not develop. There is, however, one very important fact in this association which must be strongly emphasised: after convalescence from distemper, but before the dog has quite recovered, excessive or even only moderate exercise, along with strenuous conditions, such as chills or soakings from rain, are extremely liable to be followed by the development of chorea. All dog owners would be well advised to regard cases of distemper as not cured until the lapse of at least ten days after *apparent recovery*, and during this period to continue to treat the animal as though it were still sick, so far as exercise is concerned.

Symptoms.—The characteristic symptoms are twitchings of individual muscles. of whole limbs, of the head and neck, or of practically the whole of the body, These twitchings usually commence about the lips and face, or in the extremities of one or more limbs. There may at first only be a mere quiver, best appreciated by the hand laid over the part, but as time goes on a distinct movement is seen. Later, the spasm is more apparent, and perhaps the whole head is seen continually nodding or jerking backwards and forwards, quite irrespective of the pose or position of the animal. In the early stages of the condition, apart from the twitchings, the animal remains in quite good health. It feeds, sleeps, moves about, and is apparently not in any pain or discomfort. As the condition progresses, however, there comes a time when it is unable to rest, the appetite becomes irregular, loss of condition and weakness result; and then in a short while the dog becomes moody, loses its interest in things around, frequently changes its position, and is very easily exhausted. Convulsive seizures (' fits ') may appear, or they may have appeared earlier, before the twitchings were well marked. In a few cases the spasms are intermittent, disappearing altogether during sleep, or the animal may become accustomed to the twitching and sleep well in spite of it. In the majority of instances, however, the twitching becomes progressively worse; new sets of muscles become affected. Ulceration of an affected limb, as the result of continual friction with surrounding objects, the ground, etc., is not uncommon, and sometimes the animal will persistently gnaw at a foot or other part of its body, inflicting ugly wounds, without apparently being aware of the damage it is causing or of the pain produced. Chorea is always a serious condition.

Treatment.—The twitchings may be partially controlled by the use of antispasmodics. Aim at keeping the animal's strength up by good feeding, special attention being given to an abundant supply of vitamins in the diet, and to the inclusion of good-quality proteins. It is also necessary to ensure regular evacuation of the bowels by laxatives or enemata. Dryness and comfortable surroundings are very necessary, and the animal should be protected from all sources of annoyance. 'Luminal soda', has given very encouraging results in a certain type of case, but it is by no means a specific. Parathyroid extract, with or without calcium salts, may prove successful. (*See also* ANTISPASMODICS.)

CHORION (χόριον) is the outermost of the three fœtal membranes, the others being the amnion and the allantois. The chorion is a strong fibrous membrane, whose outer surface is closely moulded to the inner surface of the uterus. Chorionic villi are the vascular projections from the chorion which are inserted into the crypts of the uterine mucous membrane. (*See also* PARTURITION.)

CHORIONIC GONADOTROPHIN (*see* HORMONE THERAPY).

CHOROID, or **CHORIOID** (χόριον, a membrane; εἶδος, form), is the middle of the three coats of the eye, and consists chiefly of the blood-vessels which effect nourishment of the organ. (*See* EYE.)

CHOROIDITIS means inflammation of the choroid coat of the eye and is always to be regarded as serious.

CHRISTMAS ROSE (*see* HELLEBORE).

CHROMOBACTER VIOLACEUM. —An organism, often regarded as nonpathogenic, which has caused a fatal pneumonia in pigs in the U.S.A.

CHRONIC CATARRHAL ENTERITIS. —A disease of horses seen in the U.K., characterised by chronic diarrhœa. It is invariably fatal.

Cause.—Unknown.

CHRONIC DISEASE is the term applied to a disease when the symptoms commence gradually with low fever, when tissue alteration occurs very slowly and a great deal of fibrous tissue is laid down, and when after a considerable period of time the disease resolves only very slowly or not at all. It is the opposite from Acute (which see). Examples are, chronic bronchitis, chronic inflammation of the kidney.

CHRONIC RESPIRATORY DISEASE of poultry.—(*See* C.R.D.)

CHYLE (χυλος) is the name given to the partly digested food as it passes down the small intestine, and also to that part of it which is absorbed by the lymphatic vessels of the intestine. It is mixed with the lymph, which, after circulating in the lacteals of the small intestine and becoming laden with tiny globules of fat, is collected, by fusion of the efferent lymph vessels, into an irregular sac-like structure in the upper anterior part of the abdomen called the 'cisterna chyli'. From thence it passes by the thoracic duct to the anterior part of the chest and is discharged into the blood-stream. (*See* LYMPH, DIGESTION.)

CHYME (χυμός, juice) is the name given to the partly digested food that is passed from the stomach into the first part of the small intestine. It is very acid in nature, contains salts and sugars in solution, and the animal constituents in a semi-liquid state.

CICATRIX (*cicatrix*) is a scar.

CILIA (*cilium*, eyelash) is a term applied to minute, lash-like processes which are seen by the microscope upon the cells covering certain mucous membranes, and which maintain movement in the fluid passing over these membranes. They are also found upon certain bacteria which have the power of rapid movement.

CILIATA (*see* PARASITES).

CIRCLING MOVEMENTS.—These may be a symptom of GID, LISTERIOSIS, or POLIOENCEPHALOMALACIA. In pigs, MENINGOENCEPHALITIS may be a cause.

CIRCULATION OF BLOOD. — **The course of the circulation is as follows.**

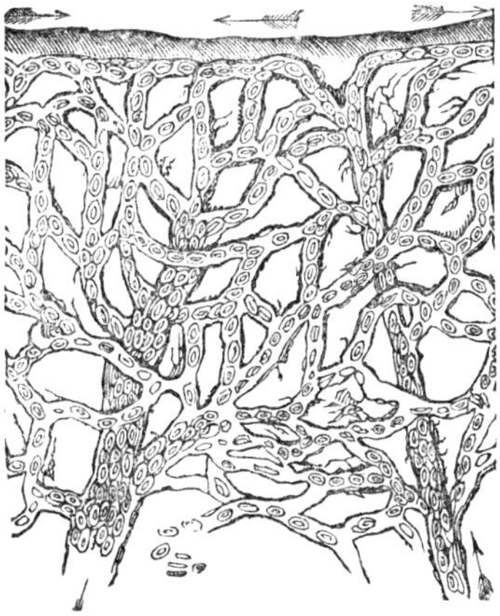

Diagram of capillaries with circulating blood. The arrows indicate the direction of the flow. (Turner's *Anatomy*.)

The veins of the whole body—head, trunk, limbs, and organs in the abdomen—with the exception of those in the thorax, pour their blood into one of the three great terminal radicles which open into the right atrium of the heart. This contracts and drives the blood into the right ventricle, which then forces the blood into the lungs by way of the pulmonary artery. In the lungs it is contained in very thin-walled capillaries, over which the inspired air plays freely, and through which the exchange of gases can easily take place. The blood is consequently oxygenated (*see* RESPIRATION), and passes on by the pulmonary veins to the left atrium of the heart. This left

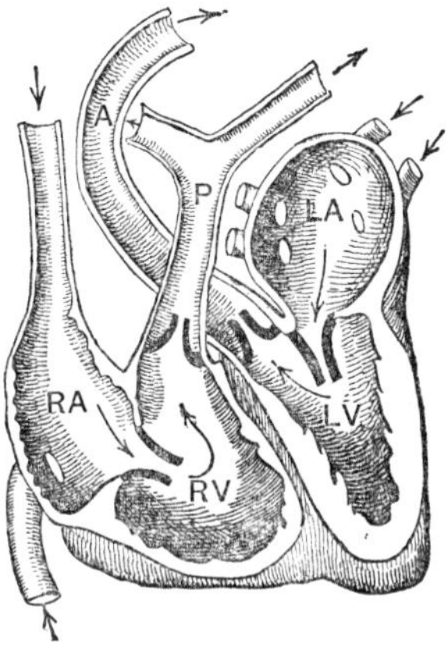

Diagram of the heart sectioned to show the course of the blood through it, and the arrangement of the valves. RA, Right atrium; RV, right ventricle; P, pulmonary artery; LA, left atrium; LV, left ventricle; A, aorta.

atrium expels it into the left ventricle, which forces it on into the aorta, by which it is distributed all over the body. Passing through the capillaries in the various organs and tissues it eventually again enters the lesser veins, and is collected into the cranial and caudal vena cava and the vena azygos (*see* VEINS), from whence it passes to the right atrium once more. Thus is the circle of the circulation completed.

In one part of the body there is, however, a further complication. The veins coming from the stomach, intestines, spleen, and pancreas, charged with food materials and other products, unite into the large 'portal vein' which enters the porta of the liver and splits up into a second capillary system in the liver tissue. Here it is relieved of some of its food content, is purified from harmful substances absorbed by accident from the digestive system, and passes to the caudal vena cava by a second series of veins, joining with the rest of the blood coming from the hind parts of the body, and so goes on to the right atrium. This is known as the ' portal circulation '.

The circuit is maintained always in one direction by four valves, situated one at the outlet from each cavity of the heart (*see* HEART), and by the presence of valves situated along the course of the larger veins.

The blood in the arteries going to the body generally (*i.e.* to the systemic circulation) is a bright red in colour, while that in the veins is a dull red ; this is owing to the oxygen content of arterial blood being much greater than that of venous blood, which latter is charged with carbonic acid gas (*see* RESPIRATION). For the same reason the blood in the pulmonary artery going to the lungs is dark, while in the pulmonary veins it is bright red.

It should be remembered that there is normally no connection between the blood

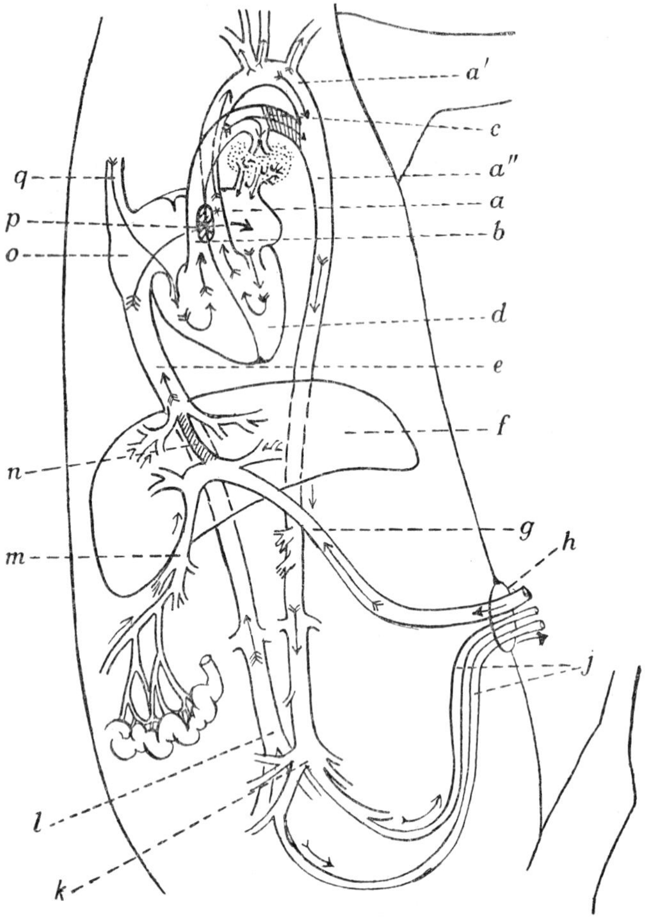

Diagram of fœtal circulation. *a*, Origin of aorta ; *a'*, arch of aorta ; *a"*, posterior aorta ; *b*, origin of pulmonary artery ; *c*, the ductus arteriosus (shaded) ; *d*, left ventricle ; *e*, caudal vena cava ; *f*, liver ; *g*, umbilical vein ; *h*, the umbilicus ; *j*, umbilical arteries ; *k*, bifurcation of aorta ; *l*, origin of caudal vena cava ; *m*, portal vein ; *n*, ductus venosus, which short-circuits blood from umbilical vein to vena cava without passing through liver ; *o*, right atrium ; *p*, foramen ovale (shaded) ; *q*, cranial vena cava. (After Bradley's *Thorax and Abdomen of the Horse.*)

in the right side of the heart and that in the left; the blood from the right ventricle must pass through the lungs before it can reach the left atrium. In the fœtus, however, before birth, the course is somewhat different, owing to the fact that no nourishment comes from the bowels nor does air pass into the lungs. Accordingly, two large arteries pass out from the umbilicus (navel), and convey blood which is to circulate in close proximity to the maternal blood in the placenta, and to receive from it both the oxygen and the nourishment necessary for the needs of the fœtus, while one large vein brings back this blood into the fœtal body through the umbilicus again. There are also communications between the right and the left atria (the *foramen ovale*) and between the aorta and the pulmonary artery (the *ductus arteriosus*), which serve to 'short-circuit' the blood from passing through the lungs in any quantity. At birth these extra communications rapidly close and shrivel up, leaving mere vestiges of their presence in adult life. There are rare instances, however, in which one or more of the passages may persist throughout life, although they do not appreciably affect the health of the animal.

CIRCULATION OF LYMPH (*see* LYMPH).

CIRRHOSIS, or **FIBROSIS** (κιρρός, yellow), is a diseased condition of various internal organs, in which the essential cellular elements of the organ are replaced by fibrous tissue similar to scar-tissue. The name 'cirrhosis' was first used by Laennec for the disease as it occurs in the liver, because of the yellow colour, but it has been applied to the same condition in the lung, kidney, etc.

Classic instances of cirrhosis are seen in the liver in chronic ragwort poisoning in cattle, in tuberculosis of the mammary gland in the cow, in chronic alcoholism in man, and in the kidneys in old dogs.

CLACKING (*see* OVER-REACHING).

CLAVICLE (*clavicula*, a twig) is another name for the 'collar-bone' in man. This bone is not present in the domesticated mammals owing to the formation of the narrow and deep chest, but it is represented in some cases by a strand of cartilage or fibrous tissue. It is present in the fowl.

CLAWS (*see* NAILS).

CLAY PIGEONS.—Eating of these has led to fatal poisoning in pigs. (*See* PITCH POISONING.)

'CLEAN' PASTURE.—It is widely assumed that resting a pasture heavily contaminated with parasitic worm larvæ of sheep or cattle for 4 to 6 weeks during dry, cold weather will render it safe for grazing by susceptible stock. This is a dangerous assumption, for such larvæ can survive on pasture rested for a whole winter.

'CLEANSING' (*see* AFTERBIRTH).

CLEFT PALATE is a hereditary defect of the roof of the mouth, generally seen in puppies of the toy breeds that have been in-bred. It consists of a gap in the structures forming the palate, often so extensive as to allow of communication between the mouth and the nasal passages. Puppies so affected are usually unable to suck, and die soon after birth unless given artificial feeding; others are able to obtain some small amount of nourishment, but never thrive as the rest of the litter. The condition of 'hare-lip', or 'split-lip', is often associated with cleft palate. The palate may also be cleft as the result of violence; for example, it is commonly seen in the cat which has fallen from a considerable height. (*See* HARE-LIP.)

CLIMATE IN RELATION TO DISEASE.—In cold and temperate areas lung diseases, kidney diseases, and certain minor ailments are commoner than they are in tropical areas, but with a few exceptions (such as tuberculosis), bacterial diseases and parasitic diseases are less common and less serious. Roughly speaking, the major contagious epizoötic diseases, which spread as scourges over large tracks of land, are mainly confined to tropical and sub-tropical climates. Parasitic worms are usually more common in hot countries than they are in colder areas, where the intermediate stages have to withstand more trying conditions.

Roughly speaking, the specific diseases which are more common in the tropics than elsewhere are as follows: Anthrax, glanders, rabies, cattle-plague, contagious pleuro-pneumonia of cattle, the variolæ, foot-and-mouth disease, the trypanosomiases and other diseases due to protozoön parasites, the hæmorrhagic septicæmias, heartwater, blue tongue, African horse-sickness, and bursatee. (*See also* RAINFALL, EXPOSURE.)

CLINCHES, or **CLENCHES,** are the turned-down portions of horse-shoe nails which appear on the outside of the wall of the shod hoof. They are formed by twisting off the point of each nail as it is driven, and afterwards hammering the projecting portion down flat against the surface of the wall, or into a little 'clinch-bed' which has been prepared by rasping previously. The clinches should be higher at the toes than at the quarters, for the wall is thicker at the former.

CLINICAL (κλίνη, a bed) means literally 'belonging to a bed', but the word is used to denote anything associated with the practical study or observation of a sick person or animal, such as clinical medicine, clinical thermometer. (*See also* SUB-CLINICAL.)

CLIPPING OF ANIMALS.—The covering of hair over the body of certain of the domesticated animals is liable at times to interfere with health if allowed to grow unchecked, and accordingly it is customary to remove it at certain periods of the year; thus in horses the long winter coat, if left to grow, hinders efficient grooming and drying, prevents the skin from excreting waste products, and causes the horse to perspire more. (*See also* SHEARING.)

Methods.—There are two forms of horse clippers, one consisting of two toothed blades working backwards and forwards across each other, and provided with handles, the second consisting of similar blades carried at the end of a flexible cable, the top one of which is made to vibrate by a rotary device, power being supplied either by hand or from an electric motor. The horse may stand without restraint other than a halter, but it is frequently necessary to twitch or blindfold refractory animals. The clippers work best when used against the flow of the hair, and should be thoroughly and frequently lubricated. It is of course essential that the blades should be sharp. For race-horses, carriage-horses, ponies, etc., it is usual to clip 'down to the ground', as it is called, *i.e.* all the hair is clipped from the body, legs, and face, the mane is 'hogged' (clipped short), and the tail is thinned. For saddle-horses a 'hunter's clip' is preferred; in this the hair is taken from the body, except for a patch on the back which corresponds with the outline of the saddle ('saddle-patch'), and the legs, which are left covered with hair below the level of an oblique line running across the middles of the fore-arms and gaskins. The mane is hogged, and the tail is thinned and cut straight across about a hand's-breadth above the level of the points of the hocks. For heavy and light draught-horses generally a 'trace-high clip' is usual. In this form a patch of hair is left covering the upper parts of the trunk, reaching down to about the level of the points of the shoulders straight back, and the hair is removed from below this level down to about half the distance between the elbows and knees in front, and stifles and hocks behind. The mane and tail are trimmed but are not cut short.

Times for clipping.—The time for clipping horses varies according to the weather, but should take place as soon as the winter coat has 'set', *i.e.* as soon as the summer coat has been fully cast off and the winter coat is well grown. It usually happens that in an ordinary autumn this condition is fulfilled about the end of October and the beginning of November, but in some years it is earlier and in some later. Sometimes horses are clipped twice during the winter, once before Christmas and once some time after; but this is only necessary in animals which have a luxuriant growth of hair.

Precautions.—Never clip a horse suffering from a cold or other respiratory trouble. Never clip during excessively severe weather. Always provide a rug when standing outside for the first week or ten days to allow the heat-regulating mechanism to become accustomed to the more rapid radiation of heat from the body surface. Thoroughly dry a newly clipped horse after coming into the stable in wet or snowy weather, by means of straw or hay wisps. Do not allow newly clipped horses to stand in draughty places in a stable without protection. Give extra bedding for a few days after clipping. Give an extra ration of hay and oats to recently clipped horses to make good the loss of heat occasioned.

Clipping of dogs.—These animals are usually clipped for medical reasons, such as to allow better dressing of the skin during treatment of mange or other skin diseases, and to stimulate a thicker growth of hair when baldness threatens. There are some owners, however, who have their dogs regularly clipped at the beginning of the summer to rid them of long matted, or thick winter, coats. In addition to this, certain breeds are clipped for show purposes, such as the French poodle and the Bedlington terrier. The dog may either be clipped by means of a pair of small hand horse clippers or an ordinary pair of scissors may be used.

CLIPS are projections drawn along the outer edges of the foot surfaces of horses' shoes which prevent the shoe from shifting on the foot. *Toe-clips* are drawn at the toes, and should be exactly opposite to the point of the frog when the shod foot is viewed from the ground aspect. They prevent the shoe from moving backwards. *Side-clips* are drawn at the sides of the toes, outer and inner, when for some reason it is not convenient or possible to draw a single toe-clip. They are put on to the hind shoes when the horse is given to forging or clacking, and on to either fore or hind shoes when sandcrack is present. *Quarter-clips* are usually drawn upon the shoes of the hind-feet, frequently on the outsides, but sometimes on the insides as well. They are situated at the quarters, about half-way from the toe of the shoe to the heel. They prevent the shoe from shifting across the foot in a lateral direction. *Bar-clips* are seldom seen at present. They used to be made on the inner edge of the web in such a position that they would fit inside the bars of the foot. Their vogue was due to an error in understanding the physiology of the movement of the horse's hoof, and except in surgical shoes for the relief of sandcrack they are never used nowadays.

The shape of a clip is of some importance. Owing to the danger of a clip penetrating the sole of the foot and perhaps causing very severe lameness, its tip should never be sharp. In turning the clip over the edge of the anvil the smith should ensure that he does not also hammer up a quantity of iron which will form a projection against the wall and necessitate the removal of a large amount of horn as a recess for the toe clip, thereby weakening the wall. A good clip should be ear-shaped or semicircular in outline, should neither be too high nor too low, and should not encroach upon the bearing surface of the shoe.

CLITORIS is a small organ composed of erectile tissue, situated just within the lower commissure of the vulva of the female. It is the homologue of the male penis, and has no important function other than acting as a sensory organ.

CLONIC (κλόνος, a tumult) is a word applied to spasmodic movements of muscles lasting for a short time only.

CLOSTRIDIAL ENTERITIS.—This is recorded as a cause of sudden death in cattle. The deaths usually, though not invariably, occur shortly after calving. The animal, usually one, is found dead. Where death is not immediate, 'milk fever' may be suspected, but the elevated temperature at once rules this out. The cow may be in considerable pain before succumbing. On post-mortem examination, acute inflammation of the intestine is found—such as might be expected with some types of poisoning. This enteritis is associated with the presence of a toxin, difficult to demonstrate in the laboratory, produced by the organism *Clostridium welchii* Type A. The same condition may account for the sudden death of pigs. *Clostridium œdematiens* may likewise be a cause of sudden death in sheep, pigs, and cattle.

CLOSTRIDIUM.—A genus of anærobe spore-bearing bacteria of ovoid, spindle, or club shape. They include ***Cl. tetani***, ***Cl. Welchii***, ***Cl. botulini***. (***See above***, TETANUS, LAMB DYSENTERY, LAMZIEKTE.)

CLOTHING OF ANIMALS.—As a general rule, only the horse, ox, and dog, of the domesticated animals, are supplied with clothing. Sheep already possess protection in the form of wool sufficient except in severe weather on the uplands; while pigs carry a deep layer of subcutaneous fat.

Horses.—Horses require clothing for the following reasons: (1) to provide protection against cold, chills, draughts, and sudden lowering of the temperature; (2) to protect parts of the body from bruises and abrasions, such as might occur while travelling by rail or on board ship; (3) to protect the coat from dust and débris, and the feet and legs from mud during exercise out of doors; and (4) to afford protection from sudden showers of rain or snow when at work in the open. For the latter purpose waterproof sheets lined with woollen fabric on the inside are usually used.

Articles used.—A full set of clothing consists of the following articles: (*a*) quarter-sheet; (*b*) breast-sheet, breast-cloth, or breast-piece ; (*c*) long hood ; (*d*) roller, or surcingle ; (*e*) tail-boot, or tail-saver ; (*f*) set of four woollen bandages ; (*g*) knee-caps and hock-boots ; (*h*) fillet-strings.

But it is seldom that a complete full set is used at the present day. More often the quarter-sheet and breast-sheet are combined into the familiar *horse-rug*, and very often a surcingle is sewn on to it, making a three-piece garment, which is handier and quite as efficient for all ordinary purposes

Materials used.—The quarter-sheet, breast-sheet, and hood are made of pure wool with leather or braided edges, for winter wear, and a mixture of woollen and cotton, or even pure cotton, is employed for summer wear, when its chief purpose is to provide protection from dust and dirt. During autumn and spring it depends upon the weather as to what kind of clothing is selected. Horse-rugs are frequently made from hempen fabric, or stout canvas lined with wool, for commercial horses. All-wool rugs are to be preferred, however ; they are warmer, allow of more regular evaporation from the skin, fit the curves of the horse's body better, and are not much more difficult to wash than those of a mixed fabric. The horse-rug and the breast-sheet are provided with a strap and buckle which fasten at the lower part of the neck, while the long hood has a single strap and buckle below the lower jaw, and a series of tapes which tie over the throat and down the neck. The roller is made of jute, string-webbing, or canvas-webbing, and is padded on either side of where it passes over the backbone, so that it does not press upon the spines of the thoracic vertebræ. One or two buckles and straps are provided, and made to fasten on the near side of the chest, in such a position that when the horse lies down it will not lie upon the fastened buckle. The surcingle is made after the same fashion, but it is not provided with padding. The tail-saver is made of either fine leather or stout cotton, and either buckles or laces around the tail. It has a strap which runs forward along croup, loins, and back, to buckle around the central part of the surcingle. This prevents the boot from shifting its position by the movement of the tail. In many instances the tail-boot is dispensed with, a long tail bandage being used instead, or a bandage and boot may be used together. Bandages for travelling purposes, or for use in a stable—*i.e.* 'stable bandages'—are made of wool. They are about 7 to 9 feet long, and 4 inches wide. On one end are sewn tapes for fastening purposes. They are applied from immediately below the knees and hocks down to the coronets ('hoof heads'), and back again, so that they fasten round the cannon just below the knee or hock. The knot of the tapes should lie on the outside or the inside of the limb for preference, *i.e.* not immediately over either the bone at the front or the tendon at the back. 'Exercising bandages' are used to give support to the tendons and to brace up the lower parts of the limbs. They are usually about 5 or 6 feet long, and 3½ to 4 inches wide. They are frequently made of Newmarket stockinette, or of some similar elastic fabric, and are applied tightly round the cannons (between the knees, or hocks, and the fetlocks), not reaching lower than the ergots. They may be used with or without a layer of cotton-wool below them. Knee-caps and hock-boots are made of leather (sometimes backed by plates of steel), and are of such a shape as will fit the respective joints. They are lined with felt or wool on the insides. Each is provided with two straps—an upper which encircles the limb above the joint and is well padded, and a lower, below the joint, which is not padded. The upper straps are fastened tightly and hold the article in position, while the lower ones are fastened loosely so as to prevent flapping while the horse is moving, and never so tightly as to embarrass freedom of flexion of the joints. The straps all buckle to the outside of the limb. Fillet-strings are made of plaited braiding or tape, and run across the buttocks from the one hind corner of the rug or quarter-sheet to the opposite one. Fillet-strings do not, as is commonly supposed, serve to keep the rug from shifting forwards on the horse's body ; a rug will never shift forwards ; it always works backwards. They merely keep the corners of the rug in position, and hinder them from doubling over the loins on a windy day, or when the horse lies down.

Cattle.—Formerly, it was only for sick cattle, and for use at agricultural shows and upon similar occasions, that clothing was provided for cattle, but of recent years Jersey, etc., cows often wear coats. A large quarter-sheet, kept in position by a surcingle, and sometimes provided with fillet-strings, is most commonly employed. An ordinary horse-rug serves the purpose, but the buckle at the neck should never be fastened for cattle. For the clothing of sick animals two or more large corn sacks are very often employed.

Sheep.—Jute coats are now on the market for ewes, and cost about 5s. per head. They were designed and introduced by Mr. William Wilson, a Carlisle farmer, who found them economic in his flock in severe winter weather on the Pennines. The idea is for the coats to be worn from mating to lambing. Five stitches secure the coat.

Rugs or coats of man-made fibre have been used in Australia to protect the fleeces of sheep, and have proved economic, since wool buyers have paid more.

Dogs.—For the dog a coat made of woollen fabrics which wraps round the body and buttons or straps together is often used. Dog-coats or rugs are made according to various patterns, but whatever variety is selected should provide protection for the front and under part of the chest, as well as for the sides of the body. The elaborate garments which are used for coursing greyhounds and whippets are excellent articles of clothing, and may be copied with advantage for other breeds of dogs. Many of them are provided with cowls or hoods which can be turned forwards so as to cover the neck and part of the head, or may be folded back over the withers, according to the weather. Some are slipped over the dog's head, and are then fastened round the body by one or more straps, while others button along the back, or to one side, the two fore-legs being slipped through holes provided for them. The choice of any particular type is mainly a matter of individual taste on the part of the owner.

CLOTTING, or COAGULATION, is a process of solidification or semi-solidification of a body fluid, which occurs when it is brought into contact with some foreign material or a particular secretion. For example, when blood is shed it clots, and milk clots on contact with the gastric juice. Coagulation of the blood is most important, because it is on account of this that the natural arrest of hæmorrhage depends. (*See* BLEEDING, ARREST OF.) In hæmophilia, from which some dogs suffer, there is an absence or an impairment of the power of coagulation of the blood. (*See* BLOOD, MILK, HÆMOPHILIA.)

In blood, the chemical processes which take place in coagulation consist of a combination of three substances normally present, *prothrombin*, *calcium*, and *thromboplastin*. These form *thrombin* which unites with *fibrinogen* to produce *fibrin*, which is essentially the clot of blood in the meshes of which the blood cells are entangled. Prothrombin and calcium are normally present in the blood and the delicate platelets contain the thromboplastin. When hæmorrhage occurs the platelets are disintegrated and the thromboplastin is released. The thrombin acts upon the fibrinogen of the blood to form the fibrils or crystals of fibrin.

The above, however, is only a part of the story, for several other factors are now known to operate first. They include the Hageman Factor, Plasma Thromboplastin Antecedent, Christmas Factor, Factor V, and Stewart-Power Factor.

Clotting time varies in different species and under different degrees of health, but normally it takes between 7 and 9 or 10 minutes after the blood is shed. After some hours the fibrin contracts and blood serum is squeezed out from the clot.

In the intact blood-vessel the smooth lining of endothelium protects the platelets from damage and clotting does not take place. If a blood-vessel is cut or injured so that the platelets are damaged coagulation can take place. If this occurs extensively a large thrombus may form which may readily cut off the circulation to the part the vessel supplies. (*See* THROMBOSIS.)

'CLOUDBURST' is a colloquial name for false pregnancy in the goat which, after an apparently normal gestation, suddenly voids from the vulva a large quantity of cloudy fluid—after which the size of the abdomen returns to normal. 'Cloudburst' is a fairly common condition. The cause is unknown. Milk yield afterwards is below normal.

COAGULATION is another name for CLOTTING (which see).

COAL-GAS is a mixture of various gases which varies according to the composition of the coal from which it is prepared, and also according to the method of manufacture. It owes its dangerous properties to the presence of carbon monoxide. The warning signs of threatened poisoning are bellowing or roaring and neighing, a rapid rate of respiration, an occasional cough, a staggering, uncertain gait; and if the animal be lying, apparently deeply asleep, actual poisoning has begun and immediate measures are necessary. Artificial respiration should be started when the animal has been dragged outside, and cold water douches may be applied to the head. Drugs other than stimulants are of little use, because the carbon monoxide forms a very stable compound with the blood, and elimination is slow. Complete recovery in a few days after the removal of the cause, provided no complications supervene, often results, but in the dog and cat temporary or permanent deafness may follow.

Coal-gas is sometimes used for the humane destruction of small animals. The gas is introduced into a closed 'lethal chamber' into which the animal has been previously placed. There is some conflict of opinion among authorities as to whether the use of coal-gas is the most humane method of destruction or not, but it is probably not inhumane.

Nowadays, town gas is often a gas from oil products.

COB is a short-legged horse, suitable for saddle work of a prolonged but not rapid nature; also used for light trade-carts. Cobs generally stand from 13½ to 14½ hands high.

The word 'cob' is also used for cubes made from *unmilled* dried grass.

COBALT is one of the mineral elements known to be essential to normal health, but only required in minute amounts. Because of this, cobalt is said to be one of the 'trace elements'. Its function is to act as a catalyst in the assimilation of iron into hæmoglobin in the red blood corpuscles. (*See* BUSH SICKNESS; PINING; ANÆMIA; TRACE ELEMENTS; MOLYBDENUM.)

Poisoning.—Overdosage must be avoided. Twelve beef stores on cobalt-deficient land died when they were not only offered a cobalt supplement in boxes, but drenched as well with cobalt sulphate 'measured' by the handful.

COCAINE, or **COCA.**—Coca leaves are obtained from two South American plants, *Erythroxylon coca*, and *Erythroxylon bolivianum*, and contain the alkaloid *cocaine*. This acts as a local anæsthetic by paralysing the nerves of sensation in the region to which it is applied. It may either be painted on to a raw surface, or on to a mucous membrane, or it may be injected hypodermically. It has now been largely displaced by synthetic local anæsthetic agents which are less toxic and do not come under the Dangerous Drugs Act regulations.

Eye-lotions for painful conditions in the eye often have cocaine added to act as a soothing agent, and to allow other substances to be applied without increasing the pain.

Cocaine ointment is used to relieve pain. It should never be used in greater strength than 5 per cent.

COCCIDIOMYCOSIS is the name given to a tumour-like swelling met with in the internal lymph-glands in cattle, sheep, dogs, cats, and certain wild rodents, caused by infection with a fungus, called *Coccidioides immitis*. This fungus sets up a purulent condition in the affected lumph-glands. It has been recognised in many parts of the U.S.A. and Canada, but has not been reported in Britain. Clinical symptoms are vague and indefinite unless an abscess in an affected lymph-gland should burst into the pleural or peritoneal cavities, when a septic infection follows. The condition is chiefly met with in abattoirs during the inspection of meat for human consumption, or in other animals at post-mortem examination. The lesions are sometimes confused with those of actinomycosis or actinobacillosis.

COCCIDIOSIS.—Under the section on PARASITES will be found an account of the life-history of the causal agent of coccidiosis in each of the susceptible domesticated animals, and a brief parasitological description is given there (p. 640).

Cattle.—In the ox this disease is also known as 'Red dysentery', and Dysenteria coccidiosa bovum. The parasite is known as *Coccidium zürnii* or *Eimeria zürnii*, and is present chiefly in the large intestine. It can be demonstrated microscopically in the fæces as a round or oval body with a small spot in the centre.

Occurrence.—The disease occurs during summer and early autumn, and is particularly prevalent in marshy districts. It is common in the mountainous regions of France and Switzerland, and is met with in Cumberland, Devonshire, Cornwall, Wales, and other parts of Great Britain. Animals are usually infected at pasture between the age when they first go out to graze and two years. It may also occur in animals kept indoors, when it reaches them through the medium of contaminated food or water.

Symptoms.—The incubation period of the disease is usually considered to be about 1 to 3 weeks. The first symptom is diarrhœa, not very severe to begin with, but becoming streaked with spots of blood in about 2 or 3 days' time. The animal strains when passing its motions —a symptom which increases in severity. Prolapse of the rectum may occur about this time, as the result of the straining. The diarrhœa may go on for some days and then gradually clear up, but more often the straining increases in intensity, the animal becomes rapidly emaciated and very weak, appetite and rumination are suspended, the pulse increases in frequency, the temperature rises or fluctuates in an irregular manner, and in the course of from five days to a fortnight or so from the beginning of the disease (sometimes less than these periods) the animal staggers and falls to the ground and dies from exhaustion. In a number of cases the animal lingers on for weeks or even months before becoming so weak and anæmic that it dies from exhaustion. The death-rate varies between 2 per cent and 10 per cent of affected, and, generally speaking, the younger the animal the more likely is it to succumb.

Treatment.—Attempts should be made to kill the coccidia by the administration of sulphamezathine, sulphaquinoxylene, or one of the other sulpha-drugs which are specific for the parasite. As soon as diagnosis is confirmed, or, better, as soon as the disease is suspected, the affected animals should be isolated from amongst the others, and a careful look-out kept for further cases. (*See* DAPSONE.)

The feeding should be carefully supervised; affected animals always do better when kept on dry food-stuffs, given plenty of good hay, and rich, easily digested concentrates, such as ground linseed cake and crushed oats in equal parts. The water-supply should be clean and not excessive in amount. If possible, pastures that are infected or believed to be infected should be put under the plough, or may be heavily limed.

Sheep and Goats.—These animals are attacked with the intestinal form of the disease as are cattle, and the same type of grazing land is blamed. Lambs sucking their mothers are very frequently affected. Diarrhœa, with progressive emaciation, is the most pronounced feature of the disease, but it usually runs a course of several weeks before the animal dies. There is no blood passed in the fæces, and it is not usually possible to find the organism in the fæces by microscopic examination, but upon post-mortem masses of white spots, or single white spots, are seen in the mucous membrane of the small intestine. The causal parasite in sheep is known as *Eimeria faurei*, which is probably identical with *Eimeria arloingi*, though some authorities maintain that the latter is found only in the goat.

Rabbits.—In the rabbit there are two forms of the disease: one attacking the intestines, and another attacking the liver and responsible for the very common 'white livers' of wild rabbits from warrens. The intestinal form is due to a parasite called *Eimeria perforans*, and the small intestine is almost solely affected. To the naked eye the lesions appear as whitish nodules massed together, and there are signs of a severe intestinal catarrh and diarrhœa. The affected rabbits pine, become weak and exhausted, and death occurs in a few days.

'*White liver*'.—Coccidiosis of the liver of wild rabbits is an extremely common disease in almost all countries. It is due to the *Eimeria stiedæ*, and may occur in the same rabbit as the intestinal form. In many cases practically all the rabbits of a warren are found to be affected after death, their livers appearing as though speckled with many whitish spots of a comparatively small size (about the size of a small pea), which when opened are found to contain creamy or cheesy material.

Symptoms.—Young rabbits are more often affected than are adults, and the disease in them is more severe. At first there are no definite symptoms: the animal is a little dull, off his food, and a gradual emaciation begins to show. The animals are weak, hop about without vigour, frequently lie up in their burrows for long periods, and when killed are extremely light. At a later stage a persistent diarrhœa begins, the visible membranes are stained a yellowish colour (jaundice), and there is a discharge from the nostrils ('snuffles'). Death occurs at a variable time from the commencement of the symptoms, mainly depending upon the speed with which emaciation occurs.

Treatment.—Tame rabbits should be treated with sulphamezathine and hutches should be disinfected.

Dogs and Cats.—Coccidiosis in carnivores is commoner than was once believed, especially in young cats, where the parasite is *Isospora felis*. The disease causes no symptoms except diarrhœa where a heavy infestation has occurred. Death is rare. The rabbit parasite may be found in fæces when diseased rabbits have been eaten.

Fowls.—The disease is caused by several different species of parasites. This is probably the reason for the great diversity of symptoms described, as all the species, although similar in appearance, affect different parts of the intestine, take different times to develop, and cause different symptoms. Some are frequently fatal, others only produce vague illness ; some affect chickens principally, others are most commonly seen in dault birds, and so on.

The accompanying figure shows the distribution in the intestine of six of the commoner species which are recognised as occurring in chickens. *Eimeria tenella* usually attacks young chickens, causing an acute disease in the cæca—in some cases attacking the large intestine and the lower small intestine. It produces a hæmorrhagic coccidiosis with a high mortality, and is the most serious form. About five days

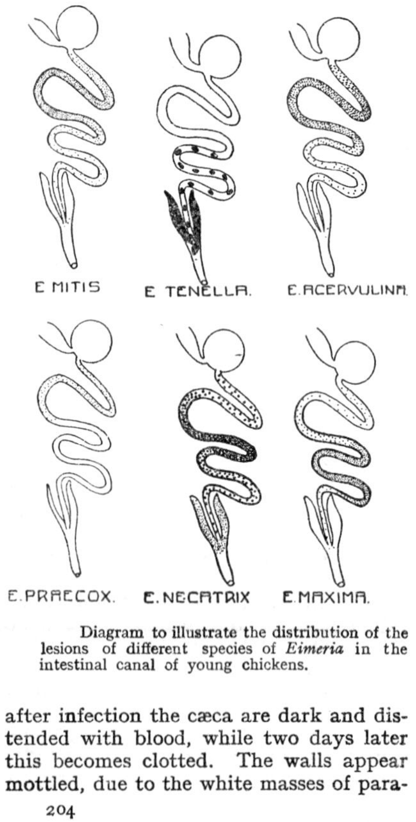

Diagram to illustrate the distribution of the lesions of different species of *Eimeria* in the intestinal canal of young chickens.

after infection the cæca are dark and distended with blood, while two days later this becomes clotted. The walls appear mottled, due to the white masses of parasites alternating with the dark blood. Development of the parasites takes place in the depth of the glands of the epithelium, and they may actually invade the underlying tissue. In adult birds this condition has a serious effect on egg production as well as on their general condition. Immunity develops fairly promptly.

Oöcysts appear in the fæces seven days after feeding. There are generally three asexual cycles before the sexual process begins ; in the absence of reinfection the parasites are eliminated in ten days, although some oöcysts may be found up to the nineteenth day.

Fowls on range harbour few parasites, and, as the disease depends on the number of cysts swallowed, they are generally free from the disease. But where large numbers are concentrated on a limited area of ground, many more cysts are swallowed at once ; the infection becomes severe, and disease results. This is especially true with young fowls, because it appears that a series of light infections produces a considerable degree of resistance to the parasite. A heavy infection may have the same result but is more likely to kill the bird in the process. Fowls which have not been previously infected are highly susceptible to the disease at all ages, and in a well-managed, healthy commercial flock, where the parasites have been absent for a time, no resistance has been built up, and so their introduction from outside may produce very severe loss. The various species produce no cross-immunity—that is, an infection with one species affords no protection against any other.

The disease, because of climatic conditions, of which moisture and warmth are the most important, is most common in spring and summer, although it is possible to have outbreaks at any time.

Control.—Efforts should be directed towards preventing birds from consuming more than very small doses of the infective cysts.

Yards, poultry houses, etc., should be regularly cleaned and disinfected, especially before young chicks are put in them. Rearing in brooders with wire-netting floors avoids much infection from fæces. Moving fold units every 2 or 3 days to fresh sites on clean ground also keeps infestation at low levels.

Faulty ventilation is a predisposing factor in poultry houses, and management can play a more important part than drugs in controlling coccidiosis. Overcrowding must be avoided, and temperature control studied.

Disinfection of buildings is best done with 10 per cent ammonia; the walls and floors being scrubbed. But the smallest amount of contaminated litter or of fæces on shoes, etc., can bring infection into a new house, with disastrous results.

Coccidiostat drugs have largely brought cæcal coccidiosis, due to *E. tenella*, under control. However, in both broilers and laying stock, coccidiosis due to *E. maxima*, *E. brunetti*, and *E. necatrix* is an increasingly serious problem.

COCCYX (κόκκυξ, a cuckoo) is the name given to the last part of the spinal column, which is composed of the coccygeal vertebra and forms the tail bones of those animals that possess a tail.

COCONUT CAKE is the residue remaining after expression or extraction of the oil from *copra*, which consists of the broken-up kernel of the coconut (*Cocus nucifera*). The cake is well digested and forms a valuable food for dairy cows especially, although at first they may not eat it with relish. Two or three pounds per head per day are given, and the butter made from the milk of cows getting coconut cake is firmer and of a better flavour than when cows are fed on linseed cake.

COCCIDIOSTATS.—Drugs used to control coccidiosis, and usually given to poultry in drinking water or, more often, mixed in the feed. Examples: zoalene, trithiadol, sulphadimidine, sulphaguanidine, sulphaguinoxaline, nitrofurazone, nitrophenide, nicarbazin, amprolium, methyl benzoquate.

CODEINE is one of the active principles of opium, which is used as the phosphate of codeine to check severe coughing in bronchitis, common cold, and in some cases of laryngitis. (*See* OPIUM.)

COD-LIVER OIL has an advantage over other oils in that some of the bile substances from the liver of the cod are incorporated with the oil, and as a consequence digestion is rendered easier, and absorption is more thorough. Cod-liver oil is one of the most valuable sources of vitamins A and D available for animal feeding. It should be purchased on a guarantee basis. The best varieties contain about 1000 to 1200 International Units of vitamin A, and 80 to 100 Units of D, per gramme. It should be stored in a dark-coloured container preferably in a cool place, and if air can be excluded until it is to be used, this will enable it to be kept longer. Both strong sunlight and oxygen cause a destruction of vitamin A. (*See* VITAMINS.)

Uses.—Cod-liver oil is useful for all young animals. It has a particularly beneficial action in warding off rachitis or rickets in young animals, and if this trouble has already started it may be checked, or cured, by the administration of cod-liver oil. For foals and calves, 1 to 2 ounces daily; for lambs and pigs, ½ to 1 ounce; and for puppies, ½ to 1 teaspoonful are usual doses. For chicks from ½ to 1 per cent of the food weight is required, and rather larger doses for ducklings and young turkeys. Synthetic vitamins are increasingly replacing cod-liver oil.

Swabs of cod-liver oil are also useful in eye injuries and in simple burns.

COD-LIVER OIL POISONING.—This may occur through the use of oil which has been allowed to oxidise or become rancid.

Associated is Muscular Dystrophy in cattle (which see, on p. 574).

CŒNUROSIS.—Infestation of the sheep's brain with cysts of the dog (and fox) tapeworm *Tænia multiceps* or *cœnurus*. For symptoms, etc., *see under* GID.

COFFEE, on account of its contained caffeine, is useful as a stimulating agent when nothing better can be obtained.

COITION (*see* REPRODUCTION).

COIT, MAL DU (*see* PARASITES, p. 634).

COLBRED.—A cross between the East Friesland and 3 British breeds of sheep (Border Leicester, Clun Forest, and Dorset Horn). The aim of Mr. Oscar Colburn, their breeder, was to produce ewes with a consistent 200 per cent lambing average and a sufficiency of milk for this.

COLCHICINE.—The alkaloid obtained from Meadow Saffron (*Colchicum autumnale*). It is used in plant and experimental animal breeding as 'a multiplier of chromosomes'. It has been possible to produce triploid rabbits, pigs, etc., by exposing semen to a solution of colchicine prior to artificial insemination. (*See* TRIPLOID.)

COLCHICUM POISONING (*see* MEADOW SAFFRON POISONING).

COLD (*see* CHILLS AND COLDS, EXPOSURE, FROST-BITE, SHEARING).

COLIC (from κόλον, the large intestine) is a vague term applied to any form of abdominal pain, or more correctly to the symptoms of abdominal pain which are exhibited by horses. Strictly speaking, it means disturbance in the colon or in the large intestine, but through common usage it has become almost entirely reserved for digestive disturbances, and is applied indiscriminately to conditions which differ widely in their causes. Popularly the terms 'gripes', 'stomach-ache', etc., are synonymous with 'colic', and to some extent indicate the nature of the condition. In order to emphasise the large number of different conditions which may produce abdominal pain, the following list is included:

1. *Acute indigestion*, resulting from the feeding of unsuitable food, the taking of poisons, crib-biting and wind-sucking, over-exertion, etc., and leading to gas formation, paralysis of the bowel, general intoxication, inflammation, etc.
2. *Spasm* of the bowel, from similar causes to the above, but usually less severe.
3. Severe digestive disorders, such as impaction of the colon, intussusception, volvulus, or strangulation of the bowel, rupture of the stomach, inflammation or enteritis of the bowel, and peritonitis, are among the serious causes.
4. The presence of large numbers of *parasitic worms, horse bots*, etc.
5. *Calculi* present in the large intestine. These may be either of the nature of dung-balls, oat-hair balls, or concretions.
6. *Calculi* present in the kidney, urinary bladder, or urethra in the male, causing irritation of these organs.
7. *Anthrax*, where one of the common symptoms is abdominal pain.
8. Approaching *parturition* in the pregnant mare.
9. Initial stages of equine *influenza*.
10. *Lead poisoning*.
11. *Diseases of the liver*.
12. *Hernia* of the abdominal contents into the scrotum or inguinal canal.
13. *Grass Sickness*.
14. *Intestinal strangulation*.

Causes.—From what has been said above it will be obvious that colic, in the widest sense of the word, is a symptom rather than a disease, but for the purpose of this description it will be considered as restricted to those conditions in which there is some disturbance in the alimentary canal.

The horse has a peculiarity in the arrangement of its alimentary canal, in that while the stomach is comparatively small, the intestines, and especially the large intestines, are of great bulk and capacity. In addition to this, the stomach itself has the peculiarity that its entrance and exit are small; the former only allows escape of gas into the gullet under exceptional circumstances, and the latter, owing to the S-shaped bend of the pylorus and first part of the small intestine, is very liable to become occluded when there is any considerable pressure of gas within the stomach. These two facts combine to make it difficult or impossible for gas collected in the stomach, as the result of fermentation, either to escape by the mouth or to pass on into the intestines. Food, therefore, which is in an unwholesome, fermented, or partially cooked condition, is liable to cause *tympany of the stomach*, associated with pain, and to induce colic. Even when the food is sound and good, if it is taken in excessively large amounts so that the stomach becomes replete to the point of distension, it may so embarrass the normal movements of the organ that evacuation is impossible and *impaction of the stomach*, with colic, occurs. In certain instances distension of the stomach with either food material or gas may be so acute as to stress the walls beyond the point of endurance, and *rupture of the stomach* results.

It has been found that the large intestines are, almost exclusively, the seat of those forms of colic that are not attributable to derangements of the stomach. The small intestine is certainly found upon post-mortem examination to be involved in certain cases of fatal twist or inflammation, but it is not often that the primary seat of the colic is in them only. The large colon of the horse, which is in the form of a sudden dilatation flexed twice upon itself, has a greater capacity than any other part, and with the cæcum, which precedes it, always contains by far the greater amount of the food material in the alimentary canal. Food can be passed into the cæcum and colon with ease; but after it has negotiated these parts its evacuation into the small colon must of necessity be slower. Should any irregularity in the food itself, in the times of feeding, or in the general life of the horse, take place, it very often happens that the muscular movements of the cæcum and colon are decreased in vigour; stasis or stoppage occurs; these organs, and especially the colon, become packed with ingesta, and *impaction of the cæcum or colon* results.

Under very similar circumstances it may happen that when the passage of food through the large intestines is slow, undue fermentation or even decomposition of the food may occur; gas collects and is unable to be expelled, and *tympany of the cæcum or colon*, accompanied by severe distention of the bowel wall and pain, is the consequence. Under the influence of several varying conditions, perhaps when there has been a considerable collection of gas in one or other part of the cæcum or colon, perhaps when the normal peristaltic movements have been over-stimulated, or from some other cause, one part of the large intestine (or occasionally of the small intestine) becomes twisted along a short length of its course, and *volvulus* or *strangulation* occurs. The blood-vessels supplying the twisted portion are involved in the process and the blood-supply to that part of the bowel is cut off, or seriously hindered. Organisms, or the toxins they manufacture, are enabled to attack the devitalised gut and *inflammation* or *enteritis* follows. In yet other cases some powerful irritant has been taken along with the food, either in large amount at one time, or in smaller quantities at frequent intervals, and inflammation of the mucous membrane of stomach or intestines results. Less commonly one piece of the gut may telescope into an adjacent portion, causing an *intussusception*.

External conditions, and errors in management or feeding, may bring about these abnormalities in the alimentary canal. In the first place, *over-work* must be mentioned. Upon returning to the stable, food is taken ravenously, and the tired organs are unable to cope with it as fast as it is eaten. In this way digestive derangements often occur. *Too little exercise*, especially when full working feeds are given, is another fruitful cause of colic. When the food is in an *unwholesome* condition, such as, for example, when mouldy hay, wet oats or other grains, sour bran, etc., are used for feeding; or when partially fermented foods, such as brewers' grains, scalded barley which has been allowed to cool, or other partially cooked foods, are given; or when a sudden change is made to new hay, new oats, or to green food, disturbances of the stomach are very likely to occur, and stomachic colic results. When the food is unduly *fibrous* in nature, or when it is *not thoroughly chewed*, longer time is required for the completion of the normal processes of digestion, and, since the greater part of the digestion of crude or fibrous material takes place in the colon, the ingesta must spend a longer time in this part of the large intestine than would be needed for food-stuffs of better quality. Food collected in the colon in this way is another source of impaction and colic.

Symptoms.—Colic is often considered as being *acute* when the pain is very intense; *subacute* when the pain is less severe and more like an ache. The so-called *true colic* is pain affecting the colon, while *false colic* means that the pain is elsewhere. For purposes of description colic will here be treated under three headings: (1) Spasmodic colic; (2) Obstructed colic; and (3) Colic with inflammation.

(1) *Spasmodic colic* is characterised by sudden and severe attacks of pain, usually of an intermittent character. The horse may be attacked while at work, or it may be seized immediately upon, or soon after, coming into the stable from work. The animal perspires; breathing is blowing and faster than usual; there is an anxious expression about the face; and the pulse is accelerated and hard. In a few minutes the attack may pass off and the horse becomes easier, or the pain may continue. In the latter case the horse lies down and rolls, after having first walked round about the box. In some cases rolling appears to afford some measure of relief, but in others the horse rises again almost at once. The bowels usually move frequently in the earlier stages, but after a time fæces are withheld, particularly when some obstruction is the cause of the colic. (*See also under* 'Obstructive Colic'.) Diarrhœa may be in evidence, particularly when inflammation sets in, or when the bowels are in an irritated condition. It is not, however, common in the early stages. Horses often stretch as though to pass urine, but generally without result. During an attack the horse may kick at its belly, or may turn and gaze at its flank.

In another form, which is often called

flatulent colic, the pain begins suddenly, but there are not such distinct periods of ease. The horse walks round and round the box, kicks at the abdomen, gazes at its sides, breaks out into patchy sweating, and breathes heavily. The pulse is hard and fast; the temperature is usually normal, although it may be elevated one or two degrees, and the expression on the face is anxious and strained. The horse frequently crouches as if to lie down, but only actually lies in the less severe cases, and seldom or never remains lying for any length of time. He does not usually roll. After a short time the abdomen fills with gas, and the hollows of the flanks fill out. Upon tapping these regions a hollow resonant sound is heard, and pressure upon them by the closed fist is painful to the horse. Attempts at the passage of urine are noticed, but, as in the truly spasmodic colic, they are seldom successful. Fæces may be passed in small quantities, and are usually accompanied by flatus. In very severe instances where relief is not obtained, the horse may suddenly rear in agony and then fall to the ground. The breathing becomes very distressed, the mucous membranes of eyes and mouth become livid, and the horse expires from asphyxia in a few minutes. The diaphragm may rupture under the influence of the pressure of gas in the abdomen, or its action may become so embarrassed that the horse is unable to oxygenate its blood; it staggers and falls; and dies from suffocation.

(2) *Obstructive colic* may arise through the partial or complete occlusion of the lumen of the bowel by a calculus, or it may be due to impaction with dry, fibrous, partly digested food material in some part of the large intestine. The symptoms develop slowly, commencing with dullness and depression, irregularity in feeding, and abdominal discomfort. If the horse is out at work, it gets easily tired, perhaps during the morning, but more often this form of colic occurs during a week-end, or when horses are standing idle in the stable. Food is picked, but the feed is not finished, and in 12 hours abdominal pain becomes manifested. No distension of the abdomen with gas is noticed at first, though it may occur later. As the intestine becomes more and more distended with impacted food-stuffs, pain increases, and the more definite symptoms develop. The horse looks round at its flank, paws with the fore-feet, and kicks at the abdomen. Attempts at micturition are frequent, and appear to be caused by the pressure of the distended gut upon the urinary bladder. The owner is sometimes misled by the attempts at urination into thinking that the seat of the pain is in some part of the urinary system. The horse generally wanders round the box, and with care chooses a position in which to lie. When on the ground it usually stretches out on one side, very often the off, and appears to derive some ease from lying in this position. Considerable grunting and groaning usually accompany recumbency, and breathing is often long and 'sighing'. In some cases acute pain is shown, the horse rolling on the ground in agony. Small amounts of fæces are passed with considerable frequency at first, but when an attack is well established the passage of both urine and dung ceases. An attitude to which some importance may be attached, since it is very strongly suggestive of impaction of the colon, is one in which the horse backs against the manger or other projection, and appears to sit upon it, sometimes with the hind-feet off the ground. In other cases a horse with obstruction in the colon or cæcum may sit with the hind-quarters on the ground, but retains an upright position with the fore-legs—somewhat similar to the position assumed by a dog.

(3) *Colic with inflammation*.—Inflammatory colics, which include such diverse conditions as rupture of the stomach, twist, intussusception, enteritis, strangulation of a portion of bowel, etc., may therefore commence with an attack such as has been described already. The horse shows a continuance of the pain, and at times severe spasms appear to pass through the body. During the height of a spasm the suffering animal may wander round and round the box, colliding with the walls, door, or dashing its head against the manger or other fitting. It appears to disregard the pain caused by such behaviour—all its attention being concentrated upon the internal agony. It may throw itself to the ground and half rising throw itself down again with great violence. It is only controlled with the greatest of difficulty, and may prove a danger to the attendant. The spasm passes off, but the continual subacute pain shows no abatement. If the temperature can be taken it is found to be raised to perhaps 105° or 106° F., or, in the later stages, it may be sub-normal. Sweating, either all over the body or in localised patches, is always a marked symptom during the earlier stages, but

some hours later the body may be quite dry. The expression is anxious and haggard; the respirations are blowing, fast, or perhaps sobbing; the nostrils are fully dilated; the eyes are injected; and the pulse is at first found to be full and hard, but when death approaches it is irregular, soft, and spoken of as 'running down'. Severe straining accompanies any attempt to inject enemata, and in some cases the rectum may be everted. Blood may be passed, or a watery diarrhœa, in which flocculi of mucus are seen, may set in. Later still, just before death relieves the suffering animal, pain ceases. The animal stands quiet and may even take a little water. Necrosis of the bowel has set in, and the part is rapidly becoming gangrenous. A little later the animal staggers, and dies in convulsions. In other cases the animal goes down sooner; it rises again, only to lie once more, and each time the attempt to rise is weaker than the last, until finally it has not the necessary strength to regain its feet. It lies struggling on the ground, and after a short while expires in convulsions. These acute symptoms seldom last more than 6 or 10 hours, although cases are met with in which spasms appear at intervals during as long as a week. When twist occurs there is usually a continuation of the acute pain right up to the moment of death, no period of ease supervening.

Treatment.—Expert assistance should be sought whenever an attack of colic persists for longer than 3 hours. The simpler cases seldom last as long as 6 hours, and when symptoms are continued for longer than that it should be an indication that the case has passed beyond the simple stage, and the sooner skilled assistance is sought the less likely is it that complications will arise. Many colics end fatally, and it is certain that many horses might have been saved if a veterinary surgeon had been summoned at the outset.

The horse should be taken from work or from the stable and put into a large, airy, well-littered loose-box, and all restraint removed. At first it may be allowed to do as it likes. There is always some danger of torsion or twisting of the bowel from rolling, but the ease that frequently follows more than counterbalances the risk. Many proprietary so-called 'colic drinks' are upon the market, and the natural tendency is for the attendant to drench the horse with the first upon which he can lay his hand, quite irrespective of the cause of the colic and of the nature of the ingredients. The folly of such a procedure can be illustrated by taking the example of the drenching of a horse with a 'colic drink' containing some compound of opium (a very favourite ingredient in colic mixtures), which certainly may allay the pain, but which has the grave disadvantage that it inhibits peristalsis, checks the natural secretions, and aggravates those colics which are caused by impaction of the bowel or obstruction. Again, the composition of but few proprietary medicines is indicated, so that the attending veterinary surgeon, who must be called in later in the majority of cases, is met with the dilemma of administering some drug which perhaps has already been administered in the proprietary medicine, or of giving one the action of which is counteracted by something already received. A safer and better course overseas, where a veterinary surgeon is not available, is to administer a drench composed of:

Medicinal turpentine .	2 tablespoonfuls.
Whisky (if available) .	1 teacupful.
Ground ginger . .	1 teaspoonful.
Olive Oil . . .	1 pint.

The proportions are for a full-sized cart-horse; for smaller animals the dosage should be reduced accordingly. They may be repeated in 3 hours if necessary, and four doses may be given provided the amount of turpentine is reduced to one-half. If possible, enemata of warm soapy water should be given in copious amounts.

If, however, the obstruction is high up in the intestine, large quantities of fluid should NOT be given by stomach tube. (*See also under* DEHYDRATION.)

Prevention.—Regular feeding; good quality foods, neither too bulky nor too concentrated, and with succulents when available; clean water in plentiful supply, and watering before feeding for working horses; regular work and regular rest; the avoidance of too sudden changes in food, work, or routine, and of food-stuffs that are dirty, contaminated, or harmful for other reasons.

COLIFORM INFECTIONS.—Examination of cattle carcases at slaughterhouses showed that coliform organisms were isolated from surface swabbings from 208 out of 400 head of cattle (52 per cent); 81 of these being resistant to one or more antibiotics. Of 400 pig carcase swabs, 331 (83 per cent) were positive for coliforms; 246 being resistant to one or more antibiotics. Chloramphenicol resistance was present in 19 pig isolates and 1 cattle isolate. (John R. Walton, M.R.C.V.S., *Lancet*, Sept. 12, 1970.) (*See E. coli.*)

COLITIS (κόλον, the large intestine) means inflammation of the colon, or first part of the large intestine.

COLLAPSE is that lowered condition of the bodily powers which often terminates severe diseases, when all the systems of the organism are in a condition of extreme weakness. The nervous system is most affected, and in consequence death may occur from failure of the heart or respiration. Blood-pressure is usually low, and may be responsible for the weakness of heart action, or this latter may cause a lowered blood-pressure. Collapse often succeeds severe injuries of a violent nature, such as runaway accidents, collisions, run-over accidents, severe crushes, kicks, etc.; conditions demanding much exertion, such as long races when unfit, parturition when some factor prevents the act taking place normally, chasing of sheep by dogs, especially in hot weather, are all apt to induce collapse in the respective animals concerned.

Symptoms.—In collapse from a debilitating disease the main symptoms are those of the disease concerned, and in addition to them the animal shows a patchy sweat, lies prostrated, takes no notice of anything, has not strength to lift its head; breathing is shallow, pulse is almost imperceptible, and temperature is generally sub-normal. Death frequently takes place during such a collapsed phase. In cases of collapse from violence, the signs vary in each instance according to whether the actual cause is nervous shock, or whether external or internal hæmorrhage is to blame. There may be rapid, irregular breathing, a tumultuous heart's action, paleness of the visible mucous membranes (*i.e.* eyelid linings, mouth, nose, etc.), cold patchy sweating, or the body may be bathed in perspiration. The temperature is almost always sub-normal, and the animal takes little or no interest in its surroundings.

Treatment.—Drugs such as caffeine, adrenalin, or camphor may be necessary. The animal should be removed from noise and disturbance, the room or loose-box should be darkened, and some clean cold water provided. A good sign of recovery is the drinking of a considerable amount of water.

COLLAR, INJURIES FROM.—'Sore shoulders', in which the hair and surface layers of the skin become rubbed away from areas under the collar, are due to the wearing of a collar which is too large for the horse, and which slips backward and forward with each step. (*See under* CHAFING OF SKIN, and SHOULDER-GALLS.)

COLLATERAL CIRCULATION (*see* ANASTOMOSIS).

COLLIE EYE ANOMALY.—A hereditary defect seen in some rough collies, smooth collies, and Shetland sheepdogs.

COLLODION (κόλλα, glue) is a thick, colourless, syrupy liquid, made by dissolving gun-cotton in a mixture of ether and alcohol. When painted on to the skin, the ether and alcohol evaporate, and leave a tough film behind. *Flexible collodion*, made by adding castor oil and Canada balsam, is more elastic and does not crack with the movements of the part, and is eminently suitable for application to regions around joints. Medicated collodion contains substances such as salicylic acid and iodoform. A collodion preparation containing a caustic is used for destroying the horn-buds of calves. (*See* DISHORNING.)

COLLOID (κόλλα, glue; εἶδος, form) is matter in which the individual particles consist either of single large molecules, such as proteins, or aggregates of smaller molecules, more or less uniformly distributed in a dispersion medium, *e.g.* water, oil. Examples: colloidal silver (used for eye infections), and colloidal manganese.

COLLUNARIUM (*collutio*, a washing; *nares*, the nose) is a nose wash.

COLLUTORIUM, or **COLLUTORY** (*colluttio*, a washing; *os*, *oris*, the mouth), is a mouth wash.

COLLYRIUM (κολλύριον) means an eye wash.

COLON (κόλον) is the first part of the large intestine. (*See* INTESTINE.)

COLOSTRUM is the milk secreted by the udder immediately after parturition and for the following 3 to 4 days. It consists of the cells (epithelia) which previous to the birth of the young animal were packed in the acini, mixed with serum and fat globules, etc. It contains 20 per cent or more protein, a little more fat than normal milk, and may be tinged pink due to blood corpuscles. It coagulates at about 80° to 85° C., and cannot therefore be boiled. This is sometimes used as a test. It is normally rich in vitamins A and D provided the dam has not been deprived of these in her food. It acts as a natural purgative for the young animal, clearing romits intestines the accumulated fæcal matter known as 'meconium', which is often of a dry, putty-like nature. In addition it has been shown that it is through the medium of the colostrum that the young animal obtains its first supply of antibodies which protect it against various bacteria and viruses.

Hookworm larvæ have been found in a bitch's colostrum (10 were recovered by experimental milking before whelping), and larvæ of *strongyloides ransomi* in a sow's milk.

COLOUR-MARKING BULLS, *e.g.* Hereford, Aberdeen-Angus, and Galloway, for mating with cows in dairy herds which are of dual-purpose type and moderate to poor milkers, in order to increase the number of store cattle suitable for fattening for beef production. (*See also* BEEF-BREEDS AND CROSSES.)

COLOURS OF HORSES.—There is a very great deal of confusion existing as to the methods of describing the colours of horses—one person calling an animal dark bay, for instance, while another would call it dark brown. Moreover, in different parts of the country local names are used. Accordingly, there will be given a brief account of the generally accepted colours and names.

There are two chief kinds of colour: *whole-colour*, and *broken-colour*. A horse is whole-coloured when the whole of its body is covered by hair of the same colour, the mane and tail excepted. Such horses are rare, but the recognised whole-colours are: black, brown, bay, chestnut, dun, grey, and white. There are those who consider that certain roans may be whole-coloured, *i.e.* when the roan is due to a uniform scattering of hairs over the body, each of which shows two colours, such as red and white. Roans are, however, nearly always composed of an admixture of individual white hairs and individual hairs of another colour such as red, brown, chestnut, black, etc. There are various shades of the whole colours, and the differentiation between them is often a matter of difficulty. A horse is said to be broken-coloured when its coat is made up of bold splashes of two different colours, each colour being separated sharply from the other by comparatively discrete edges. The recognised broken colours are: Piebalds, Skewbalds, and Roans of a certain type, such as roan and white, roan and red, etc.

Piebalds are marked in black and white, each colour being distinctly separated from the other, and the patches being large and irregular.

Skewbalds are horses with splashes of white and any definite colour except black over the body, each colour being separated from the other.

Black horses must have black muzzles. *Jet black* means that the coat has a glossy sheen; *black chestnut, black grey*, etc., means that a few hairs of the second colour are scattered through the coat.

Brown horses must have tan-coloured muzzles; they may be *brown roans, brown chestnuts*, or *brown bays*, when a few hairs of the second colour are present. *Brown-ticked grey* is a colour in which little spots of brown about the size of millet seeds are scattered over a background of grey.

Bay horses are of a light reddish-brown, suggestive of the colouring of a fox, with muzzles of the same colour. *Golden bays* are rich yellowish-red; *blood bays* are a warm, rich bronze colour; *mealy bays* are rust-coloured; *bright bay*, or *light bay*, is a light glossy tan.

Chestnuts, according to the Suffolk Horse Society, are divided into seven shades for the purpose of Suffolk horses; these are: *Dark chestnut*, a brown-black, mahogany, or liver colour; *dull dark, light mealy, red, golden, lemon*, and *bright chestnut*. For ordinary purposes, however, chestnut is usually described as being *light chestnut, dark chestnut*, or *chestnut roan*.

Dun horses are mostly either crosses from Russian ponies, Iceland ponies, Highland garrons, or Arabs. They must always carry a black stripe along the backbone, from the withers to the root of the tail, or as it is put, from the mane to the tail. *Dark dun* is the colour of a mouse; *light dun* is light colour; *silver dun* is about the colour of a mountain hare; and *yellow dun* is a light lemon colour.

Grey horses must have grey points, grey mane and tail, and be of the same shade of grey over the body. If they have black or dark grey points they are called *steel-grey* ; if there are reddish hairs through the coat they are *iron-grey*, or *rusty grey* ; *flea-bitten greys* have tiny spots of black or dark hairs throughout the coat ; *blue greys* have steely blue hairs scattered over the coat ; *mealy greys* are a sort of rusty blue ; *light greys*, and *silver-greys*, are lighter in colour, nearly white, and the latter must have white manes and tails.

White horses must have white muzzles, although a faint bluish tinge does not matter. The variations of white are described as *white with grey mane and tail*, *white with black* (*bay*, *brown*, etc.) *spots*, or as *flea-bitten white*. White horses may have white, pink, or black skins. If the muzzle, eyelids, inside of ears, and the skin of the perineal region round the genital organs and the dock are white or pink, and if the iris has no colouring matter in each eye (*i.e.* double ' wall-eyed '), the animal is an *albino* ; such horses are very rare, but they are sometimes seen among Arabs.

Cream horses must have cream manes and tails, muzzles and points, with no stripe or ' eland mark ' (*see later*). *Silver-creams* must have bright silver-coloured manes and tails.

Roans are mixtures of various colours. *Black roan* is a very dark roan with black points, mane, tail, and muzzle, although there may be a few white or roan hairs. *Brown roans* have brown points, manes, tails, and muzzles. *Blue roan* is a free mixture of blue and grey hairs, with dark mixed mane and tail. *Bay roans* have bay points, manes, tails, and muzzles. *Roan chestnut* is a colour with roan hairs as a background and chestnut or reddish hairs throughout the coat, chestnut manes and tails, and light muzzles. It is often called a ' *strawberry roan* '.

Changes of colour in horses.—Black horses sometimes become grey, due to the absorption of melanin (the colouring matter of the hair). They may turn quite white, or may remain a flea-bitten grey. In many cases the whitening commences around the mouth and muzzle, giving rise to the name ' mealy-muzzled '.

Foals very often change colour three or four weeks after birth, the change being in some cases remarkable. A light bay foal may turn black ; an apparently chestnut foal may turn brown, and so on. In most instances, however, the colour of the muzzle is an indication of what the final colour will be.

Markings.—The ' points ' of a horse are the four legs, including the knees and hocks, downward. They may be black, which is a sign of hardiness and stamina. One or more may be white, or only parts may be white ; for example, there may be ' white legs ', which means that the knees and hocks and all below them are white ; ' white fetlocks ', ' white pasterns ', ' white coronets ', etc. Irregular white markings are described as ' white splashes ', ' speckled coronets ', etc. When the fetlocks and all below are white, and when the line of demarcation from the colour above is regular, the term ' white socks ' is sometimes used. In the same way when the white extends to the knees or hocks or nearly so, the term ' white stockings ' is employed. Some hesitation should be felt in using these terms, however, for what is a ' white sock ' to one man may mean a ' white stocking ' to another. It is better to describe exactly what parts of the legs are actually white. White on the body is often due to pressure from harness and is called a ' collar- ', ' saddle- ', ' girth- ', or ' crupper-mark ' according to its position, but white splashes are met with in other parts also.

Faces are called ' white ' when the white encloses both eyes and comes well over the sides of the cheeks ; ' blaze ' when there is a broad stripe running down the nose ; and when lesser marks are present they are known as ' reaches ', ' races ', ' strips ', or ' snips ', according to their sizes. Any shaped white mark on the forehead is a ' star ', and it may be ' large ', ' small ', ' medium ', or ' faint '. A white face generally means that one or both eyes are devoid of colouring matter in the iris, and the horse is called ' ring-eyed ', ' wall-eyed ', or ' ringle-eyed ' ; contrary to general belief, such horses are not blind, but they do not withstand strong tropical sunlight as well as do those not deficient in this respect. ' Zebra-marks ', or ' tiger stripes ', are transverse parallel black stripes across the back of the fore-arms and front of the gaskins, and rarely across the shoulders and quarters. Highland garrons and Yorkshire coach-horses are often marked in this way. An ' eland mark ' is a black stripe about an inch wide running down the centre of the back from withers to dock. It is seen in dun horses. The word ' dappled ' before a colour means that there are patches of darker hairs scattered through the coat, about the size of a walnut or a little larger as a rule, and fairly regularly distributed.

'Flea-bitten' is much the same as dappled except that the areas of dark hairs are only about the size of fleas or millet seeds. 'Speckled', unless applied to the coronets, where the speckles can be of any size, usually means that the dark spots are about the size of peas or a little larger. 'Sorrel' means that the horse is the colour of the dried withered sorrel or dock, that is, a reddish-brown of a warm tinge. It is a somewhat vague word, used by the laity.

COLT.—A young male horse.

COLOUR VISION.—The absence of cones in the retina of domesticated animals led to the belief that they must be colour blind. There is now scientific evidence to show that cats have partial colour-vision, and to suggest that dogs can appreciate some colours. It is likely that cattle can likewise distinguish certain colours. (Maurice Burton, D.Sc.)

COMA (κῶμα, deep sleep) is a state of profound unconsciousness in which the patient not only cannot be roused, but there are no reflex movements when the skin is pinched or pricked, or when the eyeballs are touched, etc. The breathing is often stertorous but deep and regular, and the heart's action may be strong or weak. The cause is generally an excessively high temperature, apoplexy, or some poison. If it does not pass off in 12 or 15 hours death is imminent. Since it is always a very serious manifestation in the course of an illness, assistance should be sought as soon as it is noted.

COMB.—In healthy poultry, this should be bright red and well developed. When birds go out of lay or are caponised, the comb becomes smaller and paler. Anæmia may also cause this. A pale comb of normal size suggests internal hæmorrhage. Scurfiness is suggestive of favus, yellow scabs of fowl-pox.

COMENY'S INFECTIOUS PARALYSIS OF HORSES.—This was first described in French army horses by Comény. A suspected outbreak of this at the Evans Biological Institute, Runcorn, in 1961 was described in the *Veterinary Record* of April 3, 1965.

Symptoms.—A sudden rise in temperature to 104° or 105°, persisting for 5 days, and followed in some cases by paralysis after a period of hind-limb inco-ordination and difficulty in turning.

COMMENSALS.—Micro-organisms found on the skin or within the body which do not produce disease. (Compare pathogenic bacteria, which do.)

COMMISSURE (*committo*, I join) means a joining, and is a term applied to strands of nerve fibres that join one side of the brain to the other, to the band joining one optic nerve to the other, to the junction of the lips at the corners of the mouth, etc.

COMMUNICABLE DISEASES.—For diseases communicable *to* man, *see under* PUBLIC HEALTH. Diseases with which human beings may infect farm livestock, etc., include: tuberculosis, scarlet fever (giving rise to mastitis in dairy cows), tonsillitis (giving rise to calf pneumonia, etc.), infestation with the beef tapeworm, cow-pox (from a person newly vaccinated against smallpox). (*See also under* INFLUENZA.)

COMPARATIVE TEST (*see* TUBERCULIN TEST.)

COMPENSATION is the term applied to the method by which the body makes good a defect of form or function in an organ which is abnormal in these respects. These powers are very remarkable in certain cases, and even serious defects can be compensated for so that after a time the animal may suffer little or no handicap. The heart muscle possesses great powers of compensation to enable it to become more efficient and compensatory hypertrophy of the heart is very common especially in horses and dogs. It may occur as the result of any factor which impedes the circulating blood, such as disease of the lungs, liver, or kidneys with fibrosis.

COMPLEMENT.—This is a constituent of serum and plays an essential part in the production of immunity. Bacteria are killed by the specific antibody developed in an animal's serum only in the presence of complement. Complement is also necessary for hæmolysis.

An immune serum may contain antibodies which, together with the antigen, absorb or fix complement and are hence called *complement-fixing antibodies.* These form the basis for the Complement Fixation Test, which is used in the diagnosis of certain diseases, *e.g.* Johne's. As an indicator for the test, red blood corpuscles plus their specific antibody are used, *i.e.* the corpuscles plus the antiserum heated at 55° C. to inactivate or destroy the complement. In the test, on adding the indicator, hæmolysis will not occur if the complement has been fixed.

COMPOUND FEEDS.—A number of different ingredients (including major minerals, trace elements, vitamins and other additives) mixed and blended in appropriate proportions, to provide properly balanced diets for all types of stock at every stage of growth and development.

CONCAVE SHOE is a shoe usually used for hunters and other fast-moving horses, which is made from concave iron, *i.e.* one edge is bevelled off. The bevelled edge is situated on the inside of the shoe, so that the ground surface is narrower than the foot surface. They are especially necessary for horses which are given to over-reaching. (*See* OVER-REACHING.)

CONCENTRATES.—The bulk of these in Britain today come from highly reputable compound feeding-stuffs manufacturers, and are expert formulations related not only to the current price of various ingredients but also to the proper balancing of these ingredients. Computers are often used in the formulations. The inclusion of trace elements, minerals, and vitamins makes these compound feeding-stuffs foods complete in themselves. Suitable mixes are obtainable for every class of farm live-stock.

Farm-mixed concentrates are commonly used on large arable farms, using home-grown barley, oats, beans, etc. Very small-scale mixing is apt to be inefficient and result in a less bulky ingredient being unequally distributed. The expertise required for formulation may also be lacking, so that on the smaller farm proprietary concentrates are often to be preferred. (*See* DIET, CUBES; *also* ADDITIVES, COMPOUND FEEDS, SUPPLEMENTS.)

CONCEPTION signifies the complex set of changes which occur in the ovum and in the body of the mother at the beginning of pregnancy. The precise moment of conception is that instant at which the male cell, or spermatozoön, finds the female cell, or ovum, and fertilises it. (*See* REPRODUCTION.)

CONCEPTION RATES following artificial insemination of cattle are stated to be in the region of 65 per cent in dairy breeds, and over 70 per cent in beef breeds. In the U.K., the conception rate is usually based upon the number of animals which, on a 3-month period, do not return to the first insemination. In Denmark, the conception rate is based on the evidence of a physical pregnancy diagnosis carried out 3 months after insemination.

Conception rates are influenced by many factors. The best time for insemination is between 2 and 20 hours after 'heat' is observed; after that delay will mean a lower conception rate. Health of male and female, and inseminator's skill also influence the rate. (*See also* FARROWING RATES.)

CONCEPTUS.—The product of conception: initially a fertilised egg, later an embryo which develops into a fœtus plus fœtal membranes.

CONCRETE.—The precise nature of the ingredients of this may prove important where floor feeding is practised. Suspected iron poisoning from the licking of concrete made with sand rich in iron is described under 'WHITE PIG DISEASE'.

Concrete floors of piggeries, etc., should be made with integral air spaces in order to have some insulating effect. (*See under* FOOT-ROT OF PIGS, HOUSING OF ANIMALS, *and* BEDDING.)

CONCUSSION (*see* BRAIN).

CONDENSATION IN BUILDINGS (*see* NITRITE POISONING, CALF REARING, PNEUMONIA, SWEAT HOUSE).

CONDITION (*see under* MUSCLE).

CONDYLE (κόνδυλος, a knuckle) is the name given to the rounded prominence at the end of a bone; for instance, the condyles of the humerus are the two prominences on either side of the elbow-joint in animals, while the condyles of the femur enter into the formation of the stifle joint.

CONFORMATION DEFECTS (*conformo*, I shape symmetrically), and the names by which they are commonly known, are given below. Some of the terms used are descriptive rather than elegant.

Roman-nosed means that the face shows a convexity between eyes and nose when viewed in profile.

CONFORMATION DEFECTS

Dished or *stag face* means that there is a concavity in the line of the face when seen in profile.

Brow bump is a prominence between the eyes, as seen in profile.

Pigeon-eyed or *spectacled* means that each eyelid is devoid of colouring matter around its free margin, giving a horse the appearance of having a painted white ring round each eye.

Wall-eyed or *ring-eyed* means absence of colouring matter in the iris, so that a ring of white appears to surround the black pupil.

Turned-in ears is a term the meaning of which is obvious.

Lop ears means that the ears are flaccid and slack, and tend to fall outwards and to move to and fro with each step.

Cock-throttled means that there is an abundance of flesh below and around the jowl, giving the head a full and heavy appearance. Good size and plenty of width at the throat are good points, however.

Ewe-necked means that the upper line of the neck is concave when seen in profile.

High-crested is the opposite of ewe-necked.

Bull-necked means that the neck is short, thick, and fleshy—a quality which militates against easy control of a riding or driving horse.

High in the withers means that the withers are unduly prominent.

Low in the withers means that the withers are poorly developed.

Straight or *upright shoulders* means that there is not a good backward slope of the shoulder-blades.

Light fore-arms means a poor muscular development between elbow and knee.

Calf or *buck knees* means that the joints are shallow from front to back and that, instead of being straight when seen from the side, they tend to bend backwards as if over-extended.

Knock-knees are those which bend toward each other when seen from the front.

Bandy knees are the opposite of the above.

Over at the knees means that the joints are not fully extended when seen from the side.

Tied-in below the knees means that there is an apparent constriction of the limb immediately below the knee.

Knuckled over means that the fetlock cannot be lowered back into its normal position because of shortness of the flexor tendons.

Straight or *upright pasterns* means that there is not enough backward slope of the pasterns.

Slack or *sloping pasterns* means that there is too much backward slope.

Turned-in toes and *turned-out toes* are self-descriptive terms.

Hollow back means that the back is markedly concave.

Razor back is one in which the spines of the vertebræ are unduly prominent and appear as a ridge.

Roach back is one in which there is a convexity along the back.

Long-backed means that the back is too long for the size of the horse, and consequently weak.

Light in the middle means that the development of the trunk is poor.

Slack or *hollow at the heart* means that there is a distinct depression behind the shoulder muscles over the region of the heart.

Flat-chested means that there is not sufficient curvature along their lengths in the ribs.

Herring-gutted means that the animal is poorly developed in its middle, and that the trunk tapers from front to back, so that a girth would be difficult to keep from slipping back. Such animals are also very often flat in the chest.

Pot-bellied means that the abdomen is excessively pendulous and the lower line of the belly is markedly convex.

Slack in the loins indicates that there is a large hollow in the flank, occasioned by a great distance between the last rib and the point of the haunch bone. It is the opposite of '*well ribbed-up*'.

Ragged hips means that the points of the haunch bone are not symmetrical, and that they are irregular or excessively prominent in their outlines. (This condition often results from fracture.)

Goose-rumped means that the tail is set on low down, and that the quarters are drooped downwards.

Plain quarters means that instead of the natural nearly horizontal quarters of a good horse, there is a rounded appearance somewhat suggesting a fat pig's quarter.

Wide behind means that the hind-legs are wide apart.

Cow-hocked means that the hock joints are too close together, and also that the joints are small and weak.

Sickle-shaped or *curby hocks* means that

there is too much curve on the hock when seen from the side.

Straight or *upright hocks* means that there is not enough curve in these joints.

Tied-in below hocks is a similar condition to tied-in below the knees. (*See also* DEFORMITIES.)

CONGENITAL (*con*, together; *genitus*, begotten) deformities, diseases, etc., are those which are either present at birth, or which, being transmitted direct from the parents, show themselves some time after birth. (*See* Heredity and disease *under* GENETICS.)

CONGESTION (*congero*, I accumulate) means the accumulation of blood in a part due to overfilling of its blood-vessels.

CONJUNCTIVA (*conjungo*, I join together) is the membrane which covers the front of the eye. It lines the insides of the eyelids of all animals, both upper and lower, and from each of these places it is reflected on to the front of the eyeball. The membrane is transparent in its central portion, where it is specialised to form the covering to the cornea, which admits light into the cavity of the eye. The so-called 'white of the eye' is formed by the sclerotic, or outer coat of the eyeball, shining through the conjunctiva. This membrane is richly supplied with nerves, so that the merest touch results in the reflex closing of the eyelids. This 'corneal reflex' is of some moment as a guide to consciousness, and as an indication of certain diseases. (*See* EYE.)

CONJUNCTIVITIS means inflammation of the conjunctiva. (*See* EYE, DISEASES OF.)

CONSOLIDATION is a term applied to solidification of an organ, especially of a lung. The consolidation may be of a permanent nature due to formation of fibrous tissue or tumour cells, or temporary, as in acute pneumonia.

CONSTIPATION (*con*, together; *stipo*, I cram) is the word used to indicate that state which results from non-passage of motions for a longer period than is normal. It is a chronic condition, and should be distinguished from a sudden stoppage of the bowels, which is generally acute. The fæces are passed in a variety of ways among the domestic animals. In the horse, cow, and sheep, the excreta appears to be evacuated with very little or even no effort. The horse can defæcate perfectly and naturally when galloping in harness, and seems only partly aware of the process. In the case of the dog and pig, on the other hand, the process involves a cessation of all other occupation, the assumption of a special position of the body, and an obviously conscious effort. This attitude towards the process is more nearly that of human beings, and it is easy to understand that the more involved and particular the process, the more likely is it to become upset when circumstances arise which alter the animal's mode of living. Consequently it is found that while dogs and pigs are liable to suffer from the true form of constipation, especially after exposure to some unusual factor, horses, cattle, and sheep, although they are liable to suffer from acute obstruction of the bowels, are seldom affected with true constipation.

Causes.—Since the expulsion of waste products from the digestive system is dependent upon the proper performance of digestion, it is obvious that the most likely cause of constipation is some digestive disturbance. Anything which is likely to interfere with the normal peristaltic movements of the bowels, such as the use of too dry, bulky, or concentrated foods, overloading of the alimentary tract with unsuitable foods, tumours in the abdomen, pain originating from an enlarged prostate gland, or from obstructed anal glands, will at any rate predispose to constipation if not actually cause it. Inadequate exercise and too much food is a common cause. Changes from one owner to another, or from one district to another, in the case of nervous individuals, is a frequent cause; while a train journey immediately after a full feed is blamed for inducing constipation in pigs. In these latter animals the causes of constipation are somewhat similar to those that operate in the dog, especially in large fat sows that are unable to take an average amount of exercise, the lack of which alone is quite sufficient to produce the condition.

In the horse constipation is usually a symptom of some diseased condition either in the liver or in the intestines. (*See* INTESTINES, DISEASES OF.) It happens sometimes that the fæces are passed but that they are abnormally hard and dry and in the form of small solid balls which do not break up when gently pressed. These symptoms point to either too dry a diet with an insufficiency of fluid in the rations, or else to atony of the bowel wall, due to some other co-existing trouble, or to an insufficiency of exercise.

Symptoms.—The symptoms of constipation are familiar to every one and need only brief notice. The motions are smaller in amount and diminished in frequency, while if the condition is serious there is pain, straining, and even considerable distress. The abdomen swells in size, appetite is lost; there may be vomiting in the pig and dog; the horse shows signs of a mild attack of abdominal pain or 'colic', and frequently will be found to assume the recumbent position when left to itself. When the condition persists, the breath develops a 'taint', the pulse becomes weaker, respirations may be accelerated, and signs of absorption of the decomposing food materials are manifest.

Treatment.—This is generally a simple matter if the case has not been neglected too long and when no toxins have been absorbed. It is necessary in the first place to clear out the obstruction, and then to correct the diet or whatever was the cause. For the horse a bran mash over which has been poured ½ to 1 lb. of Epsom or Glauber's salts dissolved in warm water, will be enough to evacuate the feculent material; and if this be assisted by subsequent feeding on green food or roots for a few days, and plenty of exercise given as well, little fear need be entertained as to recovery. Obstinate cases may require one of the modern organic compound purgatives and perhaps a course of tonic medicine to follow. Cattle may be given either salts as for the horse or 1 to 1½ pints of linseed oil. For sheep and pigs a variety of drugs is available, but the former do well with a third of the dose of linseed oil that is given to cattle, with an ounce of castor oil and a teaspoonful of ginger, the whole given in gruel. Pigs may be given Epsom salts. (*See* GLAUBER'S SALTS.) For the dog there are numerous laxatives that are gentle in their action, such as syrup of buckthorn, liquid paraffin, equal parts of castor and olive oil, cascara sagrada, syrup of figs, etc. In all animals and whenever it is practicable it is advisable to assist the action of the medicine that is given by the mouth, by the administration of enemata of warm soapy water. It may be helpful to add a little glycerine to the solution in the case of the smaller animals. Errors in diet must be corrected.

CONTAGION (*contagio*, pollution by touching) means the principle of the spread of disease by direct contact between a healthy and a diseased individual; by 'infection' (*inficio*, I taint) is meant spread by the air or other more remote means.

CONTAGIOUS ABORTION OF CATTLE (*see* BRUCELLOSIS IN CATTLE).

CONTAGIOUS ACNE (*see* ACNE, CONTAGIOUS).

CONTAGIOUS AGALACTIA (*see* AGALACTIA).

CONTAGIOUS BOVINE PLEURO-PNEUMONIA, PLEURO-PNEUMONIA CONTAGIOSA BOVUM, or LUNG PLAGUE, is a contagious disease of cattle, of an acute, sub-acute, or chronic nature.

History.—This disease has decimated herds throughout Europe and in other parts of the world on several occasions, and probably has been directly responsible for the death of more cattle than any other single disease with the possible exception of cattle plague (rinderpest).

The disease was introduced into Ireland in 1839 from Holland, whence it spread all over the country, and in 1842 was brought into England and Scotland, both from Ireland and the Continent. All districts in the country were ultimately affected except the Scottish and Welsh Highlands. In the year 1860 alone, 187,000 cattle were lost from this disease in Great Britain, and between 1869 and 1894, 103,000 more succumbed to its ravages, either by being slaughtered in accordance with the policy of extermination then adopted, or as a result of deaths. From 1891 onwards the disease rapidly decreased, only one case being recorded in 1898, since when Great Britain has been entirely free; as are most countries in Europe. It is present in Asia and Africa, while in recent years outbreaks have occurred in Australia and South America. No case has been seen in the United States of America since 1892.

Cattle, buffaloes, and related species, such as reindeer, yak, and bison, are susceptible. Other animals, including man, are immune. Housed cattle are always more susceptible than those in the open.

Cause.—*Mycoplasma mycoides*.

Infection may occur by direct contact. Buildings which have housed infected cattle may remain infective for long periods.

Contagious pleuro-pneumonia has achieved a relatively greater importance in recent years, for unlike rinderpest it has proved very difficult to control. In many areas it has become the major cattle disease.

Incubative period.—3 weeks to 6 months.

Symptoms.—The first sign of illness is a rise of temperature to 103° or 105° F. In the acute disease this rise of temperature is soon followed by signs of general illness, such as dull coat, debility, loss of appetite, cessation of rumination. Shortly afterwards a dry, short, painful cough makes its appearance. This may only occur at certain times, as, for example, when the animal first comes out of a warm shed into the open air on a cold morning, drinks cold water, or when it is especially made to exert itself. In other cases the cough may soon become severe and be accompanied by a mucoid discharge. In 2 to 4 weeks from the onset the breathing is found to be disturbed, the respirations are short and 'catchy', increased in number, and expiration is accompanied by a double movement of the muscles of the abdomen. Affected animals stand with their elbows turned out (abducted) and resent being touched over the ribs. Examination of the chest by auscultation and percussion reveals the presence of pneumonia and at the same time usually pleurisy. Indigestion may accompany the disease, tympany being often present, and constipation and diarrhœa may alternate. Pregnant cows are liable to abort. As the disease gets worse, the animal becomes very weak and emaciated, has a hidebound appearance, a severe cough, tucked-up belly, the fever increases, and the heart becomes very weak. Œdematous swellings may occur on the under-parts of the body and even around the joints.

Death usually follows in 2 or 3 weeks after the symptoms have become pronounced and acute. Recovery is frequently more apparent than real, for a chronic cough remains, and the disease may again become acute and even end fatally.

The mortality varies much in different countries and in different outbreaks, but if the outbreak is left unchecked it is always high—about 50 to 70 per cent of those attacked dying.

Post-mortem appearances. Large or small areas of pneumonia in the lungs, which are often of a marbled appearance. The lesion is primarily one of interstitial pneumonia, with thickened septa dividing the lung up into lobules; some lobules show acute congestion, some are in a stage of red or grey hepatisation, while others consist of dead encapsulated tissue, known as 'sequestra'. Evidence of pleurisy with often much fibrinous deposit around the lungs is usual. The glands of the chest are found to be somewhat enlarged and hæmorrhagic.

Diagnosis.—The slaughter of suspected animals may be essential for this. Corroboration may be obtained by laboratory methods.

Treatment is not allowed in most countries, but neoarsphenamine has proved useful.

Immunisation.—There are four methods which have been practised to immunise cattle against this disease.

CONTAGIOUS CAPRINE PLEURO-PNEUMONIA.—A disease of goats, caused by one of the P.P.L.O. group, occurring in Europe, Asia, and Africa. Acute, peracute, and chronic forms occur. Mortality may be 60 to 100 per cent. Antibiotics are useful for treatment where a slaughter policy is not in force.

CONTAGIOUS DISEASES.—Certain of these are notifiable. (*See under* NOTIFIABLE DISEASES.) The responsibilities of animal owners are discussed under DISEASES OF ANIMALS ACT, 1950.

CONTAGIOUS ECTHYMA OF SHEEP is another name for orf. (*See* ORF.)

CONTAGIOUS EPITHELIOMA OF BIRDS (*see* AVIAN CONTAGIOUS EPITHELIOMA).

CONTAGIOUS PUSTULAR DERMATITIS (*see* ACNE, CONTAGIOUS and ORF).

CONTAGIOUS STOMATITIS (*see* FOOT-AND-MOUTH DISEASE; also VESICULAR STOMATITIS).

CONTRACEPTIVES (*see under* STILBŒSTROL *on page* 427 *and* EFFEMINATOR SPRINGS). (For preventing bitches, etc., coming on heat, *see under* ŒSTRUS, SUPPRESSION OF.)

CONTRACTED FOOT, or **CONTRACTED HOOF,** is a condition in which some part of the foot, very often a quarter or heel, becomes contracted and shrunken to less than its usual size. It is brought about by anything which favours rapid evaporation of the moisture in the horn, such as rasping away the outer surface of the wall ; or by conditions which prevent expansion of the hoof, such as paring away the frog so that it does not come into contact with the ground, cutting the bars, allowing the wall at the heels to fall inwards, shoeing with high calkins, etc.

Symptoms.—When the foot is viewed upon the ground it is seen to be narrowed from side to side, and the outline of the wall is uneven instead of being uniformly oval. When the foot is picked up the alteration in shape can be more easily noticed. Instead of having a transverse diameter practically equal to its length, it is found to be laterally compressed, so that it is very much longer from toe to heel than broad. The frog is misshapen and small, very narrow from side to side, and hard and dry in appearance. The wall at the heels and the bars have approached each other ; instead of being divergent the bars are almost parallel, and are usually very much overgrown, the sum total of these alterations giving the foot in extreme cases a tubular appearance. In advanced cases the condition causes lameness, or lameness may be due to navicular disease, which is very often partially the cause of the contraction, through over-use of the toe and saving of the heels ; but in the majority of simple cases the horse merely goes stiffly and more slowly than normal, thereby doing less work and doing it less efficiently.

Prevention consists in leaving the frog as large and well developed as possible ; reducing the overgrowth at the heels and bars to the same extent as at the toe and other parts of the foot, shoeing with shoes which allow the frog to come into contact with the ground, avoiding calkins and thick heels or shoeing with a bar shoe, and periodically inspecting each horse's feet to ascertain that contraction is not beginning without being noticed.

Treatment.—In severe cases a run at grass with tips on the affected feet, and leaving the heels bare, is advisable. Shoeing with bar-pads, after reducing the heels and bars to the normal level, or shoeing with rubber pads over the frog, with or without a bar or strap across the shoe, will be found beneficial in less serious cases. In the very worst instances operative treatment, consisting in grooving the wall at the heels and quarters so that it may expand, is necessary. This requires the services of a veterinary surgeon. (*See also* Hoof Repair.)

CONTRACTED HEELS (*see* Contracted Foot).

CONTRACTED TENDONS.—After a severe sprain of the flexor tendons of

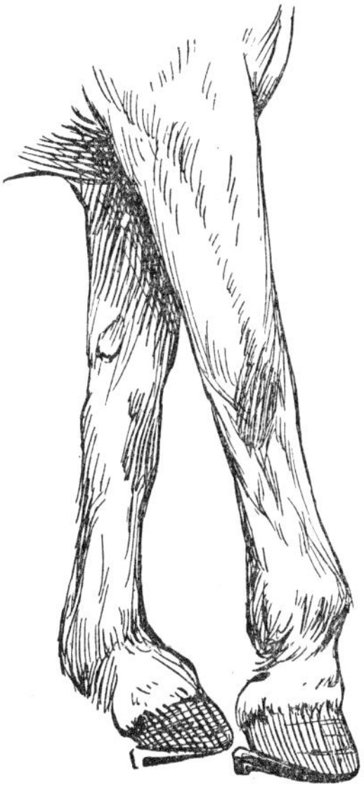

Contracted flexor tendons of the off fore-leg of horse. The thickening of the tendons at and above the fetlock, and the knuckling of this joint, can be well seen.

either a fore- or a hind-limb, and after the acute stage has passed and the pain and inflammation have subsided, there often results a thickening of the tendon at the seat of the injury and for some distance above and below it. After a time this thickening becomes complicated by a noticeable shortening of the tendon, which shows as a tendency to wear the shoe at the toe faster than at the heels, and the heels themselves are seen not to bear the same amount of weight as in the normal foot. Later still, a certain amount of knuckling forward of the fetlock-joint appears, and in severe cases the condition may become so acute that the heels are kept off the ground altogether. The condition is a difficult one to ameliorate, but by applying a bar shoe and fairly high calkins the balance may be restored to the heels, and the horse may work for some time. (*See also* Tendons, Injuries of.)

CONTRACTURE means the permanent shortening of muscle fibres, fibrous tissue, etc. 'Contraction' is the name given to permanent shortening of a tendon, muscle, etc., when a larger amount of tissue is involved.

CONTRA-INDICATION means a symptom or sign appearing during an illness which indicates the danger or undesirability of administering some particular remedy commonly used against the disease. For example, a weak heart would be a contra-indication to the use of chloroform for general anæsthesia.

CONTROL, CONTROLLED EXPERIMENT.—In any scientifically conducted experiment or field trial, the results of treatment of one group of animals are compared with results in another, untreated, group. Animals in the untreated group are known as ' the controls '.

CONTROLLED ENVIRONMENT HOUSING.—This term is applied to live-stock buildings in which temperature, ventilation, and humidity are controlled within narrow limits by means of electric fans, heaters, etc., and good insulation. Poultry, for example, are protected in this way from sudden changes in temperature, rearing can be carried out with the minimum loss throughout the year, and increased egg yields and decreased food intake can effect a considerable saving in costs of production. Some of these houses are windowless ; artificial lighting being provided. Respiratory disease may occur through overcrowding or ventilation defects.

For further information, consult *Controlled Environment*—a small handbook published by the Electrical Development Association, Trafalgar Buildings, 1 Charing Cross, London, S.W.1.

CONTUSION means a bruise. (*See* WOUNDS.)

CONVALESCENCE means that terminational period to a disease which occurs after the symptoms of the disease have ceased, but when the body is still in a weakened state and not fit for ordinary work. During this period there is an increased liability either to a relapse or to complications taking place, and measures are taken to ward off these by restricting the amount of rich food, the amount of vigorous exercise, and disallowing any exposure to extremes of temperature, etc. In many cases horses are turned out to grass to convalesce ; also cattle.

CONVEX SOLE, or **DROPPED SOLE.**—The sole of the horse's foot, instead of being arched (concave) when viewed from the ground surface, is convex and projects to a lower level than does the outer rim of the wall in many cases. It very frequently follows acute inflammation of the foot, such as laminitis. (*See* LAMINITIS.)

CONVOLUTIONS (*convolvo*, I roll up) (*see* BRAIN).

CONVOLVULUS POISONING (*see under* MORNING GLORY).

CONVULSIONS (*convulsio*) are rapidly alternating violent contractions and relaxations of the muscles which produce irregular aimless movements of the body generally, accompanied by unconsciousness. They are in reality only a symptom of some other trouble, usually associated with deranged function of the brain or of the spinal cord. Sometimes, especially in young puppies, they are not serious, but proceed from continued irritation of the gums by the cutting of the permanent teeth, or from irritation of the intestinal system by parasites, but in other cases they are of the greatest seriousness, such as when occurring during an attack of a virus disease.

Causes.—Among the conditions in which convulsions may be exhibited are the following : colic, eclampsia, hysteria, encephalitis (inflammation of the brain), affections of the ears, anthrax, milk fever, louping ill, swayback, scrapie, swine fever, swine erysipelas, brine poisoning, and various other forms of poisoning ; in dogs, extreme excitement in a highly strung animal, the presence of hard foreign bodies in the stomach, rabies, distemper, chorea, parasites in the alimentary system or in the heart, acute indigestion with absorption of toxic products, and sometimes the wedging of a piece of bone in the back of the throat.

Treatment.—First, a diagnosis as to the precise cause is necessary, and this requires the services of a veterinary surgeon. For immediate treatment the animal, if it can be moved, should be housed in some place where it will not injure itself. A sedative, such as bromide or chloral hydrate, may be given. Phenytoin sodium or methyl phenobarbitone are preferable as they have an anti-convulsant action rather than a sedative one.

When convulsions occur during the course of some other disease, they are usually but the prelude to coma (unconsciousness), which heralds death. (*See also* FITS, ECLAMPSIA, HYSTERIA, and under the headings of diseases mentioned above.)

COOPWORTH.—A breed of New Zealand sheep derived from the 'Border-Romney' cross.

CO-ORDINATION means the governing power exercised by the brain as a whole, or by certain centres in the nervous system, to make muscles or groups of muscles contract in harmony, and perform definite regulated movements.

During intoxications this part of the brain, suffering as well as the conscious regions, becomes unable to co-ordinate correctly the motions of the muscles, and the characteristic staggering gait of an intoxicated individual results. (*See also* MUSCLE ; NERVES.)

COPPER is used in veterinary medicine only as the sulphate, which is also known as 'bluestone' and 'blue vitriol'. Internally, it is astringent, irritant, and emetic, while it is sometimes used as an antidote to phosphorus poisoning, and as a remedy for the expulsion of small round worms in cattle and sheep. Externally, it is an antiseptic, astringent, and caustic.

Copper is also one of the trace elements which is essential in the nutrition of animals. It acts as a catalyst in the assimilation of iron, which is needed in the manufacture of hæmoglobin in the liver. Its absence from the food-stuffs eaten in some areas leads to a form of anæmia. In several parts of Britain copper deficiency is a serious condition. In cattle, symptoms include scouring, unthriftiness, and stunted growth, and often a greyness of the hair around the eyes. The trouble can be overcome by injecting or feeding copper salts, but the indiscriminate dressing of pastures with copper salts is liable to cause poisoning. Copper deficiency is associated with sway-back in lambs. Copper sulphate, added to the fattening ration at the rate of about 150 parts per million, has produced an improvement in the growth rate in pigs—comparable to that obtained by using antibiotic supplements. (*See* SWAYBACK ; *also* MOLYBDENUM.)

COPPER, POISONING BY.—With the exception of sheep, which may be given an overdose to expel worms, animals are not likely to be poisoned through internal administration of copper sulphate *as a medicine*. Poisoning has occurred, however, in sheep given a copper-rich supplement, intended for pigs, over a 3½ months' period ; in a heifer similarly, also in pigs given too strong a copper supplement. Poisoning also occurs when animals are grazed in the vicinity of copper-smelting works, where the herbage gradually becomes contaminated with copper, in orchards where fruit-trees have been sprayed with copper salts, and also when their food is cooked in copper boilers. Pigs sometimes suffer in this latter manner, especially if their 'brock' contains acids or fatty substances, and if the food is allowed to stand for any length of time in the copper. The symptoms are those of any irritant poison—colicky pains, diarrhœa (or perhaps constipation), and weakness ; staggering and muscular twitchings are seen in chronic cases. A fatal chronic copper poisoning may occur in pigs fed a copper supplement of 250 parts per million (the figure formerly recommended for copper supplements).

Mr. R. M. Loosmore, B.V.Sc., has pointed out that copper poisoning is almost specific to the housing of sheep. It occurs even on diets ostensibly containing no copper supplement. 'The capacity of the sheep for storing copper from the normal constituents of the diet is higher than that of other animals, and markedly higher in housed sheep.' And it is a remarkable fact that lambs reared indoors have died because their hay was made from grass contaminated by slurry from pigs on a copper-supplemented diet.

Treatment.—The antidotes are demulcents, such as white of egg, barley water, gruel, milk, after emetics have been given where they are indicated.

COPPERBOTTLE.—*Lucilia cuprina*, the strike fly which attacks sheep in Australia and South Africa.

'COPPER NOSE.'—A form of Light Sensitisation (which see) occurring in cattle.

COPROPHAGY.—The eating of its fæces by an animal. In rabbits this is a normal practice. Within 3 weeks of birth, foals will eat their dams' fæces and thereby acquire the various bacteria needed for digestive purposes in their own intestines.

CORAMINE.—Proprietary name of a solution of nikethamide ; a valuable respiratory and circulatory stimulant, given by injection.

CORN COCKLE POISONING may occur through animals eating meal, screenings, etc., made from either wheat or barley contaminated with the seeds of the corn cockle—*Agrostemma Githago*. This plant is very common in temperate countries, and is a very common weed in the corn-fields of the British Isles. Although the green plant itself contains small amounts of poisonous principle, it is not likely that animals will ever eat sufficient of it to cause symptoms ; poisoning almost always occurs through eating the seeds. These latter contain up to as much as 6·5 per cent of the glucoside *githagin*, or *Agrostemmin* (which has many other names), but the actual amount present depends upon the season and the nature of the soil upon which the corn cockle grows. The usual cause of poisoning occurs through poultry and young animals being fed upon either a mixture containing whole grains, or upon meal or flour, which have been made from grains contaminated with corn cockle seeds. Flour contaminated with cockle has a grey colour, and bread made from it is dull in colour and has a disagreeable odour. Fatal results have followed the eating of such bread by children.

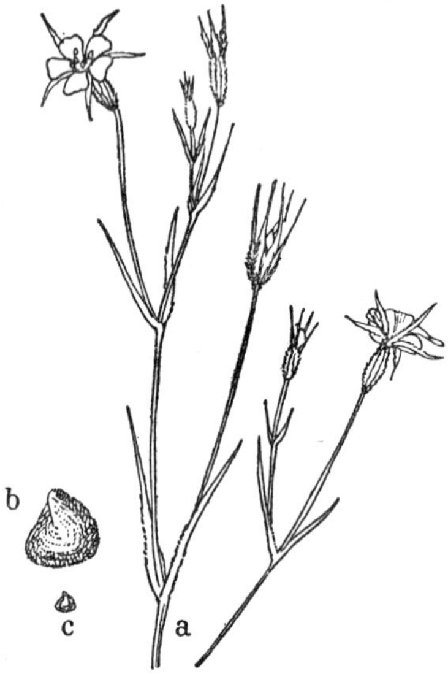

Corn Cockle (*Agrostemma Githago*). *a*, flowering heads ; *b*, ripe seed (enlarged) ; *c*, actual size of ripe seed.

Poisoning from this plant usually occurs through contamination of meals, etc., with ground seeds, as the result of the presence of these in grain for milling. The green plant also contains the poisonous principle, but is very seldom eaten by animals.

Symptoms.—It is mainly young animals and fowls which have been fed on contaminated meal that suffer. Two forms of poisoning are met with : in the first, which follows the ingestion of large amounts, death may occur in 12 hours ; in the second, which results from taking small amounts for long periods, a chronic form of poisoning occurs. In the acute cases are seen restlessness, salivation, grinding of the teeth, acute indigestion and colic, coughing and excitement, with unconsciousness following in 5 to 8 hours ; death may occur in 24 hours, or the animal becomes paralysed, is affected with an intense diarrhœa, lies groaning and distressed, and dies later. Vomiting occurs in pigs and dogs, and abortion may result in pregnant animals. In the chronic form, which is only seen in pigs, there is gradual wasting, chronic diarrhœa, loss of strength, staggering, and nervous complications. Death occurs from exhaustion.

Treatment.—Acutely affected animals should be given a drench of chlorodyne and chalk in appropriate doses, or if the means are available the stomach-tube should be passed, and the contents of the stomach removed by siphonage. The abdomen may be fomented with hot cloths dipped in warm water, or hot packs may be used. Large amounts of white of egg, starch paste, and milk may be given to calves and dogs as a drench.

CORNEA (*cornu*, horn) is the clear part of the front of the eye through which the rays of light pass to the retina. (*See* Eye.)

CORNS.—This word is applied to a bruise of the sensitive part of the horse's foot occurring in the ' seat of corn '. This latter is the angle formed between the wall of the hoof at the heel and the bar of the foot. Protecting the sensitive sole in this area is an angle of the horny sole, where the thickness of the horn is less than that in other parts of the foot, and lying immediately below, but separated from actual contact, is the heel of the iron shoe.

Causes.—Firstly, the horn of the sole in the seat of corn may so overgrow as to come to press upon the shoe ; and as the horn here is not fitted to take and bear weight, bruising of the underlying sensitive structure results. This bruise may so remain, causing no lameness, and only showing as a red staining of the horn, or it may suppurate and form pus, when a ' suppurating corn ' results. In the second place, stones, pieces of glass, etc., may become wedged between the heel of the shoe and the sole in the seat of corn, and if left in position for any time they bruise and damage the sensitive sole and even the deeper structures. The shoe itself may, when worn for too long a period, shift forward on the foot, since the wall is always growing and the shoe is not, and the result of this is that the iron of the heel of the shoe comes to press and bruise the sole in the heel of the foot, and a bruised heel or a corn is the consequence. Lastly, some corns of a severe nature appear in a foot that is perfectly shod, and when none of the previous causes have been in operation.

Symptoms.—In the majority of cases the horse goes very lame either gradually or suddenly. When made to walk he does so by using the toe of the affected foot, keeping the heels raised. Sometimes the pain is so great that he refuses to place the affected foot on the ground at all, but hops on the sound foot of the other side. In bad cases, or when the cause is not removed, the pus may burrow upwards towards the coronet and actually burst there, or it may under-run the horny sole and cause much or little separation of horn from matrix below. In these instances the lameness is most severe, and the horse may refuse to eat; it stands with the affected foot held off the ground, or resting on the toe only; it may break out in a patchy sweat if of a nervous disposition, and if the trouble is not treated it will lose condition rapidly, and the whole limb may swell.

Treatment.—The shoe should be removed as in all cases of lameness, and the hard dry outer horn pared away. Particular attention should always be paid to the region of the heels, for stones often become lodged there. If a corn is present the horse will show pain whenever the knife is applied to the affected part, and efficient paring may necessitate the use of cocaine. All the diseased horn must be removed from the surface of the bruised or suppurating area, and this latter should be cleansed. Corns that are bruised only and have not begun to 'fester', only require the removal of the cause to effect recovery. On the other hand, when a part of the sole has been under-run all the discoloured horn must be stripped from the matrix, and if the wall is affected efficient drainage must be provided below and sometimes above as well, and the tract along which the pus has burrowed must be treated as an infected wound.

Mild cases take about 5 days to a week to recover, while horses with severe suppurating corns may be as long as 6 or 7 weeks before they are fit to work. (*See also* FOOT OF HORSE.)

CORNSTALK DISEASE (*see under* PASTEURELLOSIS OF CATTLE).

CORONARY (*coronarius*, crown-like) is a term applied to several structures in the body encircling an organ in the manner of a crown. The coronary arteries are the arteries of supply to the heart which arise from the aorta, just beyond the aortic valve; through them blood is delivered with great pressure to the heart muscle.

CORONARY BAND, or **CORONARY CUSHION,** is the part of the sensitive matrix of the horse's foot from which grows the wall. It runs round the foot at the coronet, lying in a groove in the upper edge of the wall. Its more correct name is the *coronary matrix*. (*See* FOOT OF HORSE.)

CORONARY THROMBOSIS, associated with *Strongylus vulgaris*, is a cause of sudden death in yearling and 2-year-old horses.

CORONET (*see* FOOT OF THE HORSE).

CORPORA QUADRIGEMINA form a division of the brain. (*See* BRAIN.)

CORPUS LUTEUM (*see page* 618).

CORPUSCLES (*corpusculum*) means a small body. (*See* BLOOD.)

CORRIDOR DISEASE.—This affects the African buffalo and also cattle, and is caused by the protozoan parasite *Theileria lawrencei*, transmitted by ticks. It resembles East Coast Fever but is sometimes fatal in buffaloes, and has a 60 to 80 per cent mortality in cattle.

CORROSIVE SUBLIMATE, or **PERCHLORIDE OF MERCURY,** is a powerful antiseptic, disinfectant, and an irritant poison. It should not be confused with the subchloride of mercury, or calomel.

CORROSIVES.—Examples are: strong mineral acids such as sulphuric, nitric, and hydrochloric, the caustic alkalies, and some salts, e.g. the chlorides of mercury and zinc. (*See* POISONING.)

CORTICOSTEROIDS.—These comprise the *natural* glucocorticoids, cortisone, and hydrocortisone — hormones from the adrenal gland; and the *synthetic* equivalents, *e.g.* prednisone, prednisolone, and fluoroprednisolone. (For the dangers of corticosteroid therapy, see *Vet. Record*, April 23, 1966.)

Referring to their use in human medicine, the *Lancet* commented in 1970: 'Controversy about the relative merits of corticosteroids and corticotrophins continues, particularly in the treatment of asthma and rheumatoid arthritis. There seems little evidence that one is more effective than the other, but no agreement can be reached on the question of whether one causes more pituitary suppression than the other. It is accepted that natural or synthetic corticosteroids may cause suppression of pituitary function and, in turn, adrenal atrophy. This serious complication may be especially dangerous in the presence of infection or after an operation.' (*See also* CORTISONE.)

CORTICOTROPHIN.—The hormone from the anterior lobe of the pituitary gland which controls the secretion by the adrenal gland of corticoid hormones. These corticosteroids, or steroid hormones, are of three kinds: (1) those concerned with carbohydrate metabolism and which also allay inflammation; (2) those concerned with maintaining the correct proportion of electrolytes; (3) the sex corticoids, not used in medicine.

CORTISONE.—A hormone from the cortex of the adrenal gland. In medicine the acetate of cortisone is used, prepared from extracts of the adrenal cortex or partly synthetically. It is a white or cream-coloured crystalline powder almost insoluble in water.

Actions.—Cortisone raises the sugar content of the blood and the glycogen content of the liver, among other actions.

Uses.—Cortisone has been used with success in the temporary relief of rheumatoid arthritis, but when the drug is discontinued symptoms return. In human medicine, it has been concluded that long-continued cortisone treatment is not to be recommended. It has been used in the relief of navicular disease in the horse and of other forms of lameness, being given by injection into the joint involved. (*See Vet. Record*, Dec. 16th, 1961.)

Cortisone has also been used in the treatment of acetonæmia in cattle, and successful results have been claimed. It has also been used in non-suppurative inflammation of the eye and eyelid.

The healing of wounds may be delayed in animals receiving cortisone. Overdosage may give rise to wasting and diabetes. Cortisone has, when given by injection, a suppressive effect on antibody production and may increase an animal's susceptibility to viral infection. (*See* CORTICOSTEROIDS.)

CORYNEBACTERIUM.—A genus of slender, Gram-positive bacteria which includes the cause of diphtheria in man. In veterinary medicine *C. pyogenes* is of the greatest importance, causing 'summer mastitis' and sterility in dairy cattle. A generalised infection has been reported, giving rise in cattle to lameness, slight fever, leg-swellings, lachrymation, and later emaciation and death. *C. suis* is responsible for infectious cystitis and pyelonephritis in pigs.

CORYZA (*κορύζα*, a running at the nose) is the technical name for a cold in the head. (*See* CHILLS, COLDS, ROUP.)

COTTON SEEDS are the seeds of the cotton plants (*Gossypium* sp.) which contain quantities of cotton-seed oil, much used in commerce and for making margarine and cooking fats. After the oil has been removed, either by expression or by dissolving in a solvent, the residue in the form of cotton-cake or extracted cotton-seed meal, forms a very valuable animal feeding-stuff. It is rich in protein and fairly easily digested by adult animals. Two kinds of cake are sold: decorticated, in which the lint and husk have been removed, and undecorticated, in which they are present. The latter is not always suitable for feeding to calves under 6 months and lambs under 4 months of age. (*See* GOSSYPOL.)

COTYLEDONS (*see* PREGNANCY, *page* 748).

COUGH is a powerful reflex expiratory act due to a variety of causes. In the majority of cases there is some irritation of the laryngeal nerve endings, either by inflammation, the presence of foreign material — mucus, catarrhal discharge, fluids or solids entering from the mouth, etc.—or swelling of the mucous membrane such as occurs in œdema of the glottis. In bronchitis, coughing is an important symptom. Lung-worms give rise to it. The presence of pungent fumes in the atmosphere in the majority of cases induces a sneeze, but when concentrated they produce fits of coughing.

Horses with a cough but no rise in temperature may prove to be infested with the lung-worm *Dictyocaulus arnfieldi*. More common causes of coughing in horses include equine influenza; other virus infections; laryngitis and bronchitis from other causes; an allergic or asthmatic cough often heard in the autumn; strangles; and 'broken wind'.

In pigs, coughing may be due to dusty meal or to enzoötic pneumonia.

In the dog a sporadic yet persistent cough, noticed especially after exercise or excitement, may be a symptom of infestation with the common tracheal worm *Oslerus osleri*. Mortality among puppies of 4–8 months has been as high as 75 per cent in some litters, following emaciation. Less serious is infestation with *Capillaria aerophilia*, which may give rise to a mild cough.

(*See* BRONCHITIS, BROKEN WIND, TUBERCULOSIS, HUSK.)

COUNTER-IRRITANTS (*see* BLISTERS, LINIMENTS, etc.)

COWBANE POISONING.—Cowbane, or Water Hemlock (*Cicuta virosa*), is an exceedingly poisonous umbelliferous plant found in marshy, damp places. It has been estimated that a portion of the root no larger than a walnut will kill a young heifer or stirk in fifteen minutes, and the fatal dose for a horse is less than one pound. Sheep and goats are more resistant, and cattle the most susceptible, as might be gathered from its name. In man death occurs in about 45 per cent of all cases where it is eaten. In the spring, when growth is most luscious and abundant, its poisonous qualities are greatest, and the old dried stalks in autumn are less dangerous. The root in springtime contains the greatest amount of the poisonous principles, which are three in number: viz. an alkaloid, *cicutine*; an oil, *oil of cicuta*; and a bitter resinous substance, *cicutoxine*.

Symptoms.—Whether the root, stem, or leaves are eaten, either in the green state or when dry, death occurs very rapidly. In many cases animals are found dead a few minutes after eating the plant, or there may be a few hours' illness. In some cases symptoms do not appear until about two hours after the plant has been eaten, probably because in a full rumen it is mixed with the other ingesta, and no absorption of the toxic principles can take place until digestion has begun. There is salivation, indisposition, dullness, vomiting (in pigs), colic (in horses), bloating (in cattle), diarrhœa, rolling of the eyeballs, giddiness, reeling in circles, twisting of the neck, and convulsions. The mouth opens and shuts, and death occurs shortly afterwards. In cattle the limbs may be alternately extended and stiffened and then relaxed. Loss of consciousness usually precedes death.

Treatment.—Owing to the rapidity of the appearance of symptoms it is not often that treatment can be successfully carried out. Strong black coffee, tannic acid or gallic acid may be given. Veterinary advice should be sought.

COW KENNELS.—These have become popular as a cheaper (first cost) alternative to cubicle houses, though some have been developed to the point where they are almost cubicle houses, with the wood or metal partitions forming an integral part of the structure. Slurry can be a problem, and sometimes exposure to draughts and rain requires protection with straw bales or hardboard at the ends. (*See also* CUBICLES FOR COWS.)

COW-POX (*see* VARIOLA VACCINIA).

COW-POX, PSEUDO- (*See* MILKER'S NODULE).

COWS' MILK, ABSENCE OF.—In a newly calved cow giving virtually no milk, the cause may be a second calf in the uterus, and a rectal examination is accordingly advised. A normal milk yield can be expected, in such cases, to follow the birth of the second calf which may occur a few months later. (*See* SUPERFŒTATION, *also* AGALACTIA.)

COWS.—Gentle treatment.—Cows should at all times be quietly and gently treated. Hurried driving in and out of gates and doors, chasing by dogs, beating with stick or milking stool, are objectionable in every way and should not be tolerated. A cow in milk must have time to eat, chew, and digest her food in comfort, and rough treatment will not only interfere with digestion but will also disturb the nervous system which more or less controls the action of the milk-making glands, and thus lessens the milk yield. (*See* STRESS.)

Gentle treatment should begin with the calf, and be continued with the yearling, two-year-old, and in-calf heifer; where it is customary to approach and handle young stock at all ages there will be no difficulty in the management and milking of the newly calved heifer ; her milk-yield will be increased, and much time will be saved. (*See* MILKING.)

Comfort and fresh air.—The housing provided should ensure comfort. In winter sufficient litter should be provided to keep the cows warm and clean. (*See* HOUSING OF ANIMALS, RATIONS.)

COW-WHEAT is the common name of the plant *Melampyrum arvense*, which may be poisonous to live-stock when eaten in large amounts. The seeds may occur in badly screened samples of wheat and barley, and may be ground into meal. They give a bitter taste, peculiar odour, and a violet colour to flour, and their presence in cornfields is undesirable. They may produce symptoms of sleepiness and colic.

COXALGIA (*coxa*, the hip ; *ἄλγος*, pain) means pain in the hip-joint.

COXIELLA infection. (*See under* Q FEVER.

CRACKED HEELS IN HORSES (*see under* NECROSIS, BACILLARY).

CRAMP.—Painful involuntary contraction of a muscle. Cramp is of importance in the racing greyhound, which is observed to slow down and drag both hind legs, or —in severe cases—may collapse and struggle on the ground. The animal's gait and appearance are 'wooden'. The muscles of the hind-quarters are hard to the touch. Cyanosis may be present. Recovery usually takes place within a quarter of an hour, aided by rest and massage. Possible causes include: fatigue, defective heart action, bacterial or chemical toxins, sexual repression, a dietary deficiency, poor management from the point of view of exercise, and cold. (*See also* SCOTTIE CRAMP.)

CRANIAL NERVES are those large and important nerves that originate from the brain. They are twelve in number, as follows :

1. Olfactory . . .	Sensory (smell).
2. Optic . . .	Sensory (sight).
3. Oculomotor . .	Motor.
4. Trochlear or pathetic	Motor.
5. Trigemial or trifacial . . .	Mixed.
6. Abducent . .	Motor.
7. Facial . . .	Mixed.
8. Auditory . . .	Sensory (hearing and equilibration).
9. Glossopharyngeal .	Mixed.
10. Vagus or pneumogastric . . .	Mixed.
11. Spinal accessory or accessory . .	Motor.
12. Hypoglossal . .	Motor.

(*See also under* BRAIN.)

'CRAZY CHICK' DISEASE occurs in the U.S.A., and also in the U.K. It is associated with a diet too rich in fats, or containing food which has gone rancid, and Vitamin E has been used in its treatment. The term 'Crazy Chick' Disease includes not only this Nutritional Encephalomacia but also a virus disease of chicks under 6 weeks of age known as avian encephalomyelitis. Symptoms in each case include falling over and paralysis.

C.R.D.—An abbreviation for Chronic Respiratory Disease of poultry, caused by organisms similar to those which give rise to Contagious Pleuro-pneumonia. A general loss of condition and reduction in egg yield are caused. Antibiotics such as aureomycin and terramycin have been recommended. As a precaution, deep litter should not be left in a house for more than one year.

Chronic Respiratory Disease—which *E. coli* infection may sometimes resemble —is by far the commonest cause of broiler mortality in the U.S.A., and in Britain it has begun to be a serious cause of loss. Swelling of the face, with discharge from the nostrils, usually occurs in addition to distressed breathing. Outbreaks in Britain have involved broilers aged 8 to 10 weeks. C.R.D. is often referred to as mycoplasmosis.

CREEP-FEEDING. — The feeding of un-weaned piglets in the creep—a portion of the farrowing house or ark inaccessible to the sow and usually provided with artificial warmth. Creep-feeding often begins with a little flaked maize being put under a turf, and is followed by a proprietary or home-mixed meal from 3–8 weeks. Creep-feeding of in-wintered lambs and calves is good practice. (*See also* RATIONS, SOW'S MILK.)

CREEP-GRAZING is a method of pasture management, enabling lambs to gain access to certain areas of pasture in advance of their dams.

CREOSOTED TIMBER may give rise to poisoning in young pigs where the wood is freshly treated. For disease in cattle from this cause *see under* HYPERKERATOSIS.

CREPITATIONS (*crepito*, I rattle) is the name applied to certain sounds which occur along with the normal sounds of breathing, as heard by auscultation, in various diseases of the lungs or bronchial tubes. They are signs of the presence of moist exudations in the lungs or in the bronchial tubes. They may resemble the rustle of crushed tissue paper.

CREPITUS.—This word has the same meaning as crepitation, but is perhaps more commonly used to indicate the grating of fractured bones.

CRESOL SOLUTIONS.—(*See under* DISINFECTANTS.)

CRETINISM (Swiss *cretin*, a Christian), or **HYPOTHYROIDISM,** is a condition in man where there is atrophy of the thyroid gland and a myxœdematous condition of the subcutaneous tissues. In animals it affects the dog, but it is by no means a common condition. It has been seen in dingos brought from Australia and kept in captivity in zoological gardens, and it is also sometimes met with in foxhounds and beagles. When it occurs before growth is complete, there is an arrest of development of the bony parts and the brain. The limbs become short, thick, and clumsy; the neck gets thick and stout, and digestive troubles, dullness, and lack of interest in surroundings are exhibited.

Satisfactory results often (but not invariably) follow the administration of thyroid extract. (*See also* THYROID GLAND.)

CRIB-BITING and **WIND-SUCKING** are different varieties of the same vice, which are learned chiefly by young horses, and may become so severe as to constitute nervous diseases (known as neuroses). In each case the horse swallows air. A 'crib-biter' effects this by grasping the edge of the manger or some other convenient fixture with the incisor teeth; it then raises the floor of the mouth; the soft palate is forced open; a swallowing movement occurs; and a gulp of air is passed down the gullet into the stomach. A 'wind-sucker' achieves the same end, but it does not require a resting-place for the teeth. Air is swallowed by firmly closing the mouth, arching the neck, and gulping down air in much the same way. Accompanying each swallowing effort there is usually a distinct grunt. In some cases horses may rest their teeth against the bottom of the manger, the lower edge of the rack, the end of a shaft or pole, the rope of a halter-strap, or some part of the harness. In rare cases the mouth may be placed against the knees or cannons. Some horses which have been crib-biters learn to wind-suck when remedial measures are taken, and there are some wind-suckers which learn to crib-bite. Some horses indulge in these vices when alone in the stable; some when in company with other horses; some will never show any signs of vice when carefully observed, and others disregard the presence of human beings; occasionally a horse will indulge when at work, but the majority only misbehave when in the stable. Young idle animals, standing in company with confirmed crib-biters or wind-suckers, very often learn the bad habit from these latter.

Ill effects result from these vices in different ways. In crib-biters the incisor teeth of both jaws show signs of excessive wear, sometimes so much so that they no longer meet when the mouth is shut, and grazing is impossible. The muscles of the throat usually show an increase in size (due to hypertrophy from excessive use), but there is rarely any pathological change in this region. The continual swallowing of air has a very bad effect upon the digestive system. The air dilates the walls of the stomach (probably thereby giving the horse a sense of repletion which it finds pleasant), passes along the small intestine, and interferes with the normal peristaltic movement of these parts. A certain amount of indigestion and fermentation result, and the horse may be attacked by colic. Condition is lost, and the animal becomes less fit for its work than formerly. Remedial measures are not always satisfactory. The most common preventative is to fasten a strap round the throat, sufficiently tight to make arching of the neck uncomfortable, but not tight enough to interfere with respiration. Such straps usually require to be removed during feeding. In up-to-date types there is a metal 'gullet-plate' which has a recess into which the windpipe fits, and which allows the device to be worn without danger. Another preventive consists of a hollow cylindrical perforated bit, which disallows a horse making its mouth airtight so long as it is worn. A thick rubber or wooden bit which prevents the jaws from closing entails acute discomfort, and is not recommended upon humane grounds. Very often crib-biters will cease the habit if housed in a bare loose-box, being fed from a trough which is removed as soon as the feed is finished.

An operation, devised by Forssell of Stockholm has been performed with excellent results in Great Britain. This operation, however, will not prevent wind-sucking—to overcome which another operation has been devised. Known as buccostomy, it involves the creation of permanent buccal fistulæ, and results so far seem promising. It is claimed to eliminate the habit and following the operation horses have shown a considerable improvement in condition. Body-weight has increased, skin condition improves, and intermittent colic ceases. After a brief period of accommodation the horse has no difficulty in swallowing fluids. One disadvantage of the method is that the metal tube tends to collect food particles and daily cleansing may be required; however, this is a simple procedure, quickly performed. The longest period for which a horse has been under observation following buccostomy is 4 years.

CROCUS POISONING (*see* MEADOW SAFFRON POISONING).

CROP, of birds, is a dilatation of the gullet at the base of the neck, just at the entrance to the thorax. In it the food is stored for a time and softened with fluids. It acts as a reservoir from which the food can be passed downwards into the stomach, gizzard, etc., in small amounts. Some such arrangement as this is necessary since the food is not chewed, the bird is a rapid feeder, and the gizzard can deal with food-stuff only slowly.

CROP, DISEASES OF.—By far the commonest trouble affecting the crop of the bird is that known as '*crop-bound*', in which food material collects in the crop through the swallowing of bodies which cannot pass on to the stomach and gizzard, such as feathers, wool, straw, small pieces of stick, etc. Other cases are due to a lack of vitality in the walls of the crop, whereby they become too weak to force the contents onwards. The bird becomes dull, opens its beak and expels gases, wanders about slowly and in obvious discomfort, and the dilated crop can often be noticed pendulous and distended. Death occurs from exhaustion unless relief is obtained. Massage of the impacted food material from the outside, along with the introduction of warm water in small amounts through a rubber tube, may be sufficient to dispel mild impactions, but usually surgical measures are required. The feathers are removed from the front of the breast, the skin is cleansed, an incision into the distended organ is made with a clean knife, and the obstructing contents are removed. The wall of the crop and the incision in the skin are sutured up separately. *Tympany of the crop* is a condition in which gas collects in the crop and distends it to an extent even greater than in crop-bound. It is due to the presence of gas bacilli, which produce fermentation of the food in the intestines, and the gas collects in the usually empty crop. Intestinal antiseptics are necessary after the gas has been expelled by kneading and massage, or by puncture in severe cases. *Inflammation of the crop*, or catarrh, is usually caused through eating decomposing fleshy materials, poisonous substances, or actual injury. It is a serious condition in which the crop may be almost filled with a pulpy, soft, gaseous mass. It frequently leads to grave loss of condition, and death from exhaustion may result. The doughy mass should be pressed out of the crop (the bird being held by the legs, head downwards), and the crop filled with water from the mouth. Again empty the crop in the same manner. This results in washing out the crop, and afterwards gruel and an antiseptic such as salol, or bismuth, should be introduced. With regard to turkeys, *see also* MONILIASIS.

CROSS-IMMUNITY.—Immunity resulting from infection with one disease-producing organism against another. For example, rinderpest virus infection in dogs gives rise to a degree of immunity against canine distemper virus.

CROSS PREGNANCY.—Development of a fœtus in the opposite horn of the uterus to that side on which ovulation occurred. Migration from one horn to the other may occur.

CROTON POISONING may occur from the administration of too large a dose of croton oil, but more often it results from the feeding of adulterated feeding-cakes. The residue left when the oil has been expressed is sometimes utilised in the making of cattle-cakes, and if the proportion of croton product exceeds 1 per cent of the total, poisoning is likely to result when the cake is fed.

Symptoms.—No harmful effects may be

noticed for a few days after the commencement of the feeding of the adulterated cake, but sooner or later profuse diarrhœa with the passage of blood-clots and quantities of mucus, and prostration, are seen. In calves and sheep, blistering of the mouth may be noticed and salivation is excessive.

Treatment.—Starch gruels, linseed tea, barley-water, along with opium and chalk, should be given at once ; and later, hyposulphite of sodium dissolved in water should be administered. If much diarrhœa has occurred, injections of normal saline may be needed.

CROUP of the horse is that part of the hind-quarters lying immediately behind the loins. The 'point of the croup' is the highest part of the croup, and corresponds to the internal angles of the ilia. The crupper of the harness passes over the croup, and derives its name from it.

CROUP, FOWL, is another name for roup. (*See* AVIAN DIPHTHERIA.)

CRUCIAL, or **CRUCIATE, LIGAMENTS** (*crux*, a cross) are two strong ligaments in the stifle-joint which prevent any possibility of over-extension of the joint. They are arranged in the form of the limbs of the letter X.

'CRUELS'.—Actinobacillosis of sheep.

CRURAL (*crus*, the leg) means something connected with the leg.

CRUSH.—An appliance constructed of tubular steel, or wood, and used for holding cattle, etc., in order to facilitate tuberculin testing, inoculations, the taking of blood samples, etc.

A wooden crush is better than a metal one because it involves less noise ; clanging metalwork can be alarming to cattle. Collecting cattle in darkened pens or boxes an hour before testing is due to begin makes for better behaviour in the crushes.

One of the best crushes described in the *Vet. Record* ' is in a building through which the cows always come on leaving the parlour. The two ends are solid and fixed in concrete. The sides consist of iron gates hinged one on the front and the other on the back of the crush. Before an animal enters, the gate hinged on the front is opened back against the wall. This provides a wide space and she is not asked to enter a narrow confine. When she is in, the gate is shut and the neck secured with a rope. The other gate may now be opened and testing done without reaching through the side of the crush'.

A funnel-shaped pen for filling the crush is useful, and if the crush is big enough to hold two animals, the second will enter more readily. Fast working can be achieved with a race to hold 7 or 8 cows ; there being 2 men each with a rope on the side opposite to the veterinary surgeon. The whole batch is tested before release.

For testing purposes, as opposed to dehorning, the use of a rope—preferably fitted with a steel eye or ring—is far better than a yoke. Indeed, some yokes with a narrow 'V' at the bottom, are dangerous. Cattle tend to lean on them, and may lose consciousness in a matter of seconds and even die in the crush. Covering in the sides and end of a crush at the bottom tends to make cattle keep their heads up.

It is generally agreed that behaviour in crushes is partly dependent upon breed. For example, Dairy Shorthorns are generally docile, Ayrshires easily alarmed, and Friesians often more angry than frightened. Angus and Galloways seem to resent the crush rather than be alarmed by it.

Much also depends, of course, upon gentle treatment and avoiding the indiscriminate use of sticks. Some farm workers never learn to hold cattle properly by their noses, but push a thumb into one nostril and try and cram all their fingers into the other—naturally the animal struggles for breath ! Even when it is done properly, Angus and Galloways seem to dislike this form of restraint intensely.

It may save a lot of time in the end if animals are *accustomed* to being put into a crush. An experiment at the Ministry's central veterinary laboratory involved weekly weighings of 60 adult heifers, which were obstreperous in the extreme. Each was led (with a head-collar, not a halter) from its standing in a cowshed to a crate mounted on the low platform of a large weighing machine in a yard. The first weighing occupied two strenuous periods totalling 135 minutes. The thirty-seventh weighing was accomplished in 38 minutes ! The heifers not only learnt what was expected of them but seemed to relish this break in their routine ; trotting into the crate, coming to a dead stop, and standing stock still while the weighing machine beam was adjusted.

'CRUTCHING'.—Shearing of wool from

sheep's breech, tail, and back of hind-legs. It is done before May and in autumn as an aid to controlling 'Strike'.

CRYPTOCOCCOSIS.—Infection with the yeast *Cryptococcus neoformans* occurs occasionally in all species. Lungs, udder, brain, etc., may be involved.

CRYPTORCHID (*see* RIG).

CRYSTAL VIOLET VACCINE is made from the virus of swine fever attenuated by exposure to the dyestuff called crystal violet. It is used for immunising young pigs and has given good results. Its use in the U.K. has been discontinued.

Crystal violet vaccine is prepared from pig's blood and, in a *very small percentage* of sows vaccinated twice or more, its use has given rise to antibody formation leading to HÆMOLYTIC DISEASE (*which see*). Most cases of this have occurred in Essex, Large Black, Berkshire, and Wessex—very few in Large Whites or Landrace. (*See* SWINE FEVER.)

CUBES and **PELLETS.**—A cow takes about 10 minutes to eat 8 lb. of cubes : a fact of some importance in the milking parlour where time may not permit of a high-yielder receiving her entire concentrate ration. (The figure for meal is about 6 lb. in 10 minutes.)

It is sometimes suggested that cubes can replace hay for horses on pasture in winter, or for rabbits, chinchilla, etc., which are not out at grass. However, roughage is needed in addition for peristalsis and the health of the digestive system. (*See also* DRIED GRASS.)

The type of lubricant used in cubing and pelleting machines is important; hyperkeratosis can arise in cattle if an unsuitable one is used. (*See* LUBRICANTS.)

CUBICLES FOR COWS.—This is a recent development in Britain and America. The cows are free to come and go between the silage face and the cubicles, which have a concave floor (to retain the sawdust) sloping slightly backwards away from the wall. For larger breeds of cows the cubicles are made about 6 feet 9 inches long by 3 feet 9 inches. Two horizontal rails, the lower one not less than 15 inches high, divide the cubicles. The cubicles are raised 6 to 12 inches, to prevent a cow backing in and soiling the litter. Where sawdust is used, about 10 lb. is required per cow, per week, and the system is much cheaper than with straw used in conventional housing.

There are now several types of cubicle. It appears that the type of heelstones, floor, and the width are important factors in determining whether cows take to cubicles or not. (*See also* COW KENNELS.)

CUCKOO - PINT POISONING. — The Cuckoo-pint, Lords and Ladies, or Wild Arum Lily—*Arum maculatum*—is one of the highly poisonous common plants which are found at the bottom of hedgerows and on waste land in many parts of the country. The brilliant red cluster of berries as seen during summer, and sometimes eaten by children with fatal results, are the most poisonous, although all parts of the plant are dangerous. Animals do not readily eat it on account of the acrid, disagreeable smell emitted when the plant is bruised, but pigs sometimes root up the tuber-like corms (roots) and suffer from eating them. The symptoms recorded are swelling, reddening, and irritation of the mucous membranes of the mouth and throat ; profuse salivation ; difficulty in swallowing ; vomiting ; purgation and inflammation of stomach and intestines. Convulsions, exhaustion, and death from shock may result when large amounts have been taken, but owing to the very irritant nature of the plant it is rare that animals will take sufficient to cause fatal results. It is interesting to note that poisoning may occur through washing wounds with a decoction made from steeping the bruised plant in water, and death has resulted in the horse from such a cause. Treatment consists in giving soothing and demulcent gruels and milk ; administering opium and other sedatives, and withholding all solid and fibrous food-stuffs for 3 or 4 days.

CUD and **CUDDING** (*see* RUMINATION).

CUFFING PNEUMONIA.—A pneumonia of calves caused by a virus. A chronic cough is the usual symptom. It is so called because a 'cuff' of lymphocytic elements forms around the bronchioles.

CULTURE MEDIUM.—That substance in or upon which bacteria and other pathogenic organisms are grown in the laboratory. Such media include nutrient agar, broths, nutrient gelatin, sugar media, and many special ones adapted to the requirements of particular organisms. Viruses cannot be grown in such media but require living cells, *e.g.* of chick embryos.

CURARE, also known as CURARI, CURARA, WOOLRARI, WOURALI, URARI, and TRICUNAS, is a dark-coloured extract from trees of the *Strychnos* family, used by the South American Indians as an arrow poison. Such arrow-heads were used by a veterinary surgeon in 1835 in treating tetanus in a horse and a donkey.

Curare, when injected under the skin, is one of the most powerful and deadly poisons known, but by the mouth it is harmless, since the kidneys are able to excrete it as rapidly as it is absorbed, and it does not collect in the system. Its action depends on the presence of an alkaloid, *curarine*, which paralyses the motor nerve-endings in muscle, and so throws the muscular system out of action yet leaving the sensory nervous system unaffected. Consequently an animal into which the drug is injected lies incapable of the slightest action, but fully conscious of its surroundings. Finally, death results. A standardised preparation of tubocurarine is now available and is of use to ensure full muscular relaxation during anæsthesia. (*See also under* MUSCULAR RELAXANTS.)

CURB is the name given to a swelling which occurs about a hand's-breadth below the point of the hock, due to sprain,

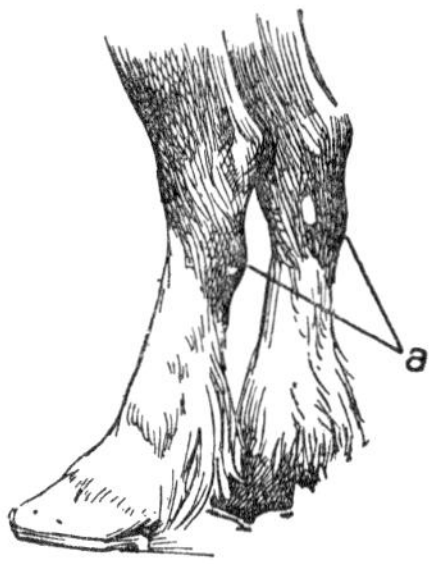

Curb (Horse). The swellings of curb are seen at *a*.

or local thickening of the calcaneocuboid ligament, or to similar conditions affecting the superficial flexor tendon, or even to a bony deposit upon the head of the lateral small metatarsal bone (when it is sometimes called 'false curb'). An unduly large head upon this small metatarsal bone, even though there is no bony deposit and consequently no diseased condition present, is also known as 'false curb' and is liable to lead to confusion with 'true curb' in the mind of the layman.

Curb is caused by slipping forwards with the hind-limbs, to sprains and strains occasioned by attempting to start too heavy loads, especially in young horses, to jumping badly in hunters, when undue strain is put upon the hocks, and to other similar causes, which produce great stress on the back of the joint. Very often curb appears without any history of strains or sprains, and in some cases reappears without any signs of discomfort or lameness. When the hind-limbs are of faulty conformation, especially when the hocks are 'sickle-like' (*i.e.* too much bent), and when the calcaneous, instead of being situated vertically, leans forwards when viewed in profile, curb is more likely to appear than in good, well-shaped hocks. (*Note.*—The line from the point of the hock down to the fetlock should be quite straight when the limb is viewed from the side.)

Lameness usually accompanies the formation of curb, but after the swelling has become established it usually disappears, and, although the joint is weakened and lameness may return, many horses with large curbs work well and never go lame subsequently. There is nothing characteristic about the lameness, except that the horse rests the toe on the ground, keeping the heels elevated, and that upon strong pressure over the 'seat of curb', particularly when the limb is raised and the foot carried forwards, pain may become evident.

Treatment includes putting shoes on to the hind-feet which have wedge-shaped heels, pattens, or calkins, and resting the horse.

CURBY HOCKS are those in which the calcaneous slopes forwards from a point about a hand's-breadth below the point of the hock to its summit. (*See* CURB.)

'CURLED TONGUE'.—A deformity occurring in turkey poults, due to feeding an all-mash diet, composed of very small particles in a dry state, during the first few weeks of life. If a change is made to wet feeding many of the poults will become normal.

CUTANEOUS (*cutis*, the skin) means belonging or pertaining to the skin. (*See* SKIN.)

CUTTER.—A pork pig weighing 140–190 lb. (liveweight) or 100–140 lb. (deadweight).

CUTTING (*see* BRUSHING).

C.V.H.—Canine Virus Hepatitis.

CYANACETHYDRAZIDE.—A drug used to rid an animal of Husk worms, which it narcotises but does not kill. Dosing on 3 consecutive days is recommended.

CYANIDES are salts of hydrocyanic or prussic acid. They are all highly poisonous. (*See* PRUSSIC ACID.)

CYANOSIS (κυάνεος, blue) is a condition of blueness seen about the tongue, lips, mucous membranes of the eyes, etc., when there is some obstruction of the circulation or in the heart. It sometimes results from a weak or overworked heart, such as after severe disease, and in animals that have been hunted or chased. It is always a serious symptom, and if there are other complications present at the same time it may be a warning of approaching death.

CYCLOPHOSPHAMIDE.—This has been used (not in the U.K.) as a chemical means of defleecing sheep, and of treating mystic dermatitis.

CYCLOPS.—This genus of minute crustaceans act as intermediate hosts of the broad tapeworm of man, dog, and cat. (*See* p. 650, DIPHYLLOBOTHRIUM.)

CYCLOPROPANE-OXYGEN ANÆSTHESIA.—A costly but otherwise useful form of anæsthesia for dogs and cats. It has also been used for horses and goats. Cyclopropane is an inflammable gas.

CYPRESS POISONING.—This is rare. A 1962 report refers to the death of two yearling heifers. They had been in a field where several cypress trees (*Cupressus sempervirens*) were felled one morning. One heifer was dead by the afternoon; the other two nights later.

CYSTIC CALCULI (*see* CALCULI).

CYSTICERCOSIS (*see* PARASITES, p. 645).

CYSTITIS (κύστις, a bladder) means inflammation of the bladder. (*See* BLADDER, DISEASES OF.)

CYSTOSCOPE (κύστις, the bladder; σκοπέω, I view) is an instrument used in human medicine for the purpose of viewing the interior of the bladder. In a modified form it has been used for dogs and the smaller animals, but the difficulties attending its use, as well as the initial expense, are so great that its use is not likely to become general.

CYSTS (κύστις, a bladder) are hollow tumours containing fluid or soft material. They are almost always simple in nature and seldom return after removal, though in the case of certain types there are apt to be several of various sizes, and in some cases they may be of the nature of a tumour.

Varieties. (*a*) **Retention cysts.**—In these some cavity which ought naturally to contain a little fluid becomes, in consequence of irritation or other causes, distended to a great extent, or the natural outlet from the cavity becomes blocked. Ranula is a clear swelling under the tongue, due to the collection of saliva in consequence of an obstruction to a salivary duct. Cysts form in the kidney sometimes, as the result of obstruction to the free flow of urine from the tiny urinary tubules of that organ. Cysts filled with altered milk sometimes form in the mammary glands of bitches, but they are not common in other animals. Cystic thyroid is a condition of the thyroid gland in which the thyroid secretion forms faster than it is absorbed, and consequently collects in little pouches, or in one large thick-walled cavity, in or around the glands.

(*b*) **Ovarian cysts** are formed when some disturbance of the normal function of the ovary occurs. They are formed from failure of a Graäfian follicle to burst and release its ovum. They may grow to a large size or may become multiple. They generally give rise to symptoms of nymphomania in mares and cows, and lead to temporary or permanent infertility. When punctured surgically they may disappear and normal breeding may become possible. If they have been in existence for some time, however, new cysts may form or the old ones may re-form and the condition of infertility persists. When chronic and incurable, one or both ovaries may require removal to overcome the intractability caused by the nymphomania.

(*c*) **Developmental cysts.**—The most important of these are dermoid cysts, which originate in early life through failure of a cleft of the skin or of an epithelial structure in the fœtus to close normally. They are met with about the corners of the eyes and between the toes of dogs, in the temporal region and in the testicles of horses, and in other parts of other animals. They contain hair, fatty material, fragments of irregularly developed bone, scraps of skin, and sometimes even scores of ill-formed teeth. (*See* DERMOID CYST.)

(*d*) **Hydatid cysts** are produced in internal organs through the ingestion of the eggs of tape-worms from other animals. They occur in the peritoneal cavity, liver, spleen, brain, etc. (*See* PARASITES, p. 653).

(*e*) **Hard tumour cysts** sometimes occur in tumours growing in connection with glands, such as the adeno-carcinomata, which may occur in the mammary gland.

(*f*) **'Interdigital cysts'** in between the toes of dogs are in reality often abscesses. (*See* INTERDIGITAL ABSCESSES IN DOGS.)

Treatment.—The only rational treatment of cysts is their radical removal by careful surgical excision, after which they do not usually recur. Failing this, their contents may be evacuated by puncture through the walls, destroying the secretory lining by scraping or the injection of irritants, and plugging the opening so that closure is effected by healing from the bottom.

D

DANISH RED CATTLE.—More than half the cattle in Jutland, and 97 per cent of those in the Islands, belong to this breed, which is a very old one, though its official name (meaning Red Danish Milk breed) dates from 1878.

Danish Reds are strong, dual-purpose animals with a good ' barrel ', teats and udders, and weigh between 1,100 and 1,700 lb. During 1959–60, recorded cows averaged 960 gallons at 4·18 per cent butter-fat. Many herds, of course, have considerably higher average milk yields. In 1955 a Danish Red gave over 2,850 gallons. (*See also* BRITISH DANE *under* CATTLE, BREEDS OF.)

' DAFT LAMBS '.—Those affected with cerebellar atrophy—a condition occurring in the north of England and Scotland. It has been suggested that the condition is an inherited one; another view is that it is comparable to swayback and due to a trace element deficiency.

' DAGGING '.—Removal of soiled wool by shepherd from sheep's hind-quarters as an aid to preventing ' Strike '.

DAIRY HERD MANAGEMENT.—Even in 1970 herd size averages only 30 in the U.K., and 80 per cent of cows are still tied up in cowsheds. There is, however, a growing movement towards larger herds, and many of those which formerly were 50 to 70 cows are now 90 to 120 in size, while there are several 300-cow units, and by the mid-seventies a few may attain a size of 600 to 800.

Increase in size has been accompanied by other changes: notably, milking in a parlour and housing in a cubicle house instead of in a cowshed. (*See* CUBICLES FOR COWS, COW KENNELS.) There has been a tendency to replace the tandem parlour by the herringbone. Parlour feeding is now, in some very up-to-date units, related automatically to milk yield; and this both makes for economy and avoids the problem of cow identification in the big herd, so far as the milker is concerned. Identification is still necessary, however, for use in conjunction with herd records and in the parlour where the milker or relief milker (who will rarely know all the cows) must feed according to yield in the absence of automated equipment. Plastic numbered collars, anklets, discs on chain or nylon, freeze branding and even udder tattooing are the methods currently used.

Feeding outside the parlour has been mechanised in many large units by means of auger feeders delivering direct from tower silos. In others, side-delivery trucks are drawn by tractor down the feeding passages and deliver into the long mangers. Self-feed silage, with the clamp face in or near the cubicle house, is another labour-saver. Batch feeding (*e.g.* of dry cows, high yielders, and low yielders) is convenient management practice but may give rise to stress (*see* BUNT ORDER).

Zero-grazing is practised on some farms where poaching is a serious problem in wet weather, or where the movement of a large number of cows presents problems. With a very large herd on a very small acreage (such as an American 550-cow herd on under 5 acres) zero-grazing obviously becomes essential.

Paddock grazing now forms an important part of dairy herd management, and includes the two-sward system in which separate areas are used for grazing and for conservation.

Dung disposal is a major problem with large herds. Basically, there are two methods, handling it as a solid or as a liquid. Straw bedding lends itself to solid muck handling, with the liquid (urine, washing-down water, rainwater) being taken separately to a lagoon or to an underground tank. Slatted floors can be used in a cubicle house, either over a dung cellar which is cleared out once a year, or over a channel leading to an underground tank. With the semi-solid method, dung may be spread on the land by tanker, or the slurry may pass to a lagoon or be pumped through an organic irrigation pipeline system.

Where this is used, cows must not be expected to graze pasture until there has been time for rain to wash the slurry off the herbage. The use of organic irrigation is not entirely free from the risk of spreading infectious diseases.

Poaching must be avoided by the use of concrete aprons at gateways, by mobile drinking troughs, by wide corridors between paddocks with an electric fence dividing the 'corridor' so that one half can be kept in reserve, or by moveable ramps as used in New Zealand.

In the large herd one of the biggest problems is spotting the bulling heifer or the cow on heat. Properly kept herd records can be a help in alerting cowmen to the approximate dates. (*See* CALVING INDEX.)

On several large units regular weekly visits by veterinary surgeons help in the detection and treatment of infertility and the application of veterinary preventive medicine. (*See* HEALTH SCHEMES.)

DAPSONE.—A bacteriostatic given by injection into the udder in cases of mastitis due to *Streptococcus agalactiæ*; and by mouth in the treatment of coccidiosis in cattle.

DARNEL POISONING.—It has been recognised for a very long time that the seeds of the grass known as 'Darnel' (*Lolium temulentum*) were harmful to both man and beast when eaten, and it has been suggested that the 'tares' mentioned in Scripture, which the enemy sowed among the wheat, were in reality intended to mean darnel. It is a common weed in cereal crops and in pastures in some parts, but it does no harm when eaten before the seeds are ripe (or almost so), and its chief danger is that the grain may not be thoroughly removed from the grains of wheat, oats, or barley during threshing operations. Many instances are on record where harmful results to man and animals have followed the use of meal or flour which contained ground-up darnel seeds, and there are numerous references in classic literature to the harmful effect produced upon the eyes as the result of eating bread made from flour containing darnel. Cornevin's conclusions in connection with poisoning by darnel are that the following amounts will produce death of the animals mentioned:

	Per 100 lb. live weight
Horse	0·7 lb.
Cattle, Sheep, Poultry	1·5 to 1·8 lb.
Dog	1·8 lb.

Pigs are resistant, while about 1 ounce of darnel flour is all that an average man can tolerate without the production of symptoms.

The presence of darnel in flour can be demonstrated by a microscopic examination of the starch grains; those of darnel being only about one-fifth the size of those of rye, and only one-eighth the size of those of maize.

Toxic principle.—Contained within the grains there is a narcotic alkaloid, called *temuline*, which is said to be present to the extent of about 0·66 per cent, but some authorities assert that a substance called *loliine*, and others that *pricrotoxin*, should be considered responsible. A fungus called *Endoconidium temulentum* is very often found present in the seeds of darnel, living a life that is to a great extent one of symbiosis (*i.e.* two species living together for mutual benefit); and according to many authorities the poisonous alkaloid *temuline* is found in the fungus.

Symptoms.—Darnel is an irritant narcotic intoxicant. It produces giddiness and a staggering gait, drowsiness and stupefaction, dilatation of the pupils in the horse, and interference with vision in almost all animals. Vomiting, loss of sensation, convulsive seizures, and death follow when it is eaten by animals in large amounts. In some cases tremblings of the surface muscles are seen, and the extremities of the body become cold. Death usually occurs within 30 hours of eating the darnel seeds.

Treatment.—Strong black tea or coffee at once. Thereafter a demulcent purge, such as linseed oil for the horse and ox, and liquid paraffin for the pig and sheep, should be administered. Hypodermic injections of caffeine, strychnine, or other powerful stimulants, are useful. The animal should be kept warm.

DARROW'S SOLUTION.—This is used for fluid replacement therapy in dehydration arising from neonatal diarrhœa in infants. It is useful in calf scours. (*See under* DEHYDRATION.)

DATURINE.—An alkaloid. (*See under* STRAMOMIUM.)

DAY-OLD CHICKS (*see* CHICKS).

DDT.—The common abbreviation for dichloro-diphenyl-trichlorethane, a valuable parasiticide, lethal to fleas, lice, flies, etc. DDT was once used incorporated in dusting powders, for applying to animals; and dissolved in solvents for use as a fly-spray. DDT-resistant insects are now found in nearly all countries, unfortunately.

DDT preparations should not be applied to animals, owing to the risk of poisoning. The use of DDT with oils or fats enhances its toxic effects, and should be avoided. Symptoms of poisoning include coldness, diarrhœa, and hyperæsthesia. Minute doses over a period result in complete loss of appetite. DDT sprays may contaminate milk if used in the dairy; and may lead to poisonous residues in food animals when applied in live-stock buildings, with consequent danger to human beings eating the contaminated meat. DDT can also contaminate streams and rivers, and prove harmful to fish.

DEAD ANIMALS, DISPOSAL OF (*see* DISPOSAL OF CARCASES).

DEADLY NIGHTSHADE is the popular name of *Atropa belladonna*, from which the alkaloid *atropine* is obtained. It is a deadly poison, and parts of the plant are sometimes eaten by stock. (*See* ATROPINE.)

DEAFNESS.—In the horse the seriousness of the affection depends to a great deal on the work for which the horse is used, and on the animal's disposition. Apart altogether from the disease itself, which causes inability to hear, a horse that is of an even, good-natured, quiet temperament, used for work of a slow variety in the country, can manage quite well without the sense of hearing, provided allowances are made in the manner of driving it. It must not be expected to stop on verbal orders, nor to alter its speed, turn, or back a load except under the control of the reins, or of a man at its head. On the other hand, a horse that has to work in fast-moving traffic and is of a nervous disposition may become absolutely useless as the result of losing its hearing. Not being able to appreciate vehicles approaching from behind until they suddenly rush past may be enough to cause the horse to swerve to the side, or even run away, with disastrous results. Generally, deaf horses have their senses of sight and smell intensified to such an extent that in time they compensate for loss of hearing, and after the preliminary uncertain stage the horse becomes a capable and reliable animal.

In the ox deafness is of little importance, and very often is not suspected until discovered by accident. The same applies to sheep and pigs.

In dogs the inability to hear is always a source of inconvenience both to the animal and its owner. Collies and sheepdogs must be able to hear acutely, otherwise their utility is confined to working within sight of their masters, a condition that only seldom obtains. Sporting dogs must be able to hear orders issued, no matter in what work they are engaged. In the household pet acuteness of hearing is not of such importance as in the previous cases, but a deaf dog is a continual source of anxiety to its owner when out of doors ; for it does not hear traffic. Congenital deafness is common in white bull terriers.

Deafness is or may be also a symptom of santonin poisoning, coal-gas poisoning (which see), of a vitamin deficiency, and, at least in humans, a side-effect of streptomycin. Other causes include damage to the internal ear, to the Eustachian tube, nervous system, etc.

DEATH, CAUSES OF SUDDEN.—In the majority of cases either failure of the heart or damage to a blood-vessel (*e.g.*, in cattle caused by a nail or a piece of wire from the reticulum) is the direct cause, but nervous shock following an accident or injury, cerebral hæmorrhage, anthrax, black-quarter, lightning-stroke, braxy, and over-eating of green succulent fodder in young cattle, are all capable of producing sudden death. In the case of pigs, sudden death has sometimes been met with from 'heat stroke'. (*See also* ŒDEMA OF THE BOWEL.) In both cattle and pigs sudden death due to *Clostridium Welchii* Type A has been reported. In cattle, hypomagnesæmia is a cause. In countries bordering the Red Sea, horses that have not been bred locally are sometimes attacked by a form of 'sunstroke' with fatal results. (*See also* POISONING *and* (*with reference to dogs*) CANINE VIRUS HEPATITIS.)

DEATH, SIGNS OF.—The physical signs of death are well known, but there are occasions when it is difficult to state whether an animal is dead or not. In deep coma an animal may have all the superficial appearances of being dead, and yet recovery is possible if effective measures are taken. In the later stage of milk fever a cow has often been mistaken for dead, has been dragged out of the byre preparatory to removal to the slaughterer's cart, has been examined by a practitioner, found to be living, has been suitably treated, and within two hours has been up on her feet again looking well. Foals have frequently been discarded soon after being born and considered dead, have been removed to the outside of the loose-box while attention was paid to the dam, and later have been found living, the fresh cold air having revived respiration and stimulated the circulation, etc.

When an animal dies, the essential sign of the cessation of life is said to be the stopping of the heart. This, however, is not strictly correct, for it is possible by massage to resuscitate an already stopped heart, and to recover an apparently dead creature. Strictly speaking, it is almost impossible to say exactly when death takes place, but it is considered that when heart and respiration have ceased, when the eyelids do not flicker if a finger be applied to the eyeballs, when a cut artery no longer bleeds, and when the tissues lose their natural elasticity, life is extinct. A few of the common tests that are applied in uncertain cases are as follows: The animal is dead when (1) a piece of cold glass held to the nostrils for three minutes comes away without any condensed moisture upon it; (2) when a superficial incision in the skin does not gape open; and (3) the natural elastic tension of the tissues disappears. Changes that follow death in a variable period depending upon the species of animal, and upon the weather at the time, are: (1) the clotting of the blood in the vessels; (2) the onset of *rigor mortis*—the stiffness of death; and (3) the commencement of decomposition of the carcase, usually first evident along the lower surface of the abdomen.

DE-BEAKING.—This is done by poultry-keepers either when feather-picking or cannibalism begins, or as a routine method of prevention when the pullets are about to be put in the laying houses. Some trim the tip of the beak; but most cut back a third of the upper beak, which gives rise to bleeding. This is usually controlled by means of a red-hot iron. Special machines are also used, incorporating an electro-cautery. Infectious sinusitis is sometimes a sequel of de-beaking, especially in turkeys. On some farms de-beaking may be so badly done that deformity or fatal hæmorrhage results. De-beaking wastes feed.

DE-SNOODING.—The removal of a turkey poult's snood, which may be pinched out or removed with a suitable instrument. De-snooding is done by turkey owners in order to reduce the risk of cannibalism.

DE-WATTLING.—The removal of a fowl's wattles. It is said to reduce the risk of frost-bite. (*See also* DUBBING).

DÉBRIDEMENT.—Removal of infected tissue from a wound surface. This may be done by enzymes. (*See* STREPTODORNASE.)

DECIDUA (*decido*, I fall off) is the name of the soft coat which lines the interior of the womb during pregnancy, and which is cast off at birth.

DECOCTION (*decoquo*, I boil down) is the name used for a preparation made by boiling various plants in water and straining the fluid.

DECUBITUS (*decumbo*, I lie down) is the name applied to the recumbent position assumed by animals suffering from certain diseases.

DECUSSATION (*decussatio*) is a term applied to any place in the nervous system at which nerve fibres cross from one side to the other, *e.g.* the decussation of the pyramids in the medulla, where the motor fibres from one side of the brain cross to the other side of the spinal cord.

DEEP-FREEZE (*see* ARTIFICIAL INSEMINATION, SEMEN: STORAGE OF).

DEEP LITTER FOR CATTLE.—This is a very satisfactory system if well managed. Straw, shavings, and sawdust can be used. Warmth given off as a result of the fermentation taking place in the litter makes for cow-comfort; and there is, of course, the added advantage of a thick layer of insulation between the cows and the concrete of a covered yard. In the 'Bed-and-breakfast' system, cows were bedded on top of a self-feed silage clamp in a covered yard.

A considerable depth—2 or 3 feet—is often attained, and the cost is much less than that of conventional straw litter as bedding; £1 to £4 per head for the winter period of housing.

DEEP LITTER FOR POULTRY.—Chopped straw, shavings, and sawdust are commonly used. Musty straw could cause an outbreak of Aspergillosis. Peat-moss is apt to be too dusty. Oak sawdust should not be used as it may discolour the egg-yolks. The depth should be at least 4 inches. The litter should be forked over, and added to from time to time. If it gets damp, the ventilation should be attended to. Many coccidia larvæ get buried in the litter, and this is an advantage. After each crop of birds, the litter should be removed and heaped, so that enough heat will be generated to kill parasites. If deep litter is returned to a house, the succeeding batch of birds *sometimes* suffer from ammonia fumes, which may cause serious eye troubles and even blindness.

DEEP-ROOTING PLANTS are valuable in a pasture for the sake of the minerals they provide. Examples of such plants are: chicory, yarrow, tall fescue.

DEER.—In Britain the following infections have been found in deer: brucellosis, Johne's disease, louping ill, tick-borne fever, tuberculosis (avian).

DEFÆCATION (*defæco*, I cleanse) means the act of opening the bowels and the evacuation of the contents of the posterior part of the alimentary canal. The act is very differently performed in the various animals, and some diagnostic importance is attached to the manner of its performance. (*See* CONSTIPATION, DIARRHŒA.)

DEFICIENCY DISEASES.—These form a group of diseases bearing no clinical resemblance to each other, but having the common feature that in each some substance or element essential for normal health and nutrition has been absent from the diet for a longer or shorter period. The essential element may be one of the inorganic mineral substances, such as calcium, phosphorus, magnesium, manganese, iron, copper, cobalt, iodine, or more than one of these; it may be a protein or an amino-acid; or it may be a vitamin. In the latter case the condition is often referred to as an 'Avitaminosis', and the particular vitamin is specified, *e.g.* A, B, or D. Starvation through inadequacy of general nutritive food intake, is not classed as a deficiency disease. Some deficiency diseases are simple, such as iron deficiency in young pigs, others are more complex, such as phosphate deficiency in South Africa, which is associated with botulism through the gnawing of bones of dead animals contaminated with *Cl. botulinus*.

DEFINITIVE HOST.—This is the host in which an adult parasite with an indirect life-history lives and produces its eggs. A definitive host is the final host, as compared with the intermediate host or hosts. For example, an ant is one of the intermediate hosts of one species of liver-fluke (*see* ANTS); the definitive host is a sheep or other grazing animal.

DE-FLEECING.—(*See under* CYCLOPHOSPHAMIDE.)

DEFORMITIES may be present at birth, or they may be the result of injuries or of disease. They are produced before birth either as the result of hereditary influence (*e.g.* bull-dog calves in Dexter cattle), on account of the abnormal processes at work in the uterus (*e.g.* monstrosities in which there are parts of two distinct creatures fused together, like Siamese twins), or through the agency of pressure upon the developing fœtus, which results in twisted or bent limbs, wry-neck, flat chest-walls, etc.

Deformities resulting from injuries or disease are of more importance to stock owners, because in the majority of cases of deformity at birth the young animal is destroyed. Indeed, many such are born dead; others die in the process. Of the deformities which result from injury those that follow a fracture of one of the long bones of the limbs are the most common and serious. The healing of a fracture is a particularly risky process in any animal, and the larger the animal the more difficult is it to secure union of the bones (*see* FRACTURES). Injuries which involve tendon or ligament are sometimes followed by deformity, which most often consists of a shortening of the damaged structure and an approximation of its extremities. This results in permanent flexion of a joint if the injured structure runs across one, such as is seen in contracted tendons in the limbs of horses. Wounds of the skin and surface muscles seldom result in any serious deformity unless some delicate structure, such as the eyelids, nostrils, lips, vulva, or anus, is implicated. Burns or scalds in which extensive areas are destroyed are generally followed by the formation of most unsightly scars, which may so draw the skin together that a marked deformity results. Of the commoner diseases which produce deformities the following are the most important: rickets, lymphangitis, laminitis, splints, side-bones, ring-bones, spavins, curbs, thoroughpins, and canker of the ears in small animals (*see these headings*).

The following sections should also be consulted: EMBRYOLOGY; REPRODUCTION; CONFORMATION, ERRORS IN ; GENETICS.

'DEG NALA' DISEASE.—This takes its name from an area in West Pakistan, where it affects mainly buffaloes and occasionally cattle in the winter months when the animals are fed on green rice fodder or fresh rice straw. Symptoms include : loss of appetite, discharge from the eyes, salivation, and dropsical swellings on the lower part of the legs and other dependent parts of the body. The legs, ears, and tail, tongue and muzzle may show ulceration, and there may be necrosis and even gangrene, with shedding of a hoof. The cause of the disease is not known.

DEGENERATION (*degenero*, I degenerate) means a change in structure or in chemical composition of a tissue or organ by which its vitality is lowered or its function disturbed. Degeneration is of various kinds, the chief being fatty (*see* FATTY DEGENERATION), and fibroid (*see* CIRRHOSIS).

DEGLUTITION (*deglutio*, I swallow) means the act of swallowing. (*See* CHOKING.)

DE-HORNING (*see under* DISHORNING).

DEHYDRATION.—Loss of water from the tissues, such as occurs during various illnesses, especially those producing vomiting or diarrhœa ; in impaction of the rumen and as a result of serious burns.

'Measurement of fæcal volume shows that by this route a scouring calf may lose as much as 100 ml. of water from each kilogramme bodyweight in a period of 12 hours. Most of the water loss is into the intestine but some is lost by respiration and minimal urine formation. Because urine formation is reduced to minimal levels in an attempt to conserve body fluids there is a marked increase in metabolic waste material in the plasma. In a calf which has diarrhœa, but has kept its plasma volume within normal limits by movement of water from the intracellular fluid phase, the blood urea concentration will usually increase from a normal 10 to 20 mg. per 100 ml. to 30 to 45 mg. per 100 ml. but, as dehydration progresses beyond the point of compensation, this accumulation of urea increases rapidly to levels as high as 120 mg. per 100 ml.'

'Irrespective of the causes of diarrhœa, several factors are common to all cases. Some degree of inanition and dehydration occurs due to the upset absorption of food; in addition to this losses of specific electrolytes occur due to the continuation of gastro-intestinal secretion. The main electrolytes secreted in the abomasum are sodium and chloride while those secreted in the intestinal tract are principally, bicarbonate, sodium, and potassium. Due to the position of secretion the main losses into the gut of a diarrhoeic calf are water, bicarbonate, potassium, sodium, and chloride in order of magnitude.'

'Diarrhœa is accompanied by a metabolic acidosis ; this is related to losses of bicarbonate in the fæces and ketone body accumulation due to starvation.'

Treatment.—Homologous plasma is the first recommendation, although dextran solutions can be used as an alternative. The object of infusing homologous plasma in the early part of fluid replacement therapy is so that the circulatory defects produced by high blood viscosity, higher than normal plasma potassium levels and lowered blood *pH* are reduced rapidly and effectively to nearer normal limits.

'Initially the rate at which the fluid is administered should be carefully supervised, lest acute venous congestion occurs with the danger of producing pulmonary œdema. The flow-rate should be increased gradually to about 6 ml. per minute (90 drops from standard drip set) but, at the first sign of respiratory distress, if necessary this rate of flow may have to be drastically curtailed. Once 150 to 200 ml. have been infused the flow-rate can be increased to the maximum capable of delivery by the apparatus under gravity flow. After 400 to 600 ml. have been infused the rate should be reduced to 2 to 3 ml. per minute and kept at this rate or slightly slower throughout the remainder of the infusion. The amount of plasma usually sufficient to return the circulation of the animal to reasonable efficiency is 400 to 800 ml.'

'Having achieved the first stage of repair the remaining problem is to hydrate the tissues and replace some of the electrolyte losses which have occurred. The simplest method of achieving this is to alternate the fluids (*e.g.* 500 ml. Darrows solution followed by 500 ml. glucose solution) from the end of the infusion of plasma and continued for 24 hours. The majority of calves do not require further fluid therapy after 24 hours' continuous drip but a few individuals are still recumbent or slow to respond at the end of this period. In these cases the procedure is simply to repeat the whole course of therapy as for the first day, having first re-assessed and re-calculated the fluid requirement.'

'The effects of infusion of plasma plus electrolyte solutions appear to be considerably greater than the effects of replacement of electrolytes alone. The reason for the increased benefit may, in part, be due to the more rapid and efficient repair of the circulation which is a feature of plasma administration. The infusion of plasma gives better perfusion of the tissues without the development of hypertension in the major blood-vessels which tends to occur when crystalloids are administered intravenously. Such hypertensions increase secretion of urine and the passage of fluid into the intestine so that a considerable part of the benefit of the infusion may be lost to the animal. It is important to promote renal function in order to eliminate the metabolic waste material which tends to accumulate in the tissues of the calf but this will be more beneficial if it is accompanied by adequate tissue rehydration.'

'The plasma used, being the pooled product of groups of at least 10 healthy young adult animals, contains most of the substances normally present in the plasma of such animals; in addition it contains some 3 per cent of dextrose which is added to the collected blood as a preservative. Thus it has nutritive properties. Also, it contains the gamma-globulin fraction of the plasma proteins of these donor animals. As yet there is little knowledge of the standard of surivval of these proteins during the processing of the plasma to the freeze-dried state but there is increasing evidence that some of their immunological properties are retained.'

(Source: J. G. Watt, B.V.M.S., M.R.C.V.S., *Veterinary Record*, Dec. 4, 1965.)

With untreated scouring calves' death probably results from acidosis and the high plasma potassium levels.

In a horse suffering from intestinal obstruction, up to 10 l. of whole blood or plasma may be required to restore the blood volume, while the total fluid deficit may be much greater.

DELIVERY means the final expulsion of the young during the act of birth. (*See* PARTURITION.)

DELNAV. — An organo-phosphorus compound used for the control of two- and three-host ticks. A brown liquid, insoluble in water, it is used for dipping or washing cattle at a strength of 0·05 to 0·1 per cent.

DEMEPHION.—An organophosphorous preparation used as an insecticide and acaricide. Live-stock should be kept out of treated areas for at least a fortnight.

DEMODECTIC MANGE, or **FOLLICULAR MANGE,** is the name of that variety of mange which is caused by the *demodectic* parasite *Demodex folliculorum.* This parasite, which is microscopic and cigar-shaped in appearance, with very short stumpy legs, lives deep down in the hair follicles, and is accordingly difficult to eradicate by dressings. (*See* PARASITES, p. 691).

In cattle *Demodex bovis* is in the U.K. responsible for mild and infrequently reported cases of demodectic mange, but in some parts of the world the disease may be severe. Fatal, generalised cases have been reported from Africa.

D. caprae infestation of goats may also be severe in the tropics.

The parasites have been recovered from the eyelids of cattle, sheep, horses, dogs, and man.

DEMULCENTS (*demulceo,* I stroke down) are substances which exert a soothing influence upon the skin or the mucous membranes of the alimentary canal, and in addition afford some protection when these are corroded or inflamed.

Varieties.—Mucilaginous substances, such as gum, mucilage in water, isinglass, etc.; oils, like olive, linseed, rape, and whale oil; starchy substances, such as arrowroot, cornflour, barley gruel, and wheaten-flour gruel; as well as glycerine, borax, most weak alkalies, and certain powders, such as the subnitrate of bismuth.

Uses.—They are used when there is any inflammation in the early part of the alimentary canal, especially in the throat or the stomach, and are given as draughts, electuaries, or mouth-washes, and occasionally as powders. They are used to protect the mucous surfaces from their own secretions, which may irritate them when they are inflamed, or they may be given to counteract the corroding effects of irritant or corrosive poisons that have been accidentally swallowed, and to soothe and promote healing in those parts that have been damaged.

DEMYELINATION.—Destruction of the myelin, a semi-fluid which surrounds the axis-cylinder of a medullated nerve fibre.

DENGUE (*see* THREE-DAY SICKNESS).

DENTINE is the dense yellow or yellowish-white material of which the greater part of the teeth is composed, and which in elephants, etc., constitutes ivory. The dentine is pierced by numberless fine tubules which communicate with the sensitive pulp in the hollow of the tooth-root, along each of which runs tiny vessels and nerves which nourish its structure. In the young newly erupted tooth the dentine is covered over with a layer of enamel, hard, dense, and brittle, which prevents too rapid wear of the softer dentine. (*See* TEETH.)

DENTITION

DENTITION (*dentio*, I cut teeth) is the name given to the study of the configuration and conformation of the teeth, with special reference to their periods of eruption through the gums.

Among domesticated stock it is possible within certain limits to estimate the age of an animal by an examination of the appearance of its teeth; but while such an estimation is reasonably reliable, it is by no means always accurate. Numerous factors influence the dates of eruption of both temporary and permanent teeth, and it is not always possible to take these factors into consideration in any given case, for they may not be known. Artificial methods of management, forced feeding upon concentrated food-stuffs, and the selection of early maturing breeding types, have combined to produce earlier and earlier eruption of the teeth, so that very considerable variations now exist between breeds of stock which are managed under an intensive system and those that are kept under more natural conditions. It appears, however, that in Great Britain the limit of early appearance of the teeth has been reached for all practical purposes, for in the British breeds of live-stock there has been but little change during the last seventy years, in this respect.

In the following description the periods of eruption given are those that are now considered to be average periods for each species of animal in Great Britain, and while variations from them will certainly be met with, the majority of animals will be observed to cut their teeth at the periods stated, or within a narrow margin of time before or after.

HORSE.—The full permanent dentition of the horse consists of the following teeth:

	Incisors.	Canines.	Molars.
Upper jaws	6	2	12, 13, or 14
Lower jaws	6	2	12, 13, or 14

The variation in the number of molars depends upon whether '*wolf teeth*' are or are not present. These are small rudimentary teeth situated in front of the first molar; one, two, three, or four 'wolf teeth' may be present in an adult horse, but in the majority of cases there are none. One other variation must be mentioned: in the mare canine teeth may be either absent or they may be small and rudimentary.

The permanent teeth are not, however, present in the young foal; the majority of them are preceded by *milk*, *temporary*, or *deciduous* representatives. The temporary dentition consists of the following teeth:

	Incisors.	Canines.	Molars.
Upper jaws .	6	0	6
Lower jaws .	6	0	6

Some authorities distinguish between molars and premolars in the permanent dentition; those teeth which are represented in the temporary dentition (*i.e.* the first *three* in either jaw, right and left, and upper and lower) being called *pre-molars*; while those which have no such representatives are known as *molars*. This may lead to some confusion, however and all the cheek teeth will be called 'molars' in this section, and will be designated by a number (*i.e.* from No. 1 to No. 6) to avoid confusion.

Incisor teeth, 'nippers' or 'pincers', are six in number in the upper and lower jaws; they are found in the front of the mouth in each jaw, and reference is made to them almost exclusively for the purpose of estimating the ages of animals; the molars are only examined when irregularities of abnormalities are present in the incisor region. The temporary incisors differ from the permanents in that while each of the former possesses a definite crown, neck, and root, the latter do not. Moreover, the temporaries are smoother, whiter, and smaller, and to some extent resemble the incisors of cattle. When there are both temporaries and permanents present in the mouth it is not usually difficult to differentiate between them, but inexperienced persons sometimes confuse temporaries and permanents in yearlings and five-year-olds, or in two-year-olds and six-year-olds. A typical unworn permanent incisor tooth from a horse possesses an *infundibulum*, or 'tucking-in' from its free edge or crown (*see* TEETH), and since this results in an infolding of the enamel, two rings of enamel, an outer and an inner, are seen in the partly worn tooth. However, as wear proceeds there comes a time when the inner ring of enamel disappears, since the level of wear has passed the depth of the infundibulum. In addition to the disappearance of the infundibulum the outline of the tooth changes from an oval to a quadrilateral, and eventually to a triangle, since the tooth is tapered from crown to root. It is upon an examination of these factors that the estimation of the age of an adult horse is based.

The incisors are named *centrals*, *laterals* or *intermediaries*, and *corners*, according to their situation in the mouth.

Canines.—'Tushes', 'eye-teeth', or 'dog-teeth' number two in each of the jaws—one on the right and one on the left side. In the horse tribe canines are only typically present in male animals, although they may be found in mares upon occasion. As a rule, if present in the mare they are either small or rudimentary. They are situated in a position between the last incisor and the first molar, one on either side, being nearer to the incisors than to the molars. The spaces between the canines and the molars are spoken of as the *bars* of the mouth, and across the bars runs the bit in the bridled horse. The canine teeth are comparatively simple, showing no folding of enamel.

Molars.—'Grinders', or 'cheek teeth', number six or seven in each of the four jaws, according to whether 'wolf teeth' are or are not present. The first three permanent molars are represented in the milk dentition and are therefore sometimes called *premolars*. Each tooth has a complicated folding of the enamel which bears some resemblance to the capital letter 'B'. The roots of the molars are long, and there is but little tapering from the crown downwards—an arrangement which allows of the maximum wear.

Eruption.—The 'eruption' means the time when the tooth cuts through the gums, and not when it comes into wear. It will be convenient to consider the eruption of the horse's teeth in tabular form. It must be remembered that in the following table allowance has to be made for the time of foaling. All thoroughbreds are dated as having their birthdays on the 1st of January each year, and all other breeds of horses on the 1st of May, so that with an early foal the teeth will appear sooner than the corresponding periods subsequent to 1st May or 1st January in any year, and with a late foal later. Allowance must also be made for the system

Time of Eruption.	Incisors.	Canines.	Molars.
Birth to 1 week.	2 temporary centrals	..	..
2 to 4 weeks	2 temporary laterals	..	Nos. 1, 2, and 3 temporary molars.
7 to 9 mths.	2 temporary corners	..	No. 4 permanent molar.
1 yr. 6 mths. to 1 year 8 mths.	..	..	No. 5 permanent molar.
2 yrs. 6 mths.	2 permanent centrals	..	Nos. 1 and 2 permanent molars.
3 yrs. 6 mths.	2 permanent laterals	..	No. 3 permanent molar.
4 years .	..	All 4 canines	No. 6 permanent molar.
4 yrs. 6 mths.	2 permanent corners	..	..

under which horses are kept; in the case of New Forest ponies or those reared on rough pasturage, for example, the teeth are slower in erupting than in animals that are bred under an intensive system.

It should be also noted that as a rule the teeth in the upper jaw erupt sooner than those in the lower jaw, although there are many exceptions to this rule.

Appearance of teeth at various ages.—To facilitate reference, although it entails some repetition, the appearance of the horse's teeth at various definite periods of its life will be described.

At birth the foal usually has the two central temporary incisors in each jaw through the gums, or just appearing. They are placed somewhat obliquely in the small mouth. In a few cases the laterals may also be showing, especially in foals carried longer than the usual gestation period. The first three molars can be felt below the gums, but they have not yet cut.

At 1 month, or soon after, the two temporary laterals erupt, whilst the two centrals are in wear and placed more nearly parallel in the mouth. At about this time the first three temporary molars cut through the gums.

At 6 months the foal's mouth has a neat, compact appearance, the centrals and laterals being well developed and in wear upon their anterior edges, although they are not all usually wearing along their posterior edges.

At 9 months the colt has the two temporary corners through the gums, but these are only touching along their anterior edges. The appearance of the mouth in profile shows an angular space between the upper and lower corner incisors. The centrals and laterals are well in wear. At about this time the 4th molars (permanent) cut through the gums, but do not yet come into wear.

At 1 year old the 4th molar is in wear. The corner incisors are still shell-like and only touching along their anterior edges.

At 1 year 6 months the corner incisors are now wearing all along their edges, and the centrals and laterals have become large and well-formed. At about this time the 5th molars (permanent) erupt, coming into wear at about 2 years.

At 2 years the corner incisors are well in wear, and all the incisor teeth have well-formed tables. There is as yet no sign of the displacement of the centrals.

At 2 years off, i.e. about 2 years and 3 months, the central incisors are often loose and the gums are receding from their necks. The teeth are only held in position by a short portion of fang or root.

At 2 years 6 months the two central temporary incisors fall out and their places are taken by the permanent centrals. At the same time the first two temporary molars (Nos. 1 and 2) in each jaw are shed, and the corresponding permanent molars are erupted.

At rising 3 years, i.e. about 2 years and 9 months, the two centrals have come well through the gums, but they do not quite meet each other until a little later. Nos. 1 and 2 permanent molars in each jaw are well up and in wear.

At 3 years old the two central permanent incisors have met their fellows of the opposite jaw, but only a slight amount of wear is showing on their tables. The infundibula are only slightly worn and the 'tucked in' appearance can be well seen. In most cases there is a little wear showing on the anterior edges, but the tables are not yet well-formed.

At 3 years off the tables of the permanent central incisors are formed and show an appreciable amount of wear. There is some indication of the replacement of the laterals, such as was noticed at 2 years off in connection with the centrals.

At 3 years 6 months some or perhaps all four of the permanent laterals have erupted, pushing out the corresponding temporaries in the process. Very shortly after this age the 3rd permanent molars are cut, the 3rd temporary molars making way for them by falling out.

At rising 4 years the permanent laterals are coming into wear. They may be touching, but an examination of their tables shows no appreciable wear. The centrals are well in wear and their tables are formed. About this time the canines of 'tushes', in the male, are beginning to show signs of eruption, the mucous membrane over them becoming bulged, white in colour, and painful on pressure. The 6th and last permanent molars are cutting through the gums, or may be already partly through, but they are not yet level with the other molars.

At 4 years the picture is similar to that at rising 4 years, but the laterals are now in wear, and the 6th molars are level or are nearly level with the other teeth.

At 4 years 6 months, or about that time, the temporary corner incisors fall out and the last permanent teeth to erupt—the corners—cut through the gums. The molars are all well in wear and level. The horse has now a 'full mouth', all teeth being cut, although they are not all in wear.

At 5 years the corner incisors have met their fellows of the other jaw along their

DENTITION

anterior edges, but their posterior corners are still rounded off and unworn. At this stage an angular space is visible when the mouth is looked at in profile with the jaws shut.

At 5 years off the corner incisors are showing more wear but they do not accurately meet until the horse is rising six years.

From this time onwards the age of the horse is estimated by a consideration of the appearance of the wear on the tables of the *lower incisor teeth,* by the changes in their outlines, and by the gradual lessening of the angle at which they meet the upper incisors.

At 6 years the corner teeth have lost their shell-like appearance and are in wear along both sides of their central cavity or 'mark'. In some cases the inner edge of the tooth is indentated (especially the upper tooth), and a small part of the margin may not be quite in wear, but this is not a uniform feature. The laterals present cavities more shallow than those of the centrals, but still easily recognisable as such. Both the rings of enamel (outer and inner) are intact, and the outline of the centrals and laterals is distinctly oval, with the long axis in line with the rest of the teeth. In the central incisors the cavity is almost worn out, but the rings of enamel are distinct. The tushes are usually well developed and are prominent features of the male animal's mouth; their points are sharp.

At 7 years the tables of the lower corner teeth are well formed and the infundibulum in each is shallow. The central rings of enamel in both the central and lateral teeth are nearer to the posterior edge of the tooth than the anterior edge, and in the centrals though the ring is present it has lost its cavity. A shallow cavity is present in the laterals. The outline of the centrals is now much broader (antero-posteriorly) than at six years old, and also broader than is that of either the laterals or corners. In fact, the outline of the central teeth is becoming triangular (with the innermost angle rounded), while the outlines of their central enamel rings are broader ovals than formerly. In addition there is formed at this age what is often known as the '7-year-old hook'. This is seen when the jaws are examined in profile. It is due to the fact that the lower corner incisor is placed somewhat farther forward in the jaw than the corresponding upper tooth, and it is not so large. There results an imperfect apposition, and the posterior corner of the upper tooth develops a notch where wear occurs, and a slight projection where there is none. Some horses with badly aligned jaws do not develop this hook.

At 8 years the central teeth are more distinctly triangular than they were, and the central ring of enamel is also becoming triangular. The cavities in the centrals and laterals are either wholly obliterated or are nearly so, but in each case the inner ring of enamel is still perfect. A shallow true cavity is generally present in the corners. If the tables of the centrals are carefully examined a brownish or yellowish-brown linear streak will be seen running transversely across the tooth between the inner and outer rings of enamel and situated just behind the anterior edge of the tooth. This is called the 'dental star', and though it may be found in all six incisor teeth at 8 years, it is usually confined to the centrals, or to these and the laterals. The teeth are meeting each other at an angle considerably less than 180° when viewed in profile. The 7-year-old hook has worn out from the upper corner teeth, or is almost gone.

Beyond 8 years the teeth of horses vary to such an extent that, while a rough estimate is possible, it is very easy to make considerable mistakes. Much depends upon the management, rate of development, quality of the food, wear of the teeth as determined by their softness or hardness, and upon other factors. The subsequent notes must therefore be understood to apply only to average horses, and to be suggestions rather than rules.

At 9 years the central and lateral teeth are no longer triangular in outline but are becoming rounded—their angles disappearing. The outline of the corner teeth is never very definite. A smaller irregular enamel ring still persists, which encloses about one-fifth of the area of the table surface. The cavity has disappeared from the corner teeth, and these as well as the centrals and laterals show a fairly definite dental star occupying practically the centre of the table surface. There is more of each tooth exposed from the gums, which appear to have receded. The teeth are more oblique in their incidence, and are less fresh-looking than at 8 years.

At 10 years the central tables are almost as broad antero-posteriorly as they are long transversely, and there only remains a small inner ring of enamel, almost circular in outline and possessing no central depression. The inner rings in the laterals and corners are, however, still irregularly oval. The dental star is distinct in all the lower incisor teeth and occupies a central position. At this age 'Galvayne's groove', which is seen as a groove just protruding from under the gum on the outer surface of each of the upper corner teeth, appears. This groove appears at 10 years, has grown about half-way down the tooth at 15 or 16 years, reaches the free edge of each tooth at about 21, and by 25 has started to disappear, the upper part of the tooth becoming once more smooth. By about 30 years the groove has quite disappeared.

At 11 to 13 years all the teeth appear longer on account of the receding of the gums. The tables of each of them gradually assume distinctly round and then square outlines. By the time 12 years is reached only a very small indistinct inner ring of enamel remains, and when the horse is 13 years old, it has typically disappeared from the centrals and laterals, but in the corners it may persist very close to the inner margin. A distinct dental star remains in all the teeth; this is small, rounded in outline, and occupies the centre of the table. The slope of the teeth in each jaw is now such that they meet at a much more acute angle when viewed in profile. A hook often appears in the upper corner teeth, similar to the 7-year-old hook but less regular.

At 15 or 16 years the tables of the teeth are becoming broader antero-posteriorly than they are long, and in the centre of the dental star a cleft or depression usually appears, due to the softer consistence of the tissue there. Galvayne's groove has grown about half-way down to the free edge in the upper corner teeth.

At 18 to 20 years the angle formed between the teeth of the two jaws is almost a right angle, and the tables of teeth are getting much smaller. In outline they are triangular, or are like quadrilaterals which have been flattened from side to side. A distinct depression appears in the centre of the dental star. Galvayne's groove has almost reached the free border.

From 20 to 30 years the teeth gradually appear older and more worn. They become smaller, and occupy a line along the gum which is no longer a definite arc, but gradually gets flatter until at about 30 years it is almost straight across, and the teeth are huddled together with no spaces between them.

As can be understood, an estimate of the horse's age can only be approximate in later life. Galvayne's groove is practically the only definite guide, and even it may be indistinct or absent.

OX.—The *permanent dentition* of the ox consists of the following teeth:

	Incisors.	Canines.	Molars.
Upper jaws .	0	0	12
Lower jaws .	8	0	12

In the upper jaw there are neither incisors nor canines, while in the lower jaw there are 8 teeth present in the incisor region. The most posterior of these (*i.e.* one on either side) are supposed to be in reality modified canines, which have moved forward in the gums and have assumed the shape and the functions of incisors.

The *temporary* or *milk dentition* is as follows:

	Incisors.	Canines.	Molars.
Upper jaws .	0	0	6
Lower jaws .	8	0	6

Incisors are absent from the upper jaws of cattle, their place being taken by the 'dental pad', a hard, dense mass of fibrous tissue developed in the upper incisor region, against which the 8 lower incisor teeth bite. Each is a simple tooth possessing a spatulate (spade-shaped) crown, a constricted neck, and a tapered root or fang. The teeth are loosely embedded in the jaw so that a slight amount of movement is normally possible. They are named *centrals*, *first intermediates* or *medials*, *second intermediates* or *laterals*, and *corners*; but it is perhaps more convenient to enumerate them from the central pair as 1st pair, 2nd pair, etc. The temporary incisors are small, brittle, and little or no trouble is likely to be met with in differentiating them from permanents.

Canines are absent unless the corner incisors are considered as modified canines.

Molars are like those of the horse in number and arrangement, except that they are smaller and progressively increase in size from first to last, so that the first is quite small, and the length of gum which accommodates the first three is only about half that occupied by the last three. One or more 'wolf teeth' may be present in rare cases.

Eruption. — In ruminants — whether domesticated or not—the eruption of the permanent teeth is subject to very considerable variations. As in the horse, but even more so, the eruption of the teeth is influenced by domestication, methods of management, and nature of the food, and what applies to the more highly specialised improved breeds does not apply to commonly-bred cattle, and what applies to these latter does not hold good for ranch cattle. It is therefore necessary to give average figures for each of these classes, and to emphasise that while in any particular type of cattle the times given are about the average for that type, individual animals will be met with whose teeth are cut at periods very much earlier or later than the times given.

The following tables have been drawn up for more easy reference :

(1) Highly-bred Stock

Time of Eruption.	Incisors.	Molars.
Birth to 1 month	All 8 temporary teeth in lower jaw.	All 12 temporary teeth.
6 months . .	. .	4th permanent
1 year to 1 year and 3 months.	. .	5th ,,
1 year 9 months .	1st pair permanents	6th ,,
2 years . .	. .	1st and 2nd permanents.
2 years 3 months	2nd pair permanents	. .
2 ,, 9 ,,	3rd pair permanents	3rd permanent
3 ,, 3 ,,	4th pair permanents	. .

(2) Commonly-bred Stock

Time of Eruption.	Incisors.	Molars.
Birth to 1 month	All 8 temporaries	All 12 temporaries.
6 months . .	. .	4th permanent
1 year 3 months to 1 year 6 months	. .	5th ,,
1 year 9 months to 2 years.	1st pair permanents	. .
2 years . .	. .	6th permanent
2 years 6 months	2nd pair permanents	1st and 2nd permanents
3 years . .	3rd pair permanents	3rd permanent
3 years 6 months to 4 years.	4th pair permanents	. .

(3) Ranch Cattle

It is difficult to obtain statistics dealing with the eruption of molar teeth, but as these latter are only seldom referred to for the purpose of estimating age their periods of eruption are not so important practically. The following table is compiled

Time of Eruption.	Incisors.
Birth to 1 month .	All 8 temporary incisors.
2 years, or a little earlier	1st pair permanents.
2 years 6 months to 3 years	2nd ,, ,,
3 years 6 months .	3rd ,, ,,
4 years 6 months to 5 years	4th ,, ,,

from literature published by the United States Bureau of Animal Industry.

Smithfield Rules.—In Great Britain at most fat stock shows where the age of an animal is of some moment from a competitive point of view, there is a series of rules drawn up which governs inclusion or exclusion of animals in certain classes ; the rules concerning cattle are as follows :

1. Cattle having their *central permanent incisors cut* will be considered as exceeding 1 year 6 months.
2. Cattle having their *central permanent incisors fully up* will be considered as exceeding 1 year 9 months.
3. Cattle having their *second pair of permanent incisors fully up* will be considered as exceeding 2 years 3 months.
4. Cattle having their *third pair of permanent incisors cut* will be considered as exceeding 2 years 8 months.
5. Cattle having their *fourth pair* (*corner*) *permanent incisors fully up* and their *anterior molars showing signs of wear* will be considered as exceeding 3 years.

Some of these rules appear to indicate that the teeth erupt earlier than according to the tables given, but they apply especially to animals that have been reared and fed under a very intensive forcing system in preparation for fat stock shows, rather than to ordinary breeding or milking stock.

Appearance of teeth at various ages.—The same system as was followed in the case of the horse will be adhered to as applied to cattle.

At birth calves are usually found to have their 8 incisors of the temporary dentition either easily palpable below the soft gums, or the cutting edges of the teeth may be through the gums. The same remarks apply to the 3 temporary molars.

At 1 month, or sooner, the 8 temporary incisors have their crowns free from the gums and the teeth are quite prominent and well-defined. However, owing to the smallness of the jaw, they are overlapping each other to some extent. The 3 temporary molars are well up and wearing.

At 6 months the teeth are well placed in the now expanded jaw and are no longer overlapping. At this time the 4th molar is cut, but it is not usually entirely free from a membranous covering posteriorly until a little later.

At 1 year the most marked alteration between this time and 6 months is the wear of the temporary incisors. They are now situated in the jaw with spaces between them, and much of their expanded crowns have become worn away through attrition. Shortly after 1 year the 5th molar erupts.

At 1 year 3 months the 5th molar is generally well up and in wear, and the incisors are showing signs of still more wear.

At 1 year 9 months the 1st pair of permanent incisors replace the corresponding temporaries, and the 6th molar is cut.

At 2 years the 1st permanent incisors are well up and in full wear, and the 1st and 2nd permanent molars push out the temporaries and cut through the gums.

At 2 years 3 months the 2nd permanent incisors cut through the gum but are not yet in wear.

At 2 years 6 months an ox has 4 broad teeth (permanent incisors) all level and in wear.

At 2 years 9 months the 3rd pair of permanent incisors erupt, the temporaries often having fallen out some time previously. At the same time the 3rd permanent molar comes through the gum, but is not level with the other molars.

At 3 years the ox has 6 broad teeth all in wear and level with each other, and the molars present a uniform ridge when the fingers are run along their free edges.

At 3 years 3 months the last (corner) pair of incisors erupt. They may appear somewhat later than this time, but signs of their eruption will be seen.

At 3 years 6 months the incisor arcade is full, there are 8 broad teeth all level, but the corners are obviously younger and less worn than the others. There is generally some overlapping.

At 4 to 5 years the teeth are slightly worn along their cutting edges, and they occupy a less crowded position than earlier.

DENTITION

At about 6 years the surface of wear has reached practically half-way across the upper surfaces of the teeth, and a portion of the root is exposed.

At 10 years the greater part of the crowns have worn from the teeth and only a little cup-shaped piece of enamel remains.

At about 12 to 14 years only the stumps of the teeth remain. These are at first widely separated from each other, but by about 16 years they have become close together again.

Cattle seldom live longer than 15 or 16 years, and when they do their age is usually of no immediate importance. In the horned breeds of cattle a rough estimate of age can usually be made by counting the number of rings round the bases of the horns. The first ring appears at about 2 years, and thereafter one ring is added annually, so that the age in years of the ox = the number of rings plus two.

SHEEP.—The terms which were used as applied to cattle, and the description of the various teeth, may be taken to hold good for sheep as well. The sheep has 8 lower incisor teeth but none in the upper jaw. There are 24 molar teeth, 12 in each jaw, of which half these numbers are represented in the temporary dentition.

Eruption.—Except that the teeth appear sooner, the periods of eruption are comparatively like those in the ox. In the case of the improved breeds the teeth erupt much sooner than in coarser bred half-wild varieties, and so considerable allowances must be made when dealing with the sheep under different conditions. The following is given as an average eruption table for improved breeds of sheep in Great Britain :

Time of Eruption.	Incisors.	Molars.
Birth to 1 month	All 8 temporaries	All 12 temporaries.
3 months . .	..	4th permanent.
9 months . .	..	5th ,,
1 year to 1 year 3 months	1st pair permanent	..
1 year 6 months .	..	6th permanent.
1 ,, 9 ,,	2nd pair permanent	1st and 2nd permanents.
2 years . . .	..	3rd permanent.
2 years 3 months	3rd pair permanent	..
2 years 9 months to 3 years	4th pair permanent	..

Smithfield Rules.—There have been rules drawn up to apply to sheep as well as to cattle, for the purpose of classes at fat stock shows, etc. These are given below.

1. Sheep having their *central permanent incisors cut* will be considered as exceeding 10 months.

2. Sheep having their *central permanent incisors fully up* will be considered as exceeding 12 months.

3. Sheep having their *second pair of permanent incisors cut* will be considered as exceeding 19 months.

4. Sheep having their *third pair of permanent incisors fully up* and the *temporary molars shed* will be considered as exceeding 24 months.

5. Sheep having their *corner permanent incisors well up* and *showing marks of wear* will be considered as exceeding 3 years.

These rules apply to sheep that have been forced for fat stock show purposes, rather than to ordinary sheep.

Appearance of teeth at various ages.—*From birth to 1 year* the temporary incisors have been in use, and the mouth of the hogg at one year shows these lamb teeth well worn, while in many cases the 1st pair of permanent incisors (broad teeth) will be cutting.

At 1 year 3 months the 1st pair of broad teeth are cut or may be well up and in wear. Hill sheep, however, may not get their 1st pair until a little later.

At 1 year 9 months the 2nd pair of broad teeth are cut and come into wear about 2 to 3 months later.

At 2 years 3 months the 3rd pair of broad teeth are cut, or will be within the next 2 months. They are in wear by the time the sheep is 2 years 6 months to 2 years 8 months.

At 3 years to 3 years 3 months the 4th pair of broad teeth are cut and come into wear by 3 years 6 months. The sheep is now 'full-mouthed'. After this the age cannot be ascertained from an examination of the teeth, unless by experts who have observed the rate of wear in other sheep under similar circumstances.

PIG.—There is probably no farm animal which shows such variation in the eruption of its teeth as the pig, but because of the demand for young pigs for killing by weight and size rather than by age, and because of the intractability of older breeding animals—sows and boars—the actual age of the pig is not of such very great importance, except perhaps for fat stock show purposes.

When the *permanent teeth* have all erupted they are distributed as follows:

	Incisors.	Canines.	Molars.
Upper jaws	6	2	14 (*i.e.* 8 and 6)
Lower jaws	6	2	14 (*i.e.* 8 and 6)

In the molar region there is one little tooth in each of the four jaws, erupting at about 5 to 6 months, which is permanent from the very beginning. It is sometimes called *the premolar*, and in some cases is never developed. The next three teeth behind it are represented in the temporary dentition, the permanents replacing them in the usual way. The last three teeth are true molars; *i.e.* permanents only.

The *temporary dentition* is as follows:

	Incisors.	Canines.	Molars.
Upper jaws	6	2	6
Lower jaws	6	2	6

Incisors.—The upper incisors are small, and are separated from each other by spaces. The 1st pair (centrals) are the largest, and converge together. The 2nd pair are narrower and smaller; while the corner pair are very small and laterally flattened. The lower incisors are arranged in a convergent manner, and point forwards horizontally in the jaw. The 1st two pairs are large prismatic teeth deeply implanted in the jaw-bones and are used for 'rooting' purposes. The corner pair are smaller, and possess a distinct neck.

Canines, or *Tusks*, are greatly developed in the entire male, and both upper and lower tusks project out of the mouth. The upper canines of a boar may be 3 to 4 inches long, while the lower ones may reach as much as 8 inches in an aged animal. Each has a large permanent pulp cavity from which the tooth continues to grow throughout the animal's life.

Molars.—These become progressively larger from first to last. Typically, they have complex, tuberculated, short crowns, with distinct necks and roots, but the first three in the upper jaw, and the first four in the lower jaw, are laterally compressed and sectorial. This means that the first few teeth are used for cutting purposes, and the latter ones for grinding purposes.

Eruption.—Eruption of the pig's teeth is in many ways peculiar. The incisors do not erupt according to their position in the jaws: the corners erupt first; then the centrals, while the last to arrive are the laterals or 2nd pair. In the molar region the first tooth in each jaw immediately behind the canines comes in at about 6 months and remains for life, while the next three are represented in the milk dentition, the temporaries giving way to the permanent teeth in the usual way. The last three teeth in each jaw are normal permanent molars.

Smithfield Rules:

1. Pigs having their *corner permanent incisors cut* will be considered as exceeding 6 months.
2. Pigs having their *permanent tusks more than half-up* will be considered as exceeding 9 months.
3. Pigs having their *central permanent incisors up*, and any of the *first three permanent molars cut*, will be considered as exceeding 12 months.
4. Pigs having their *lateral temporary incisors shed* and the *permanents appearing* will be considered as exceeding 15 months.
5. Pigs having their *lateral permanent incisors fully up* will be considered as exceeding 18 months.

In spite of the above, many pigs will be encountered in which, for some reason not well understood, the teeth are cut at times widely different from those given.

Time of Eruption.	Incisors.	Canines.	Molars.
At birth .	Corner temporaries	All 4 temporaries	..
1 month .	Central temporaries	..	Nos. 2, 3 and 4 temporaries.
2 months .	Lateral	..	..
5-6 months .	..	..	No. 1, which remains through life, and No. 5 permanent.
8 months .	Corner permanents	..	..
9 months .	..	All 4 permanents	..
10-12 months	..	..	No. 6 permanent.
12-13 months	Central permanents	..	Nos. 2, 3 and 4 permanents.
17-18 months	Lateral permanents	..	No. 7 permanent.

Appearance of teeth at various ages.—*At birth* the little pig has two pairs of sharp-pointed teeth in each jaw, top and

bottom, placed so that there is a distinct space between each pair. These are the two temporary tusks and the two temporary corner incisors. These are the only teeth present in the gums, though the temporary molars, Nos. 2, 3, and 4, can be felt below the gums.

At 1 month, or sometimes a little sooner, the two central incisors, which are broader than the laterals and tusks, are cut, and the three molars above mentioned come through the gums.

At 2 months the temporary central incisors are fully up and there are signs of the eruption of the laterals.

At 3 months the lateral temporary incisors are well up, and the temporary molars are well in wear.

At 5 months there are signs of the cutting of the premolars (*i.e.* the No. 1 molars), and the 5th molar (a permanent) is seen behind the temporaries. It is, however, not yet in wear.

At 6 months the premolars are cut and the 5th permanent molar is in wear.

At 7 to 8 months there are signs of the cutting of the corner permanent incisors, or they may already be through the gums. The permanent tusks are also often cutting through the gums at this age in forward animals.

At 9 months the corner permanent incisors are well up and the permanent tusks are through the gums, although in many cases there may be still one or two of the small temporary tusks in position. Where they are cut they are not far through the gums.

At 1 year it is generally held that the central permanent incisors cut through the gums, but there are a large number of animals which do not cut these teeth till about 13 months old. The 6th permanent molar cuts at this time, and is more reliable than the incisors for reference.

Shortly after 1 year the three temporary molars fall out and their places are taken by the permanents. They are into line with the other molar teeth 3 months later.

At 17 to 18 months, when the final changes occur, the 7th molar, the last permanent molar tooth, and the lateral permanent incisors, are cut through the gums. By this time the pig has obtained its full permanent dentition, and the succeeding changes are not sufficiently reliable to warrant estimations of age being based upon them. Great variation in the hardness or softness of the teeth is seen, and subsequently the rate of wear is irregular. In addition to this a great deal depends upon the nature of the food, whether the pigs are kept in the open where they are allowed to root, and whether the jaws meet each other with accuracy.

DOG.—Many attempts have been made to draw up a table which will roughly indicate the age of the dog as evidenced by its teeth, but owing to the very great variations in the size, rate of maturity, and shape of the skulls of present-day breeds of dogs there is no method of judging the age with accuracy. At birth the jaws of the puppy contain no teeth. From 3 to 4 weeks the temporary canines erupt and at 4 to 5 weeks the temporary incisors and the first three temporary cheek teeth erupt. About 4 months of age will generally show the eruption of the permanent premolar, and soon afterwards the fourth cheek tooth erupts. In the toy breeds, the permanent canines may appear at this time and sometimes they show before the premolar. In other dogs, the permanent canines appear at about 5 to 6 months and the corner incisors as well as the first three permanent cheek teeth erupt. The fifth cheek tooth shows very soon afterwards, and the sixth, often absent in the top jaw, shows at 6 to 8 months.

At 1 year the incisors are all in wear but they still retain their triple crown (called the 'fleur-de-lys'). By 2 years this is wearing off, or may have already disappeared. At about 4 years the cutting edges of the incisors in upper and lower jaws show a line of wear but the amount of wear depends on the shape of the jaws and the kind of food eaten.

DEPILATION (*de*, from; *pilo*, I make bald) means the process of the destruction of hair that takes place during certain skin or other diseases, or after the application of chemical or thermal substances to the surface of the body. (*See* MANGE, RINGWORM, BALDNESS, BURNS, etc.)

DEPLUMING SCABIES is a form of parasitic mange affecting the fowl, in which the feathers are eaten through close to the skin surface and fall off or break off. It is best treated with a Gammexane preparation. (*See* PARASITES, p. 691.)

'DEPRAVED APPETITE' (*see under* APPETITE).

DEPRESSOR is the name given to a nerve by stimulation of which secretion, or some other function is restrained or prevented, *e.g.* the depressor nerve of the heart slows the beating of this organ.

DERMATITIS (δέρμα, skin) means any inflammation of the skin, but is usually reserved for those cases when there is some accompanying irritation. (*See* SKIN.)

DERMATOSIS VEGETANS.—A hereditary disease of young pigs characterised by raised skin lesions, abnormalities of the hooves, and pneumonia. The semi-lethal recessive gene probably originated in the Danish Landrace. U.K. outbreaks occurred in 1958, 1964.

DERMOID CYST is one of the commonest of the teratomatous tumours. It consists usually of a spherical mass with a surrounding envelope of skin. In this there are sebaceous glands and hair follicles from which grow long hairs. These, together with shed cells, sebaceous material, form the central part of the mass.

They develop subcutaneously in various situations, and are also found in ovary or testicle. They arise through the inclusion in other tissues of a piece of embryonic skin, which continues to grow and produces hair, etc., just as does skin on the surface of the body. Owing to the cystic structure (*i.e.* the cavity being a closed one) there is no means of getting rid of shed hair, debris, etc., and these substances accumulating in the centre cause the cyst to continue slowly increasing in size.

A dermoid sinus is a common congenital abnormality of the Rhodesian Ridgeback dog.

Treatment.—No local treatment is of benefit. Surgical removal of the cyst wall and its contents, with the necessary means to obliterate the cavity, is desirable with subcutaneous dermoid cysts.

DERRINGUE.—The Mexican name for vampire-bat rabies.

DERRIS.—The powder, obtained by grinding the root of a South American plant, is a valuable parasiticide, useful against warbles, fleas, and lice. It will not kill the nits of the latter, however, and hence the dressing must be repeated. Against fleas and lice it can be used as a constituent of a dusting powder, or with soap and warm water as a wet shampoo. It is safe for cats (compare DDT) provided the normal precautions against licking are taken—*i.e.* the bulk of the powder is brushed out of the coat after 10 minutes or so, during which licking is prevented—but must be used with caution on young kittens.

Derris is highly poisonous to fish—a fact which must be borne in mind when disposing of the powder or solutions in circumstances which could lead to river pollution.

DESOXYRIBONUCLEIC ACID (*see under* ARTIFICIAL SOMATIC MUTATIONS).

DESQUAMATION (*de*, away; *squama*, a scale) means the scaling off of the superficial layers of the skin, and is applied to the peeling process that accompanies some forms of mange and ringworm, as well as to the state of the skin in dry eczema.

DESTRUCTION OF ANIMALS.—It becomes necessary for the owners of animals to destroy them upon occasion, when they are unable to secure an expert's services. It is necessary for such owners to have a correct knowledge of how to kill with a minimum of pain and suffering. Many animals are destroyed each year in a barbarous and inhuman manner, such as is a disgrace to a civilised community, not perhaps through any intention to be cruel, but rather through ignorance. The most humane agent of destruction is the firearm correctly used. Special 'humane killers' are upon the market in most countries, which are easy to use, clean, reliable, and which inflict instantaneous death, and these should be used whenever possible in preference to sporting guns, rifles, or revolvers. Instructions are given with each. Some employ a free bullet, others have a captive bolt. For horses and cattle the point aimed at is *not* in the middle of the forehead, between the eyes; a shot so placed passes into the nasal chambers or air sinuses, down into the mouth and throat, and misses the important vital centres. The correct spot is higher up than this. Two imaginary lines should be drawn, each running from one eye to the opposite ear across the front of the forehead, and the point of their intersection is the most vital spot. A shot aimed about parallel with the ground and directed at this spot enters the brain cavity, destroys the brain and the beginning of the spinal cord, and passes on into the neck, where its energy is expended. Otherwise, if for some reason this part is not accessible, the next best place to aim at is the base of one ear, the direction being again parallel with the ground. In the case of horned cattle, the presence of the horn may deflect the shot, and in them it is better to shoot into the base of the brain from behind, directing the charge downwards and forwards. When pigs have to be shot the middle line of the head is not altogether the best place, because there is a strong crest of bone running downwards in this position; the shot should be placed a little above and a little nearer the centre of the skull than the eye. For dogs and cats the centre of the forehead should be aimed at, for in these animals the brain is of relatively larger size, and more easily accessible.

Where firearms are not immediately available it is better to send for them and await their arrival in the case of the larger animals, and to use other methods for the dog and cat. Prussic acid is a violent poison, and is now not considered advisable for use unless no other agent is available. Lethal chambers have been much employed for destroying small animals such as dogs and cats, either by means of chloroform, coal-gas, or by electrocution.

The use of nembutal by intravenous injections has become a common method of destroying small animals by veterinary surgeons. This substance is used for anæsthesia before operation in graduated amounts. Larger amounts are needed to produce death. (*See also* STUNNING, ELECTRIC; and CARBON DIOXIDE ANÆSTHESIA, which is used for pigs.)

A flock of 2500 adult turkeys—affected with ornithosis—were painlessly destroyed within ten minutes by piping car exhaust fumes into two long pits covered with polythene sheeting. There was no excitement or struggling after the birds had been driven into the pits.

DESTRUCTION OF BIRDS.—For the destruction of poultry and other birds a lidless wooden box or chamber (of a size to take a polypropylene poultry crate) and a cylinder of carbon dioxide with regulating valve are useful. The box has a $\frac{1}{2}$-inch copper pipe, drilled with $\frac{9}{64}$-in. holes at 4 in. centres fitted at levels of 2 in. and 2 ft. 2 in. from the bottom and connected by plastic tubing to the regulator valve of the cylinder.

The chamber is filled with carbon dioxide to within 1 foot of the top. This is achieved by allowing the gas to flow until a lighted match held at this level is extinguished. The crate containing birds up to a weight of 45 lb. is hoisted by block and tackle, and after the chamber has been moved underneath the crate is lowered into the chamber and moved up and down through a distance of 6 to 12 inches to help displace any air pockets between the birds and the feathers. The birds become anæsthetised within 30 to 45 seconds and a very small amount of flapping which may occur is inhibited within a minute. To ensure that all birds are killed before the crate is removed it is necessary to allow five minutes to elapse from the time the crate enters the chamber. When the birds have been in the chamber for two minutes, more carbon dioxide is introduced into the chamber for 30 to 45 seconds to replace the gas which has been used for destruction. It has been observed that even though the chamber is filled with gas initially, the time taken for destruction of the first crate of birds is at least 50 per cent longer than that for the second and subsequent crates. On removal of the crate the birds are laid on the floor to allow a check to be made that all are dead.

This technique may be modified for the destruction of single adult birds or small numbers of young chicks by placing the birds in a clear polythene bag (preferably 500 gauge) and then filling the bag with carbon dioxide. A rubber band placed about the neck of the bag prevents the gas from escaping.

DETERGENTS (*detergo*, I cleanse) are substances which cleanse, and many are among the best wetting agents (*i.e.* substances which lower the surface tension of water and cause it to spread over a surface rather than remain in droplet form). Detergents include soap, washing soda, and many new synthetic compounds analogous to soap but derived from alkalies and petroleum rather than from alkalies and vegetable or mineral oils. Disinfection of food vessels, milk pails, etc., requires the use of detergents as well as disinfectant solutions or the application of steam. Examples of detergents are cetrimide and sodium lauryl sulphate.

DETERGENT RESIDUE in syringes used for spinal injections have caused serious demyelinating complications in humans. Similarly, an unrinsed ' spinal outfit ' has led to paraplegia in a dog.

DETTOL.—A proprietary non-toxic antiseptic of much value for skin lesions and obstetrical work. (*See under* ANTISEPTICS.)

DEW-CLAWS in cattle are sometimes torn off or injured by slatted floors. For dew-claws in dogs (*see* NAILS).

DEXTRAN.—A plasma substitute, for use in transfusion instead of whole blood in cases of severe hæmorrhage, etc.

DEXTRAN SULPHATE.—An alternative anticoagulant to Heparin, longer lasting in its effects.

DEXTRIN (*dexter*, right) is a soluble carbohydrate substance into which starch is converted by diastatic ferment or by dilute acids. It is a white or yellowish powder which, dissolved in water, forms mucilage. Animal dextrin, or glycogen, is a carbohydrate stored in the liver.

DEXTROSE is another name for purified grape sugar or glucose.

DIABETES INSIPIDUS, or **POLYURIA,** is a condition in which there is secreted an excessively large quantity of urine of low specific gravity. It usually occurs in horses through the eating of mouldy or damaged hay or other food-stuff, and passes off when this is discontinued. It may occur in dogs as a result of fright; symptoms including poor appetite, dull coat, and frequent urinating in the house. This may persist and require treatment, *e.g.* with pitressin tannate in oil. Feeding in the mornings only may prevent urine being passed in the house at night. (*See Vet. Record* April 25, 1964.) (*See* URINE, sub-heading ' Polyuria '.)

DIABETES MELLITUS, or **GLYCOSURIA,** is a condition in which an excess of sugar (glucose) is found in the urine. A small amount of sugar may be present in the urine without indicating serious disturbance, but when there is a large amount of water and a permanent excess of sugar, it is an indication of a serious disturbance of carbohydrate metabolism.

Cause.—Pancreatic disease in which insulin (a hormone produced by the islets of Langerhans) is deficient. Recent medical research suggests that the disease may be due not necessarily to a deficiency of insulin but to an excess of insulin-antagonist circulating in the bloodstream. (*See also under* KETOSIS.)

The function of insulin, whether produced normally from the pancreas or injected subcutaneously, is to enable proper use to be made of the sugar circulating in the blood-stream and to prevent its passage into the urine, whereby it is wasted. The chemical details involved are very complex.

Diabetes is commoner in females than in males, and in hot countries than in temperate or cold countries.

Treatment with an excessive dosage of cortisone or other steroids may give rise to diabetes.

In human medicine, viruses are now believed to be among the causes of damage to the islets of Langerhans. It was pointed out in the *Lancet* (Oct. 9, 1971) that mumps is a well recognised cause of inflammation of the pancreas, and that it may be followed by diabetes. ' However, mumps pancreatitis is rare and diabetes is relatively common. Other viruses have come under suspicion, especially some of the picornaviruses. These include foot-and-mouth disease virus, but of the picornaviruses commonly infecting man the Coxsackie group, and in particular Coxsackie–B4, appears to be linked with inflammation of the pancreas leading to diabetes.

It should be mentioned that a temporary presence of sugar in the urine, due to a metabolic disorder, involving liver and other tissues, is encountered from time to time in the course of fevered conditions some forms of poisoning or overdosage with chloroform, chloral or morphine, and when excessive amounts of sugars or starchy foods have been eaten. These cases return to normal with recovery from the exciting cause.

Symptoms.—These are vague. The affected animal, usually a dog, develops an excessive thirst, and passes larger quantities of urine than normally. Its appetite remains good, but its condition wastes. The abdomen becomes pendulous and dropsical ; there is occasional vomiting ; a cataract may develop in one or each eye ; and sluggishness in an otherwise active animal is noticed.

In all cases an examination of the urine shows the presence of large amounts of sugar, perhaps as much as 0·4 per cent or 0·5 per cent being present, three or four times the normal amounts.

Treatment.—The only effective method of treatment is the injection of *insulin*, at regular intervals for the rest of the animal's life, and attention to the diet. This is a matter which must be undertaken with expert supervision.

Unexpectedly, cats tolerate the daily injections well and owners find the routine easy. The dosage range is less variable than in the dog since bodyweight in the cat is so much more uniform ; stabilisation is often achieved in the range 5 to 10 units daily. Long-acting insulins are prone to cause hypoglycæmic crises hence zinc suspension insulin or protamine zinc insulin are recommended. Prognosis is more favourable than in dogs. Survival periods of six and seven years are known in patients which became diabetic at 9–10 years of age. (British Veterinary Association, 1968.)

DIAGNOSIS (διάγνωσις) is the art of distinguishing one disease from another, and is essential to successful and scientific (as distinct from empirical) treatment. The name is also given to the opinion arrived at as to the nature of a certain disease. It is in diagnosis that scientific skill is tested to its greatest capacity, and particularly in that branch concerned with the diagnosis of the troubles of animals and small children. Very often a diagnosis cannot be given at once, for the history of the case, the influence of ancestors, as well as the seat of the illness, and other relevant information, cannot be obtained when the case is first seen. It is obvious that where the patient—human or veterinary—is unable to give any informative assistance with regard to the pain felt, the actual duration of the illness, any previous complaints, the symptoms exhibited, or other necessary information, it is extremely difficult, and in some cases quite impossible, to form an opinion as to the cause of the trouble or to say with certainty exactly what the trouble is. Certain instruments are used for diagnostic purposes, the chief of which are the clinical thermometer, used for registering the temperature, the stethoscope, used for listening to the sounds of the internal organs (heart and lungs particularly), and for special parts there are ophthalmoscopes for the eye, auroscopes for the ears, œsophagoscopes for viewing the œsophagus, laryngoscopes for examining the throat, urethroscopes for looking at the urethra and the bladder, and specula for use in other parts of the body. The use of X-rays to illuminate the outlines of bones and dense tissues, especially in the dog and the limbs or head of horses, has made great progress during recent years and for some conditions has become almost a routine. Other uses of electricity, such as the electric cardiograph, are as yet not widely employed but have potentially an important place in future.

Very great advances have been made in the use of laboratory techniques for diagnosis of disease in animals. Microscopic examinations of tissues, body fluids or discharges, for abnormal cells or bacteria ; the inoculation of materials from diseased animals into special culture media, or into test animals ; the submission of blood, urine, saliva, milk, or the contents of abdominal organs, or various body tissues to chemical or biochemical analysis ; and the use of biological diagnostic agents, such as tuberculin, mallein, johnin, are regularly and extensively employed now as most valuable aids to diagnosis. Veterinary science is now enabled to exert a far greater influence on disease control and eradication than formerly.

DIAMOND SHOE is a shoe for horses which forge with their hind-feet. It is made in the outline of a conventional playing-card diamond, with the lower point cut off. At the toe of the shoe there is a point and on either side the iron is reduced. The shoe is fitted to the hind-foot so that there is less iron to strike against the shoe of the fore-foot just as the latter is leaving the ground.

DIAPHORESIS (*διά*, through ; *φορέω*, I carry) is another name for the process of perspiring. (*See* PERSPIRATION.)

DIAPHORETICS (from *διαφορέω*, I carry through) are remedies which promote perspiration.

DIAPHRAGM (*διάφραγμα*) is the name of the muscular and tendinous structure which separates the chest from the abdominal cavity in mammals. It is an important organ in respiration. (*See* MUSCLES.)

DIAPHRAGMATOCELE means a rupture in the diaphragm through which some of the abdominal organs, often the small intestine, stomach, and perhaps spleen and liver, have obtruded themselves, so that they become situated actually within the chest cavity. It occurs during falls, when jumping from a great height, and sometimes in cats and dogs during fighting. The breathing becomes very much disturbed and the animal usually shows an inclination to assume an upright position, whereby the organs are encouraged to return to the abdominal cavity and pressure on the lungs is relieved. Treatment by surgical means has occasionally been effected in the dog. (*See* THORACOTOMY.)

DIARRHŒA (*διαρρέω*, I flow away), or looseness of the bowels, when at all protracted, is a most serious condition.

Varieties and causes.—Diarrhœa is one of the chief symptoms of several serious diseases.

As a rule, whenever there is diarrhœa in existence for more than 3 or 4 days, loss of condition is very marked, for the absorptive functions of the bowels are interfered with, and dehydration occurs.

Catarrhal diarrhœa is the ordinary form in which the mucous membrane of the alimentary canal, and especially of the later parts of the intestine, is in a condition not unlike the condition of swelling and congestion which occurs in the nasal mucous membranes during a ' cold in the head ', and secretes a clear, viscid mucus of a similar nature. This mucus mixes with the contents of the alimentary canal and makes the whole fluid. It is produced by slight temporary disturbances, such as the taking of indigestible food, especially by young animals, nervous excitement, or it may be caused by a chill.

Occasionally it is set up by ingestion of irritant poisons of an inorganic nature, such as salts of arsenic or mercury. In this form it is a common symptom of enteritis, in which there is an inflammation of the bowel wall. Changes of food which are made suddenly are liable to set up a rather serious form of catarrhal diarrhœa for a few days, *i.e.* until the bowels can accommodate themselves to the new kind of food, and until the different bacterial forms of life, which are essential to the digestion, can assert themselves. *Other forms* of diarrhœa result from causes so diverse as infection with tuberculosis in some part of the bowel wall ; the presence of parasites such as worms, flukes, or coccidiæ ; infection with specific diseases, such as Johne's disease, lamb dysentery, white scour, etc. ; or the excessive action of purgatives given in too large doses. In all of these instances there are other symptoms which help in the diagnosis of the condition, and an examination of the diarrhœic material will often show the presence of the agent responsible.

Treatment.—The treatment of diarrhœa

from causes which are specific, is dealt with under these headings.

Chlorodyne, Dover's powder, chalk and opium powder, are useful.

(For adult cattle, *see* SCOURS, GRUEL.)

If diarrhœa persists, the mere withdrawal of large amounts of fluid from the body may itself become serious, and it becomes essential to replace this fluid. (*See under* DEHYDRATION.)

Various antiseptics like sulphaguanidine, salol, salicylate of bismuth, carbonate of bismuth, dimol, or brilliant green may be given. Irrigation of the bowel with warm saline is useful in some cases of severe diarrhœa in puppies.

In the dog, diarrhœa may be associated with distemper, toxoplasmosis, lead-poisoning, nocardiosis, kidney failure; occasionally with pyometra, with allergies; tumours, intussception.

Whenever an apparently simple diarrhœa lasts for more than 1 or 2 days in an animal it is wise to seek skilled advice rather than attempt what must at best be only empirical treatment. The temperature is a useful guide to the severity of the condition, especially in young animals such as foals and puppies, and in all cases where it is high it is an indication that there is some serious condition complicating the diarrhœa which demands immediate attention. (*See also under* SCOURS; *and* ANTIBIOTIC SUPPLEMENTS.)

DIASTASIS (διάστασις, separation) is a term applied to separation of the end of a growing bone from the shaft. The condition resembles fracture, but is more serious because of the damage done to the growing cartilage through which the separation takes place, so that the future growth of the bone is prejudiced.

DIASTOLE (διαστολή) means the relaxation of a hollow organ. The term is applied in particular to the heart, to indicate the resting period that occurs between the beats (systoles) while the blood is flowing into the organ.

DIATHERMY (διά, through; θέρμη, heat) is a process by which electric currents can be passed into the deeper parts of the body so as to produce internal warmth and relieve pain, or, by using powerful currents, to destroy tumours and diseased parts bloodlessly. The use of short-wave therapy is gaining ground in the treatment of muscle, tendon, and ligament strains. In horses with, *e.g.*, flexor tendon trouble 20-minute treatments over a period of a week are often effective—more so than the old blistering and firing which are thereby obviated.

DIATHESIS (διάθεσις, a disposition) is another name for constitution.

DIAZINON.—An anti-tick organo-phosphorus compound.

DICHLOROPHEN.—A drug of value against tapeworms in the dog. Dichlorophen ointment and a spray preparation have been used in the treatment of ringworm in cattle.

DICHLORVOS.—A parasiticide used against fowl mites on laying hens and turkeys. Strips of resin impregnated with dichlorvos have been used successfully for the control of dog fleas by attachment to the dog's collar, over a period of three months or so.

DICOUMARIN. — An anti-blood-coagulant; the precursor of WARFARIN.

DICROTIC (δίς, double; κρότος, a stroke) pulse is one in which at each heart-beat two impulses are felt by the finger that is taking the pulse. A dicrotic wave is normally present in a tracing of a pulse as recorded by special instruments for the purpose, but in health it is imperceptible to the finger. A dicrotic pulse is present in fevers when there is a nervous prostration; the heart beats fiercely but the smaller blood-vessels have lost their tone, and do not expand and contract normally. This form of pulse is met with in the horse particularly, but also recognised in the dog.

DIELDRIN.—An insecticide of particular value against the maggot-fly of sheep. Dieldrin is claimed to be ten times more powerful than DDT and also more lasting in its effects. Dieldrin is highly poisonous to birds, and fish. The symptoms of Dieldrin poisoning in foxes (which have eaten poisoned birds) are stated to resemble closely those of Fox Encephalitis. Dogs and cats have been poisoned similarly. (*See* CHLORINATED HYDROCARBONS.) Dieldrin has been suspected as a cause of infertility in sheep, and residues in the fat may be a danger to people eating the mutton or lamb. The use of dieldrin sheep dips was banned in the U.K. in 1965, following similar bans in Australia and New Zealand.

DIET AND DIETETICS

DIET and DIETETICS.—It may be taken for granted that the most important part of animal husbandry is sound feeding of the animals. This is not by any means, as might be supposed, a simple matter.

In order fully to understand rational feeding, the stock-owner must be conversant with the various food constituents and what part they play in the body, he must have an idea of the composition of the many foods that are available to him, and he must know how to make the best use of them. He should never under-rate *the importance of palatability*.

COMPOSITION OF FOODS.—By ordinary chemical analysis foods can be split up and separated into what are sometimes called their *proximate principles*; these proximate principles or constituents are: water, proteins (albuminoids), fats or oils, soluble carbohydrates, crude fibre or insoluble carbohydrates, and ash. In addition to these there are vitamins.

Water.—Water, as an essential need for live-stock, has been discussed under the appropriate heading (*see* WATER). All foods contain a certain percentage of water. It is found in greatest amount in roots, succulents, such as cabbages and kale, wet brewers' grains, silage, and pasture grasses, which contain from 75 to 90 per cent. Cereal grains, such as wheat, oats, barley, etc., average 11 per cent. Meadow grass yields from 70 to 80 per cent of water, but when it is air-dried and made into hay under favourable circumstances, this is reduced to 12 or 14 per cent.

Carbohydrates.—The carbohydrates in foods are divisible into two groups, the *crude fibre*, and the *soluble carbohydrates*. The crude fibre is the less digestible part of the carbohydrate, and its quantity in the food determines if the food is to be classed as a *concentrated food* or as a *coarse fodder*, those foods which contain less than 15 to 20 per cent of fibre being classed as concentrated, and those which contain more than 20 per cent as coarse foods. A concentrated food is one which contains much than 20 per cent as coarse foods.

Oats contain 10 per cent of fibre, and hay and wheat straw 25 per cent and 40 per cent respectively.

Crude fibre is a mixture of celluloses, lignin, cutin, and some pentosans, etc. While it is cheapest of all food materials, it is nevertheless an indispensable constituent of all properly balanced rations. Cellulose is the material that forms the cell-wall of plants. In its simplest form it is easily digested, but with the growth of the plant cellulose becomes associated with *lignin*, which gives stiffness to the parts of the plant requiring support, and also *cutin*, which is a waterproofing material. Cotton, wood, flax, etc., are all modified forms of cellulose.

The carbohydrates are made up of carbon, hydrogen, and oxygen. Foods containing much carbohydrate are called carbonaceous foods; for example, the cereal grains, potatoes, molasses, etc. The cereals contain from 60 to 70 per cent of carbohydrate. The simplest of the carbohydrates, such as the simple sugars, are absorbed directly from the gut, while the more complex sugars, and still more complex starches, have to be reduced by processes of digestion to more simple forms before they can be absorbed and be of use to the body. Starch is one of the chief forms in which food is given to animals.

Fats or Oils.—Fat is present in all foods, but the quantity varies greatly; thus in hay there is 3 per cent, in turnips there is 0·2 per cent, in cereals from 2 to 6 per cent, and in linseed as much as 40 per cent, while linseed cake, from which most of the fat has been expressed, contains on an average rather less than 10 per cent. In meals produced from fat rich foods such as cotton seed or linseed, by extraction with a solvent, all the oil except some 1 or 2 per cent is removed. The fats are compounds of glycerine with various fatty acids such as stearic acid, palmitic, and oleic.

Cakes and other foods in which the fat has gone rancid are dangerous for animals, and often cause diarrhœa. (*See* COD-LIVER OIL POISONING.)

Proteins.—The proteins or albuminoids in a food differ from the other constituents we have considered, in that in addition to having carbon, hydrogen, and oxygen in their composition, they also contain nitrogen and usually sulphur and sometimes phosphorus. They are very complex substances, and are made up of a number of much simpler bodies called *amino-acids*. (*See under that heading*.) The practical importance of all this to the stock-owner is that he feeds his animals on a mixed diet, so making sure that the animals will get the amino-acids from the various proteins that they may require.

Mineral matter or ash.—The mineral matter in a food is sometimes called its *inorganic* constituent, to distinguish it from the foregoing organic constituents. The mineral matter, like the other constituents, is taken into the plant through the roots from the soil; and as the soil differs in its mineral character in different localities, so will the mineral content of the herbage vary in character and quantity. Individual plants also have their own mineral peculiarities; for example, the leguminous plants are rich in calcium which is so necessary for animals; other foods, such as maize, are deficient in calcium, but contain phosphorus; while others again, such as the wheat offals, have an unbalanced mineral content.

Vitamins (*see under that heading*).

FUNCTION OF FOOD CONSTITUENTS.—All the constituents of foods above mentioned play an important part in nourishing the animal, and the secret of success in animal rearing and feeding lies in giving these substances not only in sufficient quantity but also in proper proportion. It is important that the stock-owner should know of what use these food elements are to the body.

Carbohydrates.—The carbohydrates are chiefly utilised for the production of energy and heat, and what is not required for immediate use is stored as fat, which is to be regarded as a reserve store of energy. It is the carbohydrates which are mainly used for the peposition of fat when animals are fattened.

Fibre.—A certain amount of crude fibre is necessary in the diet of all animals except those under 3½ weeks of age, when all young domesticated animals are on a fluid diet and most are supported solely by sucking. If animals, especially herbivorous animals, are given insufficient fibre they fail to thrive, are restless and uncomfortable, and every cattle-feeder knows that without 'bulk' to the ration the animals do not do well.

Adequate fibre is necessary to cattle for proper muscular activity of the whole digestive system. Secondly, the proportion of fibre in the diet has an important bearing upon the actual digestion done by living organisms within the rumen. Thirdly, a high-protein and low-fibre intake may lead to bloat. Fourthly, adequate fibre is necessary in the cow's rations if she is to give a high yield of butterfat and solids-not-fat.

On the other hand, if too much fibre is given in the ration the animals cannot digest enough food to get sufficient nutriment. This is the reason why wheat straw would be a very bad food for hard-working horses. Ruminants make the most use of fibre, then horses, pigs, and dogs, in the order given. Fattening pigs, though requiring a certain amount of fibre, must have the allowance strictly limited, though sows and boars can do with more.

Fat.—The fat that is digested and absorbed may be oxidised to form energy direct, or it may be built up to form body fat. Speaking generally, fat has two and a half times the value of carbohydrates or protein as energy producer. While a certain amount of fat is desirable, indeed necessary, in the daily diet of animals, an excessive amount does harm. For proper utilisation by the body, the fats have to oxidise fully; where too much fat is taken in the food, this oxidation does not proceed fully and a series of harmful substances, called ketones, accumulate in the system.

Protein.—Protein is the only constituent in a food that can be used to build up muscle or make good the wear and tear of muscular tissue. Animals are frequently expected to subsist on a diet deficient in protein: a not uncommon cause of infertility. If they are given too little the body draws on the protein of the muscles and the animals fail to remain in good health. If given too much there is undue strain on the kidneys, and also if there is a large amount of protein undergoing decomposition in the intestines it acts as an intestinal irritant, thus causing diarrhœa and may lead to the reabsorption of toxic substances into the blood-stream. (*See also* ANIMAL PROTEIN FACTOR WINTER DIET.)

Mineral matter.—Mineral matter is absolutely essential for the well-being of the animal. It is required for building up

DIET AND DIETETICS

bone in the growing animal, and it is required in solution in the blood and in the tissue fluids. Among other important duties it controls very largely the rate of absorption of the digested nutrients from the intestines. If too little of any mineral is given in the food the body draws its supply from the bones and tissues, and the same thing takes place if too much of one mineral is given and too little of another. The mineral matter in food plays a very important part in maintaining health and good growth in young animals. Animals growing quickly, such as chicks, puppies, and pigs, and cows giving large quantities of milk, are most likely to suffer from mineral insufficiency, and it is certain that they often do. This is particularly the case when pigs are fed on wheat offals which are notably deficient in calcium, without being given some compensating food such as fish-meal or meat- and bone-meal or steamed bone flour. (*See also* MINERALS; TRACE ELEMENTS; OSTEOFIBROSIS.)

Vitamins are discussed elsewhere; for information on these important substances, see, therefore, VITAMINS.

ANTIBIOTIC SUPPLEMENTS (*see under this heading*).

GENERAL PRINCIPLES OF FEEDING.—A well-balanced ration is one that contains all the nutriments, and these in proper ratio the one to the other, that the particular animal may require. Each class of animal, and each animal in particular, requires its own particular diet; there is no such thing as a well-balanced ration suitable for all animals and all needs. Every stock-owner knows in general that a store bullock requires a diet that would not be suitable for a cow giving four gallons of milk a day; that an idle horse will not be suitably served with a diet that would do for a heavy draught animal drawing a heavy load at a slow rate, and that the diet for this horse will not be suitable for a hunter.

In order that the stock-owner may make the best use of the many foods that are at his disposal he should obtain a copy of *Rations for Live Stock*, issued by the Ministry of Agriculture and Fisheries. Since only those parts of a food that are digestible are of use to the body, the tables also give the percentages of each constituent digested. Knowledge of the degree to which various foods are digested by different animals and under different conditions of combining foods is limited, so that most of the figures given in published tables are only strictly applicable to cattle.

Standards of feeding and published figures of digestible constituents in foods should be used rather as guides than as definite formulæ.

Work at the Hannah Dairy Research Institute by Dr. K. L. Blaxter and his colleagues suggests that long-accepted standards (based on work more than half a century old) need revision. 'We tend to overfeed the low-producing cow, and underfeed the high yielder,' he says.

Regularity in the times of feeding is essential for success. Only good quality food should be used; there is no economy in feeding with inferior or damaged fodder; on the contrary, the use of such food has been the cause of much illness. There should not be long intervals between meals; with horses this is one of the common causes of colic. When compounding a ration it should be remembered that a mixture of foods gives a better result than the use of one or two foods. The ration should contain a sufficiency of energy-producing constituents, sufficient protein, fibre, and mineral matter, and an adequate allowance of food rich in vitamins. The proportion of the various constituents the one to the other has also to be studied. (*See* CONCENTRATES.)

THE DIGESTIBILITY OF FOODS.—Only that part of a food which is digested is of value to an animal. The digestibility of foods varies greatly, some being easily and completely digested, while others, especially those containing much fibre, are digested imperfectly and with difficulty; and, of course, some animals will digest a particular food better than other animals will. The method of feeding is important; if it is erratic instead of at regular intervals the food will not be so well digested as when the feeding hours are regular.

An over-tired horse should be given a small feed after it has been watered and then left for a couple of hours, when it may with safety be given more.

It is a great mistake to give an overworked animal or an animal which has been kept short of food, as after a long train journey, an extra large feed; it should invariably be given less than the usual feed, not more.

PREPARATION OF FOODS.—Some foods are fed to animals in the natural state, while others are prepared in some such way as by grinding, bruising, cutting, chaffing, boiling, steaming, or soaking in water. The object of preparing a food before giving it to an animal is to increase its digestibility. Oats may be bruised for hard-working horses, for colts changing their teeth, and for calves; there is undoubtedly a slight increase in the digestibility of bruised over whole grain, but for an economic advantage the total cost of bruising should be less than 10 per cent of the whole grain. Beans should be split or 'kibbled' for horses, as the tough seed-coat makes them difficult to masticate. Maize also is more easily eaten if it is cracked.

It is important to remember that bruised or kibbled seeds do not keep well, especially if exposed to a damp atmosphere, and are liable to turn musty, owing to fermentation changes. A very important principle is involved in crushing, kibbling, bruising, etc., which stockowners should fully appreciate. So long as the grain is whole and intact it is essentially still a living entity. When crushed, etc., it is killed, and in common with all dead things, the enzymes are quite uncontrolled and so the normal processes of deterioration and decomposition commence.

Grinding grains to a meal is advisable for pigs, **but it is important that the particle size is not too small.** Absence of milk in the recently farrowed sow and bowel œdema may, it has been suggested (*Veterinary Record*, April 3, 1971), be associated with too fine meal particles.

PALATABILITY.—It is important that foods offered to animals should be palatable and appetising. Some foods are not very palatable, such as palm kernel cake or meal, but may be made more palatable by mixing with some molasses or locust bean meal. On the other hand, foods which are naturally palatable may become very unappetising if they have been allowed to get damp and musty. The inclusion of even a small quantity of musty food—such as foxy oats and mouldy hay—in a ration spoils the whole food. The greatest care should be taken to see that the food is fresh and wholesome and that food-troughs and water-troughs are kept clean.

VARIETY AND MIXTURES.—Animals benefit from variety in their rations. It is often found that while a given ration may give excellent results for a time, there is a tendency for animals to eat their food without zest. This applies less to pigs and horses than to cattle, sheep, poultry, dogs, and cats. A change, which may be quite simple, results in a return of the normal zest.

Also, as a rule, mixtures of several different foods are more palatable and are better digested than single food-stuffs. This is partly because during digestion foods of different origins actually assist to digest each other, and partly because if there is any deficiency in a particular food substance in one food, it may be made good to the animal by being present in another one of the mixture.

MAINTENANCE AND PRODUCTION RATIONS.—Rations given to animals can be divided into two parts, a maintenance and a production part. A maintenance ration may be described as that which will maintain an animal that is in a resting and non-producing condition and in good health, in the same condition and at the same weight for an indefinite period.

A production ration is that part of the daily diet which is given in excess of maintenance requirements, and which is available for being converted into energy, as in working horses, or into milk, or into fat or wool, or is used for growth.

It will be clear that a maintenance ration by itself is uneconomical, since it gives no return. It is seldom that animals are kept on bare maintenance diets except idle horses, non-pregnant sows, and young store cattle which are kept over the winter for fattening during the summer on grass.

In devising a maintenance ration it should be clearly understood that any food will not do; wheat straw does not contain sufficient protein for the maintenance of health in yearling bullocks, but wheat straw in combination with good quality hay will do so. For the composition of maintenance and production rations the reader should consult any of the well-known text-books or pamphlets on the subject. (*See* WINTER DIET.)

The most practical application of maintenance and production rations is in use where the cows are fed according to their milk yield. The average weight of the cows is found and the maintenance ration is fixed, usually of hay, straw, and succulent foods, and every cow receives the same allowance, unless very small or very big, and then to each is given an allowance of concentrates according to the weight and quality of the milk produced.

SUBSTITUTIONAL DIETING.—A farmer having fixed a daily ration for, let us say, his dairy cows, desires to change some of the constituents in the diet by substituting other foods. If foods are merely changed haphazardly pound for pound it is almost certain that the diet will be altered appreciably. For example, if 5 lb. of maize is substituted for 5 lb. of oats in a horse's ration the animal will be getting more nutriment than formerly, as 80 lb. of oats are equal to 60 lb. of maize. Again, oat straw, pound for pound, has rather less than half the nutriment found in meadow hay, and so on. Most stock-owners have a general idea of the relative values of foods, but it is only by studying them on the basis of their starch equivalent and protein content that a real idea of their energy value can be obtained and that substitution can be effected in an economical manner. (*See* STARCH EQUIVALENT, PROTEIN EQUIVALENT, RATIONS.)

When substituting one food for another it is important that the change be made gradually. Disastrous results have followed the sudden change of a diet.

DIETHYLCARBAMAZINE.—An anthelmintic, used for Husk, etc.

DIGESTIBILITY (*see* DIET).

DIGESTION, ABSORPTION, and ASSIMILATION are the three processes by which food is incorporated into the body.

In digestion food is softened and converted into a form which is soluble in the watery fluids of the body, or, in the case of fats, into very minute globules which are split up into their component parts. In absorption these soluble substances are taken up from the bowels by the blood- and lymph-streams and carried through the body. In assimilation they are deposited from the blood, united with the various tissues for their growth or repair, and become integral parts of the existing or of new body cells endowed with the property of life.

SALIVARY DIGESTION begins as soon as the food enters the mouth and becomes mixed with saliva secreted by the salivary glands. It is not very thorough in animals, such as the dog, which bolt their food without careful chewing, but in the horse during feeding, and in the ox and sheep while rumination is proceeding, it reaches a greater state of perfection, especially when starchy foods are eaten. Raw starches, which are very often enclosed in a matrix of cellulose or woody material, are not acted upon to any great extent until the cellulose covering has been dissolved, through the action of bacteria, in other parts of the system. Saliva has no digestive action upon proteins. In the domesticated dog, however, there seems little doubt that when given dry biscuits, which necessitate a certain amount of chewing, some salivary digestion does occur.

Typically, there is found in the saliva an enzyme called *ptyalin*, which actively changes the insoluble starch of carbohydrate foods into partly soluble sugars, but the process requires consummation by the enzymes of the small intestines. Ptyalin is only able to act in an alkaline medium, and its action therefore ceases as soon as the food has become permeated with acid gastric juice in the stomach. The saliva has one other very important function: it is incorporated and mixed with dry or mealy foods by the process of chewing, so that these may be formed into little coherent masses known as 'boli' and be more easily swallowed.

STOMACH DIGESTION commences shortly after the food enters the true stomach and continues till it leaves this organ. There are great differences in the domesticated animals, due to the fact that some—*e.g.* ruminants—have a compound stomach, and these must receive separate consideration.

In the horse, pig, and dog, when food enters the stomach, 'gastric juice' is secreted from the digestive glands situated in its walls. This juice contains at least one (possibly more) enzyme, *pepsin*, which, in the presence of dilute hydrochloric or lactic acid, also elaborated by these glands, acts upon the protein constituents. Before any action occurs, however, the stomach actively engages in a vigorous churning movement which has the effect of thoroughly mixing the gastric juice with the contained food, and of breaking up the latter. Actually the stomach does not prepare the food for absorption, but rather warms it up, incorporates with it the gastric juice, softens it, and converts the whole mass into a greyish-white (in pig and dog) or brownish (horse) mass of uniform consistency, in which particles of the various foods taken can be easily recognised.

In the horse, food stays in the stomach till it is about two-thirds full, and is then hurried through to the small intestine to make room for further amounts entering from the mouth, and yet in spite of this the stomach is practically never found empty after death—unless the horse has been starved. In this way the stomach of the horse may allow an amount of food two or even three times greater than its maximum capacity to pass through it during a feed, but when no more food is taken the stomach retains the last portions and only allows them to pass slowly out into the intestines. In the pig and dog food is retained in the stomach for a variable time according to the state in which it was swallowed, and is thoroughly churned and mixed with gastric juice. During this time the softer portions along with fluids and semi-fluids are squeezed through the pylorus into the intestine. As soon as any solid hard material comes into contact with the walls near the pylorus, the latter immediately closes tightly and retains the hard substance.

In the ruminating farm animals—ox and sheep—stomach digestion is complicated by the presence of three compartments before the true stomach is reached. These may briefly be said to be concerned in the preparation of the food before it enters the abomasum for true digestion. Although the rumen possesses no true digestive glands, yet a very considerable amount of digestion (if we term as digestion the splitting up of complex into simple products) takes place in it through the activity of cellulose-splitting and other organisms, which are normally present in enormous numbers. Neither the ox nor the sheep could live for any length of time without these organisms, since it is almost entirely due to their activity that coarse food materials like hay, chaff, grass, and even the husks of cereals, are broken down into soluble constituents. (*See also* RUMINAL DIGESTION.)

After the food has been subjected to the action of the organisms in the rumen, and has been chewed for a second time as 'cud', it is sent on into the third stomach or omasum for further breaking up by triturition, and then into the true stomach or abomasum, where digestive glands are present, and where a form of digestion similar to what occurs in the stomach of other animals takes place. The main function of the second stomach or reticulum is to act as a fluid reservoir from whence a supply of fluid can be sent into any compartment where it is needed for normal digestion.

INTESTINAL DIGESTION.—The softened semi-fluid material which leaves the stomach is commonly known as 'chyme'; it has an acid reaction, since it has been well mixed with the hydrochloric or lactic acid in the stomach. Shortly after entering the small intestine it meets with alkaline fluids and its acidity is neutralised. This occurs through the action of the bile from the liver and of the pancreatic juice from the pancreas. These fluids are similar in that they are both alkaline, but they differ greatly in their functions. The bile is partly composed of complex salts and pigments, and partly of waste products derived from the blood, or from the absorption of waste products which are of no use in the body economy. Its function is fourfold: it aids the emulsification of fats, dividing large droplets into tiny globules which are more easily split into their component parts by other enzymes prior to absorption; it assists in keeping the intestinal contents fluid and preventing undue fermentation and putrefaction through its slight antiseptic action against putrefactive organisms; it stimulates peristalsis to some extent, and it gives to the fæces their characteristic colour. The pancreatic juice possesses at least three powerful enzymes which are probably sufficient in themselves to ensure complete digestion of a food without other assistance. The first of these is called *trypsin*, and is concerned in the further splitting up of protein substances which have been partly acted upon by the pepsin of the stomach. It completes the work of the pepsin, so to speak. After proteins have been acted upon for a period by trypsin they are capable of being absorbed and made use of in the body. The next pancreatic enzyme is called *amylopsin*. It acts on carbohydrate constituents, splitting them up into sugars and other substances, but not carrying the process far enough to allow of complete absorption. Amylopsin has an action similar to that of the ptyalin of saliva, but it is more powerful, and it can act upon raw starch which is not able to be split up by the latter. *Lipase*, or *steapsin*, is the name of the fat-splitting enzyme of the pancreatic fluid. It acts upon the tiny globules of fat which have been emulsified by the bile, etc., and splits them into their compounds—glycerol and a fatty acid, the latter depending upon the origin of the fat.

Now, it will be obvious that there must be occasions when some of the food constituents escape action by these enzymes. But any such food is dealt with by the intestinal juice. This is produced by the intestinal glands, and is of very complex composition. It contains a number of enzymes of which the most important are: *erepsin*, *enterokinase*, *maltase*, *lactase*, and *invertase*. The first of these completes the breaking up of any protein which may have escaped the action of the pepsin and trypsin. Enterokinase is concerned with the formation of trypsin from its forerunner trypsinogen, and the last three complete the splitting up of carbohydrates into soluble sugars. Bacteria also have a most important digestive function in the intestines. In the large intestines of herbivorous animals they have a cellulose splitting action, which is somewhat allied to fermentation, and is similar to the activity of the organisms present in the first stomachs of ruminants. They act upon fats in a similar manner to the pancreatic juice; they form certain volatile obnoxious substances (indol and skatol) from proteins, which give the fæces their characteristic odour; they produce lactic acid in certain cases; and they may even destroy alkaloidal poisons which have been formed during other stages of digestion.

ABSORPTION.—Water passes through the stomach into the intestines almost immediately, and, in the horse at least, reaches the large intestine in the course of a very few seconds. It is very rapidly absorbed, and is in reality the medium through which all other food products are taken up into the body, with the single exception of fats. But it is only after subjection to digestion in the intestines for some hours that the bulk of the food is taken up into the system. The chyme which leaves the stomach is converted by the action of the bile and pancreatic fluids into a yellowish-grey or a brownish-green fluid of creamy consistency called 'chyle', containing in the herbivorous animals particles of hay, oats, grass, etc. From this the fats are absorbed (after emulsification and breakdown) by the lymph vessels or 'lacteals' which occupy the centre of each of the 'villi' of the small intestines. The villi are small finger-like processes which project from the wall of the small intestine into its lumen, and are therefore continually in contact with the food passing through it. In the lacteals the fat globules are re-formed and from these they are collected by the lymph vessels of the intestines, and are ultimately passed into the blood-stream. Sugar, salts, and soluble proteins pass directly into the small blood-vessels in the walls of the intestines, and are thence carried to the liver and so enter the general circulation.

The food is passed onwards through the various folds and coils of the intestines, each particular part of the bowel wall removing some portions of the food, and the residual, unabsorbable, useless constituents are eventually discharged from the rectum and anus during the process of defæcation, constituting the dung.

ASSIMILATION takes place slowly. After the products of digestion have been absorbed into the blood- and lymph-streams they are carried round the body, ultimately reaching every organ and tissue, and the body cells extract from the blood in the capillaries whatever nutritive products they may require for growth or repair. For instance, cells in bony tissues extract lime salts, muscles take proteins and sugars, etc. When the supply of food is much in excess of immediate requirements the surplus is stored up, perhaps as glycogen in liver or muscle, perhaps as fat deposited in the looser areas of the body, *e.g.* in the peritoneal cavity, or around various organs, or under the skin and among the muscle fibres.

DIGITALIS is the dried and powdered leaf of the wild Foxglove, *Digitalis purpurea*, gathered when the flowers are at a certain stage. The leaf contains several active agents extracted in various ways, but there are no alkaloids present. Its action is to strengthen involuntary muscular contraction, particularly that of the muscle fibres in the heart and blood-vessels. It is one of the most valuable heart stimulants when it is desired to obtain an increase in the force without any increase in the rate of the beat. In fact, it causes a greater period to elapse between each successive beat, so that the muscle of the damaged organ obtains longer periods for rest and repair. By its action on the heart, and by causing constriction of the fibres in the walls of the small arteries and veins, it raises the general blood-pressure of the body, and thus, in cases where the pressure is already low, causes an increase in the excretion of urine, and tends to stimulate the absorption of dropsical or œdematous effusions in the peritoneal or other cavities, as well as in other areas of the body.

Uses.—Digitalis is mainly employed for affections of the heart in which there is weakness and irregularity in its action. It is often given to horses and dogs during the convalescent stages following debilitating diseases, as a tonic, and it is greatly employed to hasten the absorption of fluid in cases of œdema. It should not be used indiscriminately in heart affections, because little benefit is likely to be derived when there is any fatty or other degeneration present, or when there is any valvular insufficiency. Owing to its tendency to accumulate in the system when given for long periods in full doses, it must be used with care. It is usual to alternate digitalis with strophanthus, which does not accumulate to the same extent, when long courses of treatment are necessary.

DIGITALIS POISONING may occur from the administration of digitalis over too long a period, from a single large dose, or from foxgloves in hay.

Symptoms.—The beat of the heart is at first slow and full, but soon becomes quick and irregular, and there is an accompanying murmur. Abdominal pain, purging, and vomiting in the small animals, occur; there is great salivation, disturbance of digestion, and usually pain over the region of the kidneys, which are highly inflamed.

Treatment.—Cases of poisoning are not common among animals, and when they do arise it is usually through repeated and prolonged administration. The drug should be stopped at once, and the animal should be given a dose of strong black tea or coffee. Stimulants such as caffeine and aromatic spirits of ammonia, are useful. The dog should be given an emetic when a single large dose has been taken.

DIHYDROTACHYSTEROL.—An oil-soluble steroid used to raise the calcium level of the blood, and so treat or prevent hypocalcæmia.

DIHYDROXYANTHRAQUINONE.—A non-toxic purgative, acting chiefly on the large intestine, effective in all the domestic animals, including horses. It may be given in the food, when it acts in about 24 hours.

DIMIDIUM BROMIDE.—A trypanocide effective against *T. congolense*.

DIODONE.—A contrast medium used in radiography of the kidneys.

DIPHTHERIA, CALF (*see* CALF DIPHTHERIA).

DIPHTHERIA, FOWL (*see* FOWL-POX).

DIPHTHERIA, GUTTURAL POUCH, of horses. (*See under* GUTTURAL.)

DIPLEGIA (δίς, twice; πληγή, a blow) means extensive paralysis on both sides of the body.

DIPLOCOCCUS is the name given to a genus of organisms of which the *Diplococcus pneumoniæ* is the most typical. They usually appear under the microscope as minute paired spheres.

DIPS and DIPPING.—In Britain mostly sheep are dipped, but beef cattle may also be dipped with advantage. Dipping is an important means of tick control in cattle, and is widely practised in the tropics.

Sheep are dipped in order: (1) to eradicate the commoner parasitic agents, such as keds, lice, ticks, etc.; (2) to act as a check upon the spread of mange in the sheep, commonly called 'sheep scab', and where that disease has broken out, to cure it; and (3) to prevent attack by the sheep-blowflies and consequent infestation with maggots.

In different districts there are different times for dipping according to the breeds kept and the climate. On farms in the south of England the sheep are sometimes dipped three times a year: once before clipping, once soon after clipping, and again in the autumn. In mountain districts dipping ordinarily takes place twice a year, the early spring dipping being missed. In addition to local custom, special dipping orders can still be enforced in Britain by the Ministry of Agriculture for the purpose of keeping in check such diseases as sheep scab, and for the eradication of ticks.

Precautions.—Owners should ensure that any dips they purchase carry on their labels the statement that the dip has been approved by the Ministry of Agriculture and Fisheries. The following precautions should be observed when sheep are dipped:

1. For 1 month or 5 weeks after service ewes should not be dipped lest abortion result. Pregnant ewes require careful handling to avoid injury, but with care they may be dipped almost up to the time they lamb, provided weather is favourable.

2. Early spring washing or dipping must be carried out with a solution which does not harm the wool, making the fibres brittle or stained.

3. Summer dipping should take place when there is a sufficiency of fleece to carry and hold the dip, and when parasites may most easily be destroyed, *i.e.* at from 3 to 5 weeks after clipping.

DIPS AND DIPPING

4. Autumn dipping should be finished before the first frosts of the season begin, and when the weather is so much settled that rain is not expected during the next 24 hours. This is of more importance in autumn dipping than otherwise, because the dip has to remain in the fleece during the winter, and it is more easily washed out before it has dried than afterwards.

5. Sheep should be offered a drink of water before being dipped in hot weather, as there is some risk of thirsty animals drinking the dip, with fatal results if it is a poisonous variety.

6. Sheep should be rested before actual immersion, especially if recently brought in from a hill, or when they have walked a distance to the dipper. This is particularly important in hot weather.

7. Sheep with open wounds or sores, and those that have recently been attacked with maggots or have been ill, should not be dipped until the skin is whole and until they have otherwise recovered. This is another reason why dipping should not immediately follow shearing.

8. Sheep must not be turned out on to grazing land immediately after being dipped, for the drainage from their fleeces contaminates the herbage, and the sheep being hungry may eat sufficient dip-sodden grass to produce poisoning. They should be allowed about 15 minutes in the draining pens.

9. Each sheep should be immersed in the dipper for the requisite length of time according to the instructions that are furnished with each kind of dip by the makers.

10. The dip must be carefully made up according to instructions, and fresh dipping powder and fluid added to make up the loss that occurs from the removal of a small amount upon the fleece of each sheep. It is not sufficient to add water.

11. After dipping operations are finished the dip should be disposed of in such a way that there is no danger of it contaminating water-supplies, ponds, streams, etc.

(*See* FISH, POISONING OF.)

Dipping.—This is used almost exclusively for the destruction of parasites.

In every case it is advisable to consult the local veterinary authority as to the dip to be used for any given purpose, as not only may a dip suitable for one place or for one parasite be unsuitable for another place or another parasite, but local regulations may require the use of a specific type of dip. It is important to get the dip from a good firm of known reputation, and it is essential to make it up strictly according to the accompanying instructions and to the exact strength stated.

In Britain, the ban on the use of dieldrin and aldrin-based sheep dips came into force at the end of 1965. With a view to replacing these organo-chlorine dips, a range of organo-phosphorous ones came on to the market. Dip manufacturers have emphasised that in a 'normal' season, there will be no need for a return to double dipping, but it has to be admitted that if we have a period of warm, moist weather during late August or September, it would be unwise not to treat the sheep a second time.

Before Australia and New Zealand imposed their own ban on dieldrin dips, on account of the contamination with residues of lamb sold overseas, some of their farmers had already made the change to organo-phosphorus insecticides, as blow-flies resistant to dieldrin were causing losses. Reports of experience with the newer type of dip in those countries, and of field trials carried out in Britain, are most encouraging. One good point is that, like dieldrin, an organo-phosphorus compound diffuses down the wool as it grows, so that no unprotected layer—vulnerable to the green-bottle's maggots—is left.

The new dips are generally more expensive than those based on dieldrin. They have been tested for safety in use, but must still be treated with respect. The concentrated liquid must not be allowed to come into contact with human skin. There is, too, a prescribed period, varying with the chemical, to be observed between dipping and slaughter: usually 14 or 21 days.

The bath to be used depends on many circumstances, such as numbers to be dipped, land and materials available, and so on. The best material to use is concrete, and the most popular shape is that shown in Fig. 85. The dimensions for the various animals are as follows:

	Horse.		Cattle.		Sheep.		Pigs.	
	ft.	in.	ft.	in.	ft.	in.	ft.	in.
Breadth at top .	5	9	5	2	3	3	3	3
,, at bottom	3	3	3	3	2	6	2	6
Depth . . .	8	5	7	6	5	9	5	9
Length at top .	55	0	50	0	45	0	35	0
Length of well .	30	0	30	0	30	0	20	0
Entrance slope .	7	3	6	6	5	0	5	0
Exit slope . .	16	3	13	0	10	0	10	0
Depth of dip from bottom .	6	6	5	6	4	0	4	0

DIPS AND DIPPING

These figures are only given as a general guide.

In order to avoid waste of dip, the farmer needs to know exactly how much liquid the bath will hold, and he also needs a calibrated stick or side-marking to indicate the volume of liquid still in the bath at all stages of dipping. What is sometimes overlooked is the fact that a sheep with wool 1 to $1\frac{1}{2}$ inches long will not merely remove permanently at least $\frac{1}{2}$ gallon of liquid, but will strain off additional insecticide. This necessitates ' topping up ' of the dip wash at double strength as compared with the liquid used for the first filling of the bath. Obviously, the number, size, and dirtiness of the sheep will determine the number of times that topping up is necessary for a given size of bath.

It is a false economy not to top up before the last 20 or 30 sheep are put through the dip, since any saving of money thereby could later be more than offset by those animals becoming victims of strike. Disappointing results of any dip can also follow if sheep are immersed or far short of 30 seconds ; for if they are soaking wet when they enter the bath, for then their fleeces can carry much less than the normal quantity of wash.

A sheep with a short growth of wool (1 to $1\frac{1}{2}$ inches) will emerge from the bath carrying 4 or 5 gallons of wash, and will retain $\frac{1}{2}$ gallon. If there is not to be an expensive waste of dip, it is important that the floor of the draining pens should be such as to allow the maximum run-back of liquid to the bath.

Arsenic-dipped animals should never be allowed on to pasturage until there is no risk of contamination of grass.

In all cases the animal should be totally immersed at least once (hence the abrupt commencement of the bath), and special attention should be paid to the ears and tail. Dipping must be thorough.

Lameness.—Especially in warm climates, where the dip has been allowed to remain in the tank and has become dirty, there is a danger of sheep becoming lame after dipping. This results from infection with *Erysipelothrix rhusiospathiae* (*see under* SWINE FEVER) through any cuts or abrasions. Such lameness does not follow the use of a freshly prepared dip. It has been obviated by the addition to the dip of tetramethyl thiuram disulphide. This controls any bacteria which contaminate the dip liquid. Non-phenolic sheep dips have little or no action against bacteria.

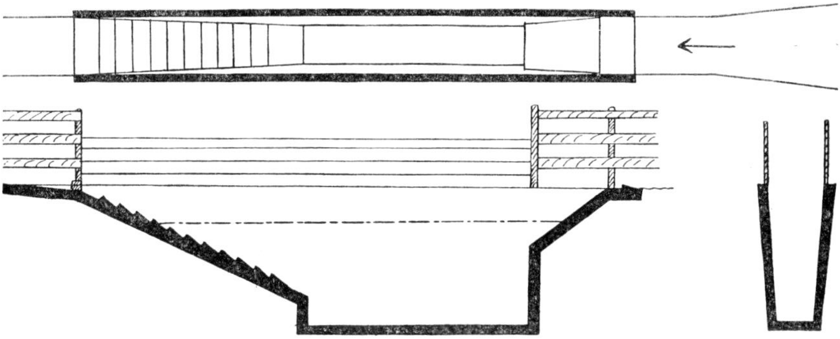

Plan of Dipping bath. (For dimensions see text.)

Dips for special purposes.—The following is a list of dips classified according to disease to be treated. The first dip is that considered to be the best for the particular parasite ; but local circumstances may indicate the use of one of the others.

Maggots . .	Any sulphur dip, BHC.
Maggot fly .	Organo-phosphorus dips.
Lice, in any animal	Derris, BHC.
Horn - fly in cattle	Any oily dip (with splash boards).
Keds in sheep	BHC, DDT, derris.
Mange, in all animals	BHC, arsenic and sulphur.
Ticks . .	BHC, arsenic (strength varies according to interval).

For tick control in Africa, see under TICKS.)

One dipping will seldom (if ever) be effective in ridding an animal of parasites, as the dip may not affect the eggs, or the young animals may not yet be on the host. The dip must accordingly be repeated at suitable intervals. Against keds, dips require to be repeated in 3 to 4 weeks, and against mange in about 7 to 10 days.

Spraying.—Dipping of all animals involves considerable trouble, expensive equipment, and in most cases is static so that animals must come to the dipper. The use of modern sprays and jets, whereby the chemical agent is directed on to the animal's skin with considerable force, has some advantages over dipping and is partly replacing dipping in some countries. (*See* SPRAY-RACE.) (*See also* JETTING.) In Britain, those who practise spraying, as opposed to dipping, would be unwise to rely on more than 3 weeks' protection against strike. This is partly because less insecticide remains in the fleece after spraying; also, the organophosphorus insecticides move down the wool but, apparently, not sideways, so that if a patch is left unsprayed it remains vulnerable to strike.

DIQUAT.—This herbicide has caused fatal poisoning in cattle, four years after the discarding of a container.

DISBUDDING is the name applied to removal of, or the prevention of growth in, the horn buds in calves, kids, and sometimes in lambs. (*See* DISHORNING.)

DISC, INTERVERTEBRAL PROTRUSION (*see under* SPINE *on page* 863).

DISCRETE (*discerno*, I separate) is the opposite of confluent. It is used to indicate that a patch of diseased tissue, or a particular colour of the body, is distinct from similar or dissimilar areas near.

DISEASE, FACTORS INFLUENCING.—(1) **Age.**—Both youth and age are responsible for modifications in disease which do not apply to animals in their prime. Thus young animals are unable to withstand attack by parasitic worms so well as the adult; old animals succumb more readily to general infectious fevers than the young in many cases, though in extensive outbreaks the latter are more often affected. Age may predispose to disease; thus young horses are affected by strangles, puppies by distemper, calves by black-quarter, and all young animals by rickets, while on the other hand tumours, heart and circulatory weaknesses, and chronic inflammations are essentially troubles of the aged.

(2) **Sex.**—The difference in the anatomy of the genital organs of the two sexes obviously accounts for the appearance of certain diseases in the one which cannot affect the other. Moreover, such conditions as œstrum in the female tend to exaggerate the symptoms of a fever which has nothing to do with the female sex organs; for example, should a mare affected with influenza come into season her temperature will rise, and a suckling mare in œstrum often results in an attack of diarrhœa in the foal.

(3) **Pregnancy.**—That pregnancy has an adverse influence upon the vitality of the dam will be obvious when one considers the great demand made by the fœtus upon its dam, especially during the later stages. It often happens that the pregnant female becomes subjected to attacks of colic, indigestion, constipation, and other abdominal troubles owing to the mechanical interference with the functions of these organs by the pregnant uterus. During pregnancy any acute disease is likely to be more serious and more fatal than otherwise. A severe attack of influenza, foot-and-mouth disease, or swine fever, will often produce abortion and death. In fact, in foot-and-mouth disease the number of abortions among cows, sows, and ewes may be as high as 50 per cent. The chronic diseases are not as a rule affected by pregnancy except that they are often kept in check till after parturition, when they reassert themselves. Thus broken wind in the mare and tuberculosis in the cow may lie apparently dormant while these animals are pregnant, but after foaling and calving their symptoms become worse. Nervous diseases and general constitutional diseases, such as chorea in the bitch and osteomalacia in the larger animals, become exaggerated by pregnancy. It has been found that the excretion of the various products of metabolism is not so thorough during pregnancy as otherwise, and the partial retention of these effete materials may possibly adversely influence the whole of the body tissues and make them less capable of withstanding attack by disease.

(4) **Temperament.**—The influence of this is very obvious. An animal that is so nervous or vicious as to resent the careful cleansing of a wound, the setting of a fracture, the application of bandages or of dressings, cannot recover so quickly as one that will allow man to materially assist Nature's reparative processes. Indeed, sometimes if an animal of the larger

variety which has fractured a limb can be persuaded to allow itself to be slung, slaughter, as is often the case, would not be necessary.

(5) **Conformation.**—A horse with well-formed feet will recover from corns, bruises to the sole, and conditions such as thrush and canker, more quickly than one with narrow, high, and contracted heels. Then again, too sloping pasterns are likely to be associated with strained tendons; hocks with too much curve in them easily develop curbs; too upright hocks are liable to bone spavins, and so on.

(6) **Colour** plays a part in some cases. Hereford cattle that have a red ring round their eyes are not so liable to go blind from the extreme glare of the sun in tropical countries as those that have all-white faces. Ayrshire cattle that have little red or roan in their coats are often attacked by an inflammation of the skin brought on by the sun in hot countries, while those that have less white escape. (*See* LIGHT SENSITISATION.) Grey horses only are attacked by melanomata.

(7) **Idiosyncrasy.**—This is that peculiar state of the whole or part of the body which renders it especially susceptible to attack by some particular disease, or, conversely, gives it some inherent resistance against it. It is the only explanation of the fact that one animal alone of a number that have been living together under the same conditions becomes attacked with disease when the others escape, or only escapes when all the others succumb.

(8) **Previous disease** may either confer a certain amount of immunity against that particular disease, or it may make the animal more susceptible. Thus cattle recovered from rinderpest do not again contract the disease, but one attack of pneumonia weakens the lungs and makes the subject more liable to subsequently become affected again. Generally speaking, the specific diseases leave an immunity in the animals that recover, while the non-specific diseases predispose to further attacks.

(9) **Exposure** to extremes of heat and cold generally has an adverse influence upon disease, for while animals can easily withstand great extremes of either when the condition is continuous, they cannot tolerate sudden changes from one to the other. This is well seen in the great frequency with which household dogs become attacked with respiratory troubles in cold weather when they are allowed to lie close to hot fires for long periods, and then are taken out into the cold. The same applies to young horses that have been used to an open-air life in the country and are sold to come into warm town stables, where many of them develop strangles, etc. (*See* SHEARING.)

(10) **Heredity** plays a very important part in the causation of some varieties of developmental abnormalities. *E.g.* hernia, cryptorchidism, achondroplasia in cattle, hare-lip and cleft palate, while many types of monstrosities in sheep and cattle especially are inherited from parents which have been bred from tainted ancestry. The degree of resistance to a particular disease may also be determined by heredity.

(11) **Food.**—A very great deal of the treatment of many of the diseases of the domestic stock depends upon the nature, amount, and frequency of the feeding. For details see under separate diseases and under DIET, NURSING OF SICK ANIMALS.

(12) **Surroundings,** including climate, are of the greatest importance to animals, and exercise a great influence upon the course of a disease. (*See* NURSING OF SICK ANIMALS.)

'DISEASE-FREE' ANIMALS.—Piglet mortality is one of the main sources of economic loss to the pig industry, and it is in the study of these very important piglet diseases that special laboratory pigs are necessary. Without such animals research work may not only be hampered or even brought to a standstill by natural infections, but complications may arise.

From the moment the piglet leaves the warm security of the womb and enters the birth-canal it becomes exposed to an infected environment. Under natural conditions it is protected against this environment, to a greater or lesser degree, by the wide range of antibodies received from its dam in the first milk, the colostrum. When deprived of colostrum piglets almost always die. But the research worker wishes to avoid the feeding of colostrum, since this substance may well contain antibodies against the disease under investigation.

The problem is, then, to rear piglets which are both disease-free and devoid of antibodies. In principle, the solution to the problem is a simple one. All that needs to be done is to obtain the piglets before they reach the infected environment and to rear them away from possible infection, so that colostrum is unnecessary. In practice, these requirements are not easily met. However, by using a technique developed in the U.S.A. at the University of Nebraska, 'disease-free', antibody-devoid pigs are now being produced at the School of Veterinary Medicine, University of Cambridge, and elsewhere.

The piglets are taken direct from the womb of the sow a day or two before the estimated farrowing date. The sow is anæsthetised, the whole womb carefully but rapidly removed and passed through a bath of disinfectant, which forms an antiseptic lock, into a sterilised hood. The sow is immediately slaughtered. The hood is supplied with warm, filtered air under slight pressure and the two operators work through long-sleeved rubber gloves. In the hood the piglets are taken rapidly from the womb, their navel cords are tied off, and they are dried with sterile towels. The piglets are then transferred, by means of a sealed carrying case, to sterile incubator units kept in a heated isolation room. These incubators, each of which holds one pig, are equipped with filter pads so that both the air entering the unit and that passing out into the exhaust system is filtered.

During the first few days of their independent existence, great care is necessary to protect the young animals from bacteria in general. The attendant wears mask and cap in addition to rubber gloves and overalls. Subsequently, masks and caps are unnecessary. The diet, which consists of pasteurised milk, eggs and minerals, is sterilised by heat for the first three days of life, but not thereafter. The piglets are fed from flat-bottomed trays three times daily—morning, midday and late afternoon. There are no night feeds. After some ten days in the incubator units the young pigs are transferred to individual open cages in another isolation pen. There they are rapidly weaned to solid food. Later, the pigs are mixed together and treated as ordinary ones except that, of course, precautions are taken to prevent accidental infection.

Pigs reared by this technique are in a state of minimal disease: they are not germ-free. In fact, non-pathogenic bacteria are deliberately introduced by feeding pasteurised, instead of sterilised, milk from the fourth day of life onwards. These pigs are not, therefore, in the same category as the germ-free animals produced with the aid of elaborate and expensive equipment by Dr. Reyniers at the University of Notre Dame in Indiana. (*See* G. NOTOBIOTICS.) Production of 'disease-free' pigs was begun at Cambridge primarily to permit the critical investigation of pig diseases, particularly diseases of suckling pigs, but such pigs have obvious advantages for nutritional and genetic studies because the technique does eliminate that unpredictable variable, disease.

Another possible use for this technique, which may be of more immediate interest to pig farmers, is in ridding valuable blood lines of such maladies as rhinitis, virus-pneumonia, enteritis, and parasitic infection. When the salvage value of the sow is taken into account the procedure comes into the realms of practical economics. This field application is being tried on a small scale in Nebraska. As expected, the results show that the artificially reared pigs, which have been freed from their disease-burden, grow better, and make better use of their food than 'normal' farm pigs. (*See also* S.P.F.)

DISEASES OF ANIMALS ACT, 1950.— This Act (and Orders relating to it) is administered by the Animal Health Division of the Ministry of Agriculture of Great Britain.

It covers the diseases listed under NOTIFIABLE DISEASES.

The Act and Orders provide for the compulsory notification of the existence or suspected existence of these diseases; for the immediate isolation or segregation of diseased or suspected animals; for the diagnosis of suspected disease by specially trained persons; for the slaughter of diseased or in-contact animals where necessary, and for the safe disposal of their carcases; for the payment of compensation to owners in certain cases; for the apprehension and punishment of offenders; for the systematic inspection of markets, fairs, sales, and exhibitions, etc., and for the seizure of diseased or suspected animals therein; for regulating the transit and transport of animals by land or water, both within the country and in the home waters; for controlling the importation of animals and things which may introduce one or other of these diseases from abroad; and for inspection at the ports and quarantine or slaughter where necessary.

The following regulations have a general application to all scheduled diseases, but in practically every case there is at least one

Order applicable to the particular disease, in which there is set out more fully regulations dealing with that disease. These Orders can be obtained from Her Majesty's Stationery Offices, and must be consulted individually if complete information is required.

Notification of disease or suspected disease must always be made by the owner of an animal, or by the occupier or person in charge, and by the veterinary surgeon in attendance, to an inspector of the Local Authority or to a police constable, and that without undue delay.

Presumption of knowledge of disease.—A person required to give notice if charged with failure to carry out his obligation shall be presumed to have known of the existence of the disease, unless and until he shows, to the satisfaction of the Court, that he had not knowledge thereof and could not with reasonable care have obtained that knowledge.

Separation of diseased animals.—Every person having a diseased animal shall, as far as is practicable, keep it separate from animals not so diseased.

Facilities and assistance to be given for inspection, cleansing, and disinfection.—Persons in charge of diseased animals are required to give every facility for the execution of the above, and must not obstruct or in any way hinder inspectors or other officers in doing their duty.

Prohibition of exposure of diseased animals.—It is unlawful to expose a diseased or suspected animal in a market, sale-yard, fair, or other public or private place where such animals are commonly exposed for sale; to place an affected animal in a lair or other place adjacent to or connected with a market, sale-yard, etc., or where such animals are commonly exposed for sale; to send a diseased animal on a railway, or on any canal, inland navigation or coasting vessels; or to allow one on a highway or thoroughfare, or on any common or unenclosed land or in any insufficiently fenced field; or to graze one on the sides of a highway; or to allow one to stray on a highway or thoroughfare or on the sides thereof, etc.

Digging up carcases.—No person may dig up the carcase of an animal that has been buried, without permission from the Ministry of Agriculture. (*See also* under each main heading of the scheduled diseases, *e.g.* ANTHRAX.)

DISHORNING OF CATTLE.—It has been found advisable to remove the horns from dairy cows housed in yards and from fattening beef cattle in yards or pens, because there is usually one that obtains mastery over the others, and if it possesses horns it is liable to inflict wounds upon others or upon the attendants. The horn is a useless weapon in cattle and if the operation is carried out scientifically no cruelty is involved in dishorning.

The most satisfactory method is that known as 'disbudding'. This consists of painting the young buds of the horns, when they first appear in calves, with caustic compound. It is best to disbud at one week of age and certainly not later than 10 days. A little vaseline or thick grease may be rubbed on the hair around the base of the bud and care is needed to ensure that no caustic gets into the eyes. The bud of the horn is first cleaned with spirit to remove grease—an essential preliminary—and a second coating of the caustic is given after the first has dried. A scab will form over the bud and drop off, carrying with it the cells which would have produced horn. Little or no pain is occasioned to the calf by caustic collodion (whereas caustic potash sticks, now largely superseded, do cause much pain) and the horn is effectively prevented from growing.

In Great Britain the operation of dishorning cattle requires the administration of an anæsthetic. (*See* ANÆSTHETICS, LEGAL REQUIREMENTS.) A saw, an electric saw, cutting wire or special horn shears may be used.

Bleeding from the matrix and horn core can usually be controlled by using a figure-of-eight tourniquet round the roots of the horns.

DISHORNING OF GOATS.—This presents several problems not encountered to the same extent in cattle. For techniques, see the *Veterinary Record* for August 1, 1964.

DISINFECTANTS may be either physical or chemical. Among the former are heat, sunlight, wind, and electricity; while among the latter are solids, liquids, and gases.

Chemical disinfectants.—At the present time these are numerous and diverse. The Ministry of Agriculture and Fisheries test them from time to time and issues its approval only to those that are maintained up to standard. Consequently, owners should examine the labels on containers and use only those that carry the official approval since this is a guarantee of potency.

The Diseases of Animals (Approved Disinfectants) Order 1970 governs the uses of disinfectants in the U.K., and specifies those approved for use in connection with foot-and-mouth disease, tuberculosis, fowl pest, and general orders relating to disease control. Dilution rates are also specified.

A full list of disinfectants approved for use in outbreaks of foot-and-mouth disease is given under that subject entry.

Disinfectants act in one of three ways: (1) as oxidising agents or as reducing agents; (2) as corrosives or coagulants acting upon the protoplasm of bacterial life; or (3) as bacterial poisons.

Most chemical disinfectants are supplied in a concentrated form and must be diluted with water before use. The water should be clean, preferably soft, and if it can be used warm the efficiency of the disinfectant is increased. After the active agent has been added the whole should be well stirred for a few moments to ensure thorough mixing. The solution must be applied so that it remains in contact with the offending material for a sufficiently long time to kill the bacterial life therein; generally ten minutes to half an hour should elapse before disinfecting solutions are rinsed away.

When two or more disinfectants are mixed together, instead of an increased disinfecting power in the mixture they often enter into chemical combination with each other and a useless compound results.

Quaternary Ammonia Compounds (*see under this heading*).

Cresol Solutions.—There are many of these, *e.g.* the cresol and soap solution of the B.P., the compound cresol solution of the U.S.A.P., lysol, isal, cyllin, creolin, cresylin, Jeyes' fluid, or one of the proprietary preparations. These are used as 3 per cent to 5 per cent solutions for practically all purposes of disinfection about a farm premises, and very often as antiseptics also. Their action is enhanced by the use of hot water instead of cold. None of them are suitable for use in connection with food, for all are to a greater or lesser degree poisonous. Cresols are not very effective against many viruses or bacterial spores.

Formalin is sometimes used as a solution for disinfecting floors, about 5 per cent strength being necessary.

Formaldehyde gas may be used for fumigation of livestock buildings where virus or other diseases have occurred. (*See under* DISINFECTION.)

Creosote is useful for disinfecting and preserving woodwork. (*See* HYPERKERATOSIS.) (*See also under* ANTISEPTICS.)

DISINFECTION.—The process of rendering stables, byres, piggeries, etc., harmless, depends upon what variety of infection has existed in the building. For example, cresol solutions are not quickly effective against the virus of foot-and-mouth disease, which is rapidly killed by a 4 per cent solution of washing soda.

Limitation of Infection.—This consists of soaking the dead animal, the stall or standing, and surrounding litter, dung, etc., with an approved disinfectant in proper strength. The men should wear protective clothing. Unauthorised persons, children, and other animals must be denied access to the infected area.

Disposal of the dead, litter, dung, etc.—Carcases of animals that have died from the disease must be removed and disposed of as given under DISPOSAL OF CARCASES (which see). If the floor is of concrete and there is not a great deal of litter and dung present, these latter are collected into a heap (either inside the building, or outside), soaked with paraffin oil, and burned. If dry they require no oil to assist combustion. The ashes are thereafter collected and may be mixed with the ordinary farmyard manure with safety. Should there be any liquid contamination, *e.g.* pus, blood, urine, fæces, etc., it should be covered and mixed with ordinary bleaching-powder (dry) of good strength, and then sprinkled with earth or sawdust, after which it can be removed and burned.

Cleansing.—The building must now be thoroughly scraped, brushed, and cleansed. Concrete floors may be power-hosed, scraped free from all dirt and debris. A hot detergent solution of 2½ to 4 per cent washing-soda is then thoroughly scrubbed onto floors, walls, stall partitions, mangers, troughs, or other fittings.

Disinfection.—Thereafter the parts of the building that have been contaminated should be soaked with a hot solution of one of the approved disinfectants, and thoroughly scrubbed. It is an advantage to block up any drains that lead out from the building if this is possible. A sack or a sod of turf is suitable. All mangers, troughs, and drinking-vessels that are fixed to the stalls, etc., should be filled with the solution and then well scrubbed.

Finally the whole building is shut up for 24 hours, no attempt being made to rinse it out with clean water till the next day. Where other animals inhabit the building, as in a byre after a case of anthrax has occurred, the disinfection is scrupulously carried out in the stall from which the dead animal has been removed, and the rest of the byre treated in a general manner. In certain cases it may be desirable to fumigate the building. All air entrances and exits are securely closed, the inside of the walls and roof is soaked with water, and formaldehyde gas generated (*e.g.* by pouring on to 250 gm. of potassium permanganate 500 ml. of formalin per 1,000 cu. ft. of air space. All doors and windows are left shut for a day, and the building is then flushed out with clean water under pressure from a hose-pipe.

Movable objects.—All pails, grooming tools, wheelbarrows, shovels, forks, etc., which have been used for the infected animals must also be disinfected before they can be considered safe for further use. They may be scrubbed with one of the disinfecting solutions before mentioned, or they may be soaked in Jeyes' fluid for six hours in a convenient receptacle (*i.e.* brushes, curry-combs, etc., may be placed in a pailful of the solution). Harness requires special treatment. When the traces or some other localised parts have become accidentally contaminated during the removal of cattle carcases it is only necessary to disinfect them; the whole harness does not require treatment; but when mange has appeared in a stable, it is necessary to take down all the harness, separating it into its component parts, rip out the padding unless it is leather-lined and intact, and immerse the whole for an hour in a 5 per cent solution of Jeyes' fluid or other solution. If there is much grease and scurf it is necessary to scrub it with soda and hot water firstly. Afterwards, the harness is removed from the solution, dried, and then oiled or treated with harness composition.

Finally, it is most essential that all attendants who have carried out cleansing and disinfection of a building should take precautions to ensure that they neither contract the disease themselves nor act as agents in its spread to other animals.

DISLOCATIONS (*dis*, apart; *loco*, I place) are injuries to joints of such a nature that the ends of the opposed bones are forced apart more or less out of connection with each other. As well as displacement there is also more or less bruising of the soft tissues around the joints, and tearing of the ligaments which bind the bones together.

Varieties.—Dislocations may be either simple or compound, and either of these may be of recent occurrence or may have existed for a long period. In simple dislocations the bones are forced apart out of position, but the skin over the joint remains intact, while in compound dislocations the end of one of the bones is forced through the skin.

Speaking generally, the ligaments or muscles which bind the component parts of a joint together are so strong in animals that a fracture is much more likely to occur than a dislocation, but there are certain joints the conformation of which renders them liable to dislocation in the young animal. Probably the most common dislocation is that of the patella, which becomes lodged on the uppermost part of the outer ridge of the patellar surface of the femur and is unable to extricate itself from this position. In fact, if the stifle-joints be excluded, dislocations or luxations are very rare in the domesticated animals. (*See* SLIPPED STIFLE.)

Causes.—The causes of dislocations are similar to those which produce fracture. Violence applied in such a manner that the structures around the joint are unable to withstand the stress results in the giving way of ligaments, tendons, or muscles, and the separation of the bones forming the joint. Whether the bones or the joint will give way depends upon the manner of the application of the force and on the relative strengths of these structures. As a rule, in very young animals, and in very old animals, the bones will fracture before the joints give way; while it is in animals that are still young though no longer *very young*—that is, in those in which the ossification of the bones is complete but the binding structures have not yet attained their maximum strength—it is in such that dislocations may occur. (For inherited abnormality in dogs, *see under* PATELLA.)

Symptoms.—The injured limb is useless, and as a rule is held off the ground in an unnatural attitude. There is generally little or no pain so long as the parts are not forcibly moved; but if a nerve trunk is pressed upon, the animal may perspire with the pain. When the limb is compared with that of the opposite side there is seen a marked difference in its contours or outline—the joint affected shows hollows or prominences where none are seen in the normal limb. There is a loss of the power of movement, but there is no grating sound heard when the joint or the whole limb is passively moved, such as occurs when a fracture exists.

Treatment.—Immediate treatment is not of such importance as in a fracture, for there is less danger of damage to nerves or arteries by the end of the dislocated bone than there is when a fracture is present. Where possible the animal should be kept still until skilled assistance arrives, for the reduction of most dislocations necessitates the use of chloroform to overcome the powerful contractions of the muscles. There are, however, some dislocations which can be comparatively easily reduced without an anæsthetic, such as that of the patella. In this instance it is often only necessary to attach a rope round the pastern of the affected limb and to pull the limb forwards, when the patella will fall back into its place with a distinct click.

It must be emphasised that skilled assistance should always be sought where a serious dislocation has occurred in any of the domesticated animals, for by an early reduction recovery is more likely.

DISPLACED ABOMASUM.—A condition encountered in cattle some weeks after calving and leading to a complete lack of appetite. (*See under* STOMACH, DISEASES OF.)

DISPOSAL OF CARCASES.—Carcases of animals may be disposed of by sending them to a knackery or destructor, or by burial or burning. It is most important that they should not be left lying for any length of time in summer weather, for within a few hours after death they are usually selected by female flies for the deposition of their eggs, and within 24 to 36 hours they are swarming with maggots. Moreover, where the cause of death has been a contagious disease there is always the risk of healthy animals becoming directly or indirectly affected, and of the disease spreading accordingly.

In most progressive countries there are Government regulations which provide for the safe disposal of the carcases of animals that have died from any one of the notifiable contagious diseases, such as anthrax, foot-and-mouth disease, cattle plague, etc., but it is important that *all* carcases should be safely and efficiently disposed of, no matter what has been the cause of death.

The safest and most expeditious manner of disposal is for the carcases to be digested in a special destructor, either by heat (burning, or by live steam) or by chemical agents. In country districts, however, such plants as these are seldom available, and it is necessary to bury or burn the carcases.

Burial of carcases.—A suitable site should be selected where there will be no danger of pollution of streams, rivers, canals, or other water-supplies, and where there is a sufficiency of subsoil to allow a depth of 6 clear feet of soil above the carcase. A pit is dug, about 8 or 9 feet deep, in such a manner that the surface soil and the subsoil are not mixed, and a clear approach is left to its edge. Roughly, about 2½ to 3 square yards of surface are required for a horse, 1½ to 2½ square yards for an ox, and about 1 square yard for each large pig or sheep. The carcase should be dragged to the pit by chains attached to the back of a cart, or pulled by a trace-horse, and if a considerable distance has to be covered it is better to roll the carcase on to a barn door or gate to avoid contamination of the ground with blood, discharges, etc. The dead animal should be arranged upon its back with the feet upwards, and if these rigidly project too far upwards, the hocks may be 'hamstringed' and the tendons round the knee divided. This allows the limbs to be folded into a more compact space. It is advisable to slash the skin after the carcase has been placed within the pit, to prevent its disinterment by unscrupulous persons desiring to salve the hide. Where the cause of death has been accidental there are no objections to the removal of the skin previously, but where a contagious disease has been the cause of death the removal of the skin is an instance of a 'penny wise, pound foolish' policy. The carcase is next covered with quicklime or a powerful disinfectant, and the pit filled in with the soil—subsoil first and surface soil last. If the weather is very wet, or if the soil is naturally loose and soft, the surface of the ground should be fenced off to prevent horses and cattle from passing over it and perhaps sinking into the loose soil. It is not safe to plough over a large burial pit for six months after it has been closed, nor should heavy implements or vehicles be allowed to pass over it.

Cremation of carcases.—Where a large coal boiler or furnace is used for heating supplies of water, there is no reason why the carcases of small animals that have died should not be burned in it, but dead horses and cattle, and large sheep and pigs, should not be dismembered and destroyed in such a manner ; they must be burned in a specially constructed cremation pit.

There are three methods of cremation : (1) The Crossed Trench ; (2) The Bostock Pit ; and (3) The Surface Burning Method.

In the first of these—the *crossed trench*—two trenches 7 feet long are dug so that they form a cross. Each is about 15 inches wide and 18 inches deep in the centre, becoming shallower towards the extremities of the limbs. The soil is thrown on to the surface in the angles of the cross, and upon the mounds so made two or three stout pieces of iron, beams of wood, or branches from a tree, are placed. Straw and faggots are piled in the trenches to the level of the surface of the ground, the carcase is placed across the centre of the trenches, and more wood or coal is piled around and above it. Two gallons of paraffin oil are poured over the whole, and the straw is lighted.

In the *Bostock pit*, an oval pit 7 feet long and 4 feet wide is dug to a depth of 3 feet to 4 feet, and a crossed trench 9 inches by 9 inches is dug in its floor. Upon the windward side of the pit a ventilation trench 4 feet long and 1 foot 6 inches wide, and a foot deeper than the main pit, and at right angles to it, is dug. A field drain-pipe is placed in a tunnel connecting the trench with the pit, and this pipe is stuffed with straw. Straw is laid in the bottom of the main pit, wood or coal is piled above it so that about three-quarters of the pit is filled, and the carcase is next rolled into the pit. More wood or coal is piled around and above it, and paraffin oil is poured over the whole. The straw is finally lighted in the bottom of the ventilation trench. A carcase cremated by this method takes about 8 to 10 hours to burn away, and requires little or no attention. When burning is complete the soil is replaced and the ground levelled.

The *surface burning method* is mainly used where there are numbers of animals to be burned. One long trench is dug about 1 foot 6 inches deep and 1 foot wide, and about 3 feet length is allowed for each cattle carcase. At intervals along each side there are placed side flues to coincide with each carcase. Fuel (straw, wood, and coal) is placed around the central trench and the carcases are drawn across it. More fuel is heaped around and between them, and paraffin oil or petrol is sprayed over the whole. The straw is lighted. More fuel requires to be added at intervals. Instead of the trench and side flues battens of stout wood are sometimes laid upon the ground, and the carcases are pulled over them. Fuel is piled around them and lighted, and more is added as required. This latter method is specially applicable where the ground is very wet, or where there is rock immediately below the soil and digging is impossible.

Precautions.—Where the carcase of an animal that has died from a contagious disease is being disposed of in one of the above ways, it is very necessary to ensure that blood or discharges are not spilled upon the ground in the process of removal. An efficient method of preventing this is to stuff tow saturated with some strong disinfectant into all the natural orifices—nostrils, mouth, anus, etc.—and to cover the surface of the improvised sleigh (door or gate) with pieces of old sacking which have been soaked with disinfectant, so that parts of the carcase do not become chafed through friction with the ground and so leave behind bloodstains. Everything that has come into contact with the carcase must be carefully disinfected before it is removed. Old ropes, sacking, and other objects used for handling the dead animal may be burned. The surface of the soil around the edge of the pit, upon which the carcase rests, should be scraped off and thrown into the fire or pit so that any blood or discharges may be rendered harmless. Finally, all attendants should be impressed with the risks they run in handling diseased carcases, and with the risks there are of contaminating other healthy cattle, and each one of them should be made to wash his hands and arms, and to dip his feet into a pailful of disinfectant, before he leaves the place of disposal.

DISTEMPER is a name applied to a specific virus disease, but was once applied somewhat indiscriminately to almost any fevered condition of animals or man. As a general rule, all members of the Canidæ and Mustelidæ are susceptible to canine distemper. These classes contain all those animals which do not have retractable claws (as opposed to the Felidæ), and include : dog, fox, wolf, ferret, mink, weasel, ermine, marten, otter, and badger.

Infection of dogs with measles or rinderpest virus confers immunity against distemper.

Canine distemper is an infectious disease mainly of young dogs, characterised in the A type by a rise in temperature, dullness, and loss of appetite, and in the later stages by a catarrhal discharge from the eyes and nostrils. The disease is often complicated by broncho-pneumonia, and in some cases nervous symptoms develop, either when the febrile conditions subside, or before this happens. The incubation period of the disease is stated to be from 4 to 21 days, though it may be longer.

Causes.—A virus of which there is **only one antigenic type,** though various syndromes (including 'Hard Pad') may be associated with various strains. The Animal Health Trust stated, in 1958:

"A study of 50 strains of distemper virus isolated from outbreaks scattered throughout England and Wales has shown that infections of dogs with the original type of Virus A ("Laidlaw and Dunkin") are in the minority (14 per cent), while type B shows 20 per cent, and type C 66 per cent—the latter being of a low virulence." Certain bacteria are responsible for secondary lesions; for example, *Bacillus coli* is responsible for the bowel disturbance that is often present. Cases of Distemper may be complicated by the coexistence of other infections such as CANINE VIRUS HEPATITIS, LEPTOSPIROSIS, and TOXOPLASMOSIS.

Although it is chiefly in young dogs that the disease is met with, older dogs are occasionally affected; as a general rule, however, young animals between the ages of 3 and 12 months are the most susceptible. The breed of the dog may act as a predisposing cause; thus, distemper is almost always serious and common in dogs that are of foreign origin, such as Japanese spaniels, Samoyedes, Chow-chows, Borzoi, etc., especially when these animals have been recently imported into Great Britain. The indigenous hardy breeds are more resistant, as also are those families of other breeds that have been born and reared in this country for generations. That the weather has an important influence on the incidence of distemper is shown by the fact that most cases are encountered during wet, moist, foggy, chilly weather during the spring and autumn, while during dry, hot, or cold frosty periods of the year it is uncommon. Sudden changes seem to favour its appearance, especially when the change is to wet, cold, or stormy weather following a period of either dry heat or cold. Bad management on the part of the owner, such as carelessness in drying after washing, exhaustive exercise when unfit, housing in unhygienic damp or draughty places, an insufficiency in the quantity or quality of the food, and early weaning, are all predisposing factors.

Symptoms.—It must be stated at the outset that while the disease usually takes from 2 to 4 weeks to run its course, everything depends upon the nature of the complications as to how long a time will elapse before the dog is fit again.

Distemper commences insidiously. In some cases a fit is the first warning to the owner of the onset of the disease. Often all that is noticed is a certain amount of dullness and lack of interest in its surroundings on the part of the dog, for a day or two. If the temperature be taken it will be found raised to 103° or 104° F., and the dog's nose will be hot and dry and its eyes congested. Food is refused or taken half-heartedly; but there is often great thirst. In a few days a small amount of yellowish-green discharge from the eyes and nose is noticed, the temperature rises, and the depression and dullness are more marked than before. The course of the disease from this stage onwards depends upon whether or not infection by secondary organisms produces complications. In some cases symptoms of bronchitis may be present, characterised by a slight cough, a further rise in temperature, and a more profuse discharge from the nostrils. On the other hand, bowel complications may ensue, manifested by diarrhœa, pain in the abdomen, and vomiting; or nervous symptoms assert themselves.

The eye lesions generally take the form of a conjunctivitis which varies in severity; the mucous membranes of the eyelids become swollen and congested, and a purulent discharge appears. This discharge collects at the inner corners of the eyes and soils the edges of the eyelids, often causing them to adhere to one another. Ulcers may form on the cornea as a result of the action of the accumulated and decomposing pus, and from the affected animal constantly rubbing its eyes. In some cases inflammation of the cornea (keratitis) producing a milk-white opacity may be present.

The nasal discharge is at first serous, and later mucoid or purulent. It varies in colour from a dirty yellow to a green, and occasionally may be streaked with blood. The discharge is always highly virulent. Sneezing and coughing are common, and the respiration is hurried.

Should *bronchitis* occur the cough becomes more frequent, harsh, dry, painful, and is accompanied by wheezing; the discharge is more profuse; breathing is easily distressed, especially upon exertion, and there is a marked rise in temperature.

Broncho-pneumonia, which so often complicates distemper, is evidenced by paroxysms of a short hacking cough which greatly distresses the animal. When the inflammation of the lungs spreads and becomes more extensive the cough generally becomes very much suppressed. The discharge from the nostrils increases in amount and is stained with streaks of blood, and extreme difficulty in breathing is seen. The slightest exertion causes the animal literally to fight for breath, and weakness and depression are very marked. (*See* BORDETELLA.)

Gastro-enteritis may occur. There may be repeated vomiting of a greenish or brownish glairy mucus, and by a coppery discoloration of the tongue and ulceration of the mucous membranes of both the tongue and insides of the cheeks. It is common to find that ulcerated areas are markedly present along the gums and round the roots of the teeth. These lesions of the mouth, along with gas regurgitated from the stomach, give rise to an extremely unpleasant odour perceptible from the whole dog, but most marked when the mouth is opened for examination. Food is refused, or, if it be taken, is followed by vomiting almost at once. Whenever alimentary complications occur the animal evinces a marked thirst; large quantities of water are taken, but the water is ejected almost at once. There is frequently diarrhœa, which produces great weakness and rapid emaciation. When bowel complications are present worms may be expelled spontaneously, and the owner may be tempted to administer a vermifuge. The presence of these parasites is not the cause of the symptoms, however; their expulsion is rather the effect of the condition. On no account should such a dog be given worm medicine.

In some cases *cerebral congestion* arises and is manifested by excitement, restlessness, or even convulsions (fits). The animal falls down as if suffering from epilepsy, screams or yelps, foams at the mouth, rolls on to its side, becomes unconscious, and exhibits spasmodic contractions of the muscles generally. The sphincters of the bladder and rectum are relaxed, and urine and fæces are passed quite involuntarily. In a few minutes there is a gradual return to consciousness and the dog manages to rise, though for some time he appears weak and dazed. When once these convulsions appear they tend to recur at increasingly frequent intervals. (*See* ENCEPHALITIS.)

Paralysis may follow the convulsions. It may be confined to certain groups of muscles, such as those of a limb, or there may be almost total paralysis of the skeletal muscles. Paralysis of the hind-quarters (paraplegia) is sometimes met with; it is accompanied by incontinence of the fæces and urine, and seldom responds to treatment.

A rash may or may not develop; when present it occurs on the abdomen and the inner aspects of the thighs.

Other localisations, such as inflammation of the kidneys, bladder, testes, uterus, liver, or heart wall may appear during the course of the disease, but they are comparatively uncommon. Abscesses may develop in the joints.

In Britain canine distemper of the 'classical type' described here is encountered much less frequently than formerly.

In rare cases the pads of the feet become visibly thickened and swollen, occasionally to such an extent that they make a tapping sound on the floor when the dog walks. (This gave rise to the name 'Hard Pad Disease'.)

Diagnosis and treatment.—An early diagnosis is important, and a veterinary surgeon should be consulted as soon as any of the above symptoms appear. Good nursing is highly important, but not enough by itself, and treatment is best left to the professional man who can advise on the use of serum, sulphonamides, penicillin, etc., as the situation demands. What follows is designed as a guide only to those living in remote places.

1. *General treatment.*—(*See* NURSING.)

If constipation be present, some mild laxative is indicated. Cascara in 2-grain doses, or Epsom salts in half-teaspoonful doses, are suitable.

2. *Local treatment.*—The discharge from the eyes may be moderated by the application of mild astringent eye-lotions, such as are sold for human use, or a 0·2 per cent solution of zinc sulphate; of such a solution 5 or 6 drops should be instilled into the eye twice or thrice daily by means of a drop-bottle, after the discharge has been removed by washing with a little warm water. In the treatment of corneal ulcers a 5 per cent solution of protargol in distilled water is useful.

If a simple cough is present some mild

soothing expectorant such as syrup of squills and honey may be given. Covering the chest with a woollen jacket will guard against the further complication of pneumonia. Should the latter arise, on account of the lessened area of lung surface available for respiration, a plentiful supply of fresh air should be ensured. Heart stimulants, may be given hypodermically. Antibiotics are usually prescribed. Many cases of pneumonia end fatally, however, in spite of all treatment.

Ulcerations in the mouth should be treated by swabbing with dilute hydrogen peroxide and followed by mouth-washes.

The principle employed in the treatment of diarrhœa and vomiting is to soothe the mucous membrane of the alimentary canal. Bismuth salts in from 5- to 10-grain doses soothe the stomach, and should be given in the switched white of an egg as a first-aid measure.

Convulsions (*i.e.* 'fits'), if present, may be checked by the administration of anti-spasmodics. As a general rule, cases that show convulsions end fatally. (For treatment of chorea, *see* CHOREA.)

3. *Convalescence.*—After recovery from distemper it is important to remember that, unless the dog is looked after with great care, relapses are liable to occur. For a week or ten days after all symptoms have *apparently* subsided the dog should be given only a limited amount of exercise and his food should be increased slowly and gradually, no matter how ravenous his appetite may be. The return to the normal diet should be slow, and abrupt changes should be avoided. He may receive some simple tonic, such as a half-teaspoonful of Parrish's Food, once daily for a week or so, with or without cod-liver oil and malt extract, mixed with a food or given on a full stomach.

4. *Prevention.*—Inoculation with an egg-adapted virus may be carried out when the puppy is 11 weeks old. If vaccine was used at 8 or 9 weeks, a second dose must be given. A booster dose is often advisable when the dog is about 2 years old.

A second type of distemper vaccine is prepared from virus not grown on eggs. The makers claim that a single dose at 7 to 9 weeks of age will give lasting immunity; though many veterinary surgeons prefer to wait till the puppy is 10 weeks old.

The distemper and CVH antigens most commonly used (1966) and which are also present in combined vaccines are:

1. *Live, egg-adapted distemper virus*
   (a) obtained from embryonated hens' eggs
   (b) obtained from cultures of avian fibroblastic tissue.
2. *Live distemper virus adapted to homologous tissue culture*
   obtained from cultures of dog kidney epithelial tissue.
3. *Inactivated CVH virus*
   obtained from organs or from cultured tissue.
4. *Live CVH virus adapted to tissue culture*
   obtained from dog or pig kidney tissue.

Distemper-CVH vaccines either contain two live viruses or live distemper and inactivated CVH virus. The properties of these vaccines depend to a large extent on the antigens selected and the manner of their combination. (O. Ackermann.)

It is of course very important to ensure that the puppy is healthy when vaccinated. If the temperature is found raised, serum alone may be used. Serum is also sometimes used to control an outbreak, the immunity it confers being reinforced by a mild attack of natural infection in dogs which are themselves not actually suffering although exposed to the virus.

Combined vaccines, against distemper, virus hepatitis, and leptospirosis, are available.

For temporary protection, a gamma-globulin preparation may be used. (*See* GLOBULIN.)

A measles virus vaccine has been introduced for use in dogs to give protection against distemper. The advantage of this vaccine is that it can be used in puppies 3 weeks old and upwards, and so tide the young animal over a danger period—one in which immunity conferred by the maternal antibodies is waning and when distemper virus cannot be used effectively. Immunity is usually established in 72 hours, and lasts 5 months at least. Ordinary distemper vaccination is not interfered with.

DISTOMIASIS means infestation with liver flukes.

DIURETICS (διά, through; οὐρέω, I pass water) are substances which produce diuresis, that is, which cause a copious excretion of urine.

Varieties.—Non-irritating watery fluids, such as barley-water, hay-tea, etc. Substances which dilate the kidney arteries, such as alcohol, nitrous ether, salts of the alkalies, especially the potassium compounds which upset the composition of the blood and are quickly discharged, all have a diuretic action. Substances which irritate the kidneys act, in small amounts, as diuretics ; for example, oil of turpentine, oil of juniper, caffeine, and diuretin. Substances which increase the force of the heart, and consequently the pressure of the blood, act under ordinary circumstances in this way also ; such are digitalis, squills, strophanthus, and strychnine.

Uses.—Diuretics are given to increase the amount of fluid excreted from the body, and consequently to diminish the amount that remains behind. They are not always satisfactory, since disease of the kidneys, which may be the cause of the dropsy, will prevent these organs exercising their function, and in such cases they must not be used. They are generally given in fevers to accelerate the discharge from the body of waste products of metabolism and to clear away the poisons that are formed during the course of fever. For this purpose the saline substances are most useful.

DIURETIN is the salicylate of theobromine and soda, and being a powerful diuretic, is used for the treatment of dropsy in old dogs due to kidney insufficiency.

DIVERTICULUM (*diverto*, I turn aside) is a small pouch formed in connection with a hollow organ. There are certain diverticula which are normally present in the body, *e.g.* the *diverticulum of the duodenum*, which is found at the point of entrance of the bile and pancreatic ducts, or the *post-urethral diverticulum*, a little pouch behind the opening of the female urethra into the posterior genital tract in the sow and cow ; while there are others which are found as the result of injury or disease, *e.g.* in the œsophagus, in the rectum, and sometimes in the intestines.

DNA.—Desoxyribonucleic acid. A constituent of some viruses, especially bacteriophages. (*See also under* ARTIFICIAL SOMATIC MUTATIONS.)

DNOC. — Dinitro-*ortho*-cresol, a yellow crystalline substance employed in agriculture as a weed-killer spray solution, acts as a powerful cumulative poison. In man the symptoms are excessive sweating, thirst, and loss of weight. Poisoning in domestic animals might well be encountered following contamination by the spray or residue.

DNP.—A product somewhat similar to DNOC (which see).

DOCKING is the name applied to the operation of removing the tail or a part of that organ. In Great Britain, docking of the horse (excluding amputation of the tail by a veterinary surgeon for reasons of disease of the tail) is now illegal. Certain breeds of dogs are docked under Kennel Club rules, and others must not be docked. Docking of puppies is usually carried out when they are 3–5 days old. It can legally be done without anæsthesia by a layman up to the time the eyes open. Late docking should be done under anæsthesia by a veterinary surgeon.

It is customary for sheep of lowland breeds to be docked, for if the tail is left long it accumulates dirt and fæces, and these predispose to the attacks of blowflies. Many mountain breeds of sheep are left undocked ; the long woolly tail helps to keep the hind parts protected from frost and wind. Lambs are usually docked by the use of a long sharp knife, the bleeding being negligible if the lambs are not more than a month old. The rubber-ring method is also used sometimes within 48 hours of birth.

The operation is performed as follows: A local anæsthetic solution is injected under the skin at the root of the tail, after first cleansing the part. The hair is clipped (or shaved in dogs) from about 1½ inches over the part that will become the end of the tail after docking, and a tape ligature is applied above this. The skin is rendered aseptic (or nearly so), by painting with iodine or spirit, and when this is dry the preparations are complete. After the tail is severed the wound is closed by drawing the skin together by means of two or more stitches which are removed in 4 or 5 days' time.

(See **ANÆSTHETICS, LEGAL REQUIREMENTS.**)

DOCKS, POISONING BY.—Although poisoning by docks is not at all common, yet there have been a few cases of it recorded, and losses of sheep have been occasionally ascribed to eating either the common Sorrel dock (*Rumex acetona*) or to Sheep's Sorrel (*Rumex acetosella*), both of which contain oxalates. A condition of staggering with dilated pupils, muscular tremors, and later, convulsions and prostration, has been noticed in horses which have eaten large quantities of sheep's sorrel. In sheep, there is a loss of appetite, rapid breathing, exhaustion, sometimes constipation and at other times diarrhœa, with an uncertain, drunken gait and occasionally death. The milk of cows that have eaten docks is made into butter only with difficulty.

Treatment.—Purgatives should be given along with doses of baking soda, and the animals taken into a shed and fed on demulcent and laxative foods for a few days.

DODDER, POISONING BY.—It seems possible that the parasitic dodder, which may attack clover or hay crops, may, when fed to horses and cattle, cause digestive troubles. The progressive farmer, however, will always take the precaution of having patches of dodder (*Cuscuta europœa* and *C. epithymum*) cut with a scythe from amongst a green fodder crop and burned before any seeds have been produced which will contaminate his samples, or before the parasitic plant has attained serious dimensions.

DOG-POX (*see* VARIOLA).

DOG-SITTING POSITION.—In pigs this may be a symptom of pantothenic acid (Vitamin B) deficiency.

DOG TICKS.—In Britain these include Ixodes hexagonus (common on suburban dogs and cats) ; *I. ricinus* (the sheep tick, commonly found on country dogs ; *I. canisuga* (' the British dog tick ') ; and *Dermacentor reticulatus* (which may infest also cattle and horses). *I. canisuga* may establish itself in buildings, as may *Rhipicephalus sanguineus*, which has infested houses in Denmark as well as quarantine stations. Modern central heating may facilitate the survival of this tick in northern latitudes.

DOGS, BREEDS OF.—The reader is advised to consult text-books on this subject, such as *Keeping a Dog*, by R. F. Wall, M.R.C.V.S., *Dogs of To-day*, by Harding-Cox, both published by A. & C. Black.

DOGS, DISEASES OF.—These include distemper, rabies, virus hepatitis, tuberculosis, leptospirosis, nephritis, hysteria, mange, eczema, ringworm, blastomycosis, disease of the pancreas, ' fading ' of puppies, canine herpes virus, ' haemorrhagic disease ', hookworm infestation, pyometra. (*See also under* TINNED FOOD, BLACK TONGUE.)

DOLICHOCEPHALIC SKULL is one which is long and narrow, as distinct from one which is short and broad. Examples of the former are skulls of the greyhound and collie, and of the latter (*brachycephalic*), those of the pug and bulldog.

DOMINANT.—That member of an allelic pair of genes which asserts its effects over the other dissimilar member (recessive) of a gene pair.

DOSAGE.—The quantity of medicine that is given in one dose varies very considerably with certain circumstances. Many drugs produce one effect when given in small amount, and quite another effect when given in larger doses ; thus, ipecacuanha wine is expectorant in small doses, and causes vomiting when given in large doses to the dog. Certain drugs are suitable for administration to one species of animal, but are quite useless when given to another ; for example, the dog reacts to morphine very well, but cattle and cats, instead of being soothed, are driven into a state of acute delirium when it is given to them. Climatic conditions alter the actions of some drugs. Among other factors which influence the amount of a drug that must be given are the following : weight, age, sex, habitual previous administration, disease, fasting, combination with other drugs, individual idiosyncrasy, and the form in which, as well as the method by which, the drug is administered.

Weight. With greater accuracy and purity of manufacture, most modern drugs are best given strictly upon the basis of the weight of the animal in pounds or kilograms. This applies in particular to those drugs which are chemical entities themselves, rather than preparations from plants or plant substances.

For ordinary purposes the weight of an animal may be roughly guessed, but with powerful drugs it is very advisable to know the weight precisely, and the animal should be weighed.

Age is an important factor to take into consideration when adjusting doses of medicines for animals.

Habitual previous administration of a drug may either give an animal a tolerance against the substance, or it may make it more susceptible to its action; *e.g.* repeated administration of arsenic will allow an animal to take a dose much larger than could ordinarily be given with safety; and the continued administration of strychnine or digitalis results in the accumulation of these drugs in the system and makes their further administration dangerous.

Disease very greatly modifies the dose of certain medicines, for their tendency to produce poisonous effects diminishes in circumstances that urgently require their administration.

Fasting aids the rapidity of the absorption of, and also makes the system more susceptible than otherwise to, the action of most remedies.

Combinations of different drugs possessing a similar action are generally made use of when writing prescriptions, and frequently this enables the total dose to be more effective, and undesirable effects are eliminated. This is especially the case with purgatives, as well as with powerful drugs such as atropine and morphine.

Form of administration is also highly important, for active principles when separated and given by themselves in solution in water produce more rapid and intense effects than when the crude drug is given. Moreover, the means employed to introduce the agents into the body are also influential; *e.g.* if the dose given by the stomach (through the mouth) is taken as 1, the dose by rectal injection is 2, by subcutaneous injection it is about $\frac{1}{8}$th, by intratracheal injection $\frac{1}{20}$th, and by intravenous injection it is $\frac{1}{25}$th to $\frac{1}{50}$th. (*See also* APOTHECARIES' WEIGHTS, PRESCRIPTION.)

DOUBLE PREGNANCY.—A term applied to the existence of two sets of fœtuses, of different ages and born with a corresponding interval between litters, in the sow, cow, etc. (*See* SUPERFŒTATION *for further information.*)

'DOUBLE SCALP'.—A condition seen in older lambs and young sheep, mainly on hill grazings, in autumn and winter. There is unthriftiness associated with a thinning of the bones of the skull. In advanced cases the animal cannot eat or close its mouth. The cause is believed to be related to phosphorus-deficient pastures, but feeding bone-meal will not prevent the disease.

DOUCHE (*see* IRRIGATION).

DOURINE is a venereal disease of horses due to a trypanosome called the *Trypanosoma equiperdum*, which is transmitted by sexual intercourse among breeding horses, asses, and mules. It occurs in Africa, Asia, parts of Europe, and in areas in both North and South America. (*See* PARASITES, p. 634.)

DOVER'S POWDER, also known as COMPOUND IPECACUANHA POWDER, is made up from 10 per cent each of powdered opium and ipecacuanha, with 80 per cent of sulphate of potassium.

DRAINAGE (*see* SANITATION).

'DRENCHING'.—The giving of liquid medicine to animals. It must be done slowly, and with care, especially in the pig and horse—and in all animals suffering from bronchitis and consequently liable to cough. Pneumonia is a common sequel to liquid medicines 'going the wrong way'.

Another danger is associated with the use on pigs of a drenching gun intended for sheep. Unless these appliances are used with care, severe injury may result. In a series of cases reported in Australia, 24 pigs suffered rupture of the pharyngeal diverticulum—part of the throat—and 12 died.

DRESSED SEED CORN.—Any surplus should *not* be fed to farm livestock owing to the danger of poisoning. Pigs have been accidentally killed in this way after being given corn treated with a mercury dressing. Dieldrin dressings kill birds.

DRIED GRASS has for long been incorporated by compounders into feeding-stuffs for poultry and pigs, but now an increasing quantity is being fed to dairy cows as part of a ration together with some roughage (straw, hay, silage) and some other concentrate feed, such as barley. Dried green crops are also being fed on a small scale to sheep and beef cattle.

Grass drying is not an alternative to hay- and silage-making, since it needs a planned programme to give a succession of crops for cutting. Today this is possible, and a succession of grass or lucerne crops can be cut at the correct stage of growth and processed economically by modern factory-size drying plants.

The dried grass can either be milled and made into pellets or cubes; or left unmilled and pressed into cobs or wafers, which saves the high cost of hammer-milling. Unmilled material may have other advantages, too, for it has been shown that hammer-milling and pelleting decreases the digestibility of the product and, while increasing the efficiency with which digested nutrients are used by non-lactating animals, depresses butterfat production of those in milk.

The hardness of pellets and cobs is an important factor; if too hard, they can give disappointing results. Particle size is also important.

Minimum protein content of dried grass for use without supplementary protein is considered to be 18 per cent; minimum digestibility figure about 60 per cent. ADAS work has shown that crude protein analysis is of little help in indicating digestibility. This (and hence energy equivalent) mainly determines milk production, not protein.

DROPPED ELBOW (*see* RADIAL PARALYSIS).

DROPPED SOLE (*see* LAMINITIS).

DROPSY, or **HYDROPS** (ὕδρωψ), means an accumulation of watery fluid below the skin, or in one or more of the body cavities. The term is a general one, the accumulations in special localities having special names; *e.g.* dropsy below the skin is called *œdema*; if it is widespread it is known as *anasarca*; dropsy affecting the abdominal cavity is known as *ascites*; in the chest it is *hydrothorax*, and in the head *hydrocephalus*. A normal physiological form of œdema occurs in the pregnant mare and cow a short time before parturition and disappears spontaneously a few hours or a day or two afterwards. This is variously referred to as 'udder œdema', 'udder nature', or 'udder dropsy'. It is seen to a less extent in other animals. It should not be confused with pathological dropsy or œdema.

Causes.—It is a mistake to assume that because a part of the body becomes dropsical there is some diseased condition at work in it, for dropsy is in every case merely a symptom of some or other of several diseased conditions. As a rule, œdema of the surface of the body, *i.e.* where there is fluid located in the tissue spaces immediately below the skin, is due to a local disturbance of the circulation, such as may be produced by too tight a girth in the horse, or the application of bandages that are causing pressure upon the blood-vessels; but it may also arise through weak heart action, with stagnation of the blood in the lowermost veins (along the lower line of and the chest abdomen). Such cases are especially common after debilitating diseases, such as influenza, mastitis; lack of exercise and food in old animals are also contributory causes. Anasarca is a condition of widespread dropsy affecting the whole of the surface of the body. It is chiefly seen in fœtuses that have died during or previous to delayed parturition, in which fluid and gas collect below the skin and puff it out to its fullest extent. Ascites is perhaps the most common and important form of dropsy occurring among animals. An excessive amount of fluid collects in the abdominal cavity, causing a fluctuating swelling and entailing disturbances of digestion, nutrition, and heart action, and sometimes of respiration. It is not uncommon in dogs and cats affected with tuberculosis, a failing heart, or some degenerative process in the liver or kidneys, and occasionally with diabetes. It affects animals of other species at almost any age, *e.g.* in sheep which harbour large numbers of liver flukes (*Fasciola hepatica*, and other species), when it is popularly described as a 'pot belly'. It is associated with a stagnation of blood in the veins of the abdomen and peritoneum, whereby an oozing of the fluid constituents of the blood into the peritoneal cavity can occur. This stagnation may be caused through a faulty heart action, or through some obstruction to the free flow of blood in the abdominal veins, such as pressure from a tumour, enlarged mesenteric glands, verminous aneurysm in horses, dense fibrous tissue laid down in the liver as the result of previous inflammation, swelling and inflammation of the kidneys, growths on the valves of the right side of the heart; or it may arise when an animal is heavily infected with worms, or seriously affected with coccidiosis or tuberculosis. Hydrothorax is frequently associated with either an acute but more commonly a chronic pleurisy (*see* PLEURISY). Hydrocephalus occurs mainly in the unborn fœtus.

Symptoms.—Œdema occurring under the skin is manifested by a diffuse painless swelling, which feels like dough to the touch and pits on pressure. Anasarca appears as if the body had been blown full of gas by inserting a tube below the skin. There are usually obvious signs of decomposition. Ascites usually develops slowly, and as the fluid collects, the abdominal wall enlarges to accommodate it. The abdomen becomes slowly more and more pendulous, and very frequently the owner may be led to imagine that a female animal so affected is pregnant. After some time, however, the fluctuation of the fluid present becomes obvious; a tap upon one side of the abdomen being conveyed through the walls to the opposite side. Breathing may be laboured on account of the fluid pressing the diaphragm forwards, limiting the action of this structure, and compressing the chest cavity. Later still, the affected animal commences to lose condition, and in a short while the spines of the vertebræ become prominent. Food is taken, but without relish. At times there may be attacks of diarrhœa, but these usually pass off without treatment. Less and less desire for exercise, or even movement, is shown; and if the animal is made to work it very soon becomes tired. Afterwards, exhaustion, emaciation, and death occur.

Treatment.—Before treatment can be undertaken it is necessary to discover the actual cause of the dropsy, whether local or general. Such cases of œdema as are due to artificial pressure require nothing more than removal of the cause. In dropsy of the abdomen it is nearly always only possible to effect a temporary improvement, for the fluid re-forms afterwards, and is less tractable with each subsequent recurrence. It is customary to tap such as occur in animals that show no serious symptoms and withdraw the fluid. Internally, drugs which hasten absorption and stimulate the heart and circulation, such as potassium iodide and digitalis, are given, and the animal is put on to rich, easily digested food, while its exercise is arranged so that it does not become too tired. Where worms or other parasites are present they must be expelled.

In very many cases, however, immediate destruction is the more humane and economical course, and is in the interests of public health where dropsy is of tuberculous origin.

DROPWORT POISONING (*see* WATER DROPWORT POISONING).

DROUGHTMASTER.—A breed of cattle developed in Australia from Brahman and British (mainly Shorthorn) ancestors. It is claimed to be 10 times more tick-resistant than British breeds, and a more efficient beef producer under the relatively harsh grazing conditions of North Australia.

DROWNING.—*Submersion* in water for a period of about 4 minutes is sufficient to cause asphyxia and death, but shorter periods, while they may cause apparent death, usually only produce a collapse from which recovery is possible. Practically all animals, even the very young, are able to swim naturally, so that *immersion* in water for this period does not necessarily result in drowning. The specific gravity of an animal's body is slightly greater than that of water, so that if a severe injury has occurred before entering the water, whereby swimming does not take place, the body sinks and death may occur quickly. Animals falling into water are drowned from one of several causes: they may be exhausted by struggling in mud; they may be carried away by a swift current, *e.g.* during floods; they may be hindered by harness or other tackle from keeping their nostrils above the level of the water; or they may become panic-stricken and swim away from shore. Remarkable instances of the powers of swimming that are naturally possessed by animals are on record; one example being that of a heifer, which, becoming excited and frightened on the southern banks of the Solway Firth, entered the water and swam across to the Scottish side, a distance of over seven miles, and was brought back next day none the worse!

Recovery from drowning.—As soon as the animal has been rescued from the water, it should be placed in a position which will allow water which has been taken into the lungs to run out by the mouth and the nostrils. Small animals may be held up by the hind-legs and swung from side to side, and larger ones should be laid on their sides with the hind-quarters elevated at a higher level than their heads. If they can be placed with their heads downhill, so much the better. Pressure should be brought to bear on the chest, by one man throwing all his weight on to the upper part of the chest wall, or kneeling on this part. When no more fluid runs from the mouth, the animal should be turned over on to the opposite side and the process repeated. No time should be lost in so doing, especially if the animal has been in the water for some time. (*See* ARTIFICIAL RESPIRATION.)

After-treatment.—As soon as possible the animal should be removed to warm surroundings and dried by wisping or by vigorous rubbing with a rough towel. Clothing should be applied, and the smaller animals may be provided with one or more hot-water bottles. The danger that has to be remembered is that of pneumonia, either from the water in the lungs or the general chilling of the body, and the chest should be specially well covered. Sometimes the ingestion of salt water leads to salt poisoning in dogs, or to a disturbance of the digestive functions, and appropriate treatment is necessary.

DRUG RESISTANCE (*See under* ANTIBIOTIC RESISTANCE).

DRY FEEDING of meal may give rise to PARAKERATOSIS in pigs; to 'CURLED TONGUE' in turkey poults; and to 'SHOVEL BEAK' in chicks. (*See under these headings.*)

DRYING-OFF COWS.—After milking out completely, the teats should be washed and 300,000 i.u. of penicillin inserted in each teat. Do not milk again unless it becomes necessary.

The cows should be inspected daily and if any quarter becomes much enlarged, it should be milked, treated with penicillin and reported for treatment. The quarters should swell up equally for about three days and then gradually subside.

A more recent recommendation is to replace the penicillin with a Cloxacillin preparation.

If possible, keep the cows on dry food or very short pasture for three days after drying off.

DRY PERIOD.—In cattle it is considered advisable on health grounds that the body should have a rest from lactation for about 8 weeks.

DUBBING.—This is an operation performed with scissors by poultry-keepers, and involves removal of a crescent of comb—about $\frac{1}{16}$-inch deep—in day-old chicks. It is credited with increasing egg production by 3 to 4 per year. It is also advocated in intensive rearing, where a floppy comb may be a disadvantage if pecking and cannibalism are rife; and in order to reduce the risk of frost-bite.

DUCK VIRUS HEPATITIS causes up to 90% mortality among ducklings under 3 weeks of age, but in ducklings a month or more old losses are slight. Resistant ducks can be bred. A vaccine has proved successful. A notifiable disease.

DUCT is the name applied to a passage leading from a gland into some hollow organ, or on to the surface of the body, by which the secretion of the gland is discharged; *e.g.* the pancreatic duct and the bile duct open into the duodenum, and the milk ducts open at the end of the teats. Some glands, *e.g.* the thyroid, pituitary, and adrenal glands have no ducts, but their secretions are received by the blood-vessels or lymph channels in their neighbourhood.

DUCTLESS GLANDS (*see* ENDOCRINE GLANDS).

DUNG-FOULED PASTURE.—(*See* PASTURE MANAGEMENT.)

DUNG HEAPS.—Blades of grass growing near these often harbour large numbers of Husk worm larvæ. (*See* HUSK.) Dung heaps are best fenced in. Care should be taken over the disposal of pig manure, as otherwise trichomoniasis might be spread from pigs to cattle.

DUODENUM (*duodenum*) is the first part of the small intestine immediately following the stomach. Into it open the bile and pancreatic ducts. (*See* INTESTINE.)

DURA MATER (*durus*, hard; *mater*, mother) is the outermost and the strongest of the three membranes or meninges which envelop the brain and spinal cord. In it also are found the blood-vessels that nourish the inner surface of the skull. (*See* BRAIN.)

DURAZNILLO BLANCO.—A poisonous plant of South America. (*See* ENTEQUE SECO.)

DUROC.—A breed of pig, varying in colour from a light golden-yellow to a very dark red, originating from the eastern states of the U.S.A.

DUSTING POWDERS form most convenient applications for wounds in animals. They may be used for an antiseptic effect, to control infection, or for astringent and protective effects to dry up superficial lesions and encourage scab formation.

Dusting powders containing parasiticides are used to destroy fleas and lice on animals.

Varieties.—Some of the most satisfactory for animal treatment are compounds of sulphathiazole and amino-acridines, such as 'Flavazole' powder. Formerly iodoform was much used.

Parasitic dusting powders contain derris or BHC, for example.

DUSTY ATMOSPHERE.—In piggeries, this can be a cause of coughing, etc., simulating Virus Pneumonia. (*See* MEAL FEEDING.) Inoculations should not be carried out in a dusty shed. (*See* ANTHRAX.) Material in dust may give rise to an allergy (*see* FOG FEVER, BROKEN WIND) and to abortion if fungi are present (*See* UTERINE INFECTIONS).

DYES, ANILINE (*see* ANILINE).

DYS- (δυσ-, badly) is a prefix meaning painful or difficult.

DYSENTERY (from the prefix δυσ-, and ἔντερον, the intestine) is a condition in which blood is discharged from the bowels with or without diarrhœa. Dysentery is most commonly encountered in certain specific diseases such as anthrax, cattle plague, hæmorrhagic septicæmia, purpura hæmorrhagica, lamb dysentery, swine fever, and winter dysentery, although it may occur when there are large numbers of strongyle worms or coccidiæ present in the bowels. Dysentery in young pigs may be due to *Clostridium welchii* infection, which causes death within 36 hours of birth. (*See also* SWINE DYSENTERY.)

DYSPEPSIA (δυσ-, with difficulty; πέπτω, I digest) means literally, as its derivation would suggest, digestive difficulty. The word is practically synonymous with indigestion, and should be used to include every condition which results in pain or discomfort during the process of digestion in all parts of the alimentary canal, and not such as have their origin in the stomach only; for instance, inflammation of the walls of the stomach, collections of gas in stomach or intestines, the presence of parasites in the stomach or n testines, improper food or methods of feeding, imperfect mastication of food by the teeth, and various factors, may give rise to dyspepsia. (*See* STOMACH, DISEASES OF; PARASITES, COLIC; TEETH; INTESTINES, DISEASES OF; etc.)

DYSPHAGIA means a difficulty in swallowing. For one cause in horses, *see under* GUTTURAL POUCH DIPHTHERIA.

DYSPNŒA (δύσπνοια) means a difficulty in breathing, and is seen in cases of pneumonia, during anæsthesia, etc.

DYSTOKIA (δυσ-, difficult; τόκος, birth) means difficulty during parturition. (*See* PARTURITION.)

DYSTROPHY (δυσ-, badly; τρέφω, I nourish) means defective or faulty nutrition, and is a term generally applied to some developmental change in the muscles occurring independently of the nervous system. (*See* MUSCULAR DYSTROPHY.)

DYSURIA means an absence of uri ne (*See* URINE.)

E

E. COLI.—This is an abbreviation for *Escherichia coli*, formerly known as *Bacillus coli*. This bacterial family is a large one, comprising many differing serotypes which can be differentiated in the laboratory by means of the agglutination test.

E. coli scours are common in newborn lambs and often fatal.

In the pig, one serotype gives rise to œdema of the bowel, another to the death of piglets within a few days of birth. Another serotype is responsible for white scour in calves. In poultry, a serotype produces a septicæmia in broiler chickens, especially during the winter and often associated with faulty ventilation. This disease is known as Coli Septicæmia or Coliform Pericarditis. Symptoms may resemble those of C.R.D.

Pigs in apparently good health are, to a greater or lesser extent, extremely sensitive to certain types of *E. coli* which occur in small numbers in their intestines. 'The multiplication of any of these serotypes will result in a sudden increase in the absorption of polysaccharide from the intestines and cause an anaphylatic reaction. Whether this reaction leads to the symptoms and lesions of hæmorrhagic gastro-enteritis, œdema disease, or mulberry heart disease will depend upon the degree of hypersensitivity of the individual animal as well as to the amount of polysaccharide absorbed. . . . Necrotic enteritis probably occurs as a later manifestation of the same disease process.' (Dr. J. R. Thomlinson.)

EAR.—Sound, which consists of waves of vibration radiating through the ether from a point of origin, is appreciated through the intricate mechanism of the outer, middle, and internal ears. The waves are collected by the funnel-like external ear and transmitted down into an external canal, across the bottom of which is stretched the ear-drum or *tympanum*, and against which these waves strike. The impact of sound-waves causes a vibration of the tympanum, and the wave of ether becomes transformed into a wave of movement. This movement is transmitted through a chain of tiny bones, called *auditory ossicles*, in the middle ear, and then to fluid contained in canals excavated in the bone of the internal ear. The vibration of this fluid stimulates the delicate hair-like nerve-endings which are found in the membranous walls of the canals, and impulses pass to the brain, whereby an animal is able to appreciate external sounds literally by *feeling* them.

Structure.—The middle and inner ears are essentially the same in all animals, but the external ears present certain differences in different species, and each merits a separate consideration here. The aural cartilages have been described under their appropriate heading, and should be referred to in this connection.

External ear.—*Horse.*—In this animal the external ear is relatively small and has the shape of a narrow, incomplete funnel with a very oblique opening. This opening may be directed straight forward, to the side, or straight backward, as well as to any intermediate position, so that sound-waves may be caught when coming from any direction—the right ear collecting waves from the right side of the body, and the left from the left side, and both ears gathering all those sounds which reach the horse from immediately in front or immediately behind. Each ear is composed of a rigid supportive structure of cartilage covered over by delicate skin on both the outside and the inside. The outer surface is uniformly covered with fine dense hairs, while the inner cavity possesses a number of longer densely arranged hairs around the margins of the opening, but in the deeper parts the skin is bare. These internal hairs serve to prevent particles, etc., from becoming lodged within the cavity, where they would set up irritation. A large number of muscles actuate the ear and are responsible for its extraordinary mobility in the horse. The position of the ears serves to some extent as an indication of the state of the horse's emotions—anger or viciousness being shown by laying the ears flat back against the head, and surprise, anticipation, or pleasure being indicated by 'pricking' the ears. At the base of the ear a complete cartilaginous tube is formed, and this leads into the bony canal or *external auditory meatus.*

Ox.—The external ear is inclined outwards; the middle part and the tip are wider and flatter than in the horse, and the whole ear is relatively larger. It is mobile, but not to the same extent as in the horse, and it is not so expressive. The *sheep's* ear is like that of the horse, but relatively longer and narrower. It possesses considerable mobility.

Pig.—The appearance and size of the pig's ear varies with the breed: in some it is small and carried vertically; in others it is larger and inclined inwards or downwards; while in the Cumberland breed it hangs downwards over the face almost to the tip of the nose.

Dog.—In the various breeds of dogs also there is a large number of different varieties of ears, varying from the small loose ears of the bulldog or pup to the long loose ears of the spaniel, and from the small prick ears of the Schipperke to the large erect ears of the Alsatian. In most breeds the tip is curled over forwards, but nearly all dogs, except those of the spaniel type, are able to erect their ears to a greater or lesser extent when alarmed or surprised.

Middle ear.—The tympanic membrane, forming the 'drum', is stretched completely across the outer passage at its innermost extremity. In the horse it is an oval disc which lies at a slope of about 30°. It is about one-half inch across its greatest diameter, and is about the thickness of a gold-beater's skin in its central parts with edges slightly thickened. It is white or pale pink in colour, and partly transparent. The cavity of the middle ear is a compartment excavated in the hard mass of the petrous part of the temporal bone which lodges the ossicles. Although important structures pass around the cavity it is chiefly important on account of its contents; these are the small auditory bones which carry impulses across its cavity and are called the *malleus* (hammer), *incus* (anvil), and *stapes* (stirrup), and two small muscles which regulate their movements, as well as certain nerves, such as the chorda tympani. The auditory ossicles are of great importance. The malleus has a long spicule of bone, the 'handle', embedded in the substance of the drum, while its 'head' is in contact with the incus. The incus, suspended by one process of bone, has another affixed to the stapes, and between the two bones there is another tiny little bone which is sometimes called the *os lenticulare.* The stapes fits, by what in a real stirrup would be the foot-piece, into one (*fenestra vestibuli*) of the two openings which lead through the inner wall of the middle ear into the internal ear. Accordingly these little bones form a chain across the middle ear, connecting the drum with the internal ear. Their function is to convert the air-waves, which strike upon the drum, into magnified mechanical movements, which can affect the fluid in the internal ear, because air-waves can produce but little effect upon fluid directly. The middle ear has two connections which are of great importance as regards disease: in front, it communicates by a passage about 4 inches long with the upper part of the throat; this is called the *Eustachian tube*; while below and behind the fenestra vestibuli there is a closed foramen which leads to the cochlea and is known as the *fenestra cochleæ.* The Eustachian tube admits air from the throat, and so keeps the pressure on both sides of the tympanum equal. When it becomes closed through a swelling of its lining membrane, or through collections of pus, such as occasionally occurs during strangles or influenza in the horse, or distemper in the dog, the animal becomes definitely deaf. In the animals of the horse tribe there is a peculiar dilatation of each Eustachian tube known as the 'diverticulum of the Eustachian tube' (*guttural pouch*), which is situated between the atlas and the pharynx. The function of these pouches, one on either side, is not very well understood, but certain authorities hold that they act as resonating chambers whereby the horse increases the intensity of the voice. Upon occasions they may become filled with pus or purulent material, *e.g.* when an abscess bursts into their cavities. In such cases they may cause a kind of false roaring when the horse is put to fast paces. The other opening (fenestra cochleæ), which is normally closed by a delicate membranous layer, may serve as an entrance for pus into the inner ear. This is especially the case when the middle ear becomes filled with pus during acute inflammations, and the pus destroys the membrane over the fenestra cochleæ. In all such cases incurable deafness results, and if the process continues the brain cavity may become affected.

Internal ear.—This consists of a complex system of hollows in the substance of the temporal bone enclosing a membranous duplicate. Between the membrane and the bone is a fluid known as *perilymph*, while the membrane is distended by another collection of fluid known as *endolymph.* This *membranous labyrinth*, as it is called, consists of two parts. The posterior part, comprising a sac, called the *utricle*, and three *semicircular canals* opening at each end into it, is the part probably concerned with the preservation of balance; the anterior part consists of another small pouch, the *saccule*, and of a still more important part, the *cochlea*, and is the part concerned in hearing. In the cochlea there are three tubes, known as the *scala tympani*, *scala media*, and *scala vestibuli*, placed side by side (the middle one being part of the membranous labyrinth), which take two and a half spiral turns round a central stem, somewhat after the manner of a snail's shell. In the central one (*scala media*) is placed the apparatus known as the *organ of Corti*, by which the sound impulses are finally received, and by which they are communicated to the auditory nerve, which ends in filaments to the organ of Corti. The essential parts of the organ are a double row of rods and several rows of cells furnished with hairs of varying length. This organ runs the whole length of the scala media. Different musical notes are probably appreciated by the hair-like processes and by different cells.

The act of hearing.—The main function of the movement of the ears is that of efficiently collecting sound-waves emanating from different directions, without the necessity of turning the whole head, although in some animals the ears may be moved for the purpose of dislodging flies or other irritating particles. When sound-waves in the air reach the ear, the drum is alternately pressed in and pulled out, in consequence of which a to-and-fro movement is communicated to the chain of ossicles. The foot of the stapes communicates these movements to the perilymph in the scala tympani, by which in turn the fluid in the scala media is set in motion. Finally these motions reach the delicate filaments placed in the organ of Corti, and so affect the nerve of hearing, which conveys the sensations to the auditory centre in the brain. The vibrations in the fluid of the internal ear are prevented from doing damage to the delicate structures therein by the fact that the scala vestibuli, which communicates with the scala tympani at the apex of the cochlea, is separated at its other end from the cavity of the middle ear only by a membrane closing the fenestra cochleæ, and this bulges out as the stapes is driven in, and *vice versa*.

EAR, DISEASES OF.—Diseases of the ears of animals should never be neglected, for although in the early stages most are fairly easily amenable to treatment, in the later stages they are often very difficult to cure. Very often the first signs of inflammatory troubles escape notice or are disregarded, and the sense of hearing is permanently destroyed before treatment is attempted. From what has already been said under EAR it will be obvious that this organ is extremely intricate and not easily accessible; moreover, the connections with the throat and with the brain make the spread of inflammatory conditions easy from the former and to the latter.

Syringing is carried out by means of a syringe with a very short nozzle, not longer than half an inch, for the dog and cat, and by means of an ordinary rubber enema syringe for the larger animals. A steady stream of solution at blood heat is directed against one of the walls of the external canal, and allowed to run out when the cavity is full. The nozzle should never be pressed down into the ear so that the escape of fluid is prevented, for by so doing there is danger of bursting the drum.

General symptoms.—The following are some of the chief symptoms of ear disease:

Deafness (*see* DEAFNESS).

Shaking the head is often performed persistently for a few moments at a time, especially after the head or ear has been handled. The animal usually carries its head to one side, *i.e.* with the affected ear lowermost, and it may walk round in circles, stumbling or falling against objects in the vicinity, vigorously shaking its head meanwhile. This behaviour is occasioned by some irritation in the ear, such as the presence of parasites, wax, or mild inflammations.

Discharge from the ear is a condition often popularly alluded to as 'canker', and it is often a sequel to a neglected case of parasitic otitis in the dog and cat. The lining skin of the ear is reddened and painful to the touch, and there is a constant discharge of purulent materila with a foul smell from the lower part of the external opening which soils the skin of the side of the head and causes matting of the hair. In many animals discharge is accompanied by a greater or lesser amount of scratching with the hind paws, but when there is a painful irritation the head is cautiously shaken instead.

WAX in the ear is one of the commonest conditions which leads to diseased conditions later. It is especially common in dogs which have large ear flaps, when discharge of the wax does not take place naturally. An excess of it should always be suspected when a dog is noticed scratching at its ears when lying before a fire. It should be removed by syringing with warm water containing about two teaspoonfuls of bicarbonate of soda to the half-pint.

FOREIGN BODIES, such as pieces of gravel, hay seeds, sand, pieces of glass, wood, peas, or parasites may become lodged in the ears of animals and give rise to irritation occurring very suddenly.

HÆMATOMA, or 'blood blister' of the flap of the ear, may occur as the result of continued irritation, such as scratching or continual shaking of the head. It is common in dogs with large ears like spaniels, and in cats which are affected with ear mange, but it may occur in almost any animal. A large fluctuating swelling appears upon the flap of the ear and causes the animal to hang its head towards the same side. In many cases little or no pain is experienced once the swelling has appeared, and, in fact, a small swelling becomes larger in many cases through the continued shaking of the head even after its original formation. The swelling is caused by bruising of the skin and the blood-vessels which lie between it and the cartilage, with a consequent extravasation of blood or serum under the skin. The condition is treated by opening the hæmatoma under conditions of surgical cleanliness, evacuating the fluid contents, and suturing the skin in such a way that the collection of more fluid is prevented.

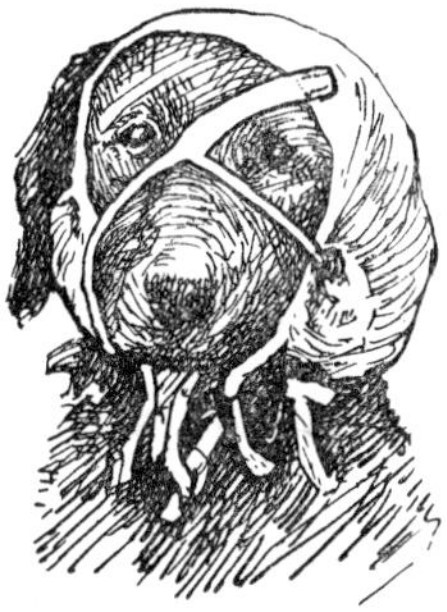

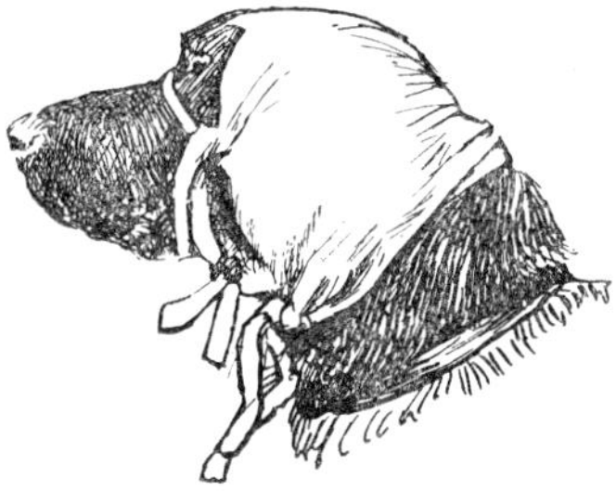

Method of improvising an ear bandage for the dog. A piece of cloth is cut to fit over the head as shown, the tapes are tied below the jaw, and the sound ear left outside the bandage as in the upper diagram.

WOUNDS of the flaps of the ears are usually caused by bites from dogs or horses, or from barbed wire, nails, etc., in the larger animals. They are usually difficult to treat in the dog, because of the persistent shaking of the head and the consequent interference with the union of the torn or damaged tissues, as well as on account of the comparatively poor blood-supply. The hair should be clipped from round the edges of the wound, and an antiseptic applied. If it will allow of suturing it is usually better to bring the edges into apposition by this means rather than allow it to heal as an open wound. In dogs it is always necessary to prevent further damage, tearing out of the stitches, etc., by the use of an ear cap. This may either be made from a wide 'many-tailed' bandage, or a leather helmet may be strapped over the head after the wound has been covered with cotton-wool and a simple bandage. In some cases slight abrasions of the edges of the ear flaps are very intractable, since each time a scab forms over the surface it is almost immediately removed by scratching or shaking. Such an abrasion may persist for a long period of time, becoming partially healed at times, only to be opened up afresh later on. There is generally a considerable amount of thickening and ulceration of the skin, and in bad cases the cartilage below may be affected. Such conditions are best treated by the removal of a portion of healthy tissue from around the diseased area, scarification or cauterisation, and subsequent protection.

EAR MANGE in the goat is not uncommon. Gammexane preparations are used in treatment of this form of Psoroptic mange.

'CANKER' is a popular term applied somewhat indiscriminately to any inflammation of the lining of the external ear, including the simple excess of wax already referred to, the presence of parasites (ear-mange), or a purulent discharge. The term is, perhaps, more often reserved for the purulent form. It is most common in the dog and cat. It is often due to the irritation set up by the presence of an excessive amount of wax in the external meatus, which leads to superficial inflammation, infection with germs, and later to ulceration of the cartilage. In some cases parasites, such as *Otodectis cyanotis*, in the cat and dog, are the predisposing cause. (*See* PARASITES.)

Symptoms.—The affected animal shakes or scratches at its ears, is frequently noticed rubbing its head along the ground, and shows signs of pleasure when the ears are rubbed by the hand. When the inflammation is very acute it cannot bear to have its ears touched, and will scream or snap when they are accidentally handled. If the interior of the affected ear or ears be examined there is seen a greater or lesser amount of discharge of a dirty brownish or greyish colour which usually has a characteristic foul odour. The lining delicate skin of the ear is inflamed and reddened, and areas may be visible where the skin has been destroyed and the underlying tissues are exposed. If the animal has been scratching a great deal the hair around the outside of the ear will be thin and the surface of the skin will be scratched or torn, while inside the ear there may be also slight abrasions. In very severe cases there may be some hæmorrhage from the inside of the ear, and the matted or clotted blood will be seen at the lower part of the external opening. In old-standing cases the head may be carried with the affected ears at a lower level than the sound ear, where only one is affected; while where both are diseased to the same extent the dog moves its head stiffly and cautiously, and it may be completely deaf.

In the simple, uncomplicated case of parasitic otitis, shaking of the head and scratching of the ears occur. A brownish powdery material is visible inside the ear-flap.

Treatment.—It is advisable always to obtain professional treatment. Ear mange parasites can be killed by a 1 per cent solution of gammexane in medicinal liquid paraffin.

As a first-aid measure in all the forms of 'canker', the ear may be syringed out with a cleansing solution, such as liquid soap solution, 1 in 5 parts of warm water; or a solution of Cetrimide may be used. Soapy water, to which has been added a pinch of washing-soda to every breakfastcupful, is also useful where other agents are not available. This will usually alleviate the condition, but professional treatment is desirable if the condition is not to become persistent. Cotton-wool should never be forced down the ear with orange sticks, etc., nor boracic acid or other powders used.

In some cases, dressing the inner parts of the ear is difficult or impossible because of the thickening and perhaps distortion. For these an operation, in which the cartilages at the lower parts are opened or resected, has been devised. Operation may also be needed where deep-seated ulceration of one or other of the aural cartilages has occurred, and even the mere initial cleaning of a very inflamed and painful ear may have to be done under an anæsthetic.

TUMOURS are occasionally found affecting the ears of all domesticated animals. Warts are especially common in horses and cattle, and almost any kind of tumour may affect the ears of dogs.

EARLY WEANING (*see under* WEANING.)

EARS AS FOOD.—Ears from beef-cattle which had been receiving sex hormones have been fed in breeding kennels with disastrous results.

EARTHWORMS are of veterinary interest in that they act as intermediate hosts to stages in the life-history of the gape-worm of poultry (*see* GAPES) and of lung-worm in pigs. Indirectly, they may also harbour viruses which cause disease in pigs. Earthworms can live for as long as 10 years. Earthworms can often be found at night in drains outside piggeries, and in crevices and cracks in the cement inside piggeries. (*See also* INFLUENZA.)

EARTHING of electrical apparatus on farms, and especially in the dairy, is often done in such a way that in the event of a short-circuit, the water-pipes supplying the cows' drinking-bowls become 'live'—leading to the electrocution of the cows.

EASING THE HEELS is a phrase used in two different senses: it may mean rasping away the lower edge of the horn of the wall and bar of one heel of the horse's foot so that these do not bear upon the shoe—a method employed at times in the treatment of corns or bruised heels; or it may be used to indicate the operation of dividing the connection between the wall and the bars of the heels so that continuity is destroyed. This latter malpractice, which is also called ' opening the heel ', is sometimes carried out under the supposition that it induces an enlargement of the posterior part of the foot producing a ' wide open heels ' ; actually it leads to contraction of the heels through doing away with the natural elasticity of the foot.

EAST COAST FEVER, which has many other names, such as East African coast fever, Rhodesian red-water or tick fever, bovine Theleriasis, etc., is an acute specific disease of cattle enzoötic in certain parts of Africa, especially in the eastern provinces of Soulth Africa, in Kenya and in Northern Rhodesia. In these areas the native cattle attain a certain amount of natural immunity, and only imported animals are affected. Animals which recover are commonly known as ' salted ', but the mortality is very high (*e.g.* 90 per cent) in new outbreaks of the disease.

Cause.—*Theileria parva,* which spends part of its life-history in cattle and part in ticks. Ticks feeding from infected cattle take into their systems some of the parasites, which undergo sexual multiplication in the ticks' bodies. Spore-like forms are formed which are then inoculated into a fresh ox when the tick next sucks blood. At first the spore-like forms invade the lymphatic glands and spleen, where they infect the white blood corpuscles and undergo non-sexual division, and later they break out from the white cells and attack the red blood corpuscles, in which they are again taken up by the ticks. There is no great diminution in the numbers of the red cells, and there is but little destruction of these, even although as many as 75 per cent of them are attacked. The injury to the host appears to be brought about through the action of toxic substances produced by the parasite. It is believed that in animals which recover the parasites die out, and that such an animal becomes incapable of spreading the disease further.

Symptoms.—The average time from the date of infection until death occurs is 30 days. For the first ten days there are no symptoms shown and there is no rise in temperature, but after the 12th day the spore forms can be found in the white blood cells in lymph glands and the spleen, and a distinct rise in temperature occurs. On or about the 16th or 17th day a very high temperature is registered, sometimes as high as 107° or 108° F., and a few days later the parasites can be found in the circulating blood, and the animal becomes obviously sick. The symptoms manifested are vague, except that the usual signs of fever are present. There may, however, be heaving of the flanks, running at the eyes and nose, a husky cough, weakness, and a staggering gait, and there is almost always constipation followed by diarrhœa. The typical appearance of the dead animal (death occurring about 30 days after infection, or from a week to ten days after the rise in temperature is noticed) is in some respects similar to what is seen in anthrax ; there is a frothy straw-coloured or blood-stained discharge from the mouth and nostrils, and there is often a blood-stained discharge from the rectum. Upon opening the carcase the 4th stomach is usually found to be inflamed, and blood-spots are found throughout the intestines. Small white or yellow areas, varying in size from a pin's head to a pea, are found upon the surface of the liver and kidneys ; they are known as infarcts, and are almost diagnostic.

Transmission.—The disease is not contagious from animal to animal, but is spread through the agency of one or other of the ticks which belong to the class *Rhipicephalidæ* (*see* PARASITES). These ticks are extremely tenacious of life, since they may be able to survive for as long as 14 months upon an infected farm from which cattle have been removed, and they have been kept alive in the laboratory for as long as 630 days.

Prevention and Treatment.—East coast fever may be to a great extent prevented by systematic dipping of all newly purchased cattle, and quarantining them for at least five weeks before they are mixed with the rest of the stock. The dippings are directed towards the eradication of ticks with which the cattle may become infected, before they are able to take into their bodies any of the parasites with which the newly bought animals may be affected. The tick can only prove dangerous if it bites an infected animal during the latter stages of the disease, when the parasites are present in the red blood cells, and therefore ailing cattle whose temperatures are high, and which show signs of the disease otherwise, should be separated from the others and destroyed, their bodies being disposed of in such a way that the ticks present on them are also killed.

Where the disease has broken out on a

farm the 'short-interval' dipping system first devised by Watkins-Pritchford has proved of immense benefit in eradicating it. (*See under* TICK CONTROL.)

Since ticks responsible for the spread of east coast fever can live for some time on other domesticated animals, it is advisable to dip sheep, goats, and horses at suitable intervals.

Artificial immunisation is also carried out. Spleen or lymph-gland pulp in peptone solution is injected intravenously. After about 14 days from inoculation the cattle are exposed to natural infection; about 80 per cent become immune. The method has given good results in Kenya, where animals 2 to 4 years old are thus treated. It is not successful with calves.

EAST FRIESLAND MILK SHEEP.—This breed comes from N.W. Germany, and in England has been used to produce the COLBRED (which see). East Friesland ewes average 120 gallons at 6 per cent butterfat in a lactation, rearing their lambs, and a yield of 220 gallons is not unknown. The lambs have a high growth rate and early maturity.

EASTON'S SYRUP.—A tonic containing strychnine hydrochloride ($\frac{1}{60}$th grain to a teaspoonful) with iron phosphate and quinine. It should never be given to puppies, and even with adult dogs must be used with the greatest caution.

ECBOLICS (ἐκβάλλω, I throw out) are drugs which cause contraction of the muscle fibres of the uterus, such as ergot, pituitrin, etc. They are used in cases of inertia at parturition.

ECCHYMOSIS (ἐκ, out of; χυμός, juice) means the collection beneath the skin of blood which has escaped from the vessels in the neighbourhood, as in a bruise.

ECHINOCOCCOSIS (ἐχῖνος, hedgehog; κόκκος, a berry) means infection with the cyst stages of the tapeworm called *Taenia echinococcus*, and it may also be applied to the symptoms produced in an animal affected with the adult tapeworm itself. The former type mainly occurs in cattle, but may also be encountered in man; while the latter is a disease of the dog. (*See* PARASITES, p. 651.)

ECLAMPSIA (ἐκλάμπω, I explode) is a condition where an animal, in which there is no obvious diseased condition of the brain, becomes suddenly seized with severe convulsions or fits. These are usually of peripheral origin unlike epilepsy, and while epilepsy is hereditary, eclampsia is not.

Causes.—Very often the cause cannot be determined, but in other cases some form of irritation, such as that which is present during the cutting of the permanent teeth, or that due to the presence of parasitic worms in the intestines, or to hard foreign bodies in the stomach, is the cause. A special form is sometimes seen in bitches, cats, sows, and goats, and also in the mare and cow, following parturition, when it is probably due to irritation in the uterus or udder. This variety is known as *parturient eclampsia*. (*See also under* 'MILK FEVER'.)

Symptoms.—There is usually first noticed some abnormality in the behaviour of the animal. It becomes restless, dazed-looking, and moves uncertainly. In a very short while muscular spasms occur, and the limbs become rigid. The animal lies on its side and may perform the movements of walking or galloping, which are punctuated every now and then by sudden severe spasmodic seizures involving the whole body. Consciousness is generally suddenly lost in the ordinary form, but in parturient eclampsia the animal may retain consciousness. After a few minutes the attack may pass off, only to be repeated a short while later. One attack may succeed another with only brief intervals, until the animal dies from exhaustion or falls dead during an attack.

Treatment.—It is necessary to ascertain the cause of the condition in the first place, and to remove it. The animal should be placed in a quiet room or loosebox by itself, and may be given a dose of some sedative. Nembutal may be required for highly strung dogs, in either the ordinary or in parturient eclampsia.

ECRASEUR.—A surgical instrument used for castration of the larger domestic animals. Hæmorrhage is largely prevented by crushing of the blood-vessels of the spermatic cord.

ECTASIS (ἐκ, out; τείνειν, to stretch) means a dilatation of a hollow organ, such as an artery or the stomach.

ECTHYMA (ἐκ, out; θύειν, to rush) is a localised inflammation of the skin characterised by the formation of pustules. (*See* ACNE, IMPETIGO.)

ECTO- (ἐκτός, without) is a prefix meaning on the outside.

ECTOPIC (ἐκ, out of; τόπος, place) means out of the usual place. For instance, it is not uncommon to find the heart situated below the lower jaw in some kinds of monsters, resulting from errors in development; the heart is said to be ectopic in such cases.

Ectopic pregnancy means that the young animal (or animals) has developed outside the uterus.

ECTROMELIA means literally absence of a limb or limbs. The word is also used to describe a contagious disease caused by a Rickettsia, which affects laboratory mice, and by causing a disturbance in the circulation of the fore- or hind-limbs causes one or more of these to become necrotic and slough off. Outbreaks are usually very severe at the outset, killing many of the affected mice, but later on the mortality becomes less, and the outbreak gradually fades and disappears.

ECTROPION (ἐκ, out of; τρέπω, I turn) is a condition of the eyelids, upper or lower, in which the skin is so contracted as to turn the mucous membrane lining of the lid to the outside. It is much more rare than the opposite condition where the edge of the eyelid is turned inwards, and as in the latter, is remedied by a particular operation. A congenital or perhaps hereditary form is sometimes seen in lambs.

ECZEMA (ἐκζέω, I bubble up) is a superficial disease of the skin of an inflammatory nature, which is characterised by the formation of a scaly and fissured condition of the surface layers, a watery or serous discharge, and sometimes a considerable amount of irritation or itchiness.

Causes.—Idiosyncrasy or allergy which renders the animal especially liable to inflammation of the skin through the action of foreign substances (often of a protein nature) with which it comes into contact. There is evidence to show that certain families of dogs are more liable to attacks of eczema than others, and it is supposed that in such there is some hereditary transmission of an eczematous predisposition from one generation to another. An allergy or sensitisation to flea-bites is undoubtedly one cause.

There is one fact which is of great importance in the causation of some forms of the disease: *i.e.* that an absence or a diminution in the supply of vitamins in the food, along with an excess of cooked protein or carbohydrate and an insufficiency of exercise, is particularly liable to be associated with an attack of eczema in the dog and cat. In these animals, disease of the kidneys may sometimes be an accompaniment, if not a cause.

Lesions resembling eczema, and in some cases almost indistinguishable from it by the naked eye, are occasionally caused by the presence of mange parasites, so that before the owner of an animal is certain that it is affected with eczema the possibility of infection with one or other of the various forms of mange should be eliminated by microscopic examination.

Symptoms.—There are several different forms of this disease, but the classification is by no means satisfactory; for practical purposes it may be divided into a moist and a dry form.

Moist eczema is more common than the dry variety and attacks each of the domesticated animals to a greater or lesser extent. It consists essentially of the outpouring of a serous discharge from the skin surface, which causes cohesion and matting of the hairs, and it is usually associated with itchiness or irritation. It is not uncommon for this form to become infected with organisms and for pus to form upon the surface of the eczematous patch, giving rise to a very considerable amount of pain. Moist eczema is very common upon the backs and sides of the long-haired breeds of dogs and cats, and it is also seen in horses about the flexures of the knees and hocks, and behind the pastern joints. The affected dog or cat scratches or licks the diseased area if accessible, often giving rise to severe abrasions, and sometimes lacerating large patches around the primary sore. As a rule the area can be easily noticed, since the hair over it is gummed together; and if it is examined the surface of the skin is found to be moist, sticky, reddened, and inflamed. The dog resents any one handling the part. Another form of moist eczema occurs between the digits of the dog, especially in the folds of delicate skin between the pads. A dog affected with this form becomes markedly lame, spends considerable time lying on the ground with the affected foot so placed that it can lick it, and generally objects to having the affected foot examined. Occasionally, when a dog so affected has been licking at its foot for perhaps three or four days, a similar form of eczema commences around the mouth, particularly along the margins of the lips, and both forms in such cases are difficult to treat. Still another form of moist eczema is sometimes seen around the eyes of long-haired or other breeds of dogs; it is often called 'eczematous conjunctivitis,' because the lining membranes of the eyelids are frequently inflamed. 'Scrotal eczema' occurs in some dogs; in this case the area is not always moist; often there is a dry scab formed over the affected area, which gives rise to a marked amount of irritation, the animal drawing himself along the ground and sometimes producing large inflamed or ulcerated areas. Moist eczema in the horse often affects areas on the limbs or body which are covered with white hair; the skin in these regions being devoid of pigment matter, is perhaps adversely affected by the rays of the sun, or by light. In the flexures of limb joints (knees and hocks) eczema in the horse usually becomes scaly, and the condition is called mallenders or sallenders. (*See* MALLENDERS.) In cattle, sheep, and pigs there is a form of eczema which affects the tender skin between the claws. It often becomes infected with the *Actinomyces necrophorus*, and the condition is indistinguishable from 'FOUL-IN-THE-FOOT', *which see.*

Dry eczema, which mainly affects the dog, appears as an area of the skin where the hairs fall out, the surface becomes covered with a number of dry greyish scales, and after some time there is noticed a thickened and wrinkled condition, very similar to what is seen in some forms of follicular mange. These lesions are especially seen on the limbs, neck, and head. In typical dry eczema only the surface of the skin is affected, and if there should be a small amount of discharge it dries up or is absorbed by the surface epithelium. Care is needed to differentiate this form from ringworm, which may be very much more serious than eczema if neglected.

Treatment.—It is always necessary to change the food of any animal that suffers from eczema, because in a great many cases the system has become overloaded with the products of one particular variety of food, and it is necessary to allow time for the excess of these to be eliminated. In fact, external treatment alone does not always suffice to effect a cure, but when the feeding is altered there is immediate improvement. Herbivorous animals should be fed upon green food, mashes, etc., and the amount of their concentrates should be reduced. Dogs and cats should get a supply of minced raw turnip or carrot, cabbage, cauliflower, lettuce, chopped up fine and added to the food, and a fish diet should be avoided. Antihistamines may be tried. Externally, the affected areas should in every case be carefully clipped and cleansed. Hot water containing a trace of washing-soda should be used in preference to soaps, which are themselves liable to irritate delicate skins. After thorough cleansing, the areas should be dressed with one of the following agents: in mild cases of moist eczema, calamine lotion, a weak astringent lotion of alum (3 per cent to 5 per cent), or sulphate of zinc (5 per cent); in cases where there is pus formation, sulphanilamide powder may be used. Some of those drugs mentioned as useful for moist cases may be used for the dry cases, and frequent changes should be tried.

In all cases of eczema it is advisable to obtain skilled assistance, for very often parasitic mange is mistaken for eczema by the owner, who cannot carry out a microscopic examination of the scrapings from a lesion. (*See also* 'FACIAL ECZEMA'.)

EDEMA is another form of the term œdema. (*See* DROPSY.)

'EFFEMINATOR' SPRINGS.—These are inserted by means of a special instrument into the cervix and prevent it from closing. They are used in India, and occasionally in Britain, as a contraceptive in cattle.

EFFERENT (*efferens,* carrying out) is the term applied to vessels which convey away blood or a secretion from a part, or of nerves which carry nerve impulses outwards from the nerve-centres.

EFFUSION (*effundo,* I pour out) means the pouring out of a fluid from the vessels in which it is normally enclosed, into the substance of the organs, or into a body cavity, and is generally the result of inflammation or injury. There are effusions into joints, pleuritic and peritoneal effusions, and effusions of blood in various parts of the body.

EGG-BOUND is the name given to that condition in laying poultry in which an egg (or eggs) may be formed in the oviduct, but, owing to weakness or overwork, the hen is unable to discharge it.

It may result in breaking of the shell of the egg, or the wall of the oviduct may rupture, death usually resulting in either case. The bird shows obvious discomfort, stands straining and pressing, and the abdomen is usually markedly drooped.

The egg should be manipulated by the fingers, which fix it in front and gently exert a backward pressure until one of its poles appears at the cloaca or vent.

The regulation of exercise by providing adequate runs, scratching-grounds, etc., will do much to prevent the condition; and the too-rapid forcing of the heavy egg-laying strains of poultry, especially the young pullets, should be avoided.

EGG EATING. — Among intensively housed poultry, this may be a sign either of boredom or of pain.

EGG YIELD.—In Britain, the average is approximately 130 eggs per bird per year. An annual yield of 200 is obtained in well-managed batteries; about 190 on deep litter; 170 in fold units. A Honegger has laid 305 in 350 days.

ELASTIC BANDS (*see* RUBBER BANDS).

'ELASTRATOR.'—An instrument used to stretch a strong rubber ring so that it may be placed over the neck of the scrotum for the purpose of castration.

ELBOW is the name given to the joint formed between the lower end of the humerus and the upper ends of the radius and ulna.

ELDER POISONING.—Both the Common Elder (*Sambucus nigra*) and the Dwarf Elder (*S. ebulus*) have been blamed for poisoning stock, but their poisonous properties are not great, and they are unlikely to be eaten to any extent in Britain on account of their odour. The ripe black berries, used by country folk for making 'elderberry wine', have been the cause of severe diarrhœa in turkeys, pigs, and human beings, when taken in large amounts. The symptoms are purgation, passage of large amounts of urine, great depression, vomiting in the pig, and the passage of blood in severe cases. The first-aid treatment consists of large draughts of strong black tea or coffee. No effort should be made to check vomiting or diarrhœa at first, since by these means the berries are hurried out of the system. Easily digested demulcent foods should be given for a few days subsequently.

ELECTRIC FENCES (*see under* PASTURE MANAGEMENT).

ELECTRIC SHOCK, ELECTROCUTION.—Lightning is not uncommonly responsible for the sudden death of cattle, etc., which may also be electrocuted in their stalls owing to short-circuits and the faulty earthing of electrical equipment.

Electrocution is used for purposes of euthanasia in the case of dogs and cats, but recent research has shown that if the apparatus in use is to be humane in its effects—not causing paralysis initially without loss of consciousness—certain safeguards must be fulfilled.

ELECTRO-CARDIOGRAM is the term applied to a record of the variations in electric potential which occur in the heart as it contracts and relaxes. This record is obtained by placing electrodes on either side of the chest wall or on the two fore-legs, the skin being first wetted with salt solution; these are then connected with one another through an instrument known as the electro-cardiograph, which records on to a moving photographic film. The normal electrogram of each heart-beat shows one wave corresponding to the activity of the auricle, and four waves corresponding to the phases of each ventricular beat. Various readily recognisable changes are seen in cases in which the heart is acting in an abnormal manner, or in which one or other side of the heart is hypertrophied. This record, therefore, forms a useful aid in many cases of cardiac disease.

ELECTRO-CAUTERY.—This is frequently exceedingly useful for operations where space is restricted, such as removing small tumours, etc., in mouth, nose, or throat, and to check hæmorrhage in the deeper parts of wounds, and sometimes for disbudding.

ELECTRO-THERAPY.—**High-Frequency currents.**—By these no muscular contractions are brought about, but the effect is expended probably as a kind of individual cell massage, although some authorities claim that the current remains too superficial to effect any such action. There is, however, an increase in the output of CO_2, and in the total amount of urine excreted during passage of the current. Elimination of nitrogen and phosphates is hastened and there is an increased production of body heat.

This form of electro-therapy has had probably most application to treatment of animals. It has advantages that it is painless in application; no control measures are necessary other than means to hold the animal reasonably quiet. The duration of treatment is usually about 5 to 20 minutes daily or for shorter periods twice daily.

Good results are claimed in the treatment of various forms of paralysis in dogs and horses, muscular atrophy, chronic skin diseases of a non-parasitic nature, enlargements of joints and painful conditions in the limbs due to ligamentous or tendinous adhesions following injury, arthritis, rheumatism, and various inflammatory changes in peripheral nerves.

A modification of high-frequency treatment is known as diathermy. In this, electric currents pass into the deeper tissues and can be made to produce internal warmth. (*See* DIATHERMY.)

Faradic currents are used to produce rhythmic muscular contractions in the treatment of muscle, tendon and joint injuries in the horse, etc. (*See also* LIGHT TREATMENT, X-RAYS, IONIC TREATMENT, STUNNING.)

ELECTROLYTE.—Any compound which, in solution, conducts an electric current and is decomposed by it. (*See under* IONIC MEDICATION, NORMAL SALINE, DEHYDRATION.)

ELECTRON MICROSCOPE.—These costly and complex instruments have made it possible to study and photograph viruses, bacteriophages, and the structure of bacteria. The instrument makes use of a high-voltage 'electron gun', with electro-magnets taking the place of lenses. The 'specimen' is prepared in the form of a finely divided suspension on a cellulose supporting film, mounted on metal gauze, and the electron microscope subjects it to a high degree of vacuum. The electron image is focussed on a fluorescent screen, which is then replaced by a photographic plate. Magnification may be of the order of $\times$60,000; photographic enlargement bringing this up to $\times$150,000 or $\times$250,000.

ELECTROPHORESIS.—Starch gel electrophoresis is a method of separating certain constituents of blood serum in such a way that they form visible and identifiable patterns which can then be 'read' and recorded.

It has been used in the investigation of infertility in cattle. The mating of animals presenting certain serum patterns resulted in a higher rate of fœtal mortality than the mating of other animals. This technique, therefore, may become valuable in planned breeding of the future in order to avoid incompatibility and wastage. (*See* BLOOD SERUM PROTEIN.)

ELECTUARY, or **CONFECTION,** is a soft paste made by compounding drugs with treacle, sugar, or honey. It is used as a convenient method of applying drugs to the throat and pharynx of animals, and has much the same effect as lozenges in human beings. In pigs, where dosing is very difficult and often dangerous, purgative or other medicines are often given as electuaries, and antiseptic mouth applications are sometimes made up in the same way for all animals. To relieve sore throat in the horse an electuary of extract of belladonna, potassium chlorate, and aniseed, made up into a paste with treacle, is much used and serves to soothe the inflamed surface. The electuary is applied by means of a flat stick, and is smeared upon the back of the tongue, upon the teeth.

ELEPHANTIASIS is a condition met with in the human subject due to the attacks of parasitic filarial worms in the lymph vessels chiefly of the lower limbs. Applied to animals it is used to indicate the immense thickening that often results from repeated attacks of lymphangitis in the legs of horses. (*See* LYMPHANGITIS.)

ELIXIR (*elixio*, I boil) is a diluted tincture made pleasant to the taste by the addition of aromatic substances—sugar or glycerine.

ELIZABETHAN COLLAR.—Usually made of cardboard, the shape of a lampshade, and designed to fit over the dog's head and to be attached to its collar, with the object of preventing the animal interfering with wounds, skin lesions, or dressings.

EMBOLISM (ἔμβολον, a plug) means the plugging of a small blood-vessel by a piece of some material that has been carried into it from larger vessels. It is generally due to fragments of a blood-clot which has formed in some other part of the body, and have been carried by the circulation. Bacteria, worm larvæ in the horse, air-bubbles, tiny parts of the heart valves (which sometimes separate), and masses of fat, are other causes of embolism. The importance of the embolism depends upon the situation. In the brain it may cause a localised softening and consequent paralysis of some part of the body, or even death from apoplexy. If the embolism is of large size affecting the arterial trunks it is much more serious, but is then called a thrombus. (*See* THROMBUS.) In other organs the area that was supplied by the little vessel before it became blocked by the embolism ceases to function, and if the blood-supply is totally cut off it dies, or degenerates into fat. Such fatty masses in an organ are known as 'infarcts'. When the plug is a mass of bacteria, an abscess results. If it be a piece of a malignant tumour a secondary tumour develops. (*See* METASTASIS.) When an air-bubble enters the circulation it is very liable to be accompanied by a tiny clot from the wound whence it entered; and if air in large amounts gains entrance, such as from carelessness at bleeding, or when administering an intravenous injection, bursting of the heart valves is often the consequence.

EMBROCATIONS (ἐμβρέχω, I soak in) are mixtures, usually of an oily nature, that are applied to sprains, some forms of bruises, and other painful conditions. They act partly by virtue of the massage that is applied when they are rubbed in, and partly by the mild counter-irritation of the substances of which they are composed. (*See* LINIMENTS.)

EMBRYO (ἔμβρυον) means the fœtus in the womb early in pregnancy before the various parts are visibly recognisable. (*See* FŒTUS.)

EMBRYOLOGY (ἔμβρυον, an embryo; λόγος, a discourse) is the study of the development of the embryo within the body of the female. Strictly speaking, it includes the various stages concerned in the whole process of reproduction, but under REPRODUCTION will be found a description which carries its consideration up to the fertilisation of the female ovum by the male spermatozoön.

Segmentation.—After the fusion of the male and female germ cells (fertilisation) has taken place the two nuclei lying within the envelope of the ovum coalesce. Each carries half the number of chromosomes peculiar to the particular species of animal, and in the fusion of the two nuclei a new nucleus (the *segmentation nucleus*), carrying the complete number of chromosomes, is formed. This almost immediately commences to divide under the influence of the small body carried by the spermatozoön and known as the *centrosome*, and the single cell gives rise to two daughter cells. Each of these new cells possesses the full number of chromosomes, since each of the chromosomes of the segmentation nucleus splits into two new chromosomes. It is an ascertained fact that the chromosomes are greatly, if not entirely, responsible for the transmission of hereditary qualities from parents to offspring. When once segmentation, which is a process in which each cell splits to form two new cells, has commenced, it proceeds very rapidly, so that in a short while a solid mass of cells results. This is known as a *morula*. Up till about the time the morula is formed the process has been taking place in the oviduct, the developing embryo being gradually passed down this tube until it finally comes to rest in the horn of the uterus, where the embryo develops into the fœtus. The cells on the outside of the morula are different from those found inside the mass and grow much more rapidly than the latter. In a short while a hollow cavity is formed, known as the *segmentation cavity*, and the whole structure is now called the *blastoderm* or the *blastodermic vesicle*. The cavity contains broken-down yolk, and at one part there is found a small disc of cells which is composed of the cells which formerly occupied the centre of the morula. These spread over practically the whole of the inner surface of the outermost layer of cells, so that in time a hollow ball is formed composed of two single layers of cells—the outer of which becomes known as the *epiblastic layer*, and the inner as the *hypoblastic layer* or *endoblastic layer*. At one part there is a concentration of cells to which the name *germinal area* is given, for it is from this area that the embryo develops. An invagination of the epiblast occurs over the germinal area, giving rise to the *primitive streak*, and then the edges of the streak deepen and the *primitive groove* is formed. The process of invagination continues until the primitive groove has become a canal, the *neural canal*, from which develop the various parts of the central nervous system. About this time, between the epiblast and the hypoblast, there develops another layer of cells known as the *mesoblastic layer*. There are thus three layers—epiblast, mesoblast, and hypoblast—arranged in this order from without inwards, and it is from these three layers that all the tissues of the future young animal are formed. In the following table the structures which these layers give rise to are mentioned :

From the epiblast :

The whole of the nervous system.

The skin and its appendages—hair, hoof, claws, horn.

The lining epithelium of all glands opening on to the skin—mammary, sebaceous, and sweat.

The lining epithelium of the mouth (not the tongue) and glands opening into it, the enamel of the teeth, and the epithelium of the anus.

The epithelium of the nasal passages and the sinuses of the skull.

The epithelial sense end-organs—taste buds, touch corpuscles, the organs of smell, the retina and the lens of the eye, the organ of Corti in the ear, and the nerves of the special senses.

From the mesoblast :

The bones, cartilages, and the connective tissues (fibrous tissues) of the whole body.

The muscles, both voluntary and involuntary.

The entire blood and lymph systems, blood corpuscles, spleen, and serous membranes.

The generative organs and the generative elements.

The urinary organs.

From the hypoblast :

The epithelium of the alimentary canal and the ducts of all glands opening into it.

The epithelium of the larynx, trachea, and lungs.

The epithelium of the bladder, uterus, thyroids, and part of the thymus gland.

The cells of the liver and pancreas.

The details of the formations of these structures are too complicated to be discussed here ; suffice it to say that two tubes are formed, one above the other, the upper of which is the neural canal, and the lower of which is to be the alimentary canal, and it is by the growth of these and developments from them, along with the laying down of special structures in certain parts, that the young animal is eventually formed.

Nutrition of the embryo.—In the mare up to the 7th week or thereabout the young embryo has derived its nourishment from the yolk sac—which is in turn filled by ' uterine milk ' secreted by the crypts of the uterus. When this supply ceases the developing embryo is brought into communication with the maternal blood circulating in the uterine wall, by means of the fœtal membranes or the *placenta*. There are three of these membranes enveloping the fœtus and protecting it, each being attached to the fœtus in the region of the *umbilicus* (navel). They are called amnion, allantois, and choroin.

1 **Amnion.**—Immediately enveloping the fœtus, but separated from it by a fluid, there is a membranous sac called the amnion. It is, practically speaking, an outgrowth from the area of the abdominal wall which surrounds the umbilicus. In the mare it possesses epithelial tufts on its inner surface. The amniotic fluid, or *liquor amni*, is alkaline in reaction, contains proteins, mucin, urea, sugar, lactic acid, salts, keratin, and portions of solid waste matter derived from the hoofs, hair, fœtal fæces, etc. It acts as a water bed in which the fœtus is immersed, and in which the delicate tissues of the embryo are protected from pressure, shocks, etc., and it allows some movement of the limbs, head, etc., when ' *quickening* ' occurs some time later during pregnancy. During parturition it assists in the dilatation of the cervical canal of the uterus, and acts as a lubricant for the passage of the fœtus through the maternal genital canal.

2. **Allantois.**—The second membrane is called the allantois, and is also directly connected with the embryo at the umbilicus. Unlike the amnion, however, it has no connection with the skin of the abdominal wall. It is best described as being an outgrowth of the embryonic urinary bladder, which is protruded from the abdominal cavity to the outside of the body of the embryo, passing through the umbilical ring, where it is called the *urachus*, both the outer part and the inner part (*i.e.* the urinary bladder) being in communication with each other. The extra-fœtal part forms a double-walled sac whose innermost layer lies on the outside of the amnion, and whose outermost layer lines the inside of the stout outer membrane —the chorion. These two walls are not distinct ; they are really but parts of a continuous whole. The space between

them is filled by fluid, some of which is fœtal urine secreted by the fœtal kidneys. The urinary bladder could not accommodate all the urine secreted before birth, and the cavity of the allantois acts as a kind of reservoir in which the overflow from the bladder may be stored. The rest of the allantoic fluid, or *liquor allanti*, is formed of water containing urea, albumin, lactic acid, certain salts, and a substance called ' allantoin '. Floating in this fluid there are often found peculiar bodies of a jelly-like nature to which the name *hippomanes* is given. They are met with in the mare and cow, and in some cases are attached to the wall of the allantoic membrane. Their origin and functions are obscure ; but it is certain that they do not obstruct the mouth and nostrils of the fœtus, according to popular supposition.

3. **Chorion.**—The outermost membrane of the fœtus is thus named. It is a very large sac, completely closed, and when developed is moulded to the inner surface of the uterus, possessing two horns and a body in the larger animals. The external surface is studded with large numbers of small red projections called *villi*, which are inserted into the crypts of the mucous membrane of the uterus. The inner surface of the chorion is lined by the outermost layer of the allantois, to which it is closely adherent. On this surface the branches of the umbilical veins and arteries ramify, and their minutest branches pass to the villi. It is through the walls of the villi and the delicate membrane lining the uterus that the blood of the fœtus receives oxygen and nutritive products from the maternal blood. In the cow and ewe the whole outer surface of the chorion is not covered with villi, but these are concentrated into areas which correspond with the surfaces of the cotyledons of the uterus ; for in ruminants the attachment of the fœtal membranes is not diffuse but localised to the cotyledons.

Umbilical cord, or ' navel string ', is the tube connecting the fœtus with the fœtal membranes. It is composed of two umbilical arteries, the umbilical vein, which is sometimes double the urachus, and the remnants of the yolk sac or umbilical vesicle, which are embedded in a soft jelly-like connective tissue, known as ' Wharton's jelly ', and ensheathed in a part of the amnion which is usually twisted somewhat like a rope. The two umbilical arteries are given off from the internal iliacs, and carry blood which has been circulating in the fœtus, and is therefore loaded with carbon dioxide and devoid of oxygen. Each artery passes out through the umbilical cord, and gives off a large number of branches which are distributed to the chorion, and ultimately end in the villi as tiny capillaries. In the villi the blood comes into contact with the maternal blood, and there is an exchange of gases similar to what occurs in the lungs of an adult. Nutritive products are also absorbed from the maternal blood, and waste products of fœtal metabolism are given up to some extent. The blood now returns through the umbilical veins, and is eventually collected into the single umbilical vein which enters the fœtus at the umbilicus and passes to its liver. In the substance of the liver it opens directly into the vena cava of the young animal, and its blood in this way is once more returned to the fœtal circulation. It is extremely important to ensure that during parturition no infection shall gain entrance into the umbilical cord, because through the umbilicus there is for some time a direct entrance for germs into the body of the young animal. It is in this way that the infection of joint-ill in foals often gains the body. The methods of dealing with the cord are discussed under PARTURITION (which see). (*See also* CIRCULATION.)

EMESIS (ἔμεσις) means VOMITING (which see).

EMETICS (ἐμετικός, provoking sickness) are drugs or other agents which produce vomiting. Of the domesticated animals only the dog, cat, and pig are able to vomit in the ordinary sense of the word. The horse may at times expel fluid food-stuffs, which have been swallowed, out through its nostrils (not through the mouth), but this indicates serious disease or injury, such as poisoning or rupture of the stomach. The ox, sheep, and goat *ruminate*, whereby food materials are brought up into the mouth, there to be re-chewed, but the process is not the same as vomiting. In none of these animals can discharge of food-stuffs which have been swallowed be effected through the mouth by the agency of drugs. If emetics are given to them violent pains may be experienced, but the drug eventually passes along the intestinal canal or is absorbed.

Varieties.—Emetics are divided into two classes : (1) direct emetics, which being taken in through the mouth, irritate the stomach and so cause vomiting ; and (2) indirect emetics, which will cause vomiting, even when injected into the bloodstream through an action upon the nerve centre in the brain which controls the processes of vomiting. Examples of the first are sulphate of zinc, mustard and water, salt and water, washing-soda (carbonate of soda), sulphate of copper. Into the second class fall apomorphine, ipecacuanha, tartar emetic, and in dogs ordinary doses of morphia if the stomach contains any food material.

Uses.—Emetics are made use of when it is desired to expel from the stomach some harmful poisonous or indigestible material which has been taken.

EMETINE is one of the alkaloids or active principles of the drug ipecacuanha.

EMMETROPIA (ἔμμετρος, in proper measure; ὄψις, vision) means neither short sight nor long sight, and is the normal state of vision in which the rays of light fall exactly upon the retina of the eye. (*See* VISION.)

EMOLLIENTS (*emollio*, I soften) are substances that have a softening and soothing effect upon the tissues of the body to which they are applied. They are chiefly used upon hard dry skin. The chief are ointments, glycerine, soap, lard, oils, and fats.

EMPHYSEMA (ἐμφύσημα) means an abnormal presence of air in some part of the body, generally the lungs. There are two main types of the condition, one affecting the lungs, and another that may affect any part of the body, usually above a wound which serves to admit air to the subcutaneous tissues.

PULMONARY EMPHYSEMA: **Horse.**—

Chronic alveolar emphysema, or Broken Wind, is described under BROKEN WIND.

Interstitial emphysema or interlobular emphysema is a condition in which the walls of the air alveoli not only become stretched, but actually rupture so that a single irregular ragged wall bounds what once was two or more separate air-cells. This is more frequently encountered in cattle than among horses, but it is met with in these latter when from any cause there is a sudden increase in the alveolar pressure.

Causes.—Forced inspiration made by the animal to overcome aerial insufficiency such as occurs in broncho-pneumonia, over-exertion, careless drenching, violent struggling during falls and accidents, obstructions in the air passages such as tumours, enlarged glands, etc., are all causes which may operate so as to produce the interstitial form.

Symptoms.—Owing to the reduced space available for the necessary exchange of gases in the lungs, there is a tendency to respiratory distress upon exertion, accompanied by an anxious expression; crepitating sounds are heard over the surface of the chest and the normal sounds are altered; swelling of the base of the neck is sometimes seen, and constitutes a very reliable symptom of the condition. Death may take place in 24 or 48 hours after the onset of the distress. In other cases this latter passes off with rest and quietness, but will recur if violent exercise occurs again.

Cattle.—These animals suffer from acute and chronic pulmonary emphysema in regions where they are used for draught purposes. The acute form is brought on by conditions similar to those that produce the interstitial form in horses: violent struggling and extreme exertion, careless drenching, the presence of foreign bodies in the trachea, broncho-pneumonia, tuberculosis when accompanied by constrictions or dilatations of the bronchi, flatulence of the rumen which causes distress in breathing by pressure on the diaphragm, and it has been seen in difficult parturition when it is induced by the violent labour pains. Ephysema in cattle grazing aftermath might possibly be caused by a fungal toxin. Several outbreaks of emphysema with associated heart trouble have been encountered recently in Yorkshire among calves 3 to 4 months old. Most of them had never been out. On some farms there has been a 100 per cent mortality among the animals showing symptoms. Lungworms and other infective agents had been ruled out.

Symptoms.—These resemble those met with in the horse.

An infectious form of the disease has been reported from the swampy districts of the Netherlands to which the name 'pneumatosis' is applied.

Chronic pulmonary emphysema, such as is somewhat common in horses under the name of 'broken wind', is very rare in cattle.

Pigs.—Interstitial emphysema is often seen in slaughter-houses, but during life it is not recognised. It follows bronchial catarrh, or pneumonia, especially that which is associated with swine fever and parasitic bronchitis.

Dog and Cat.—An acute and a chronic form of pulmonary emphysema are seen in the dog and cat.

Acute form.—This occurs in connection with broncho-pneumonia or any lesions that diminish the calibre of the trachea. It may suddenly arise during a fit of coughing such as takes place during chronic bronchitis, as well as from respiratory distress resulting from a weak heart. Exertion will produce it, especially if violent and when the animal is old or obese.

Symptoms.—A persistent cough with difficulty in breathing, irregularity of the pulse, and a whining or whimpering when the cough allows, are seen. These symptoms, mild and not always noticed at first, become progressively worse, and, in the majority of cases, a fatal termination ensues in the course of a few months.

Chronic form.—This is often associated with eczema of a very intractable nature in aged and fat dogs. Such are little inclined for exertion, and are frequently affected with chronic bronchitis, often popularly known as 'asthma', but so called erroneously. It is generally associated with a dilatation of the right side of the heart from overwork. The symptoms are those of chronic bronchitis (*see* CHRONIC BRONCHITIS), to which must be added an extra liability to a coughing fit whenever the animal is changed from a warm to a cold atmosphere or *vice versa,* and upon slight exertion.

Treatment.—Absolute recovery is impossible, for it is not within the recuperative powers of the lungs to rebuild the damaged walls of the air-sacs, and without this the condition must persist. Treatment, therefore, must be directed towards protection from exertion, from chills, draughts, and sudden changes in temperature.

EMPIRICAL (ἐμπειρία, experience) treatment is that school of treatment which is founded simply upon experience. Because a given remedy has been successful in the treatment of a certain group of symptoms, it is assumed by those who uphold this principle that it will always be successful in other cases presenting similar groups of symptoms, without any inquiry as to the cause of the symptoms, or the reason underlying the action of the remedy. It is the contrary of 'rational' or 'scientific' treatment. Sometimes a course of treatment must perforce be empirical, through lack of knowledge.

EMPYÆMA (ἐμπούς, suffering from an abscess) is a term used in medicine to denote a collection of purulent fluid within the cavity of the pleura. (*See* PLEURISY.)

EMULSIONS (*emulgeo,* I milk out) are mixtures contan ing oily substances in a very fine state of division. This division is effected, and the oil kept in suspension in the fluid, by means of alkalies and sticky ingredients such as albumin, glycerine, and mucilage. Milk is a good example of a perfect emulsion of fat globules each surrounded by an envelope of albumin. The various preparations of cod-liver oil are usually emulsified by the aid of glycerine. The oil is in this way rendered more palatable, and digestion and absorption are made easier by the emulsification of the fatty ingredient.

ENAMEL is a thin, hard, transparent, or white layer which covers the outer surface of the teeth and is, in some cases, reflected or invaginated into the substance of the tooth, whereby its durability is increased. It is composed almost entirely of earthy salts such as are found in bone, and is the hardest tissue in the animal's body. (*See* TEETH.)

ENCEPHALITIS (ἐγκέφαλος, the brain), or BRAIN FEVER, is rarely met with as a primary condition; rather is it secondary to some other inflammatory process, or else it is associated with meningitis.

Causes.—Inflammation of the brain may be brought about through the activity of bacteria such as those of glanders, strangles, listeriosis, but especially during infection with viruses, such as those of rabies, canine distemper.

Symptoms.—There is usually a preliminary stage when all the blood-vessels of the brain are engorged with blood (active hyperæmia), and associated with this there are periods of excitement and irregular movements. The temperature rises, and remains high throughout the course of the disease. In the early stages of some cases the affected animal may become wild with excitement; cattle rush to and fro bellowing and roaring; pigs squeal and roll over on their sides; the dog utters piercing yells and has a wild, staring expression; sheep often perform circus movements, turning round and round in circles and eventually falling to the ground, from which they cannot rise.

Later on a stage of depression supervenes. The animal becomes quiet, lies with a vacant expression in its face, or stands resting its head upon some convenient object; it does not respond to external stimulation, and finally it becomes unconscious. Paralysis of one side of the body, of a group of muscles, or even of practically the whole of the muscular system, may precede death.

Treatment.—Inflammation of the brain is a notoriously difficult condition to treat. Accordingly, it is often better to destroy the animal as soon as the diagnosis is established, so as to minimise suffering and salve the carcases of food animals. Where treatment is adopted, the animal should be put into a dark, quiet place away from other animals and protected from noise and sources of excitement. Cold packs should be arranged over the skull, and ice-bags may be applied when they can be obtained. Internally a sedative should be given. Foods should be easily digested and easily swallowed. Recovery is not common.

In the dog, treatment of encephalitis will often depend largely upon the identity of the virus believed to be responsible. (*See* RABIES, DISTEMPER, RUBARTH'S DISEASE, JAPANESE B ENCEPHALITIS, EQUINE ENCEPHALITIS.)

ENCEPHALOMALACIA.—A group name for the degenerative diseases of the brain. Causes include the copper deficiency of swayback, horse-tail and bracken poisoning, metallic poisoning, and mulberry heart disease of pigs.

ENCEPHALOMYELITIS means inflammation of the nervous tissues in both the brain and the spinal cord.

ENCEPHALOMYELITIS, VIRAL, OF PIGS.—This term covers the group of diseases known as Teschen disease, Talfan disease, and *Poliomyelitis suum*, which may possibly be all caused by the same virus, though this remains uncertain.

Believed to have originated in Czechoslovakia, Viral Encephalomyelitis of pigs is now encountered throughout most of Europe. In Britain and Denmark, only a small percentage of pigs become infected, and illness is far milder than in some other countries.

Symptoms include fever, stiffness, staggering gait, paralysis, and those of encephalitis generally.

ENCHONDROMA (ἐν, in; χόνδρος, cartilage; *-oma*, termination meaning tumour) means a tumour formed of cartilage. (*See* TUMOURS.)

ENCYSTED (ἐν, in; κυστις, a bladder) means enclosed within a bladder-like wall. The term is applied to parasites, collections of pus, fluid, etc., which are shut off from the surrounding structures by a ring of dense fibrous tissue or by a membrane.

ENDARTERITIS (ἔνδον, within; ἀρτηρία, an artery) means inflammation of the inner coat of an artery. (*See* ARTERIES, DISEASES OF.)

ENDO- (ἔνδον, within) is a prefix meaning situated inside.

ENDOCARDITIS (ἔνδον, within; καρδαί, the heart) means inflammation of the smooth membrane that lines the inside of the heart. It occurs especially over the heart valves. (*See* HEART DISEASES.)

ENDOCRINE GLANDS (ἔνδον, within; κρινω, I separate): or 'ductless glands'. Their secretion is added to the bloodstream and circulates all over the body, producing its effects in distant parts rather than locally. Included among these endocrine glands are the following: thyroid, parathyroid, thymus, adrenals, pituitary, and pineal bodies. There are, moreover, tissues incorporated among the cells of other glands which produce *internal secretions* or hormones; *e.g.* in the ovary, testicles, and pancreas.

Thyroids, which produce a hormone called *thyroxin*, were the first of the ductless glands from which an extract was made and used. The hormone of the thyroid has the property of stimulating many chemical changes in the body, acting like the draught of a furnace in bringing about combustion. A superabundance of thyroxine circulating in the blood-stream leads to exophthalmic goitre or Graves's disease, which is common among human beings but is of little importance among animals. A deficiency of thyroxine leads to a condition known as myxœdema in adults, and cretinism in the young. Both of these latter conditions can be remedied by the use of thyroid extract. (*See* THYROID GLAND.)

Parathyroids are small structures situated either wholly within, or upon the surface of, the thyroid gland. Their secretion has been provisionally named *parathyrine*; its absence is responsible for a condition known as tetany, in which convulsive movements occur. The parathyroids regulate the metabolism of calcium and of nitrogenous materials; and although preparations from them are upon the market, their action cannot yet be said to be fully understood. That they are essential to life, however, is proved by the fact that if they are removed death follows. (*See* CHOREA.)

Adrenals produce two kinds of hormone. The glands consist of an outer or cortical and an inner or medullary part, and it is the latter of these which is engaged in the production of the comparatively well-known and very useful *adrenaline*. This has a most pronounced function of stimulating and increasing the contractions of all involuntary muscles of the body, but most especially that which is present in the walls of the smaller arteries. (*See also* section on ADRENALS.) It is used to check capillary hæmorrhage and oozing of blood during detailed operations, and it has a valuable action of raising the blood-pressure and so warding off shock. The function of the cortex or outer layer of the adrenals is not so well understood, but it is associated with a peculiar condition in man in which bronzing of exposed parts of the body occur, along with great muscular weakness (called Addison's disease), since it is found diseased in all such cases. Several complex steroid hormones are produced by the cortex among them one known as D.O.C.A. or desoxycorticosterone acetate, which has profound effects and is essential to life. The cortisone compounds also belong to this class, and the cortex is also associated with the production of a hormone concerned in the functioning of the reproductive system.

Pituitary body is a small gland in the skull at the base of the brain which has two distinct parts each possessing different functions. The posterior lobe, which is of nervous origin, produces an extract to which the name *pituitrin* is given, and it is also responsible for producing a hormone concerned in milk secretion, called the lactogenic hormone. Pituitrin when given by hypodermic injection, has a pronounced effect in stimulating the contraction of involuntary muscle in the hollow organs, particularly the uterus. (*See* PITUITRIN.) Pituitrin has other functions; if it is injected into a lactating animal it causes an increased secretion of milk, but this is not a permanent effect. It also stimulates the circulation, its action being less pronounced but more lasting than that of adrenalin. The anterior lobe has recently been shown to be of great importance in controlling the functions of ovary and testicle. It produces gonadotropic hormones which activate the ovary and stimulate it to produce female germ cells. It also produces a hormone which controls body growth, including fœtal growth in pregnant females. When hypertrophied in the young it causes gigantism in which a great increase in size occurs. Hypertrophy or increased function in adults results in acromegaly, in which there is a sudden growth of extremities of the body. If it be atrophied, injured, or removed in the young creature, growth ceases, and a condition of infantilism results. In this there is a pronounced lack of development of ovaries and testes and of secondary sex characters, together with deposition of fat, and a general sluggishness and lack of development. In the male there is a tendency towards reversion to female characteristics, but the opposite effect in the female is not observed. Anterior lobe extract is used to correct such atrophic conditions. During pregnancy in the mare, the ovary-stimulating hormone (called the follicle-stimulating hormone, or F.S.H.) continues to be produced up to about the 120th day, and large amounts accumulate in the blood-stream. By removing blood from pregnant mares at the correct stage, large amounts of this hormone can be prepared for use in animals which require it to correct certain forms of sterility. (*See also* TWINNING.)

Pancreas is engaged in the secretion of the pancreatic fluid for digestive purposes, so far as the greater part of the gland is concerned, but here and there lying among the secretory cells there are little 'cell-islets', which are engaged in the production of *insulin*, which regulates the sugar metabolism of the body, and prevents its excretion in the urine. When these cells are diseased, or when the pancreas is experimentally removed, the condition of the body rapidly wastes, and there are large amounts of sugar excreted from the kidneys into the urine. When insulin is injected, however, this excretion of sugar ceases, and health is restored. It must not be understood that insulin will *cure* the condition, but rather does it bring into the body a power of preventing such waste as occurs when the sugar is eliminated. This discovery of insulin was made by Dr. Banting in 1923, and since then the use of insulin to correct diabetes has been one of the greatest advances of modern treatment.

Testicles are normally engaged in the production of the male germ cells or spermatozoa, but lying between the tubules which produce these germ cells there are 'interstitial cells' which have an important effect upon the production of the accessory sexual features of the individual, such as the arched neck and aggressive propensities of the stallion, the massive horn formation and general masculine appearance of the bull and ram, and beard of the billy-goat, the spurs and large wattles of the cock, etc. When the testicles are removed or diseased these features disappear and the appearance of the animal reverts to a position similar to that of the female of the species.

Ovaries, like testicles, are chiefly concerned in the production of female germ cells, from which the young of the species is developed. There is a very special arrangement in connection with their function, for information upon which *see* OVARY. In addition to the production of ova, the ovary produces a hormone called *œstrone*, which is largely responsible for the effects seen during œstrus upon the uterus, vagina, and mammary glands. This is produced by the Graäfian follicles and is sometimes called the follicular hormone. Another hormone, *progesterone*, is elaborated by the corpus luteum, which develops in the old follicle after rupture. This hormone has an important function to play in stimulating the glands in the uterus to proliferate and secrete, and so aid in the nidation (or 'nesting in') of the fertilised ovum which is to become the embryo and develop into a young animal. In this way the ovary through its hormones has a very profound influence upon the other genital organs in the female. It has other effects, not so well understood but concerned with growth and development of uterus vagina and udder and also with the behaviour of the animal. Thus if the ovaries are artificially removed when a cow is in full milk she will continue secreting milk for 2, 3, or even 4 years, and there will be but little diminution during this period. The influence of the ovaries upon the temperament of an animal is considerable. In certain cases cysts may form in the ovaries and the pressure may cause (or perhaps the stimulation they give to the hormone-secreting cells results in) a disturbance of the temperament, and viciousness, irritability, and intractability follow. The removal of the ovaries in many instances improves or eradicates such conditions. In addition to these functions there appears to be some control exercised by the ovarian hormone over the consumption of oxygen. This may be a provision of Nature whereby the female can take into her body sufficient oxygen for the needs of the fœtus as well as for her own use, whenever the occasion arises.

Pineal body is regarded as the vestigeal remains of what once was a central eye in remote ancestry. It is small and composed of modified ocular tissue, some of whose cells would suggest by their appearance that they may be concerned in the production of a hormone. There is not much known concerning the functions of this body, but in the young animal it is especially well supplied with blood, and after puberty it degenerates and changes to a mass of little more than fibrous tissue, which indicates that it is concerned in growth and development of the sexual organs.

Thymus gland is another structure which is only well developed in the young and the fœtus, for before an animal has attained maturity the thymus has in most cases become very small. It is composed of modified lymphatic tissue not unlike what is found in lymph glands, but there are also bodies known as the 'concentric corpuscles of Hassal' present. Little is known of its functions, but it has been noted that the process of atrophy is much slower in the castrated than in the uncastrated animal, and that its rapid absorption is associated with a rapid development of testicles.

(*See also* HORMONES *and* HORMONE THERAPY ; MAMMARY GLAND.)

ENDOMETRITIS (ἔνδον, within ; μήτρα, the womb) means an inflammation of the mucous membrane that lines the womb or uterus. (*See* UTERUS, DISEASES OF.)

ENDOTHELIUM (ἔνδον, within ; θηλή, nipple) is the term applied to the membrane lining various vessels and cavities of the body, such as the pleura, pericardium, peritoneum, lymphatic vessels blood-vessels, and joints. It consists of a fibrous layer covered with thin flat cells, which render the surface perfectly smooth and secrete the fluid for its lubrication.

ENDOTOXINS.—Are those toxins which are retained within the bodies of bacteria until the latter die and disintegrate.

ENDOTRACHEAL ANÆSTHESIA.—This technique, used in dogs and cats to a limited extent, depends upon the introduction into the trachea of a tube which connects with the outside. The tube is passed via the mouth under a narcotic or anæsthetic, such as nembutal, given into a vein, and may then be used as the route for an inhalant anæsthetic mixture. The method ensures a clear airway throughout the period of anæsthesia, and thus obviates the danger of laryngeal obstruction (*e.g.* by the tongue falling backwards), which sometimes causes death. The method has several other advantages, *e.g.* it permits an unobstructed operation field during lengthy major operations, obviates excessive salivation, achieves better oxygenation, more even anæsthesia, and permits of positive pressure ventilation of the lungs in the event of respiratory failure.

Endotracheal anæsthesia is administered in one of two ways. *Insufflation anæsthesia* involves the use of air and a volatile anæsthetic vapour delivered into the tube by means of a pump or, more commonly, a mixture of gases supplied from cylinders (and sometimes bubbled through a volatile anæsthetic liquid in addition). *Auto-inhalation anæsthesia* involves the use of a wide bore endotracheal tube through which the animal inhales the anæsthetic mixture by its own respiratory efforts. A ' rebreathing bag ' may be used. (*See also* ANÆSTHESIA.)

ENDRIN.—A highly toxic insecticide of the chlorinated hydrocarbon group. It has caused fatal poisoning in cattle, dogs, fish, and birds.

ENEMA (ἔνεμα) means an injection of a fluid into the bowel.

Uses.—*Purgative enemata* are given for the distension of the rectum so that accumulated fæces may be expelled with greater ease than otherwise. They are most often required in dogs and cats, especially when these are suffering from some condition associated with constipation, such as high fever, impaction of the bowel with foreign bodies, etc. About 2 pints of soapy water, or glycerine and water (tablespoonful to the pint), used either cold or warm, are usually needed.

For the horse two or four pailfuls of soapy water are necessary (but see under COLIC, treatment). In all cases enemata should be introduced very slowly at first so as to allow time for the bowel wall to expand and accommodate the fluid. For the dog, foal, and calf, a rubber Higginson's syringe is the best appliance, and for the larger animals, either a special continuous flow force-pump or a length of hose-pipe with a petrol-filler or other large funnel attached to one end.

Vermifuge enemata are made up with common salt (2 ounces to the pint), or an infusion of quassia chips may be used. They are useful for expelling the small oxyurid worms that, by causing irritation of the anus, often induce a horse to rub its tail, and in the dog they assist the action of doses of worm medicine given by the mouth.

Enemata are also useful in certain special cases where there has been injury to the posterior part of the bowel, such as after a prolapse of the rectum ; they may contain drugs such as acriflavine (1 : 1000), common salt, or other antiseptic. Occasionally *anæsthetics*, or *narcotics*, such as chloral hydrate, are administered by the rectum when for some reason it is not advisable to give them by the mouth.

ENSILAGE (*see* SILAGE).

ENTÉQUÉ SECO.—A wasting disease of cattle, sheep and horses. It occurs mainly in Argentina, but also in Uruguay and possibly Brazil. It may be identical with Manchester wasting disease (Jamaica) and Naalehu disease (Hawaii).

Cause.—A plant, common on wet land, known as duraznillo blanco (*Solanum melacoxylon* or *glaucum*). Poisoning may arise from the deliberate eating of the leaves or the accidental consumption of dead, fallen leaves during grazing of the underlying pasture plants. It is particularly dangerous when growing in association with white clover. The toxic substance has been extracted but not (1968) identified.

It produces an arteriosclerosis, with calcification in heart, aorta, lungs, etc.

Symptoms.—Emaciation occurring over weeks or months, and an abnormal gait.

ENTERALGIA (ἔντερον, the intestines ; ἄλγος, pain) is another name for colic.

ENTERITIS (ἔντερον, the intestines) means inflammation of the intestines. (*See* DIARRHŒA *and* INTESTINES, DISEASES OF, *also* SCOURS; *and* CHRONIC CATARRHAL ENTERITIS of horses.)

ENTERITIS, SPECIFIC FELINE (*see* FELINE ENTERITIS).

ENTEROCELE (ἔντερον, the intestine; κήλη, a tumour) means a hernia of the bowel. (*See* HERNIA.)

ENTEROLITHS (ἔντερον, the intestine; λιθος, a stone) are stones that develop in the intestines, being formed by deposition of salts round a hard metallic or other nucleus. (*See* CALCULI.)

ENTEROSTOMY (ἔντερον, intestine; στόμα, mouth) means an operation by which an artificial opening is formed into the intestine.

ENTEROVIRUSES.—A group of smaller viruses pathogenic to animals.

ENTERO-TOXÆMIA.—**Sheep.**—There are two forms of this acute disease, each caused by a different type of the organism *Clostridium welchii* (also responsible for lamb dysentery and pulpy kidney disease). One form of entero-toxæmia, due to *Cl. welchii*, Type D, is widespread in Great Britain, and affects sheep of any age, though principally those under 2 years of age. Losses generally occur when sheep are grazing on rich pasture, particularly if they have just come from a poor one. Similarly, when folded sheep are attacked, it is usually shortly after having been moved on to a new and highly nutritious crop. The illness is short, an animal seeming perfectly well one day and being found dead the next.

When the disease appears in sheep recently folded on a fresh crop or recently turned out on to vetches, clover, stubble, etc., or on to an improved grass pasture, the sheep should, if possible, be removed from the place where losses occur and later returned for an hour or two each day until accustomed to their new diet. Where it is not convenient to carry out this procedure, use may be made of an antiserum.

The second form of entero-toxæmia, due to *Cl. welchii*, Type C, is apparently very restricted in its distribution, occurring on the Romney Marsh—where it is known as 'struck'—and in isolated valleys in North Wales. It usually occurs during the late winter and spring. Sheep of 1 to 2 years old are affected, and are usually found dead, though in a few cases symptoms of dullness and unnatural posture are observed.

This infection was reported (1968) in unweaned **lambs** in Northumberland, and also occurs in lambs overseas. Five to 10 per cent of sheep may die in one season on a particular portion of land, while on adjoining fields the diseases may be entirely absent. A vaccine is available for preventive purposes, and it is advisable to give two doses at an interval of at least 14 days.

Goat.—Entero-toxæmia is also of considerable importance in goats. Two forms are recognised: acute, and sub-acute or chronic. The symptoms of the acute form, which is invariably fatal within 36 hours, include: sudden drop in milk yield, loss of appetite, diarrhœa (blood-stained), persistent straining, convulsions.

The sub-acute type lasts 7 or 10 days is followed by recovery, and characterise, by attacks of diarrhœa and dullness.

Diagnosis may be confirmed in the laboratory by identification of *Cl. welchii*, Type D, and its toxin E, provided the last few feet of small intestine (tied at both ends) is submitted before putrefaction has taken place.

Treatment consists in the administration of large doses (up to 100 c.c.) of Type D antiserum (except to the all-white Saanen which appears to have an idiosyncrasy in this respect). Sulphamezathine has proved effective. In-contact animals should received 20 c.c. of serum. and subsequently 'pulpy kidney' vaccine,

Cattle.—Cases have occasionally been reported in Australia.

ENTROPION (ἐν, in; τρέπω, I turn) means a condition in which, as a result of disease, the edge of the eyelid is turned in towards the eyeball, and the eyelashes irritate and inflame the surface of the cornea. (*See* EYE, DISEASES OF.)

ENURESIS (ἐν, in; οὐρέω, I make water) means the unconscious or involuntary passage of water. (*See* URINE.)

ENZOÖTIC (ἐν, in; ζῶον, animal) is a term applied to an outbreak of disease among animals in particular areas or districts, or among certain breeds or species of animals. Thus rabies is enzoötic on the continent of Europe, braxy and louping ill are enzoötic among sheep in the south and west of Scotland and the north of England, and anthrax is enzoötic among horses in many parts of Asia Minor.

Enzoötic diseases are liable to become epizoötic under certain circumstances, in which case animals are attacked in large numbers in many parts or all over a continent at about the same time.

For Enzoötic Abortion of Sheep, *see under* ABORTION, ENZOÖTIC.

ENZOÖTIC PNEUMONIA OF PIGS.—This was formerly erroneously described as Virus Pneumonia of Pigs (V.P.P.), but the cause is *mycoplasma hyopneumoniæ.*

Fifty per cent of pigs reaching the bacon factories are affected with some degree of pneumonia, so that the matter is of the very greatest economic importance.

Symptoms.—When the disease is first introduced into a herd pigs of all ages (from 10 days upwards) go down with it, and many die. Where the disease is already present, deaths are few. Symptoms, which may easily be overlooked or ignored, then consist merely of a cough. There is, in addition, a certain degree of unthriftiness which in extreme cases may amount to stunted growth. In all cases one may expect the liveweight gain to be reduced, and it has been estimated that in many cases it costs £2 more to fatten a pig with this pneumonia than one free from the disease. Sometimes pigs which contract the disease earlier in life quite suddenly develop acute pneumonia at nineteen to twenty-six weeks of age, known as 'secondary breakdown'. Affected animals lose their appetite and often become prostrate; breathing rapidly with a temperature over 105° F. A number die if left untreated, but the majority have a fluctuating fever for a few days and then recover.

Treatment.—Aureomycin and terramycin have been used, but it is difficult to overcome the initial infection, and to prevent animals from becoming or remaining carriers.

Prevention.—An attack of this Pneumonia is not followed by immunity, and there is no means of preventive inoculation. All that can be done is to try to avoid buying in infected stock. Litters are best kept in arks on pasture, and any sows showing a cough eliminated. Weaned pigs should not be brought into a fattening house where pigs with Pneumonia are present. (*See* DUSTY ATMOSPHERE, SWINE INFLUENZA.)

A health-control scheme for pig herds claiming freedom from enzootic pneumonia was introduced in 1959. The scheme is privately financed, is independent of Government agencies, and is under veterinary supervision both centrally and locally. By the end of 1966, 241 herds had participated for varying lengths of time, a population of about 400,000 fattening pigs had been screened for respiratory disease and the lungs from about 140,000 of these pigs had been examined *post mortem.* In January, 1967, 91 herds were registered as free from enzootic pneumonia.

Two main observations have been made. First, there has been a constant need for differential diagnosis, because so many herds free from enzootic pneumonia contain pigs that have other forms of pneumonia. Secondly, the reinfection rate has been high. Consequently, although the benefits of an enzootic-pneumonia-free herd are now well established, there seems little hope of extending the scheme beyond its present voluntary basis until these two questions are more fully understood. In the meantime, the continual veterinary supervision of this population of pigs provides an excellent medium for studying the diagnosis, epidemiology and control of respiratory disease. (*Veterinary Record,* Dec. 16, 1967.)

Diagnosis.—A complement fixation test has been devised.

ENZYME (ἐν, in ; ζύμη, leaven) is the name given to a chemical ferment formed within the body. Enzymes are complex organic chemical compounds which possess the power of splitting up compounds of food-stuffs into simpler compounds which may be absorbed into the system. Some are formed by the secreting glands or cells of the body, and some are elaborated by the normal bacillary inhabitants of the intestinal canal, while certain food-stuffs contain their own ferment (auto-enzyme), which is only liberated in the warm and moist conditions of the alimentary canal, or in circumstances where similar conditions obtain. Each of them has a specific use in splitting up either proteins, carbohydrates, fats, or crude fibre. The best known are the ptyalin of saliva and diastase of the pancreatic juice, which break down starches into soluble sugars, pepsin from the gastric juice and trypsin from the pancreas, which break complex proteins into simple amino-acids, and lipase in the intestines which attacks fats. (*See* DIGESTION.) Enzymes are used in the cleaning of badly infected wounds. (*See* STREPTODORNASE.)

EOSINOPHIL is the name given to white cells in the blood-stream containing granules which readily stain with eosin, a histological dye. As well as these white corpuscles, eosinophils are found in the pituitary and pineal glands.

In a normal horse, one cubic inch of blood contains between 5 and 8 million eosinophil white cells—compared with about 160 million other white cells, and 128,000 million red corpuscles.

Work by the Animal Health Trust has shown that eosinophil white cells contain a very powerful anti-histamine. By a special technique, the cells have been separated from the blood of a horse, and an extract made which has potent anti-inflammatory properties. This research work may lead to more successful treatment of shock, inflammatory conditions, and allergies.

EOSINOPHILIA means that an abnormally large number of eosinophils are present in the blood-stream. This may occur during severe parasitic infestation in horses and dogs, in certain wasting conditions, and in disease of the lymph system.

EOSINOPHILIC MYOSITIS (*see under* MUSCLES, DISEASES OF).

EPERYTHROZOÖN PARVUM.—A recently discovered blood parasite of the pig, which gives rise to fever, anæmia, and sometimes jaundice. It can be transmitted from pig to pig by lice. It occurs in Britain and U.S.A.

Other species of this parasite affect sheep, and cattle in Africa.

EPERYTHROZOÖN FELIS.—A blood parasite found in cats in Britain, and first reported in 1959. (*See* FELINE INFECTIOUS ANÆMIA.)

EPHEDRINE is an alkaloid derived from the Chinese plant *Ma Huang*, or prepared synthetically. It stimulates the heart and central nervous system and relaxes the bronchioles. It is used for asthma in dogs and sometimes given to horses with broken wind.

EPHEMERAL FEVER (*see* THREE-DAY SICKNESS).

EPI- (ἐπί, upon) is a prefix meaning situated on or outside of.

'EPIDEMIC TREMORS' is the colloquial name for a virus disease of poultry characterised by an unsteady gait. (*See* AVIAN ENCEPHALOMYELITIS.)

EPIDIDYMIS (ἐπί, on; δίδυμος, testis) is the name of the structure from which the deferent duct takes origin. (*See* TESTIS.)

EPIDIDYMITIS (ἐπί, on; δίδυμος, testis) means inflammation of the epididymis.

EPIDIDYMITIS and VAGINITIS, CONTAGIOUS ('Epivag').—A venereal disease of cattle in Kenya and Southern Africa, and an important cause there of infertility and sterility.

Cause.—Possibly a double infection with a virus and *Vibrio fœtus*.

Symptoms.—There may be a yellowish discharge from the vagina, or merely a redness of the mucous membrane. In the bull, enlargement of the epididymis occurs over a period of months.

Prevention.—Slaughter of infected bulls, and use of A.I.

EPIDURAL ANÆSTHESIA is a form of spinal anæsthesia induced by the injection of a local anæsthetic solution into the spinal canal, but not into the cerebrospinal fluid. That is to say, the needle of the syringe does not penetrate the meninges, the anæsthetic solution remaining outside the *dura mater*. This technique is extensively employed in obstetrics, etc., in cattle. The injection is made through the space between the arches of the 1st and 2nd coccygeal vertebræ. Between 10 and 150 c.c. of 1 per cent to 2 per cent procaine hydrochloride solution are injected, according to the size of the animal and the area to be anæsthetised. (*See also* ANÆSTHETICS, ANALGESICS.)

EPIGASTRIUM (ἐπί, upon; γαστήρ, the stomach) is the region lying in the middle of the abdomen, immediately over the stomach. (*See* ABDOMEN.)

EPIGLOTTIS (ἐπιγλωττίς) is a leaf-like piece of elastic cartilage covered with mucous membrane, which stands upright between the back of the tongue and the entrance to the glottis, or larynx. It plays an important part in the act of swallowing, preventing solids and fluids from passing directly off the back of the tongue into the larynx.

EPILEPSY (ἐπίληψις) is a chronic nervous disorder characterised by a sudden complete loss of consciousness, associated with muscular convulsions. This is particularly a disease of the dog, although other domesticated animals may be affected upon rare occasions.

Cause.—The cause of epilepsy is not fully understood. Attacks of the convulsions, etc., may be brought on by shock, fright, injuries, sexual excitement, or from severe pain or stress (whelping, inoculations, anæsthesia, etc.). Large feeds of certain kinds of food, especially minced liver, will bring about repeated attacks in some cases; a sudden change of atmosphere, as from a warm room to out of doors on a frosty night, will induce the fits in others, but there are a large number of cases in which no factor can be pointed to as an actuating cause.

In a series of 260 cases of suspected central nervous system lesions, studied by Dr. Phyllis Croft (*Veterinary Record*, April 17, 1965), 167 were shown by electro-encephalogram to be examples of epilepsy.

Secondary epilepsy may be the result of a head injury, and can occur whenever scar tissue is formed in the brain.

'Fits', practically indistinguishable from true epileptic seizures, frequently occur when puppies are cutting their permanent teeth about the ages of 2 to 6 months, and also when there are large numbers of round or tape worms present in the intestines. (*See also* FITS, HYSTERIA, ENCEPHALITIS, POISONS, HEART DISEASE.)

Symptoms.—Attacks usually commence without any warning, the animal falling to the ground unconscious and becoming seized with violent convulsions. The limbs are sometimes held out rigidly, and sometimes moved as if the animal were running or galloping. The neck muscles are stiff and the head is held tensely. The animal champs its jaws; the eyes are fixed and staring, or the eyeballs may roll, and the pupils are dilated. There is usually a good deal of salivation from the mouth, and the dog often utters piercing shrieks incessantly. The rectum and the bladder are usually evacuated involuntarily. The dog regains consciousness in one to two minutes; in a few cases consciousness may not be completely lost. The first fit often occurs between the age of 1 and 3.

Treatment.—During an attack all restraint should be released and the animal should be so placed that it will not injure itself. Some recommend that a dog be held by the back of its head, so that the animal will not dash it against the ground or other objects, and that a cold water douche be applied to the skull.

After consciousness returns the dog should be placed in a quiet room away from other dogs or human beings, provided with a blanket or rug, and allowed time to recover from the great exhaustion which always follows a fit. Medicinal treatment should be left to a veterinary surgeon. (*See* LARGACTIL, MYSOLINE.)

EPIPHORA (ἐπί, upon; φέρω, I carry) means a condition in which the tears, instead of passing down the tear-duct to the inside of the nose, run over on to the cheek. It is due to a blocking of the tear-duct, generally from inflammation of its lining membrane. (*See* EYE.)

EPIPHYSEAL FRACTURE is one which occurs along the line of the epiphyseal cartilage, and results in the epiphysis of a bone becoming separated from the shaft or diaphysis. These fractures may occur n any young animal before complete ossification has occurred. (*See* FRACTURES.)

EPIPHYSIS (ἐπίφυσις) means the spongy extremity of a bone which is attached to the shaft for the purpose of forming a joint with the similar process of the adjacent bone. An epiphysis is covered on its surface by cartilage, is developed from a separate centre of ossification, and in a young animal is connected with the shaft of the bone by a plate of cartilage that disappears in the adult, being replaced by bone.

EPISPASTICS (ἐπί, upon; σπάω, I draw) are substances which produce blistering on the skin. (*See* BLISTERS.)

EPISTAXIS (ἐπί, upon; στάζω, I drop) means bleeding from the nose. (*Se* GUTTURAL POUCH DIPHTHERIA, HÆMORRHAGE.)

EPITHELIOMA (ἐπί, upon; θηλή, the nipple; *-oma*, meaning tumour) is a tumour of a malignant nature arising in the epithelium covering the surface of the body. (*See* CARCINOMATA AND SARCOMATA.)

EPITHELIUM (ἐπί, upon; θηλή, the nipple) is the name given to the cellular layer which covers the skin forming the cuticle, forms the inner layer of the walls

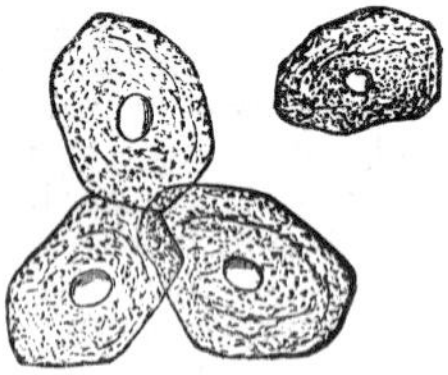

Scaly epithelium from the roof of the mouth. (Turner's *Anatomy*.)

of the bowels and forms the lining of ducts and hollow organs generally, such as the bladder, uterus, etc. It consists of one or more layers of cells which adhere to one another, and is one of the simplest tissues of the body. It takes several forms, *e.g.* that of the cuticle is scaly epithelium,

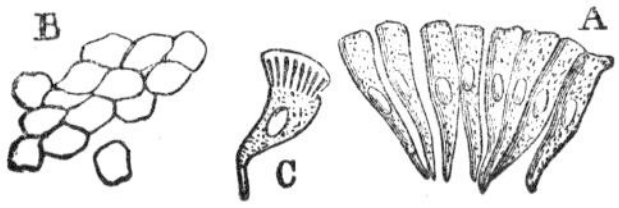

Columnar epithelium. *A*, side view of a group of cells; *B*, surface view of the ends of a group of cells; *C*, a columnar cell from the mucous membrane of the small intestine. (Turner's *Anatomy*.)

the cells being in several layers and more or less flattened (*see* SKIN); the bowels are lined by a single layer of columnar epithelium, the cells being long and narrow in shape; the air passages are lined by ciliated epithelium—that is to say, each cell is provided with lashes

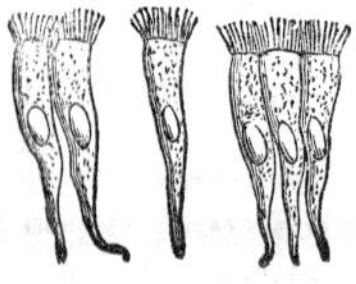

Ciliated columnar epithelial cells from the respiratory tract. (Turner's *Anatomy*.)

which drive the fluid or particles or mucus, etc., upon the surface, in an upward direction, by a continuous undulating or lashing motion; the inner surface of the bladder and the urinary channels are lined by a form of epithelium the cells of which are intermediate in shape between those of the skin and those of the bowels.

'EPIVAG'.—A venereal disease of cattle in Kenya and Southern Africa; Contagious Epididymitis and Vaginitis. (*See* EPIDIDYMITIS.)

EPIZOÖTIC (ἐπί, upon; ζῷον, animal) is a term applied to a disease which affects a large number of animals in a large area of land at the same time and spreads with great rapidity. An epizoötic is not the same as an *enzoötic*, where the disease affects animals in a smaller area, and is practically always present there; but an enzoötic may develop into an epizoötic; for instance, foot-and-mouth disease is enzoötic in many tropical countries, but is always liable to become epizoötic.

Generally, an epizoötic disease is contagious from one animal to another, but that is not essential, for spread may occur by means of intermediate objects, such as straw or forage or by insect carriers.

Among the agents known to be responsible for the introduction of epizoötics from time to time may be mentioned infected food-supplies, fertilisers, and other articles of commerce which are contaminated; pollution of the drinking water; possibly movements of game or wild animals and bird migration; seasonal factors are responsible for certain disease outbreaks, such as African horse sickness. where cases are only seen when the weather is mild and warm and none occur after the first frosts of the autumn, and 'grass sickness', which is encountered only in the spring and summer; insects are also very important factors in the spread of epizoötics, for the tick-borne diseases are always commoner when ticks are numerous, and the incidence of cattle trypanosomiasis exactly coincides with the situations of the 'fly belts' of tsetse flies in many parts of Central Africa. In addition to these recognised factors there are others, as yet unknown, which operate to originate epizoötics in certain areas.

EPIZOÖTIC CEREBRO-SPINAL MENINGITIS (*see* BORNA DISEASES).

EPIZOÖTIC LYMPHANGITIS. — Synonyms: Lymphangitis epizoötica, 'African glanders', 'Japanese farcy', and 'Neapolitan farcy'.

EPIZOÖTIC LYMPHANGITIS

This is a chronic contagious disease of the horse family (*Equidæ*), only characterised by a purulent inflammation of the superficial lymphatic vessels and of certain of the lymphatic glands, with a tendency to abscess formation.

Distribution.—It occurs widely in Asia, in Africa, and has also been described in America. In Europe it was at one time common in certain regions. It was unknown in Great Britain until 1902, when it was brought into the country by army horses returning from the South African war. The disease was made a notifiable one by the Epizoötic Lymphangitis Orders of 1904 and 1905, after which it was rapidly eradicated. Apart from very occasional reports following the Great War of 1914–18, it has not occurred in Britain for over fifty years.

Cause.—The disease is produced by a fungus *Histoplasma* (Cryptococcus) *farciminosus*. Infection can only occur by the fungus gaining access to the system through a wound, either on the skin or of a mucous surface. The disease is spread by harness, grooming tools, such as curry combs, brushes, scrapers, or by any materials which have come into contact with diseased animals or their infective discharges, and by wrong methods of dressing wounds by means of cloths, sponges, etc., which have been used on infected animals previously. The parasite shows considerable vitality outside the animal body, and may even be spread by using the same antiseptic solution in a pail to dress several cases.

Incubative period.—Under natural conditions at least one month, but more commonly three or more, may elapse from the time of contamination of a wound till the onset of the symptoms. Even by means of experimental inoculation, incubation takes one month.

Symptoms.—The first signs of the disease are often thickenings or ' cording ' of a lymphatic vessel and the enlargement of the adjacent lymphatic glands. The commonest situations of the lesions are on those places liable to be abraded or wounded, such as the shoulders, withers, knees, etc. The fore-limb, from the shoulder to the knee, is perhaps the most usual seat; in fact, a sore shoulder or a broken knee may be the point where the fungus first gains entrance. Tumour-like masses may be seen at or around the point of the shoulder, and a cord about the thickness of an ordinary lead pencil, or even broader, may run down the limb. The inside of the limb is a more common position than the outside. The tumefied masses on the shoulder may each reach the size of a hen's egg, or even a small orange, and here and there small hard tumours occur along the course of the thickened lymphatic, in size from that of a pea to a bean. These small nodules or ' tumours ' soften and burst; the smaller they are the quicker they become ' ripe '. The larger ones may sometimes not burst at all if left alone. In those that burst, the hair usually falls off at the ' point ', as is usual in any ' pointing ' abscess. The pus is yellowish and somewhat oily. After discharging the nodules give rise to ulcers which have raised, red, granulating edges, with but little tendency to heal. Although the fore-limb is the commonest seat of the lesions, a hind-leg may become affected, and the small characteristic pustules may be found at any part of the limb, even down to the hoofs. ' Brushing ' sores may be the primary cause of infection on the fetlocks in some cases. The affected limb may swell and become ' gummy ', and later on be chronically thickened.

Lesions of a similar nature may occur on the body, sides of the neck, or on the face, and there is often a tendency for chains or groups of these nodules to occur. From the point of the shoulder, the lymphatics running down the breast between the fore-legs may be involved, and in this case the corded condition may reach the size of a man's arm with here and there a softening taking place which leads to abscess formation. This cord may extend as far as the umbilical region. Ulcers may be found on the mucous membrane of the nose, and must not be mistaken for those due to glanders. The course of the disease is slow, lasting for months; a few cases may recover naturally, but there is always a tendency for lesions to form again at some later date. Most cases if left alone gradually become worse, and the animal may finally die as the result of the extension of the lesions internally. During the course of the disease there is practically no loss of flesh, no rise of temperature, no constitutional disturbance, nor does the appetite fall off.

Diagnosis.—An early recognition of the disease is of paramount importance, and when prevalent, any sore that shows a tendency to suppurate or a reluctance to heal should be considered as suspicious and skilled advice sought. The great danger is that the lesions are so slight—perhaps consisting of only one small ulcer no larger than a pea—that the lay horse-owner does not appreciate the necessity of the drastic measures necessary to prevent its spread. Neglect of these precautions often results in serious loss in Eastern countries. The condition is most likely to be mistaken for glanders or ulcerative lymphangitis; but by taking a smear of pus on a microscopic slide, a trained veterinarian can at once diagnose epizoötic lymphangitis should it be present. From glanders it can easily be distinguished by the use of the mallein test. (*See* GLANDERS.)

Treatment.—In the United Kingdom this is not allowable, as all cases must immediately be destroyed. Destruction of affected horses and mules is the general rule in the army, as it is found to be uneconomical and too risky to treat them.

EPIZOÖTIC PULMONARY ADENOMATOSIS (*see under* JAAGSIEKTE).

EPSOM SALTS is the popular name for sulphate of magnesium, which is one of the most frequently used saline purgatives. (*See* PURGATIVES.)

EPULIS (ἐπουλίς, a gumboil) is a term applied to any tumour connected with the jaws.

EQUINE ANIMALS (IMPORTATION) ORDER 1969 prohibits the importation of horses from Africa and the Near and Middle East, and was amended in 1971. (*See* EQUINE ENCEPHALITIS.)

EQUINE BILIARY FEVER (*see under* PARASITES, p. 637).

EQUINE COITAL EXANTHEMA.—A venereal disease of horses caused by a virus.

EQUINE CONTAGIOUS PLEURO-PNEUMONIA.—A disease encountered where large numbers of horses are crowded together under bad hygienic conditions. The cause is a virus but secondary bacterial invaders (*e.g. Streptococcus equi*) are important. A high mortality results.

EQUINE EHRLICHIOSIS.—The tentative name given to a transmissible disease of horses first recognised in California. The causal agent resembles that of tick-borne fever of cattle. Œdema of the extremities is a symptom.

EQUINE ENCEPHALITIS.—A virus disease occurring in North America, South America, Russia, Far and Middle East. It affects horses, but chickens, pheasants, etc., act as a reservoir of infection. Man can be infected. Four or five viruses are known to exist. Paralysis of the head and neck muscles is a feature. Treatment consists in the use of anti-serum in large doses. Mosquitoes transmit this disease, or group of diseases; the horse is an 'accidental' host. (*See also* NEAR EAST ENCEPHALITIS, VENEZUELAN.)

The deaths of thousands of horses in Mexico and the U.S.A. in 1971 led to further restrictions on the import of horses into the U.K.

EQUINE FILARIASIS.—Infestation of horses with the filarid worm *Seturia equina*, the larvæ being carried by mosquitoes and biting flies. It occurs in South and Central Europe, and Asia.

Symptoms.—Malaise and anæmia, or fever, conjunctivitis, and dropsical swellings.

EQUINE INFECTIOUS ANÆMIA.—Synonyms: pernicious equine anæmia, swamp fever, horse malaria, etc.

A contagious disease of horses and mules during the course of which changes occur in the blood, and rapid emaciation with debility and prostration are evident. It occurs chiefly in the Western States of America and the North-Western Provinces of Canada, as well as in most countries of Europe, and in Asia, and Africa.

Causes.—The disease is caused by a virus. The method of infection is by contamination of the food or water with blood or urine from an infected case; or by stabling healthy horses in premises that have recently housed affected animals and have not been disinfected subsequently. Foals suckling infected dams are liable to contract the disease, although in some instances they escape. It may be transmitted from an infected stallion to a healthy mare, but not in the reverse direction. The disease is most prevalent in low-lying swampy parts of the countries mentioned, during wet, mild weather, and most of the cases occur between July and early October. It is suspected that the disease is spread by biting insects such as flies.

The virus may cause illness in man (who may infect a horse); also in pigs.

Symptoms.—There are three types of

the disease—acute, sub-acute, and chronic, but these may merge into each other.

Acute type.—In this the cases occur suddenly, run a short severe course of from 3 to 14 days, and are terminated by death. The animal becomes dull and unfit for work; it shows weakness of the hind-legs and rapid respirations. Food is refused, and the lining membrane of the eyelids becomes swollen and œdematous, and tears may flow. The temperature rises to about 105° F. and remains high. The lower parts of the body swell and become dropsical, due to a weakened heart's action. The urine is increased in quantity, and generally of a high colour. Inflammation of the bowels often takes place, and a blood-stained diarrhœa with colicky pains is then seen. An important symptom: hæmorrhages on the underside of the tongue. Death occurs in up to 70 per cent of cases. In the final stages of the disease paralysis of the two hind-limbs with an inability to rise from the ground may be noticed. Relapses are common in cases which appear to recover and are put back to work too soon.

Sub-acute type.—The symptoms presented in this form of the disease are similar to those already mentioned but much less severe. The horse may live for weeks or even months before death occurs. Periodically, remissions are exhibited when the horse becomes to all outward appearances normal.

Chronic type.—In this form the commencement of the trouble is insidious in nature. The affected animal becomes dull at times, it tends to lose its condition, the coat stares, eyes and mouth assume a yellowish colour, the appetite is capricious, and the horse is easily distressed when made to work. Accidental wounds bleed profusely, the blood clotting very slowly, and healing processes are long delayed. General weakness and emaciation become more and more marked, until finally the animal dies from exhaustion. Some few cases do recover with care and attentive nursing, but these act as carriers of the disease for some considerable time.

Treatment.—All doubtful cases must be isolated until a definite diagnosis is established. Horses obviously affected should be destroyed. The fæces and urine from all infected cases, as well as contaminated litter, discharges, etc., must be disposed of in such a manner that healthy horses will have no access to them, while thorough disinfection of the premises must be undertaken. The water-supply, especially if from a stream, must be carefully guarded; affected horses must be watered from buckets, etc., and not allowed access to the running water.

No treatment has so far been proved to be efficacious, and recovered animals become carriers. Vaccines are ineffective.

EQUINE INFECTIOUS BRONCHITIS.—This is a virus infection, also known as 'Newmarket Cough' or Equine Epidemic Cough or Influenza.

EQUINE INFLUENZA.—A common and highly infectious disease of horses. Provided that they have not been worked while ill, mortality from influenza is usually nil, except in foals infected during the first few days of life. There is surely a danger in referring to equine influenza as 'The Cough' or 'Newmarket Cough' if those colloquialisms give rise to the idea that it is only a cough and not an illness. Owners should appreciate that influenza viruses need to be treated with respect; also that there are many other causes of coughing in horses. (*See* COUGH.)

Cause.—A virus was first isolated in Prague in 1957. One of a similar type was isolated in the 1963 outbreak in Britain, and is now known as A/Equi/1. Also referred to as the Cambridge strain, it was also found in the U.S.A. In the 1963 outbreak in the U.S.A., another virus, believed to have come from South America, was isolated. This is called A/Equi/2 or the 'Miami strain'. This virus appeared in Britain for the first time in the 1965 outbreak, and is expected largely to replace the A/Equi/1 virus here. It is not unlikely that other myxovirus types will be isolated from cases of equine influenza in the future.

Symptoms.—The temperature rises to a degree or two above normal, or even as high as 106° F. Often the first symptom observed by the owner is the cough, at first of a dry type but later becoming moist. Coughing may last for 1 week, or persist for 3 weeks. In mild cases there may be virtually no other symptoms and —if rested—the horse makes an uneventful recovery.

In less mild cases the animal has a dejected appearance and very little appetite. Sometimes there is probably pain in the muscles, for the horse may show difficulty or clumsiness in lying down and getting up, or may appear stiff.

A foal born to a mare during the course

of an attack of influenza, or as the first symptoms are beginning to appear, will appear normal for 4 or 5 days; but then the temperature rises to 105° or more, the foal ceases to feed, and within a couple of days its breathing becomes very laboured. Death can be expected when the foal is about 9 or 10 days old.

Treatment.—First-aid measures call for rest, warmth and, if appetite fails, several small feeds a day. Professional advice should always be obtained. Antibiotics may be used in order to prevent any complications caused by bacteria.

In the foal, hyperimmune serum has proved effective in saving life **when given between 60 and 80 hours after birth.** Antibiotics may also be used liberally during the first 3 or 4 days of life in order to try to avoid complications arising from secondary infection.

When the disease has already appeared in a stable, it is wise to rely upon the thermometer rather than the cough as the first sign of infection in a horse. The temperature may be up 12 hours before coughing starts, and if the fever is detected early the animal can be rested with all the greater chances of the influenza remaining mild.

Prevention.—A reliable vaccine, containing both A/Equi/1 and A/Equi/2 viruses, is available. It is reommended that foals are vaccinated when between 3 and 6 months old. In-foal mares should be vaccinated at least 3 weeks before they foal. Horses should be vaccinated 3 weeks before they go to sales, etc., where they are likely to be exposed to infection. Newcomers to a stable, especially 2- or 3-year-olds, should also be vaccinated. Immunity is developed in 98 per cent of vaccinated animals within 2 or 3 weeks, and should last for about a year.

EQUINE PIROPLASMOSIS is another name for biliary fever of the horse, which is due to one of two protozoön parasites, *Piroplasma* (or *Babesia*) *caballi*, or else *Nuttallia equi*. (*See under* PARASITES, p. 637.)

EQUINE VIRAL ARTERITIS.—As its name suggests, this is a disease in which damage is caused to the arteries, especially the smaller ones. Hæmorrhagic enteritis, with abdominal pain and diarrhœa, occurs; and distressed breathing results from œdema of the lungs. Abortion is common in the affected mare. Death is common.

EQUINE VIRAL RHINOPNEUMONITIS.—A disease recognised in America and Europe. It gives rise to symptoms associated with the common cold of Man. What gives the disease its alternative name of 'Equine Virus Abortion', is the fact that pregnant mares exposed for the first time to the infection may abort.

Indeed, the term 'abortion storms' has been used, since 40 to 60 per cent. (or even more) of the mares in a stud may abort. Usually such an occurrence is a sequel to an outbreak of severe and extensive nasal catarrh when the in-foal mares were between 4½ and 7 months pregnant.

It must be emphasised, however, that these 'abortion storms' are exceptional, and have become more so, both on the Continent and in the U.S.A., in recent years.

Abortion may occur at any time from 4½ months of pregnancy right up to the normal foaling date, but 8½ to 10 months is the most common period. Mares show no other symptoms at this time. Subsequent foaling is nearly always normal.

The virus is present in the aborted fœtus, fluids, and membranes. It cannot survive more than a fortnight in the absence of horse tissue. On straw, concrete floors, etc., it dies within a week. But when dried on to horse hairs, it has been shown to be infective for up to six weeks. The stallion is not, it is believed, involved in the spread of the disease—first reported in the U.K. in 1961.

EQUISETUM POISONING (*see* HORSETAILS, POISONING BY).

EQUIVALENTS, TABLES OF.—In Great Britain the metric system of weights and measures has been adopted as the more accurate and convenient manner by which drugs and medicines can be dispensed.

Measures of Length.

1 inch = 2·5399 centimetres (= 2·54 approx.).
1 foot = 30·4794 centimetres (= 30·48 approx.).
1 yard = 91·4383 centimetres or 0·914 of a metre.

To convert inches to centimetres, multiply by 2·54.

1 centimetre = 0·3937 inches.
1 metre = 1 yard 0 feet 3·37 inches.
To convert centimetres into inches, multiply by 0·39.
To convert metres into yards, multiply by 1·09.

Measures of Weight.

1 grain = 0·0648 grammes (or grams).
= 64·8 milligrammes.
1 dram (Apothec.) = 3·888 grammes.
= 3888·0 milligrammes.
1 ounce (Avoir.) = 28·35 grammes.
1 pound (Avoir.) = 453·592 grammes.
= ½ kilogramme (roughly).
To convert ounces (Avoir.) into grammes, multiply by 28·35.
To convert pounds into grammes, multiply by 453·6.
To convert pounds into kilogrammes, multiply by 0·454.
To convert ounces (Troy) into grammes, multiply by 31·104.
1 milligramme = 0·0154 grains.
1 gramme = 15·4323 grains.
= 0·0321 ounces.
1 kilogramme = 2·2046 lb. (Avoir.).
To convert grammes into ounces (Avoir.). multiply by 0·0352.
To convert grammes into grains, multiply by 15·432.
To convert kilogrammes into pounds (Avoir.), multiply by 2·2046.

Measures of Capacity.

1 fluid dram = 3·544 cubic centimetres (c.c. or mil.).
1 fluid ounce = 28·412 cubic centimetres.
(1 ounce (Troy) = 31·1034 grammes).
1 pint = 567·933 cubic centimetres (0·568 litres).
1 gallon = 4·54 litres.
To convert fluid ounces into c.c., multiply by 28·412.
To convert pints into c.c., multiply by 568·0.
To convert gallons into litres, multiply by 4·54.
1 cubic centimetre (c.c. or mil.) = 1 gramme of distilled water at 4° C.
= 0·061 cubic inches.
= 0·352 fluid ounces.
= 16·896 minims (Imper.).
1 litre = 61·0 cubic inches.
= 1·7607 pints.
= 35·196 fluid ounces.
To convert cubic centimetres into ounces, multiply by 0·352.
To convert litres into pints, multiply by 1·76.
To convert litres into fluid ounces (Imperial), multiply by 35·196.

Other Equivalents.

1 cubic centimetre = $\frac{1}{1000}$ litre = 1 millilitre (or 1 mil.) = the amount of distilled water which weighs 1 gramme at 4° C. or 39° F.
1 gallon of water weighs 10 lb., and occupies 277·274 cubic inches (4·54 litres or 4540·0 c.c.).

EREPSIN, or **EREPTASE,** is a ferment secreted by the intestine which breaks up peptones into amino-acids and other products of digestion.

ERGOMETRINE is the most powerful of the active constituents of ergot in producing muscular contractions of the uterus. It is used to stimulate a sluggish uterus during parturition and to control uterine hæmorrhage following parturition.

ERGOSTEROL is a sterol obtained from ergot of rye, yeast, and other sources, which, under the action of sunlight or ultra-violet rays, produces vitamin D_2. The substance changed in this way is known as calciferol, and is used for the prevention and cure of rickets and other bone diseases. A similar change in the sterols of the skin is produced when the body is freely exposed to sunlight. (*See* VITAMINS.)

ERGOT is the name given to the small mass of horn which is found amongst the tuft of hair which grows from the back of the fetlocks of horses. It is produced by cells which are similar to those which form the horn of the hoof, and it is considered by some authorities to be the remains of what once was the hoof of another digit which the horse has now lost.

ERGOT OF MUNGA, the bulrush millet, is in Southern Rhodesia an important cause of loss to the pig industry. The sow's udder fails to enlarge and become functional, and piglet mortality is heavy as a result of the absence of milk or *agalactia*. Sows show no other signs of ill health. The alkaloidal composition of this ergot is believed to differ from that of *Claviceps purpurea*.

ERGOT OF RYE is the name of a fungus which attacks the seed of rye or other cereal, subsists upon it, and finally replaces it. The fungus is called *Claviceps purpurea*, and is artificially cultivated on account of its medicinal properties. Its medicinal preparations are used to stimulate the wall of the uterus during parturition when there is inertia, and are also useful for checking hæmorrhage by causing constriction of the arterioles. Purified products from ergot, especially *ergotoxine*, *tyramine*, and *ergometrine*, induce abortion, and are sometimes used for this purpose. The crude ergot is unsafe to use. In parturition the active principle ergometrine is employed both in human and animal work to increase the force and efficiency of labour pains.

ERGOT POISONING occurs through eating cereals upon which the fungus is parasitic, such as rye and various kinds of maize, etc., and through taking foods made from plants so affected (*e.g.* ground rye or maize meals). Extensive outbreaks have occurred in various parts of the United States of America, in Germany, Austria, and other parts of Europe. Abortion and gangrene of the extremities in cattle have been seen in Britain.

Symptoms.—The characteristic feature of poisoning due to *Claviceps purpurea* is that there is irritation and pain in the extremities of the body, and later, areas of the skin of these parts become gangrenous, and may slough off. There are two forms recognised: in the first, spasmodic symptoms due to stimulation of the nervous system are seen; and in the second, gangrene occurs. Horses that have eaten large amounts of ergotised hay develop symptoms during the first 24 hours after feeding. The animal becomes dull and listless, a cold sweat breaks out on the neck and flanks, the breathing is slow and deep, the temperature is below normal, the pulse is weak and finally imperceptible, and death occurs during deep coma. When less amounts have been taken over a longer period there may be diarrhœa, colic, vomiting, and signs of abdominal pain. Pregnant animals may abort, and lose condition. From this stage the symptoms may pass on into one or other of the two forms mentioned above. If spasmodic symptoms develop, the animal shows contractions of the muscles of the limbs, trembling, general muscular spasms, loss of sensation of the extremities, convulsions and delirium. Death in such cases arises from secondary complications. In the gangrenous form there is coldness of the feet, ears, lips, tail, combs and wattles of birds, and other extremities, a loss of sensation in these parts, and eventually dry gangrene sets in. After a day or two the hair falls out, teeth drop out, the tips of the ears and tail may slough off, and the skin of the limbs, or even the whole of the feet, may be cast off. Death occurs from exhaustion, or from septicæmia. (*See also under* ERGOT OF MUNGA.)

ERYSIPELAS, SWINE (*see* SWINE ERYSIPELAS).

ERYSIPELOID.—Human infection with *Erysipelothrix rhusiopathiæ*, the cause of swine erysipelas.

ERYTHEMA (ἐρύθημα) is a general term denoting a red eruption on the skin, the surface blood-vessels of which become gorged with blood, and often considerable pain is evinced in the affected parts. It is a symptom of several diseases, being almost always present in digestive disorders in pigs, in swine erysipelas, and in mange and ringworm in all animals.

ERYTHROCYTE (ἐρυθρός, red; κύτος, cell) is another name for a red blood corpuscle.

ERYTHROCYTE MOSAICISM.—The mixture of 2 blood types in each of non-identical twins.

ERYTHROLEUCOSIS.—This is a transmissible virus-associated type of cancer occurring in poultry. It is associated with the fowl paralysis group of diseases. It was described and named in 1908, three years before the Rous sarcoma made history. (*See under* LEUCOSIS COMPLEX.)

ESCHAR (ἐσχρα, a slough) is an area of body tissue that has been killed by heat or by caustics. (*See* CAUSTICS.)

ESCHERICHIA COLI.—This is the modern name for *Bacillus coli*. For further information *see* E. COLI.

ESCUTCHEON.—The anal region of an ox, with especial reference to the direction of growth of hair.

ESERINE is another name for PHYSOSTIGMINE, *which see*.

ESSENCES are strong solutions of active substances. They are made either by solution in water, such as essence of rennet or of pancreas, or in the case of aromatic essences, such as essence of peppermint, in rectified spirit.

ESTER.—A compound formed from an alcohol and an acid by elimination of water, *e.g.*, ethyl acetate.

ETHER, or **ETHYL OXIDE,** is a colourless, volatile, highly inflammable liquid formed by the action of sulphuric acid upon alcohol, with the aid of heat. It boils below the body temperature, and when sprayed over the skin rapidly evaporates. It dissolves many substances, such as fats, oils, resins, better than alcohol or water, and is used accordingly in the preparation of many drugs.

Uses.—Externally it is used as a cleansing agent before operations upon parts where the skin is liable to be greasy, because it dissolves fats which often protect bacteria from the action of antiseptics used afterwards. By inhalation it is a general anæsthetic, relatively non-toxic. High concentrations of ether cause coughing and spasm of the larynx, especially after the administration of barbiturates. Salviation and bronchial secretions are increased by ether. (*See* ANÆSTHETICS.) Internally, it is similar to alcohol and chloroform in many of its actions. It stimulates gastric secretion, and increases the vigour of the stomach movements. Injected hypodermically it is useful for stimulating the heart and warding off threatened collapse.

ETHIDIUM BROMIDE.—A trypanocide given by intra-muscular injection. This drug is also used in the treatment of 'Heather Blindness' (Contagious Ophthalmia) in sheep and Bovine Keratitis.

ETHMOID (ἠθμός, a sieve; εἶδος, form) is the name of a bone which separates the nasal cavity from that of the brain. It is spongy in nature and contains numerous cavities, some of which communicate with the nose and serve to carry the nerves of the sense of smell.

ETHYL BROMIDE and ETHYL CHLORIDE are clear, colourless liquids, produced respectively by the action of hydrobromic and hydrochloric acids upon alcohol. Both are extremely volatile, and rapidly produce freezing of the surface of the skin when sprayed upon it. They are used to produce insensibility for short surface operations, such as the removal of warts or small tumours, the lancing of painful abscesses, the removal of thorns or foreign bodies, etc. They are put up in glass or metal tubes provided with a fine nozzle, from which the liquid is forced by warming the tube with the hand. Ethyl chloride is sometimes used as a general anæsthetic for the extraction of teeth. Insensibility is easily induced, but is of only short duration, and rapidly passes off when the administration ceases.

ETHYLENE is a colourless inflammable gas which is sometimes used as an anæsthetic in small animals.

ETIOLOGY (αἰτία, a cause; λόγος, a discourse) is the study of the conditions which cause disease.

ETORPHINE (M99 Reckitt).—This is an analgesic and immobilising agent, originally used for the capture of elephants, rhinoceroses, zebra, antelopes, and other animals in Africa, and for facilitating handling of 'zoo' animals.

A combination of etorphine with the tranquilliser methotrimeprazine has been shown to produce effective immobilisation of dogs when given intramuscularly. Analgesia, immobilisation, sedation, and muscle relaxation are adequate for a wide variety of diagnostic and therapeutic procedures including setting of fractures, suturing of wounds, dentistry, and minor surgery.

The drug does not, like morphine, cause excitement, vomiting or defæcation.

When required, immobilisation was reversed by intravenous administration of the specific etorphine antagonist diprenorphine.

It would appear that the drug is of great value in the horse but must be used with extreme caution in the pig.

EU- (εὖ, well) is a prefix meaning satisfactory or beneficial.

EUCAINE is a substance closely resembling cocaine in action and composition, but it is less depressant to the heart.

EUSTACHIAN TUBES are the passages, one on each side, which lead from the throat to the middle ear, and serve to maintain an even atmospheric pressure upon the inner surface of the 'ear-drum' or tympanum. They open widely in the act of swallowing, and during a yawn. Each has a sac or diverticulum connected with it in the horse, and in certain conditions these become filled with pus from a strangles abscess or from some other suppurating source near, when operation becomes necessary to evacuate the pus and prevent it doing damage by burrowing into the middle ear or surrounding parts. (*See* EAR.)

EUTHANASIA (εὖ, well; θάνατος, death) as applied to animals, is the name given to the process of producing death free from associated ante-mortem fear or suffering. The term has chiefly an application to dogs and cats and other pets, although, strictly speaking, the humane slaughtering of animals for food purposes, and the humane destruction of horses or other animals kept for working purposes, should also fall within the meaning of the word. (*See also* DESTRUCTION OF ANIMALS.)

EVERSION OF BLADDER is an accident in which the bladder becomes turned inside out through the urethra and hangs to the outside of the body. It is only possible for it to occur in the female, for the length of the urethra in the male precludes the possibility of the bladder being able to pass through it. In the female it is almost always associated with eversion or prolapse of the uterus as the result of difficulty during parturition. (*See* UTERUS, DISEASES OF.)

EVERSION OF UTERUS (*see* UTERUS, DISEASES OF).

EXANTHEMATA (ἐξ, out; ἀνθέω, I blossom) is an old name used to indicate those diseases that are characterised by a rash or eruption. (*See under* VESICULAR.)

EXCHANGE TRANSFUSION (*see* BLOOD TRANSFUSION).

EXCIPIENT (*excipio*, I mix with) means any more or less inert substance added to a prescription in order to make the remedy as prescribed more suitable in bulk, consistence, or form for administration.

EXCISION (*excisio*) means literally 'a cutting out', and is a term applied to the removal of any structure from the body, when such removal necessitates a certain amount of separation from surrounding parts. One speaks of the excision of a tumour, of a gland, or of a joint, but when a prominent part or member is removed the operation is called 'amputation'. If a simple opening is made into the part, one speaks of 'incision'.

EXCITING CAUSE of a disease is the name given to the direct or immediate cause of that disease, as opposed to an indirect or 'predisposing cause', which merely renders the body specially liable to the disease in question. Thus, overcrowding of cows in a badly ventilated byre, with an insufficiency of food, is a predisposing cause of pulmonary tuberculosis, but the exciting cause is the presence of the bacillus of tuberculosis in the lungs.

EXCORIATION (*ex*, out of; *corium*, the skin) means the destruction of small pieces of the skin or of mucous membrane often by chafing. (*See* CHAFING.)

EXERCISE is a matter of the greatest importance in the preservation of health among all classes of animals. It is obvious that the methods of domestication, which have made such enormous modifications in the characteristics of horses, cattle, sheep, pigs, dogs, and cats, to mention only the commoner domesticated animals, have also so altered their modes of life that exercise is a matter over which they themselves often have little or no control, and it is essential that the owners of these animals should have an intelligent idea of the need for exercise, and of the amount necessary.

Effects of exercise.—Upon the muscles of the body exercise produces a loss of watery and fatty materials, and stimulates the formation of new fleshy material, the muscles gradually growing in size as the demand made upon them increases. Upon the blood-vessels and lymph-vessels the alternate contraction and relaxation of the muscles exerts a pumping action, so that blood and lymph circulate more freely, the waste products carried by them are expelled faster, and the general blood supply of the whole of the tissues of the body is increased. This results in an increased activity in the heart, lungs, kidneys, liver, and other vital organs, with resulting benefit to the animal as a whole. Further, the increased circulation results in more vigorous movements by the respiratory muscles (chest walls, diaphragm, and abdominal muscles), and the organs of digestion are compressed and relaxed more often and more vigorously, so that digestion is aided and sluggishness of the bowels, or constipation, is prevented.

Want of exercise.—When an animal is compelled to do without a minimum of exercise for long periods of time the bad effects become obvious, but when the exercise is merely insufficient they are not so easily noticed, although they will be seen sooner or later. Lack of sufficient exercise is most serious in young animals, especially calves, pigs, and puppies. They do not grow and develop as they should; their bones do not fully ossify, and malformations of the limbs are common; the abdomen becomes pendulous ('pot-bellied'), and rickets is encouraged. (Some doubt exists as to the actual relationship between rickets and exercise, but the fact remains that under-exercised animals contract rickets more readily than those living out of doors and able to move about at will. The effect of radiation of the body with ultra-violet rays from the sun in preventing rickets is of course a major factor in the difference in incidence between young animals kept indoors and out of doors.) Other effects of an insufficiency of exercise in the young are delayed maturity, irregularity in the occurrence of œstrus, and a weakened constitution which predisposes to disease. In foals and lambs the method of rearing usually ensures that they receive a sufficient amount of exercise, for all animals in health will take exercise of their own accord if allowed a free range, and the energy expended by young animals out at pasture, especially lambs, is proverbial.

Very many of the diseases to which tied-up cattle are liable, especially digestive disturbances, are directly traceable to lack of exercise. In the horse, kept for working purposes, the amount of exercise it gets while performing its work is usually sufficient for its needs, but during holidays, week-ends, or when the weather is bad and work on the land impossible, it may happen that exercise is neglected. In such cases bad effects do not as a rule result if the feeding is reduced accordingly and if the rest is not prolonged; but otherwise such a horse is liable to become attacked with colic, lymphangitis, azoturia, and various foot troubles. Females of all species must receive a regular amount of exercise during pregnancy, for otherwise the tone of the uterine wall and other muscles of the body is lost, and there is a risk of trouble occurring at parturition. In all these respects what applies to the larger animals also applies to the smaller animals, and especially to sows kept in small, inadequate pens, and to the house-dog in cities and large towns.

Over-exercise, especially if an animal is not in a fit condition, is, on the other hand, equally bad. As the result of excessive exertion certain muscles become at first over-developed, but later they waste. Excessive efforts beyond the animal's strength are apt to bring about dilatation of the heart, broken-wind in horses, roaring, sprains or ruptures of muscles or tendons, particularly in the limbs of horses which are hunted or raced when unfit, etc. Occasionally an animal making a supreme effort drops dead through heart failure, rupture of a large artery, or through sheer exhaustion, but death from over-exercise is much more likely to occur the following day, through complications.

Amount of exercise.—Individual animals vary to a great extent in the amount of exercise required, and it is not necessary to state that the race-horse needs more exercise than does the milking cow, so that absolute figures cannot be given for every case. On an average, a light horse used for saddle purposes should get about an hour's walk with a short gallop or trot in the middle of it daily when it is to be idle for any length of time, but if only one day's rest is taken no exercise needs to be given. Heavy draught horses should get a short walk for 10 or 15 minutes twice daily when standing idle, or they may be turned out into a paddock or yard for the greater part of the day. Cattle tied up in stalls should receive a minimum of 10 to 20 minutes' exercise out of doors twice daily. When shut in loose-boxes they do not require to be let out every day, for they can move about to a certain extent in the box, and get some exercise in that way. Breeding sows and boars kept in pig-houses where space is limited always thrive better when allowed into a yard for some part of the day, or when allowed into a paddock to graze. House-dogs need different amounts of exercise according to their breeds and ages. Young dogs of the sporting breeds never do well unless they receive at least one hour's sharp walk morning and night when on the leash, or about half this period when allowed to range at liberty. Older dogs and those of pet breeds need less, but, generally speaking, the more exercise the dog gets the better health will it enjoy. (*See also* SHEEP-DOGS, MUSCLE, sub-heading 'Condition'.)

EXERCISING HORSES.—Horses must be gradually introduced to exercise or work, because over-exertion of an unfit or of a partly fit horse may have serious and permanent consequences. To get a riding horse fit it is usual to commence with daily walking exercise, with only an occasional trot for the first month or so. As the horse becomes fitter the duration of the exercise is lengthened, and the animal is made to walk at the commencement, then given a sharp trot or a short gallop, and finally another walk home each day for a further 2 to 4 weeks.

From this stage it proceeds to one when the gallop is of longer duration on alternate days, and then, later, the horse gets a stiff gallop every day for perhaps half an hour or so. In some stables there is a system of morning and afternoon exercise for each horse, but much must be left to the individual requirements of each animal, and to the judgment of the trainer. After a time, varying up to four months or more in some cases, the horse arrives at its maximum pitch of perfection, and then begins to 'go stale'. The art of the race-horse trainer enables him to judge the length of time it takes for each individual horse to arrive at his best at such a time as will allow him to enter for the race for which he is being trained. Every horse-trainer has his own individual methods, and as these are by no means hard-and-fast rules, nothing more than the merest outline can be given here.

The 'condition' of a horse, by which is meant its capacity for doing work, cannot be retained indefinitely; there comes a time when it begins to perform less and less well, and is said to have 'gone stale'. This is an indication that a rest is required.

EXFOLIATION (*ex*, out of; *folium*, a leaf) means the separation in layers of pieces of dead bone or of skin.

EXOMPHALOS is the name used for a hernia of abdominal organs which have escaped from the abdominal cavity through the umbilicus, *i.e.* an umbilical hernia. It is common in some breeds of dogs, and may be seen in any species.

EXOPHTHALMOS.—Bulging of the eyeballs. In America it has been observed as a hereditary defect in certain Jersey cattle in the U.S.A.; and in Britain in certain Shorthorn herds—the condition being preceded by a squint. (*See* EYE, DISEASES OF.)

EXOSTOSIS (ἐξ, out of; ὀστέον, a bone) means an outgrowth from a bone, usually the result of some form of inflammation. Splints, high and low ring-bones, bone spavins, and bony enlargements of the knees and hocks of horses, are of this nature. (*See* BONE, DISEASES OF.)

EXOTOXINS.—Toxins which diffuse readily from the bodies of bacteria during their lifetime. Examples: tetanus and botulinus toxins.

EXPECTORANTS (*ex*, out of; *pectus*, the chest) are drugs which assist the removal of secretions from the air passages. They include syrup of squills, ipecacuanha, Friar's balsam.

EXPOSURE to intense cold can usually be well tolerated by the animal which is well fed. More food is required during very cold weather in order to maintain the body temperature, and when snow is on the ground good hay should be taken to outwintered stock. The provision of windbreaks is important, but the tendency is for their number to decline in the interests of larger fields and units more suited to mechanisation. Animals denied shelter from very cold winds, and at the same time inadequately fed, are most liable to disease of one kind or another. (*See also* SHEARING).

EXTENSION is the term applied to the process of straightening or stretching a limb or other part of the body. In the case of a fracture, extension is applied to bring the two severed parts of the bone into apposition, and to prevent movement and separation of these when a splint or fixing bandage is being applied. Extension, along with flexion (*i.e.* bending), is made use of in the diagnosis of lameness.

EXTRACT OF MALE FERN, or **EXTRACT OF FERN ROOT,** is an oleo-resin prepared by percolating the rhizome ('root') of male fern (*Dryopteris filixmas*) with ether, and evaporating. It contains two active constituents known as *aspidinal* and *filicic acid* respectively. Male fern is an anthelmintic used for the destruction of tapeworms. For the dog more modern preparations which obviate fasting and are tasteless are to be preferred.

EXTRACTS are preparations, usually of a semi-solid consistence, containing the active parts of various plants extracted in one of several ways. In the case of some extracts the juice of the fresh plant is simply pressed out and purified; in the case of others the active principles are dissolved out in water, which is then removed to a great extent by evaporation or distillation; other extracts are made similarly but alcohol is used instead of water, while in others ether is the solvent.

EXTRAVASATION (*extra*, outside of; *vas*, a vessel) means an escape of a fluid from the vessels or passages which ought to contain it. Extravasation of blood is found in apoplexy and in bruises on the surface of the body, when tearing of the walls of the smaller vessels is the cause. Extravasation of urine occurs when the bladder is ruptured from a fall, blow on the abdomen, or from a run-over accident, or, as happens in some cases, from a fracture of the pelvis, when the sharp parts of the bones tear the organ.

EXUDATION (*exudo*, I sweat) means the process by which the fluid constituent of the blood passes slowly through the walls of the vessels in the course of inflammation, and also means the accumulation of fluid in cavities resulting from this process. Often other constituents pass out along with the fluid portions, and not infrequently the whole exuded material coagulates into a semi-solid or solid rough deposit, as in pleurisy and diphtheritic enteritis, which is often seen in cases of swine fever.

EYE

EYE.—The eyes are set, one on either side, in deep cavities known as 'bony orbits', whose edges are prominent and form a protection to the eyeball. In the pig, dog, and cat the edge of the bony orbit is not complete posteriorly, but in the other domesticated animals it forms a complete circle. The two orbits are separated from each other in the middle line of the skull by only a very small space, and posteriorly the nerves leaving each eye (optic nerves) converge and meet each other on the floor of the brain cavity, so that each eye is intimately associated with its fellow behind, though they are set on opposite sides of the skull when viewed from the front Lying inside the orbit but around the eyeball proper there is a large quantity of 'peri-orbital fat' upon which the eye rests as though upon an elastic cushion, and by virtue of which it is endowed with great mobility. The eye is protected by two main eyelids and in many cases by a small rudimentary 'third eyelid', 'haw', or *nictitating membrane*, which is found at the inner corner. The eyelids meet at the outer and inner 'canthi'. The external canthus is rounded, but the internal canthus is narrowed to form a ⊂-shaped bay or recess, called the 'lacrimal lake'. Just within the inner canthus and attached to

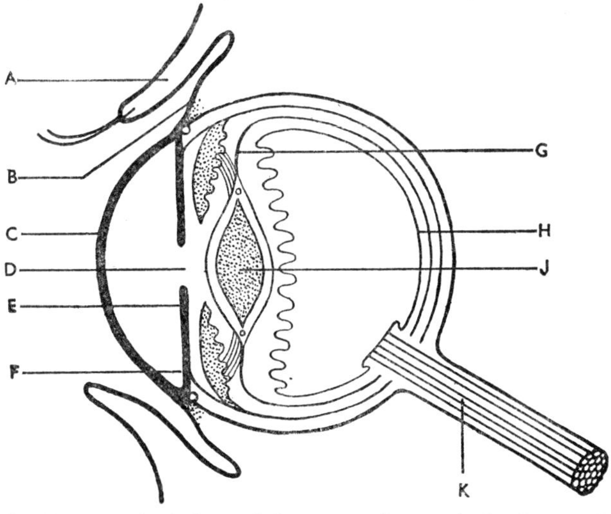

THE EYE: a sectional view. A indicates the eyelid, B conjuctiva, C cornea, D pupil, E iris, F ligament of the iris, G ligament of the lens, H retina, J lens, K optic nerve. Next to the retina (H) comes the hyaloid membrane, then the choroid coat and (the outermost) the sclerotic coat.

the nictitating membrane of which it forms a part, is a small rounded pigmented prominence known as the 'lacrimal caruncle', which is formed of modified skin, and which often bears one or two tiny hairs. (*See also* HARDERIAN GLAND.)

Eyelids.—Each of the two main eyelids consists of four layers: on the surface there is skin similar to that which covers the adjacent part of the face, but thin, loose, pliant, and bearing extremely fine hairs; below this is a layer of thin subcutaneous tissue, and then comes the second or muscular layer which is instrumental in opening and shutting the eyelids; the third layer is fibrous, and along the free edge of the lid this layer is denser and forms the 'tarsus' of the eyelid, in the substance of which is embedded a row of glands, called the 'tarsal glands', numbering 45 to 50 in the upper and 30 to 35 in the lower lid of the horse (small cysts are occasionally formed in connection with these glands which appear as rounded, painful swellings upon the surface of the lid); the fourth layer consists of the delicate mucous membrane called the 'conjunctiva', which rubs over the surface of the eyeball (also covered by conjunctiva) and tends to remove any dust, particles of debris, etc., that may collect on the moist surface. The two layers of conjunctiva are continuous with each other, being reflected off the eyelid on to the anterior surface of the eyeball, and forming little pockets (upper and lower) in which oat-chaffs sometimes lodge and are difficult to remove; normally these pockets should contain small amounts of fluid, forming tears. Any excess secretion of tears reaches the nasal cavity by the 'lacrimal duct', the two openings of which can be seen towards the inner canthus along the free margins of each of the lids. The third eyelid is situated at the inner angle of the eye, consisting of a semilunar fold of the conjunctiva, which is supported and strengthened by a small roughly crescentic plate of cartilage. Ordinarily this eyelid covers only a very small part of the surface of the eye, but in certain diseases, such as tetanus, the pressure by the muscles of the eyeball upon the orbital fat displaces the third eyelid, and it may reach across the eye to the extent of almost one inch.

In the cat, the appearance of the third eyelid (nictitating membrane), like a curtain partly drawn across a window, is a common sign of general ill health and is due to absorption of fat in the vicinity and is not usually a disease of the eye. Both in the cat and dog given to sitting close to, and staring into, a gas or electric fire, however, the condition may arise from drying of the surface of the cornea.

Front of the eye.—If the lids of a horse's eye be separated widely the 'white' of the eye comes into view. The white appearance is due to the sclerotic coat, composed of dense white fibrous tissue, shining through the translucent conjunctival covering. In the centre of the white is set the transparent oval 'cornea', through which the rays of light pass on their way to the inner parts of the eye. (In the pig, dog, and cat the cornea is practically circular in outline.) Behind the cornea lies the beautifully coloured 'iris', with a hole in its centre, the 'pupil', which looks black against the dark interior of the eye. The edge of the pupil is often irregular in outline, owing to the presence of 'nigroid bodies', the function of which is not well known. The shape of the pupil and the colour of the iris vary in each of the domesticated animals, and in individuals of the same or different breeds. In the horse and ox the pupil is roughly oval, or even egg-shaped, with the larger end inwards, and the colour of the iris is either a warm chocolate brown, greyish-blue, very dark or almost black, or else appears variegated with patches of white. In some horses, though rarely in cattle, there may be an absence of pigment matter in the iris, and the horse is then said to be 'wall-eyed' or 'ring-eyed'. In the pig, dog, and cat the pupil is rounded when fully dilated, but in the cat the contracted pupil (*e.g.* during the day or in a strong light) resolves itself into a vertical slit; the contracted pupil of the dog and pig is round. The colour of the iris in the smaller animals varies, but, generally speaking, it is some shade of brown, or dark blue, in the dog, greenish of greenish-grey in the pig, and a pale emerald green in most cats. In pure white cats it is occasionally some shade of pink, and such animals are of tenblind. Lying between the anterior surface of the eye, the cornea, and the iris, in a space known as the 'anterior chamber' of the eye, which is filled with a clear lymph-like fluid known as the 'aqueous humour', If one attempts to look straight in through the pupil of an animal's eye one sees nothing, because the light entering the eye is obstructed by one's head, just as in a camera, and only a very little enters at the sides. If, however, one holds a mirror in front of the eye into which one wishes to look, thereby reflecting a bright beam of light into the eye, and if one then looks from behind the mirror, or through a small hole in its centre, one sees the interior of the eye brightly lighted up. The ophthalmoscope is an instrument constructed upon this principle. By its help one sees the interior of the eye as a brilliant clean background, shaded in certain places to yellowish, and stippled over with brownish dots, while at one point is a pale rounded area, the end of the optic nerve, from the centre of which small reddish thread-like arteries and veins can be seen branching out over the surface of the back of the eyeball. The signs of various diseases of the eye can be diagnosed by the skilled expert noting alterations in the appearance of the picture presented through an ophthalmoscope, used in this way.

Coats of the eyeball.—The eyeball, as already mentioned, rests upon a pad of fat within the cavity of the orbit, where it is held in position partly by the action of the eyelids, and partly through the agency of seven ocular muscles and the optic nerve around which they are arranged. There are three layers forming the ball of the eye :

(*a*) **The sclerotic coat,** which is outermost, is composed of dense white fibrous tissue, which gives its appearance to the white of the eye in front. This coat completely encloses the ball, except for a small area through which emerges the optic nerve, while in front it is modified so as to form the transparent cornea. It maintains the shape of, and gives strength to, the ball of the eye. The cornea, which has a greater curvature than the rest of the ball, bulges out in front, and is formed of fibrous tissue arranged in layers so as to be quite transparent. In front of and behind these layers there are thin protective membranes, and both surfaces, back and front, are covered by a transparent layer of cells, so that the whole cornea is somewhat like a window let into the front of the sclerotic coat.

(*b*) **The choroid**, or vascular coat, lies within the sclerotic, and consists of three parts. The choroid membrane, which forms more than two-thirds of a lining to the sclerotic, consists mainly of a network of vessels which nourish the sclerotic coat and the interior of the eyeball. Its general colour is bluish-black, but an area a little above the level of the end of the optic nerve has a remarkable metallic lustre and is known as the ' tapetum '. The colour of the tapetum is variable, but generally it has a brilliant iridescent bluish-green colour shading almost imperceptibly into yellow. It was formerly thought that this area acted as a luminescent surface which enabled animals to see in the dark, but this is now known not to be the case. Its function is unknown. The choroid membrane is prolonged forwards into the ' ciliary body ', a very complex structure which forms a thickened ring opposite the line where the sclera merges into the cornea. To this line of junction the ciliary body is firmly attached by the ciliary muscle, which by its contraction and relaxation moves the ciliary body to and fro over the sclerotic, so as to allow the lens of the eye which is suspended from, or rather, ' set into ', the ciliary body, to alter its shape in such a way that it is able accurately to focus rays of light, coming from an object before the eye, on to the retina. The farthest forward part of the choroid coat is known as the ' iris ', and, as already stated, it may be seen lying in front of the lens and behind the cornea. The iris consists partly of fibrous tissue and partly of muscle fibres, arranged radially and circularly, with pigment cells interspaced throughout. These fibres by their contraction serve to narrow or dilate the pupil, according to whether the light entering the eye is strong or weak, and according as the animal looks at a near or distant object. The iris and ciliary muscle are powerfully acted upon by certain drugs ; thus, when atropine or belladonna is instilled into the eye or is taken internally, the pupil becomes widely dilated, while when eserine or pilocarpine is dropped into the eye the pupil becomes contracted almost to a pin-point. These actions are made use of in the treatment of diseases where there is a tendency towards adherence of the iris to surrounding structures.

(*c*) **The retina**, or nervous coat, is the innermost of the three coats of the eyeball. After the optic nerve has pierced the sclerotic and choroid coats, it ends by a sudden spreading out of its fibres in all directions to form the retina, which also contains some blood-vessels and pigment cells. The retina, in microscopic sections, is seen to consist of no less than ten layers. Of these, that outermost, *i.e.* nearest to the choroid, is composed of a layer of absorptive pigment cells which prevent the diffusion or reflection of light from one part of the inside of the eye to another. The layer next inside this is the very important layer of the rods and cones, by which rays of light are received, and from which sensations of light are conveyed by the optic nerve fibres to the brain, where they are registered in such a way that the animal becomes acquainted with what it is looking at. The rods are of a purple colour containing a substance known as the 'visual purple', which fades after a time when the eyes are subjected to a very strong light. They are excessively minute, being less than $\frac{1}{400}$th of an inch long and only about $\frac{1}{10,000}$th of an inch thick. The cones are still shorter, but they are slightly thicker. It is believed that the cones are the agents by which light sensations are perceived, but it is also possible that the rods play some part in this as well. Towards the bottom of the sphere of the eye, and slightly towards the inner aspect, there is the 'optic papilla', or 'blind spot'. Over it there are no rods or cones, and so light sensations are not appreciated. Owing to the fact that a startled horse which wishes to concentrate all its visual powers upon a particular object raises its head and brings the face almost horizontal in many cases, it is probable that an area of the retina, upon which the light may be focussed by this procedure, is specially sensitive and capable of more acute perception than the remainder of the retina. Microscopic examinations, however, reveal no difference in structure at any part of the retina which would account for this supposed area of clearer perception.

Contents of the eyeball.—A word or two descriptive of the contents of the eyeball, viz. aqueous humour, vitreous humour, and crystalline lens, is necessary. Occupying the space between the iris and the cornea, *i.e.* the anterior chamber of the eye, there is a clear watery, lymph-like fluid which serves to maintain the contours of the cornea. It is being constantly secreted and drained away, and eventually reaches the veins of the eye. Behind the iris lies the 'crystalline lens', which acts as does the lens of a camera, with the exception that it can alter the curves of its surfaces and therefore is able to change its refractive powers. It is composed of layers arranged like the leaves of an onion to some extent. The lens is held suspended by its capsule, which is attached to the ciliary body already mentioned. Behind the lens the cavity of the ball of the eye is filled with a viscid, jelly-like, tenacious fluid called the 'vitreous humour'. It maintains the intra-ocular pressure by which the eyeball retains its shape.

The lacrimal apparatus is an attachment whereby the eye surface is maintained free from dust and other foreign material. It consists of the lacrimal gland which secretes the clear fluid popularly known as 'tears'; excretory ducts, from 12 to 16 in number; and the two lacrimal ducts which open into a lacrimal sac from which begins the naso-lacrimal duct which carries the secretion down into the nose. The gland lies towards the upper outer aspect of the orbit, measuring about 2 inches long and 1 inch broad. It secretes the clear salty, watery fluid which flows out through the excretory ducts to reach the conjunctival sac and bathe the surface of the eye. The secretion is finally received by the two lacrimal ducts, the openings of which lie one in each eyelid about a third of an inch from the inner canthus. These open into the lacrimal sac, from which takes origin the long naso-lacrimal duct which conveys the secretion down into the lower part of the corresponding nasal passage, just within the nostril.

Accommodation.—All the rays of light proceeding from a distant object may be looked upon as being practically parallel, while those coming from a near object are divergent. The difference between *distant* and *near* in this connection can be taken as about 20 feet from the animal. A 'near' object can be seen anywhere between 20 feet and 4 to 5 inches from the eye, but nearer than this it loses its distinction. Parallel rays of light do not require any focussing on the retina other than is provided by the surface of the cornea, and when an animal looks at a distant object the lens capsule which is attached to the ciliary process retains the lens in a temporarily flattened condition and the ciliary muscle is relaxed, so that no great strain is put upon the eye. Rays of light from an object near at hand, however, which are divergent, require to be brought to a point of focus upon the retina, and as they pass through the lens their direction is changed on account of the convexity of the lens. The amount of this convexity is determined by the divergency of the rays, and is automatically provided for through the pull of the ciliary muscle upon the ciliary body. As the function of the muscle is to pull the ciliary body forwards, the tension upon the ligament of the lens is lessened and the capsule of the lens slackens, so that the lens, by its inherent elasticity, is allowed to bulge with a greater convexity upon its anterior surface. The greater the convexity, the more are the rays of light refracted, and the more convergent do rays which pass through it become. (*See also* VISION.)

EYE, INJURIES AND DISEASES OF

EYE, INJURIES AND DISEASES OF.—The delicacy of the eye renders it liable to a number of diseased conditions in animals, but the importance is only great in animals which must work, such as horses and dogs. A horse with defective vision, or even one that is quite blind, may be able to do good work in slow draught, but in one that is used for riding purposes or fast draught work on the roads it is a serious matter. Sporting dogs are practically useless unless they possess good vision, but the household pet, although it experiences great inconvenience, may live a long time after becoming quite blind. Cattle, sheep, and pigs may be blind without their usefulness being greatly diminished, either as breeding stock or as food producers, but with animals which must seek for their food in the open, blindness is something of a handicap. The subject of PERIODIC OPHTHALMIA is considered under that heading; while under VISION, DEFECTS OF, are considered astigmatism, emmetropia, hypermetropia, and myopia; others will be briefly mentioned here.

CONJUNCTIVITIS, or inflammation of the conjunctival membranes, is an extremely common condition among animals, and probably constitutes the commonest trouble to which the eyes are subject. As a rule it is not in itself a serious condition, but it may give rise to a number of very grave complications, such as ulceration of the cornea, which may be incurable and lead to loss of sight.

Causes.—A very large number of factors may give rise to conjunctivitis, among the commoner of which are injuries by external violence, such as blows, falls, or the presence of foreign bodies, infection with specific germs, such as in strangles, glanders, tuberculosis, etc.; and it may occur during the course of other diseases, such as sheep-pox, cattle plague, distemper, influenza, etc. The presence of dust, sand, pollen, seeds, lime, irritant gases, pieces of chaff or corn husks, in the atmosphere of a stable or field, is probably one of the commonest acuses in the larger farm animals, but such agents as flies, worms, and ticks, must also be noted in addition to the above. In any case, whatever be the exciting cause, the direct cause of the inflammation is the activity of the organisms which are already present upon the moist surface, or are blown on to it from the air.

In the cat two infections which cause conjunctivitis—*Hæmophilus parainfluenzæ* and *Moraxella lacunata*—are transmissible to man, in which illness may also be caused.

Symptoms.—The first signs of conjunctivitis are redness and swelling of the lining membranes of the eyelids, excessive discharge of tears, and a tendency on the part of the animal to keep its eyelids shut. A little later, perhaps within 12 hours, these symptoms become aggravated, and a discharge of serum, mucus, and later purulent material, is seen. The eye may be kept completely closed, or it may be slightly opened. The discharge blisters the skin of the face down which it trickles, and mats the hair together in this region. Generally, cases of conjunctivitis remain sporadic, but in certain circumstances they assume an enzoötic nature, attacking numbers of animals in a district, and spreading from the affected to the healthy.

Treatment.—It is essential in the first place to clean away the discharges by

EYE, INJURIES AND DISEASES OF

bathing in warm water to which a little baking soda (bicarbonate) has been added, and to search for any foreign body that may have lodged in the eye. The animal usually requires to be controlled, since it resents having the painful organ examined. After removal of the irritant body, if such exists, the eye should be irrigated with warm water. In many cases no further treatment is necessary, but if the infection is severe, with much discharge of pus, an antiseptic eye lotion will be required. The best ways to apply these solutions, whether to the horse, dog, or other animal, is to use a perfectly clean piece of cotton-wool soaked in the solution and squeezed above the eye so that the drops trickle into it. Cases of conjunctivitis should never be neglected, for what appears as a simple inflammation of the surface membranes often develops into the deeper-seated keratitis, which frequently leads to blindness.

BLEPHARITIS (βλέφαρα, eyelids) means inflammation of the edges of the eyelids, and usually accompanies conjunctivitis. Its causes, symptoms, and treatment are similar to those of that disease.

SCLEROTITIS, or 'blood-shot eye', is the name given to inflammation of the sclerotic coat of the eyeball. It often accompanies conjunctivitis when the latter is at all severe. It is treated as for conjunctivitis.

FOREIGN BODIES in the eye have been already referred to under CONJUNCTIVITIS, but they deserve some special consideration. The commonest objects which get into the eyes are the husks of oats, wheat chaff, hay-seeds, flies, eyelashes, and long hairs. For some reasons the eye of the dog seems able to accommodate itself to the presence of some of these, especially hairs; but if they gain entrance into the eyes of horses or cattle, inflammation and trouble result. For the first few hours pieces of chaff will move about with the movements of the eyelids made to dislodge them, but lymph soon begins to exude from the surface of the cornea, and the objects become fixed in the eye. The cause of this fixation is that the foreign body has become, as it were, glued to the surface of the cornea, and the eyelids move over it without shifting it. Pain is caused to the corneal surface and to the inner surface of the eyelid, for each of these surfaces is possessed of large numbers of sensory nerves. After a few hours more, round the edge of the foreign body will be seen a ring of whitish material, which is often referred to as a 'film' by the uninitiated, but which actually is simply a clotting of the lymph that has exuded or is still below the corneal conjunctiva. At this stage the animal keeps its eye half shut, tears are copiously produced and run down the face, and the membranes of the eye swell. It is about this stage that the condition is usually first seen, and that an attempt is made to remove the object. If, however, nothing is done, the condition becomes rapidly worse, until by the next day practically the whole of the cornea is a dull white, and the swelling has so increased that the eye is kept closed. Later still an acute inflammation spreads over the eye, suppuration may occur, the eyeball may burst, and in any case the sight is usually eventually destroyed, or a permanent white spot remains on the eye.

Treatment.—Occasionally the object may be removed by taking the corner of a clean handkerchief, winding it into a point, and lifting the offending body out with it. In other cases a little treacle or syrup may be smeared upon the finger, and the latter is brushed quickly across the eyeball when the animal has its eyelids open. These are, however, crude first-aid measures and it is always best to seek professional assistance and have the foreign body removed under a local anæsthetic by means of a camel-hair brush or special forceps. The use of a suitable eye-lotion will be helpful afterwards.

PROGRESSIVE RETINAL ATROPHY, or so-called 'Night Blindness', is a hereditary condition which was common in some strains of Irish Red Setter. The nervous elements of the retina undergo progressive atrophy and the animal suffers from impaired vision in consequence. To endeavour to correct this the pupil dilates widely, even in daylight, and the dog's expression becomes staring. At night or at dawn or dusk, the dog is unable to avoid objects and blunders into them, but during full daylight it appears to see quite well.

No treatment can arrest the progressive degeneration and the dog becomes steadily more and more blind. In severe cases puppies may show first symptoms soon after weaning, but it is more common for the disease to develop at 3 to 5 months of age.

The disease is definitely hereditary and neither dogs nor bitches which show the condition should be used for breeding. Breeds affected include Collies, Griffons,

EYE, INJURIES AND DISEASES OF

Poodles, Retrievers, Sealyhams, Cocker and English Springer Spaniels.

CORNEAL OPACITY, or KERATITIS, is a condition brought about in a large number of different ways, in which the surface of the cornea, instead of remaining transparent and translucent, becomes opaque through the coagulation of the lymph by which it received its nourishment. The cornea is not nourished by blood, for if it were, light could not pass through to the deeper parts of the eye, but it possesses large numbers of tiny spaces between the cells which compose it, in which flows clear lymph ; it is the coagulation, or clotting, of this lymph which leads to corneal opacity. Popularly the condition is often spoken of as 'a film over the eye', but really the film is *in the substance* of the cornea, rather than upon its surface.

Causes.—The cause of corneal opacity is, in every case, some inflammation of the cornea, *i.e.* keratitis.

Keratitis may be caused by injuries to the eye from external violence—kicks, blows, falls on to the side of the head, contact with objects in the dark, the lash of a whip, etc. ; from foreign bodies—pieces of chaff, seeds, pollen grains, thorns, grit, small stones, glass, etc. ; from burning with chemical substances—quicklime, acids, or irritant skin dressings which run into the eyes ; from burning with sparks (*see also page* 320) ; through the inflammatory processes of conjunctivitis spreading to the cornea ; it may arise during the course of certain diseases, such as distemper in dogs and influenza in horses ; it can be produced by the presence of round worms in the eyes, or by various kinds of flies ; chills, colds, or draughts may bring it about ; frost-bite is very frequently the cause of it in ewes on hills during severe weather, when it is called 'snow blindness' ; turning-in of the eyelids (*entropion*) may give rise to it ; and any severe disturbance which lowers the general bodily vitality may occasion it. In some cases it spreads from animal to animal, as may conjunctivitis, assuming a contagious nature, but as a rule it only affects single animals and does not spread.

Contagious ophthalmia ('Heather Blindness') in sheep begins as a conjunctivitis which is rapidly followed by a keratitis. The cause is *Rickettsia conjunctivæ*. *Moraxella* (*Hæmophilus*) *bovis* is responsible for a contagious keratitis in cattle often called 'New Forest Disease'. This is becoming more common—perhaps partly due to greater movement about the country of calves and store cattle.

Where trough space is too restricted, cattle may flick their ear-tips into the eyes of their neighbours, setting up a condition resembling contagious ophthalmia.

A verminous ophthalmia has been reported in the U.K. (*See Vet. Record* for Feb. 12, 1966.) The species of worm involved was stated to be probably *Thelazia gulosa*. Host : cattle.

Phenothiazine may set up keratitis in calves, especially if they are exposed to strong sunlight during the 24 hours after dosing. (*See also* HYPERKERATOSIS.)

Symptoms.—In the early stages, inflammation of the cornea results in symptoms very similar to those seen in conjunctivitis ; the production of tears, closing of the eyelids, pain and swelling, being noticed. When the eye is examined, however, the surface of the cornea is found to be duller than usual (although in the very early stages little change may be seen), the dullness varying from a mere haze to a dense bluish appearance, and the blood-vessels around the margins of the cornea are congested and the white of the eye appears 'blood-shot'. When severe there is always suppuration and a discharge of the pus. In the mornings the affected eye may be closed through the gumming effect of the pus upon the eyelids, expecially in cases which arise during distemper in the dog. When the surface of the cornea is examined it may be found to be quite smooth, or there may be the irregularities associated with an injury, or with ulcer. In some cases a small projection, varying from the size of a pin's head to that of a grain of wheat or slightly larger, may be seen apparently protruding from the surface of the cornea ; it is usually greyish in colour, or tinged with pink. In such cases the process of ulceration has destroyed the wall of the cornea, and the pressure of the contents of the eyeball has pressed outwards the delicate membrane which lines it on the inside. If this membrane becomes ruptured the aqueous humour escapes through the hole in the cornea, and the front of the eyeball collapses. Where a foreign body has caused the keratitis this will be seen when the eyelids are separated, or the place where it has lain will be obvious. When the dullness is a mere haze over the eye the term *nebula* is applied to the condition ; when there is an opaque, dense, white appearance, it is called *leucoma* ;

EYE, INJURIES AND DISEASES OF

when there is a black or dark-brown deposit in chronic cases in old dogs the condition is one of *melanotic keratitis*, and it is usually quite impossible to effect absorption and restore translucency. When the condition of inflammation spreads from the cornea and affects the whole of the structures of the eye, so that the organ is eventually completely destroyed, the term *panophthalmitis* is used. *Pannus* is a complication of keratitis in which blood-vessels bud out from the margins of the cornea and run in towards the centre of the eye, stopping at the edges of an ulcer if such exists. Pannus is a condition which always takes a long time to clear up, and even months after there may be seen a dullness of the cornea, due to the tiny vessels that still exist but are invisible to the naked eye.

Treatment.—In those cases where a foreign body has been the cause of the keratitis, it should be removed and the eye treated as already mentioned under ' Foreign Bodies ' in this section. Otherwise warm fomentation, or the application of warm compresses to the outside of the eye, should be first carried out to allay the pain. Any pus or discharge should be carefully removed by a piece of clean cotton-wool dipped in salt and water—a dessertspoonful to the pint. Thereafter the eye should be treated as given under ' Conjunctivitis ', in this section. Where ulceration occurs during a severe keratitis it is sometimes necessary to cauterise the surface of the ulcer before healing takes place. Skilled advice should be sought in good time, so that the diseased processes are not allowed to progress to a stage which is likely to be followed by serious consequences. Boracic and similar eye lotions are useless in treating Infectious Ophthalmia or ' Heather Blindness ', but chloramphenicol is of value. Ethidium bromide, used twice daily for 5 days, can save the sight, and is as effective as chloramphenicol in the disease of cattle.

IRITIS means inflammation of the iris, a condition which is very often associated with inflammation of the ciliary body, when the term *irido-cyclitis* is used. It is a common complication of specific ophthalmia of the horse, and it also sometimes occurs during distemper or influenza, or during high fevers ; it may arise during conjunctivitis or keratitis, when it is due to a spreading of the inflammatory reaction from the conjunctiva or cornea to the iris and its associated structures. The chief symptoms are dullness of the iris, congestion of the blood-vessels around its margin, a lessened response to varying intensities of light, and usually a firmly contracted pupil. Occasionally, especially during inflammation of the cornea, the iris adheres to this structure—a condition known as *anterior synechia* ; while more frequently the iris adheres to the lens, which lies behind it, and the condition is spoken of as *posterior synechia*. The aqueous humour is often cloudy and may appear purulent, little flocculi of lymph being seen floating in the anterior chamber or sticking to the posterior surface of the cornea. There is always great pain, fear of light (*photophobia*), and the animal hangs its head and is dull and listless.

Treatment.—Rest is essential for the diseased eye, and the animal should be placed in a darkened room or loose-box. A bandage may be applied over the eye when only one is affected, but it is unwise to blindfold both eyes in bilateral cases. Solutions of atropine, which paralyse the muscles of accommodation and give them rest and dilate the pupil, are dropped into the eye at intervals, and these are sometimes alternated with agents which contract the pupil, such as pilocarpine or eserine. The alternate contraction and dilatation serves to prevent adhesions between the iris and surrounding structures, which are the most common sequels of iritis. In addition to local treatment it is advisable to give a purgative and keep the bowels moving by laxatives afterwards, and to give general tonics.

GLAUCOMA is a condition the cause and pathology of which are obscure, in which the tension of the fluid contents of the eyeball is greatly in excess of the normal. It is associated with obstruction to the drainage system of the eye, in which fluid continues to be secreted but the excess is not removed. It may follow cases of progressive retinal atrophy. It eventually results in swelling and bulging of one or both of the eyes, and blindness results. It is sometimes treated by the operation of iridectomy, in which a portion of the iris is removed and the aqueous humour is drained away through an opening in the cornea. In other cases, extirpation of the eyeball has to be undertaken. (*See also under* EXOPHTHLAMOS.)

DISLOCATION OF THE LENS is a condition in which, probably on account of a hereditary disability, the crystalline lens becomes displaced forwards into the

EYE, INJURIES AND DISEASES OF

anterior chamber. It occurs in dogs, especially Sealyhams and Rough-haired terriers, and at first is very hard to recognise. The dog runs into stationary objects without any obvious reason. Casual examination of the eyes reveals no change and the condition may not be suspected for many months. Later, the owner becomes aware that sight is failing in the dog and careful examination reveals a peculiar change in the eye. Operation may do much to restore some degree of vision and save the eye, but neglect almost invariably results in the development of glaucoma (*see* GLAUCOMA) and the affected eye may have to be surgically removed.

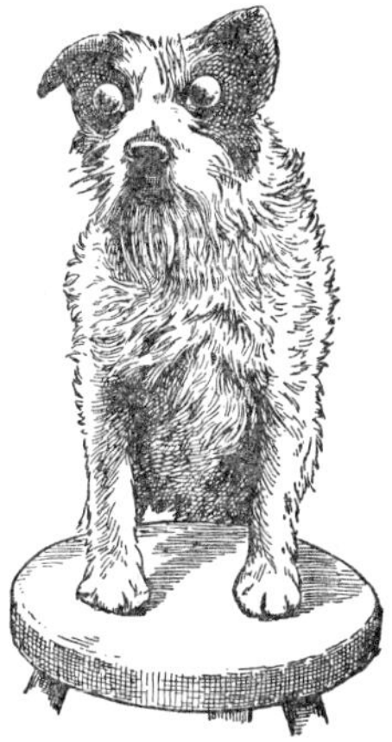

Drawing from a photograph of a dog suffering from glaucoma. The blank, unseeing but bulging eyes are characteristic of this condition.

EPIPHORA is another name for what is commonly called 'watery eye' or 'overflow of tears'. It is generally due to some obstruction to the drainage of tears through the lacrimal duct to the nose, but it is also an accompanying symptom of most forms of mild inflammation of the conjunctiva or cornea.

PTOSIS is an inability to raise the upper eyelid, usually associated with some general disease, such as distemper in dogs or 'grass sickness' in horses. It may also arise after injuries when the nerve supplying the muscles of the upper lid (3rd cranial nerve) is paralysed. (*See* GUTTURAL POUCH DIPHTHERIA.)

TRICHIASIS means turning-in of the eyelashes, and is very often brought about by chronic inflammation of the conjunctiva, although it may be hereditary. It is treated by removal of the lashes, and by an operation in which an elliptical piece of skin is removed from the outer surface of the eyelid, and the edges sutured together. This causes the lashes to turn outwards, where they will not irritate or inflame the cornea.

ENTROPION means turning-in of the eyelid, usually the lower, in such a way that the lashes irritate the cornea and often set up keratitis. It frequently follows inflammatory conditions of the eyelids or the cornea, and causes the animal great trouble. It also constitutes an inherited abnormality, occurring in 27 breeds of dogs. It is treated by a plastic operation such as is performed for trichiasis.

ECTROPION means a turning-out of one or both eyelids, so that the conjunctiva is exposed. It is a common condition in bloodhounds and St. Bernards, and is in them regarded as practically normal. It also is treated by operation, but a part of the conjunctiva from within the edge of the lid is removed instead of part of the skin from the outside, as in entropion.

RETENTION CYSTS are produced in the thickness of the eyelid owing to a small collection of pus in a tarsal gland, or more correctly, to a collection of tarsal secretion which has not made its escape. The swelling produced varies from the size of a barley-grain to a small hazel-nut. It is treated by excision.

STYE, or **HORDEOLUM,** is a condition in which a small amount of pus collects in the follicle around the root of one of the eyelashes. One after another may form in succession, owing to the spread of infective material from follicle to follicle.

HARDERIAN GLAND, DISPLACED.—In the dog this gland sometimes becomes enlarged and displaced, owing to blockage of its ducts or to a nearby swelling, when it becomes visible at the corner of the eye as a reddish lump. It may then require surgical removal.

DERMOID CYSTS are, strictly speaking, not 'cysts', but tumours, when they arise in connection with the eyes. They are usually found in the horse, ox, and dog, attached to the margin of the sclerotic where it joins the cornea, and from their free surfaces grow hairs of variable length. The dermoid is really a piece of skin which has become displaced during the formation of the embryo before birth. It gives rise to irritation, an excessive flow of tears, and may spread over the cornea so that it interferes with vision. It is removed under anæsthesia by careful dissection from the underlying corneal or sclerotic tissues.

WARTS occur in connection with the eyelids comparatively frequently in horses, cattle, and dogs, but they are less common in other animals. They sometimes become malignant, spreading at a rapid rate and causing interference with sight or the movements of the eyelids. Owing to the malformation which they may cause when numerous, warts should always be removed before they attain a large size or before they have time to spread.

TUMOURS, either of sarcomatous or carcinomatous nature, are sometimes found in connection with the conjunctiva, where they appear as red hard swellings, painless when small, but not when large. They often grow at a rapid rate, and may infiltrate the surrounding tissues, sometimes affecting the bones of the orbit. Cancer of the eye is a common condition in Hereford cattle. In Australia, Dr. D. J. Richards, B.V.Sc., has commented: 'It has been suggested that several factors may contribute to the development of cancer eye in cattle. These include age, irritation of the eyes by dust, sand, insects or chemicals, sunlight, lack of eyelid pigmentation and virus infection. Some authorities believe that cattle may be genetically prone to the condition, while others feel that poor nutrition is another factor as the condition appears to occur more frequently following a drought.' (*See* TUMOURS.)

CATARACT.—The condition is by far the most common in the horse and dog in old age, although it is also met with in other animals, and it may occur at almost any time of life. It actually consists of first a coagulation of the plasma of the cells in the lens followed by a degeneration and shrinking at the centre, hardening, and finally loss of transparency.

Causes.—Any condition which interferes with the nutrition of the lens, such as inflammation of the iris, pressure from tumours, glaucoma, etc., may give rise to a cataract, and it also occurs in connection with diabetes, with injuries to the eyes, such as severe blows, and with naphthalene and other forms of poisoning. Cataract must also be looked upon as a change characteristic of old age.

Symptoms.—In horses it is frequently between the ages of 18 and 24 years that it makes its appearance, and it gradually progresses until in from 1 to 2 years after its first appearance the horse is blind. At the outset there is nothing further than a faint bluishness or cloudiness to be seen, and the horse enjoys practically normal vision; but as time goes on the opacity becomes denser and the animal begins to make obvious mistakes. In dogs it may appear first at the age of 9 or 10 years, and its progress is usually more rapid.

Treatment.—In human beings an operation, in which the entire lens is removed or its capsule is scraped, is very frequently undertaken with considerable success. It necessitates the use of spectacles afterwards, however. In animals the same operation is sometimes performed, but the results are less encouraging. The animal cannot be provided with spectacles, and as the lens is the main focusing apparatus of the eye, the animal which has lost its lens is only able to appreciate objects with any accuracy at a certain fixed distance away from it.

BLINDNESS.—There are many causes of this, including disease of the retina, of the optic nerve, and of the brain. Blindness may be congenital or acquired, temporary or permanent. Vitamin A deficiency may be responsible, and also poisoning by rape and other plants, and by substances such as lead. (*See also under* QUININE.) Opacity of the cornea will, of course, prevent light rays reaching the retina, as happens in keratitis, so that partial or complete blindness results. Similarly, partial or complete blindness may result from a cataract. Other causes have been mentioned on the preceding pages, *e.g.* dislocation of the lens, glaucoma, etc. In cattle and sheep, cerebrocortical necrosis. In sheep, other causes of blindness include: infectious keratitis or contagious ophthalmia (' Heather Blindness '); pregnancy toxæmia; and possibly the effects of eating bracken, as described under BRIGHT BLINDNESS of sheep. (For an African disease *see* BLOUWILDEBEESOOG.)

In poultry, blindness may be the result of excessive ammonia fumes from deep litter, or it may be associated with fowl paralysis, salmonellosis, aspergillosis, etc. Cataract, followed in some cases by liquefaction of the lens, occurs during outbreaks of avian infectious encephalomyelitis.

TRACHOMA.—A term used in human medicine for a granular conjunctivitis, often followed by keratitis and pannus.

MYIASIS (*See* UITPEULOOG, a disease occurring in South Africa).

EYELIDS (*see under* EYE).

F

FACE FLIES.—These 'raven flies' (*Musca autumnalis*) plague beef and dairy cattle at pasture, feeding on watery secretions from nostrils and eyes. (*See* NANKOR.)

'FACIAL ECZEMA' is a synonym used overseas for light sensitisation in cattle and sheep. In New Zealand it is associated with the fungus *Stemphylium botryosum.* Ryegrass favours attachment of fungus spores; sweet vernal and clovers are antagonistic to the fungus. The mould *Pithomyces chartarum* has more recently been quoted as a cause and this has been found in the U.K.; *Sporidismium bakeri* is a synonym. (*See* SPORIDISMIN.)

FACIAL NERVE is the seventh of the cranial nerves, and supplies the muscles of expression of the face. It is totally a motor nerve. (For facial paralysis, *see under* GUTTURAL POUCH DIPHTHERIA.)

FACTORY CHIMNEYS.—Smoke from these may contaminate pastures and cause disease in grazing animals. (*See* FLUOROSIS, MOLYBDENUM.)

'FADING'.—The colloquial name for an illness of puppies, leading usually to their death within a few days of birth. Symptoms include: progressive weakness which soon makes suckling impossible; a falling body temperature; and 'paddling' movements. Infected puppies may be killed by their dams. One cause is canine virus hepatitis; another is a canine herpes virus; a third may be a blood incompatibility; a fourth, Bordetella; a fifth is hypothermia or 'chilling' in which the puppy's body temperature falls.
(*See also under* PUPPIES, HERPES.)

FÆCES (*fæx*, dregs) is another name for the evacuations from the bowels.

FAINTING FITS, or **SYNCOPE** (*συγκοπή*, fainting), means a sudden failure of the heart's action producing prostration and unconsciousness. It is generally due to cerebral anæmia occurring through weakened pulsation of the heart, sudden shock, or severe injury. It is most commonly seen in dogs and cats, especially when old, but cases have been seen in all animals. The horse sometimes falls to the ground when going uphill with a heavy load, but instead of lying unconscious it attempts to rise again in a minute or two. In such instances the fault is usually in the harness, either the throat-lash or more often the collar being too tight and interfering with the circulation to the head. A horse sometimes falls to the ground as though in a faint, due to diseased condition of the brain.

Ordinary fainting fits are treated by laying the animal flat out upon the ground, preferably with the head at a lower level than the rest of the body so that the blood may be assisted to the brain by gravity, by removing all harness or apparatus which may impede the circulation, and by douching cold water over the poll and face. The animal should be allowed to lie quiet for a time. Subsequently a course of tonics should be administered, and the animal rested.

FALCONS, DISEASES OF.—Avian pox has been found in imported peregrine falcons, giving rise to scab formation on feet and face and leading sometimes to blindness. Tuberculosis is not uncommon, and may be suspected when the bird loses weight. (A tuberculin test is practicable and worth carrying out, owing to the risk of infection being transmitted to other falcons and to people handling them.) Frounce and inflammation of the crop are two old names for a condition, caused by infestation with *Capillaria* worms, which can be successfully treated. Frounce causes a bird to refuse food, or to pick up pieces of meat and flick them away again, swallowing apparently being too painful; there is also a sticky, white discharge at the corners of the beak and in the mouth.

FALL-OUT, RADIO-ACTIVE (*see under* RADIO-ACTIVE FALL-OUT).

FALLOPIAN TUBES are tubes, one on each side, that run from the extremity of the horns of the uterus (or womb) to the region of the ovary, where they end in a funnel-shaped structure, which lies close to the corresponding ovary. The opening next to the ovary is large, but from there the tube narrows until at the attachment to the extremity of the horn of the uterus it only has the calibre of a hair. These tubes carry extruded ova from the ovary down to the uterus, where they meet the male germ cells.

FALSE MEMBRANE is the name given to the deposit which forms upon the walls of the air passages in calf-diphtheria, and upon the surface of the intestinal walls in some forms of enteritis, particularly that occurring in swine fever. It consists partly of fibrin derived from the blood, partly of the destroyed surface of the mucous membrane upon which it rests, and it contains large numbers of bacteria.

FALSE PREGNANCY (*see under* PSEUDO-PREGNANCY).

FAM.—A useful disinfectant approved for use in outbreaks of fowl pest, foot-and-mouth disease, and tuberculosis.

FARASE (from farcy) is the name given to a suspension of killed organisms of glanders in glycerine, which are subsequently dried and powdered and used for producing immunity in healthy horses. Good results have been obtained in some countries by this method, but it can only be recommended where the disease is rife. (*See* GLANDERS.)

FARCY and FARCY BUDS (*see* GLANDERS).

FARM CHEMICALS.—(For dangers of poisoning, *see under* SPRAYS USED ON CROPS, INSECTICIDES, FERTILISERS, WEED-KILLERS, RAT POISONS, POTATO HAULM, FISH POISONING, GAME BIRDS.)

FARROWING.—The act of parturition in the sow.

Farrowing quarters should be rigorously disinfected before the sow goes into them, and she should have been previously de-wormed and washed with a preparation to destroy lice or mange parasites. Otherwise, her litter of piglets will be infested by her parasites. Thiabendazole is recommended for worming. (*See* PIG, EXTERNAL PARASITES OF).

FARROWING CRATES.—The use of these is helpful in preventing overlying of piglets by the sow, and so in obviating one cause of piglet mortality; but they are far from ideal. Farrowing rails serve the same purpose but perhaps the best arrangement is the circular one which originated in New Zealand. (*See* ROUND HOUSE.)

Work at the University of Nebraska suggests that a round stall is better, because the conventional rectangular one does not allow the sow to obey her natural nesting instincts, and may give rise to stress, more stillbirths and agalactia.

FARROWING RATES.—In the sow, the farrowing rate after one natural service appears to be in the region of 86 per cent. Following a first artificial insemination, the farrowing rate appears to be appreciably lower, but at the Lyndhurst, Hants, A.I. Centre, a farrowing rate of about 83 per cent was obtained when only females which stood firmly to be mounted at insemination time were used. In 1966 the national (British) average farrowing rate was 65 per cent to a first insemination.

FASCIA is the name applied to sheets or bands of fibrous tissue which enclose and connect the muscles.

FASCIOLIASIS means infestation with liver flukes.

FASTING.—If food and water are withheld two results follow with great rapidity: the animal becomes thinner and lighter as it draws upon its reserves, and the temperature falls below normal. If food only is withheld and water supplied in large amounts, the process of using up the stored fat is much more thorough, the animal lives longer, becoming extremely emaciated before death, and the falling of the temperature is not so rapid as when no water is allowed. If the animal must withstand great cold or exposure, or if it must make continued muscular efforts during the period of fasting, it dies in a short while.

The fasting animal subsists first of all upon the fat that has been deposited in various parts of the body, *e.g.* in the abdominal or thoracic cavity, under the skin, between the layers of muscles in the limbs and trunk. After this store is exhausted the glandular organs supply enough food materials for the maintenance of life, losing in the process as much as 56 per cent of their previous bulk. Next, the skeletal muscles are drawn upon for their stored animal starch and then for the substance of their fibres. Finally, just before death, the blood begins to give up its food materials, and the percentages of its food products fall. The heart and the central nervous system show no very appreciable loss of weight, although the muscle of the heart undergoes an alteration in appearance.

Horses have been known to live for 3 weeks without food or water, and dogs for 4 weeks. With a supply of water but no food horses have survived for 30 days and dogs for 6 weeks. Carnivorous animals withstand fasting better than do herbivores, but sheep are an exception to this rule. It has been reported that in a case in Scotland 18 sheep were buried in the snow for 6 weeks and only one died, and in another case 7 sheep were buried for 8 weeks and 5 days; all were recovered alive, and eventually did well. In another case the writer knows of two newly born twin lambs which were buried by a fall of snow for 17 days, and when the thaw set in an ear was found sticking up above the snow at the back of a dyke, and the two little creatures were brought out alive and able to stagger for a few feet. They eventually recovered and did well. In this case they probably sucked at the snow and provided themselves with a certain amount of water, and they would be kept comparatively warm by the snow.

In many zoological parks it is customary to fast the carnivorous animals one day each week, and experience proves that this procedure is beneficial, especially to the large carnivores.

Fasting must also be mentioned in connection with medicines for the purpose of expelling worms. With certain of the more modern anthelmintics, however, fasting is not necessary; particularly is this the case with carbon tetrachloride in the horse, with sodium fluoride in the pig, and with arecoline hydrobromide in the dog.

FAT (*see* Adipose Tissue).

FAT SUPPLEMENTS in poultry rations can lead to Toxic Fat Disease (which see).

FATIGUE (*see* Exercise, Muscle, Nerves).

FATTY DEGENERATION is the name given to that condition in which globules of fat become deposited in the cells of a tissue. It is common in the liver, kidneys, heart, and in muscles which have sustained serious injury. In nerve trunks which have been divided fatty degeneration occurs beyond the line of section, *i.e.* distant from the nerve cells from which the fibres take origin. In many cases the cause of fatty degeneration is obscure, but it is known to follow mild inflammations, when it is usually preceded by a condition known as *cloudy swelling*, and it is also very often seen in organs from animals which have been affected with chronic tuberculosis and glanders. Certain poisonous substances, such as arsenic and phosphorus, and in birds tartar emetic, also bring about fatty degeneration when given for long periods in considerable doses. It is a common condition in old age, when it very often affects the heart and kidneys.

FATTY LIVER/KIDNEY SYNDROME OF CHICKENS.—The above name has been suggested for a condition in which excessive amounts of fat are present in the liver, kidneys, and myocardium. The liver is pale and swollen, with hæmorrhages sometimes present, and the kidneys vary from being slightly swollen and pale pink to being excessively enlarged and white.

Cause.—Unknown.

Symptoms.—A number of the more forward birds (usually 2 to 3 weeks old) suddenly show symptoms of paralysis. They lie down on their breasts with their heads stretched forward; others lie on their sides with their heads bent over their backs. Death occurs usually within a few hours. Mortality seldom exceeds 1 per cent. The best birds appear to be affected and the duration of an attack is short, usually lasting for only a few days. Birds that show symptoms usually die, but unaffected birds grow normally.

FAUCES (*fauces*) is the name given to the narrow opening which connects the mouth with the throat. It is bounded above by the soft palate, below by the base of the tongue, and the openings of the tonsils lie at either side.

FAVUS (*favus*, a honeycomb) is another name for 'honeycomb ringworm'. (*See* Ringworm.)

FEATHER EATING, or **FEATHER PULLING.**—This condition is recognised amongst poultry and in cage birds, particularly parrots. It is in many cases a vice and occurs from a variety of causes. It is often due to the irritation caused by lice or to the ravages of the depluming mite. In such cases the necessary anti-parasitic measures must be taken. It occurs in birds penned up, due to a lack of exercise and facilities for scratching, to keep them occupied. Errors in nutrition also play a part, a monotonous diet predisposing to this vice. Lack of adequate animal protein in the diet of young growing chicks, especially when kept under intensive conditions, may cause the vice. Once the birds start pulling the feathers they sooner or later draw blood, and an outbreak of cannibalism results. Treatment consists in isolating the culprit if it can be found at the beginning and feeding the birds a balanced diet containing green food. The addition of blood meal in the mash in many cases acts as a specific. The use of blue-glass in intensive houses has stopped the habit in some cases, but is not always effective. In dealing with cage birds, variation of the diet, salines in the drinking water, and keeping the birds in the dark for a time sometimes has the desired effect, but once the habit is confirmed it is very difficult to control. (*See also* CANNIBALISM, DE-BEAKING.)

FEATHERS, PROCESSED.—At packing stations it has become the practice to collect and process *together* feathers and poultry offal. In order to obtain feather protein in a form useful as food, such a high temperature has to be employed that the feeding value of the offal is destroyed. Accordingly, this material should not be sold as 'meat meal' or bought as an ingredient for rations on account of its alleged protein value.

FEBRIFUGES (*febris*, a fever; *fugo*, I drive away), or **ANTIPYRETICS**, are remedies employed to reduce temperature during fevers. Among the chief are antipyrine, aspirin, quinine, salol, and salicylate of soda. (*See under* each of these headings.)

FEED ADDITIVES.—(*See* ADDITIVES.)

FEEDING (*see* DIET).

FEEDING-STUFFS.—These must be stored separately from fertilisers, or contamination and subsequent poisoning may occur.

Poultry and rats and mice must not be allowed to contaminate feeding-stuffs, or SALMONELLOSIS may result in stock eating the food. If warfarin has been used, this may be contained in rodents' urine and lead to poisoning of stock through contamination of feeding-stuffs.

Unsterilised bone-meal is a potential source of salmonellosis and anthrax infections.

(*See also* ADDITIVES, CONCENTRATES, DIET, CUBES, SACKS, *and* LUBRICANTS.)

FELINE ENCEPHALOMYELITIS.—This has been reported in Sydney, Australia, and is characterised by non-fatal cases of hind-leg ataxia, and sometimes by side-to-side movements of head and neck. On *post-mortem* examination, demyelinating lesions and perivascular cuffing involving the brain and spinal cord were found. The cause is thought to be a virus, but efforts to transmit the disease failed.

FELINE ENTERITIS, SPECIFIC (INFECTIOUS FELINE ENTERITIS).—Also known in the U.S.A. as Panleucopenia or agranulocytosis. This is a highly contagious disease of cats, caused by a virus. Cats of all ages are susceptible. Survivors appear to acquire lifelong immunity, but the mortality is about 90 per cent.

Symptoms.—Loss of appetite, vomiting, intense depression, and prostration; the animal prefers to lie in cold places, cries out, and rapidly loses weight. The temperature, at first 105° F. or more, becomes subnormal in 12 to 18 hours, and death commonly occurs within 24 hours. The cat may pass no motions throughout its illness. In a few cases (which often recover) the tongue becomes ulcerated.

It seems that a mild form is common as many older cats have immunity without previous severe illness.

Diagnosis may be confirmed by laboratory means—examination of bone marrow and blood smears.

Prevention.—A vaccine is available.

Treatment consists in good nursing, normal saline and glucose given subcutaneously, and the use of penicillin and sulphapyridine. Penicillin has given good results. Chloramphenicol has also been used with success. If available, antiserum should be used. In a cattery, isolation of in-contact animals and rigid disinfection must be practised. (*See* also FELINE DISTEMPER; NURSING.)

FELINE HERPES VIRUS.—See FELINE VIRAL RHINO TRACHEITIS and INFLUENZA.

FELINE INFECTIOUS ANÆMIA.—This disease, caused by parasites of the genus Perythrozoon, has been reported in the U.K., U.S.A. and S. Africa. It is treated with antibiotics.

Infection with *Hæmobartonella felis* has been described in the U.S.A. in cats 1 to 3 years old, and successfully reproduced experimentally. It is believed that many adult cats carry the parasite and that the disease lies dormant until some debilitating condition lowers the cat's resistance. In Britain, the causal agent has been named *Eperythrozoon felis*.

The symptoms may include: fever, anæmia, loss of appetite, depression, weakness, and loss of weight. Anæmia may be severe enough to cause panting.

For diagnosis and staining techniques, see *Veterinary Record*, Sept. 12, 1970. Blood smears are essential, and must be repeated. The parasites are in blood only 10–15 days after infection.

FELINE INFECTIOUS PERITONITIS.—This disease was first described in the U.S.A. in 1966, and has been encountered also in the U.K. It is a slowly progressive and fatal disease of young cats, and sometimes of older ones also, caused by a virus.

Symptoms.—A poor appetite, gradual loss of weight, depression, weakness, and distension of the abdomen. There may be distressed breathing and, towards the end, jaundice.

Post-mortem findings.—The abdominal cavity contains fluid and its lining membrane is inflamed. Whitish flakes of fibrin may be present in the fluid, and the liver may show white spots.

FELINE INFLUENZA.—This name is loosely applied at present to respiratory infections involving more than one virus. It commonly occurs in cat-breeding and boarding establishments, and in cats which have been taken to a show; the infection(s) being highly contagious. Secondary bacterial invaders account for many of the symptoms. It was suggested by R. C. Povey, B.V.Sc. (*Veterinary Record*, 1969 **84** 335), that

'Cat flu' = Feline herpes virus infection (F.V.R.) and/or + Secondary bacteria
Feline picornavirus infection (F.P.I.)

Symptoms.—Sneezing and coughing. The temperature is usually high at first; the appetite is in abeyance; the animal is dull; the eyes are kept half-shut, or the eyelids may be closed altogether; from the nose there is a certain amount of discharge, thin at first and thicker and creamy later on; the condition is rapidly lost. If pneumonia supervenes the breathing becomes very rapid and great distress is apparent; exhaustion and prostration follow, and death usually takes place in from 3 to 6 or 7 days.

Treatment.—Isolation under the best possible hygienic conditions is immediately necessary in every case. There should be plenty of light and fresh air, and domesticated cats need to be kept fairly warm. A woollen or flannel coat or body bandage may be necessary in highly bred and delicate cats, and the use of thermogene on the chest will often ward off threatened pneumonia. Cats lend themselves very well to medicated inhalations of steam, and this form of treatment will be found very satisfactory in the simpler forms of the disease. Medicinal treatment is not to be advocated unless the symptoms warrant it. Cats are difficult animals to dose, except by skilled persons, and very often the struggles occasioned by attempts at administration of medicines do more harm than the medicines do good.

Often one of the sulpha drugs given twice daily in butter or small amounts of fish or meat, gives satisfactory results. Food should be light and easily digested; milk foods and invalid articles of diet, such as proprietary infant foods, etc., are good. Meat jellies, raw minced rabbit, liver, chicken, etc., in very small amounts, or these same substances stewed in milk, fish boiled in milk, will often be taken when all other food is refused.

After the acute symptoms have subsided cats need to be fed with care lest a relapse occurs. (*See* NURSING, HYDROLISED PROTEIN.)

Owing to the very highly contagious nature of feline 'flu, disinfection after recovery must be very thorough before other cats are admitted to the premises; and where death has occurred, at least 6 weeks should be allowed to elapse before a new cat is purchased. (*See* F.V.R. below.)

FELINE JUVENILE OSTEODYSTROPHY.—This is a disease, of nutritional origin, in the growing kitten. (It may occur, too, in young wild feline animals reared in captivity.)

Cause.—The disease has been reproduced by feeding a diet deficient in calcium and rich in phosphorus; *e.g.* kittens fed exclusively on a diet of minced beef or sheep heart have developed the disease within 8 weeks.

Symptoms.—The kitten becomes less playful and reluctant to jump down even from modest heights; it may become stranded when climbing curtains owing to be unable to disengage its claws; lameness, sometimes due to a greenstick fracture; pain in the back, making the kitten bad-tempered and sometimes unable to stand. In kittens which survive, deformity of the skeleton may be shown in later life, with bowing of long bones, fractures, prominence of the spine of the shoulder blade, and abnormalities which together suggest a shortening of the back.

FELINE PANLEUCOPÆNIA (*see under* FELINE ENTERITIS).

FELINE PICORNAVIRUS INFECTION.—A disease virtually indistinguishable from FELINE VIRAL RHINOTRACHEITIS.

FELINE VIRAL RHINOTRACHEITIS.—This disease was discovered in the U.S.A. and first recorded in Britain in 1966. Severe symptoms are usually confined to kittens of up to 6 months old. Sneezing, conjunctivitis with discharge, coughing and ulcerated tongue may be seen. Bronchopneumonia and chronic sinusitis are possible complications. Cause: a herpes virus.

FEMUR is the bone of the thigh, reaching from the hip-joint above to the stifle-joint below. It is the largest, strongest, and longest individual bone of the body, and at times has enormous strains passed through it, *e.g.* in the horse pulling a heavy load, or rearing or kicking. The bone lies at a slope of about 45 degrees to the horizontal in most animals when they are at rest, articulating at its upper end with the acetabulum of the pelvis, and at its lower end with the tibia. Just above the joint surface for the tibia is the patellar surface, upon which slides the patella, or 'knee-cap'. The femur is clothed with powerful muscles arranged practically all around, and is accordingly protected from blows and injuries. It is, however, very frequently fractured in dogs, especially when young, when they are run over by heavy vehicles. (*See* BONES.)

FERN-ROOT (*see* EXTRACT OF MALE FERN).

FERNS (*see* BRACKEN POISONING).

FERTILISATION (*see* REPRODUCTION).

FERTILISERS should not be stored near feeding-stuffs, as contamination of the latter, leading to poisoning, may occur. In Australia, 17 out of 50 Herefords died after gaining access to the remains of a fertiliser dump. A crust of superphosphate and ammonium sulphate had remained on the ground.

For the risk associated with unsterilised bone-meal, *see under* ANTHRAX and SALMONELLOSIS.

Hypomagnesæmia is frequently encountered in animals grazing pasture which has received a recent dressing with potash. (*See also* BASIC SLAG.)

FERTILITY (*see* CONCEPTION RATES FARROWING RATES, INFERTILITY).

FESCUE.—In New Zealand and the U.S.A. a severe hind-foot lameness of cattle has been attributed to the grazing of *Festuca aruníncea*, a coarse and unpalatable grass which grows on poorly drained land or on the banks of ditches, and being tall stands out above the snow. In typical cases, the left hind-foot is affected first, and becomes cold, the skin being dry and necrotic. Symptoms appear 10 to 14 days after the cattle go on to the Tall-Fescue-dominated pasture. Ergot may be present, but is not invariably so.

It was suggested in 1971 in Australia that 'fescue foot' may be associated with a potent toxin produced by the fungus *Fusarium tricinctum*.

FESTER (*see* ABSCESS, ULCER, SINUS).

FETLOCK-JOINT is the joint in the horse's limb between the metacarpus or metatarsus (cannon bones) and the first phalanx (long pastern bone). At the back of this joint are situated the sesamoids of the first phalanx. (*See* BONES.)

FEVER (*ferveo*, I burn) is one of the commonest symptoms of disease in general, and serves to make the distinction between *febrile* and *non-febrile* ailments.

Examples of *specific fevers*: equine influenza, distemper, braxy, black-quarter, or swine fever. (Note: 'Milk fever' of dairy cows is not a fever at all. *See* MILK FEVER.) Many of these diseases depend upon the growth of bacteria in the blood or tissues of the body, the toxins being formed as the result of the activity of these organisms. The amount of fever is estimated by the degrees of elevation of the temperature above the normal standard. When it reaches an excessively high stage, *e.g.* 107° F. in the horse or dog, the term *hyperpyrexia* (excessive fever) is applied, and it is regarded as indicating a condition of danger ; while if it exceeds 108° or 109° F. for any length of time, death almost always results. Occasionally, in certain fevers or febrile conditions, such as severe heat-stroke or tetanus, the temperature may reach as high as 112°. (*See also under* TEMPERATURE.)

Symptoms.—At the commencement of any ordinary fever there is usually a certain amount of shivering, to which the term 'rigor' is applied, but this is very often not noticed by the owner. It may exist only as a slight shivering fit in which the hair stands on end and the animal shakes itself and trembles, or it may be severe when the whole body is convulsed by violent tremors. The stage of rigors is followed by dullness, the animal standing about with a distressed expression or moving sluggishly. Later, perspiration, rapid breathing, a fast, full, bounding pulse, and a greater elevation of temperature are exhibited. Thirst is usually marked ; the appetite disappears ; the urine is scanty and of a high specific gravity ; the bowels are generally constipated, although diarrhœa may follow later ; intense injection of all the visible mucous membranes, *i.e.* those of the eyes, nostrils, mouth, vagina and rectum, occurs, their appearance in high fever being somewhat suggestive of beef-steak ; and general torpor and lassitude are marked. In horses the hoofs and the extremities of the ears, as well as the muzzle in many cases, are cold ; in cattle the horns and the ears are cold ; in dogs the muzzle is dry and often hot, while in fevers of considerable duration its surface may become fissured, and the skin may assume an irritable condition with considerable scurfiness ; in pigs there is often a rash present upon the skin over the sides of the body and along the belly, and perhaps behind the ears, the rash slightly resembling what is seen in swine erysipelas. These symptoms are common to most fevered conditions, whether specific or non-specific. (*See also* BILIARY FEVER, MALTA FEVER (*i.e.* Mediterranean fever), RED-WATER FEVER, SWAMP FEVER, SWINE FEVER, TEXAS FEVER, etc.)

Clinically, certain types of fever are recognised, such as *remittent fever*, in which there are short intermittent periods of fever with normal times between them ; *relapsing fever*, in which the chief characteristic is that after about a week's duration the fever comes to a *crisis* and the symptoms then recommence all over again.

The term *crisis* is applied when there is a sudden termination of the symptoms, often accompanied by some form of discharge from the body, such as the passage of large amounts of thick, heavy urine, copious evacuation of fluid fæces, or a profuse nasal discharge ; while *lysis* means that the fevered condition gradually subsides, getting less and less each day for a week or so, by the end of which it has disappeared.

Treatment.—The treatment of fever aims at reducing the high temperature, stimulating the action of the heart and nervous system, and placing the animal in surroundings where it will be comfortable and supplied with plenty of fresh air.

In practically all severe fevers from whatever cause, loss of water from the body occurs more rapidly than normal. This is particularly so when sweating is severe, but it also occurs from excessive respiration, panting or gasping, and from diarrhœa or the excessive passage of urine. In time the body tissues and later the blood-stream become seriously depleted of water and this must be replenished. Thirst is usually excessive, and contrary to former belief, it is now known that it is not dangerous to allow animals access to as much water as they will drink. Tissue fluid can also be replenished by giving normal saline by stomach tube and by subcutaneous or intravenous injection where, because of disease or injury, it may be inadvisable to fill the stomach. Best results are generally obtained when the normal saline solution is given at blood heat.

The great majority of febrile conditions are due to infection with bacteria or viruses, and where specific sera are available, the use of these will counteract or control the infection and the natural healing processes of the body will eliminate the fever soon afterwards. Similarly, the use of specific antibiotics, such as penicillin, streptomycin, or other compounds which attack the causal organisms is often the first step in controlling the fevered condition.

FIBRE, IMPORTANCE OF (*see under* DIET).

FIBRILLATION, or **FIBRILLARY TWITCHING**, means contraction of individual bundles of muscle fibres without relation to the whole. The condition is well seen in wounds which involve muscular areas of the body, immediately after infliction. The raw living muscles are seen quivering and twitching, but the muscle does not move as a whole. The term is also sometimes applied to the contractions of the auricles or ventricles of the heart, when, instead of a uniform wave of contraction spreading from the auricles downward to the apex of the heart, the muscle contracts in small irregular areas. This condition in the heart may be serious. In the mildest form it may cause only irregularity of the pulse, *e.g.* in racehorses which have made a supreme effort during a race, and it may pass off with rest and proper management. In more severe cases, when much or all of the auricular and ventricular muscle is affected, the heart may be unable to maintain the circulation of the blood through the body and death results. (*See also* CHOREA, TREMBLING.)

FIBRIN is a substance upon which depends the formation of blood-clots. It is produced immediately before the process of clotting starts by the union of thrombin with a substance called *fibrinogen*, that is found dissolved in the circulating blood, and takes the form of minute threads. When tissues are injured a substance called *thrombokinase* is liberated. This acts upon the *prothrombin* in the blood-stream to form the enzyme *thrombin*. Thrombin, so formed, acts upon fibrinogen circulating in the blood plasma to form the fibrin threads of the blood-clot. The process is an elaborate one depending upon the presence of calcium salts in the blood and for the formation of prothrombin, also upon the presence of vitamin K. Coagulation of the blood can be prevented by a variety of means, such as cooling of the blood to freezing-point, a deficiency of lime salts, or by the precipitation of these by the addition of certain chemicals, etc. After the threads have formed a close network through the blood, they contract and produce a dense felted mass in which are entangled the blood corpuscles. Fibrin is found not only in coagulated blood, but in lymph shed from its vessels, and consequently it is present in all inflammatory conditions within serous membranes like the pleura, pericardium, and peritoneum, and forms a coating upon the surface of these membranes. It is also found in inflamed joints, in the lung as the result of pneumonia, etc. Its deposition in the body may result in one of two things: it is either dissolved again by, and taken up into, the blood, or is 'organised' into fibrous tissue.

FIBROMA is a tumour consisting of fibrous tissue. (*See* TUMOURS.)

FIBROUS TISSUE is one of the most abundant tissues of the body, being found in quantity below the skin, around muscles and to a less extent between them, and forming tendons to a great extent; quantities are associated with bone when it is being calcified and afterwards, and fibrous tissue is always laid down where healing or inflammatory processes are at work. There are two varieties: white fibrous tissue and yellow elastic fibrous tissue.

White fibrous tissue consists of a substance called 'collagen' which yields gelatin on boiling, and is arranged in bundles of fibres between which lie flattened star-shaped cells. It is very unyielding and forms tendons and ligaments; it binds the bundles of muscle fibres together, is laid down during the repair of wounds, and forms the scars which result; it may form the basis of cartilage, and it has the property of contracting as time goes on and may cause puckering of the tissues around.

Yellow fibrous tissue is not so plentiful as the former. It consists of bundles of long yellow fibres, formed from a substance called 'elastin', and is very elastic. It is found in the walls of arteries, in certain ligaments which are elastic, and the bundles are present in some varieties of elastic cartilage. (*See* ADHESIONS, SCARS, WOUNDS.)

FIBULA is one of the bones of the hind-limb, running from the stifle to the hock. It appears to become less and less important in direct proportion as the number of the digits of the limb decreases. Thus in the horse and ox it is a very small and slim bone which does not take any part in the bearing of weight, while in the dog it is quite large, and, with the tibia, takes its share in supporting the weight of the body.

FILARIASIS (*filum*, a thread) is the name given to a group of diseases caused by the presence in the body of certain small thread-like Nematode worms, called filariæ, which are often found in the blood-stream. Biting insects act as vectors. (*See under* HEARTWORM for the Canine Filariasis, and EQUINE FILARIASIS.)

FILTERABLE.—As applied to viruses, this term is nowadays somewhat vague, since it does not imply any particular type of bacteriological filter (such as the Berkefeld). Pleuro-pneumonia organisms, spirochætes and vibrios may all be classified as filterable, in addition to viruses, for all pass through filters which hold back ordinary bacteria.

FILTERS (*see* BACTERIOLOGY, WATER SUPPLY, and also below).

FILTERS, BACTERIOLOGICAL.—These include the Berkefeld Filter—made from kieselguhr (a fossil diatomaceous earth)—having relatively large pores, and a Chamberland Filter which is made of unglazed porcelain, and allows only the smallest viruses to pass. (But *see* FILTERABLE.)

FINGER AND TOE is a term that is applied to two conditions, one affecting animals, and due to the presence of finger-like tumours in various parts of the body (*see* TUMOURS); the second is a disease of turnips, mangels, and other root crops, and is due to the fungus *Plasmodiophora brassicæ*. When roots which are badly affected with 'finger and toe' are fed to stock in quantity, they are liable to set up a simple indigestion, and have been blamed for the death of cows in certain cases.

FINNISH LANDRACE SHEEP have been imported into the U.K. for experimental and commercial breeding programmes. They are remarkable for very high prolificacy, triplets being common, and 4 or 5 lambs not rare.

FIRES, GAS OR ELECTRIC (*see under* EYE, *page* 320, for effect on cat or dog sitting *with eyes open* too close to fires).

FISH MEAL is largely used for feeding to pigs and poultry, although it is also added to the rations for dairy cows, calves, and other farm live-stock. It is composed of the dried and ground residue from fish, the edible portions of which are used for human consumption. The best variety is that made from 'white' fish—known in the trade as white fish meal. When prepared with a large admixture of herring or mackerel offal it is liable to have a strong odour, which may taint the flesh of pigs and the eggs of hens receiving it.

Fish meal is rich in protein, chlorine, calcium, phosphorus, and contains smaller amounts of iodine and other elements useful to animals. It contains a variable amount of oil. It forms a useful means of maintaining the amount of protein in the ration for all breeding females and for young animals during their period of active growth. From 3 to 10 per cent of the weight of food may consist of white fish meal. When pigs are being fattened for bacon and 'fattening-off' rations are fed, the amount of fish meal is reduced, and during the last 4 to 6 weeks it is customary to discontinue it entirely. Pigs may, however, continue to receive an amount of white fish meal up to one four-hundredth of their live weight without producing any recognisable taint in the flesh.

Many investigations have emphasised the very great economic value of fish meal for animals fed largely upon cereal by-products. It serves to correct the protein and mineral deficiencies of these and enable a balanced ration to be fed. It serves a very useful purpose by enabling more home-grown cereals to be fed and largely replaces protein-rich imported vegetable products. (*See also* ANIMAL PROTEIN FACTOR.)

FISH OILS.—Livestock owners should beware of feeding inferior fish oils, which often cause illness owing to their quickly becoming rancid, in place of good quality cod-liver oil. (*See* RANCIDITY.)

FISH, POISONING OF.—This may occur through liquor from silage clamps seeping into streams, etc. The following, in very small concentrations, are lethal to fish: DDT, Derris, BHC (Gammexane), Aldrin, Dieldrin, TEPP, Toxaphene, Heptachlor. Many agricultural sprays may, therefore, kill fish; and likewise snail-killers used in fluke control.

FISH SOLUBLES.—Concentrated and purified stickwater, the liquid which is pressed out of fish during oil-extraction and meal-making processes. Fish solubles vary in quality but the best contain four times more vitamin B_{12} than ordinary fish-meal, and also the Animal Protein Factor. They are for this reason a valuable supplement to pig and poultry rations. (*See also* ANIMAL PROTEIN FACTOR.)

FISTULA (*fistula*, a pipe) is an unnatural narrow channel leading from some natural cavity, such as a duct of the mammary gland, or the interior of the bowels, to the surface. Or it may be a communication between two such cavities, where none should normally exist, as, for example, a direct communication between the bladder and the bowel as the result of damage sustained during difficult parturition.

Causes.—Occasionally a young animal is born with a fistula; such as in the case of pervious urachus, where there is an opening between the urinary bladder and the outside through the umbilicus, from which urine trickles, or in fistulous thyroid in puppies, where there is a communication between the surface of the skin and the thyroid gland. But fistulæ much more frequently result from accidents in which the patency of a duct is compromised, and the secretion eventually bursts out through the side of the canal; it is in this way that salivary fistulæ, and anal fistulæ in dogs, are formed. Direct injury, in which the wall of the tube or the substance of a gland is involved, is also a very common cause of the condition. In cows, treads by neighbours, tears by thorns or barbed wire, bites or other injury to the teats, frequently cause laceration and tearing, and milk escapes from a fistula in the side of the teat thereafter. Ulcerating diseases of the bowels sometimes causes fistulæ between the two adjacent or superimposed parts of the gut, or between the cavity of one part of the intestine and the surface of the body. In these cases an abscess forms in one part of the bowel wall and on bursting opens up a communication between the cavity of the bowel on the one hand and the skin surface, through the abdominal wall, on the other. In anal fistula, the abscess primarily forms in the small scent gland that lies just within the anal ring of the dog. In certain cases a dog or cat may swallow a small fish-bone or a pin, and this becomes lodged in the throat. Owing to the movements of swallowing, the point of the object sometimes penetrates through the wall of the pharynx or œsophagus to the outside, and a fistula results. In a similar manner a large pin or a needle may cause a fistula in connection with the stomach or intestine. In dental fistula, which occurs in cats and dogs most commonly, but is also seen in the horse, an abscess develops at the root of a molar tooth, and the pus burrows upwards and bursts through the skin on to the surface of the face.

Treatment.—As a rule a fistula is extremely hard to close, especially if it has persisted for some time. The treatment consists in an operation to restore the natural channel, be it salivary duct, bowel, bladder, or teat canal.

FISTULOUS WITHERS is the name given to that condition in which a sinus develops in connection with the withers of the horse. It is generally due to an external injury which has become infected with bacteria, when, on account of the poor blood-supply, local necrosis (death) of the ligaments above the vertebræ, or of the summits of the spinous processes, with suppuration, sets in. The causes are very varied, and range from injuries which result from passing below the lower branches of trees in pastures, to such abrasions as are caused by a badly fitting collar, blows from sticks, bites from other horses, etc. Organisms identical with those causing abortion in cows—*Brucella abortus*—are often found, and numerous pus-forming organisms can generally be identified. In other cases, filarial worms have been found embedded in the ligament, and are responsible for those cases which arise without any previous history of injury to this part of the body.

Symptoms.—At first there is noticed pain and swelling over the withers, perhaps more obvious on one side than the other, and working horses resent the application of the collar, or show a lessened inclination for work. Later on the swelling usually bursts, but it may appear to subside in a few cases. The openings which are left when the purulent material is discharged may heal over in time, but other swellings form and burst as before. In many cases one or two openings remain permanent and a thin stream of sanious pus is constantly discharged. This runs down over the shoulders and scalds the skin, causing the hair to fall off. As a rule there is not a great deal of pain so long as the sinus remains open, and the horse is not usually affected to any great extent in his general health. In very severe forms the pus may burrow downwards below the shoulder-blade and lie in a pocket at or near the level of the elbow; or it may burrow under the skin on the outside of the shoulder muscles and form a bulging pocket on the outside of the shoulder.

Treatment.—Fistulous withers is always

a serious condition which should be treated by a skilled surgeon before great and perhaps irreparable damage has been done to the tissues involved. Old-standing cases are notoriously difficult to treat, and many have to be destroyed.

The application of poultices and blisters to the outside is absolutely useless. Penicillin has not proved very efficacious; better results may follow the use of the sulpha drugs. 'S.19' vaccine is useful. Otherwise, it is necessary to have the horse operated upon and all the diseased tissues—fibrous tissue, ligament, cartilage, and even bone—removed through large openings, which will provide good drainage and allow antiseptics to reach the depths of the cavities made. The treatment generally takes from two weeks (in very slight cases) to as long as three months or more, where the sinuses are deep and bone is involved, and cases are always better if they can be sent to a veterinary hospital for treatment.

FITS is another name for convulsive seizures accompanied usually by at least a few seconds of unconsciousness. Dr. Phyllis Croft, Ph.D., M.A., F.R.C.V.S. has commented: 'Typically, the dog is relaxed or even asleep at the time when the fit occurs, and the first phase consists of a tonic spasm of voluntary muscle with arrest of respiration; this lasts 30 to 40 seconds and is succeeded by clonic contractions of limb muscles ("galloping"). After this the dog usually appears to be exhausted for a period varying from a few seconds to a few minutes, with a gasping form of respiration. Some dogs then get up and appear normal almost immediately, while others wander restlessly for half an hour or more, bump into furniture and eat greedily if they find any food. The pattern of the fit is reasonably consistent in any one dog, but varies considerably from one dog to another. In between these fits, the dog appears to be entirely normal.'

Fits may be associated with epilepsy—the most common cause in adult dogs. They may occur during the course of a generalised illness such as canine distemper or rabies; may follow a head injury; be associated with a brain tumour; or follow some types of poisoning. In puppies, hydrocephalus is a cause of fits. (*See* CONVULSIONS, EPILEPSY, HYSTERIA.)

FITZWYGRAM SHOE is a horseshoe in which the toe is rolled on the foot surface and lifted from bearing on the ground, The branches are made from iron which is triangular in cross-section, being markedly concaved so that even the nail-holes have to be stamped through the concaving. The actual ground surface is a mere rim in the unworn shoe. These shoes were sometimes used for horses which were given to stumbling through shuffling their feet forwards an inch or two before they come to rest on the ground. They are not commonly used nowadays.

FLAGELLA.—Whip-like processes possessed by certain bacteria and protozoan parasites and used for purposes of movement.

'FLAT PUP' SYNDROME.—A condition in which puppies can, at two to three weeks, use their front legs normally, but the hind legs are splayed out sideways.

FLATULENCE (*flatus*, a blowing) means a collection of gas in the stomach or bowels. In the former, which is only seen to any extent in cattle and sheep, the gas is expelled from time to time in noisy eructations from the mouth; in the latter case it may produce unpleasant rumblings in the bowels and be expelled from the anus. Gas in the alimentary canal in large amounts is always due to bacterial fermentation. (In the rumen of cattle, sheep, and goats, much gas is formed during normal digestion, the excess being evacuated through the mouth in these animals.)

FLAVINE COMPOUNDS, among which are acriflavine, euflavine, and proflavine, are derivatives of aniline. Acriflavine, the hydrochloride of diamino-methyl-acridinium, is an orange-red crystalline powder, soluble in water and forming a powerful antiseptic solution in strengths of 1 in 1000. It stains horn and skin tissues bright yellow, but does not stain dead or diseased tissue in a wounded area. It is of use in operations on horses' feet to indicate healthy and diseased tissue, but its chief use is as an antiseptic solution to control bacterial infection and stimulate healing in open wounds. It can also be used as a douche for the mouth and throat and for vagina, udder, and uterus, when weaker strengths (*e.g.* 1 in 10,000 or 15,000) are used.

FLAVOMYCIN.—A feed antibiotic. (*See* ADDITIVES.)

FLEAS are members of the Order *Siphonaptera*, and are degenerate forms of two-winged insects. They infest the dog and cat primarily, and other animals to a less extent.

Dogs in Britain may harbour the flea-borne tapeworm (*Dipylidium caninum*) and the rabbit-borne tapeworm (*Tænia pisiformis*). Cats are subject to the mouse-borne tapeworm (*Hydatigera tæniæformis*). (*See* PARASITES AND PARASITOLOGY, *also* ECZEMA, DICHLORVOS, DERRIS, BHC.)

FLEXION (*flecto*, I bend) means bending, and is a term applied either to the bending of joints or to an abnormal shape of internal organs. It is the opposite of 'extension', which means straightening or stretching of a part.

FLIES are mostly, but not exclusively, members of the Order *Diptera*—the two-winged flies. Those of importance to the owners of animals are the following: Mosquitoes, Gad flies, Clegg flies, House flies, Stable flies, Blow flies of various varieties, Screw-worm flies, Flesh flies, Horn flies, Tsetse flies, Bot flies, Nostril flies, Warble flies, Macaw worm flies, New Forest flies, and the Sheep ked. (*See* PARASITES AND PARASITOLOGY, p. 668; FLY CONTROL, and INSECTICIDES.)

FLOOR FEEDING OF PIGS.—This practice is attractive to the pig farmer since it saves the cost of troughs and also saves space; the normal feeding passage becoming a catwalk over the pigs' sleeping quarters.

From a health point of view, the precise composition of the concrete floor may prove important. In an outbreak of illness among pigs in Eire, with anæmia, gastric ulceration, and hæmorrhage, the cause was thought to be the 'pit sand' (with a high iron content) with which the concrete was made, giving rise to iron poisoning once the surface layer had been licked off.

More important is the fact that loss of appetite in pigs—a common symptom of many diseases—may not be noticed. With trough-feeding, it is easy to see which pigs are uninterested in food.

Feeding pellets instead of meal may also cause trouble—digestive upsets. The method may involve more stress than conventional systems.

FLOOR SPACE.—As a rough guide, the following *minimum* figures may be given: bacon pig, 6 square feet; veal calf, 12 square feet; laying hen on deep litter, 2½ square feet.

FLOUR (*see* AGENE PROCESS).

FLUCTUATION (*fluctus*, a wave) is a sign obtained from collections of fluid by laying the fingers of one hand on one side of a swelling and tapping the opposite side with the fingers of the other hand. The thrill or impulse which is set up is communicated through the fluid to the second hand and establishes the presence of fluid in the part. It is a useful way of determining the presence of fluid in ascites (dropsy of the abdomen), in a tendon sheath, or in a joint cavity.

FLUID REPLACEMENT THERAPY (*see under* DEHYDRATION).

FLUKES and FLUKE DISEASE (*see* LIVER FLUKES and PARASITES, p. 645).

FLUORESCIN is a useful diagnostic agent in injuries and ulcers on the cornea of the eye. A weak solution is dropped into the eye and the injured area can be seen clearly demarcated from the surrounding healthy cornea.

FLUORESCENT (*see under* TETRACYCLINES which make bone fluoresce, and *under* WOOD'S LAMP which shows ringworm-affected hairs fluorescing). For the fluorescent antibody test, *see under* RABIES *and* IMMUNOFLUORESCENT MICROSCOPY.

FLUORINE.—The presence of this element in a concentration of about one-half part per million in drinking water is claimed to be beneficial to children under 10 drinking it; the incidence of dental caries thereby diminishing to a slight extent. In compulsory fluoridation of public water supplies, 1 p.p.m. of sodium fluoride is used. This is a costly and wasteful practice, and may harm farm livestock if the latter have other sources of fluorides. Excess of fluorine causes mottling of the teeth. (For fluorine poisoning, *see* FLUOROSIS.)

FLUOROACETATE POISONING.—Sodium mono-fluoroacetate ('1080') is used to kill rats and mice, and it is in this connection that poisoning in domestic animals and man may arise. The drug causes distress, yelping, sometimes vomiting, and convulsions in the dog. Treatment consists in the administration of nembutal. The dose of '1080' which was found to kill one dog in two was 0·066 mg. per kg.

In 1963, two outbreaks of fatal poisoning involving numerous dogs, cats, cattle and a pony were attributed to the agricultural insecticide fluoroacetamide.

FLUOROSIS or chronic fluorine poisoning is of economic importance in cattle, sheep, etc., grazing pastures contaminated by fluorine compounds emanating from iron and steel works and other industrial plant. It has also been reported in dairy cattle receiving two mineral supplements with a high fluorine content.

Symptoms.—There is severe lameness, and a resulting loss of condition; milk yield is greatly reduced. The teeth may become mottled, and the bones become particularly liable to fracture. Cows may stand with their legs crossed.

Antidote.—Calcium aluminate is of some *limited* value as an antidote to fluorine poisoning.

FLUOTHANE.—A volatile anæsthetic, which has been used with success in dogs, cats, and laboratory animals; and to a less extent, in horses and cattle. 'It is a potent respiratory depressant. One of the more important properties is its effect on the vasomotor centre, which is markedly depressed, causing a degree of hypotension. This fact is of considerable importance in that the lowered blood pressure may help to prevent shock. Fluothane should therefore not be used in conjunction with other hypotensive drugs (*e.g.* chlorpromazine).' (J. R. Campbell and D. D. Lawson.)

FLUSHING OF EWES is the term applied to the process of inducing a condition of rising metabolism in breeding ewes some 6 to 3 weeks before service, by putting them on to protein-rich foodstuff. The practical effect of this is to intensify subsequent heat or œstrus and thereby ensure that each ewe is in fit condition to breed.

There is a wide choice of food-stuffs, each of which may be used to 'flush' ewes. Some prefer split or kibbled beans or peas and crushed oats; others use linseed or earthnut cake; crushed oats and linseed meal is used in some flocks where ram-lamb production is the main object; in other parts, sheep-owners prefer to graze a green legume crop such as tares, lucerne, or red clover.

Very good results have followed the addition of blood and bone-meal to a mixture of crushed oats, flaked maize, and hay chaff, and on physiological grounds some such additions as these are logically necessary to supply the maximum stimulation to the generative organs.

In some recent experiments, doubt has been cast on the efficacy of flushing.

FLY CONTROL MEASURES.—These include dipping, spraying, and in the tropics the use of simple fly traps (*e.g.* a water-filled gulley around manure heaps into which maggots fall and are drowned). Inside buildings, such as cowsheds and dairies where the spraying of insecticides is not always desirable, other methods may be preferable. Blue glass roof windows are said to help, and flies are said to be much less numerous near ultra-violet emitters used in buildings for inhibiting the multiplication of bacteria and fungi. Electric fly traps have been used with success, mainly in North America. An automatic sprayer, operated by a photo-electric cell, has been successfully used at Pennsylvania State University, both on range and in cowshed doorways. The release of sterile male flies from aircraft has been used on a large scale in the U.S.A. in an attempt to control the screw-worm fly. A suitable insecticide may be used on cattle. (*See* NANKOR.) (*See also* INSECTICIDES.) A method of fly control which has proved successful in Denmark is the application to walls of a varnish containing a phosphorous insecticide together with a sweet bait. Three to five applications are necessary each season. No accidental poisoning of farm live-stock whatever has been reported in Denmark, and official approval has been given for the method. It is, of course, wise to use it on surfaces out of reach of domestic animals. The varnish, called Tugon, is now on the market in Britain (*see* DDT).

FOALING (*see* PARTURITION).

FOALS are young horses of either sex until the time they are one year old. Male foals are known as 'colt foals', and female foals are called 'filly foals'. Most foals are born between March and June in Britain, although quite a number (especially thoroughbreds) are dropped earlier than this. Thoroughbreds are conventionally aged as from 1st January of the year in which they are born, and all other horses from the 1st May, irrespective of whether they were actually foaled before or after these dates.

Generally speaking, foals run with their dams at grass during the summer, and are weaned at from 4 to 6 months of age. With weakly foals, however, and in the case of highly bred pedigree animals, it is not uncommon to allow them to run with their dams until nearly Christmas-time, so that they may get an exceptionally good start in life.

As a rule, foals will begin to eat grass when they are between three weeks and a month old, although some start earlier and some later than this. At about 6 weeks to 2½ months they will begin to eat dry corn from mangers along with their mothers.

FOALS, DISEASES OF.—Of the lesser ailments constipation and diarrhœa are important.

Constipation is due to a number of different causes, such as failure of action of the colostrum in very young foals, errors of diet in foal or dam, high fever, and indigestion. It appears dull and drowsy, sucks in a half-hearted manner or not at all, and frequently stands with the tail lifted endeavouring to pass fæces. If neglected, death may result. Some gentle laxative, such as 3 to 4 ounces of castor oil, or 6 to 8 ounces of medicinal paraffin, should be given in a pint of warm newly drawn mare's milk, and an enema of warm soapy water with a small amount of glycerine added should be administered with an ordinary rubber enema syringe.

Diarrhœa.—The foal frequently suffers from a condition similar to, though less dangerous than, white scours in calves. It often appears when the foal is about 9 days old ; a transient diarrhœa continuing during the second week of life. A single dose of castor oil may be given in an attempt to check the trouble. In persistent cases advantage is taken by veterinary surgeons of the sulpha drugs. (*See* Paratyphoid, etc., below.)

Simple diarrhœa may also occur as a result of changes in the mare's milk, due to metritis or laminitis, for example ; or as a result of the dam grazing avidly upon rich spring grass, etc.

In other instances, acidity of the mare's milk, due to eating unwholesome foodstuffs, causes diarrhœa in the foal. In fevers such as mastitis or laminitis, and even more so in acute inflammation of the uterus (metritis), the same thing occurs.

Paratyphoid.—This is more serious than simple diarrhœa. It is caused by *salmonella* germs, which cause food-poisoning in man and are excreted by infected rats and mice. The attack may be comparatively mild or very severe, ending in death. Symptoms include : loss of appetite, fever, thirst, restlessness, severe straining, and prostration. In fatal cases, death is usually preceded by 4 to 6 days' illness. Prevention of paratyphoid—energetic measures to keep down rats and mice in the vicinity of stables—is easier than treatment.

Hernia, which is frequently referred to as ' rupture ', is not uncommon in foals, especially if there was some difficulty during foaling. Part of the muscular abdominal wall ruptures and allows bowel or omentum to protrude outside the cavity. The skin remains intact, but there is a prominent swelling, either around the navel or in the inguinal region. (*See* Hernia.)

Hæmolytic Disease.—This results from an incompatability between the blood of sire and dam, and the consequent production of antibodies which reach the foal in the colostrum and break down the foal's red blood corpuscles. These become so reduced in number that not only is there jaundice but often also a fatal anæmia. If trouble from this cause were anticipated, the use of a foster-mother might save the situation but, obviously, this is seldom practicable. Moreover, unless the mare has previously had a ' jaundiced foal ', there will be no inkling of what is in store. If she has, however, it is possible to test her blood against the sire's during pregnancy and obtain a fairly good idea as to their incompatibility or otherwise. Treatment must be undertaken quickly and consists in exchange transfusion—the removal of up to 5 pints of the foal's blood and the simultaneous injection of up to 6 pints of a compatible donor's blood, previously bottled. The transfusion requires special apparatus and takes about 3 hours to complete. Recoveries following this treatment have been spectacular.

Worms.—Both strongyles (red worms) and ascarids may cause trouble in foals. The former give rise to malaise, cough, unthriftiness, tiredness, and sometimes abdominal pain ; the latter to diarrhœa and intermittent colic, among other symptoms. Phenothiazine and thiabendazole are effective against strongyles ; sodium fluoride against ascarids. The

Animal Health Trust recommends that foals be dosed every 4 weeks, alternately for ascarids and strongyles, until the age of 1 year.

NAVEL-ILL and JOINT-ILL.—These are popular and rather vague terms used to describe a form of 'blood-poisoning' which may be generalised, or be localised with involvement of joints, tendon sheaths, kidneys, navel, and other parts. So far, three germs have been shown to be involved: *B. coli*, *streptococci*, and *B. viscosum equi*. Symptoms vary and may include diarrhœa. The streptococcal form shows itself when the foal is about 10 to 14 days old; rarely at, or shortly after, birth. The young animal is obviously ill, with fever, weakness, swelling and pain at the navel itself, and usually enlargement of the hock and stifle joints. In many cases, indeed, the condition is first suspected on account of the swollen joints; involvement of the navel not being obvious until later. Urination is frequent. There is a severe loss of condition which may be followed by death after an illness lasting as much as 2 or 3 weeks. *Streptococci* also produce, not infrequently, a subacute or chronic infection of the joints, with little evidence of general illness. While death does not, as a rule, occur, recovery is not always complete; some of the damage to tendons or joints remains.

SLEEPY FOAL DISEASE is the name often given to the illness produced by *B. viscosum equi*. It occurs within the first three days after birth, as a rule; and often a healthy-looking new-born foal is dead within 12 hours. Sudden onset, extreme prostration, and early death are characteristic of this illness, which is also a septicæmia. The few affected foals which survive more than a week often show inflammation of the joints and tendons, with abscesses involving muscles. At one time it was thought that 'navel-ill' was invariably the result of germs gaining entry through the stump of the navel cord after birth, but these infections occur in stables where the standard of hygiene is of the highest, and it appears that some mares may transmit the infection to their offspring. Precautions include dressing the navel-cord with tincture of iodine or other suitable antiseptic, washing the mare's hind parts after the afterbirth has come away, and transferring her and her foal to another loose-box, avoiding breeding from suspected carriers. Treatment: the sulpha drugs and antiserum are of service when the infection is a streptococcal one; against *B. viscosum equi* antiserum or streptomycin may be tried. Professional services should be obtained early.

PNEUMONIA, due to *Corynebacterium equi*, is common in the United Kingdom. Treatment is difficult; control involves attention to hygiene and to the mares, some of which may be carriers.

SALMONELLOSIS has been responsible for cases of septicæmia in young horses in Britain. The organism involved is *Salmonella typhimurium*. (*See also* SALMONELLOSIS.)

STREPTOCOCCAL SEPTICÆMIA is nearly always caused by beta-hæmolytic streptococci.

PERVIOUS URACHUS, or 'leaking at the navel', is a condition in which the communication between the urinary bladder and the umbilicus or navel outside, which should close at the time of birth, remains patent and allows urine to dribble from it. The urine blisters the skin around, becomes decomposed and gives rise to a foul odour, and ultimately results in considerable swelling and suppuration around the navel. It should be treated by operation as soon as it is noticed, and kept clean by the application of antiseptics. (*See also under* 'BARKERS'.)

FODDER BEET (*see* FODDER POISONING, p. 736).

FŒTAL RESORPTION.—In a pregnant animal, illness may result in the fœtus being absorbed, so that at full term only a tarry fluid may be passed. This condition occurs, for example, in cows and bitches; and in sows which had Aujeszky's disease.

FŒTUS (*fœtus*) is the name given to the young animal while it is still in the uterus. (*See* EMBRYOLOGY, REPRODUCTION.)

FOG (*see under* SMOG *and below*).

FOG FEVER.—The colloquial name for a condition, probably of an allergic nature, encountered in adult cattle which have been grazing 'fog' (the second crop of grasses on a pasture that has been mown once that season), and characterised by the rapid onset of severe respiratory systems and a high mortality rate. It is now known that a syndrome identical with Fog Fever can be produced by immature Husk parasites. It has also been suggested that a fungal toxin might be a cause. There is a marked similarity between some cases of 'fog fever' and 'farmer's lung'. In both, exposure to mouldy hay infested with *Thermopolyspora polyspora* may be involved. In a survey (1965) 71 per cent of cows with fog fever showed reactions to farmers' lung antigens.

Symptoms.—Abnormal and rapid breathing, protrusion of the tongue, and a characteristic loud expiratory groan or grunt. A painful cough may also be present. Collapse and death may occur within a very few hours, or the symptoms may continue for a matter of days. The temperature seldom rises above 104°, and is subnormal in those animals which are the subject of an acute attack. Appetite is lost and rumination ceases.

Œdema of the lungs occurs, the lung tissue being waterlogged, and the mucous membrane of trachea and bronchi shows, on post-mortem examination, damson-coloured staining due to hæmorrhage.

Treatment.—The administration of adrenalin by injection; oxygen. The animal must be spared exertion.

FOGGAGE.—Aftermath, 'fog'. Grass grown for winter grazing.

FOLIC ACID.—One of the vitamins of the B-complex. (*See* VITAMINS.)

FOLLICLE (*folliculus*, a little bag) is the term applied to a very small sac or gland, *e.g.* small collections of lymphoid tissue in the throat and the small digestive glands on the mucous membrane of the intestine. The hair follicle is the depression in the skin in the lowest part of which is situated the hair papilla from which it grows. The Graäfian follicle is the little sac in the ovary which encloses an ovum. (*See* SKIN; OVARY.)

FOLLICULAR HORMONE (*see* HORMONES.)

FOLLICULAR MANGE is another name for demodectic mange due to the parasite *Demodex canis*, which lives in the hair follicles of the skin, and causes mange in dogs particularly. (*See* PARASITES, p. 691.)

FOMENTATION (*foveo*, I keep warm) is an application of flannel, cloth, or other soft material wrung out of hot water and applied over an injured or diseased part. (*See* POULTICES AND FOMENTATIONS.)

FOMITES (*fomes*, tinder) is a term used to include all articles that have been in actual contact with a sick animal, so as to retain some of the infective material and be capable of spreading the disease. Thus bedding material, fodder, mangers, stable or byre utensils, clothing, grooming tools, the clothes of an attendant, or even the attendant himself, may all be fomites.

FOOD CONVERSION RATIOS.—These express the number of pounds of food required to obtain a liveweight gain of 1 lb. For bacon pigs, the period taken is usually that from weaning to slaughter.

If F.C.R.s are to be used as a basis of comparison as between one litter and another, or one farm's pigs and another's it is essential that the same meal or other food be used; otherwise the figures become meaningless.

FOOD INSPECTION in countries such as Denmark and the U.S.A., is carried out entirely by members of the veterinary profession. In Britain this is not the case, with the exception of certain cities and districts where veterinary officers are responsible for the safety of meat, milk, vegetables, cheese, etc., and are assisted by other veterinarians or by Health inspectors. Meat inspection duties include pre-slaughter inspection of food animals, and the examination of organs and tissues as well as inspection of the dressed carcase. Laboratory facilities are desirable if not essential. For conditions which render meat dangerous as food, *see* TUBERCULOSIS, SALMONELLOSIS, ANTHRAX, TRICHINOSIS, ECHINOCOCCOSIS, etc.

FOOD-POISONING IN MAN (*see* SALMONELLOSIS; *also* BOTULISM).

FOODS AND FEEDING (*see* DIET AND DIETETICS, NURSING OF SICK ANIMALS; RATIONS; *also* TINNED FOODS).

FOOL'S PARSLEY POISONING.—Although a member of the Natural Order *Umbellifera*—very many of the members of which are poisonous (*e.g.* Water Hemlock, Water Dropwort, and Hemlock)—the extremely common Fool's Parsley (*Æthusa cynapium*) is not a frequent cause of poisoning of animals. It is dangerous when fed to rabbits, if it is pulled in the early green succulent stage before the flowering tops are formed, for it forms a common food for tame rabbits.

Fool's parsley is said to contain an alkaloidal substance similar to but not identical with *coniine*.

Under ordinary circumstances herbivorous animals do not readily eat fool's parsley, for at the time when its growth is most luxuriant (*i.e.* in spring) there is generally an abundance of grass, which they prefer.

Symptoms.—In cows, there have been seen a loss of appetite, salivation, fever, uncertain gait, and paralysis of the hind-quarters. In horses, an instance has been recorded in which a number of animals ate the plant in quantity; those which had white muzzles and feet became attacked with diarrhœa and all white areas of the body became severely inflamed, but other horses of a whole-colour remained unaffected. This is an instance of the very interesting condition of sensitisation of a non-pigmented area of the body. In other cases stupor, paralysis, and convulsions have been noticed. (*See* LIGHT SENSITISATION.)

Treatment.—Where possible, animals that have eaten fool's parsley should have their stomachs emptied by a stomach-tube, or by the operation of rumenotomy. Large drenches of strong black tea or coffee should be given so that the tannic acid in them may combine with the alkaloids of the plant and form inert substances. Warmth and general stimulants are also necessary.

FOOT-AND-MOUTH DISEASE, which is also called ECZEMA EPIZOÖTICA, EPIZOÖTIC APHTHA, MALIGNANT APHTHA, and APHTHOUS FEVER, is an acute febrile disease of cattle, sheep, goats, and pigs, which is characterised by the formation of vesicles in connection with the mouth and feet, and sometimes on the skin of the udder or teats of females.

Human beings are rarely susceptible to the disease, but, except in children, the symptoms are mild. Hedgehogs may be affected, and may spread the disease to stock; also rats. Chickens can be infected experimentally, develop the disease, and pass on the infection. It has occurred in almost every country in the world where cattle are kept. The continent of Europe and the countries of South America have the disease almost constantly present, and there can be no doubt that most British outbreaks trace to one or other of these sources. It is also indigenous in many parts of Africa and Asia and sometimes a strain of greatly increased virulence crosses the Mediterranean to invade south Europe and sweep over large areas with extreme rapidity. It affects not only domesticated animals, but very many of the wild herbivores as well, having been seen in deer, antelope, buffalo, bison, yaks, etc., and sometimes been introduced into Zoological Gardens. The disease is not, as a rule, fatal in the adult animal, but when it affects breeding stock as many as 85 per cent of young animals born from affected or in-contact dams die. It causes great economic loss on account of the reduction in milk secretion in dairy herds, severe loss of condition in fat stock of any species, interference with trading in live stock, and loss of calves, kids, lambs, and piglings. In countries where there is legislation against it, it also necessitates heavy expenditure in compensation to owners, quarantine, and isolation measures.

Cause. — Foot-and-mouth disease is caused by a virus which is only from 8 to 12 millemicra in size (*i.e.* 8 to 12 twenty-five millionths of an inch). Seven types of the virus are now recognised—the three, known as O, A and C, which cause outbreaks of the disease in Britain, and four more which so far have been confined to Asia and Africa—Asia and Sat 1, Sat 2, and Sat 3. In 1960 the type Asia 1 virus caused serious outbreaks in Israel, the Lebanon and Syria, and fear was expressed that it might invade Europe. Sat 1 virus appeared in Israel, Syria, Jordan, and Turkey during 1962. In 1966 the A22 strain, which had been causing disease in Turkey and Iraq, appeared in Sussex. The sub-type O_1 was responsible for the great epidemic in Britain during 1967–68.

Each strain is immunologically distinct, but the type of lesion produced in the animal is similar. The strains can only be distinguished by special laboratory tests upon animals. Recovery from attack by any one strain confers an immunity against further infection by that particular strain, but not by the others, nor by massive infection or artificial injection of the same strain of virus.

The virus is present in the vesicles and in the discharges which come from them when they burst; and since there is nearly always an excessive secretion of saliva from an animal affected with lesions in the mouth, it is through the medium of contamination with saliva that the disease is perhaps most readily spread. As well as this, however, the urine, fæces, and small amounts of serum from lesions in the feet, are also very important factors in the spread to other animals. The virus can easily retain its vitality for very considerable lengths of time, and may be spread by a host of intermediate objects which have been in contact with affected animals: Hides, hair, wool, hay, straw, sacks and packing fabrics generally, milk, manure, animals (especially cats and dogs, hares, rabbits, rats, mice, and birds). Migratory birds in their flights from one country to another may act as carriers. Spread by wind, watercourses, tourists and their vehicles, are all possible means of spread. Much of the spread of the disease during the 1967–68 epidemic has been attributed to wind. Rain and snow are also considered important too.

Bulk collection of milk was also implicated. The virus may be excreted in milk before symptoms in the cow have appeared or become obvious.

People who handle infected cattle and do not take the precautions to disinfect their hands and change their clothing afterwards, will distribute the virus.

Experiments at Pirbright, have shown that when examining infected pigs some of the foot-and-mouth virus reaches the human nose, and may remain there for 24 hours, or even 48 hours. During this period the virus may be transferred to any other (uninfected) pigs which the person is handling or examining. In other words, the nose of man can be a hazard in the spread of the disease.

The virus can survive in frozen liver or kidney for 4 months or more. The use of swill containing scraps of meat, bones, or other animal tissue for feeding to pigs is a very important factor in the spread of foot-and-mouth disease, and because of the number of outbreaks traced to swill, the Ministry of Agriculture imposes a requirement upon those who use swill that it shall have been boiled for at least 1 hour before being fed.

The virus can survive in bull semen stored at low temperatures.

The period for which the disease lies latent after infection (*i.e.* the incubation period) varies from 1 to 15 days, but the majority of cases show symptoms between the 2nd and the 6th day after having been exposed to infection. Infection usually takes place through the alimentary canal, but it is possible that the disease may also be contracted by inoculation and inhalation.

An important feature of the disease in relation to its spread is the excretion of virus before symptoms become evident to the owner of the animal.

This is characteristic of the O_1 virus. With pigs, experimental work at Pirbright has shown that 10 days may elapse between excretion of virus and the development of lesions. With cattle and sheep, the figure may be 5 days; or an average of $2\frac{1}{2}$ days.

Symptoms.—At first, animals are noticed to become dull, refuse their food, lie about in a sluggish manner, and milk cows suddenly give a lessened flow of milk. Their temperatures rapidly rise to 104° or 105° F. in the case of cattle, and fever is maintained until the crop of vesicles form, after which it subsides. A few hours after the initial dullness has been noticed affected animals usually commence to salivate profusely—long ropes of stringy saliva hanging from the mouth. This salivation is caused by the pain occasioned through the vesicles, and its appearance coincides with the formation of the blister or bleb stage of the lesions. During this time the animal frequently smacks its lips in a characteristic manner, yawns, and

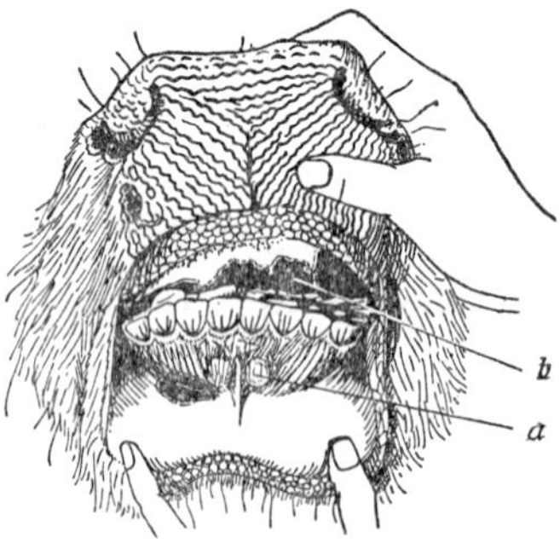

Mouth lesions of foot-and-mouth disease. *a*, unopened blisters or vesicles; *b*, ruptured vesicles.

protrudes its tongue. As a rule the combination of these symptoms leads an owner to examine his cattle, particularly their mouths, and the blisters are found in all stages of development. Some are just forming, some are well formed, some have recently burst, but the mucous membrane that formed their covering is still adherent, and in the oldest the mucous membrane has been cast off from their surfaces and shallow ulcer-like areas are left. The commonest situations are on the dental pad and in the upper incisor region, on the tongue, especially around its tip, and on the insides of the cheeks and gums. The blisters each run a similar course; for a few hours they gradually rise, then they burst, liberating a small amount of yellowish, straw-coloured serum (which should be regarded as highly infective and as containing the virus), and there remains behind a shallow, eroded, red, raw, ulcer-like area, to the edges of which little pieces of mucous membrane remain adherent for a short time until they are removed by the movements of the mouth. In from six days to a fortnight or so these areas heal, and the lesions disappear. As a rule adjacent areas become confluent, and in bad cases large irregular, ragged, red patches form, from the surfaces of which the mucous membrane has disappeared. The lesions are always extremely painful, and on this account the animal is prevented from feeding. Generally, it can still drink, and it will often take liquid or very soft food, but it refuses dry food entirely. The appetite usually returns in a few days. During these developments there has been a great loss of condition, which is especially marked in adult fat cattle, and in milking cows in good condition. Young store animals, and those in only ordinary condition, are less affected. A differential diagnosis has to be made between foot-and-mouth disease and vesicular stomatitis. What was diagnosed as the latter disease in Saskatchewan, Canada, in November 1951, proved to be foot-and-mouth disease, which was not recognised as such for 2½ months. Foot lesions generally appear 4 or 5 days after the vesicles form in the mouth. In these, blisters form around the coronets, between the claws, and practically wherever there is a junction between skin and the horn of the foot. These blisters very soon rupture, discharging a quantity of infective material, and a red, inflamed, raw area remains behind. Lameness is present, and the animal frequently kicks and shakes the affected foot as if it were endeavouring to dislodge a stone or piece of glass from between its claws. In some cases the serous exudate burrows down between the horn and the sensitive parts of the foot, and the whole of the hoof is shed.

In sheep and pigs, mouth lesions are not so common as in cattle, although they are occasionally found. Foot lesions are the commonest, and in them the disease usually begins either at the front of the coronet or at the heels instead of between the claws as in cattle. In the pig the muzzle and end of the snout may show lesions.

Animals in milk—cows, ewes, and sows—may develop characteristic lesions upon their teats or upon the skin of the udder. The lesions are similar to those forming in the mouth, but they take longer to mature. In some cases the whole of the tip of the teat shows a single large blister, which is soon burst by milking or sucking. Subsequently an eroded appearance remains, until healing is established. Milk secretion rapidly diminishes in such cases, and the animal refuses to allow any one or anything to touch its teats. The pain is usually acute, and the milk—contaminated with the exudate and with discharges from the lesions—is highly infective to young animals.

In the majority of cases the disease runs its course in from a fortnight to three weeks or so, but small individual lesions may heal in about a week. In a herd it takes from about 1 to 2½ months before the disease has spent its infective powers and the lesions in the last few cases have healed. The actual time depends upon the size of the herd and the intimacy of the animals. As already stated, the mortality in adult animals is low in most outbreaks, but in very malignant outbreaks it may be as high as 50 per cent of the affected. In all instances the mortality in young animals is high, ranging between 70 per cent and 85 per cent of those affected. In fatal cases an intense superficial inflammation of the mucous membranes of the 4th stomach and the intestines may be found upon post-mortem examination.

When the animals upon a premises are treated instead of being slaughtered, foot-and-mouth disease very often leaves behind it some permanent adverse effects, *e.g.* a drop in milk yield, mastitis, lameness.

In animals which have had foot lesions where the hoof was not cast off, a little of the infective virus may become imprisoned below the wall of the hoof, and as the hoof grows further and further downwards and wears away upon its lower surface, eventually this infective material is liberated, and another outbreak of the disease may occur in the same animals. The time when the second outbreak may arise is anything up to about six months, depending upon the rate of growth and of wear of the hoof concerned.

After recovery from infection by one strain of the virus, animals obtain immunity against further infection by that strain, but not by infection by the other strains. The duration of immunity in recovered animals is very variable.

Control.—Considerable attention is being paid to methods of preventive inoculation, and vaccines are much used on the European mainland, in S. America, and Africa. Up to the present, however, no method has been used in Europe which will give an animal immunity to more than one or two of the several strains of virus which can cause the disease. Also, as a rule, immunity lasts only 6 months. Vaccination, in fact, is practised in countries where a slaughter policy is unworkable ; not *vice versa*, as might be thought by those who condemn the slaughter policy without having studied the reasons for it.

A vaccination policy, without slaughter, is adopted in the Argentine, Belgium, France, Western Germany, Italy, and Spain, in all of which countries the disease is endemic and its incidence high. ' Overall ' vaccination is seldom practicable for reasons of cost and supply, so ' frontier ' vaccination or ' ring ' vaccination (of all susceptible animals within a given radius of an outbreak) are usually practised. A combined Vaccination And Slaughter Policy is adopted in Denmark, Sweden, Switzerland, Holland, and Mexico.

A slaughter policy obtains in Great Britain, Canada, U.S.A., Norway, Eire and Northern Ireland—countries where the disease is not endemic. Such a policy, involving compensation to owners of compulsorily slaughtered animals, is normally far less costly than vaccination.

Prevention can be attempted by rigorously excluding any direct *or indirect* contact with diseased animals.

Control Measures in Britain.—In Great Britain this disease is scheduled under the Diseases of Animals Acts, and all outbreaks must be promptly reported to the Local Authorities and to the Ministry of Agriculture. Strict isolation is at first ensured, and the affected animals are slaughtered and burned or buried. In-contact animals are slaughtered and their carcases, if otherwise satisfactory, are used for human food. The premises are carefully cleansed and disinfected under supervision, and re-stocking is not allowed for at least 28 days after the last animal was slaughtered ; the time actually varies with local conditions. During the time the cattle are being slaughtered and while disinfection is proceeding, no unauthorised person is allowed upon the premises, and every one leaving the farm (Infected Place) is required to disinfect himself as thoroughly as possible. Straw soaked with strong disinfectant is laid at the gateways.

Meanwhile, in a radius of about 10 miles around an infected farm an Infected Area is declared. No susceptible animals are allowed to leave the area, and no movement is permitted except under licence for slaughter within 96 hours ; no animals are allowed to be driven across a public highway within the radius ; no markets, fairs, shows, sales, etc., are allowed to take place within the area ; fox-hunting and other field-sports are forbidden, and owners of animals are advised to confine themselves upon their own premises as much as possible and to prevent the entrance of unauthorised persons.

Normally, the Infected Area remains as such for 21 days, being contracted to a radius of 5 miles after 14 days. Hunting is forbidden ; footpaths may be closed.

When the disease has spread, or threatens to spread over a wide area, the Ministry may declare a Controlled Area. In this, animals may be moved only under licence, and only into an Infected Area. Markets are banned (except for animals to be slaughtered immediately).

To prevent the introduction of foot-and-mouth disease into clean countries, there is usually an embargo upon the importation of cattle, sheep, and pigs from areas in which the disease is indigenous, and the importation of fodder and litter is strictly forbidden. In Great Britain pig carcases from certain European countries are also forbidden entry, since at least one outbreak of foot-and-mouth disease was traced to infection from imported pig carcases landed at the port of Leith. It is also most advisable that hides, wool, hair, horns, hoofs, bone-meals, and animal manures from foreign parts, should be effectively sterilised either before leaving the country of origin, or else upon arrival at the ports of those countries free from the disease.

Northumberland Committee Report.—Following the disastrous epidemic of 1967–68, which involved 2,397 outbreaks and payment in compensation, to owners of compulsorily slaughtered animals, of about £27m., a committee was appointed under the chairmanship of the Duke of Northumberland to review the policy and arrangements for dealing with the disease (which, in this epidemic, had resulted in the slaughter of over 211,000 head of cattle ;

108,000 sheep; and 113,000 pigs; and 50 goats).

The Northumberland Committee recommended continuation of the slaughter policy; but that this should be reinforced by a ring vaccination scheme if a meat import policy, calculated to reduce substantially the risks of primary outbreaks, were not implemented.

Treatment.—The sulpha drugs are of value in treating secondary infection; likewise the antibiotics.

Disinfectants.—The following disinfectants have satisfied the test requirements for use against foot-and-mouth disease:

Name of disinfectant	Parts of water to be added to one part disinfectant
Action approved disinfectant	240
Castrol Solvex ICD 109	50
Citric acid BP	500
Combat	240
Compass lysol BP	9
Crown special detergent disinfectant	240
Dairy Iodicide	250
Delta farm disinfectant	240
Disteola	240
FAM	240
Famosan	160
Famosan Mark II	139
Formalin BP (containing not less than 34 per cent formaldehyde)	9
GR 250	10
Hygasan	20
Iodel X	130
Iodet	240
Ortho-phosphoric acid (technical grade)	330
Resiguard F	80
Ropolik	240
Sani-Squad	5
Sodium carbonate (decahydrate) complying with BS 3674 of 1963	24

For the current list *see Diseases of Animals (Approved Disinfectants) Orders.* H.M.S.O.

FOOT-BATHS FOR CATTLE.—A foot-bath with 1¼-inch pipes laid horizontally 2 inches apart, even if filled with plain water, will help to detach mud; the pipes forcing the claws apart.

FOOT-BATHS FOR SHEEP are used for the purpose of curing or preventing certain foot diseases, especially foot-rot and the foot lesions of orf. The bath consists of a shallow trough made of concrete or wood, measuring about 6 to 9 inches wide, 4 to 6 inches deep in the middle and tapering at each end to about 1 inch depth, and about 10 to 15 feet long (or more). It is built in connection with a sheep-pen or fold, in which the sheep may be first collected, and from which they may be driven one at a time through the bath. Hurdles or a fence along each side of the trough prevent the sheep from leaving it while being driven through. No drying pen is necessary, as the small amount of poison carried out on the feet is not sufficient to impregnate the pastures to any serious extent

The solutions most often used for foot-baths are 5 per cent formalin solution; or copper sulphate, 4 to 8 per cent. As a preventative of contagious foot-rot a three-weekly run through a foot-bath gives excellent results. (*See* FOOT-ROT.)

FOOT OF THE HORSE.—Without a good foot, no matter how excellent a horse otherwise may be, it is of little or no use to man. There is a very great deal of truth in the old saying, 'No foot, no horse', although at first sight this may seem picturesque exaggeration. From the horse, man demands a capacity for movement, and this of necessity entails sound organs on which movement depends, and of these the feet are not the least important.

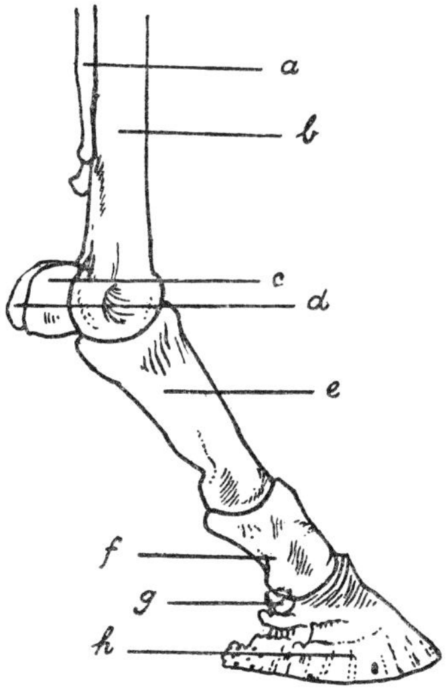

Bones of horse's foot. *a*, Splint bone *b*, cannon; *c* and *d*, sesamoids of first phalanx *e*, long pastern bone; *f*, short pastern bone *g*, navicular bone; *h*, pedal or coffin bone.

It will be the aim here to give some account of the anatomy and physiology of the normal foot; an account of the commoner diseases will be found under their respective headings, such as CORNS, QUITTOR, LAMINITIS, SANDCRACK, SEEDY

TOE, BRUISED SOLE, INJURIES FROM SHOEING, CANKER, THRUSH, etc.

Skeleton of the foot consists of the lower part of the second phalanx, the whole of the third phalanx, and the sesamoid of the third phalanx or 'navicular bone'. (*See under* BONES.) From the posterior angles of the third phalanx (coffin-bone) project two roughly quadrilateral plates of cartilage, one on either side, which are known as the 'lateral cartilages'. These are important structures in the absorption of shock and in preserving the elasticity of the foot as a whole. Under certain conditions they become ossified, when the name 'side-bones' is applied. The three bones above mentioned are bound together by a series of ligaments which, while they allow free mobility in normal directions, prevent unnatural movements which might rupture the capsules of the coffin-joint. Lying between the two lateral cartilages and behind the third phalanx there is a fibro-elastic structure known as the 'plantar cushion' or *digital torus*, which, although, strictly speaking, it is not part of the

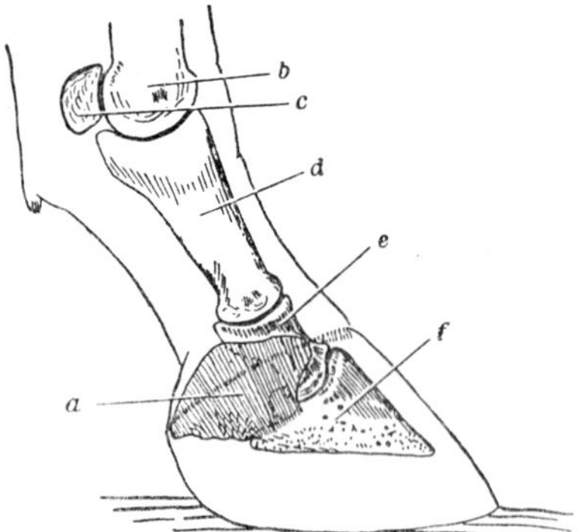

Relationship of the bones of the horse's foot to the surface. *a*, lateral cartilage; *b*, lower end of cannon bone; *c*, sesamoid of the first phalanx; *d*, long pastern or first phalanx; *e*, short pastern or second phalanx; *f*, coffin bone or third phalanx. (After Bradley's *Anatomy*.)

skeleton of the foot, will be considered here for convenience. This plantar cushion is composed of extremely elastic, dense, fibrous tissue, poorly supplied with blood-vessels and not greatly sensitive, and is one of the chief shock-absorbing structures of the foot. From above it is pressed upon by the descending deep flexor tendon, when the foot comes to the ground; from below it is pressed upwards by the horny frog; it cannot expand forwards to any great extent, because of the presence of the coffin-bone; and since it is practically a rubber-like buffer, it expands backwards and sideways. On either side of it, however, are the lateral cartilages, and these are pressed outwards in the process and carry with them the

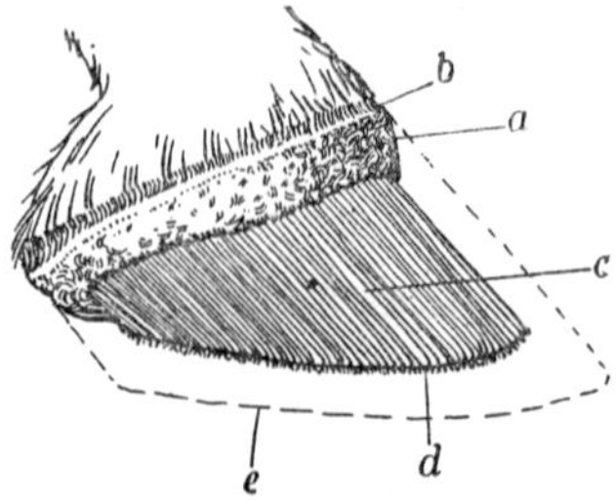

Diagram to show the sensitive parts of the foot. The dotted line, *e*, indicates the outline of the hoof. *a*, coronary matrix or coronary cushion; *b*, perioplic matrix; *c*, laminar matrix, showing the sensitive laminæ; *d*, the edge of the solar matrix, or the sensitive sole. (After Bradley's *Anatomy*.)

horny wall at the heels. These structures collectively can be likened to the bare foot of man.

Sensitive structures.—Covering the part above described and accurately moulded to them (just as the sock of a man is moulded to the foot) are the sensitive parts which nourish the horny hoof. These are, around the hoof-head above the coronary band, a *perioplic matrix*, from fine projections on the surface of which is nourished the *periople*, a layer of hard

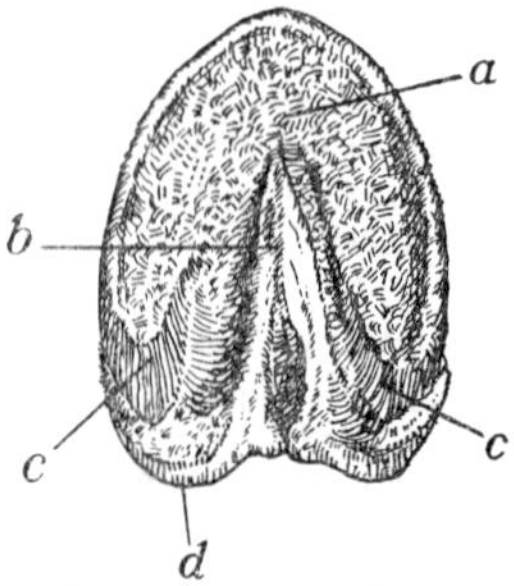

Lower aspect of foot with the horny parts removed. *a*, solar matrix; *b*, matrix of frog; *c*, laminar matrix; *d*, a small portion of the coronary matrix. The reflection of the laminar matrix forwards at either heel to form the sensitive portions of the bars can be seen.

varnish-like horn which prevents undue evaporation from the wall; around the coronet, from one heel to the other, a bolster-like structure about $\frac{4}{5}$ths of an inch wide known as the *coronary band*, or *coronary cushion*, which nourishes and from which grows the horn of the

FOOT OF THE HORSE

wall; running down the inside of the wall all the way round and turning inwards and forwards at the heels, a *laminar matrix*, which is provided with laminæ or 'leaves' which interdigitate with corresponding laminæ on the inside of the wall; covering the lower surface of the coffin-bone, and nourishing the sole of the hoof, a *solar matrix*, or *sensitive sole*, and covering the lower surface of the plantar cushion and nourishing the frog, a *furcal matrix*, or *sensitive frog*. The term *pododerm* is applied collectively to these sensitive structures, which are all continuous with each other, and bear some resemblance to the sock of a human being, as already noted. They are well supplied with blood-vessels and nerves, provide nourishment for, and produce, the horny parts of the foot. The pododermic tissues are in reality modified skin, but instead of growing hairs as does the skin in other parts of the body, they produce numerous minute tubular horn fibres which are firmly united to each other by a kind of cementing substance, the whole forming horn as we know it. When exposed, the sensitive parts are soft, red in colour, easily bleed, are extremely sensitive to the touch, and constitute what is generally known as the 'quick' of the foot.

Horny structures.—Considered collectively the horny parts of the foot form what is known as the 'hoof'. The hoof is more or less analogous to the boot of man,

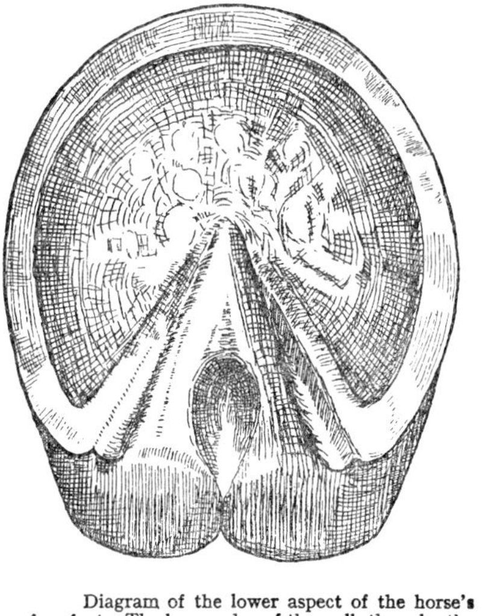

Diagram of the lower aspect of the horse's fore foot. The lower edge of the wall, the sole, the frog, and the bars, can all be seen. The white line is not well shown. Compare the oval outline of the fore foot with Fig. 100, which shows the hind foot.

the sensitive tissues being like the sock, except that the boot and sock are separable, while the hoof grows from and is nourished by the sensitive parts. The horny hoof—composed of practically the same material (keratin) as the horns or claws of other animals, and being in reality modified skin—is a protective, slightly elastic casing which protects the softer parts of the foot from concussion, friction and injury. It is composed of the wall, the sole, and the frog.

The wall is all that portion which can be seen when the foot rests upon the ground. It gives the foot its form. Its horn is hard, solid, only slightly elastic, and affords protection to the sensitive laminar matrix below it. The wall is arbitrarily divided into toe, quarters, and heel. The toe is the highest part at the

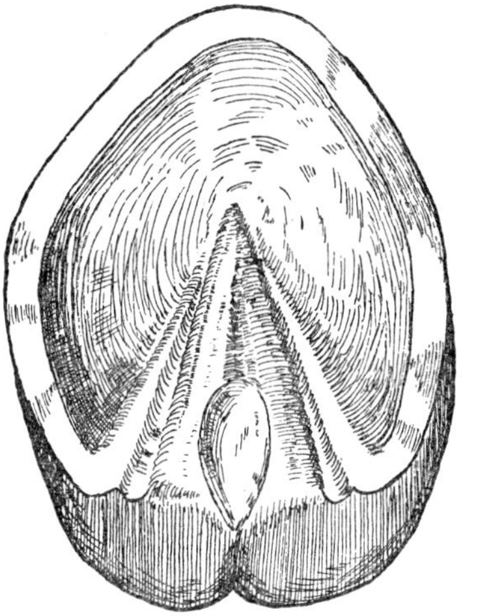

Diagram of the lower aspect of the horse's hind foot, showing the same features as in Fig. 99.

front; from it backward the wall gradually decreases in height, passes around the bulbs of the heels, and turns forward and inward to form the *bars*, which are finally lost in the edge of the sole towards the apex of the frog. In this way the wall forms an angle at each heel, and to these angles the name *buttresses* is applied. Each buttress encloses a branch of the horny sole. The inner surface of the wall presents about 600 horny leaves or *laminæ*, which dovetail with the sensitive laminæ forming a firm union between wall and matrix, which makes it very difficult to separate the two. The upper edge of the wall is thin, flexible, and grooved for the

FOOT OF THE HORSE

lodgment of the coronary cushion. The lower edge is called the 'bearing surface', and is the part to which the shoe is fitted. At the toe the wall is thickest; as the quarters are approached it gets considerably thinner, and at the heels it is only about half the thickness at the toe. It requires about 12 months for the wall to grow from the coronet to the ground at the toe; 6 to 8 months at the quarters, and from 3 to 5 months at the heels.

The sole is that part of the hoof which is nourished by the sensitive tissue covering the solar surface of the coffin-bone. It is divided into a body and two branches, and is roughly crescent-shaped. The sole is markedly vaulted in normal feet, especially in hind-feet, but in very many old horses it becomes flat or even convex;

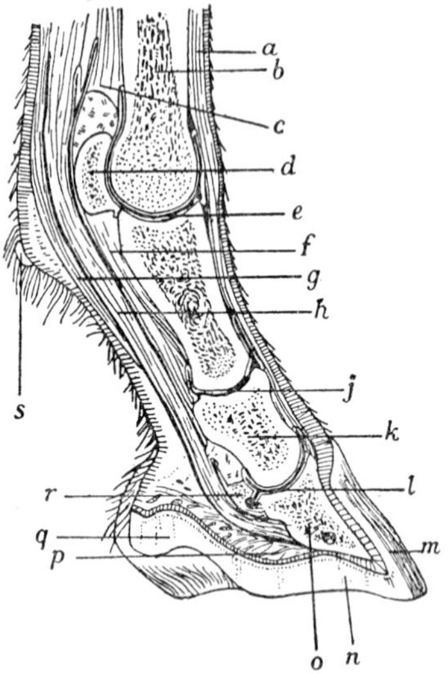

Section of horse's foot. *a*, extensor tendon; *b*, lower end of cannon bone; *c*, branch of suspensory ligament; *d*, sesamoid; *e*, fetlock joint; *f*, sesamoidean ligament; *g*, superficial flexor tendon; *h*, deep flexor tendon; *j*, pastern joint; *k*, short pastern bone; *l*, coffin joint; *m*, wall of hoof; *n*, sole of hoof; *o*, coffin bone; *p*, plantar cushion; *q*, frog of hoof; *r*, navicular bone; *s*, ergot.

when excessively convex it is called a 'dropped sole'. The horn of the sole is friable, brittle, flaky, and is shed from the lower surface in flakes from time to time. These should not be pared away with the knife during shoeing, unless for some reason they are not being cast off naturally. The outer border of the sole is bevelled to correspond to the slope of the wall, but is separated from it by the *white line* of soft horn which acts as a kind of cementing substance between the wall and the sole. This line is of great importance in shoeing, as it indicates the thickness of the wall, and is used as a guiding line through which the nails can be driven with safety. In the posterior part of the sole there is a V-shaped notch, between the branches of which lie the bars and the frog.

The frog is an exact mould of the lower surface of the plantar cushion which it protects. It is a roughly triangular wedge-shaped mass filling up the space between the bars and the V-shaped notch of the sole. It projects downwards more than the sole, and receives the greatest amount of the concussion in the normal foot; it is only seldom injured, however, for its horn is of very elastic consistency. The ground surface presents a very well-marked *median cleft*, which corresponds to an elevation in its upper (inner) surface which is commonly known as the 'frog stay', and which aids in the attachment of the frog to the overlying parts.

Movements of the hoof.—With the alternate lifting and placing of the foot the hoof is continually undergoing a variation in its shape. Even when the horse is standing still its foot is bearing different amounts of weight at different times, and its shape is altering accordingly. The main changes of form are as follows: (1) An expansion or widening of the whole of the posterior part of the foot from the coronet down to the bearing surface at the quarters and heels, which occur when the weight of the horse descends upon the foot, and alters back to normal when the foot is lifted from the ground. The variation in transverse measurement is between $\frac{1}{15}$th and $\frac{1}{10}$th of an inch according to the size of the horse; (2) a narrowing of the front half of the foot, measured at the coronet; and (3) a sinking of the heels and a flattening of the vault of the sole. These changes are more marked in horses which have well-developed feet, good sound, elastic horn, and especially in the unshod hoof. They play a very important part in the circulation of the foot, the alternate expansion and contraction causing variations in the pressure upon the arteries and veins enclosed within the hoof, and encouraging the free movement and circulation of blood. When a horse is allowed to stand in a stable for some days without getting any exercise the blood tends to stagnate, the circulation is slow, a certain amount of passive congestion of the vessel of the

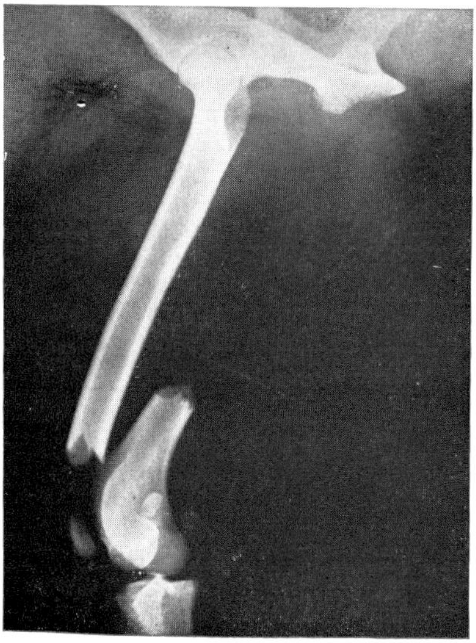

1

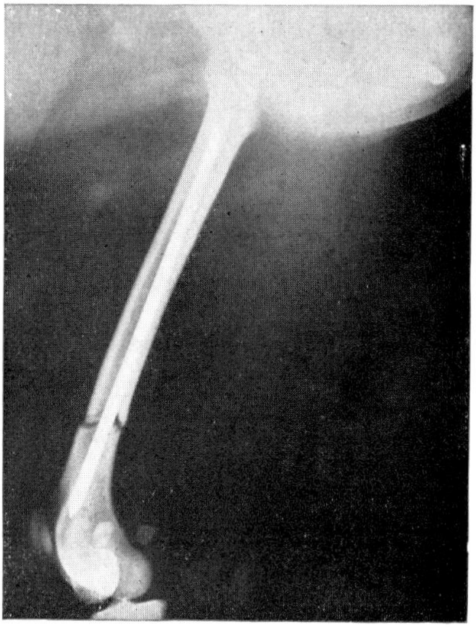

2

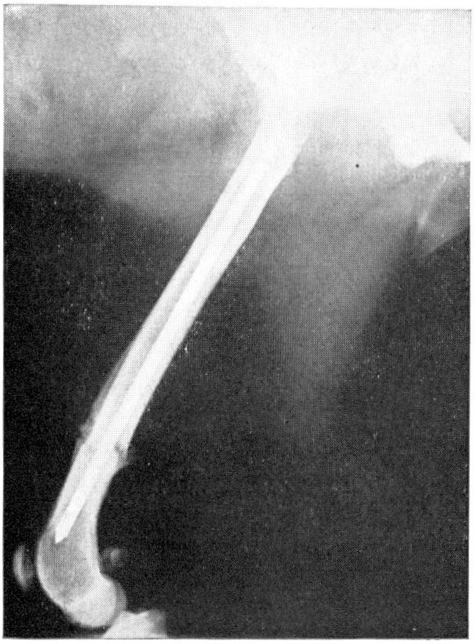

3

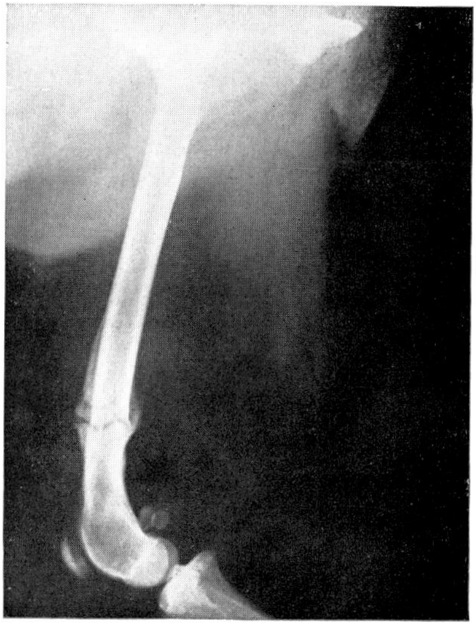

4

INTRA-MEDULLARY PINNING

1. Fracture of the femur in a dog. Note the extent of the displacement of the lower third of the bone.
2. After reduction of the fracture and the insertion of a metal pin down the narrow cavity of the bone.
3. This radiograph shows callus formation.
4. The intra-medullary pin has been removed; repair of the femur is now complete.

(*Radiographs: Royal Veterinary College.*)

PLATE 6

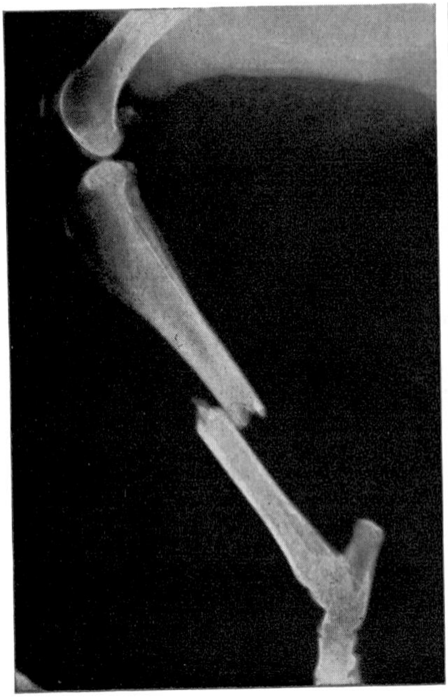

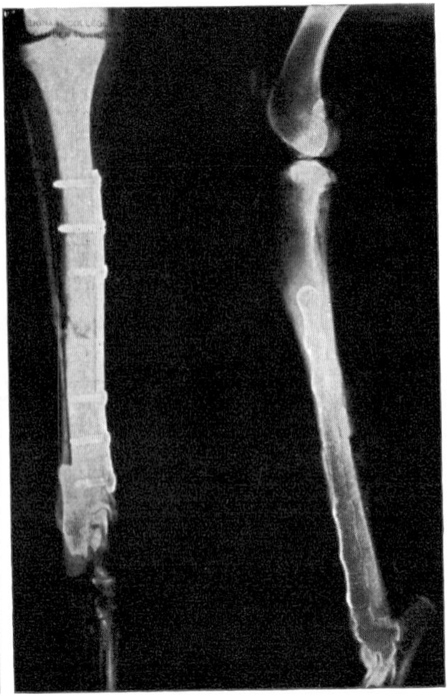

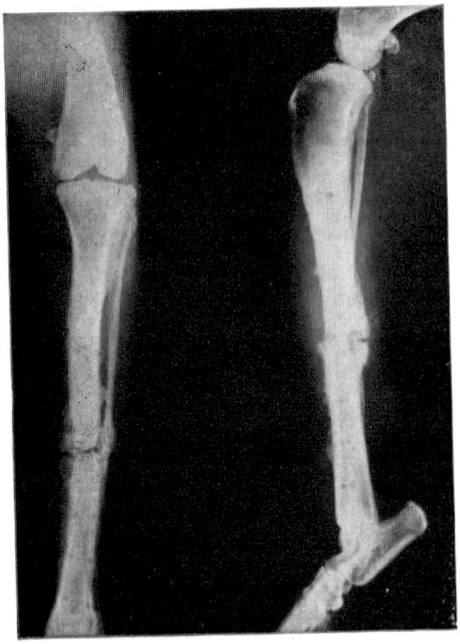

PLATING

This is another technique used in veterinary practice. The radiographs show a fracture of the tibia in the dog and the use of a metal plate screwed into the bone. Below is seen the result (from two angles) after removal of the plate. The dog was using the leg well.

(*Radiographs: Royal Veterinary College.*)

foot takes place, and the nutrition is not so perfect.

FOOT-ROT OF PIGS.—A survey (1964) suggests that in the southern counties of England, the incidence of foot lesions in pigs up to bacon weight is around 65 per cent. Most of these lesions were mild, probably causing the animal little inconvenience ; while others could be very severe indeed.

In a survey carried out at one of the slaughter houses, and involving just under 6800 pigs, 30 per cent of the lesions were erosion of the heel, 24 per cent erosion of the toe, 21 per cent erosion of the sole. Separation of the hard horn of the wall from either the very soft horn of the heel or the flaky horn of the sole, accounted for another 21 per cent of the lesions, and varied from little more than a shallow crack to a deep fissure with enlargement and deformity of the claw, and the formation of excessive 'proud flesh'. 'False sand-crack'—varying from a fine crack to a deep fissure with a series of secondary branches—made up another 2·7 of the lesions.

Trouble was encountered mostly in the outside claws, and it was commonly found that inside claws were smaller than the outer ones—especially in the hind-feet. It is suggested that this discrepancy in size is a hereditary one, and that the inner claws suffer less damage because they take less weight and are, to some extent, protected by their position.

'Many claws with white line or false sand-crack lesions were excessively worn', and housing on concrete has been put forward as an important cause. The feeding of large quantities of skim milk has been suggested as a contributory cause.

As to the erosion mentioned earlier, it is likely that damp, dirty conditions soften the horn and predispose the foot to bruising, injury, and excessive wear on concrete. Infection may follow. 'Foot conditions often flare up in heavily pregnant or lactating gilts and sows, which suggest that there may be other predisposing factors, possibly nutritional.'

'Thirty per cent of casualty pigs at one slaughter house showed abscess formation, a common reason for the condemnation of meat, and 12 per cent of these abscesses were on the feet.'

Work in 1965 suggests that excessively rough concrete is a likely cause, and that some concrete may be virtually abrasive.

A foot-bath containing a 5 to 10 per cent solution of formalin is recommended for prevention and treatment ; the bath being used twice weekly. (*See also* 'BUSH FOOT'.)

In the abattoir, the effects are seen in the condemnation of portions of leg, or of whole legs, where a chronic arthritis is involved, with up to total condemnation where pyæmia follows the primary infection.

FOOT-ROT OF SHEEP is a disease of the horny parts and of the adjacent soft structures of the feet of sheep. The organism primarily responsible is *Fusiformis nodosus.* The disease is commonly prevalent on wet, marshy, badly-drained pastures, in old folds or sheep pens, and upon land that is heavily dressed with farmyard manure. Wet soil, however, does not cause foot-rot but merely facilitates infection. This is a mixed one, with *Fusiformis necrophorus* causing sufficient damage to permit the entry of *F. nodosus.*

In Australia two forms of footrot are recognised, in both of which *Fusiformis nodosus* is always present. The type of footrot which develops depends upon the proteolyptic capacity of the infecting strain of *Fusiformis nodosus.* In **benign** footrot the infecting strain is of low proteolytic activity and the resultant disease is limited and does not spread under the hard horn, although it might cause lifting of the sole of the foot. In **virulent** footrot the infecting strain is of high proteolytic activity and results in extensive separation of the hard horn, with the clinical appearance of classical footrot. (Dr. D. F. Stewart.)

It appears that transmission of footrot infection from cattle to sheep is possible.

The *Fusiformis nodosus* cannot survive in the soil or on pasture for more than a fortnight.

Overgrowth of the horn of the feet. caused through an insufficient amount of wear, is an important contributory factor, The wall of the hoof at the toes grows longer and longer, throwing the weight of the sheep back on to the heels and increases the leverage on the toes during walking, with the result that a small amount of separation between sole and wall takes place, and an entrance for the organisms is provided. Grit, stones, thorns, and other pieces of foreign material which may penetrate the horn of the claws, or become wedged between the two digits, also may open a portal of entry for the germs, and in some cases injuries to the coronets are responsible.

Symptoms.—Lameness is the first noticeable feature. At first the sheep manages to put the foot to the ground, but after a time it goes on three legs only, the pain having greatly increased.

When the foot is examined there will either be found a swelling over the coronet or an area of the horn of the hoof is found to be soft, painful on pressure, 'rotten-looking', and a variable amount of foul-smelling discharge is present.

If neglected between the 20th and 30th day the horn will begin to separate from the underlying sensitive tissues, and will eventually be shed. Sometimes the disease penetrates into the foot, affecting the ligaments or even the bone. One, two, three, or all four feet may be affected. If only the two fore-feet are attacked the sheep very often assumes the kneeling position for feeding, and will only rise to its feet when being driven. If the two hind-feet, any three feet, or all four are affected, standing becomes an impossibility, and the sheep, still retaining its appetite, will feed from the sitting position, crawling forward a few inches at a time to a new piece of grazing. Untreated cases begin to lose flesh after the duration of the disease for two months or more, and eventually become so emaciated that they die from exhaustion. Seldom or never does a case recover spontaneously without treatment.

Prevention.—Foot-rot can be eradicated. Leave contaminated pasture free of sheep for 3 weeks. Isolate and treat all infected or suspected sheep. The feet of heavy sheep should not be allowed to get overgrown during wet weather; turning on to a bare fallow or stubble field, or walking along a hard road, is advocated by some to wear away the feet, but is not a very practicable proposition. The better way is to round up the sheep and pare each foot individually once every six weeks or two months.

Research initiated in Australia led to the development of a vaccine, which is now commercially available, and is prepared from cultures of *Fusiformis nodosus*.

Treatment.—It is advisable to separate the infected from the healthy, passing the latter through a foot-bath and changing the pasture to as high ground as possible. If the lame sheep can be shut up in a strawed yard, in pig-courts, or in pens, given hand-feeding and individual attention daily, they recover much better than if they are left out in the open and only attended to occasionally. The feet should be carefully trimmed, all necrotic horny material removed, and the natural shape of the foot restored as much as possible. It is essential that all the diseased horn shall be removed before any dressings are applied. Care should be taken to avoid paring too deeply and making the sensitive tissues bleed unduly, or even injuring the bone. When all the 'rotten' substance has been removed the foot should be cleansed in a solution of an antiseptic, and an astringent antiseptic dressing applied. The use of footrot vaccine may obviate much time-consuming work on treating diseased feet.

The modern treatment, for which a striking success has been claimed, consists in the application of an antibiotic preparation—either a tincture or other liquid preparation of chloramphenicol, or an ointment containing Terramycin. One or two applications usually suffice, except in very bad cases. The animal is kept on a hard, dry surface for an hour or so after treatment, and then returned to pasture which has not carried sheep for 14 days.

A foot-bath containing 5 to 10 per cent formalin in water has been used with success in Australasia and, more recently, in the U.K.

If the disease is extensive a bandage should be applied to keep out dirt and afford protection, or a rubber or leather boot, specially made for the purpose, should be applied.

The shepherd should take care to ensure that he does not spread the disease to other sheep through the medium of his hands or knife; he should wash both after dealing with each case, and all parings, diseased tissue, and infected swabs should be collected in a pail and burned. Neglect of these precautions often results in a continuance of new cases in a flock.

In the treatment of foot-rot in a flock, the trouble, time, and expense are greatly reduced if the first few cases are vigorously dealt with before the disease gets a hold on the flock, and if the healthy sound sheep are put through the foot-bath and moved to clean pastures.

FORAGE POISONING (*see* BOTULISM *and* FODDER POISONING, p. 736).

FORAMEN is the Latin name for a hole or opening. It is applied particularly to holes in bones through which pass nerves or blood-vessels. The *foramen magnum* is the large opening in the posterior aspect of the skull through which passes the spinal cord to enter the *foramina* in each of the vertebræ of the spine. The *nutrient foramina* are the holes in the shafts, etc., of the bones which penetrate to the marrow cavity, by which blood and lymph vessels and nerves pass to and from the marrow cavity.

FOREIGN BODIES.—This term includes a grass seed in the ear, nose, beneath the skin between the toes or beneath the eyelid; a needle embedded in the tongue; a chop bone wedged in a dog's mouth; a piece of bone lodged in the gullet; a piece of wire in the reticulum; pebbles in a dog's stomach. (*See under* STOMACH, DISEASES OF, etc.)

FORGING (*see under* OVER-REACHING).

FORMALIN, or FORMIC ALDEHYDE, is a gaseous body prepared by the oxidation of methyl alcohol. For commercial purposes it is prepared as a solution of 40 per cent strength in water. Formalin is a powerful antiseptic, and has the quality of hardening or fixing the tissues. The solution in water gives off gas slowly, and this has an irritant action on the eyes and nose.

Uses.—Owing to its high price formalin is sparingly used as a disinfectant for animal houses or for fumigation purposes, but it is very useful for disinfecting incubators, brooders, and small cages which have been used for birds, cats, or dogs affected with virus diseases. It is used as a spray of 3 to 5 per cent strength, or is wiped over the surfaces after preliminary cleansing. A 10 per cent solution of formalin has been used in a foot-bath in the treatment of Foot-rot in sheep. It has also been used for canker of the horse's foot and, at one time, for indolent ulcers. Its application, however, may cause considerable pain if it reaches sensitive tissues. (*See also under* DISINFECTION.)

FORMALISED VACCINES are prepared by subjecting the viruses of various diseases to the action of a weak solution of formaldehyde for a given length of time. After treatment, the virus becomes attenuated, so that while it can still stimulate the production of antibodies to render the animal immune, it cannot reproduce the disease. Formalised vaccines are employed for vaccination against various virus diseases, such as rinderpest, distemper, louping ill, rabies, etc.

FOSSA (*fossa*, a ditch) is an anatomical term applied to a depression in a bone which lodges some other structure, such as part of the brain in the skull. It is also used to describe grooves or pockets in soft tissues, such as the renal fossa of the liver in which is lodged the right kidney.

FOUL-IN-THE-FOOT is a term that may mean a number of different conditions. Used in its widest sense it indicates any suppurating or necrotic lesion affecting the space between the claws of cattle, or extending to the skin of the bulbs of the heels, or the coronet at the front, but it is often restricted to mean a necrotic condition of the interdigital space, due to an injury previously, in which a 'boil', with a necrotic core, forms.

Causes.—In most cases the direct cause is the *Actinomyces necrophorus*, which has gained entrance to the tissues either through a wound or through devitalisation of the skin from frost, mud, decomposing urine or fæces, or other irritants. A mild inflammation of the skin, very often called 'scald', is occasionally brought about by feeding upon brewers' or distillers' grains or bean-meal in excess; it appears as an area of reddened swollen skin about the heels or between the claws. Whatever the predisposing cause, the necrosis bacillus gains entrance to the tissues, and, as in other cases, produces its effects through the elaboration of a toxic material which kills the cells of the parts around. A necrotic patch or 'core' results, and round the edges of this there is usually some amount of suppuration. The diseased process may spread superficially to the skin around, or it may penetrate deeply into the foot, producing a sinus from which small amounts of pus escape.

Symptoms.—There is nearly always well-marked lameness, which is as easily noticed out at grass as on hard ground about a steading or in the byre. Hind-feet are more often affected than fore-feet, probably on account of their greater proximity to the dung channel, and to their greater liability to soiling from urine and fæces, in which the necrosis bacillus can generally be easily found. In many cases a cow will suddenly stop walking, and shake the affected foot as though she desired to dislodge a stone or other hard object which has become wedged between the claws. Sometimes the lameness disappears after a few days although the disease has not altered in any way, and is certainly not cured. The lameness will again appear when the necrotic process spreads.

There is also a contagious form of the disease in which several cattle show symptoms at about the same time. They are all affected to about the same extent, and very often the lesions bear a great similarity in different animals. In the majority of instances, however, the disease remains confined to one animal in a herd. If the affected foot is examined it is noticed that there is pain when the claws are separated and when any pressure is put upon the skin of the interdigital region between the claws. There is usually a foul, sour odour, not unlike what is noticed in foot-rot in sheep. A definite localised swelling or 'boil' may be found in the tissues below the skin, either between the toes or at the coronet, and in the centre of this is a very painful spot which has partly separated from the healthy skin nearly and from around which pus oozes, which is commonly called a 'core'. Or in other cases little more than a diffused thickened area of skin is found, which is wet and purulent, and which has caused some separation of the horn of the hoof at its edges. In very severe old-standing cases there may be a greatly swollen and deformed foot, showing at some part a deep irregular wounded area around the edges of which there is a great deal of 'proud flesh' formation. Lameness always accompanies severe cases, and in the worst forms the animal may be quite unable to bear any weight upon the diseased foot, but progresses by a succession of hops, or 'goes on three legs'.

Treatment.—This calls for professional aid. The intravenous injection of 'M. and B. 693' or sulphamezathine is the modern method. Apart from this the cleaning and dressing of the affected parts is desirable, and bandaging to keep dry and protect the lesions is desirable. (*See* FOOT-BATHS.)

FOUNDER (*see* LAMINITIS).

FOWL CHOLERA.—Synonyms: Cholera gallinarium, Avian pasteurellosis, Pasteurellosis of the fowl, Hæmorrhagic septicæmia of the fowl.

Definition.—A virulent, inoculable, and contagious disease of fowls, usually epizoötic in type and characterised by sudden onset, high fever, extensive blood extravasations into the different organs, and severe diarrhœa.

Distribution.—The disease occurs all over Europe. It occurs both in North and South America, is found in most parts of Africa, and in Asia.

Susceptibility.—All common fowls, including domestic poultry (chickens, ducks, geese, guinea-fowl, turkeys, pigeons, pheasants, and fancy birds), are susceptible. Most common wild birds are also liable to infection and serve to spread the disease. Rabbits and mice may also contract it under special circumstances.

Cause.—*Pasteurella multocida.*

Incubative period.—This is usually short, about 2 to 4 days, but in some outbreaks is said to be longer.

Symptoms.—In the most acute form of the disease, death may occur suddenly without any premonitory signs being noticed; the birds may be seen to stagger and fall down, or more commonly are just found dead. In the less acute type, which perhaps is the more common, the birds are seen to look ill, to stand apart from the rest, droop their wings, refuse both food and water; the combs, wattles, and ear lobes become discoloured, and there is great nervous prostration. A discharge comes away from the eyes and nose, a frothy saliva from the mouth, and there is usually severe diarrhœa, the fæcal matter being yellowish at first but later becomes greenish or red and gives off a very fœtid smell. The respirations become altered and rapid; the temperature is found to be elevated and may reach as high as 110° F. or 111° F. The feathers are very much ruffled and draggled, and those of the hinder parts of the body are soiled with fæcal discharges. Vomiting may take place, and in from 1 to 3 days the affected birds usually die. In other cases the symptoms are more sub-acute, and the disease may run on for from 7 to 9 or 10 days, but as a rule ends fatally.

In the more chronic type it may take several weeks before death ensues.

Fatality.—In acute outbreaks from 90 to 95 per cent may die, although in others the death-rate may be only 20 per cent.

FOWL LEUKÆMIA (*see under* LEUCOSIS COMPLEX).

FOWL-PARALYSIS (*Neuro-lymphomatosis*), (*See* MAREK'S DISEASE).

FOWL PEST.—This term usually refers to NEWCASTLE DISEASE (which see), but also includes FOWL PLAGUE.

FOWL PLAGUE (*see* AVIAN PLAGUE).

FOWL-POX (AVIAN CONTAGIOUS EPITHELIOMA and AVIAN DIPHTHERIA) is a virus disease in which wart-like nodules, varying in size from that of a pea to a robin's egg, appear on the comb, wattles, eyelids, and openings of the nostrils and ears, or on other parts of the head that are scantily covered with feathers.

In this disease the epithelial cells of the lesions show large inclusion bodies, known as *Bollinger bodies*, which themselves are made up of aggregations of smaller bodies, known as *Borrel bodies*.

Fowl-pox must be differentiated from contagious catarrh of fowls and nutritional roup.

The disease attacks the fowl most often, but other domesticated birds are all susceptible, and it is liable to attack both wild and domesticated pigeons. It occurs in almost all parts of the world.

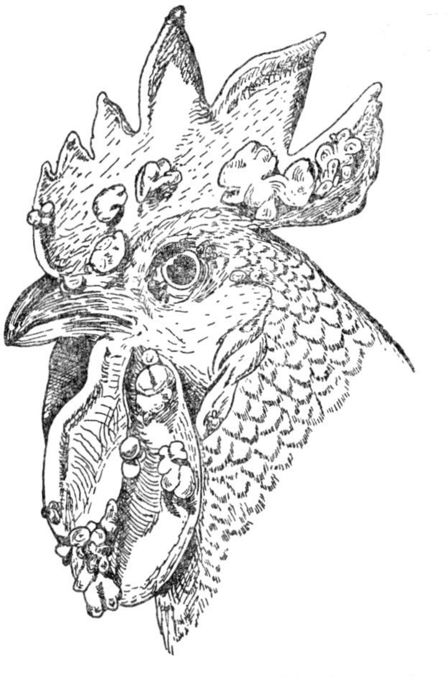

Head of cock affected with avian contagious epithelioma. Wattles and comb are mainly affected.

The virus infects the skin through abrasions, and may be transmitted by insect vectors (especially mosquitoes). Various secondary organisms are usually responsible for deaths.

Symptoms.—There are three types of lesions: (i) nodular eruptive lesions on comb and wattles; (ii) a cheesy, yellowish membrane in the mouth and throat; (iii) oculo-nasal discharges. Nodules are usually quite distinct from each other, but in some cases assume a cauliflower-like aspect. They contain either fatty material or else are watery and pus-like. Occasionally these nodules are found on other parts of the body than the head, in which case they have probably been caused by contamination of an abraded part of the skin with some of the exudate from a lesion in another part. The disease in this form is usually benign, but when diphtheritic deposits are found on the mucous membranes of the mouth, pharynx, etc., it is more serious.

In the same bird, or in different birds of the same flock, any two or all three types of lesions may be found. In the early stages of an outbreak the lesions found are sometimes all of the nodular variety, but after a time the more severe cheesy membranous deposits appear in the mouth and pharynx. The period of incubation is usually between 3 and 12 days, and bad housing conditions, severe weather, and poor feeding serve to lower vitality and render an outbreak much more serious.

In the oculo-nasal form, after a watery nasal discharge has been evident, a change to a purulent discharge is seen. Later this becomes thickened and gummy, and inflammation and swelling of the eyes and of the sinuses of the head occur. The sinuses become filled with inspissated material with considerable bulging of the side of the head, below and in front of the eye-sockets.

Sick birds stand about with a dejected appearance; move without vigour; droop their wings and tail, which become soiled with fæces; the comb and wattles are soft and become bluish or purplish in colour; the birds eat little, swallow with difficulty, are unable to breathe easily, especially when the disease has advanced to the upper air passages; hens cease to lay; and loss of condition in all varieties is very marked. In some cases there is a white diarrhœa, which has a putrid odour.

Upon catching and examining the affected birds, one is invariably struck with the often complete absence of resistance and struggling, although they may emit hoarse, woeful cries. If the mouth be examined the lesions are easily seen in almost every case. The mucous membranes show patches of a greyish, fairly firm, cheesy-looking material, which is of considerable thickness, and not easy to detach. This is the 'false membrane'. In many cases the entrance to the trachea is partially blocked with these deposits, and the breathing is consequently obstructed. The smell from the mouth is always foul. Eyes and nostrils are often similarly affected, the lids of the former being sometimes adherent to each other and much swollen.

It should be noted that all of these deposits, and any discharges from membranes that are thus affected, as well as the droppings from a diseased bird, are highly infective.

Treatment.—It has been proved that curative treatment is economically unsound. The best measures consist of the slaughter of all affected birds and the inoculation of the healthy ones with 'pigeon-pox vaccine'. This confers immunity to infection with fowl-pox virus, although it is not possible to distinguish between the two except by experimental inoculation. Any birds which recover develop an immunity against further infection. (*Note.*—Pigeon-pox vaccine does not render pigeons immune to infection and must not be used for them.)

Prevention.—Newly purchased birds should be isolated for 3 weeks before being added to the flock, and after returning from shows, laying trials, etc., the same procedure should be adopted.

Vaccination can be done at 6 weeks of age; or, more usually, between 3 and 4 months of age.

Emphasis must be laid on the fact that when only a limited number of birds are kept upon a premises where the disease has appeared it is invariably cheaper in the long run to clear out the whole flock, allow a period to elapse after disinfection, and to restock with a completely new flock of birds. The apparently healthy members of such a flock that have been killed may be used for human consumption without any risks, but those that show lesions should be burnt or buried in quicklime.

FOWL TYPHOID.—This disease is also known as 'Klein's Disease', after Klein, who first investigated it in Wales in 1886. It is an acute infectious disease of fowls (also of ducks, geese, turkeys, game and wild birds) caused by the *Salmonella gallinarum.*

The disease has a world-wide distribution, and in Great Britain it has caused losses in Wales, Yorkshire, and neighbouring counties.

Most outbreaks occur in pullets near point of lay, but birds of all ages are susceptible—even chicks. The disease is usually introduced into a flock by the purchase of 'carrier' fowls, and thereafter spreads by contamination of food and water with the droppings of such birds. The incubation period is from 4 to 6 days.

Symptoms are not always characteristic. There is generally marked drowsiness, loss of appetite, and great weakness. The fowls prefer to sit about in dark corners. The comb and wattles are sometimes pale and anæmic; but they may in other cases be markedly congested. A greenish-yellow diarrhœa is usually present. Death, following progressive weakness, results in from 4 to 14 days after the onset of the symptoms. The percentage mortality varies from about 20 to 80 per cent, and many or most of the recovered birds become 'carriers', which serve to spread the disease to other birds.

Treatment.—Fowl typhoid is a dangerous disease, and if it is suspected immediate measures should be undertaken. It is desirable to obtain an early and accurate diagnosis, and to this end a dead fowl should be sent to a reliable poultry research laboratory, where a bacteriological examination will be carried out.

If fowl typhoid is diagnosed, samples of blood from the surviving and apparently healthy birds should be submitted to the agglutination test, and all reactors should be isolated and destroyed; the carcases being burned or buried in quicklime. The remaining birds should be treated with furazolidone for 10 days, moved to fresh premises, and re-treated

Prevention.—'9R' vaccine.

After removal of the reacting birds, the houses, utensils, etc., should be disinfected.

FOX, DISEASES OF.—In North America and other parts of the world, wild foxes occasionally become victims of rabies, and spread this disease to farm live-stock which they may attack. A history of aggressiveness and the frequenting of populated areas does not, however, point conclusively to rabies; distemper may be the reason. (*See also* FOX ENCEPHALITIS *below, and* CHASTEK PARALYSIS.)

The fox acts as host of the roundworm

TOXOCARA CANIS and of the *Toxascaris leonina*, and if silver fox cubs are reared by a cat, they may become infected with *Toxocara mystax* of the cat. The fox harbours the dog tapeworms *Tænia serialis*, and *T. multiceps*, and *Echinococcus granulosus*. Leptospirosis occurs in foxes in the U.K., and may be spread to farm livestock. (Five strains have been isolated.) Flukes may infest foxes.

FOX ENCEPHALITIS.—This disease is of veterinary interest and commercial importance on the fox ranches of North America, where these animals are bred for their fur. The disease is considered identical with Rubarth's disease of dogs.

Symptoms.—Young foxes in good condition are most frequently affected. A violent convulsion is followed by a lethargic or 'sleep-walking' state. This may be followed by excitability and more convulsions—during which the slamming of a door or any loud noise may prove fatal. The illness runs a very rapid course, from 1 hour to 3 days, 24 hours being the average duration.

Control.—By means of serum and preventive inoculation.

This disease, or one caused by a similar virus, accounted for the deaths of (wild) foxes in Britain in 1959 and 1960. During this period, many young foxes are believed to have died as the result of eating birds poisoned by Dieldrin. Symptoms are similar.

FOXGLOVE POISONING (*see* DIGITALIS POISONING).

FOXY OATS are oats which have been allowed to become wet, have fermented, and then have been dried. They have a mouldy or musty smell, which is said to be like the characteristic odour emitted by the fox, and can be easily recognised. They are generally stained a reddish-golden colour on the outside of the husks—a fact which also may be partly responsible for their name. When chewed they have a bitter unpleasant taste, quite unlike the normal pleasant taste of oats. Horses very often will refuse to eat foxy oats when they have been well fed previously, but they usually eat them without objection when the general level of the feeding is low.

When suddenly fed to horses in full quantities they are very frequently the cause of an outbreak of severe diarrhœa in which large amounts of mucus are passed. They also cause the horse to pass larger quantities of urine than usual (*polyuria*). It is not often that are they responsible for deaths.

FRACTURES (*frango*, I break) are defined as being 'sudden and violent solutions in the continuity of bones, produced by external or internal violence'.

Varieties.—It is possible to divide fractures up into a large number of different classes, but the two great and important divisions are those which are simple and those which are compound.

Simple fractures are the commonest variety, and consist of those in which the bone is broken clean across, with or without much tearing and laceration of the soft parts surrounding it, but without any wound leading from the fracture through to the skin. They are spoken of as being transverse, longitudinal, or oblique, according to the direction of the break.

Compound fractures are those in which the skin is injured, so that a direct or indirect communication between the fracture and the outside air exists. In them the broken end of one bone very often penetrates through the skin and is found exposed. They are extremely serious for a number of reasons: the bleeding is apt to be very severe; infection of the ends of the bones with organisms of a dangerous nature may occur, whereby healing is greatly retarded or made impossible; replacement of the severed ends into apposition is difficult or impossible; and great deformity results in the few cases which eventually do heal. For all these reasons the greatest care is necessary in the handling of an animal's fractured limb lest a simple fracture be converted into a compound one.

Complete fractures are those in which the bone is broken completely across and no connection remains between the pieces.

Incomplete fractures are those in which the bone is broken only partly across, or in which the tough periosteum (the tissue covering the bone) is not torn. This variety occurs mainly in the shin-bones (tibiæ) of horses which have been kicked, and in the bones of young animals. In some cases the bone cracks like a twig half-way across, and then splits for some distance along its length, just as does a branch which has been cut half-way through and then bent; these fractures are known as 'greenstick fractures'.

Fissured fractures are mere cracks in the bone which are found in the skull and face bones after blows or falls. They are usually not serious unless hæmorrhage accompanies them and the blood-clot presses upon a nerve or on the brain itself.

Deferred fractures occur when the bone has actually been fractured, but owing to the presence of powerful muscles, or to a strong covering of periosteum, the fractions do not separate until or unless some extra severe strain is put upon the part. They sometimes follow kicks on the insides of the fore-arms and thighs of the horse. No fracture is apparent at the time of the injury, but when the horse next lies down or rises, or is made to turn sharply, the fractured portions are torn apart.

which there is much splintering, the term *sequestra* being applied to those splinters of bone which are separated and eventually die.

Impacted fractures are those in which, after the break has occurred, one fragment is jammed inside another, usually at an angle.

Ununited fractures are those in which, after the usual time has elapsed for the fracture to heal, it is found that union has not taken place. The failure to unite may be simply due to 'delayed union', in which the process of repair is actually proceeding, though it is slow on account of debility or other illness (especially septic

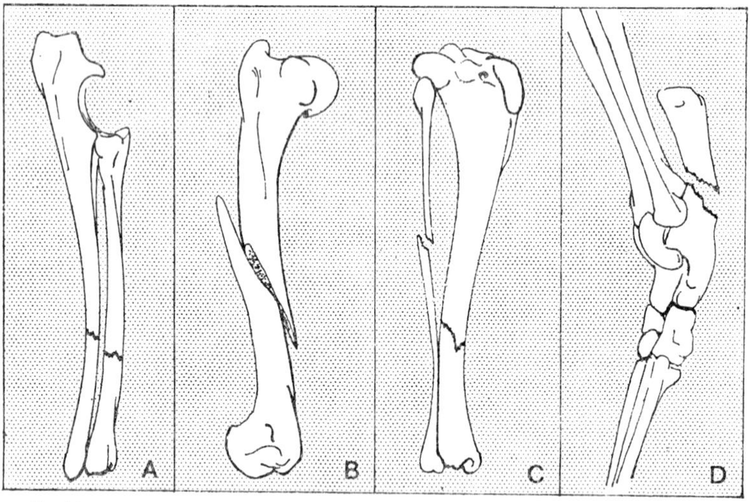

Classification of fractures. A. Transverse fracture with excellent stability after reduction. B. Oblique fracture with no stability after reduction. C. Slightly oblique fracture which, by virtue of the irregularity of the fracture line, provides a useable degree of stability after reduction. D. A typical distracted fracture. (*With acknowledgements to the British Veterinary Association.*)

Distracted fractures are those in which muscular contraction causes the detached fragment to be drawn away from the main body of the bone.

Depressed fractures also occur in the skull bones as a rule, and consist of fractures in which a fragment of bone is forced in below the level of the surrounding surface. They may give rise to very serious symptoms when the depressed portion presses upon the brain substance.

Complicated fractures are those in which there is some other serious injury produced in addition to the fracture, *e.g.* dislocation of the dog's hip along with fracture of the shaft of the femur, tearing of a large nerve, etc.

Comminuted fractures are those in

absorption) or on account of damage to the main artery which supplies the bone with blood (*nutrient artery*) ; or it may be due to the fact that the limb or other member is not kept at rest sufficiently for the process of healing to occur. In other cases of ununited fracture a piece of muscle or other tissue becomes placed between the broken ends of the bones and effectively prevents their union. It is only possible to remedy such by operation. In a few cases in old animals, no matter for how long the limb is kept bandaged, signs of healing never begin to show themselves ; after weeks of treatment the limb is as useless as when the fracture took place. Where the animal is of some value it is usually possible to bring the ends together by wire sutures or by a silver plate through which screws pass into the bone, but actual bony union in such cases is usually incomplete.

Causes.—In a number of cases some bony disease in which there is a reduction in the density of the bone, such as osteomalacia, is a cause of fracture on account of the lessened tensile strength of the bones, but by far the greater number of fractures among animals is due to external violence of an accidental nature. The violence may be applied direct to the bone, and the bone may break at the part where the force is applied, or it may break at some distant part. A certain number of fractures result from muscular action, and will be considered later.

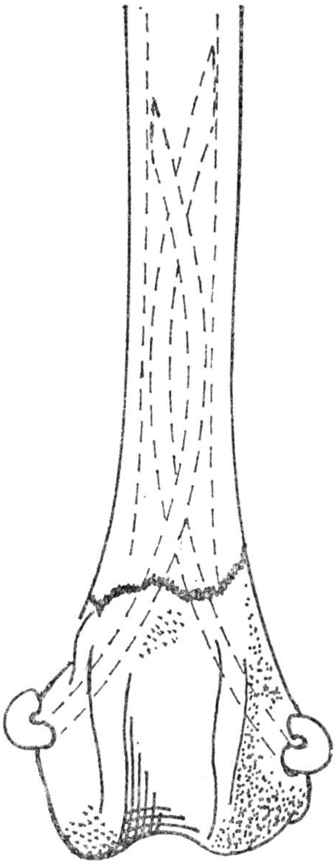

Two Rush-type intramedullary pins used to repair a supracondyloid fracture of the femur.

Direct violence.—The nature of the external violence determines to some extent what form the fracture will take and how serious it will be, but it is generally impossible to diagnose the kind of fracture from a consideration of the injury only.

Among the commoner of the agents causing fracture may be mentioned the following :

In *Horses*.—Kicks, falls, blows, errors in judgment during jumping, accidents when the animal collides with some stationary object, or is struck by a vehicle. Upon active service fractures frequently result from injury from rifle-bullets, shrapnel, or high-explosive shells, and they are then usually of a very serious nature, since there is nearly always much splintering.

In *Cattle*.—Fractures result from injuries during fighting, slipping, and falling when struggling, running, or during service, from jumping fences, hedges, ditches, from crowding accidents at markets, fairs, sales, etc., and from crushes in cattle-trucks on the railway. Cattle may be kicked by a horse and sustain serious fractures of the shoulder-blades or pelvis, or they may have limbs broken in the same way, and blows from heavy or large objects may have a like effect.

Fracture of the third phalanx in a medial front claw is commonly associated with fluorine poisoning, and causes cattle to stand with their legs crossed. (*See also* SHOEING.)

In *Pigs* and *Sheep*.—The causes are usually similar, but much less force is required to effect the fracture, and their legs are broken more easily. Such things as thrown stones, sticks or other objects, and the careless use of the shepherd's crook, are responsible for many. Falling over precipices and getting a limb fast in a gate, fence, or hurdle, may also result in a broken bone.

In *Dogs* and *Cats*.—The limbs, pelvis, or vertebræ are often fractured through being run over by vehicles. Falling from heights (especially in puppies and kittens), being tramped upon by human beings or animals, as well as getting injured by agricultural implements, and in greyhounds, injuries during racing, are other causes.

Indirect violence results from force applied to a part of the limb, but instead of the bone breaking in the immediate vicinity it snaps at the weakest part. It results from causes as mentioned under the previous heading, as well as from such occurrences as horses or cattle putting their feet into rabbit-holes when galloping and breaking their legs high up, and from dogs or cats caught by the paws in rabbit-traps and sustaining fractures of the femur.

Muscular action in a few instances produces fracture. When a horse becomes cast in its stall, or is cast for operation, it sometimes sustains a fracture of the lumbar vertebræ (*i.e.* ' breaks its back ') through struggling; this is due to the powerful action of the loin muscles which contract too vigorously. When a horse is galloping along the seashore, where the sand does not provide a firm surface from which to ' push off ', it may suddenly go dead lame from a split pastern caused by excessive muscular flexing action.

Symptoms.—The chief signs of a fracture are *uselessness of the part, crepitus of the fragments,* and sometimes *unnatural mobility* and *deformity*. If a limb is affected there is usually an unnatural mobility, inability to sustain weight, distortion or deformity, shortening of the length, a thickness or swelling at the seat of the fracture (due to overlapping of the fragments), and a variable amount of pain. Pain is by no means a certain characteristic of fracture; very often little or no pain is shown so long as the parts remain at rest, but it appears upon movement or manipulation; while in many cases showing very great pain damage has been sustained by the softer tendons or ligaments but the bones are intact. Where the pelvis is fractured there is usually some deformity, inability to stand (not invariable), a greater or lesser degree of paralysis of the hind parts, and pain on pressure or on manipulation of the hind-limbs. When the vertebral column is broken there is always both motor and sensory paralysis of the parts behind the seat of the injury, an inability to rise from the ground or to stand when lifted, and great general distress, the horse breaking out in a patchy sweat, and the dog crying and moaning, or shrieking when moved. In fractures of the skull it depends upon whether the brain cavity is involved, or whether the fracture merely affects one or more of the facial bones. In the former cases, death usually results in a short time, or before it occurs there may be unconsciousness, paralysis, unusual movements, convulsions or other symptoms of mental derangement. If the bones of the air sinuses are fractured little may be noticed beyond the actual injury and the deformity in contour resulting, but if the bones of the nose or jaws are involved, the breathing may be stertorous, hæmorrhage may be excessive, and feeding may be impossible.

The diagnostic feature of all fractures is the grating sound (*crepitus*) heard or felt when the broken fragments are passively made to rub against each other, but crepitus is by no means always in evidence. In parts where the bone is covered by large masses of muscle it is often quite impossible to evoke it; where the bones are ' over-ridden ' (*i.e.* overlapping), muscular action may effectively prevent it, and where a portion of a torn muscle or other tissue has become insinuated between the broken ends it is not possible to produce it. It should only be sought for by skilled hands, for a considerable amount of tearing and laceration of soft tissues, arteries, nerves, etc., may result from the sharp ends of broken bones being carelessly moved about by inexperienced hands.

Healing of fractures.—When the bone breaks, many vessels, both in its substance and in the periosteum, are torn, and accordingly a large clot of blood forms around the ends, between them, and for some distance up the inside of the bone. Later, great numbers of white blood corpuscles find their way into this clot, which becomes ' organised ', blood-vessels and, later, fibrous tissue being formed in it (*soft callus*). Next, lime salts are gradually deposited in this fibrous tissue, which thus develops into bone (*hard callus*). In this process a thick ring of new bone forms round the broken ends, filling up all crevices; and when union is complete, this thickening is again gradually absorbed, leaving the bone as it was before the injury. When the fragments have not been properly set, but allowed to remain overlapping, a considerable thickening remains, the ring of new bone becoming permanent for the sake of strength.

Treatment.—After it has been ascertained that an animal has sustained a major fracture, whether of a limb, pelvis, shoulder-blade, or skull, it should be taken with all care to a veterinary surgeon if it can be moved, or one should be sent for if it is badly injured. No attempt should be made on the part of the owner or an unskilled person to set and bandage the part. There is a very great liability that serious (perhaps irremediable) damage may be occasioned to the animal, and with dogs especially the kindly-intentioned but skill-less person may possibly be bitten. No matter how quiet an animal is naturally, it is not always tractable when it is suffering acute pain from the movement of a fractured part.

Generally speaking, the treatment of fractures consists of reduction, apposition, and immobilisation. Reduction and apposition are brought about by manipulation of the fractured bones under an-

FRACTURES OF SPECIAL PARTS

æsthesia. Immobilisation is then effected by means of plaster of Paris, and various proprietary mixtures impregnated into bandages. Splints of metal, leather, wood, or cardboard, padded with cotton-wool, are useful, especially with dogs and cats. Recently special types of extension splints, having transverse pins which transfix the bone, have been used with success in appropriate cases. Medullary pins, driven down the marrow cavity of long bones; wiring; and plating, have all been used with success. (*See* BONE-PINNING.)

Whenever splints, plaster, or other bandages are being applied to fractured limbs it is essential to ensure that the surface of the skin is well padded with cotton-wool, and that the pressure is evenly distributed. Failure in this respect may result in parts of the skin becoming gangrenous through obstruction to the blood-flow.

As a rule it takes about 3 to 5 weeks for a fracture of one of the long bones of a dog's limb to set, 2 to 3 weeks for a small bone in the foot, and a variable time for the pelvis or shoulder-blade. In horses where the treatment of fractures is limited in application the time needful varies from three weeks to about two months before healing is complete. In cattle it is about the same.

FRACTURES OF SPECIAL PARTS.—

1. **The cranium.**—Commonest in horses, but may occur in any animal; results from direct or indirect external violence, and often proves serious. Great swelling and bruising of the skin; pain on pressure always marked; hæmorrhage may be external or internal into brain cavity; sometimes symptoms of brain injury. Treatment consists of rest, antiseptic applications if necessary, protection from further injury, elevation of any depressed plates of bone, and protective plasters, charges, etc., later.

2. **The face bones.**—Common in all animals from external violence; may be simple or serious according to bones involved. Nasal bones, often fractures from accidents, and accompanied by swelling, pain, hæmorrhage, difficulty in breathing, much watering of the eyes. Jaw-bones broken from falls, kicks, etc., and usually interfere with feeding. Lower jaw fractures usually result in an open hanging mouth, escape of saliva, altered expression, and frequently loose teeth, torn lips, and hæmorrhage are in evidence. Bones of orbit fractured by falls on to side of head, collisions, etc.; interference with vision and with movements of lower jaw, in most cases serious. Treatment necessitates operation usually; removal of broken pieces, elevation of depressed portions, removal of loose teeth, wiring or plating broken parts together; removal of eye, etc. Feeding must be carefully undertaken when jaws are injured; sloppy food, mashes, etc., for horse, hand-feeding for dog.

3. **The vertebræ.**—May occur in all animals: commonest in horse and dog through accidents, *e.g.* getting cast in stall, casting for operation (muscular action), run-over accidents in dogs, falls from heights, blows from sticks. Result in paralysis, if whole vertebra is fractured, or in local disturbance if only a process is affected. Often a fatal termination, or necessitates destruction. Otherwise treatment consists in rest, protection, restraint from vigorous exercise, lying down, etc. Slinging the horse upon occasion. In small animals usually advisable to employ X-rays. Tail-bones often broken in dogs and cattle through getting caught in doors, gates, fences, etc. Very often compound, the skin being burst. Frequently necessitates amputation.

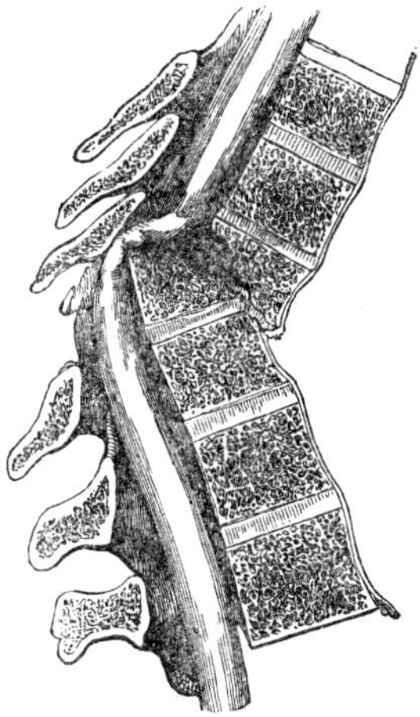

Fracture of vertebræ causing pressure on the spinal cord and paralysis of the parts behind the fracture. (Miller's *Surgery*.)

4. **The ribs.**—Seen in all animals. Due to external violence usually, but first rib of horse sometimes broken through muscular action in a side-slip and violent recovery, when it often results in radial paralysis. (*See* RADIAL PARALYSIS.) Otherwise broken ribs show little or

nothing characteristic except local pain and deformity, unless many involved, when breathing may be short and difficult. When severe and many broken pieces present, some may penetrate lungs, setting up pleurisy or pneumonia, with discharge of blood from nose or mouth (blood bright red and frothy). Air may gain entrance to chest (pneumothorax) and complicate recovery. Treatment depends on case and extent of injury. Destruction often necessary eventually.

5. **The pelvis.**—Always severe, and frequently fatal in any animal. Due to external violence, falls, collisions, run over accidents, etc. Occurs sometimes during service in bull and stallion when their hind-feet slip from under them and they fall backwards on to buttocks. Least serious when only external angle of ilium ('point of hip') involved. Lameness and stiffness always seen; sometimes paralysis of hind-quarters, inability to retain urine and fæces, and loss of sensation in hind parts, are seen. Treatment depends on case. Destruction sometimes necessary.

6. **The shoulder-blade.**—Not common. May occur in any animal. Mostly occur through neck of bone, or on the projecting spine. Clothing of muscles impedes diagnosis but assists recovery, acting as natural bandage.

7. **The humerus.**—Met with in all animals, due to external violence, muscular action when turning quickly in horses. Lameness intense in all animals; usually limb quite useless. Horses and cattle do not make good recoveries except when young, but other animals more satisfactory. Absolute rest essential; horses may be slung; bandaging usually useless except in dog; muscles act as natural bandages in many simple fractures; destruction often most humane course. (*See* BONE-PINNING.)

8. **The radius and ulna.**—Met with in horses and dogs mostly. Due to external violence—kicks and falls. One or both bones may be broken; fracture of ulna less serious unless elbow-joint involved. In dogs, if one broken the other acts as a natural splint. Lameness always marked, and pain on pressure. Local swelling usually noticed, and deformity. Bandaging useful and advisable. Young horses placed in slings. Frequently bones are fractured in horses but do not separate because of powerful periosteum. Known as a *deferred fracture*; always liable to become a complete fracture if movement is not restricted and lying, or turning sharply, prevented. Usually large callus formation follows recovery, which takes months to disappear. Bone-pinning has been carried out successfully in the dog and in the horse.

9. **Bones of knee.**—Seldom fractured except from shrapnel, bullets, etc. Impossible to bring about recovery without stiffening of joint (ankylosis). Occurs rarely in dogs, from very severe crushes; in such cases recovery very problematical, and so limb usually amputated just above injury.

10. **The metacarpals.**—Most often seen in horse and dog from external violence, but may occur in former through muscular action or twist when galloping on soft ground. In horses all three bones usually fractured; in dog may be only one or two. Generally not very serious in latter animal. In horse good recoveries made when fracture is clean across without complications or splinters. Those occurring in middle of cannon most satisfactory. Limb bandaged; horse slung; bandages left in position for at least six weeks. In dog simple bandage left on for 2 to 3 weeks. Usually little or no resulting callus or blemish when well set.

11. **The pastern bone.**—Comparatively common in fast, light horses, due to slips, falls, false steps, and sometimes to blows. May be transverse, oblique, or longitudinal ('split pastern'), often comminuted. Severe lameness always seen, but diagnosis often difficult without X-rays. Recovery or otherwise depends upon case; simple transverse fractures satisfactory if temperament of horse will allow rest and slinging; oblique, longitudinal, and all comminuted cases unsatisfactory, and if recovery occurs usually some deformity or blemish left. Bandaging in strong plaster or pitch, without hard splints, but with plenty of cotton-wool, and bandages applied tightly, best for most cases.

12. **The 2nd phalanx, coffin- and navicular bones.**—Fractures in these bones are rare; caused by direct violence, and sometimes follow operation of neurectomy (un-nerving). Fracture of coffin-bone if simple and joint surfaces not involved makes good recovery as a rule, since hoof acts as splint and bandage. Fracture of 2nd phalanx (short pastern bone) usually very unsatisfactory. Fracture of navicular bone also unsatisfactory and difficult to diagnose; sometimes happens during course of navicular disease. Prolonged

rest necessary, and great danger of large exostosis or hard callus remaining after apparent recovery.

13. **The femur.**—May occur in all animals; very common in dogs after street accidents. Nearly always results from external violence, direct or indirect; shaft, neck, or one of the trochanters may be involved. Frequently in dogs dislocation of the hip-joint accompanies fracture. Diagnosis in small animals most satisfactory by X-ray examination. Extreme lameness, shortening of the limb, local swelling, and great pain on movement usually seen. There may or may not be crepitus. In horse, fracture of pelvis very often accompanies fractured femur and makes diagnosis difficult. Usually necessitates destruction in large animals, but in small animals recovery more likely. In the latter the fracture will very often heal by expectant treatment, but a special extension splint to prevent over-riding and consequent shortening of the limb is very often required. Persistent lameness or stiffness for many months after fracture has healed is common.

14. **The patella.**—May be split across from a fall or rifle-bullet in horses and cattle. Is a very serious condition. Results in a lowering of the affected stifle and inability to advance the limb. There is great pain and much swelling over the stifle. Only treatment is union of the fragments by wire sutures; difficult to perform, and seldom does complete recovery follow.

15. **The tibia.**—Common in all animals; very often results from kicks on the inside of the hind-leg, and from slips or false steps on uneven or slippery surfaces when going at fast paces. Deferred fractures on inside of limb about half-way between stifle and hock very often result from kicks in horses. In pigs and dogs run-over and other accidents are often the cause, and in them the fibula may be fractured as well or either bone may remain intact. Deferred fractures in cattle and horses very often become complete through the extra strain put on leg when rising or lying down, and in treatment it is necessary to prevent this as far as possible by slinging. Many fractures of tibia become compound from sharp points of broken bones penetrating through the skin, and except in dogs destruction is generally necessary when this occurs Treatment must be according to case—plaster charges, bandaging with or without splints in foals, calves, sheep, and dogs, but not usually advisable in adult horses and cattle unless fracture is low down. Extension apparatus often necessary to prevent over-riding of the bones. Adult horses sometimes do well in slings with no other appliances except short sawdust bedding to prevent entanglement of feet. (*See* BONE-PINNING which has been used successfully in dog, cat, and horse.)

16. **Bones of hock.**—Fracture of os calcis (point of hock) through falling backwards when rearing or through the hind-limbs of heavy horses slipping forwards when backing loads on hard surfaces, pavements, etc. The same fracture also sometimes seen in young cattle shut up in damp yards and being forced for show or sale purposes; in these the epiphyseal summit becomes torn away from the rest of the bone by an undue pull of the Achilles' tendon (hamstring). Fractures of other bones of hock are less common (with the exception of the SCAPHOID in the racing greyhound) and very difficult to diagnose without the use of X-rays. (*See* SCAPHOID; BONES, ARTIFICIAL; WIRING.)

17. **The lower bones of the leg.**—What has been said as applied to the fore cannons, pasterns, and coffin-bones, etc., is almost equally applicable to the hind-limbs, but in a hind-limb a similar fracture is more serious than in a fore-limb.

FREEMARTIN.—A sterile heifer born twin to a normal bull calf. Blood typing can determine whether an animal is a freemartin or not. In one series, 228 freemartins were found out of 242 sets of twins. For an explanation of how freemartins are caused, and blood circulation diagram, *see* p. 383.

Pig freemartins may occur.

FREEZE-BRANDING (*See* BRANDING).

FREMITUS (*fremitus*, a low noise) is the name given to a sensation which is communicated to the hand of an observer when it is laid across the chest in certain diseases of the lungs and heart. Friction fremitus is a grating feeling communicated to the hand by the pleura or pericardium when it is roughened as in pleurisy or pericarditis.

FROG (*see* FOOT OF HORSE).

FROG-PADS are cushions made of either rubber or leather and composition, which are affixed to a leather sole, and used for preventing or minimising shock to the feet of horses. They are applied below the shoe, the leather sole to which they are attached being nailed on along with the shoe, and are of most service where the natural frog of the foot is not well developed. Whenever they are applied they

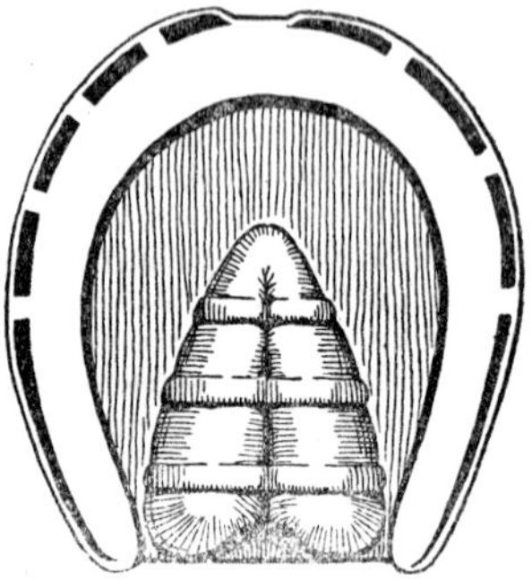

Shoe with leather sole and frog-pad.

should be stuffed with tar and tow to prevent the feet from becoming brittle; while the pad of tow prevents small stones from working in below the leather sole and perhaps damaging the sole of the foot.

FRONTAL BONE is the bone of the skull which lies immediately in front of the parietal in the region of the forehead. It is a roughly quadrilateral plate-like bone which forms part of the roof of the cranium and passes forward between the eyes to meet the nasal bones. In the horned breeds of cattle and sheep it is extended laterally to form the horn cores. (*See* BONES, *also* SINUSES OF SKULL.)

FRONTAL SINUS (*see* SINUSES OF SKULL).

FROST-BITE results from the action of extreme cold upon extremities of the body for some time. Local areas may be frozen for a short time without suffering any serious effects, and this use is made of freezing in the production of anæsthesia for small surgical operations in some cases. The condition affects all animals which are exposed to severe cold for long periods, and generally affects those parts of the body most severely which are at a distance from the heart, such as the feet of horses (especially the skin of the coronets and bulbs of the heels), the tips of the ears of sheep and lambs, the tails of lambs and dogs, the horns of cattle (seldom) and the tips of their tails. It is not uncommon in the comb and wattles of poultry, and in these parts may be severe, resulting in death and sloughing of the areas affected. It has also been recorded in the tail and ears of pigs in northern countries.

Symptoms.—Actually what happens in frost-bite is that the blood of the vessels becomes frozen, there is a disturbance of nutrition, and the parts supplied by the blood die, and finally gangrene sets in. There are two distinct forms: in the more severe, the circulation never returns to the part; it shrivels up and dry gangrene sets in without any inflammation, the part being eventually cast off from the rest of the body. In the less severe and more common variety the area is frozen but the tissues are not so completely injured; in a short while the blood-flow is re-established, the frozen blood becoming thawed, and the circulation proceeds. A severe inflammation follows, however; the area becomes extremely painful, moist gangrene sets in, suppuration occurs, and after a time the injured tissues are sloughed off. It is said that the greater the redness of the skin during frost-bite the poorer the chances of recovery.

Treatment.—The condition is not usually noticed until it has passed to a stage of moist or dry gangrene. In instances where an animal is found with a part stiffly frozen it should be first well rubbed with snow or immersed in cold water, and never plunged into warm or hot water. Stimulants should be avoided, but if possible the animal should be made to walk to restore the general circulation. Alcohol increases the danger of sloughing by dilating the frozen arteries and encouraging swelling. A little oil should be rubbed into the frozen parts as soon as they have begun to feel softer, or they may be massaged with vaseline or petroleum jelly, and if necessary they may be bandaged in cotton-wool. The treatment of gangrene which follows, and which is often in evidence as soon as the condition is noticed, is the same as given under GANGRENE.

FROST STUDS, FROST COGS, or **FROST CALKS,** are anti-slipping devices which are used for application to horses' shoes. They are made either with tapered shanks or with shanks which have a thread-cut round them. In either case they are inserted into complementary recesses in the heels or toes of the shoes. Such as are made with a thread to screw into the shoe are not so liable to become loose and work out when the horse is walking, but they necessitate the use of a blank cog during ordinary weather to preserve the thread in the recess, so that it does not become burred over as the shoe wears. Those made with a tapered shank are driven into the tapered recess whenever they are required. Both kinds should be removed every night, since they are liable to inflict damage when the horse lies down. The heads of frost studs are made in some pattern which will give a good grip and not quickly wear blunt if a thaw sets in ; some are conical, some pyramidal, chisel-shaped, H, T, N, or O-shaped, while others are made in the form of a cross, etc. They are probably the best form of anti-slipping device for use in countries where the roads may be frozen for only a few days at a time.

FULLERING consists in making a groove on the lower (ground) surface of horses' shoes, in which the heads of the nails can be accommodated. The fuller also gives a better grip upon turf or roads than is the case with a flat, plain shoe. The groove which constitutes the fuller is made by a ' fullering-iron ' which presses the hot iron when struck by a hammer when the shoe is being made.

FUMIGATION (*fumigo*, I smoke) is a means of disinfection by the use of the vapour of powerful chemicals. (*See* DISINFECTION.)

FUNCTIONAL DISEASES are disorders in which some part or organ does not act properly, although after death no change can be found to account for the condition. Thus functional paralysis may affect a part, yet the nerves, muscles, and associated areas of the brain show no change from the normal. The heart may beat weakly or irregularly, although the valves and heart muscles are quite sound. It is in connection with the nervous system that functional diseases are most often associated, and the amount of knowledge upon them is limited. The opposite condition to ' functional ' disease is ' organic ' disease, where there is some cause for the symptoms, such as a tumour, inflammation, degeneration of tissue, etc., and where the connection between the abnormal conditions and the symptoms is plain. Probablv all functional diseases are really organic in nature, but scientific methods of sufficient delicacy and detail have not yet been devised to enable even the most skilful to appreciate the changes.

FUNDUS (*fundus*) is the base or innermost part of a hollow organ distant from its mouth or opening. The fundus of the bladder is its innermost deepest cavity, and the fundus of the eye is the part behind the lens occupied by vitreous humour.

FUNGOID GROWTHS are ulcerating tumours which grow very rapidly and assume a mushroom-like appearance.

FUNGOUS DISEASES.—These include ASPERGILLOSIS, RINGWORM, ACTINOMYCOSIS, MUCORMYCOSIS, BLASTOMYCOSIS, MONILIASIS, MYCOTIC MASTITIS.

FURAZOLIDONE.—A drug used in the treatment of Blackhead and Hexamitiasis.

FURFURACEOUS (*furfur*, bran) is a term applied to skin diseases which produce a scaliness resembling bran.

FURUNCLE (*furunculus*, a little thief) is another name for a boil or abscess.

FURZE, or **GORSE** (*Ulex europæus*), which is a very common and plentiful shrub in waste lands in Great Britain, was often cut and used as fodder after chaffing or bruising. The plant contains a very small proportion of a poisonous alkaloid which is called *ulexine*, and is practically identical with *cytisine* from broom. It is a nerve and muscle poison, but it is not present in the plant in dangerous amounts, although there is more in the seeds. In many parts of the country furze is sown out on hill land and the young plants are eaten by sheep without ill effects. It is quite safe used in this way and also as a fodder when chaffed, provided it is cut before the seed-pods are full of ripened seeds. Preferably it should be cut before flowering.

The chief symptoms are the same as in broom poisoning. (*See* BROOM POISONING.)

G

GAD-FLY, 'GADDING' (*see* WARBLES).—In Britain, warble flies are on the wing from late May onwards. Bot-flies appear a little later.

GALACTOCELE (γάλα, milk; κήλη, tumour) is the name of a cyst-like swelling in the mammary gland caused by the obstruction of the milk-duct which normally carries the milk from the area to the milk sinus at the base of the teat. The condition is seen in sows and bitches, but is rare in cows.

GALENICAL PREPARATIONS are preparations of drugs that are sanctioned by the Pharmacopœia, or list of drugs and remedies published under Government regulations. The term 'official' is often used in the same sense, while 'officinal' (*officina*, a shop) means that the drug is procurable in ordinary shops.

GALL is another name for bile. (*See* BILE.)

GALL-BLADDER is the name of the little pouch-like sac in which bile produced by the liver is stored until it is required during the process of digestion. It is a hollow pear-shaped organ lying in a depression on the posterior surface of the liver, and connected by a short duct with the chief bile-duct, into which all the bile eventually finds its way. The gall-bladder is not present in the horse and in animals of the horse tribe, but is found in the other domesticated animals.

GALL-BLADDER, DISEASES OF.—Under heading LIVER will be found an account of the diseases of that organ; the gall-bladder is very often affected along with it.

BILIARY CONGESTION is, practically speaking, another name for obstruction to the flow of bile and reabsorption into the system. It results in jaundice (*see* JAUNDICE), the visible mucous membranes of the body becoming stained some shade of yellow or brown, and the general health of the animal suffering.

Causes.—Biliary congestion very frequently results from a catarrhal inflammation of the lining membrane of the gall-bladder and of the bile-ducts. This inflammation may be due to bacterial diseases such as tuberculosis or bacterial necrosis, or it may be due to one of the inorganic poisons, such as phosphorus or mercury. In some cases the presence of liver flukes or other parasites in the lower bile-ducts gives rise to an obstruction in the outflow of bile, and congestion results. Otherwise, practically any condition in which there is an obstruction to the free flow of bile down the bile-ducts into the small intestine causes a damming back of the bile in the gall-bladder and liver, and a gorging of all the little bile vessels. No further bile can be produced by the liver cells, and what has already been elaborated is very apt to be reabsorbed into the general circulation.

Symptoms.—The distension of the gall-bladder and the congestion of bile in the smaller bile-ducts results in pain over the region of the liver, sudden or gradual jaundice, and intestinal disturbance.

Treatment.—The general lines of treatment are given under jaundice, and depend upon the cause. The food must be of an easily digestible nature, fluid or semi-fluid as far as possible, and exercise should be encouraged unless the temperature is high.

GALL-STONES, which are also known as BILIARY CALCULI, are concretions which are formed in the gall-bladder or in the bile-ducts of the liver. They usually consist of bile salts deposited around something which acts as a nucleus. A small mass of bacteria, a piece of shed epithelium, which has become detached as the result of catarrhal inflammation of the ducts, or other solid particle, may act as a nucleus, but often the nucleus is only of microscopic size. Anything which results in an obstruction to the flow of bile into the intestine predisposes to gall-stone formation, such as the presence of flukes or other parasites in the lower ducts, but in some cases it is unknown how or why they form. As a rule they are hard, brownish in colour, coated with mucus, and of a more or less rounded shape.

They may be composed of cholestrin, cholestrin and bile pigments, or of pigment and lime salts. One or several may be present, as many as hundreds of small stones sometimes being found. They often cause no symptoms during life, and it is only in the abattoir or knackery that they are discovered, but in other cases they set up biliary congestion, jaundice, digestive disturbances, and even acute abdominal pain. In the latter case, generally occurring when small pointed stones are being passed down the bile-ducts into the intestines, they produce an acute attack of what is known as 'hepatic colic'.

Treatment.—The only rational treatment is the surgical removal of the gall-stone, after an accurate diagnosis has been established by X-ray examination.

GALL SICKNESS is another name for anaplasmosis of cattle. (*See under* PARASITES.)

GAME BIRDS, MORTALITY.—This may be considered under two headings:

From farm chemicals.—The most important of these are dieldrin, aldrin, and heptachlor, used as seed dressings; some of the organo-phosphorus insecticides such as schradan; dimethoate; the 'nitro-type' of weedkillers such as DNC, which stains the carcase yellow.

Even the relatively safe insecticides DDT and BHC can, if used in too high a concentration, prove lethal. Pheasant poults have died as a result of being treated for lice with a 5 per cent gamma benzene hexachloride dusting powder.

The organo-phosphorus insecticides, mentioned above, do not necessarily act quickly. Death may occur eight weeks after eating the poisoned food. The symptoms shown by poisoned birds include: ruffled feathers, saliva around the beak, high-stepping gait or unsteadiness on the legs, distressed breathing, and paralysis.

Spraying an orchard with either DDD or DDT has caused heavy game bird losses. A partridge was found dead in a field where blackcurrants had been sprayed with the insecticide Endrin. It was reported from the farm that eight or nine partridges died within a few hours of eating earthworms which came to the surface of the soil soon after spraying. Rat poisons may perhaps be included in the term 'farm chemicals'. Phosphorus and zinc phosphide have killed birds. Owls die after eating poisoned rodents.

From natural causes.—Impacted gizzard, roup, tuberculosis, aspergillosis, swine erysipelas, fowl-pox, fowl cholera, fowl typhoid, infectious sinusitis. 'Gapes' is another cause of death; in the U.S.A., Equine Encephalomyelitis. Deaths from Fowl Pest (Newcastle disease) have been reported in the U.K. Blackhead has been reported in pheasants and partridges. Experimentally, louping-ill is capable of killing grouse, and a natural infection is known to occur.

Moniliasis causes lethargy, stunted growth and a heavy mortality in partridges. Treatment with formic acid, sprayed on food, has proved successful in treatment. (*See also* BOTULISM.)

GAMETES (*see* GENETICS).

GAMGEE TISSUE is a dressing for wounds composed of a layer of cotton-wool between an upper and a lower layer of gauze or cheese-cloth. It is usually sterilised and may be impregnated with antiseptics. It has the advantage over cotton-wool that it can be removed from a wound intact, and does not leave small fragments adherent to the wound.

GAMMA GLOBULIN is a preparation of the protein fraction of the blood serum which contains the antibodies against certain bacteria or viruses. It can be prepared in a concentrated form and can be used to give protection against infection. (*See under* GLOBULIN.)

GAMMEXANE products contain the gamma isomer of benzene hexachloride, a highly effective, persistent insecticide, (*See* BENZENE HEXACHLORIDE.)

GANGLION (γάγγλιον, a swelling) is a term used to signify a concentration of nerve cells occurring upon the course of a nerve. In ganglia an alteration or an association of nerve impulses takes place, which are generally concerned with the sensory system as distinct from the motor, although motor stimuli may arise in ganglia and result in involuntary muscular action.

GANGRENE (γραίνω, I gnaw) means the death (necrosis) of a part of the body accompanied by putrefaction. In *primary gangrene* the germs which cause the necrosis also bring about the putrefactive changes. In *secondary gangrene* the putrefaction is caused by organisms which have invaded dead tissue (*e.g.* following a burn). There are two varieties of gangrene, *dry* and *moist*; dry gangrene is a condition of mummification in which the circulation stops and the part withers up, while in moist gangrene there is inflammation accompanied by putrefactive changes. The dead part, when it is formed of soft tissues, is known as a 'slough', and when it is a piece of bone it is called a 'sequestrum'.

Causes.—Certain diseases which lower the vitality of the body generally, or reduce the vital resistance of localised areas, predispose to the production of gangrene in parts which are subjected to pressure or strain. Thus, heart disease in thin animals, paralysis of the hind-quarters in cattle and horses, advanced tuberculosis in any animal, etc., are very liable to be complicated with gangrene of the skin covering bony prominences of the body; *e.g.* over the points of the hocks, hips, or elbows, and along the line of the sternum. Hard work in horses with an insufficiency of good food and badly fitting harness produce 'harness galls', which are local areas of dry gangrene in many cases. (*Note.*—These should not be confused with 'harness chafes', in which the surface of the skin is rubbed away by friction.) 'Sitfasts', which are patches of dry, leathery-looking skin with pus below them, found under the saddle when it is not well padded, are other examples of gangrene. 'Bed-sores', resulting from continued pressure against the ground when an animal is paralysed and cannot rise or turn on to the opposite side and so relieve the pressure, are in reality patches of gangrene. Otherwise, gangrene may be caused by almost any direct injury, such as a limb being crushed, or frozen, or burned by heat or powerful chemicals, or merely wounded in a simple manner and neglected afterwards. Malignant œdema produces gangrene of the skin and superficial tissues, usually about the head, and poisoning by ergot results in the same condition in the most distant parts of the body, *e.g.* the feet, tip of tail, ears, and the combs and wattles of poultry.

Symptoms.—There is at first a degree of pain when the affected part is handled, and in a short time it becomes reddened and swollen. Later it turns blue or black, the hair falls from it, and there is a distinct line of demarcation between the gangrenous and the healthy surface. Around the dividing line there is usually some degree of inflammation, and separation with pus production frequently occurs; this is especially the case in sitfasts in the horse. Once the area dies the pain usually subsides except when pressure is put upon it. In some cases a distinct foul odour is noticeable, particularly when there is oozing of pus from the edges of the gangrenous part. In the course of time complete separation between the healthy and the dead part takes place, and the latter is cast off as a slough, the remaining wound healing in the ordinary way.

Moist gangrene is perhaps commoner than the dry form, and is considerably more serious, since it is accompanied by putrefaction and the absorption of the poisonous products into the general circulation. The area becomes swollen, livid, and if on tender parts of the skin it is covered with blebs or blisters containing fluid. In a short while the whole patch turns black or greenish, the hair falls out, an offensive smell is evident, and much fluid exudes from the decomposing tissues. There is not usually a great deal of local pain, but general symptoms of fever, a high temperature, disturbed heart's action, and rapid breathing, are manifested. This form of gangrene always tends to spread to the surrounding parts, both superficially and deeply, and no line of demarcation can be distinguished. Shortly afterwards 'blood poisoning' sets in; there is a great deal of absorption of decomposing and decomposed fluids into the blood-stream, and the animal usually sinks into a weak state and dies in the course of from a week to a fortnight after the gangrene began.

Treatment.—In the dry form, immediate excision a little beyond the line of demarcation is necessary. All the dead portions are removed, and the underlying surface is scraped with a surgical spoon, to enable a new fresh healing surface to form, and the part closes as an open wound afterwards. In the moist form, free incision and antiseptic irrigation is often practised with success, but each case must be treated upon its merits. In many cases, *e.g.* the lower parts of the limbs of the smaller animals, immediate amputation before there has been any time for absorption to occur, is best. General treatment, in which the animal's strength is kept up, the heart's action is stimulated, and penicillin or sulphonamides are administered, must also be carried out. In advanced cases humane destruction becomes necessary. (*See also* FROST-BITE.)

GAPES is a disease of young chickens and turkeys particularly, although all the domesticated and many wild birds may also be affected, which is due to the presence of small worms in the bronchial tubes. The worms are called *Syngamus trachea*, or *Sclerostoma syngamus*, although another allied species, *Syngamus bronchialis*, which is slightly larger, is also sometimes found.

The presence of worms in the bronchial tubes and trachea of the bird causes it to gasp for breath or ' gape ', from which the name of the disease originated. Part of the life-history of the worm is passed in the body of the earthworm, and young chickens eating earthworms become affected. (*See also under* PARASITES, p. 667.)

Thiabendazole, given in the feed, is an effective method of treatment.

GARDEN CHEMICALS.—Birds, dogs, and cats may be poisoned as a result of the use of pesticides. For the poisoning of birds, *see preparations listed under* GAME-BIRDS. Dieldrin is highly toxic for cats, and like DDT, should not be used on them or in their vicinity. In fact, all the CHLORINATED HYDROCARBONS are best avoided in places where small domestic animals or their food may become contaminated. Pyrethrum is safe. For the dangers of slug-baits, *see* METALDEHYDE POISONING. (*See* ORCHARDS for the dangers of fruit-tree sprays. For seed dressings, *see under* SEED CORN.)

GARDEN NIGHTSHADE POISONING results from animals eating the exceptionally common Garden Nightshade (*Solanum nigrum*), which is found in practically all parts of the world except the extreme north and south, and has more than forty common names. Its toxicity appears to vary in different localities, for amounts which would prove fatal under ordinary circumstances are sometimes eaten by animals without ill effects. As a general rule, although exceedingly common, it is not very frequently eaten, partly because of its objectionable taste, and partly because it is more often found on arable and waste land than in pastures. The berries of this plant, or of species allied to it, which are variously called ' wonder-berries ' or ' huckleberries ', contain an active alkaloidal glucoside called *solanine*, which is readily converted into sugar and the poisonous *solanidine* by the action of the gastric juices in the stomach. It requires considerable amounts of this glucoside to be taken before fatal results follow. The symptoms are given as stupefaction, staggering, loss of sensation and consciousness, cramps and spasms, and sometimes convulsions. The treatment should consist of the administration of stimulants and strong black tea or coffee, the tannic acid which is present in them acting as a neutralising agent for the alkaloidal glucoside.

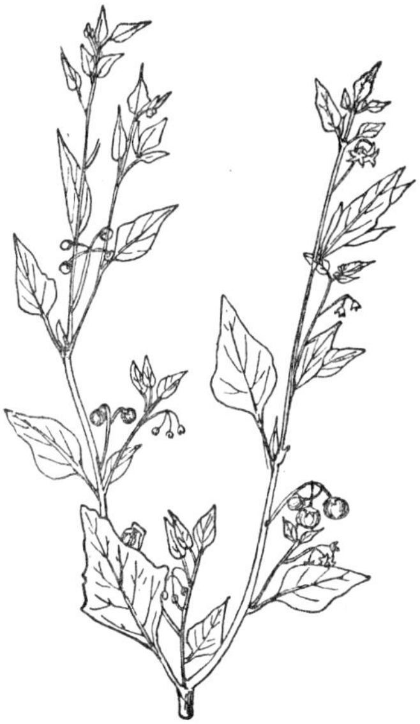

The Garden Nightshade, or Black Nightshade (*Solanum nigrum*). The leaves are ovate with central vein; flowers are small and bell-shaped, droop on short stalks and are of a dark purple colour; the fruit is a large shining-black, globular berry, several being attached to the one stalk. All parts of the plant contain proportions of the active alkaloidal glucoside *solanine*, of which large amounts are poisonous.

GARRON.—A useful type of horse for hill-farm work and carrying deer. Garrons do not constitute a separate breed, but were a cross between Western Island ponies and the Percheron. Nowadays, the Garron is regarded as a larger version of the Highland pony.

GAS (*see* ANÆSTHETICS, COAL-GAS, TYMPANY; etc.).

GAS GANGRENE is an acute bacterial disease due to the inoculation of wounds with organisms belonging to the 'gas gangrene' group. This group comprises anærobic organisms, most of which produce a gas when living in the animal body, and all of which are associated with decomposition of the tissues invaded. Some of these organisms possess the power of splitting up muscle and other tissues, and are called 'sarcolytic', while others decompose the sugars of the blood and are called 'saccharolytic'; both produce gas, and it is possible that organisms belonging to each group work together to produce their effects in the body. It includes the causal organisms of such diseases as black-quarter, braxy, lamb dysentery, and botulism.

Gas gangrene may attack any of the domestic animals and man. The horse is least resistant and the ox least susceptible. The bacilli are of world-wide distribution, being mainly present in the surface layers of soils that are intensively manured and cultivated. They are plentifully found in the digestive systems of the herbivorous animals, but in this position they are usually harmless unless the body vitality is lowered. After death they invade the walls of the intestines and the arteries and veins, where they produce decomposition and form gas, being materially responsible for the tumefaction of a carcase in the summer months.

Causes.—Gas gangrene is produced by the *Clostridium œdematiens, Cl. welchii, Cl. septique, Cl. Chauvei* gaining access to the tissues of an animal through a small wound. The disease germs may be introduced into the skin by an unclean hypodermic needle, through injuries inflicted by agricultural implements which are contaminated with soil, dung, etc.; they may enter the body through the wounds of castration or docking, through the abrasions that may be inflicted in the uterine mucous membrane after difficult foaling, and through other accidental injuries.

Symptoms.—A few hours after the germs gain entrance the area of invasion is found swollen, hot, painful on pressure, and may crackle when handled. This latter effect is due to gas formation below the skin. The skin and underlying tissues rapidly become discoloured and unhealthy-looking. If a wound is present the discharge from it becomes frothy and after a short time possesses a fœtid odour. Meantime the temperature rises, the pulse becomes fast but small and difficult to feel, the animal generally appears to be seriously distressed, and is extremely weak. In some cases the local areas swell to an enormous size, and the animal assumes a most unusual appearance; thus, when some part of the head is affected it may swell out of all proportion to the body, and somewhat resembles that of a hippopotamus. When following castration, the horse stands with its hind-limbs apart and has difficulty in moving; a large œdematous swelling appears in the scrotal region and spreads forwards along the lower line of the belly. The discharge from the wound is fœtid and may be blood-stained, and there is often an intense diarrhœa. Usually, death occurs within from 12 to 48 hours after the swellings appear.

When following parturition the symptoms are similar in general, with particular variations according to the area of invasion, *i.e.* the uterus or vagina. (*See* UTERUS, DISEASES OF, and its sub-heading 'Metritis'.)

Prevention consists in scrupulous attention to cleanliness such as is discussed under WOUNDS and ANTISEPTICS, in dealing with even the apparently slightest wounds in the horse. Immunisation can be effected by using sera, formalinised whole cultures of the organism. For cattle, cultures of *Cl. chauvœi* are often added. (*See also* BRAXY.)

GASSERIAN GANGLION is a nervous ganglion situated upon the course of the sensory division of the 5th cranial nerve at the point where it passes out of the cranial cavity through the foramen lacerum. The ganglion is crescentic in outline and about an inch in length.

GASTRALGIA (γαστήρ, the stomach; ἄλγος, pain) means pain in the stomach. (*See* DYSPEPSIA.)

GASTRECTASIS (γαστήρ, the stomach; ἔκταδις, stretching) means dilatation of the stomach. (*See* STOMACH, DISEASES OF.)

GASTRECTOMY (γαστήρ, the stomach; ἐκ, out; τέμνω, I cut) means an operation for the removal of the whole or part of the stomach.

GASTRIC (γαστήρ, the stomach) means anything connected with the stomach, *e.g.* gastric ulcer, gastric juice.

GASTRIC ULCERS.—In cattle, ulceration of the rumen may be associated with lesions in the liver caused by *Fusiformis necrophorus*. Ulcers in the abomasum are referred to on p. 886.

GASTRIC ULCERS IN PIGS.—Ulcers in the stomach occur, as is well known, during the course of swine fever. They have also been found in piglets, under a fortnight old, in association with a fungous infection. This is called MUCORMYCOSIS; the fungus itself being known as *Rhizopus microsporus*. This was isolated from the stomach ulcers and the pigs' bedding.

Concurrent with the Mucormycosis was another fungus infection, Moniliasis, caused by a yeast-like organism, *Candida albicans*, which was isolated from sores in the piglets' mouths and gullets, from bedding, drinking water, and the air in the pens.

Scouring was the only symptom observed in some of the piglets, apart from stunted growth in one or two which did not die during the early days of the attack. In others vomiting was also observed. Diagnosis was dependent upon laboratory methods following discovery of the ulcers at post-mortem examination.

Gastric ulcers may also be produced by the toxin of *Aspergillus flavus* (aflatoxin), and in copper poisoning.

GASTRITIS means inflammation of the stomach. (*See* STOMACH, DISEASES OF.)

GASTROCNEMIUS (γαστροκνημία, the calf of the leg) is the large muscle which lies behind the stifle-joint and the tibia and fibula, and ends in the tendon Achilles or 'hamstring' which is attached to the 'point of the hock'.

GASTRO-ENTERITIS means inflammation of the stomach and intestines. It is an acute condition commonest in young animals. It may be specific or due to irritant organic or inorganic poisons.

(*See also* HÆMORRHAGIC, PARASITIC, and TRANSMISSIBLE GASTRO-ENTERITIS.)

GASTRO-ENTEROSTOMY (γαστήρ, stomach; ἔντερον, intestine; στόμα mouth) is an operation performed in order to relieve some obstruction to the outlet from the stomach, such as the presence of a tumour, and consists in making one opening into the lower part of the stomach and another into a loop of the small intestine in the vicinity, so as to enable food to pass from the stomach into the intestine by means of the artificial opening when the two incisions are approximated and stitched into position.

GASTRORRHŒA (γαστήρ, the stomach; ῥέω, I flow) means an excessive secretion of gastric juice.

GASTROSCOPE.—An instrument for viewing the interior of the stomach. It has been used in the dog, under general anæsthesia—which is essential.

GASTROSTOMY (γαστήρ, the stomach; στόμα, mouth) means an operation on the stomach by which food can be directly introduced into the organ from an opening in the anterior part of the abdomen.

GAULTHERIA, or **WINTERGREEN,** is an American evergreen plant (*Gaultheria procumbens*) containing an oil with a peculiar smell and an aromatic taste. The oil consists almost solely of methyl salicylate, and is used externally to allay the pain in rheumatic conditions.

GEL is a colloid substance which is firm in consistence, although it contains much water; *e.g.* ordinary gelatin.

GELATIN is the name applied to various albuminoid materials derived from animal tissues. It forms a colourless transparent substance hard and brittle when dried, and becoming jelly-like when moistened. It is used in pharmacy. Mixed with about two and a half times its weight of glycerine, it forms glycerine-jelly used as the basis for capsules, pastilles, and suppositories.

A solution of gelatin has been used in transfusion work following severe hæmorrhage.

GELATIN SPONGE is prepared as a hæmostatic, and can be left in a wound; complete absorption taking place in 4 to 6 weeks. The sponge may be sterilised by dry heat, and applied either dry or moistened with normal saline, an antibiotic solution, or a solution of thrombin. Absorbable Gelatin Sponge complies with the requirements of the British Pharmacopœia.

GENETICS AND HEREDITY

INTRODUCTION.—The science of genetics (which means literally the science of being born or of the coming into being of an individual) seeks to account for the similarities and dissimilarities in characterisation exhibited by individuals related by a common ancestry, and to define the exact relation between successive generations. It deals with the physiology of heredity, the mechanism by which resemblance between parent and offspring is conserved and transmitted, and with the origin and significance of variation, the mechanism by hich such resemblance is modified and transformed. It seeks to define the manner in which the hereditary characters of the individual are represented in the fertilised egg in which the individual has its beginning, and to demonstrate the way in which these characters become expressed as the development of the individual proceeds.

Stock-breeding is a craft which is concerned with the maintenance of the desirable qualities of a stock, the improvement of these qualities generation by generation, and the elimination through breeding of qualities which are held to be undesirable. Since the stock-breeder deals with characters that are known to be transmitted from one generation to another by some mechanism, it is essential for intelligent breeding that there should be a knowledge of the manner in which these characters arise in a stock, are lost, or are modified. The problems of the geneticist and of the stock-breeder are identical though their interests are dissimilar.

The geneticist has made a point of studying those characters the hereditary transmission of which promised to be comparatively straightforward, and the materials he has used have been among animals, the inexpensive, quickly maturing, very highly fertile forms such as the mouse, rat, guinea-pig, rabbit, and above all the fruit fly *Drosophila*. But out of this work (with material that the stock-breeder would not regard as animals at all) results have provided interpretations and theories that can account for the phenomena of hereditary transmission encountered in the course of practical stock-breeding.

Even to-day much more is known of the craft of breeding than of the science of genetics. The principles of heredity were in operation long before they were disclosed by the scientist, but there can be no doubt that the success of the great improvers of the modern breeds was achieved by practices that were essentially in accord with these principles.

Advance in our knowledge of the hereditary phenomena was rendered possible by the birth of the new concept that the individual as a whole was not the unit in inheritance, but could be regarded as a definite orderly combination of independently heritable units. For the first time it became possible to appreciate the fact that, for example, the difference between red and black coat colour in Aberdeen-Angus cattle depended fundamentally on the same causes as in the Galloway, Kerry, or Dexter. There was no longer a peculiar Aberdeen-Angus black or Galloway black or Kerry black differing among themselves and also in relation to their respective reds, but there was a black and a red commonly possessed by many breeds of cattle.

Breed was now interpreted as signifying different combinations of unit or independently heritable characters all drawn

GENETICS AND HEREDITY

from the common source of the stock in which modern domesticated cattle had their origin, just as different arrangements and combinations of letters make different words, though all words are made up of letters derived from a common source—the alphabet.

The breeder has employed the methods of hybridisation and in-breeding associated with selection in the creation of the modern breeds. He has practised in-breeding with selection in order that the desired characters of his stock may be maintained and improved, and he has sought hybrid vigour in out-crossing. The geneticist has employed these very same methods in his studies. The method of genetics is character-analysis. The object of the breeder is character-synthesis. There is no need to stress the fact that there should be complete analysis before synthesis is undertaken.

Instead of the hereditary mechanism being a simple affair as was first thought, it is one of the most complicated. It also became evident that genetical knowledge cannot always be applied to the business of economic animal breeding. For example, in order that the facts of inheritance may be disclosed in a clear-cut way it is necessary to raise large numbers of individuals, and this is not always possible in the case of the larger domesticated stock. Again, it has been shown that animals which look exactly alike may be remarkably different in their hereditary constitution, and that the only method of demonstrating this difference is to use them for the raising of further generations. Among the more slowly maturing domesticated stock such a test as this is only possible in exceptional circumstances. It is a far more difficult task to improve the highly developed breeds of to-day than to improve the scrub.

Genetics has given an exact meaning of in-breeding, out-breeding, and prepotency. It has demonstrated beyond doubt that certain abnormalities and diseases are truly heritable, and has shown the way in which they may be prevented. It has shown that such characters as fecundity, fertility, and longevity have a definite hereditary basis. It has probed the mysteries of sex-determination. It has shown how the poultry breeder may employ sex-linkage to his economic advantage. It has given to purity and to hybridity an exact meaning, and has perfected the methods by which any character, structural or functional, which is shown to be hereditary, can be subjected to genetical analysis and made available for incorporation into a breed.

In order to illustrate the rôle of the genetics in relation to stock-breeding it is proposed to interpret in genetical terms certain problems in breeding; we will deal first with the *significance of the appearance of a red calf in a herd in which the fashionable coat colour is black, and in which all red animals are eliminated.*

Black-and-red coat colours in cattle constitute a typical pair of Mendelian characters, black being the dominant and red being the recessive member of the pair. A red calf can only be produced by black parents when both of these are heterozygous in respect of their coat-colour character, Every calf, male or female, black or red, has its origin in the union of an ovum, the reproductive cell or gamete elaborated by the maternal parent, and a sperm elaborated by the male. It is impossible on examination of the recently fertilised ovum or zygote to predict the future characterisation of the individual which arises therefrom. It is impossible to distinguish between a fertilised egg which will at the end of its development be a black individual from one which will be a red, and yet the first inevitably becomes a black and the other inevitably becomes a red. Characterisation is expressed as development proceeds. It is assumed that for all the hereditary characters that are exhibited by an individual there are corresponding determiners or factors in the fertilised egg, brought thereto by the gametes, the egg and the sperm, at the time of fertilisation. For the character black-coat colour there is thus a determiner or factor. This factor may be present in the zygote in the duplex state, having been conveyed thereinto by both egg and sperm. When the factor for black is present in the duplex state the individual that arises from that zygote is spoken of as being homozygous for the character black-coat colour. On the other hand, into the zygote there may have been brought a factor for black from one parent and a factor for red, the alternative character, from the other parent. Under these circumstances, for reasons that are not yet known, of these two factors, that for black and that for red, it is the former alone that determines what the coat colour shall be. Black is said to be dominant in its relation to red. Homozygous and heterozygous blacks will be indistinguishable on inspection.

GENETICS AND HEREDITY

If two heterozygous blacks are mated there will occur on the average in every four, 3 black calves to 1 red. To explain this 3 : 1 ratio it is assumed that *half of both male and female gametes* of such heterozygous individuals (*i.e.* sperm and ovum) carry the factor for the dominant character *black*, and the other half the factor for the alternative recessive *red*, and the two sorts of egg and of sperm occur in equal numbers. It is assumed also that the factor for the dominant is not adulterated in any way by its association with the factor for the recessive. If it is assumed that for every pair of factors that correspond to a pair of characters only one can pass into the ripe gamete, it follows that a 3 : 1 ratio in the next generation will be obtained, and of the individuals exhibiting the dominant character one will be homozygous for that character and two heterozygous, whilst the individual exhibiting the recessive character must of necessity carry the factor for that character in the duplex state, since if in its hereditary constitution it carries a factor for the dominant, it will exhibit the dominant character. It is possible by examining the records of the coat colours of he offspring to define the hereditary constitution of the parent in respect of the coat colours black and red. The following matings are possible :

Homozygous black to homozygous black will give none but blacks, all homozygous.

Homozygous black to heterozygous black will give all blacks, of which 50 per cent will be homozygous and 50 per cent heterozygous.

Homozygous black to homozygous red will give all heterozygous blacks.

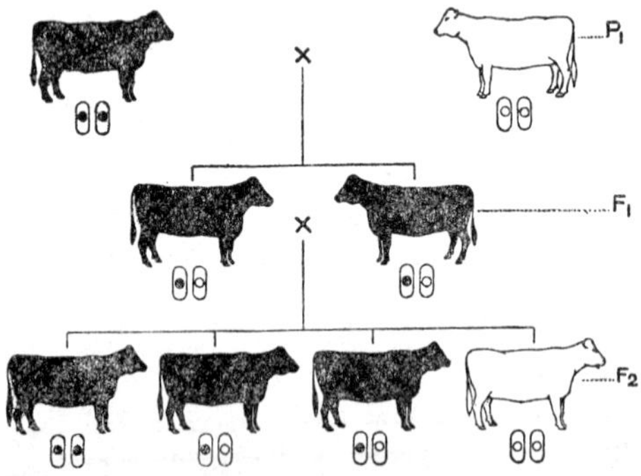

Black × Red.
(Red is necessarily white in the diagram.)

Heterozygous black to heterozygous black will give 25 per cent homozygous blacks, 50 per cent heterozygous blacks, and 25 per cent reds.

Heterozygous black to red will give 50 per cent heterozygous blacks and 50 per cent reds.

Red to red will give all reds, of necessity homozygous. The only mating of blacks that can yield a red calf is that of two individuals heterozygous in respect of this coat-colour character. (*See* Fig. 106.)

Purity can now be given an exact meaning. The coat-colour character has to be considered quite apart from all the rest of the characters that in their association make the animal what it is. An individual is a pure black when it is in respect of this character homozygous, when in its hereditary constitution the determiner or factor for this character is present in the duplex state, having been received from both its parents.

The occasional appearance of a red calf in an Aberdeen-Angus herd, or Galloway, Holstein, Kerry, or Dexter, can be accounted for if it can be shown that at some time during the formative period in the history of these breeds ared individual was employed. This, unfortunately, is not always possible, for the earlier part of the history of most breeds is not accurately recorded. From what is known of the behaviour of these coat-colour characters, however, it is perfectly legitimate to postulate that the appearance of a red calf in a black herd is a sure indication that at some time or other a red animal was used, probably at a time when coat colour was a matter of no great concern. If red was introduced and if black was chosen later as the standard coat colour, red would only exceptionally be seen, because, as has been said, black is dominant to red, and homozygous and heterozygous black are indistinguishable on inspection. If there exist in a stock a male and a female which are heterozygous blacks, sooner or later the appearance of a red calf is inevitable.

There have been red Aberdeen-Angus herds, and, as far as is known, a red Angus is as typical a specimen of the breed as is a black. A red is homozygous for this coat-colour character, and it certainly is as pure bred and as pure breeding as a black, and there is no critical evidence that suggests that it is not as valuable as its black relative. The elimination of the red is a matter of no great importance in the case of the beef breeds, but it is a most reprehensible state of affairs that in the milk breeds a potentially most valuable specimen should be disposed of merely because it happens to be born with an unfashionable coat colour. There is no reason whatsoever for suggesting that a Holstein-Friesian is not so good a Holstein-Friesian biologically because its coat colour is red-and-white instead of black-and-white, yet a red-and-white is not eligible for registration in the American herd-book. It is a fact that up to about 1859, before the importation of black-and-white Jutlands, the majority of Holstein-Friesians were red-and-whites; in Holland red-and-whites are eligible for registration and are relatively common. Since it has not been shown that an animal with a red coat colour is less valuable as a producer than a black-and-white, there is no biological justification for the elimination of what merely is unfashionable. It may be expected that a more liberal-minded attitude shall follow a spread of knowledge and that a red-and-white calf will not be slaughtered but will be disposed of to a dairy farmer to whom colour is a matter of quite secondary importance. Fashionable standards are not always true reflections of economic values.

THE UNFIXABLE HETEROZYGOTE—ROAN.—Dominance such as that of black over red is an unessential feature of Mendelian inheritance. What is essential is the orderly reappearance of the characters of the parents of the hybrid (the heterozygous black in this case) and the hybrid itself in the second hybrid generation in definite numerical proportions. The red roan behaves as though it were a hybrid in respect of coat colour out of a red by a white. A similar case is that of the blue roan, which is the hybrid out of a black by a white. Roan by roan gives on the average in every four 1 red, 2 roan, and 1 white. This 1 : 2 : 1 ratio is reminiscent of the ratio in the black second cross-bred generation of the black-red mating in which 1 homozygous black, 2 heterozygous blacks, and 1 red were obtained, and the difference between the two cases is merely a matter of the degree of dominance. Roan may be regarded as a compromise between red and white, neither of these being dominant in relation to the other. If this explanation is a satisfactory one the following results may be expected:

Red by red will give none but reds.

Red by white will give none but roans.

Red by roan should give equal numbers of reds and roans.

Roan by white should give equal numbers of roans and whites.

Roan by roan should give 25 per cent reds, 50 per cent roans, 25 per cent whites.

White by white should give none but whites.

These are the results usually obtained, and the explanation is satisfactory in the great majority of cases. It is a sound working hypothesis. Exceptional coat colours are sometmes obtained, however, in one or other of the above matings. It must be remembered that this analysis is not based upon results of critical experiment. It is based upon data obtained from the herd-books and breed registers, and it can be stated at once that the records are not in all cases trustworthy. What one breeder would call roan another might call red-and-white, and so on. It is possible that all Shorthorns are red animals fundamentally, but that in their different hereditary constitutions there may be factors of two sorts and in different combinations: (1) some that determine that the pigment shall be restricted to certain parts of the body; and (2) others that determine that the pigment shall be restricted in its distribution in the hairs, so that it is possible to get an animal with a white ground and patches of red or of roan, or a red animal with patches of roan.

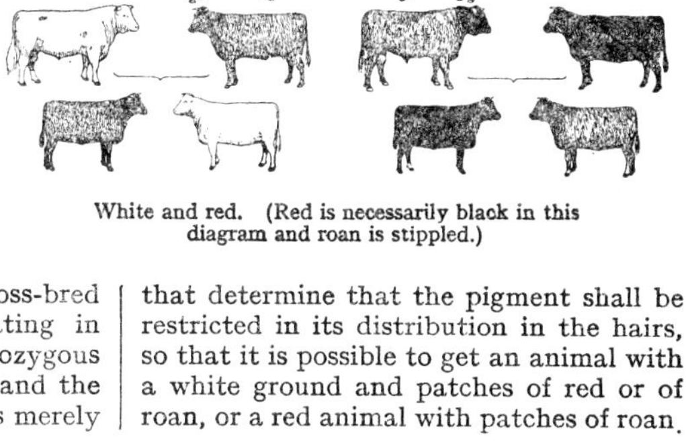

White and red. (Red is necessarily black in this diagram and roan is stippled.)

GENETICS AND HEREDITY

Be this as it may, it is impossible to give an absolutely trustworthy interpretation of the significance of roan until controlled experimentation has been undertaken. In the meantime it is enough to regard the roan as being heterozygous for its coat-colour character. It is a matter of interest to note that the blue-grey has, since the first quarter of the 19th century, been held to possess many desirable qualities to an exceptional degree—vigour and rapid growth, for example. Now, the blue-grey in those days was always the cross-bred offspring of a Galloway or an Angus and a Shorthorn. It is well known that the first cross out of two pure-bred and dissimilar parents exhibits to a remarkable degree what is known as hybrid vigour, and this hybrid vigour came to be regarded as a peculiar virtue of the blue roan and invariably associated with this colour. This first cross is heterozygous, not only for its coat-colour character but also for the very considerable number of characters in respect of which its parents differed. Hybrid vigour is not inevitably associated with a roan coat colour. It may be expected that a roan which is the first cross-bred out of a red and a white, its parents not being related or only distantly so, will exhibit the qualities of hybrid vigour. It will do so, however, not because it is a roan, but because it is heterozygous for many other characters than its coat colour.

THE INHERITANCE OF MILK YIELD.—The conclusion that inheritance accounts for much of the permanence in the milk production of a cow from one lactation to another is justified. It is established that the size of the cow is partially responsible for her milk yield, and that size is inherited in the same way as other body characters. It has been shown that conformation plays only a minor part in determining the milk production of a cow at any age. Conformation has no relation to the butter-fat percentage a cow is able to give in her milk. It is known that both sire and dam influence the production of the offspring, and also the butter-fat percentage is controlled in inheritance by a series of factors. High milk yield appears to be incompletely dominant to low milk yield, and the factors for high milk yield can be transmitted by the male. The study of the inheritance of such a character as high milk yield is one of the most difficult a geneticist can be asked to tackle. Differences in husbandry, differences in climatic conditions, and ill health, all tend to complicate genetical analysis. Environment can condition the expression of the factorial constitution of the animal. The best breed cannot excel in performance if husbandry is wrong.

The development of progeny recording, whereby a bull's value is assessed in the herd on the basis of the performances of his daughters compared with their dams, has put into the breeders' hands a method of improvement of practical application and one that can be recommended as having a scientific basis. By means of the practice of artificial insemination the progeny of a bull may well run into thousands or even tens of thousands instead of but little more than 100 by natural service. Analysis of the performance of the daughters of such a bull in comparison with their dams' performances in essentially the same environment is already showing that some bulls are capable of raising milk yields, some of lowering them, and others of altering butter-fat percentages. The genetic methods available upon which selection of dairy stock can be made, and the aids to such selection as must still remain part of the art and craft of the breeder, are now comprehensive and can be defined more precisely. They are being employed by practical breeders to an increasing extent. Much still remains obscure, but acquisition of genetic knowledge and its application to breeding for milk and butter-fat is making slow but certain progress.

THE PEDIGREE AND THE ADVANCED REGISTRY SYSTEMS.—The effort to obtain some method by which the breeding performance of an animal can be gauged in advance has resulted in the pedigree system, which is based upon a recognition of the facts of heredity. The superior animal descended from a long line of superior animals will be more likely to beget superior offspring than will another animal equally good but of mixed ancestry, for the reason that the chances are that the former will be homozygous for many of its characters, the latter heterozygous; with the result that the former will breed true for these characters whilst the latter will not. The pedigree system, while it is being of great use in breed improvement, has not been altogether free from abuses; and a knowledge of the biological principles on which it is based cannot fail to be of value in the cultivation of the sense of proportion in this matter. It is known, for example, that for all

GENETICS AND HEREDITY

practical purposes the inheritance from sire and dam is not far from equality, and the same remark applies to each generation. The 'family name' may be a useful system of pedigree as long as it is realised that the direct maternal line possesses no special importance and is of no more value than any other portion of the pedigree.

Of late years the progeny test has received more and more attention and is worthy of the greatest possible encouragement. In conjunction with a rational pedigree system and a system of line breeding it gives as much certainty in breeding methods as can be expected. It is possible to gain an idea of the factorial constitution of the parents from a review of the characterisation of their offspring; this is true not only of the structural characters but also of the functional. However, it is much more difficult to identify the latter; the use of the eye or the calipers is often far simpler than that of the milk pail.

GENETICAL INTERPRETATION OF THE VARYING RESULTS OF IN-BREEDING.—The evidence that is to be obtained from the study of the modern breeds of domesticated stock during their formative periods shows plainly that some degree of narrow breeding is an essential to the attainment of outstanding success in animal breeding. In-breeding is, therefore, not necessarily harmful, but can be definitely advantageous, leading to the development of a uniform and true breeding stock. It is true, however, that benefit does not always follow the practice of in-breeding, for in certain cases there is disappointing regression, diminution of vigour, lowered powers of resistance, decreased fertility, even reduction in size. A critical examination of the situation shows quite conclusively that the effects of in-breeding depend not upon any pernicious attribute of this method of breeding, but upon the genetic constitution of the individuals concerned. In-breeding has but one demonstrable effect upon the individuals subjected to this action, and this is the isolation of homozygous types. The ordinary specimen of the domesticated animals exhibits a great multitude of characters, and corresponding to these characters there are factors which may be in the simplex or the duplex state. It may be safely said that no animal is homozygous for all the characters that it exhibits. In point of fact the ordinary animal is homozygous for but a very few of the characters which it exhibits. In-breeding leads to a rapid increase in homozygosity, and when this state has been achieved, stability and uniformity will be reached; but as this process proceeds there is a re-shuffling of all factors, and individuals will appear which are homozygous for characters which are definitely deleterious to their possessor. The weak, sterile, and abnormal individuals which appear amongst the offspring of an in-bred line are but the individuals which have received during this process the factors for undesirable characters in the duplex state; and whilst these become eliminated there will be, on the other hand, individuals which, thanks to this process, now come to possess the factors for desirable characters in the duplex state—for such characters as fertility, longevity, early maturity, and so on, and rigorous selection from amongst these types will isolate strains which will compare very favourably indeed with the original stock. Consanguinity in itself is not a bar to a mating. If in-breeding results in disappointment all that has happened is that recessive characters previously hidden have been brought to light. In-breeding in this way purifies a stock. The process may be disastrously expensive if the ingredients of hereditary combinations which will result in undesirable or non-viable types pre-exist, but, on the other hand, those individuals which have been made homozygous for the desirable characters will be far more valuable material in the hands of the breeder than the stock with which he started, for in virtue of their hereditary constitution they must now breed true for these desirable characters.

GENETICAL INTERPRETATION OF HYBRID VIGOUR.—Hybrid vigour, usually most clearly demonstrated by increase in size and in the earlier attainment of sexual maturity, is the property of the first cross-bred generation out of the mating of two widely dissimilar pure-bred parental stocks. Hybrid vigour is an indication of heterozygosis. The two parental breeds must be within reason as dissimilar in their characterisation as possible, because they differ so markedly in their characterisations. In this way it follows that their factorial constitutions must be correspondingly different; then in the pooling of those hereditary constitutions there will be a very considerable degree of heterozygosis in the first cross-bred offspring; the desirable characters

GENETICS AND HEREDITY

are pooled, and in respect of those characters exhibited by the two parents the offspring will be heterozygous. If the first crosses which exhibit this hybrid vigour so markedly are interbred, the heterozygosis will become diminished and their offspring will not exhibit this vigour to the same extent. It is not a sound commercial proposition to pursue hybrid vigour further than the first cross-bred generation yielded by the mating of two dissimilar, more or less closely line-bred, parental stocks.

THE FUSION OF TWO IN-BRED LINES.—It has been clearly demonstrated by practical breeders who have been trained in genetics, that by in-breeding for a specific character, and by practising rigid selection for two, three, or more generations, a strain of relatively homozygous individuals for the selected character can be created. If two such strains are developed separately but simultaneously for two different but highly desirable characters, and if these two strains are then crossed, the resulting progeny can be guaranteed to possess both desirable characters to a marked degree. The mechanism has been notably successful in producing strains of poultry with large egg size and high annual yields, and in the U.S.A. has been exploited commercially to an extraordinary degree. Among cattle, there has been some success in combining high milk yield with high butter-fat percentage, but whereas the poultry-keeper may be content to reap the benefits from one generation of birds only, the dairyman wishes to have 5, 6, or more lactations from each of his cows, and the problem of mating them so that their calves can form herd replacements is difficult. When the generation in which the two desirable characters are expressed is bred from again, an immediate re-assortment of characters occurs, and only in a small percentage of the individuals will the desirable characters be expressed. The others are most likely to be useless.

GENETICAL INTERPRETATION OF PREPOTENCY.—If a certain character is dominant then its possessor will prove to be prepotent when mated with individuals exhibiting the corresponding recessive. Thus, for example, a homozygous black Aberdeen-Angus will be completely prepotent in respect of this dominant character, whereas a heterozygous black will not. This explanation, though satisfactory in the simplest cases, cannot possibly explain all the facts of prepotency. As yet, however, very little more relating to this established phenomenon is known. Bearing upon this subject is the phenomenon known as *nicking*. Two individuals not remarkable in themselves beget superior offspring. This fact can be explained on the assumption that the mating brings together the chance association of factors which are complementary or supplementary, and that these in conjunction determine characters that are greatly esteemed.

GENETICAL INTERPRETATION OF THE EFFECTS OF SELECTION.—Selection undoubtedly has been one of the greatest agencies in the permanent improvement of domestic stock. Breeders have always selected the characterisation that appealed to them most. To-day this selection by characterisation has given place rapidly to selection by factorial constitution. The sire of the milking herd is judged by the performance of his daughters ; his possible value is estimated from a consideration of the performance of his ancestors ; so also in the mating of other kinds of stocks. The individual is judged by the characterisation of his descendants, and his qualities are estimated in advance by the characterisation of his ancestors. The aim of selection is the isolation of individuals homozygous for the desirable characters. Selection does not in any way change the hereditary constitution of a stock. It merely chooses out of the best stock those individuals which are becoming homozygous for those characters for which the breeder is aiming. He alters the characterisation of a stock by altering the proportion of the different character-classes within it.

THE INHERITANCE OF TWINNING.—It is possible by the selection for mating of individuals which themselves are twins to build up a stock in which twinning is the rule. Twinning, of course, demands that at one and the same time there shall be more than one ovum available for fertilisation at the time of service, and hereditary basis of twinning must, therefore, take the form of habitual extrusion of more than one ovum from the ovary during the period of heat. The question as to whether it is desirable to develop a stock homozygous for this character is not a problem in genetics but in husbandry. It is easier to give birth to twins than to rear them in many kinds of environment. It should be mentioned in connection with this subject that it has to be recognised that the conditions of husbandry in the broadest

GENETICS AND HEREDITY

sense condition the expression of this character. A ewe may be homozygous for this character, but whether she will exhibit it depends on many things—on climatic conditions, on the abundance and kind of food, and so forth. The effects of flushing upon fertility in the sheep show how the quality and quantity of nutriment condition the character of fertility. In an entirely suitable country it is possible to develop a flock of sheep that habitually give twins, and, moreover, it is possible by the same methods of breeding to equip the ewes with extra mammary glands.

THE MECHANISM OF SEX-DETERMINATION AND SEX-DIFFERENTIATION.—A male can be distinguished from a female not only by external appearances

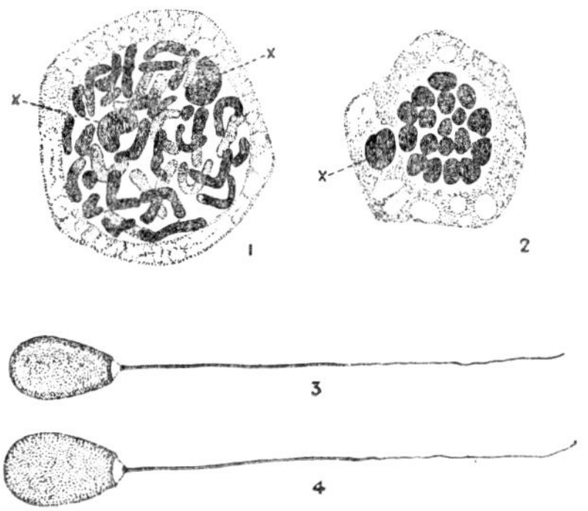

1. The chromosomes in the immature ovum of the cow—30 pairs.
2. The reduced number of chromosomes in the ripe sperm of the bull—30 single chromosomes.
3 and 4. Spermatozoa of the bull. There are two kinds according to the length of the head.

and by differences in the architecture of the reproductive system, but also by differences in the organisation of the cells of which their bodies are composed. A cell, any cell, consists essentially of a vesicular spherical body, the nucleus, lying in a viscous substance, the cytoplasm. The nucleus of the resting cell appears in stained microscopic preparations as a vesicle containing a network of delicate threads upon which are borne, like beads upon a tangled skein, minute masses of a deeply staining material known as chromatin. As the cell proceeds to divide into two—and it will be remembered that the whole of the body of anything is built up entirely of cells that have been produced by the division of the zygote—it is seen that this tangled mass of fine threads resolves itself into a constant number of filaments of definite shape and that these become progressively shorter to assume the form of stout rods known as chromosomes. The number of chromosomes is usually some multiple of two, and is constant and characteristic of the species to which the individual belongs.

The gametes, egg and sperm respectively, differ remarkably in size and form, but they are alike in that each contains half the number of chromosomes that is characteristic of the body of the individual that elaborates them. If, for example, the characteristic number of chromosomes in the cells of the body generally and in the unripe gametes is 36, then in the ripe gamete elaborated by such individual there would be but 18. Examination of

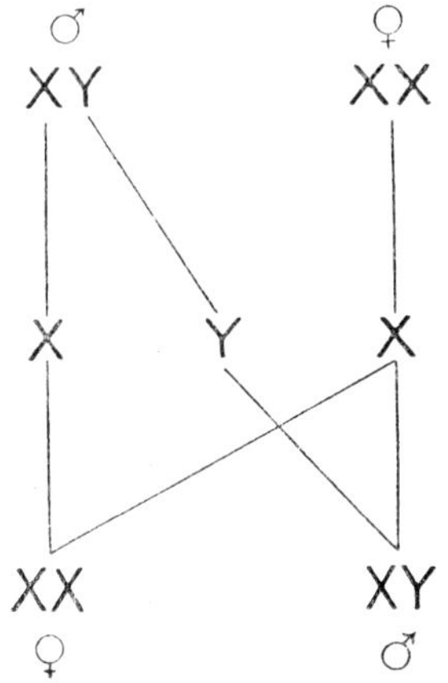

The sex-chromosome sex-determining mechanism.

cases in which there are few chromosomes, and in which these are of different sizes and shapes, has made perfectly clear that they are present in the body cells of unripe gametes in pairs, and that in each pair one member passes into the ripe gamete. When gamete unites with gamete in fertilisation, the characteristic number is restored, and in the case of each pair one member is derived from one parent, the other from the other. In the distribution of the chromosomes one finds a mechanism by which offspring may inherit from both parents if it is assumed that the factors for the hereditary characters are resident in the chromosomes.

It is possible to distinguish male from female by differences in the chromosome content. While all other pairs of chromosomes consist of two chromosomes exactly

GENETICS AND HEREDITY

alike in size and shape, one pair differs in the two sexes. For this reason these chromosomes are referred to as the sex-chromosomes. In many cases there is a pair of sex-chromosomes in one sex and a single chromosome representing this pair in the other. For example, in the female of a particular species there may be 17 pairs of autosomes and 1 pair of sex-chromosomes, whilst the male has 17 pairs of autosomes and a single sex-chromosome. In other cases the total number is similar in the two sexes; but whereas in the female the sex-chromosome pair consists of members of similar size and shape, in the male the two are unequal. For purposes of description these two types of difference in the sex-chromosome content are referred to as follows: the sex-chromosomes that in size and shape are similar are known as the X-chromosomes. The female in the illustration used above would then possess a chromosome content of 34 autosomes+XX, the male 34 autosomes+XO; or if the chromosome total is the same in the two sexes, the female would be 34+XX and the male 3+4XY. Y signifies the unequal mate of the X in the male. A bull possesses the XO type of sex-chromosome constitution. The ripe eggs of a female possessing 36 chromosomes of which 2 are sex-chromosomes would contain 18, and of these one will be an X; but in the case of the XO male half the sperm will contain 18 chromosomes, one of which is an X, whereas the other half will contain 17 autosomes and no X. An X-bearing egg can be fertilised by an X-bearing sperm to form an XX individual, a female in this case. An X-bearing egg can equally well be fertilised by a sperm that carries no X chromosome to give an XO individual, a male. The same scheme holds true for the case of the XY type of male. This XY : XX (or XO : XX) sex-chromosome mechanism ensures the automatic production of males and females in equal numbers in each generation, and through it sex is determined at the moment of fertilisation. One sex in the case of the domesticated mammals, the female, is homogametic, elaborating but one kind of gamete, as far as the components of the sex-chromosome sex-determining mechanism is concerned, whilst the male sex is heterogametic, elaborating two kinds of gametes, those leading to the production of males and those leading to the production of females.

In the case of cattle the bull elaborates two sorts of sperm, and if he produces these in equal numbers, if each sort is quite functional and if fertilisation is random, then the primary sex-ratio—the numerical proportion of male and female zygotes at the time of conception—should be equality. If, on the other hand, there is a differential production of the two sorts, or if one is relatively less active than the other, or if there is a selective mortality among the zygotes, then the secondary sex-ratio at the time of birth will be more or less profoundly disturbed.

In the bull it has been possible by measuring the length of the heads of numbers of spermatozoa to show that there are two size classes, a large sperm, presumably the X-chromosome-bearing, and a smaller sperm, presumably without the X.

The physiology of sex-differentiation.—The zygote is either a 'determined' male (XO or XY) or a determined female (XX), but much must happen before the zygote can become a functional male or, on the other hand, a functional female. The complicated processes of sex-differentiation during which the sexual organisation of the individual assumes one or the other type, male or female, must be pursued before one sex can be distinguished from the other by differences in anatomical structure and physiological functioning. It is assumed that there are male-determining and female-determining factors present in every zygote, and are borne on the chromosomes (both sex-chromosomes and autosomes), and that these factors elaborate sex-differentiating substance enzyme-like in nature, and that in the male-determined (XO or XY in constitution) the male sex-differentiating substances are effectively in excess over the female sex-differentiating substances during that period of development when the sexual organisation becomes differentiated. This period of sexual differentiation occurs quite early during the development of the fœtus, and begins after a preliminary phase of growth and of general organ formation. At the beginning of this period of sex-differentiation the reproductive system consists of paired gonads (neither ovarian nor testicular in structure), a rudimentary accessory sexual apparatus of two ducts, the Wolffian and Müllerian; and external genital organs which have the form of a cleft, the urogenital sinus, and a rudimentary erectile organ, the phallus. As differentiation proceeds, it is seen that

GENETICS AND HEREDITY

either the gonads become testes, the Müllerian ducts atrophy and the Wolffian ducts continue their development to become the functional deferent ducts of the male, and the phallus and urogenital sinus become the penis and scrotum; or else the gonads become ovaries, the Wolffian ducts atrophy, whilst the Müllerian ducts fuse to become the uterus and vagina, and the phallus and urogenital cleft develop into a clitoris and vulva. One or other type of sex-organisation is developed from embryonic structures commonly possessed by all individuals, determined male and determined female alike. Sex-differentiation is alternative. The effects of castration or implantation of ovary and testis in gonadectomised individuals (individuals from which the gonads have been removed by operation) of the recent rejuvenation work, show quite clearly that in the case of the domesticated mammals such as cattle the gonads play an important rôle in this process of sexual differentiation. It is definitely established that for the appropriate differentiation of the male type of differentiation of the accessory sexual apparatus, external genital organs, and those characters of body form that distinguish male from female, the presence of a functional testis is essential during development, and that for the appropriate differentiation of a female type of sex organisation a functional ovary must be present.

It is assumed that the undifferentiated gonad develops into a testis in a determined male because the male differentiating substances direct its differentiation, whereas in an internal environment (the embryo itself) of 'femaleness' the gonad becomes an ovary. When the gonad has thus differentiated it is seen on microscopical examination of stained preparations that it consists essentially of two sorts of tissue, that which is concerned with the elaboration of the gametes, and another kind—the so-called interstitial tissue—which is held to be the source of a specific sex-hormone, a chemical substance which, circulating in the blood, is concerned with the differentiation of the remaining parts of the sexual organisation. There is thus a male sex-hormone and a female sex-hormone, and these are specifically different.

The Bovine Freemartin.—The part played by the sex-hormones in the differentiation of the sex-organisation is well illustrated by the case of the bovine freemartin, which is now known to be a 'determined' female, co-twin to a normal male, the reproductive system of which becomes abnormal during intra-uterine life. A male (XO) and a female (XX) zygotes are concerned. The two fertilised ova pass into the bicornuate uterus and become attached to its walls. As they increase in size the embryonic membranes of the two fœtuses meet, adhere, and usually fuse. If fusion occurs, developing blood-vessels pass from membrane to membrane and a common blood communication becomes established. Thus the situation arises in which the sex-hormone of the male can pass into the body of the developing female and that of the female into the body of the developing male. The sexual differentiation of both individuals will be pursued under the direction of that sex-hormone which is exhibited earlier or

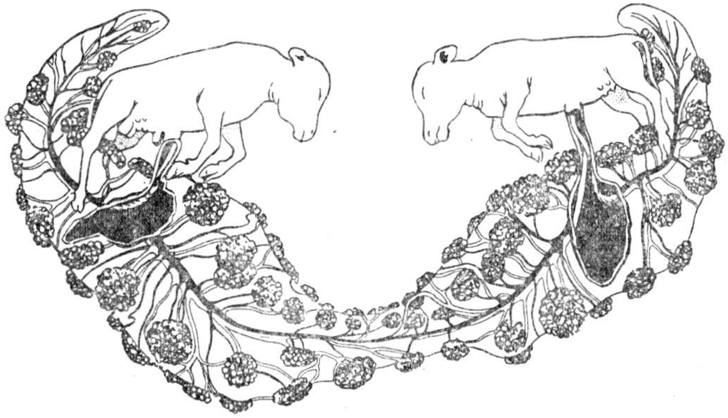

The bovine freemartin.

GENETICS AND HEREDITY

is the more potent. The testis of the male becomes differentiated at an earlier stage than the ovary, and so the sex-hormone of the male is liberated into the blood-stream before that of the female. The result is that the differentiation of the sexual organisation of both male and female is pursued under the direction of the sex-hormone of the male. The female thus comes to possess more or less completely the male organisation. It would not be expected that she should become completely possessed of the male type of sexual organisation, because her tissues are all female in chromosome-constitution. Her internal reproductive organs are more or less completely male in type, her external genital organs more or less completely female. The external genital organs of the freemartin may be obviously abnormal, or they may appear to be normally female, but she may never come on heat owing to the gross abnormality of her internal reproductive organs. But every heifer calf born co-twin to a bull is not a freemartin —it is estimated that about one in eight is normal. It is only when fusion of the embryonic membranes occurs that abnormality of the female follows.

It would appear, then, that in cattle the male is heterogametic, possessing a constitution represented by the formula XO; that sex is determined at the moment of fertilisation; that in the XO type of individual the embryonic gonad becomes a testis; that in the XX type it becomes an ovary; that ovary and testis elaborate specific sex-hormones, and that under the direction of these the differentiation of the rest of the sex-organisation is pursued.

The problem of the control of the sex-ratio is that of the differential production of the two sorts of sperm by the bull. When measures have been devised to secure such a differential production it will be possible to obtain a calf of the desired sex. It is known that in the case of certain sires there is such a differential production; it is established that the sex-ratio varies with the season of the year, with the general physiological condition of the parents. To a slight extent it is already possible to control the sex-ratio. In the case of cattle the most profitable line of research in this field would appear to be the development of methods of separating the two sorts of sperm and of performing artificial insemination with one or the other sort. There is some reason to maintain that such measures will be devised and made available to the breeder. (*See* 'Sex Determination', *under* ARTIFICIAL INSEMINATION.)

A normal calf must be either a male or a female and the chances that a calf will be a male rather than a female are as 118 : 100—practically an even chance.

Most of the cases that seem to support the contention that the cow is the heterogametic sex are to be explained on the assumption that certain sires habitually (or seasonably ?) produce more X-bearing sperm than no X-bearing, or that in certain cases the conditions within the reproductive passages of the cow are such as to favour fertilisation by one rather than by the other sort of sperm.

THE GENETIC INTERPRETATION OF VARIATIONS IN THE SEX-RATIO.—It has been shown that the sex-chromosome mechanism is one that should produce equal numbers of males and females in each successive generation. However, the *secondary sex-ratio*, that which obtains at birth and which is measured by taking the number of males per hundred females born, is never equality. The difference between the *primary sex-ratio*, which obtains at the time of fertilisation and the secondary provides an indication of the pre-natal survival value of the sexes. The difference between the secondary sex-ratio and the *tertiary* which obtains at maturity is an indication of the post-natal survival of the sexes. It is known that the secondary sex-ratio varies with the species, and that for each species it is more or less constant. It varies with the race, the breed, the strain; and there are reasons for holding that the production of a profoundly unusual sex-ratio is characteristic of a particular individual. Quite a number of instances are known in which a male has produced in different matings none but female or conversely none but male offsprings. There are females which in any mating habitually produce a preponderance of one sex. It is definitely established that in the case of the rat, which produces many offspring at a birth, it is possible by continual selection of individuals for breeding out of a line in which there is a preponderance of one sex to build up a strain which will habitually produce a preponderance of that sex. It is possible by such selection to develop lines which habitually will give a preponderance of females or of males.

The sex-ratio varies with the season of the year. It is low for births resulting from conceptions at the seasons of greatest fertility, and is high at the time of the

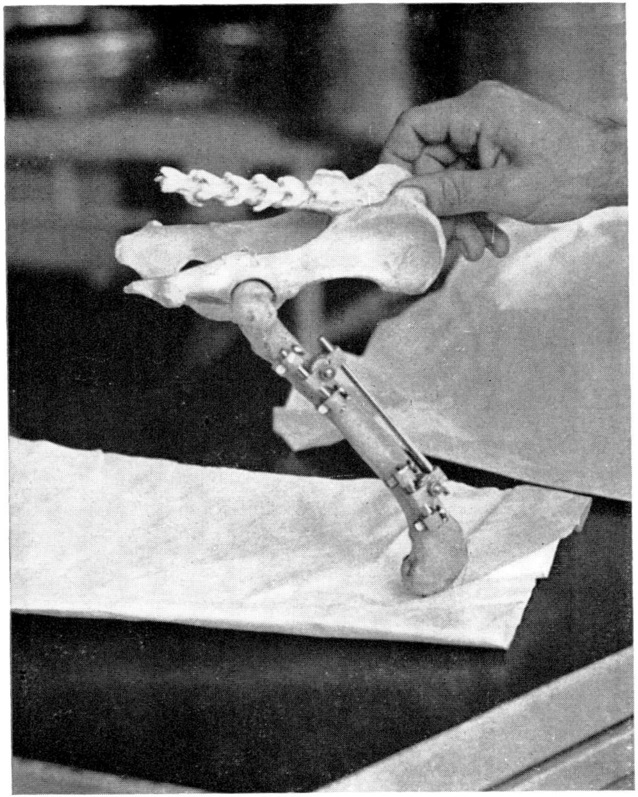

Metal splints which have transverse pins to penetrate and fix the bone are used in treating fractures in small animals, and have succeeded in cases where the older methods would have been of no avail.

See FRACTURES.

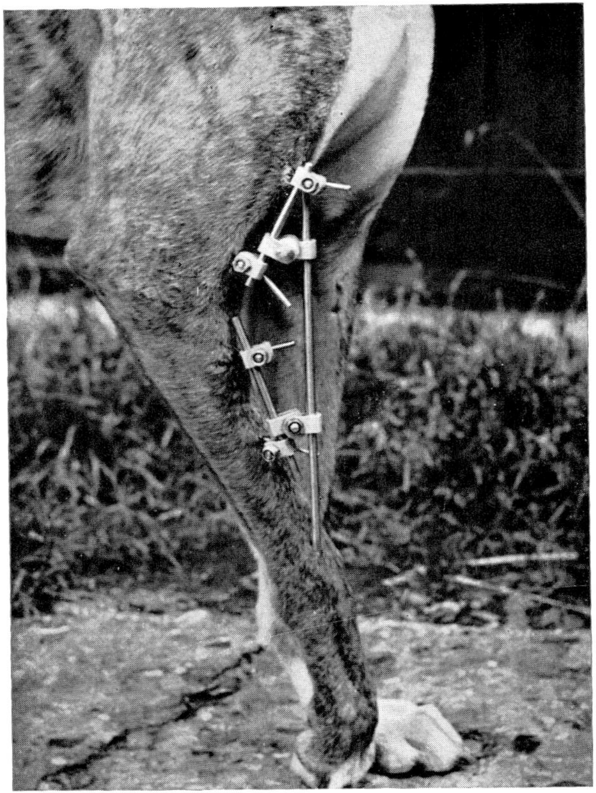

A greyhound wearing a Kirschner-Ehmer splint after sustaining multiple fractures in the region of the elbow joint. The patient made no attempt to interfere with the splint.

See FRACTURES.

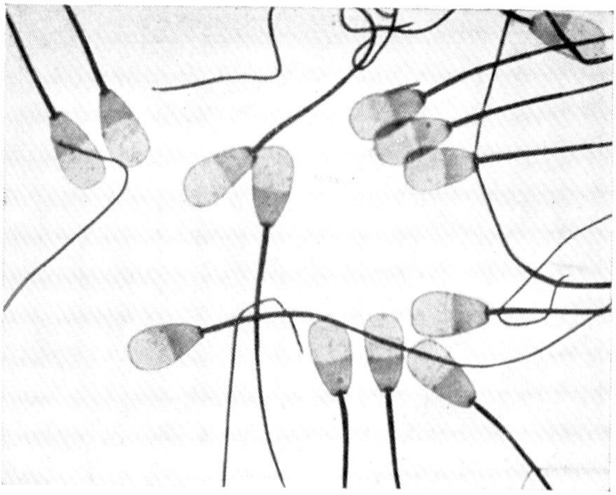

Spermatozoa from a healthy bull, highly magnified. In artificial insemination work five to ten million of these sperms are regarded as the minimum to ensure getting a cow in-calf. Bull sperms such as these can be stored at a temperature of minus 193 degrees Centigrade.

See REPRODUCTION *and* SPERMATOZOA.

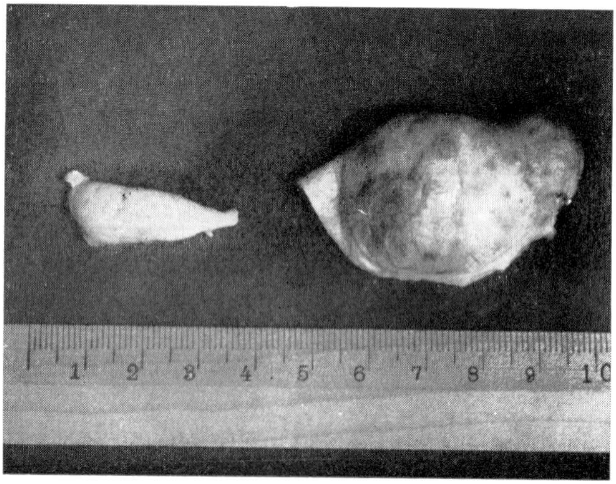

Hypoplasia of the left ovary of a cow of the Swedish Highland breed. Compare its size with that of the normal right ovary from the same animal. (*The ruler is graduated in centimetres.*)

See INFERTILITY.

lowest birth-rate. In the case of the fowl, in one experiment critically conducted, it was shown that when every egg laid by a hen was incubated, at the beginning of the laying season there was a high proportion of males, whereas at the end of the season the proportion of males had dropped by 50 per cent. There is no critical evidence which supports the conception that the sex-ratio is affected by the relative ages of the parents or by the relative vigour of the parents. It has been shown that there is no relation between the sex-ratio and the time of service during the heat period in the case of cattle. There is no evidence which supports the suggestion that there is a relation between the sex-ratio and the size of the litter, but it appears to be a fact that the sex-ratio varies with the chronological number of the pregnancy, for in many cases it has been shown that there is a continuous drop in the sex-ratio at each succeeding pregnancy. There is no evidence, as has already been suggested, which supports the contention that the sex-ratio varies with the time relation of successive conceptions. It is not the case that one ovary of the cow elaborates only male-producing ova, the other only female-producing, and that the ovaries function alternately. The sex-ratio is profoundly disturbed as a result of inter-specific crosses. It is known that in any such cross one sex is commonly absent, rare, or sterile, and that this sex is the heterogametic, the male in the case of the mammals, the female in the case of the bird.

An unusual sex-ratio may be the result of a differential production of the two sorts of gametes by the heterogametic sex. It has been possible in certain cases to control this differential production, though not yet in the case of domestic animals. The primary sex-ratio can also be affected by differential attraction on the part of the eggs towards the sperm, and by a greater activity or a greater susceptibility in unfavourable conditions on the part of the two sorts of sperm. The difference between the primary and secondary sex-ratios may be the result of the differential mortality of males and females during early embryonic life. In the case of cattle the fœtal sex-ratio is about 123 : 100, the sex-ratio at the time of birth is about 107 : 100, and this would seem to indicate that many of the males are aborted or die and are liquefied and resorbed during fœtal life. In the case of those animals which produce more than one young at a time the seasonal variation of the sex-ratio is to be explained on the assumption that there is a seasonal differential production of the two sorts of gametes. In the mammal small litters are those which have been depleted pre-natally, large litters are those which have not, and amongst the larger litters there has been a conservation of the males. The influence of the number of the pregnancy on the sex-ratio is one of selective post-conceptional elimination of fœtuses, for the number of abortions and of still-births increases with the age of the mother and with the serial number of the pregnancy.

THE GENETIC ASPECTS OF FERTILITY.—Fertility is the term used to define the ability of a mated pair to produce living offspring, and is measured by the rate at which these are produced compared to the standard of the average fertility of the stock to which these individuals belong. Fertility is based primarily on fecundity, the potential reproductive capacity of the individual measured by its ability to elaborate functional gametes, ova or sperm, as the case may be. (But see table below.) Different species exhibit a true breeding difference in the frequency of the periods of special reproductive activity during which conception may occur. There are monœstrous species in which during the year there is but one heat period, and there are polyœstrous species which exhibit during the course of a breeding season several such periods of heat. While it is certainly possible to increase the number and the intensity of the heat periods in the polyœstrous animal, there is no evidence which shows that special treatment of any kind can transform the constitutional monœstrous into the polyœstrous. Different species have markedly different durations of life, and it is known that longevity is a character in the Mendelian sense; and since the reproductive period bears a definite relation to the whole life, it follows that the fertility of the long-lived cannot be judged by the same standard as that of the short-lived. Further, some species are *polytocous*, producing several offspring at a birth, whilst others are *monotocous*, producing but one, and the standards of fertility in the two sorts must be different. In the case of the polytocous female it is known that the size of the litter is affected by the general physiological constitution of the mother during pregnancy. All fertilised eggs do not complete their

GENETICS AND HEREDITY

development. Atrophic embryos are commonly found in the uterus, and more corpora lutea than fœtuses. In the case of the pig it is estimated that about 10 per cent of the ova, though fertilised and in healthy surroundings, do not segment, that another 10 per cent degenerate before implantation, and yet another 5 to 10 per cent degenerate during implantation in the subsequent course of pregnancy. The evidence is that this pre-natal death may be due to hereditary causes.

The size of the litter is limited by the number of ova available for fertilisation by the always abundant sperm. It has been shown that litter size is a hereditary character. It is to be remembered also that the possibility of conception following sexual congress is affected by the difference in the mechanism of ovulation. In the mare, cow, ewe, sow, and bitch, ovulation has no relation to coitus, whereas in the cat, ferret, and rabbit it is coitus that determines the onset of ovulation. The size of the litter varies with the number of the pregnancy. It increases with successive pregnancies to a maximum and thereafter falls again. In the case of the pig the first litter is often the smallest and the fourth the highest. Grades of fertility are definitely racial and breed characters and are transmitted in inheritance (but see the table below).

It has already been stated that the offspring of interspecific crosses are commonly sterile. The cases of the mule and of the cattalo are noteworthy in this respect. The bulk of opinion regards the mule and the hinny as sterile, and it is suggested that this sterility is based upon a different chromosome content of the parental types. The mare has 60 chromosomes, so that each ovum will have 30. The jack probably has 65, so that each sperm would have either 32 or 33. It is when the chromosomes endeavour to pair during the elaboration of the gametes by the hybrid that their distribution is embarrassed, and as a result of this embarrassment functional gametes are not produced. In the case of the cattalo the first crossbred male if born at all is sterile. The cause of this sterility has not been conclusively demonstrated, but in all probability it is of the same nature as that of the mule.

HERITABILITY OF CERTAIN TRAITS.—The following table, compiled at the Animal Breeding Research Organisation, shows the degree of heritability of certain traits sought by the pig breeder.

Trait	*Heritabiliy*
Litter size at weaning	7%
Average weaning weight	8
Daily gain, after weaning	30
Food conversion	35
Average backfat	50
Percentage of lean meat	45

It will be seen that litter performance has a low heritability, and must be achieved by suitable crossbreeding. The crossbred sow has a marked superiority in this respect.

HEREDITY AND DISEASE.—'DISEASES exhibit a spectrum according to the genetic influence. Canine hæmophilia is entirely genetic. Swedish gonad hypoplasia is mainly genetic, mastitis is mainly environmental and injuries are entirely environmental. Simply dividing diseases into genetic and non-genetic is, therefore, inaccurate.

Recessive Inheritance.—Many diseases are inherited as autosomal recessives. Neither parent is usually affected, but the disease comes from both; the sexes are affected equally, inbreeding is often being practised, the incidence is generally low and exact genetic ratios are obtainable. Few diseases, however, fulfil all the criteria of simple recessives.

Diseases due to sex-linked recessives, *e.g.*, canine hæmophilia, are uncommon in domestic mammals and, not being transmitted by unaffected males—the carrier female transmits the disease to half her male offspring—are unlikely to be a major problem. In poultry, however, sex-linked abnormalities such as familial cerebellar degeneration are transmitted by the male to half his female progeny and are relatively common.

Diseases like cryptorchidism and intersexes are sex-limited and sometimes regarded as due to recessives, the homozygote only expressing itself in one sex. While both parents are probably involved their exact inheritance is unknown and cryptochidism is certainly subject to environmental modification.

Irregular Inheritance.—Many defects have a complex inheritance. Sporadic abnormalities, which increase on inbreeding, such as chicken "crooked toes" or pig "kinky tails", are called phenodeviants, and are probably caused by recessives exhibiting a threshold of manifestation.

Dominant Inheritance.—The disease usually comes from one affected parent, and half its offspring are affected. Few dominant diseases are known in live-stock, except in poultry. Irregular dominants, exemplified by " curved limbs ", where an unaffected male transmits defective offspring out of unrelated females and less than half are affected, do, however, occur. Environment or modifying genes may effect the genes' penetrance.

Semi-dominant Inheritance.—Several diseases are due to semi-dominants, the heterozygote being distinguishable from both homozygotes. A single dose of a semi-dominant gene produces a Dexter, a double dose a bulldog calf, and the homozygous normal allele produces a long-legged Dexter. Some American dwarfs are due to semi-dominants.' (Dr. G. B. Young, Animal Breeding Research Organisation, 1967.)

THE INHERITANCE OF LETHAL AND SEMI-LETHAL FACTORS.—Lethal factors are perhaps best defined as genes, which when present in the homozygous condition cause the death of the embryo, and when present in the heterozygous condition cause a serious impairment in the individual often leading to non-survival. Reference to a list of lethals later may serve to illustrate the position better.

Lethals may be dominant or incompletely dominant, but many are certainly recessive. They are not always recognised since they may cause death of the embryo early in development, and the mating may be regarded as having been infertile—another illustration of the difficulty of defining the genetics of infertility.

Several lethals are met with in cattle, such as parrot-mouthed, in which calves die at a few hours of age ; amputated, in which calves are born dead with legs and lower jaws absent.

Semi-lethals include over-shot jaws in calves ; closure of the intestine in horses ; cerebral hernia in cattle ; muscular atrophy and fibrosis of joints in sheep and cattle ; mummification of the fœtus, occurring at about 8 months, in cattle ; paralysis of the limbs in sheep (lambs only live a few days) ; imperforate anus, and in females vagina, in pigs ; leglessness in pigs ; cleft palate in puppies, whereby they are unable to suck ; and a number of rare conditions in man.

MODES OF INHERITANCE OF SOME CHARACTERS OF PRACTICAL IMPORTANCE.—The following brief notes may serve for reference in connection with queries that arise in breeding practice. It must not be thought that there are not exceptions to the general rules given, for in many cases the parents concerned may not themselves be of true stock, but they will be found generally to apply.

Coat colour in Horses.—The series of colours—grey, bay, brown, black, chestnut—form what is known as an epistatic series. This means that grey is dominant to the colours after it in the list, bay to the colours following it, but not to grey, and so on. Chestnut is recessive to the other colours, so that chestnut × chestnut will always give chestnut, but chestnut × any other colour will give the other colour. Creams (or whites) are of two kinds, dominant and recessive, and there is no way of differentiating them except by test matings.

Cattle.—The polled condition is dominant to horned ; black colour is dominant to red, and black and white is dominant to red and white ; white face is dominant to coloured face; and pattern-colours (*e.g.* red and white) are dominant to whole colours. High milking ability and good beef conformation are incompletely dominant to poor qualities in these respects. White × black gives blue-grey.

Pigs.—' Mule-foot ' (single toed-feet) is dominant to normal feet ; white coat is typically dominant to coloured coat, though the dominance may be incomplete ; saddle-back is dominant to whole colour ; good pork or bacon conformation is at least partially dominant to poor shape.

Sheep.—White fleece is dominant to other colours ; black is dominant to brown ; horns are variable, in some breeds they are sex-limited, only the rams possessing them ; in others both sexes are polled, while in others both sexes are horned, but the horns are of larger size in the rams. Inheritance of horns, therefore, is complicated and depends upon what types are used in the mating.

Poultry.—A great deal of the genetics of the fowl is now known accurately, and the reader is referred to text-books on poultry genetics, which deal with matters in the necessary amount of detail.

GENTIAN, which is mainly used in medicine as the dried and powdered root of the Yellow Gentian plant (*Gentiana utea*), although a compound tincture and a watery extract are also employed, is a bitter tonic, stomach stimulant, and is slightly astringent. It is very frequently incorporated in tonic powders for horses and cattle when the appetite is capricious or in abeyance. Sometimes an infusion or tincture of gentian is used for similar purposes given with nux vomica and bicarbonate of soda. For dogs the tincture is usually employed.

GENTIAN VIOLET.—A stain used in microscopical work and a valuable antiseptic, of use against fungous and bacterial skin infections. (*See also* CRYSTAL VIOLET *under* ANTISEPTICS.)

GERMS (*see* BACTERIOLOGY).

GESTATION (*gero*, I bear) is another name for pregnancy. (*See* PREGNANCY.)

GID, or **STURDY,** is a condition in sheep, and occasionally in cattle, due to the presence of a 'worm cyst' in some part of the brain. *Tænia cœnurus*, a tapeworm of the dog, is the adult worm which develops from the cyst. The eggs of this worm are passed out with the fæces of an infected dog, and some of them cling to grass and other herbage and are eventually ingested by a sheep. In the sheep's stomach they hatch into tiny embryos, which burrow through the tissues and eventually come to rest under the membranes which envelop the brain (meninges). In this situation each one develops and soon forms a little cyst filled with fluid and containing one tapeworm head. As time goes on, the cyst increases in size and more heads are budded from the lining membrane of the cyst wall. Eventually there may be as many as 50 or 60 heads present in one cyst, each one projecting into the cavity of the fluid-filled cyst and protected from pressure. Under natural conditions a sheep so affected dies in the course of 3 or 4 months. If its head should happen to be eaten by a dog, each of the tapeworm heads contained in the cyst fastens on to the lining mucous membrane of the bowels and forms a new adult tapeworm. The presence of the cysts in the brain cavity of the sheep at first gives rise to no definite symptoms, but as the cyst enlarges and fills with fluid it presses upon the important brain cells, and more or less definite symptoms are shown. The sheep begins to stagger, and loses control of its limbs when excited. If startled it becomes unable to follow a straight course, but wheels to one side or the other in a wide circle. When caught it struggles in a 'sturdy' manner and becomes very excited. At a later stage the sheep is unable to walk for even a short distance with any degree of directness, but gives the impression that it is giddy (hence one of the names). The circles become smaller and smaller with increasing excitement, and eventually the sheep falls to the ground and is unable to rise. It is noticed that the circles are always in one direction in any one animal, and upon this fact is based the diagnosis of the seat of the cyst. As a rule the cyst is situated on the side which is towards the inside of the circle, but this is not always the case. In another variety of the condition the sheep stands with its head either lowered or elevated above the normal position; it may stand with its head between the fore-legs, or it may rest its head against some convenient object and appear loth to move it; or it may turn backward somersaults. After a time the symptoms become so marked that the sheep is unable to feed or move about, and death from exhaustion follows.

Treatment.—Operative treatment is possible in a number of cases. Sometimes a softening of the bone over the affected part occurs, and such softening gives a clue to the position of the cyst. An opening is made through the skin and a small hole bored through the bone, or a trephine hole is made. The cyst is then punctured and either removed in its entirety or the contained fluid is drained away, after which the cyst wall shrivels up and the sheep recovers. Such a procedure, however, is only advisable when the value of the sheep for breeding purposes greatly exceeds its value as mutton, for there are considerable risks with operative treatment, and only about 50 to 60 per cent of cases operated upon fully recover.

Preventive measures should aim at the expulsion of worms from shepherds' dogs at regular intervals by the administration of a suitable dose of worm medicine. During the action of the medicine the dogs should be shut up in an enclosure, and the voided worms and fæcal matter should be destroyed by burning. A periodic dose of worm-expelling medicine three or four times a year should be given to each of the affected dogs. Finally, dogs should never be allowed to infect themselves with the adult tapeworms by eating the heads of sheep that have been killed or have died at pasture. All abattoir refuse should be satisfactorily disposed of. (*See also under* PARASITES, p. 653.)

GILCHRIST'S DISEASE.—Infection in man with *Blastomyces dermatitidis.* (*See* BLASTOMYCOSIS.)

GILT.—A female pig intended for breeding purposes and up to the time she has her first litter.

GIMMER (*see under* SHEEP).

GINGIVITIS (*gingivæ*, the gums) means inflammation of the gums.

GIZZARD (*see under* GRIT).

GLANDERS may be defined as a specific, contagious, and inoculable disease of the horse family (equidæ), but also liable to be contracted by certain other mammals, including man himself, and characterised by the formation of nodules in the lungs, liver, spleen, or other organs; ulcerations of the mucous membranes, especially those of the upper air passages, accompanied by changes in the lymphatics and also by skin lesions. It is due to the entrance and growth in the body of the glanders bacillus (*Pfeifferella mallei*).

History.—Glanders has been known as a serious scourge since about 450 B.C., when it was mentioned by Hippocrates, and its contagious nature was pointed out by Vegetius (a veterinary writer) in the fourth century. Loeffler and Schütz first isolated the causal organism in 1882.

Distribution.—Glanders has been distributed to practically every country in the world at some time or other, and has been a usual concomitant of wars, which probably have done more to spread it than any other single factor. It is especially a disease of armies and of towns, where animals are liable to be crowded together into a small space, and it has always been rare in country districts. It became very prevalent, both in the United Kingdom and in South Africa, after the South African war. In the year 1892 there were more than 3000 cases of glanders recorded in Great Britain, in 1904 between 2000 and 3000, while only nine outbreaks were recorded in the year 1923, and none since 1926.

Susceptibility.—The donkey is the most susceptible to the disease and always suffers from the acute form, from which it dies in from 2 to 3 weeks.

In the horse, glanders occurs in an acute or a chronic form, the latter existing for months or even years before it finally kills its victim; however, under modern conditions it is rare to allow the disease to run its natural course. The mule is intermediate in susceptibility between the donkey and the horse, but usually shows the acute type.

Of other animals, the carnivora are the most likely to be affected, instances having occurred of menagerie animals such as lions and tigers contracting the disease from feeding upon glandered horse-flesh. The dog and the cat do not take the disease unless fed upon glandered flesh. Sheep, goats, and pigs are said to be liable to artificial infection, but for all practical purposes may be considered to be immune, while the ox is completely so. The camel is susceptible, though natural cases are very rare. Of experimental animals the guinea-pig is the most susceptible, while white rats are immune. Glanders in the human subject is a very distressing and nearly always fatal disease, and may be contracted by stable-men. Laboratory workers handling infected material or pure cultures of the organism are especially liable to infection, so that every precaution against this contingency has to be taken; in fact, the glanders bacillus is amongst the most dangerous of all disease-producing germs cultivated.

The causal organism is present in all the lesions, though it does not—except the rare cases—circulate in the blood-stream. It is found in the nodules in the lungs; is present in the ulcerations produced on the nasal mucous membranes, so that it is always present in the nasal discharge of affected animals; it may be coughed up, and is always discharged in the pus coming away from the abscesses of the skin. Thus, mangers and water-troughs (and so the food and the water), stall fittings, bedding, manure, or in fact anything which comes into contact with diseased animals, may become infective and be able to spread the disease. The organism can live for long periods in dark, damp, and ill-ventilated stables. Healthy horses can be infected naturally by three different channels:

1. By the digestive tract, through the medium of infected food and water. This is by far the commonest method of spread.
2. By inhalation (rarely) when some abrasion of the respiratory passage is present.
3. By skin infection.

The commonest means of spreading the disease is by the introduction of an infected animal into a stud ; and when it is realised that a horse may be glandered and yet show no signs even to a careful observer, it will be understood that in countries where the disease is prevalent no new animal should be introduced without being first examined by a veterinary surgeon, who could submit it to the mallein test.

Incubative period.—Under normal conditions the shortest period is about a fortnight, but in the case of the horse many months may elapse between the entrance of the infection into the body and the onset of any signs of disease. By direct inoculation or other experimental means of infection the incubative period ranges from 3 to 5 days only.

Symptoms.—The signs of glanders in the horse are very varied. The disease may run an acute course of only 2 or 3 weeks, but by far the greatest number of cases met with are of a sub-acute or chronic nature. A horse may be affected and show no outward sign of disease, and yet perhaps it may have a few, or even many, small nodules in one or both lungs. Such cases are said to be 'latent', and are really of the most dangerous type, inasmuch as they are unsuspected. Sooner or later the resistance of the subject to the disease breaks down.

Glanders may be of the nasal, pulmonary, or glandular form, of the type producing skin lesions (farcy), or an admixture of these, and it may also become generalised. One of the dangers of the disease is that a horse may work for weeks or even months with 'open' lesions—not losing a great deal of flesh nor appearing very ill—and so spread the disease to healthy horses with which it comes into contact.

The general signs are some unthriftiness, dullness of the coat, sluggishness while at work ; the horse easily becomes tired, may have a slight cough (especially on coming out of its stable or drinking cold water on a cold morning), or may give an occasional grunt when turned round sharply. There may be a slight nasal discharge, 'filling' of one or more of the limbs, and the passage of an excessive quantity of urine (polyuria).

The temperature.—This varies in the more acute cases from 103° to 104° F., but may occasionally be as high as 107° F. In such cases the pulse and respirations become accelerated.

Glandular enlargements.—The commonest superficial gland to be affected is the sub-maxillary, which is found to be hard, nodular, firm, and may reach the size of a hen's egg. Suppuration is rare, and but slight pain is evinced on palpation. This condition is always present when ulcers occur on the nose, but frequently it may be seen when no nasal ulcers are apparent. When farcy is present the glands inside the axilla or inside the groin may be somewhat enlarged and even painful to the touch. In entire horses the testicles often become enlarged and painful, or even the seat of glanderous abscesses.

Nasal symptoms.—There may be a nasal discharge, thin and watery in the early stages, but later becoming thick, greyish, or yellow and oily. It is more commonly one-sided than bilateral, and the left nostril is the one more frequently involved. In severe cases the discharge may become blood-stained and mixed with pus. The nostrils often become coated with a sticky mass, which may partially block up the orifices. On looking into the nose the lining membrane may be congested or of a greyish colour, but this soon gives place to the formation of ulcerating sores. These vary in size and extent, and may be covered with a dirty loose scab, or may show exuberant, red, granulating edges, from which there may be slight bleeding. In severe cases the whole septum of the nose may be one ulcerating sore, and perforation of the cartilage separating the two nostrils may take place. In other cases no ulcers may be seen at all, although they may be present in the upper part of the nasal chamber and over the turbinated bones. When this state of affairs is present breathing becomes very fast and is accompanied by a noisy snoring which is characteristic. Examination of the nose in these cases is dangerous, as man may easily contract the disease by this means.

FARCY.—In this form of the disease the skin is involved. It is usually chronic in nature, but farcy buds and subcutaneous swellings may complicate the most acute form of the disease shortly before death. This complication is especially common in the mule, which often succumbs to the disease before the farcy buds have time to burst. In chronic farcy there is usually swelling of one or more limbs, more frequently a hind one. The lymphatic glands of the affected limb become enlarged, the lymph vessels corded, and usually a chain of farcy buds develops along their course. These 'buds' com-

GLANDERS

mence as nodules, but soon soften and burst, giving off a sticky, yellowish pus, and evince but little tendency to heal. 'Open' buds have red and exuberant edges. They vary in size from that of a hen's egg on the shoulder or groin to the size of a pea, and they show a liability to occur in consecutive crops. Similar lesions may be present on the lymphatics of the body, or even occasionally on the face and under the jaw, while lesions on the neck may also be found. As a general rule farcy is secondary to lesions in the lungs, but it may occur alone.

In acute glanders there may be all the signs of an acute broncho-pneumonia, a high temperature, a rapid loss of flesh, rapid and sometimes noisy breathing, followed by death in a few weeks; in fact, this is the common form seen in the donkey and often in the mule, with or without the complication of farcy.

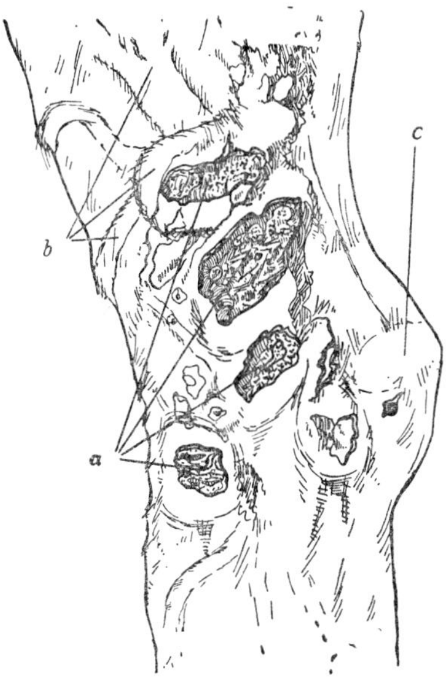

Farcy lesions, or the skin form of glanders, on the inside of the hind leg of a horse. At *a*, there are shown open raw lesions from which highly infective purulent material is discharged; *b*, swollen and corded lymphatics; *c*, point of the hock.

As glanders is in most countries a notifiable disease, any suspicious case should be shown to the nearest veterinary practitioner, or the local police notified.

According to law, the carcase of a glandered animal must be disposed of by the Local Authority in some manner as laid down in the Glanders and Farcy Order. (*See* DISPOSAL OF CARCASES.)

Diagnosis.—The following diseases may be confused with glanders:

1. *Common cold.*—In this the nasal discharge is bilateral and is less sticky, the glands are less involved, but in cases of doubt the mallein test will settle the matter.

2. *Strangles.* — This disease usually occurs in young horses; the swelling under the jaw is diffuse, more painful, and usually suppurates; the nasal discharge is profuse, bilateral, and comes away in flake-like masses and does not adhere to the nostrils in the same way as in glanders; the temperature in glanders is not usually so high as it tends to be in strangles.

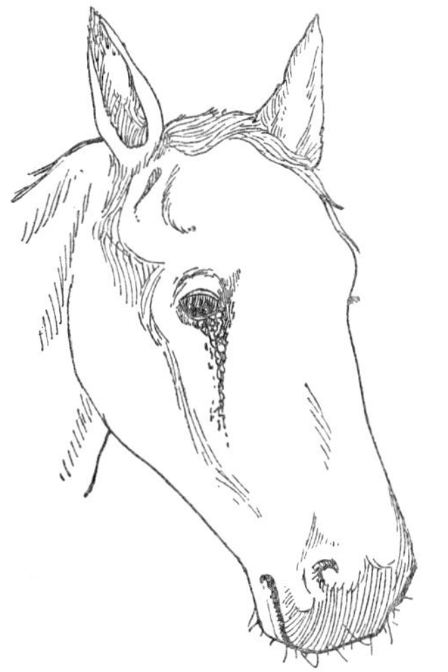

Diagram to illustrate a positive reaction to the ophthalmic mallein test. From the tested eye a muco-purulent discharge is poured out from between swollen and inflamed eyelids. The other eye is unaffected.

3. *Epizoötic lymphangitis.*—This disease is not accompanied by nasal or pulmonary lesions. Only an expert veterinarian is qualified to differentiate this condition, which he does by the examination of the pus for the causal organism of this disease (*see* EPIZOÖTIC LYMPHANGITIS) and by submitting the animal to the mallein test.

4. *Ulcerative lymphangitis.*—In this disease, which also may be mistaken for farcy, the ulcers heal up more readily and there are neither general nor nasal lesions. The mallein test is, however, indicated.

5. *Nasal gleet.*—In this condition there

is a chronic nasal discharge, which is often evil-smelling and purulent, but the application of the mallein test will definitely differentiate it from glanders.

Mallein is prepared from a pure culture of the glanders bacillus, and consists of a glycerin extract made from the dead bodies of the organisms. It does not contain the organisms, either dead or alive, and cannot under any circumstances produce glanders when injected into the body.

Mallein is usually injected under the skin, and a reaction consists of a rise of temperature at a given time and the production of a local swelling at the injection seat. The application and reading of the test should not be attempted by amateurs. Mallein may also be instilled into an eye, or injected into the thickness of the skin, but a specially prepared mallein is necessary for these tests.

Treatment.—The law in most civilised countries does not admit of any form of treatment being tried, as all diagnosed cases must be destroyed as soon as possible. In Yugoslavia, however, success has been reported with Sulphathiazole.

GLANDS is a term loosely applied to a number of different organs, such as the liver, pancreas, kidneys, udder, etc., which produce a secretion, and to the smaller structures concerned in the excretion of some substance from the body, or in the production of some substance needful for its proper working. A description of the larger so-called 'glands' will be found under headings such as KIDNEYS, LIVER, MAMMARY GLANDS, OVARIES, PANCREAS, SALIVARY GLANDS, TESTIS, etc. The smaller glands which will be considered here are divisible into two distinct groups: (1) glands which produce some formless secretion or excretion, and (2) lymphatic glands.

(1) **Secreting or excreting glands** comprise glands in almost all parts of the body, which vary in character, in size, and in the nature of the substance produced. The skin, for example, is richly supplied with sebaceous glands which secrete an oily material, and, in most animals except the dog, with sweat glands. The lining membrane of the digestive parts of the stomach is made up of long, tubular glands set as closely as possible side by side, and in these the gastric juice is formed. The structure of the mucous membrane in the intestine is much the same. In all these mucous membranes there are situated other glands, generally formed each of a small mass of twisted tubules, which secrete a clear, shining, thick fluid, known as mucus, which gives to these membranes their soft smooth appearance and their name. The glands so far mentioned are all of microscopic size, but there are many of large dimensions. The parotid gland, situated below and behind the ear; the submaxillary gland, situated just within the angle of the lower jaw; and the sublingual gland, which lies below the tongue, are all occupied in the production of saliva, and are known as salivary glands. The mammary glands are large

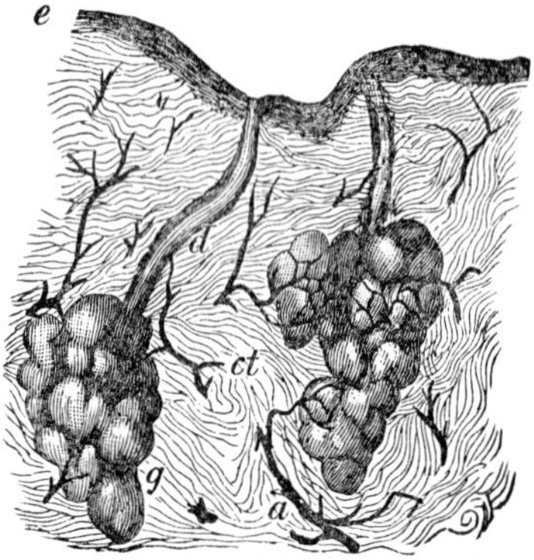

Section through the mucous membrane of the throat to show two of its mucous glands. *e*, Epithelium of surface; *ct*, connective tissue; *g*, gland; *d*, its duct; *a*, artery ending in small vessels and capillaries around the gland. Magnified ×40. (Turner's *Anatomy*.)

glands situated in the skin of the under part of the abdomen, or in the inguinal region between the thighs; they secrete milk. The thyroid gland, situated around the first ring of the trachea or windpipe, has no outlet to the exterior, but produces a very important secretion which is absorbed by the blood and carried throughout the body. The adrenal glands, which are situated at the anterior end of each kidney, and the pituitary gland, attached to the lower surface of the brain, behave similarly. Many of the glands which have a definite outlet for their secretions, such as the pancreas and testes, also produce what is called an 'internal secretion', or *hormone*, which is absorbed by the bloodstream and exerts a profound effect upon the bodily economy and upon the general nutrition of the body. (*See* HORMONES.)

(2) **Lymphatic glands** are scattered all through the body in connection with the system of lymphatic vessels, which carry

the lymph. (*See* LYMPH.) They vary in size from microscopic masses to structures as large as walnuts, but they have essentially the same structure everywhere. Round each gland is a fibrous-tissue capsule, from which partitions and bands run into the gland to join one another and give it cohesion. In the meshes of these lie enormous numbers of lymph corpuscles, which ultimately form the white corpuscles of the circulating blood. These corpuscles are arranged in masses round which the lymph circulates freely. Numbers of lymph vessels (afferent vessels) pierce the capsule of the gland, and the lymph, after passing from them, percolates through the gland and leaves the central end (carrying with it many corpuscles), by entering one of the larger outgoing lymph vessels (efferent vessels). As a rule the lymph glands are arranged in a chain one after the other, so that efferent vessels from one gland become afferent to another a short distance farther on.

In the limbs the lymph vessels pass upwards to the region of the elbow and stifle respectively before they meet any lymph glands. A few glands are situated in the bends of these joints, and the vessels passing from them reach the large chain of glands in the axilla of the fore-arm and the groin of the hind-limb. From here the vessels, carrying lymph which has been, so to speak, filtered through the various glands, pass into the thorax and abdomen respectively. At the back of the throat and down the lower part of the neck there are chains of glands which deal with lymph which has been formed in the head and neck. Inside the abdomen small lymph vessels, known as 'lacteals', collect certain substances from the food of the intestines, and pass their contents up through the 'mesenteric glands', situated in the mesenteries of the intestines. From these mesenteric glands large efferent lymphatics eventually pour their contained lymph into a large cistern, called the 'cisterna chyli', which lies high up in the abdomen close to the lower part of the spinal column. The 'thoracic duct' runs forward from the 'cisterna chyli' into and through the chest cavity, receiving as it passes lymph from the lungs, which has passed through the 'bronchial glands', situated at the root of each lung, and collecting the lymph from the fore-limbs, eventually emptying into a large vein at the root of the neck. In this way the lymph, which originally was derived from the blood-stream, is again returned to the blood-stream, and the white corpuscles formed in the lymph glands are enabled to enter the blood circulation. Beyond forming these corpuscles the glands have another function, acting as a species of filters for the lymph circulation, and keeping back organisms and other dangerous impurities from entering the blood circulation. (*See also* HARDERIAN GLAND.)

GLANDS, DISEASES OF.—The diseases of the large and important glands of the body will be found under their various headings, and reference is only made here to diseases of lymph glands. Most of the diseases which affect these glands are of an inflammatory nature, and in very many cases the cause is the trapping of some variety of pathogenic organism in the gland, or of the poisonous products of bacterial activity, with consequent localisation of a diseased focus in the gland itself.

SIMPLE ENLARGEMENT AND SUPPURATION is perhaps the commonest diseased condition to which glands are liable. Owing to the covering of hair over the animal's body this condition is very frequently not noticed by the owner until a hot, tense, painful swelling forms and the gland bursts. In other cases the swelling and inflammation subside, and it is perhaps only by accident that the condition is discovered. The condition usually depends upon the presence of a wound or other source of infection in the area drained by the lymph vessels going to the gland. For example, a severe wound of the foot may give rise to a swelling of the glands on the inside of the groin, or a diseased tooth or other suppurating area in the mouth of a horse may cause the gland at the corner of the jaw to enlarge in size, and even pass on to suppuration and acute abscess formation.

Treatment.—It is necessary to eliminate the original cause of the infection, by treating wounds in a rational manner, extracting diseased or suppurating teeth, etc. The actual gland itself is usually best left alone, but if the pain and swelling are very severe, hot fomentations may be advisable. When a gland suppurates and bursts it should be treated exactly like an acute abscess, which, in fact, it is.

TUBERCULOSIS of one or more of the glands in various parts of the body is a very common condition in pigs and cattle which are affected with this disease in other parts of their bodies. It is an important fact, from the meat inspector's point of view, that whenever tuberculosis invades a tissue, sooner or later some of the germs become imprisoned in the lymph glands which lie in the vicinity, and set up disease there. As a rule the retropharyngeal (at the back of the throat), prescapular (in front of the shoulder-blade), the precrural (just outside the fold of the stifle), the mediastinals, which drain the lungs, the mesenterics, which receive lymph from the intestines, and the mammary lymph glands are the most commonly affected. They are painless, hard, and cold to the touch, and the swelling develops slowly. They are an indication of tubercular disease in the animal's body. On rare occasions it may be advisable to remove those that are situated superficially surgically.

STRANGLES very commonly manifests itself in the horse as a swelling and suppuration in the submaxillary lymph gland, situated just inside the angle of the lower jaw. (*See* STRANGLES.)

LYMPHADENITIS is another name for the comparatively rare condition which is often known as Hodgkin's disease. (*See* PSEUDO-LEUKÆMIA.)

TUMOURS of lymph glands are not uncommon.

GLASSER'S DISEASE.—An infection and swelling of the hock or knee joints, or both, in the pig. There is fever, lameness and a disinclination to move. Death is usually a sequel, unless early treatment with *e.g.* penicillin is undertaken. Glasser's disease is differentiated from 'Joint-Ill'. Pigs of 5 to 14 weeks old are chiefly affected. The cause is *Hæmophilus suis*, or a mycoplasma, or both.

GLAUBER'S SALTS is the popular name for sodium sulphate, a saline purgative, given in doses of from ½ to 1½ lb. to horses and cattle, and 2 to 4 ounces to sheep, dissolved in treacle water. As a febrifuge it is often prescribed in small doses given in the food or drinking water. It is an antidote to carbolic acid poisoning, forming with it sulphocarbolate of soda, which is non-poisonous. A dose of 4 ounces is said to be dangerous in the pig, and fatal poisoning has occurred with Glauber's salt given in three daily doses.

GLAUCOMA (*see under* EYE, p. 326).

GLENOID CAVITY (γληνοειδής) is the shallow socket on the shoulder-blade into which the humerus fits, forming the shoulder-joint.

GLIOMA (γλία, glue) is the name given to a tumour which forms in the brain or spinal cord. It is composed of neuroglia, which is the special connective tissue found supporting the nerve cells and the nerve fibres. (*See* TUMOURS.)

GLOBIDIOSIS.—A disease characterised by enteritis and closely resembling coccidiosis. It occurs in Africa, S.W. Europe, the U.S.A., and Australia. The cause is (species of) *Globidium*. Cysts may be formed in the skin or underlying tissue. Horses, cattle, and sheep are affected.

GLOBULIN is the term applied to a class of proteins which are insoluble in water and alcohol but soluble in weak salt solution. Antibodies may be regarded as a modified form of serum globulin. A gamma globulin preparation has been introduced to give passive immunity to Distemper, Hard Pad, Rubarth's disease, and various secondary bacterial invaders; the single product being more stable and less bulky than antiserum. (*See also under* GAMMA GLOBOLIN.)

GLOMERULUS (*glomus*, a ball) is the term applied to a small knot of blood-vessels about the size of a sand grain, of which an immense number are found in the kidney, and from which the excretion of fluid out of the blood into the tubules of the kidney takes place. (*See* KIDNEY.)

GLOSSITIS (γλῶσσα, the tongue) means inflammation of the tongue.

GLOSSOPHARYNGEAL NERVE (γλῶσσα, the tongue; φάρυγξ, the throat) is the 9th cranial nerve, which in the main is sensory. It is the nerve of taste for the back of the tongue, of sensation in a general way for the upper part of the throat, as well as for the middle ear, and it supplies the parotid gland.

GLOTTIS (γλωττίς) is the narrow opening at the upper end of the larynx. (*See* AIR PASSAGES, CHOKING, LARYNX.)

GLUCOSE is the form of sugar found in honey, grapes, fruits, etc., and in diabetes mellitus it is passed in the urine. It is the form in which sugar circulates in the blood-stream, and is very useful as an injection or drench when there is a deficiency of circulating sugar in the blood or an excess of ketones. (*See* ACETONÆMIA.) Glucose is a most valuable food to give during the course of acute illnesses, since it puts no strain upon the digestive system yet provides fuel for the muscles, etc. Glucose saline is given as a drink or administered *per rectum* or by subcutaneous injection during the course of jaundice, gastro-enteritis, etc. (*See* SUGARS.)

GLUCOSIDES are crystalline bitter compounds of sugar and a non-sugar residue. They are commonly found in plants, and some such as strophanthin and digitalin are used therapeutically. Others, on being acted upon by a specific ferment produce hydrocyanic acid. These are known as cyanogenetic glucosides; some are found in linseed, laurel, and Java beans.

GLUTEALS (γλουτός, buttock) is the scientific name applied to the region of the buttocks, and to structures associated with that region, such as gluteal arteries, muscles, nerves.

GLUTEN (*gluten*, glue) is the constituent of wheat and some other flours which forms an adhesive mixture upon the addition of water. It can be separated from the starch of flour, and being rich in protein it is used for feeding purposes, that from maize flour being known as 'maize gluten feed'.

GLYCERIN, or **GLYCEROL,** is a clear, colourless, odourless, thick liquid of a sweet taste, obtained by decomposition and distillation of fats. It dissolves many substances and has a great power of absorbing water, in consequence of which, in the pure state, it is slightly irritant to moist living surfaces with which it comes in contact.

Uses.—Given by the mouth, diluted, it has been used with success in the treatment of pregnancy toxæmia in ewes and of acetonæmia in cattle. Internally, glycerin acts as a laxative to the dog in moderate doses, and as a purge when large amounts are given. It is soothing and antiseptic to inflamed mucous membranes in the mouth and throat. In amounts of ½ to 1 ounce it is useful as a rectal injection to induce passage of impacted fæces in obstinate constipation in the dog, and it may be used for the same purpose in foals and calves. For these purposes it may be given diluted with a little water, or it may be used in the pure state. It is also used as a basis for the compounding of various electuaries for the horse and dog, and it is sometimes incorporated into cough mixtures for the smaller animals. It forms a basis for certain skin dressings when it is desired to soften the skin surface and encourage the absorption of other drugs.

It is also used as a diluent for semen. (*See under* ARTIFICIAL INSEMINATION.)

GLYCEROPHOSPHATES of lime, iron, etc., are compounds of glycerin with the respective phosphates. They are supposed to be specially useful for debility following a serious or wasting disease, because glycero-phosphoric acid is present in nerve tissue.

GLYCOGEN (γλυκύς, sweet; γεννάω, I beget), or **ANIMAL STARCH,** is a carbohydrate substance found specially in the liver as well as in other tissues. It is the form in which carbohydrates taken in the food are stored in the liver and muscles before they are converted into glucose as the needs of the system require.

GLYCOSURIA (γλυκύς, sweet; οὐρέω, I make water) means the presence of glucose in the urine. It is seen in diabetes mellitus (*see* DIABETES), and in some other conditions, such as after dogs have been fed to excess upon sweet, sugary pastries, fruits, etc., and in all animals after severe shocks. (*See also under* URINE, ABNORMAL CONDITIONS OF.)

GLYCYRRHETINIC ACID.—Obtained from liquorice, it has been used for reducing inflammation and is cheaper than cortisone preparations.

GNOTOBIOTICS.—The name given to germ-free laboratory animals reared according to techniques developed by Professor J. A. Reyniers of Notre Dame University, Chicago. Such animals have been used in the investigation of certain diseases. (*See also* S.P.F., DISEASE-FREE.)

GOADS, ELECTRIC.—These are preferable to the use of carelessly or sadistically wielded sticks, and are a help. The points should be spring-loaded, as otherwise they can be jabbed into the animal—when the purpose and object of an electric goad are defeated.

GOATS, DISEASES OF.—Milk Fever (Hypocalcæmia), acetonæmia, pregnancy toxæmia, rickets, mastitis, tuberculosis, Johne's disease, infection with *Brucella melitensis* (causing Malta Fever), variola

(Goat Pox), contagious pustular dermatitis, parasitic bronchitis, parasitic gastro-enteritis, coccidosis, infestation with liver-flukes, tapeworms, sheep nostril fly, sheep keds, harvest mites, mange mites, licc, ticks, infective pneumonia, contagious agalactia, caseous lymphadentitis, enterotoxæmia, ' Cloudburst ', salmonellosis, swayback, etc.

GOITRE (from *guttar*, the throat), is a condition, associated with an iodine deficiency, in which the thyroid gland enlarges in size. It is seen in puppies, foals, and lambs, and also in calves, and it appears to be commoner in some districts than in others. Swellings may appear below the larynx, usually one on either side, and beyond the local enlargements there may be no definite symptoms shown. Some cases respond to the administration of thyroid extracts, and iodine internally, while some clear up spontaneously without treatment. Some pastures and foodstuffs may give rise to goitre. (*See* GOITROGEN.) Goitre seems particularly common in Dorset Horn sheep.

Exophthalmic Goitre (Grave's Disease) is rarely seen in the dog and is characterised by enlargement of the thryoid gland, together with exophthalmos (bulging eyeballs) and excitability. There is excessive secretion of thyroxine. Treatment may include the use of X-rays, ligature of the anterior arteries of the gland, or the administration of sodium fluoride (used in human medicine), or of methylthiouracil. (*See* IODINE DEFICIENCY.)

A number of cases of supposed ' goitre ' prove upon careful examination to be tumour growth in some part of the throat, not necessarily in connection with the thyroid gland.

Cystic goitre, so-called, is a condition sometimes met with in the dog, in which there is an enlargement of the thyroid gland and the formation of a large cyst in connection with it.

GOITROGEN, GOITROGENIC FACTOR is one which gives rise to goitre. Both kale and cabbage contain goitrogens and must therefore not constitute too large a proportion of an animal's ration over a period. The same applies to turnips. Iodine licks may be advisable. (*See* IODINE DEFICIENCY.)

GONAD is a gland which produces a gamete, *i.e.* the ovary or testis.

GONADOTROPHIC (γονη, semen ; τρέφω, I nourish) indicates something which stimulates the gonads—testes and ovaries. (*See below and* HORMONES.)

GONADOTROPHINS are hormones which have a gonadotrophic effect in the body. (*See* HORMONES.)

Chorionic gonadotrophin effects luteinisation and is used in the treatment of functional uterine hæmorrhage, cases of habitual abortion, and to induce descent of the testes in cases of cryptorchidism.

Serum gonadotrophin contains a follicle-stimulating hormone which affects the gonads of both sexes. It is used in the treatment of sterility, anœstrus, and hypoplasia of the gonads.

' GOOSE-STEPPING.'—In the pig this can be a symptom of a deficiency of pantothenic acid, one of the B group of vitamins.

GOSSYPOL POISONING affects calves fed upon undecorticated cotton-cake in any quantity. Formerly it was thought that the harmful effects resulting from feeding young calves upon such cake were due to the indigestible husks and adherent cotton collecting into a mass and forming a concretion in the 4th stomach (hair-ball), but lately it has been held that the adverse effects are due in part to *gossypol*, a substance present in these indigestible remnants of the cotton seeds. This agent is most probably one of the class of plant-poisons (phyto-toxins) which are able to exert far more powerful effects in young animals which are not receiving optimum amounts of vitamin A in their food.

Symptoms.—Severe watery diarrhœa passed with painful straining, loss of appetite, frequent gritting of the teeth, a staring coat, and rapid emaciation. Calves under three months are mainly affected, especially when allowed to feed with their mothers from the trough, and when the cows are getting undecorticated cotton-cake.

GOUT is in man now regarded as one of the rheumatic diseases. It may occur in the dog and the fowl.

Symptoms.—There is progressive tenderness over the joints of one or more limbs to begin with, and later some swelling can be detected. The animal becomes lame and may be unable to place the limb on the ground. In time the swellings become very marked, perhaps attaining the size of a walnut, and there is distortion of the limb. The general health suffers after a time, animals becoming weak, easily exhausted, emaciated, and anæmic.

GOUT, CALCIUM.—(*Calcinosis circumscripta*). This has been recorded in dogs and monkeys as well as in man, and involves the deposition of calcium salts and the appearance of fibrous tissue around the deposits. Firm, painless nodules occur under the skin of the limbs and feet and at the elbow. Ulceration, with a gritty discharge, may occur. The cause is unknown. Diagnosis may be assisted by radiography. Calcium-gout occurs mainly in large breeds of dog, *e.g.* Alsatians.

G.P.D. (*See under* GUTTURAL POUCH DIPHTHERIA).

GRAÄFIAN FOLLICLE.—The mature ovarian follicle. (*See* OVARIES.)

GRAINS, BREWERS'.—Brewers' grains are a by-product of brewing, consisting of the exhausted malt, and are used wet in some cases, where they can be easily obtained from a near-by brewery, or as dried grains. They are useful as a feeding-stuff for cattle, pigs, and sheep, but must be introduced gradually into the ration. Wet grains are almost entirely used for feeding milk cows. They must be used fresh as they deteriorate on keeping. Dried grains keep well, and are suitable for horses, about 5 to 10 lb. daily, and to sheep, up to ½ lb.

GRAINS, DISTILLERS'. — Distillery grains are produced as a by-product during the manufacture of whisky in a manner somewhat similar to brewers' grains in the manufacture of beer. They are sold either wet or dry, but are much to be preferred dry, since the wet grains are liable to contain considerable amounts of raw alcohol, which may lead to intoxication of animals eating them. The amounts and uses are similar to brewers' grains.

GRAMICIDIN is an antibiotic made from a Gram-positive organism *Bacillus brevis*, which is capable of destroying certain other organisms such as staphylococci and pneumococci which produce disease.

GRANULAR VULVOVAGINITIS (*See under* VULVOVAGINITIS).

GRANULATIONS are small masses of cells of a constructive nature containing loops of newly formed blood-vessels which spring up over the surfaces of healing wounds. What is commonly called ' proud flesh '.

GRANULOMA.—A granular tumour.

GRASS DISEASE, or **GRASS SICKNESS,** is a disease of horses which has been recognised in the central and eastern areas of Scotland since 1907, and has spread to Wales and to many parts of England; also in Sweden. It occurs in horses after they are put on to the grass between the months of April and September, being commonest in May, June, and July, and decreasing in gravity as the autumn approaches. In certain years a few sporadic cases may occur at other times. Heavy draught horses were formerly most often attacked, but of recent years practically all breeds of horses have been affected, including ponies.

Cause.—After some 40 years' or more extensive research work the exact cause is still unknown. Recently it has been suggested that a neurotropic virus could be responsible. This is suggested by the degeneration of certain ganglia of the sympathetic nervous system.

Symptoms.—The disease may be (1) *per-acute*, with death occurring in 8 to 16 hours, and periods of great violence being shown when the animal may be a danger to people looking after it; (2) *sub-acute*. The horse becomes dull and listless and off its food. It may have an anxious expression, and roll from pain. Later there may be a discharge from the nostrils, and an excessive amount of salivation. Swallowing is difficult, although the animal makes valiant attempts to chew his food and ingest it. The muscles of the shoulder show localised twitching, and patchy sweating occurs over the body, especially round the tail, where the perspiration is soapy in appearance. The bowels are quite inactive, and no fæces are passed after this stage. The food material becomes impacted in the large colon, and the bowel distension is so great that the gut feels distinctly hard when examined per rectum. The breathing alters, and a soft but indistinct snore is heard. Attempts to vomit are frequent, but only particles of food material and fluids are ejected from the nostrils. Horses with this form appear to get some relief by pressing their hindquarters firmly against a wall or manger (on which they may appear to be trying to sit). The pulse becomes weaker and weaker until it can scarcely be felt. The illness lasts for from 2 to 5 days, when death or the chronic stage supervenes. The mortality is high.

(3) *Chronic.*—Here again the animal is dull and disinclined for food, but there is not the marked impaction of the bowel that is seen in the acute variety. Some fæces are passed, of a semi-fluid nature, coated with mucus. Dribbling of saliva is not so marked but is still present, while the discharge from the nostrils is more obvious. Dry food is not easily swallowed, but soft, moist food is taken slowly. The food is very well chewed, but portions are dropped from the mouth in the process. Spasmodic attempts are made to vomit, and fluids and ingested food-stuffs are ejected from the nostrils as in the acute type. Twitchings over the shoulder are also seen, and the muscles of the back become hard and board-like. The croup falls to a lower level, the hind-legs are kept well under the body, and the tail is often elevated. During all this time the horse has been getting progressively thinner, until in the later stages it has a tucked-up 'greyhound' appearance. The horse may live for a variable period in this state; some last only a few weeks, but others linger on for six months or more. Many are killed after they have been treated for some time, owing to the unprofitableness of keeping them till better or till they regain some of their former condition. A few recover, but a long period elapses before they are able to stand up to their accustomed work. Complications due to the inspiration of vomited food-stuffs into the trachea and lungs, such as bronchitis or pneumonia, are responsible for the death of a number.

Apart from the nerve findings in this disease perhaps the most characteristic is spasm of the pylorus by which the outlet of foods from the stomach is prevented. Fluid in very large amounts collects in the stomach distending it greatly and causing distress. At the same time, fluids are absorbed from the colon and cæcum and the contents of these become very dry and doughy.

Treatment.—Most of the usual purgatives have at various times been tried, but even though very large doses were administered they failed to produce evacuation of the overloaded bowel.

No medicinal treatment is of any avail so far as is known at present. The only measures that can be recommended are those that concern the animal's comfort.

'GRASS TETANY' (*see under* HYPOMAGNESÆMIA).

GRASS, TURNING OUT TO (*see under* YARDED CATTLE).

GRASSLAND MANAGEMENT (*see under* PASTURE MANAGEMENT).

GRAVEL is the name applied to any sediment that falls down in the urine, but particularly to small masses of uric acid crystals, which in time, and if the causal conditions are not checked, will result in the production of stones or calculi. (*See* CONCRETIONS and HYALURONIDASE.)

GRAVES'S DISEASE is another name for exophthalmic goitre.

GRAZING BEHAVIOUR.—A study, made at Cornell University, of Aberdeen-Angus and Hereford cows at pasture (receiving no supplementary feed) showed that:

1. The average grazing time was 7 hours and 32 minutes, of which 4 hours and 52 minutes were spent in actual eating, and the balance in walking and selecting herbage during the process of grazing. During the hours of darkness the cattle grazed for 2 hours and 28 minutes.

2. In a pasture of six acres the cow travelled 2·45 miles, of which 1·96 were during daylight and 0·49 hours during darkness.

3. The cows lay down for 11 hours and 39 minutes, but this was divided into nine periods ranging from less than one hour to more than six hours. The time spent in chewing the cud averaged 6 hours and 51 minutes.

4. The calves, which were about three months old, were suckled three times a day at intervals of eight hours, and for 15 minutes at a time.

5. Droppings were deposited on an average twelve times a day and urine nine times.

6. Under the conditions prevailing, the cows drank water once a day only. This may be accounted for by the luxuriant

pasture herbage consisting of Kentucky bluegrass and wild white clover with an average water content of 72 per cent.

7. The cows showed no inclination to extend the grazing period beyond eight hours even when the amount of herbage consumed fell to 45 pounds a day. 'It is evident that a mechanical factor is involved in grazing management and that one of the basic principles of good pasture management is to provide the livestock with pastures in a condition which will permit them to gather the optimum amount of food within a normal period of eight hours' grazing.

'We may speculate upon the potential productivity of British pastures if we ever achieve a degree of efficiency in grazing management which will permit mature cattle to consume daily the normal maximum of about 150 lb. of green herbage. This should be sufficient for maintenance and the production of about 50 lb. of milk or possibly for the production of 5 lb. live-weight increase daily.' (Professor D. R. Johnstone-Wallace.)

Recent work, however, and especially that in New Zealand, has proved that the time dairy cattle graze and ruminate is very flexible, and that the feed intake varies much less from day to day than the time spent in grazing. The cow has, in fact, a capacity to change her grazing habits to suit both her environment and her own bodily needs.

The quartering of a field by horses into parts for grazing and parts for defæcation has been described by E. L. Taylor, who adds that cattle avoid the grass in the proximity of fæcal parts. 'The fineness of this perception of contamination is shown by a helminthologist's observation that cattle were able to detect minute traces of fæces such as he was not able to see.'

GRAZING MANAGEMENT (*see* PASTURE MANAGEMENT).

GREASE, which is also called SEBORRHŒA and STEARRHŒA, is a form of chronic inflammation of the skin of the region of the fetlocks and pasterns of horses' legs.

Cause.—Grease is usually associated with horses of a slow lymphatic temperament which have thick, coarse legs, kept in dirty, damp, dark stables, the frequent wading in muddy, stagnant ponds, and other conditions of uncleanliness. In some cases, however, grease appears in horses with clean legs, kept under good conditions of management, and it is liable to affect almost any variety of horse. It is considered by some to be due to an excessive protein content in the food, but it may appear out at grass when no hand-feeding is being given, so that while feeding may influence the condition it is not the sole cause. Various organisms, especially a *spirillum*, have been found in the discharges from greasy legs, but they are probably all accidental invaders —the result of the grease, not the cause.

It is notable that since Shires especially have been bred with less feather and with finer limbs, grease has become less frequent.

Symptoms.—The first stages of grease are very often not noticed, owing to the 'feather' which covers the areas where it usually first appears, but when they are seen they are found to be swelling and reddening of the skin, with a certain amount of itchiness. There is an excessive secretion of the natural sebaceous material over the patch, which subsequently appears wet, reddened, painful to touch, and upon the surface of the area there is found a certain amount of thick, greasy, gummy, yellowish discharge, possessing a very persistent characteristic smell. The hair over the patch stands up, and the individual hairs are usually gummed together by the discharges. As the condition advances there is a thickening and hardening of the skin and a rapid proliferation of the surface tissues. These degenerate in time and add to the discharge. When the condition has become chronic, after perhaps six months or so, there are very often found wart-like growths over the affected area. In very old-stand ng cases of this kind there may be little or no skin discharge at all, but in the centre of each bud there is a depression from which a little of the foul-smelling material exudes. Very often grease low down towards the heels of the hind-feet is associated with canker of the hoof, but whether or not there is any relation between the two conditions is not certain.

Grease most commonly affects the hind-feet, but the fore-feet may also be attacked, and in bad cases all four feet may be diseased. In very bad cases it may cause lameness, especially when large growths form in the flexures of the pasterns, but, except in the early stages, it is usually not accompanied by great pain. It is always noticed that the discharge is worse after the horse has stood in the stable at rest during a week-end or other holiday, and that when regular work can be arranged the discharge may practically cease.

Treatment.—Clip all the hair away from the affected areas, and thoroughly wash the leg with soap and water containing washing soda, or bicarbonate of soda if the pain is severe. After the skin is dry the leg should be soaked in a strong solution of an astringent antiseptic, such as 3 ounces each of copper sulphate, alum and zinc sulphate to the gallon of water. Thereafter the limb should be dressed daily at half strength. In cases where there are profuse vegetations, it is necessary to remove all the wart-like excrescences under general anæsthesia. Internally, tonics are very often given.

Prevention.—Good hygiene. The erection of a water-trough and the prevention of wading in muddy ponds, will often prevent further cases on farms where previously they occurred frequently.

'GREASY PIG DISEASE'.—This is a form of seborrhœa, sometimes labelled 'eczema', occurring in piglets. It was thought to be associated with a vitamin B deficiency, and many cases were claimed to respond dramatically when treated accordingly. It is now regarded as a staphylococcal infection. Bites, abrasions, tattooing, and lice infestation may facilitate entry of the organism through the skin.

Often only some piglets in a single litter on the farm are affected. Symptoms include dullness, loss of bloom, and soft, greasy spots on the reddened skin of the snout, ears, around the eyes, and sometimes on the abdomen. The spots join up and spread, and after a few days the piglet may have a largely greasy and brown body, with thickened and cracking skin. Severely affected cases die within a few days; survivors are seldom an economic proposition as recovery takes several weeks and may be incomplete.

Prevention.—Clipping the teeth of piglets, boiling tattooing instruments, and providing concrete which is smooth (and preferably not bare). To be successful, veterinary treatment with a suitable antibiotic has to be undertaken very promptly if it is to succeed. Long-standing cases are best slaughtered. There is no vaccine available.

'GREEN-BOTTLE' FLY (*see* PARASITES, p. 672).

GREENSTICK FRACTURE is one in which the bone fractures incompletely somewhat similar to the break of a green stick. They mostly occur in young animals. (*See* FRACTURES.)

GREYFACE.—The term often applied to a Border Leicester × Scottish Blackface cross.

GRISEOFULVIN.—An antibiotic, which can be given by mouth, effective against ringworm and other fungous diseases. Dosing over a 3-week period may be necessary in the treatment of ringworm in calves.

GRIT FOR POULTRY.—Insoluble grit—sand, flint grit, tiny pebbles—is necessary for the grinding of the food in the gizzard; poultry possessing no teeth. Flint grit should be provided at the rate of 1 lb. per 100 birds, and is best broadcast with the grain every 2 or 3 months; except for battery birds, which require a monthly ration. Where gravel is available, no special flint grit need be provided.

Soluble limestone grit is given in order to supply calcium for bone formation and egg-shell production, and it dissolves in the gizzard within 48 hours. It is not necessary for chicks, growers or birds in early lay if they are receiving commercial mash or pellets without corn Too much limestone grit can be harmful.

GROOMING.—The objects of grooming horses, cattle, and dogs, especially when kept shut up in buildings, are fourfold: it is undertaken for the purpose of cleanliness, for the prevention of disease of the skin, to stimulate the skin circulation, and to remove waste products of metabolism.

Relation to work, etc.—To many people the reason for grooming does not appear to be obvious when they consider that horses out at grass, for example, are frequently not groomed at all for months at a time, that their coats do not suffer to any marked extent, and that their health often actually improves. The reasons for this are that when the same horses are at work they are receiving a much more highly concentrated ration which makes greater demands upon the excretory organs; that tissue wear and tear are invariably heavier at work than when the horse is only taking such exercise as is necessary for him to find his food at pasture; that grass is a laxative and tends to encourage excretion of waste products through the bowels, and that hay and corn feeding have the opposite effect; and that when at work the body tissues, and especially the muscular system, are keyed up to a high pitch of efficiency, while at grass the condition soon becomes 'soft', the functions of the body only working at a 'maintenance rate' instead of at a 'productive rate', and that the higher the condition the greater is the demand made upon the skin by the rest of the body.

Quartering.—This consists of going over the horse's body with a dandy-brush and removing the coarse adherent particles of bedding, dried dung, etc., as a preliminary before the horse leaves the stable for morning exercise. At the same time a cloth and a pail of water are used to wipe away discharges from the eyes, nose, and dock, in this order, and to remove any urine stains from other parts of the body. Quartering is usually only carried out in high-class stables, where the horses go out for a short walk before the men have had their breakfasts, or when a horse is not going to work but is to be turned out to grass for the day. (*See* SPONGES.)

Dandy-brushing.—The dandy-brush is made of stiff, coarse, whisk fibre, generally of the yellow variety, with the bristles not close together. It removes the coarser particles of matter from the coat, and stirs up the finer debris, as well as disentangling matted hairs. Owing to its stiffness it is not usually used over the head, but each side of the neck, the whole of the body, and the four quarters are well brushed. It should be used in the left hand for the near side of the animal, and in the right hand for the off-side. It is advisable to make short, vigorous sweeps, turning the wrist at the end of each sweep, so that the material collected in the bristles is thrown out of the coat. Care is necessary when the under-sides of the body and the insides of the legs of thin-skinned or ticklish horses are being groomed with the dandy, for they may kick if the rough brush is used carelessly.

Body-brushing and curry-combing.—The body-brush is made from finer whisk fibre than the dandy, the bristles are set much closer together, and they are softer and more flexible. There is usually a strap across the back of the brush into which the hand is thrust, so that a better grip can be obtained. The curry-comb is made of metal, either in the form of a square plate with a series of alternately toothed and smooth ridges set across it, or it may be oval with crenated ridges running round it. The former variety is provided with a handle, and the latter has a strap across its back like the body-brush. The body-brush is used all over the horse's body, head, and neck. It picks up the finer particles of matter left behind by the dandy-brush and holds them between the fine bristles. To clean the brush it is necessary every three or four sweeps to draw it across the face of the curry-comb and transfer the dirt to the latter. The body-brush should be used in long firm sweeps, without any turn of the wrist. While grooming the near side, the body-brush is held in the left hand and the curry-comb in the right, and for the off-side the positions are reversed.

Wisping.—A wisp is a small mat of plaited straw or hay, which is used to beat out fine dust from the coat, scour and polish the surface hair, and to promote a better skin and superficial circulation. When properly applied it acts as massage to the surface of the body, and gives the coat a fine shine.

Combing the mane and tail.—For this purpose a bone or metal comb is used, fashioned after the familiar manner of a toilet comb, with stouter teeth. The mane is combed a few strands at a time, both from the outside and also from the inside (with the teeth through the whole thickness of the mane), so that the hairs may be laid straight and all tangles removed. Afterwards the tail is treated similarly. When a few unruly strands will not lie in position it is usual to damp the fibres of the water-brush (which is not unlike a small, fine dandy-brush pointed at each end) and lay the strands with the damp brush. Neither the mane nor the tail, however, should be soaked with water, for repeated soaking tends to rot the hairs and make them dry and brittle, so that they fall out by the roots or break off short.

Rubbing or shining is carried out either with a stable-rubber, which is a piece of towelling about 18 inches square, or with a chamois leather. During this process the hairs of the coat are laid straight all over the body, any loose pieces of hay or straw from the wisp are removed, and the final gloss is put on to the coat. It was customary to sprinkle a few drops of ordinary paraffin oil on to the rubber, to give an added shine and to keep away flies for a time during summer.

Cleaning out the feet.—The last operation of grooming consists of picking up each of the feet and removing any adherent dung, etc., by means of a hoof-pick, and brushing out the sole of each foot with the water-brush. If desired, the walls of the hoofs may also be blackened or oiled at this time. This operation should be left till last, just before the horse leaves the stable, for otherwise he may collect fresh dung in his feet. It is an important matter not to neglect this cleaning out of the feet, for if there is a cake of dung in the soles of each foot, not only is it extremely untidy, but small stones are liable to be picked up and may cause injury to the soles.

Parts often neglected.—When examining a horse to discover the thoroughness or otherwise of the grooming it is usual to take a white handkerchief and to rub it along the coat; the size of the particles of grey debris which adhere to its surface are in inverse ratio to the efficiency of the grooming—*i.e.* the larger the particles the less efficiently has the horse been groomed. The following parts should be carefully examined: under the forelock, the poll, jowl, under the mane, between the fore-legs, behind the elbows, along the belly, inside the thighs, in the hollows of the heels, and around the dock and between the buttocks.

To dry a wet horse.—When a horse returns to a stable soaked with rain, snow, or sweat, it is very advisable that it be dried to avoid the risk of chill through too rapid evaporation of the moisture in the coat. First of all it should be given a warm gruel or meal drink, to which a little whisky or ale may be added, if the horse is very exhausted, *e.g.* after a hard day's hunting. The harness is next removed and the surface of the body scraped down with a sweat-scraper. This is a flexible ribbon of copper provided with a handle at either end. The scraper removes the excess water from the coat, and may be used to scrape away adherent mud from the legs and belly, but it should be used with care over bony prominences, owing to the danger of abrading the skin. Two or three hay wisps are made ready, and the horse is vigorously wisped down all over. As one wisp becomes wet it is discarded and another taken. Sometimes a coarse, rough towel is used instead of a wisp. In about ten minutes all the moisture that can be removed by this means will have been removed, and the rest must be allowed to evaporate. An armful of straw is arranged across the horse's back, and a rug is thrown over all, and girthed up. The straw allows a certain amount of ventilation under the rug, and prevents too rapid cooling and chilling. In about two hours' time the rug should be removed, a second wisping should be given, and a new dry rug should be applied. If the feet and legs are very wet, especially if there is much feather, they should be bandaged with woollen stable bandages, and a little bran or sawdust may be sprinkled on to the wet hair below the bandage. Sometimes a horse's feet are washed immediately after coming in from work, especially if they are coated with mud; when this is carried out, care should be taken to see that they are well dried again afterwards, for frequent washing predisposes to grease, eczema, and other skin conditions, through maceration of the surface epithelium.

The grooming of milk cows.—The general principles as given for the horse apply almost equally to cattle, and especially to milk cows kept in byres, where they are unable to lick and clean themselves as they do in Nature. As a rule the process is not so thorough as for horses, only a dandy-brush and a curry-comb being used.

The grooming of dogs.—When grooming it is always advisable to commence by combing and brushing the coat in the wrong direction (against the lie of the hair), so as to remove pieces of dirt, débris, etc., which have become lodged under a lock of the coat and to finish by brushing and combing in the direction in which it is desired that the hair shall eventually lie.

In the spring, and again in the autumn, when the coat is changing, both dogs and cats require more careful grooming than they do at other times of the year, for at these times when they are casting their coats there is always a good deal of dead and loose hair to be removed to make way for the new young coat.

GROOTLAMSIEKTE.—A disease of sheep in S.W. Africa, associated with a prolonged gestation period, and caused by a poisonous shrub (*Salsola tuberculata.*)

GROUNDNUT MEAL.—During 1960 many turkeys fed in Britain on proprietary feeding-stuffs died, and the cause was traced to Brazilian groundnut meal—

not all samples of which, however, proved harmful. Calves and pigs also died. In calves, groundnut poisoning resembles that of ragwort.

The toxic factor has been identified as the toxin (called Aflatoxin) produced by the common mould *Aspergillus flavus*, and may contaminate groundnuts from other countries also.

'The mould can grow on decorticated groundnuts when their moisture content exceeds about 9 per cent, or on meal at about 16 per cent. It usually develops on the nuts after they are harvested, particularly if drying is delayed and the shells damaged. However, if harvesting is delayed the nuts may become toxic in the ground, and if the nuts are stored at a moisture content in excess of 9 per cent they can also become toxic.'—(*World Crops*.

Pigs of from 3 to 12 weeks are particularly susceptible, and pregnant sows to a less extent.

It was found that cows fed on hay and a concentrate ration containing 20 per cent toxic groundnut meal excreted a toxin in the milk which produced the same biological effect in ducklings as aflatoxin. There is evidence strongly suggesting that aflatoxin may be a carcinogen, giving rise to cancer of the liver. A 100 per cent incidence of carcinoma of the liver was found in pigs in Morocco in 1945 which survived illness following the feeding of a mixture of oil-cakes. The same effect has been observed in rats.

Groundnut meal contains an alkaloid Arachine, which can cause a fatal hepatitis in dogs, and temporary paralysis in frogs and rabbits.

GROWTHS.—Any formation of new or unusual tissue in the body is termed a growth. Thus tumours, aneurisms, warts, and granulations are frequently referred to as 'growths'. (*See* TUMOURS, etc.)

GRUEL is the name given to a thin paste or thick fluid made of oatmeal or maize meal and milk or water. Gruel is made by mixing 3 or 4 tablespoonfuls of meal with 1 pint of cold milk or water, allowing to stand for 15 to 20 minutes, then straining and boiling for 15 minutes, and finally adding salt or sugar. Gruels are useful during illness when ordinary food is refused, or during convalescence from debilitating diseases. They serve as convenient media for the administration of medicines. (*See also* STARCH.)

GUARNIERI BODIES (*see* INCLUSION BODIES).

GULLET, or **ŒSOPHAGUS,** is the tube down which the food passes from the mouth on its way to the stomach. The gullet begins at the throat, runs down the lower part of the neck along with the trachea, enters the chest cavity, and passing over the base of the heart and between the two lungs, it enters the abdomen about the middle of the diaphragm, to terminate in the stomach.

GUM is a complex viscid substance which exudes from the stems, branches, or roots of various plants and trees. It principally consists of *arabin* and *bassorin*. The two best-known gums are gum acacia and gum tragacanth, used in pharmacy to form emulsions.

GUMBORO DISEASE.—This takes its name from a town in Delaware, U.S.A. It affects broiler chickens of 1 to 5 weeks of age. The disease has been recorded in Britain. Listlessness and diarrhœa are the main symptoms. At the beginning of an outbreak, deaths are numerous. Nephritis is stated to be one of the principal findings at *post-mortem* examination.

Cause.—Probably a virus.

'GUT-TIE' is a condition occurring in young castrated male cattle in which a piece of bowel becomes imprisoned or entangled in the spermatic cord, or in a part of the mesentery of the spermatic cord. The condition is found in hilly districts, especially when castration has been performed carelessly. The piece of bowel becomes gangrenous owing to hindrance or stoppage of the circulation, and death usually follows in 4 or 5 days. The treatment is entirely surgical, and must be undertaken before any extensive gangrene has set in; it consists in opening the abdomen, freeing the imprisoned piece of gut from its encumbrances by cutting through the spermatic cord, and suturing the wound in the abdominal wall. This condition of gut-tie always occurs on the right side of the body, because the rumen on the left disallows the presence of intestine in the region of the spermatic cord.

GUTTURAL POUCH DIPHTHERIA.—This was described as a disease entity by W. H. Cook in the U.K. in 1966. He states that it is characterised by diphtheritic membrane formation in the guttural pouch. It is probably the cause of most cases of bleeding from the nose and paralysis of the pharynx. Some cases of 'roaring' due to laryngeal hemiplegia, paralysis of the soft palate, and facial paralysis may also be associated with G.P.D. This has been encountered in horses from 2 months to 18 years old—in ponies, cobs, hunters, and thoroughbreds. It may prove fatal within a week, or may be chronic, with symptoms shown over a period of 7 months or more.

Cause.—No specific organism has so far been implicated.

Symptoms.—Epistaxis (nose bleeding) was present in 17 out of the 22 horses examined by Cook. 'Hæmorrhage in every case occurred spontaneously while the horse was at rest in the stable. It is generally recurrent and may be mild, severe, or fatal.' In the latter case it is most likely to occur from erosion of the internal carotid artery. The internal maxillary artery and vein may be involved. 'Blood escapes from one of these vessels into the guttural pouches, from where it flows into the pharynx or down one or both nostrils.'

Pharyngeal paralysis. 'Ten of the 22 horses have shown difficulty in swallowing. Attempts to eat solid food result in coughing and the discharge of food material from mouth and nostrils. Drinking may be difficult. Water is conveyed back into the bucket via the nostrils.' It seems that parts of the vagus in particular are prone to damage, either by the inflammation associated with the presence of the diphtheritic lesion in its active stage, or by the scar tissue and fibrosis following healing of the lesion.

Laryngeal hemiplegia. 'Evidence of this was present in 10 out of the 22 horses. Five of the survivors made an abnormal inspiratory noise when exercised.'

Nasal catarrh. Discharge from one or both nostrils sometimes precedes the bleeding or difficulty in swallowing, but it is not alarmingly copious or purulent.

Drooping of the upper eyelid (ptosis) on one side may occur; also congestion of the nasal mucous membrane on the same side.

Soft palate paresis. In racehorses this is shown by the sudden onset of respiratory obstruction during a race. The horse makes a gurgling sound, 'like a death rattle'. A complete paralysis does not, apparently, usually follow the paresis (partial paralysis).

Unilateral facial paralysis. This is an occasional symptom which may develop a year after apparent recovery.

Diagnosis.—This involves an examination of the guttural pouches by endoscope.

Treatment.—Irrigation may be tried, and antibiotics used systemically.

GYRUS (γῦρος, a ring) is the term applied to a convolution of the brain.

H

HÆMANGIOMA (*αἷμα*, blood ; *ἀγγεῖον*, vessel ; *-ωμα*, tumour) is a tumour composed of blood-vessels. In the liver of adult cattle small hæmangiomata are not uncommonly found, but they are seldom of any practical importance. Upon rare occasions they may burst and give rise to internal hæmorrhage, but since the blood-vessels which form the tumour are all small and arranged in an intricate network, the hæmorrhage is seldom serious.

HÆMATEMESIS (*αἷμα*, blood ; *ἐμέως* I vomit) means vomiting blood. When the blood is from an injury to the stomach or œsophagus it is bright red in colour, but when it has been exuded from the blood-vessels as the result of some inflammation in the stomach, and has lain in that organ for some time, and has become partly digested, it is in the form of small brown granules, resembling coffee-grounds. It is always a serious symptom.

HÆMATIDROSIS (*αἷμα*, blood ; *ἵδρωσι*, sweating) and **HÆMATOPEDESIS** are words which indicate the presence of blood in the sweat. The condition is not common among animals, but it sometimes occurs when horses which are in soft condition are suddenly called upon to make some violent or prolonged effort, and it may be brought about through the agency of various biting insects, such as flies and ticks, as well as during the course of severe debilitating diseases like purpura. A few drops of blood ooze out through the skin and stain the sweat a pink or red colour.

HÆMATOCELE (*αἷμα*, blood ; *κήλη*, a tumour) means a cavity containing blood. The term is generally applied to the testicle, and is due to an injury which ruptures the smaller blood-vessels, from which the blood escapes to collect in the cavity of the scrotum, in the loose cellular tissue, or in the outer coat of the testicle itself.

HÆMATOCRIT VALUE.—This means the percentage by volume of whole blood that is composed of erythrocytes. It is determined by filling a graduated hæmatocrit tube with blood—treated so that it will not clot—and then centrifuging the tube until the erythrocytes are packed in the lower end. As a rough guide,values range as follows : sheep, 32 ; cow, 40 ; horse and pig, 42 ; dog, 45.

HÆMATOIDIN and HÆMIN are crystalline bodies derived from shed blood when it is allowed to dry. The former is produced where blood is effused in internal hæmorrhages, such as in apoplexy, and then is partly absorbed. By chemical analysis it is proved to be the same as bilirubin, the chief colouring matter of the bile. It produces the lemon-yellow colour noticed in a bruise in the human being, when the blood is being absorbed and the bruise is fading away. *Hæmin* is of great importance, because it can be recovered from blood-stains that have been long dry, and it is useful in criminal investigations whether concerning man or animals.

HÆMATOMA (*αἱματόω*, I make bloody) means a collection of blood forming a definite swelling. It is found upon parts of the surface of the body that have been exposed to blows, kicks, or great pressure, as well as to parts that are the subject of continued irritation. Thus hæmatomata are seen on the muscular parts of horses which have been kicked, on the flanks, sides, quarters, etc., of cattle that are injured in railway boxes, in the ear-flaps of dogs and cats which are suffering from irritation in the external passages of the ear, causing continued scratching or shaking of the head, and they are sometimes seen on pigs that have been beaten with a stick. They may be treated by opening surgically and draining away the collected blood.

HÆMATOPEDESIS (*see* HÆMATIDROSIS).

HÆMATOTHORAX (*αἷμα*, blood; *θώραξ*, the chest) means an effusion of blood into the pleural cavity.

HÆMATOZOA (*αἷμα*, blood ; *ζῷον*, animal) is a general name applied to the various parasites of the blood. (*See* PARASITES).

HÆMATURIA (*αἷμα*, blood ; *οὐρέω*, I make water) means any condition in which blood is found in the urine. (*See* URINE, ABNORMAL CONDITIONS OF.)

HÆMIN (*see* HÆMATOIDIN).

HÆMO-CYTOMETER (*αἷμα*, blood; *κύτος*, cell; *μέτρον*, measure) is an instrument for counting corpuscles in the blood.

HÆMOGLOBIN produces the red colour of blood and muscle. It contains much iron, and when separated from the red blood corpuscles which contain it, is crystalline in nature. It exists in two forms, *carboxyhæmoglobin*, found in venous blood, and *oxyhæmoglobin*, found in arterial blood that has been in contact with oxygen. This oxyhæmoglobin, a weak compound of hæmoglobin and oxygen, is broken down in the tissues, yielding to the cells its oxygen, and becoming once more hæmoglobin. The oxygen is utilised by the tissues for the purposes of combustion. In some forms of anæmia there is a great deficiency in hæmoglobin. (*See* RESPIRATION.)

HÆMOGLOBINURIA.—The presence of hæmoglobin in the urine, such as occurs in azoturia, Red-water fever, leptospirosis of calves, poisoning by an excess of kale or cabbage.

HÆMOLYSIS (*αἷμα*, blood; *λύσις*, setting free) means the destruction of red blood corpuscles and the consequent escape from them of hæmoglobin. It occurs gradually in some forms of anæmia and rapidly in poisoning by snake venom. Some chemicals and bacterial toxins cause hæmolysis.

HÆMOLYTIC.—Relating to hæmolysis. For Hæmolytic Disease of foals, *see* FOALS, DISEASES OF. Hæmolytic Disease in pigs and dogs is similar in its effects. In pigs its cause has been related to two or more injections of CRYSTAL VIOLET VACCINE (which see). In cattle, it may account for some cases of abortion.

HÆMOPHILIA (*αἷμα*, blood; *φιλία*, affection) is a peculiar disease sometimes met with among dogs, in which the affected animal bleeds upon the slightest provocation, and in which the hæmorrhage is very difficult to control. It is a well-recognised disease in human medicine, where there are interesting hereditary facts concerning its transmission. Only male subjects are affected, but the disease is passed on to succeeding generations by the females only, who themselves do not show the abnormality.

HÆMOPHILUS INFECTIONS.—See ROUP of poultry; infectious ophthalmia in cattle (*under* EYE, DISEASES OF). In pigs in the U.K. *Hæmophilus parasuis*, *H. parainfluenzæ* and *H. parahæmolyticus* are often associated with chronic respiratory disease.

HÆMOPTYSIS (*αἷμα*, blood; *πτύω*, I spit) means the expulsion of blood from the lower air passages, generally by coughing. The blood so expelled is bright red in colour and is frothy, thus differing from that which has been expelled from the stomach. It is seen in tuberculosis.

HÆMORRHAGE (*αἱμορραγία*) (*see* BLEEDING, THE ARREST OF; PROTHROMBIN; INTERNAL HÆMORRHAGE; *and* (HÆMORRHAGIC DISEASE' OF FOWLS).

'HÆMORRHAGIC DISEASE' OF DOGS.—A highly fatal disease occurring in Singapore, S.E. Asia, Virgin Islands and elsewhere. Cause: possibly *Ehrlichia canis*.

The symptoms include bleeding from one or both nostrils, loss of appetite, distressed breathing, and weakness.

'HÆMORRHAGIC DISEASE' OF FOWLS.—Next to coccidiosis, probably the major cause of mortality in broiler plants, is still something of a mystery. The birds huddle together, shiver, may pass blood in their droppings, and die. Sometimes hæmorrhages are observed, sometimes they are all internal; and, in fact, the birds may die without symptoms. Mortality rises rapidly after the first few cases, and may reach 50 per cent, gradually subsiding after 10 days or so. Within 2 or 3 weeks there is often no further trouble.

Present advice is to stop giving anticoccidiosis drugs, and to avoid—especially during hot weather—an excessive intake of medicated water. It seems that Blackhead and stress factors, such as caponisation, may precipitate the disease. Toxic fungi, other poisons, and drug overdosage are suggested as other causes.

HÆMORRHAGIC ENTERITIS OF TURKEYS.—This disease or syndrome has appeared in the U.K., U.S.A., Australia, Rhodesia, and South Africa. There is an increased incidence during hot weather. Causes are believed to include coccidiosis, vitamin K deficiency, and *E. coli* infection. Possibly the causes mentioned above, referring to a similar diseases in fowls, also apply.

HÆMORRHAGIC GASTRO-ENTERITIS, of unknown cause, has been seen in store and adult pigs, in East Anglia especially. Sudden death of one or two pigs in a herd occurs. The large intestine (and often other parts) is deep red and contains whole blood. The abdominal cavity contains a straw-coloured fluid.

Outbreaks involving severe hæmorrhage into the digestive tract, including the stomach, have been associated with whey feeding.

In Northern Ireland the condition is often referred to as 'whey bloat', and despite several deaths it is still found economic to feed whey, which is cheap. But there is no doubt that this disease is a serious cause of loss, and that it merits further research, which may incriminate an allergy from the milk solids in the whey, an excess of water, an allergy unconnected with whey, or some poisonous substance which occasionally finds its way into pig meal. (*See also* GASTRO-ENTERITIS.)

HÆMORRHAGIC SEPTICÆMIAS.—This term is generally used to include a group of diseases occurring in several of our domesticated and in many wild animals, due to an infection by certain micro-organisms belonging to the Pasteurella group. (*See* PASTEURELLOSIS.)

HÆMORRHOIDS (*αἱμορροίδες*) (*see* PILES).

HÆMOSTATICS (*αἷμα*, blood; *στατικός*, standing) are means taken to check bleeding, and may be either drugs applied to the area, or mechanical devices, etc. (*See* HÆMORRHAGE, GELATIN SPONGE.)

HAIR (*see* SKIN).

HAIR-BALLS often give rise to indigestion in calves, especially those aged about 6 weeks to 4 months. The hair may be in the form of a ball or in loose masses, sometimes mixed with milk curds, sand, binder twine, etc. Bad management encourages calves to lick their own or other animal's hair. The condition sometimes proves fatal both in calves and pigs.

Symptoms.—Are usually vague, but may include grinding of the teeth, an unnatural gait, and in chronic cases a general loss of condition, although the appetite remains fairly good. Convulsions may also occur.

Prevention.—Ensure a well-balanced diet, adequate minerals and roughage, and attend to any skin disease.

Treatment is surgical and often successful if carried out early.

HAIR, CLIPPING OF THE (*see* CLIPPING OF ANIMALS).

HAIR, DISEASES OF (*see* BALDNESS, RINGWORM, SKIN DISEASES).

'HAIRY SHAKER' DISEASE.—This is a transmissible disease of lambs in New Zealand, resembling Border Disease (which see).

HALF-BRED.—This term usually means the cross from a Cheviot ewe × Border Leicester.

HALIBUT-LIVER OIL is nowadays much used instead of cod-liver oil for vitamin therapy in cases of rickets, etc. Smaller doses suffice, and the vitamin content is usually standardised.

HALOTHANE. — An anæsthetic, described under its proprietary name of FLUOTHANE.

HALOXON.—An organo-phosphorus compound used against gastro-intestinal nematode worms.

HAMPSHIRE.—A black pig with a white belt, from Kentucky, U.S.A. The origins of the breed were probably 19th century Old English. Their import was sanctioned on a limited scale in 1962 and again in 1966.

'HARD PAD DISEASE' (PARADISTEMPER).—This is one syndrome in dogs, caused by the Distemper virus, and not a separate disease entity as was at one time thought.

The reader is referred to the information given under DISTEMPER

HARDERIAN GLAND.—A sebaceous gland which, in some animals, acts as an accessory to the lacrimal gland. Normally, the Harderian gland is completely covered by the third eyelid, but in dogs obstruction to the flow of material from the gland not uncommonly causes its enlargement and projection beyond the third eyelid, when it appears as a red, roundish mass. In such cases it may be necessary for the gland to be removed under local or general anæsthesia. (*See also* EYE, DISEASES OF.)

'HARDWARE DISEASE'.—The colloquial American name for traumatic pericarditis of cattle caused by metal objects, such as pieces of baling wire, nails. (*See under* HEART, DISEASES OF.)

HARE-LIP is an error in the formation of the upper lip, in which there is an absence of continuity between the two halves. These normally grow together in most animals, but in some cases, for various reasons, union does not take place.

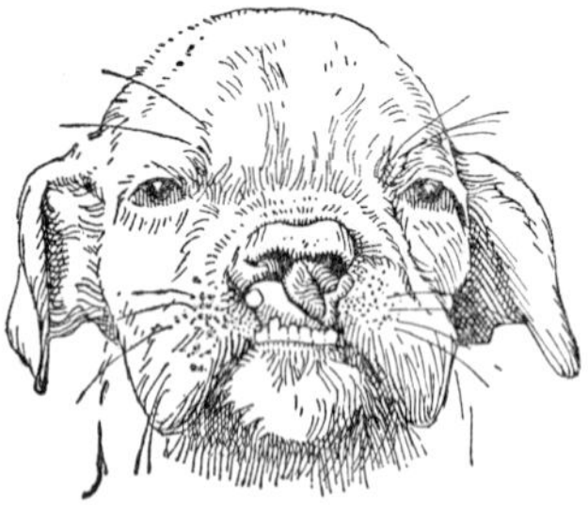

Hare-lip in a young bulldog puppy, showing a complete cleft in the upper lip, which effectively prevents successful sucking.

The condition is seen in puppies of the toy breeds and in sheep. When the cleft in the lip is wide, sucking is impossible, and the young puppies often die from starvation. In less severe cases they obtain some nourishment, but never thrive as well as the others in a litter. The malformation is generally associated with 'cleft palate'. (*See* CLEFT PALATE.)

HARES.—These may harbour the liver fluke of sheep, *Fasciola hepatica*, and the cystic stage of the tapeworm *Tænia multiceps packi* of the dog, and of *Tænia pisiformis*.

In some countries (*e.g.* Denmark), hares are a source of *Brucella abortus suis* infection to pigs. Some European hares also harbour *Br. melitensis*. In the U.K., Orf-like lesions have been seen (and confused with myxomatosis). Other diseases include aspergillosis, streptococcal endocarditis, toxoplasmosis, and coccidiosis. Louping-ill virus and/or antibody has been found in English hares, and also Q fever antibody.

In order to prevent the introduction of *Brucella suis* and also of *Pasteurella tularensis* infections, the Hares (Control of Importation) Order 1965 was enacted in the U.K. (*See* TULARÆMIA.)

HARROWING.—For its effect on the survival of lungworm larvæ on pasture *see under* HUSK.

HARVEST MITES (*see* p. 692).

HAULM DESTROYER. (For the danger of poisoning, *see under* POTATO HAULM.)

HAW (*see end of section headed* EYE).

HAY is a very important, but nowadays perhaps a somewhat under-rated, article of diet for cattle. (*See part in heavy type under* FIBRE, p. 252.) Hay is sometimes put down on very lush pasture where bloat is anticipated. As well as assisting in bloat prevention, it will help to obviate hypomagnesæmia and acetonæmia also. The feeding of hay together with green fodder crops is said to reduce the risk of scouring, especially when large quantities of the fodder are being eaten and during wet weather. When kale or rape are being fed in quantity hay is most necessary in the diet. Hay made from leys is evidently not very palatable, for it is refused by the sick cow which will often relish even not very good hay made from old pasture.

As a rough guide, 2 lb. ordinary hay = 1 lb. cereals = 7 lb. average silage for energy or 4 lb. average silage for protein.

'Tripoded hay has four or five times as much carotene as good hay made in the swathe, and barn-dried hay is even better. On the other hand, swathe hay has more vitamin D than other types if made in good weather. Badly-damaged swathe hay is deficient in both carotene and vitamin D, and there may well be a case for adding vitamins A and D as well as minerals to any cereals used to make good the losses in poor hay.'—T. H. Davies.

It must be said that the nutrient value of much hay of indifferent quality may be over-estimated. Protein value can vary from 5 to 15 per cent, and energy value from 20 to 50 per cent. (Total digestible nutrients.)—K. Harker.

Mouldy hay can be dangerous on account of the risk of ASPERGILLOSIS.

HAY-BOX BROODERS.—These are often 12 feet long by 3 feet wide. Of this, an area of 9 feet × 3 feet is merely a grass run, while the remaining area of 3 feet × 3 feet is enclosed and forms the sleeping compartment, in the roof of which two bags of hay are placed in order to act as an insulator and retain the natural heat of the chicks. Such a brooder will take about 50 chicks (from 3 or 4 weeks of age) until they are ready to go into arks or houses at 8 weeks old.

' HAYFLAKES '.—In appearance, hayflakes resemble chopped hay but retain the quality of dried grass. They are not chopped so short that the fibrous quality of grass is destroyed, nor so long that storage space becomes difficult. They can be stored loose in the barn for self- or easy feeding ; or they can be baled.

HAYLAGE is intermediate between grass and silage, made in tower silos from chopped and wilted grass.

' HEAD GRIT ' (*see* ' YELLOWSES').

HEALING OF WOUNDS (*see* WOUNDS).

HEALTH SCHEMES FOR FARM ANIMALS.—These can lead to increased profitability, especially in the large units which are becoming commonplace today. Such schemes are not altogether new. In a limited form, they were in operation during the last war and the years immediately following it. Then the emphasis was on controlling brucellosis, other aspects of infertility, mastitis and Johne's disease. Now the central core for any dairy herd scheme is usually minimising infertility, and around that can be arranged a comprehensive programme of preventive medicine covering a wide range of diseases.

As Professor C. S. G. Grunsell, of the University of Bristol Veterinary School, wrote recently: ' At the outset it is necessary to consider the definition of health. In the case of farm live-stock it can no longer be accepted as simply a state in which disease is absent, and is now more accurately regarded as a state of maximum economic production.' Similarly, in the same context, infertility could be defined as a failure to breed as often or as regularly as the farmer would wish. In financial terms, such failure has been costed by the Milk Marketing Board ; for example, missing a single heat period can mean a loss of nearly £4, 10s., and missing two costs £10, 7s.

Reference is made elsewhere to the PIG HEALTH SCHEME, confined to MLC's nucleus and reserve herds, and to the Enzootic Pneumonia Scheme introduced in 1959. The latter is a privately financed scheme, independent of government agencies, and under veterinary supervision both centrally and locally.

In Iowa, U.S.A., a pig health scheme, operated by veterinary surgeons in private practice, has found favour among producers and costs the equivalent of 14s. 6d. per pig weaned. This can include worming sows ; spraying against external parasites; vaccination against swine fever, erysipelas, and leptospirosis ; and boar fertility.

Already on farms in the U.K. health schemes are in operation. For example, a few large dairy units receive weekly or fortnightly visits, when cows are presented to the veterinary surgeon for pregnancy diagnosis and treatment. He will also advise on preventive measures.

(*See also* POULTRY HEALTH SCHEME).

HEART is a hollow muscular pump with four cavities, each provided with a valve at its outlet, the function of which is to maintain the circulation of the blood through the body. The two upper cavities are known as the *atria* (or *auricles*, although, strictly speaking, the auricle is only a part of the atrium), and the two lower chambers are called *ventricles* (*ventriculus*, a little stomach). Certain large vessels are connected with these chambers; some serve to bring blood to the heart (*anterior* and *posterior venæ cavæ*—from the systematic circulation of the body, and five or six *pulmonary veins*—from the lungs), and others carry blood away (*aorta*, to the general circulation, and *pulmonary artery*, to the lungs).

Position.—The heart lies in the lower anterior part of the chest cavity between the lungs, but projecting more to the left side than to the right. As a general rule, when an animal is standing with its two fore-feet together, in a position of attention, the heart lies roughly between its two elbows or a little above ; and a line joining the points of the elbows would pass through the apex of the heart. Its base lies opposite the 3rd to the 6th ribs inclusive, and its apex lies above the last segment of the sternum, in the horse, and in the other domesticated animals its position is somewhat similar. It lies in close contact with the diaphragm at the time of maximum expiration, but when the diaphragm recedes during the filling of the chest this close contact disappears. In other animals than the horse the heart and stomach are only separated from each other by a very small space, and diseased conditions of the stomach are liable to exert an influence upon the heart, *e.g.*

when an ox swallows a foreign body like a three-inch nail, it may become lodged in the 2nd stomach and eventually puncture the heart wall.

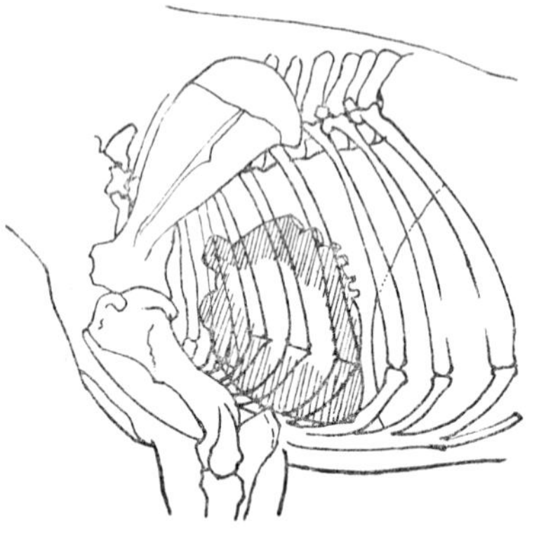

Diagram of the position of the horse's heart in relation to the bones of the chest.

Shape and size.—One end of the heart, the most posterior, is pointed and is called the *apex*, and the opposite end is broad and wide and is called the *base*. The latter is deeply cleft at the division between the right and left atria, and connected with it are the various vessels carrying blood. Dividing one ventricle from the other in a longitudinal manner is a groove in which lie the blood-vessels which nourish the heart muscle, and dividing the two atria from the two ventricles is a circular for *coronary groove*, also carrying blood-vessels. Both of these grooves are usually partly filled with fat in well-nourished animals, and in very stout individuals the amount of fat present may be so great as to embarrass the section of the heart very considerably. The weight of the horse's heart is between 6½ and 9 lb., and that of the ox 5 to 7 lb., but in different individuals the weight varies beyond these limits upon certain occasions. The pig's heart weighs between 2½ and 4 lb., and the large dog's is about 2 to 3 lb.

Structure.—The heart lies within a strong fibrous sac known as the *pericardium*, and since the inner surface of this sac and the outer surface of the heart wall are lined by a smooth glistening membrane containing fat cells and a little serous fluid, the movements of the heart are accomplished almost without friction with the surrounding organs. The main thickness of the heart wall consists of bundles of muscle fibres, which run, some in circles round the heart, others in loops first round one cavity and then round the corresponding cavity of the other side, some longitudinally, and others in an oblique manner.

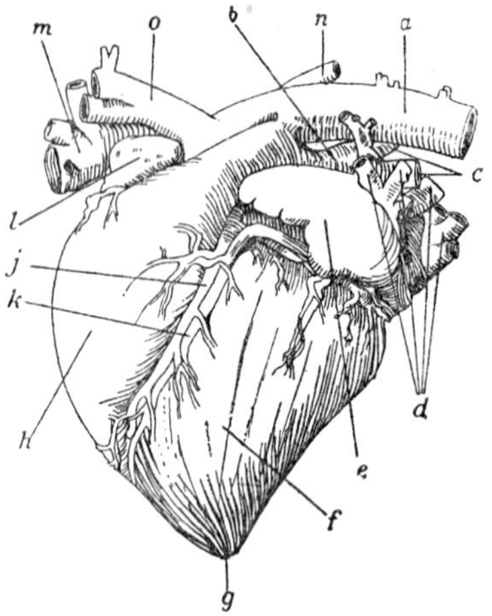

Diagram of the horse's heart and its associated structures, viewed from the left side. *a*, Aorta; *b*, pulmonary artery dividing into right and left branches; *c*, to the respective lungs; *d*, pulmonary veins; *e*, left atrium; *f*, left ventricle; *g*, apex of heart; *h*, right ventricle; *j*, descending branch of left coronary artery; *k*, the great heart vein; *l*, auricle of right atrium; *m*, cranial vena cava; *n*, azygos vein; *o*, brachiocephalic arterial trunk, which leaves the aorta to be distributed to the head and neck and the fore-limbs. (*After* Bradley's *Anatomy*.)

Within all the cavities is a smooth lining membrane which is continuous with that of the blood-vessels opening into the heart, and serves to prevent friction between the blood and the walls of the heart and vessels, and to prevent coagulation of the blood during life. This smooth inner lining membrane is called the *endocardium*, the heart muscle is *myocardium*, and the outer investing muscle is the *epicardium*.

A special band of muscle fibres, which is usually known as the ' atrio-ventricular bundle of His ', runs from the right auricle down into the septum between the two ventricles, and is believed to be the muscular connection which times the ventricles to beat immediately after the atria have finished their beat and force the blood down into the ventricles.

Openings.—There is no direct communication between the chambers on the right side and those on the left in the healthy adult (although there is a passage between the right and left atria in the fœtus) ; but the right atrium opens into the right ventricle by a large circular opening, and there is a similar opening between the left atrium and ventricle. These two openings are known as the *right atrio-ventricular* and the *left atrio-ventricular orifices* respectively. Into the right atrium open four veins, the *anterior* and the *posterior venæ cavæ*, the *vena azygos*, and the *coronary sinus*, which drains the blood from the heart muscle itself, and into the left atrium open the *pulmonary veins*, which may number almost anything between 4 and 9, but are usually 6 or 7 in the horse. One opening leads out of each ventricle, to the pulmonary artery in the case of the right, and to the aorta in the case of the left. Before birth, when the lungs are non-functional, and when the aeration of the fœtal blood is provided for through the medium of the placenta, the blood is short-circuited through an opening between the two atria which is called the *foramen ovale*, and in a few instances this remains through life. Normally, however, when the young animal draws its first breath this opening begins to close, and later it is only represented by a depression known as the *fossa ovalis*.

Valves.—As already mentioned, there are four valves. Two of these are placed at the openings leading from atrium into ventricle, and are known as *atrio-ventricular valves*, that on the right often being referred to as the 'tricuspid valve', and that on the left as the 'bicuspid' or the 'mitral valve'; their function is to prevent blood from passing upwards from the ventricles into the atria when the former contact. Two more, the *pulmonary valve* and the *aortic valve* (often known collectively as *semilunar valves*), are placed at the entrance to these vessels, and serve to prevent regurgitation into the ventricles of blood which has been driven from them into the vessels. The noises made by these valves in closing, and also partly by the heart muscle in contracting, are known as the 'heart sounds', and can be heard by any one placing his ear over the chest wall of an animal immediately behind the left fore-leg. Variations in the rhythm, intensity, or sequence of these sounds, as well as the indication of accompanying 'murmurs', heard between them, are the most important means of diagnosing heart diseases in both animals and man. Their recognition, however, requires much skill and practice.

Action.—At each heart-beat the two atria contract and expel their contents into the ventricles, through the respective valves, and at the same time they stimulate the ventricles to contract together. Blood is forced through the semilunar valves into the arteries, and from them passes to the general circulation by the aorta, and to the lungs by the pulmonary artery. After negotiating these areas of the body it returns again to the heart, and is emptied into the atria once more. Between each beat and the next the heart goes into a state of what is called *diastole*, which is a process of dilating and refilling its various chambers with blood, while the beating stage is known as *systole*. The former stage lasts about twice or three times as long as the latter, and during diastole the heart muscle gets a small amount of rest. It is the absence of this diastole, or the reduction of its duration, which acts adversely when the heart's action is rapid and strong at the beginning of acute fevers. The wear and tear of the heart muscle and the energy expended are too great to be able to last, and yet the body makes excessive demands for more and more blood to enable it to counteract the effect of disease processes; after a period of very strong, rapid beating there always comes a stage during which the force of the beat becomes weaker and weaker, and it is the rapidity of the onset of the weakening in the beat which very frequently results in death from heart failure in the early stages of severe diseases.

In the horse the normal rate of heart-beat, and therefore of the pulse, is between 32 and 40 per minute; in the ox it is 45 to 60 per minute; in the sheep, 70 to 80; in the pig, 70 to 80; and in the dog, 90 to 100. In each animal it is somewhere between 3½ and 5 times faster than the respirations.

The heart is to some extent regulated by a nerve centre in the medulla, closely connected with those centres which govern the lungs and the stomach, and from this medullary cardiac centre nerve fibres pass down through the 10th cranial nerve, the vagus, to the heart. Impulses passing down one set of these nerve fibres stimulate the heart to beat more strongly, while those in other fibres slow down the action or may even cause it to stop altogether; and it is in accordance with the needs of the body as to whether the heart is stimulated or inhibited. If this cardiac centre be injured by violence, or if it be poisoned by chemical agents like prussic acid, or by the toxins of bacteria, the heart stops beating in most of the higher mammals, although in some of the lower animals, *e.g.* frogs, fishes, and reptiles, the heart may be removed from the body and, under suitable conditions of moisture, oxygen supply, etc., it may go on beating for hours or even days.

HEART DISEASES

HEART DISEASES can be recognised only by the highly trained observer, though their presence may at times, at least, be suspected by an owner. Their treatment, and a true estimation of their gravity or otherwise, belong to the realm of the veterinary clinician, and it is only after much practice that accurate diagnosis and rational treatment are possible. Moreover, owing to the economic value of individual animals, and upon humane grounds, treatment of the majority of heart diseases of any gravity, even where it is possible, is not usually advisable.

Varieties. — Many general diseases, specific or otherwise, affect the heart, but, considering the arduous work which this organ performs, and the fact that it never completely rests from the time of its formation before birth till death ensues, it is subject to remarkably few disorders. It is usual to classify its diseases according to the part of the heart affected or to the nature of the changes produced. *Inflammatory affections* are divided into pericarditis, myocarditis, and endocarditis, according as the pericardium or outer enveloping membrane, the myocardium or muscular substance, and the endocardium or lining membrane, are affected. Myocarditis may be of bacterial origin, or associated with a vitamin deficiency. *Valvular diseases* form one of the most important groups, there being eight conditions in this class; each of the four valves may be 'stenosed', *i.e.* its opening narrowed, or may be incompetent, allowing a certain amount of blood to flow through in the wrong direction. *Hypertrophy*, in which the heart is enlarged and its wall thickened, and *dilatation*, in which one or more of the cavities is dilated, form another group very often associated with valvular diseases. *Degeneration* of the muscular tissue, producing an enfeeblement of the heart's action, may occur; it may be either a 'fatty' change, in which there are globules of fat found in the muscle fibres or between them, or it may be a 'fibroid' change, in which fibrous tissue is present in excess. Finally, there is a class of *functional changes* in which—without apparent diseased change in the structure of the heart—palpitation, rapidity, slowness, or great irregularity may appear. As would be expected, such conditions as these latter may exist in an animal, and yet no symptoms may ever be shown; the condition is only perhaps accidentally recognised when the heart is being examined in a routine manner during the course of some other coexistent disease.

Causes.—A strenuous life in which continual strains are placed upon the heart leads to hypertrophy, and when the animal gets too old to perform its accustomed work the heart is liable to undergo some form of atrophy or degeneration. This is sometimes seen in hunters, race-horses, and sporting dogs; after their more active life is over and they retire from the fields of sport, it is not uncommon for fatty degeneration, fibroid degeneration, or even ossification of the right auricle, to occur. Another condition in which fatty degeneration may arise is the feeding of bulls and cows for show purposes year after year, with little or no exercise. The enormous amount of fat carried by them when in full showyard condition becomes virtually pathological; it is a case of lipomatosis for all practical purposes, and among other organs affected is the heart. Such animals are liable to become breathless when compelled to make any vigorous movement, owing to the incompetence of the heart to supply sufficient blood to the lungs for aeration, occasioned by the deposition of fat around the heart and among its muscle fibres, the fat interfering with its contraction and relaxation.

All the febrile diseases, especially such as are due to, or associated with, bacteria in the blood-stream, have an adverse effect upon the action of the heart. Those that are particularly important in this respect are as follows: Influenza, strangles, pneumonia, and glanders in the horse; tuberculosis, septic metritis, and mastitis in cattle; swine erysipelas in pigs; distemper and tuberculosis in dogs; but almost any disease which is associated with a high temperature, in addition to those mentioned, markedly alters the beat of the heart, and throws extra strain upon it. Chest troubles, affecting other organs than the heart, and diseases of the stomach, owing to their proximity, are liable to involve either the heart itself or the pericardium, directly or indirectly; of these, pleurisy and pneumonia, causing pericarditis and perhaps myocarditis, and gastritis and the presence of penetrating foreign bodies, may be mentioned.

Disease of the heart may be set up through pressure from a tumour upon the large arteries, or by pressure from an enlarged lymphatic gland; the heart itself on rare occasions may be the seat of tumours; or the vagus nerve may be involved so that the heart action is disturbed.

General symptoms.—Because of the great powers of 'compensation' possessed by the heart, the early symptoms of heart disease are either unnoticed, or are so slight as to be disregarded. Moreover, it is an extraordinary fact that many animals, which are found upon post-mortem examination to possess grossly diseased hearts, have never shown any symptoms whatever. They have performed their legitimate work, have remained in good health, have kept their condition, and it was only when accident or other unassociated disease overtook them that death occurred and the condition of the heart was discovered.

As in man, heart troubles are very much more common in old age than in youth, and the fact that most of the animals used as food for human consumption never reach old age, reduces the incidence of heart disease in them very considerably. Again, the immunity animals enjoy from such conditions as chronic alcoholism, syphilis, generalised arterio-sclerosis, etc., *i.e.* conditions which in man predispose to heart troubles, reduces still further the percentage of heart disease in relation to other troubles.

Marked irregularity in the heart-beat, some difficulty in breathing without obvious changes in the lungs or pleura, breathlessness when compelled to exert themselves, a tendency to swelling of the dependent parts of the body (*e.g.* along the lower line of the chest and abdomen and 'filling' of the limbs), and in severe cases lividity of the tongue and congestion of the membranes of the eyes and gums, are the chief general symptoms exhibited by animals affected with heart disease. Faintness and giddiness are seen at times; dropsy of the abdomen is sometimes an accompanying condition, when the heart is very weak; digestive disturbances with occasional vomiting in dogs and cats is another not uncommon symptom.

Particular Diseases :

PERICARDITIS is an inflammation of the membrane covering the exterior of the heart. It may be 'idiopathic', when its cause is not always known; or it may be 'traumatic', when it is due to a wound: the former of these conditions is usual in animals other than the ox, but in the ox pericarditis is very often traumatic. Either variety may be 'dry', in which case the two opposing surfaces of the membrane are covered by a layer of fibrin worked up by the movements of the beating heart into little ridges, not unlike those formed upon the surfaces of two slices of bread and butter forcibly separated one from the other; or 'effusion' may accompany this condition, in which case fluid fills up the pericardial sac and, when no more distension of the sac can occur, presses upon the outside of the heart itself. The causes of the idiopathic form are diverse, but the following may be mentioned: pleurisy and pneumonia, in which the inflammatory process spreads from the adjacent pleura and lungs direct on to the pericardium; tuberculosis, strangles, and glanders, when lesions of one of these diseases occur in the region of the heart, and the diseased process spreads to its outer covering; many septic conditions, such as metritis, 'picked-nails' in horses, feet, severe suppurating wounds in distant parts of the body, pyorrhœa in dogs' mouths—become complicated with pericarditis; and in other cases it may arise in a true idiopathic sense, without any apparent reason. In a majority of cases it is due to the presence of organisms, particularly *streptococci* and *staphylococci*.

The symptoms are not always characteristic, but they include breathlessness, fixation of the chest wall during breathing, pain on pressure of the left side of the chest, a jugular pulse (seen along the jugular furrow with each heart-beat), and dropsical swellings, which are collections of fluid under the skin, on the lower part of the chest and abdominal walls. The temperature is usually higher than normal, but this rise may be due to other associated disease. On listening to the heart a variation in the normal sounds may be heard, or they may be altogether masked by the presence of the fluid. A tinkle is sometimes audible over the region of the heart; friction sounds indicate the presence of dry pericarditis; and irregularity or even palpitation may be noticed. As a rule little or nothing can be done for the heart, but when the acute symptoms have subsided it may be possible to tap the sac and withdraw the excess fluid.

Pericarditis has been reported in very young pigs at grass. 'The piglet, often in good condition and not anæmic, dies suddenly at about two to three weeks of age.'

Traumatic pericarditis of cattle is of such common occurrence that it is necessary to give special attention to it. In very many cases where the animal is thought to be suffering from simple digestive disturbance, it is found that the real cause of the trouble is some foreign body, very often a nail, or a small piece of metal shaped like a nail. Cattle have a notoriously erratic appetite, and many peculiar and unusual objects are often found in their stomachs; among these there are very often metal objects. The shape of the foreign body causing traumatic pericarditis is very often that of a pointed object about 3 inches long and not thicker than a lead pencil; accordingly, nails, pieces of wire, hair-pins, parts of hat-pins, broken cutlery forks, knitting-needles or large sack-needles, etc., have been found. These are swallowed, fall into the 2nd stomach (reticulum), and through the movements of that organ during digestion, become fixed in the wall comparatively low down. If they are pointed, sooner or later they are forced through the reticulum wall, and penetrate the diaphragm. Their movement is due to the physiological processes of digestion and respiration, in which the stomach and the diaphragm are constantly changing their positions, and to the vigour of the heart. A small distance of only about 2 inches separates the heart from the 2nd stomach in normal cattle, so that once the point of the object has passed through the wall of the latter, it is not long until it meets the wall of the former. To reach the heart wall, however, it must pass through the pericardium, and this sac is, therefore, usually first affected.

Symptoms are in many ways characteristic. In the first place there is disturbance of the stomach, which becomes sluggish and very often distended with gas on the left side. Attacks of pain may be seen, the appetite is irregular, but after a time the animal regains its normal health, since an adhesion has occurred around the hole in the reticulum wall, and the inflammation subsides. Thoracic symptoms are next shown. Breathing becomes shallow, there may be some localised pneumonia with coughing and distress, and the temperature rises well above normal. Later still the heart becomes affected, and the symptoms of pericarditis are seen. It is not necessary for the foreign object actually to penetrate the pericardium, for the organisms from the stomach which accompany its travels are in themselves usually responsible for the inflammation of the membranous sac.

When the inflammatory condition attacks the pericardium death usually follows in a short time, but there are cases in which the heart is not involved at all; the foreign body, after a course through the lower part of the lungs, reaches the chest wall, usually in the region of the dewlap, forms an abscess there, and, when the pus bursts through the skin, allows the object to escape or be removed. These cases are, however, not at all common. In other instances an animal affected with a traumatic pericarditis drops dead in her stall before there have been noticed any symptoms such as are described here.

Treatment is sometimes possible either by opening the rumen and removing the foreign body, nail, wire, or whatever it may be, or by severing two or more ribs and removing the foreign body from the chest cavity. These are often difficult and always serious operations and justified only in animals of considerable value. In others, slaughter is advisable.

MYOCARDITIS is inflammation of the heart muscle. In the pig it is seen in HERZTOD disease, for example; in cattle, in MUSCULAR DYSTROPHY (which see).

ENDOCARDITIS is an inflammation of the membrane lining the heart, and, since the part most subjected to friction and strain is that which covers the valves, so these valves are the most commonly affected parts, those on the left side being more frequently affected than those on the right. The inflammatory process consists in the appearance of small groups of nodules upon the valves. These unite to form wart-like growths, upon which fibrin from the blood is deposited and forms little pendants. This condition is known as a 'simple endocarditis', and occurs very commonly in connection with chronic swine erysipelas in middle-sized and adult pigs, in association with nephritis, and in chronic conditions in which organisms are present in the blood-stream.

Bacterial endocarditis is a cause of death in cattle, especially in South Wales. (*See* HEART WORM for another cause of endocarditis in the dog.)

The nodules result in an incomplete closing of the valves, and since the fibrin deposited upon them tends to become converted into fibrous tissue (*organised*), the growths slowly increase in size. They may attain considerable dimensions, as large as a man's thumb in the horse, and owing to their lobulated appearance they are very often known as *verrucose* or *vegetative growths*. Another form of endocarditis, in which small ulcerations occur upon the valves, and from which tiny portions of tissue may be torn away by the circulating blood, is known as 'malignant' or 'ulcerative endocarditis'. It is a very much more serious form than the simple, since the small particles broken away from the vegetations are liable to become carried away to other parts of the body, and ultimately to block up small blood-vessels, perhaps in important organs. This form is always fatal, and death usually occurs very soon. The symptoms of endocarditis by itself are vague and irregular, but the insufficiency of the valves is capable of diagnosis by competent observation. Little can be done for the condition beyond rest.

VALVULAR DISEASES form a most important and common group of heart disorders, and although the power of compensation already referred to may so neutralise the ill-effects of a narrowed valve, or one which leaks, it is not possible to foretell how far this change will be affected by future diseased conditions, severe strains or exertion, or even trying conditions such as parturition or exposure to adverse circumstances. Very often when an animal 'drops dead', perhaps after running a race, or while undergoing some departure from its normal mode of life, the actual cause is afterwards found to be a diseased heart valve, with perhaps clotting of the blood in the heart as the immediate cause of death; so that an animal affected with valvular disease is usually not suitable for any kind of life which imposes great strains upon the heart. The various disorders of the heart valves which have already been indicated almost invariably cause first of all an increase in the size of the heart, and later, a certain amount of dilatation. The general symptoms they produce are not characteristic, and in many cases are not referable to the heart at all. There may be a general sleepiness of the animal, due to lack of a sufficiency of blood circulating in the brain. Fainting fits are not by any means rare in incompetence of the tricuspid valves, in which condition dropsy of the abdominal cavity is also encountered. Passive congestion of the lungs may be brought about by incompetence of the auriculo-ventricular valve on the left side of the heart (mitral insufficiency), due to regurgitation of blood back into the left atrium, where it hinders the exit of blood coming through the pulmonary veins from the lungs. This same condition may lead to a chronic asthmatical cough in old dogs, which is occasionally mistaken for bronchitis.

All of these conditions are only able to be diagnosed by carefully noting the alterations in the pulse and heart sounds.

HYPERTROPHY, or enlargement of the heart, is of two types: dilatation of the cavity with thickening of the walls (true hypertrophy), and dilatation of the cavity with thinning of the walls (false hypertrophy). The first takes place as the result of some constant simple strain, such as occurs in race-horses, hunters, and sporting dogs; or as the result of backward pressure from a diseased valve, and which entails the 'compensation' of valvular disease; or it may be due to resistance to the flow of blood in some diseased organ or tissue, which results in high blood-pressure.

Hypertrophy of the left ventricle, leading to heart failure, may in the dog follow *Leptospira canicola* infection.

False hypertrophy, which is really an enlargement of the heart without any hypertrophy at all, is more correctly called 'dilatation'. Dilatation may precede hypertrophy, *i.e.* when it occurs before the heart muscle has had an opportunity to increase to meet the extra demands upon it, and it very frequently follows hypertrophy, especially when there is some devitalising process at work which hinders the proper nutrition of the organ. Hypertrophy may be a very beneficial condition in any animal, and, except when it is due to valvular trouble, need not cause any worry to the owner. It is sometimes excessive in horses; in some instances the heart may weigh as much as 25 lb. instead of the 7 or 8 lb. of the normal, and the enlarged condition can be determined from an examination of the pulse and heart sound even by an inexperienced observer. There is always, however, a tendency for degenerative changes to follow hypertrophy when the subject gets old and ceases active work. Dilatation of the heart is always a bad thing. It results from some excessive sudden strain, such as hard galloping when not in good sound condition, and it may also follow the working of animals which are poor in bodily condition and anæmic. It is sometimes associated with fatty degeneration, and it occurs occasionally through the presence of tumours or parasites in the heart. It is also liable to arise after recovery from a severe fevered condition, when the animal is put to work, or is violently exercised too soon after the symptoms have subsided.

DEGENERATION of the heart occurs mostly in old animals, the common form being a change of the muscle fibres into fat. Where the fat is deposited actually inside each of the fibres in a patch of the heart, the condition is known as *fatty degeneration*, and when the deposition occurs amongst the bundles of fibres, but not actually inside their sheaths, it is known as *fatty infiltration*. The former is the more serious, but both are troublesome conditions, from which recovery is not usual. Neither condition can be diagnosed with certainty during life.

RUPTURE of the heart is most likely to occur from the giving way of a local patch of degeneration in the heart wall. It may result from violent exertion, falls, or crushes over the chest, or it may follow puncture by a sharp instrument, such as the tine of a stable-fork, the splintered point of a broken shaft, or in cattle from a nail or other sharp object having passed from the reticulum and entering the heart. The symptoms are those of rapid internal hæmorrhage ; there is trembling, difficulty in breathing, almost leading to suffocation, prostration, convulsive seizures, and death in a short time. Before death the visible mucous membranes are pale in colour, and horses often emit a sobbing sound a few moments before death actually takes place.

FUNCTIONAL DISORDERS.—**Palpitation** is a condition in which the heart beats fast and strongly, due to some nervous disturbance brought about by errors in feeding, sudden frights, or unusual and terrifying surroundings.

Bradycardia is a condition of unusually slow action of the heart which may be practically a normal condition in that it causes no distress to the animal, but in some cases it is due to some functional disturbance following upon severe disease or fever. With time the normal rate may be restored. **Intermittency** or **irregularity** is an exceedingly common condition among animals, and as a rule appears to cause them no inconvenience whatever. In some horses at rest in the stable the heart constantly misses every third, fourth, or fifth beat, a long pause taking the place of the pulsation, but when at exercise or work the normal rhythm is restored.

The heart muscle has in itself, independently of nervous control, the power of contracting rhythmically when excited to do so, of conducting the impulse to contract from one part of the muscle to another, and of maintaining itself in moderate tension or tone. When any of these properties is affected by disease some change in the force, nature, or rhythm of the heart-beat is apt to appear. **Heart-block** is a condition in which the conducting mechanism between atrium and ventricle (atrio-ventricular bundle of His) is damaged in whole or in part, so that the two beat independently of each other.

Rapid heart (with a pulse of 80 or 90 per minute in the horse) may be due to some temporary irritability in the heart muscle ; it is distinguished from the rapid pulsation of a fever, by the absence of high temperature and by the normal strength of the pulse.

Cardiac flutter and fibrillation are conditions of great irregularity in the pulse, due to the atria emptying themselves, not by a series of regular waves, but by an irregular series of flutters or twitches instead, which fail to stimulate the ventricles properly.

For the correct interpretation of the many variations in the heart-beats of the domesticated animals much experience and careful observation are necessary, and the owner of animals is advised to consult a veterinary surgeon rather than to attempt diagnosis himself, whenever any of his animals exhibit deviations in heart action.

HEART-WATER, also known as BUSH SICKNESS (Boschziekte), VELD SICKNESS, and INAPUNGA, is a specific disease of cattle, sheep, and goats transmitted by the ' bont-tick ' (*Amblyomma hebræum*), in South Africa, and *A. variegatum* in Kenya. The disease is characterised by the accumulation of a large amount of fluid in the pericardial sac and certain nervous symptoms.

Cause.—Heart-water is due to infection

with *Rickettsia ruminantium* which possesses an ultra-visible stage which is taken into the body of a feeding bont-tick, and is transmitted to other animals upon which the tick feeds at a later stage of its life-history (*see* PARASITES, p. 686).

Incubation.—After sheep and goats have been bitten by infected ticks, a period of between 11 and 18 days (usually about 15) elapses before any symptoms are shown; in cattle the disease appears between 20 and 25 days after infestation with ticks. These periods are influenced by the stage of the disease in the animal supplying the infected blood to the ticks, and also by individual susceptibility, which is less in native-bred cattle than in those imported from other countries, and especially those brought from Great Britain.

Symptoms.—(1) *Sheep and Goats.*—As would be expected heart-water is commoner in the summer, when the ticks are numerous, than at other seasons. Sheep and goats at first show nothing more than a rise in temperature (which gradually increases to about 107° F., falling each evening 2 or 3 degrees lower), a general dullness, prostration, and lack of appetite, and as these conditions are common to many other diseases the difficulty of diagnosis is great. The affected animals isolate themselves from the rest of the flock, lie about in secluded spots, cease to ruminate, and when handled or driven are very easily tired and lie down.

Many animals show peculiar nervous symptoms, which vary considerably in different individuals; some may bleat almost continuously; others champ the jaws as if feeding, moving the tongue backward and forward between the lips; others lick the ground; some turn in circles until they finally fall to the ground and lie prostrate or perform galloping movements with their limbs; others develop a pronounced squint; while others, still, produce a profuse foamy salivation which clings around their lips and mouth. Convulsions are not uncommon, especially when the animals are handled, and if a sheep in a 'fit' is caught, the convulsive seizure is very much more violent and lasts longer than otherwise. Death usually follows soon after convulsions make their appearance.

(2) *Cattle.*—The symptoms in cattle are very similar to those seen in sheep, and the temperature variations are especially well pronounced. The nervous form in which peculiar masticatory movements are made by the mouth is common. Muscular tremors are better marked than in sheep, probably because they are more easily seen below the finer skin of the ox. Some animals show a tendency to bite at their feet or legs, especially when lying on the ground, and biting the ground is also seen. A number of animals in the early stages may show a dangerous tendency to charge any human being approaching them, but this is seen in other diseases, where excitement is a pronounced feature, as well as in heart-water. In cattle the disease is usually at its height about the fourth day after the first rise in temperature, and death usually occurs about the sixth day. A number of hyperacute cases occur in cattle, and the animal is suddenly found dead on the veld.

Fatality.—In sheep and goats the mortality appears to be between 50 and 60 per cent of those attacked by heart-water, while in cattle it varies very much in different years. In some as many as 80 per cent of the affected die; but usually not more than 40 per cent of the diseased animals succumb.

Autopsy.—Fluid in the pericardial sac surrounding the heart (hence the name—heart-water); but while this is usually found in sheep and goats, it may be absent in the case of cattle. In typical instances there is also a collection of similar fluid in the thoracic and abdominal cavities. Both the pericardium, and the endocardium which lines the heart, may show several small or a few large 'petechiæ', *i.e.* areas where a slight amount of hæmorrhage has taken place below the membrane. In addition to these lesions there may be dropsy or œdema under the skin, in the stomach, intestines, and lungs.

Prevention.—Entirely successful results have followed measures taken against the ticks which transmit the disease. These consist in '*five-day dippings*'.

Antibiotics and sulphadimidine are used in treatment.

HEART WORM.—*Dirofilaria immitis* is a common parasite of dogs in Central Europe, Russia, Australia, America, and Asia, and the worm larvæ are transmitted by various mosquitoes and gnats. The adult worms reach a length of up to 12 inches (females) and inhabit the right side of the heart, causing some degree of endocarditis and a variety of symptoms, *e.g.* cough, hind leg weakness, collapse on exercise, laboured breathing, anæmia, emaciation. Diagnosis is by blood smear, but these must be taken at different times of day. There is no altogether satisfactory treatment at present. Caparsolate sodium will kill the adult worms.

This infestation is known as canine filariasis or Dirofilariasis.

'HEAT' (*see* Œstrus. For the suppression of 'heat' in the bitch, *see* Œstrus, Suppression of.)

'HEATHER BLINDNESS' in sheep is a form of contagious ophthalmia, described under Eye, Diseases of.

HEAT-STROKE is a condition associated with excessively hot weather and great exertion. It occurs in domestic animals when taken to tropical countries from temperate countries, especially when recently unloaded from transport ships and subjected to great excitement in unfamiliar surroundings; it is seen in cattle, sheep, and swine travelling by road or rail, and it frequently occurs at agricultural shows; dogs may be affected when they have been lying out in the sun for some time, and poultry may be attacked during very hot oppressive weather. It is supposed to be due to the action of the high temperature upon the brain cells rather than to the direct action of the rays of the sun, for it may occur at night as well as during the day.

Symptoms.—The animal is usually suddenly attacked with a great lethargy and inability for work or movement. The gait is staggering, and if the animal is made to move it falls to the ground. Convulsions of a violent nature are seen, and if the temperature is taken it is found to be very high, perhaps as much as 108° F. in the horse. Death often takes place in a few hours, but some cases last as long as 3 days. When recovery occurs great dullness for a number of weeks is very liable to follow.

Treatment.—Removal to a cool place, douching the head and neck with cold water from a hose-pipe. Internally, a dose of pholedrine sulphate.

HEDGEHOGS are of veterinary interest in that they are susceptible to natural infection with foot-and-mouth disease, which they may transmit to other animals. They may also transmit leptospirosis.

HEIFER.—A year-old female up to her first calving.

HEINZ BODIES in red corpuscles are seen in cases of hæmolytic anæmia caused by, *e.g.* an excess of kale in dairy cattle.

HELENINE.—An antiviral substance derived from *Penicillium funiculosum.*

HELLEBORES.—There are three hellebores of importance to the owners of animals, and the three are liable to some confusion. **Black hellebore** is the dried rhizome and rootlets of the Christmas rose, or bear's-foot, *Helleborus niger*. This plant is cultivated in Great Britain in gardens, etc., and is found indigenous in many parts of Europe. It was formerly used in the powdered form to add to blistering ointments and liquids, but owing to its uncertain and often very violent actions it is no longer used for this purpose. It may be eaten by live-stock when garden trimmings are thrown out on to fields to which live-stock have access. It contains two very irritant glucosides—*helleborin* and *helleborein*. **Stinking hellebore** (*Helleborus fœtidus*) and **Green hellebore** (*H. viridis* or *Veratrum viride*), which latter is also called 'Indian poke' or 'poke root', are sometimes the cause of live-stock poisoning. The latter, along with **White hellebore** (*Veratrum album*), plants of the United States of America, contain several alkaloids, such as *jervine*, *veratrine*, and *veratroidine*, and were at one time used in medicine as powdered rhizomes, a preparation which was known as veratrum. They are depressants of the motor nervous centres, allied in action to aconite and tobacco. (*Note.—Veratrum* should not be confused with *Veratrine*; *see* Veratrine.)

Poisoning by hellebores.—At the present time the only danger of poisoning by hellebores in Great Britain is from animals eating parts of the plant which have been discarded from gardens, although formerly powdered roots and the chaffed leaves of the Christmas rose were frequently given by empiricists in bran mashes to both horses and cattle for the expulsion of worms. The symptoms produced are stupor, convulsions, and death when large amounts have been taken, and purgation, salivation, excessive urination, attempts to vomit, great straining and the evacuation of a frothy mucus, when smaller amounts have been eaten. Cows give milk which has a bitter taste and is liable to induce diarrhœa or purgation in animals and man drinking it. The treatment consists in keeping the animal's strength up by stimulants; eliminating the parts of the plant that have been eaten by the use of the stomach-tube or by performing rumenotomy in cattle and sheep; and in giving demulcent soothing drenches of gruels, milk, linseed tea, etc.

In Idaho, U.S.A., ewes eating *Veratrum californicum* give birth to lambs with hare-lip and hydrocephalus.

HELMINTHES (ἕλμινς, a worm) is a name for the great class of parasitic worms. (*See* PARASITES).

HEMIPLEGIA (ἡμιπληξία) means paralysis limited to one side of the body only. (*See under* GUTTURAL POUCH DISEASE for facial and laryngeal hemiplegia in horses.)

HEMLOCK, or CONIUM, is the leaves and young branches as well as the fruit of *Conium maculatum*, the hemlock plant. It has a paralysing action upon the endings of the motor nerves.

HEMLOCK POISONING.—As a rule

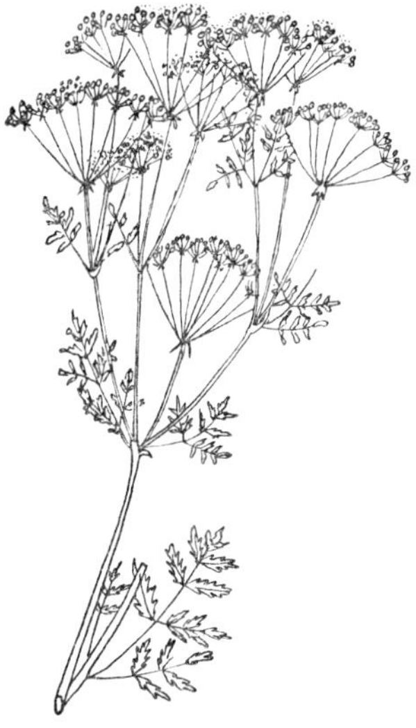

Hemlock (*Conium maculatum*) stem and flowering head. This plant is distinguished from other umbelliferous plants most easily by reference to the stems, which are spotted with a number of dull plum-coloured spots. The flowers are creamy white and arranged in the form of compound umbels. All parts of the plant are poisonous, the berries especially so.

animals will not eat Hemlock on account of the mousy odour and disagreeable taste, but in the spring, when green herbage is scarce and when the fresh shoots of the plant are plentiful, young cattle are sometimes affected. Sheep and goats are believed to be resistant to the poison, while horses require large amounts to produce symptoms of poisoning.

Symptoms.—The poison acts on the motor nerves, causing cessation of digestion, collections of gas in the stomach, salivation, dilatation of the pupils, acceleration of the pulse and respiration, in the early stages; later, paralysis, shown by an unsteady gait or an inability to rise from the ground, difficulty in breathing, and finally death from the paralysis of the respiratory muscles.

Treatment.—Large doses of tannic or gallic acid, stimulants such as alcohol, ether, or strychnine, should be administered, and some authorities recommend atropine.

HENBANE, or HYOSCYAMUS, is a plant found in the British Isles, especially in Ireland, called *Hyoscyamus niger*, from which the leaves are collected and dried, and from which the drug hyoscyamus is prepared. Hyoscyamus has actions and uses similar to belladonna. It allays irritation in the sensory nerve endings, it diminishes the secretions from all the glands of the body, and it raises the blood-pressure. In addition it is a urinary sedative, and is used to allay pain in the bladder in combination with alkaline salts.

HENBANE POISONING is rare, owing to the disagreeable odour of the plant.

Symptoms.—The animal becomes excited; breathing and pulse are hurried at first, and the former becomes difficult later. Salivation is excessive, pupils are dilated, and the muscles of the neck are thrown into a state of spasm, resulting in a stiffness and awkwardness of the head and neck. The abdomen becomes distended, and death occurs sooner or later according to the amount of the drug taken.

Treatment.—The antidotes are hypodermic injection of pilocarpine, stimulants; and artificial respiration.

HEN YARDS (*see under* POULTRY).

HEPARIN.—A naturally occurring anticoagulant.

HEPATISATION (ἧπαρ, the liver) means the solidified state of the lung that is seen in pneumonia, which gives it the appearance and consistence of the liver.

HEPATITIS (ἧπαρ, the liver) means inflammation of the liver. (*See* LIVER.) A virus is responsible for hepatitis in ducklings which sometimes show nervous symptoms or die suddenly when a few days old. The disease appeared in the U.K. in 1954 and is notifiable. (*See also under* DUCK VIRUS HEPATITUS.)

Hepatitis in horses occurs after Infectious Equine Encephalomyelitis, especially where vaccines or sera have been used, and it may correspond to viral hepatitis of man—though this is not supported by existing evidence.

Hepatitis in dogs.—(*See* CANINE VIRUS HEPATITIS.)

HEPATITIS CONTAGIOSA CANIS (*see* CANINE VIRUS HEPATITIS).

HEPTACHLOR.—A constituent of chlordane, a chlorinated hydrocarbon, and used also as an insecticide on its own. It is stored in the body fat, and in the tissues is converted into heptachlor-epoxide, 4 times as toxic to birds as Heptachlor itself.

HEREDITY (*hereditas*, heirship) (*see* GENETICS).

'HEREFORD' DISEASE.—Another name for hypomagnesæmia of cattle.

HERMAPHRODITE ('Ερμῆς, Mercury; 'Αφροδίτη, Venus) is the name applied to animals which exhibit either sexual organs so defectively formed that it is difficult or impossible to differentiate the sex, or else to those that possess some of the sexual organs of both sexes. It is not uncommon in any of the domesticated animals, but it is perhaps most often seen in goats, sheep, cattle, and pigs.

HERNIA (*hernia*) means the protrusion of any organ, or part of an organ, into or through the wall of the cavity which contains it. The term 'hernia' is usually reserved for protrusion of some of the organs or parts of them from the abdominal cavity through an accidental or a physiological opening in its walls. The term 'rupture' is popularly applied to herniæ.

Parts of a hernia.—In a typical abdominal hernia there is always the following parts: a 'ring', or opening in the muscular wall of the abdomen, which may have been brought about as the result of an accident or may have been present at birth; and secondly, a 'swelling' appearing below the skin, composed of the 'hernial sac' and its contents. The ring may be of almost any shape, but it is very often rounded or oval; and it may be of almost any size, from a small hole which will only with difficulty admit the finger, to a large opening capable of allowing the pregnant uterus to escape from the abdominal cavity and become localised under the skin (ventral hernia in the mare). The swelling is usually rounded or oval in appearance, so that the internal tension may be evenly distributed. It is composed of the skin on the outside, a few strands of fibrous tissue and perhaps some bundles of muscular fibres below the skin, then more fibrous tissue, and very often the layer of peritoneum which normally lines the inner surface of the abdominal wall, but this latter may have ruptured in company with the muscles and not be present; these form the hernial sac. The contents vary according to the situation, size, and nature of the hernia, but the following organs or parts of them are most commonly herniated: a loop of bowel with its attached mesentery; omentum, either the whole or a part (very common in dogs); the stomach; the urinary bladder; the spleen or liver (through the diaphragm); the uterus, either when non-pregnant or with its contained fœtus or fœtuses; and sometimes a kidney in the cat. In stout animals a layer of adipose tissue may be included as well.

Varieties.—A hernia is usually described according to the position at which it protrudes. There are certain weak spots in the walls of the abdomen, and herniæ are very prone to occur at these spots. In the region of the groin there is a natural canal leading from the cavity of the abdomen, in an oblique manner through the abdominal wall to the external inguinal region, where lie the scrotum in the male and the mammary gland in the female of the larger animals. This canal is normally occupied by the spermatic cords in the male and by mammary vessels in females; but upon occasion it may become so enlarged as to allow a portion of gut or omentum to descend to the outside. Such a condition is known as *inguinal hernia*, when the structures still remain in the canal; and *scrotal hernia*, when they have come to the outside and are situated in the scrotum. This condition is not uncommon in the stallion and gelding; it occasionally occurs in cattle; it is sometimes seen in the bitch (when the uterus is herniated through the canal), but it is not common in the other domesticated animals. Lying behind and to the outside of the inguinal canal on the inner aspect of the thigh is another canal, shorter and smaller than the inguinal, which is called the 'crural' or 'femoral canal'. Hernia may occur into this canal, when a swelling appears on the inside of the thigh; it is known as a *femoral hernia*, but is rare in the domesticated animals. An *umbilical hernia* is one in which bowels or omentum or both protrude from the abdominal cavity by way of an open umbilical ring. Normally, this opening should close soon after birth, but very commonly in almost any animal the ring in the muscle does not close, and internal organs find their way through it to the outside. A hernia which protrudes through some accidental opening in the abdominal wall, as, for example, through the scar of an operation wound in the dog, or through a large rent in the muscle of the abdomen in the horse occasioned by a severe fall, is known as a *ventral hernia.* Some of the abdominal organs, very frequently the bladder, may insinuate themselves between the rectum and the floor of the pelvis and pass through to the posterior aspect of the animal in the perineal region; a swelling appears below the anus, usually to one side more than the other, and causes the animal a considerable amount of discomfort; such is a *perineal hernia*, commonest in the dog. In addition to these forms, which are all obvious from the surface of the animal, various kinds of *internal herniæ* may occur. The chief of these are: *diaphragmatic hernia*, in which a rent occurs in the diaphragm and some of the abdominal organs are pushed through into the thoracic cavity and embarrass the lungs; *pelvic hernia*, in which organs which normally occupy a position in the abdomen become displaced and find their way into the pelvic cavity (*e.g.* the pelvic flexure of the double colon of the horse sometimes becomes displaced into the pelvis below the rectum); and the so-called 'gut-tie' in cattle, in which a part of the small intestine becomes imprisoned between the wall of the abdomen and the remains of the spermatic cord. It occurs in castrated males always upon the right side of the body. (*See* GUT-TIE.) A hernia may also be considered as *congenital*, that is, existing at birth, or *acquired*, when it occurs later in life. The only herniæ that are congenital are those in connection with the umbilicus and the inguinal canal. In the latter case, which occurs in the male, the herniated structures descend into the scrotum along with the testicle on one or both sides of the body.

A very important classification of hernia is made according to the condition of the protruding structures. A *reducible hernia* is one which is so freely movable that its contents may be pushed back into the abdominal cavity through the hernial ring, though it comes down through the same opening as soon as the retaining pressure is released. An *irreducible hernia*, on the other hand, is one which cannot be returned, either because it has become adherent to its new surroundings, because it has enlarged after emerging (perhaps through interference with the blood-supply), because fat has been deposited inside the abdomen in positions previously occupied by the herniated organs, or for some similar reason. An *obstructed hernia*, or an *incarcerated hernia*, is one in which, a part of the bowel being protruded, some of its contents become imprisoned inside the hernial sac, and the passage of food material down the gut is obstructed. A *strangulated hernia* is by far the most serious and most important form of hernia, because of its immediate danger to the life of the animal. In this form the circulation of blood in the herniated organ (usually bowel) becomes cut off by the margin of the opening through which the loop of bowel has passed; and if an operation be not immediately performed or its relief, the bowel will become gangrenous, and death will follow. The danger attending all forms of hernia, and especially those in which bowel is protruded, is that they may remain simple for a time and then suddenly become 'strangulated'.

Causes.—Speaking very generally, it may be said that two chief factors enter into the causation of herniæ. Firstly, there is some defect, weakening, or injury of a portion of the abdominal wall; and secondly, some increase of pressure within the cavity. With regard to the herniæ which form at the umbilicus, there is usually some imperfection in the closing of the rounded ring in the abdominal wall through which the umbilical cord passes before birth, and through this opening a loop of bowel, or, more commonly, a portion of the omentum, is forced either during the process of parturition or in consequence of some unusual strain in very early life, such as in constipation, diarrhœa, or playful gambolling.

Inguinal hernia, which is practically the same as scrotal hernia, but at a less advanced stage, is almost wholly confined to the male sex in all animals, except the bitch, where a horn of the uterus may, upon occasion, come down through the inguinal canal. There may be a wide oblique passage from the abdomen into the scrotum (scrotal hernia), through which bowel and omentum can pass with ease; or there may be only a small pocket in the peritoneum over the internal inguinal ring, which allows organs to pass into the canal but not through it (inguinal hernia). Inguinal and scrotal forms of hernia may be either congenital or acquired; congenital forms (most common in young animals) result through some failure of the inguinal canal, through which the testicle descends, to close properly; while acquired forms (commoner in adults) result from such accidents as slipping sideways with the hind-feet, injuries to the abdomen from falls, blows, and kicks, from dilatation of the inguinal canal, such as when the testicles are very large and heavy, from very vigorous copulation, etc. It may occur in the gelding and bullock following careless castration, and it sometimes suddenly appears when a horse is rolling in the agonies of a colic. In such cases as these it usually becomes strangulated and fatal results follow.

Femoral hernia is very rare, but sometimes occurs in performing dogs which have been trained to walk upon their hind legs for considerable periods of time. The vertical position of the body imposes an unusual strain upon the muscles at the fold of the thigh, and they give way. It is always acquired.

Perineal hernia is almost exclusively confined to the dog. It may occur in either sex, usually as the result of much straining occasioned by constipation or diarrhœa, chronic coughing or asthma, bronchitis, etc., and it is fairly common in old male dogs suffering from enlarged prostate glands.

Ventral hernia is almost invariably the result of a serious injury to the muscular portion of the abdominal wall. It is commonest in mares, especially those used for breeding purposes. Very often there is little or nothing to be noticed if the mare is injured when non-pregnant, but when pregnancy follows and the tension upon the abdominal wall increases, the muscular part gives way and a large mass appears along the lower line of the abdomen. In cows it very often results from horn-gores from neighbours; in such, the skin remains intact but the muscle is torn and a swelling appears at the seat of the injury. Hernia due to a gore is probably commonest in the region of the flank, where the muscle is naturally thin.

Diaphragmatic hernia may occur in any animal, but is commonest in the dog and the cat. It usually results from jumping downwards from a great height—an act which throws the full weight of the abdominal contents forwards against the diaphragm when the animal lands on its feet; but it may also occur in the horse through falling forwards, backing a very heavy load, or throwing itself about on the ground during an attack of colic. Sometimes it results from a broken rib tearing the diaphragm. The position of the rent may be in the muscular or tendinous portion of the diaphragm, but it very frequently involves one or other of the natural openings (*hiati*), giving passage to the œsophagus, the vena cava, or the aorta, although a hernia through an enlarged aortic hiatus is very rare on account of the powerful nature of the diaphragm in its upper parts.

For a case of **hiatus** hernia, involving incomplete closure of the cardia of the stomach, and dilatation of the lower end of the œsophagus, in a dog, see *Veterinary Record* for May 2, 1964, p. 501. 'The vomitus flowed out without force, and regurgitation could readily be induced by the drinking of water.'

Symptoms.—The symptoms vary much, depending upon the particular organ which is protruded, upon the size of the opening, which may or may not compress the hernia, and upon the condition of the latter. In very many cases among animals herniæ contain either omentum or a loop of bowel, or both. The swelling may be present at birth, or it may appear suddenly or gradually at almost any time during life. To the touch it may present one of several sensations: (1) in the simple form it feels soft, fluctuating (as if it contained fluid), painless, neither hot nor cold, and causes no discomfort to the animal when being handled; if it be pressed upon it can usually be returned to the abdominal cavity, though it will reappear as soon as the pressure is released; in small animals it will disappear when they are laid upon their backs, and remain out of sight until they regain their feet; the ring in the muscle through which the organs have escaped can be easily felt with the fingers; during a cough or when straining while passing fæces the swelling increases in size, as long as the abdominal muscles are tense; no general symptoms of fever, inappetence, or other disturbance are shown; (2) when the structures are adherent to the skin which covers them, return to the abdomen is impossible, no diminution in size can be appreciated with manipulation, no definite ring can be determined as a rule, and there is no increase in size with exertion, but otherwise an *adherent hernia* presents the same appearances as a simple one; (3) in the strangulated form, which may

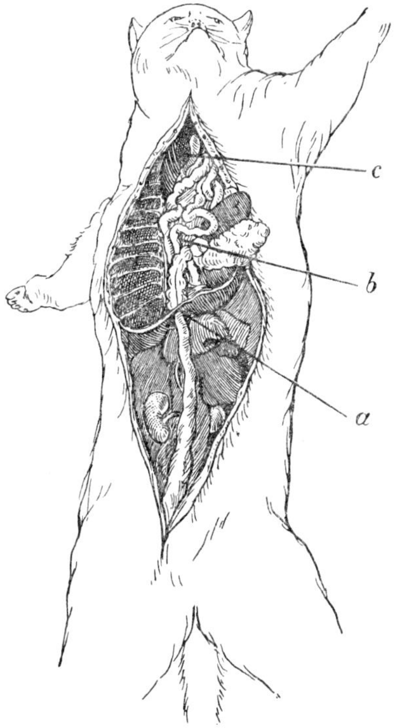

Diagram of diaphragmatic hernia in a cat. The body has been opened to expose the thoracic and abdominal contents. At *a* is seen the rupture in the diaphragm, through which certain of the abdominal organs, shown at *b*, have passed into the chest cavity. The compressed and embarrassed lung is shown at *c*.

supervene upon a hitherto simple hernia, there are very definite and serious symptoms of general disturbance; the animal is fevered, temperature is high, breathing is fast and distressed, an anxious expression is visible on the face, and the swelling shows a marked tenseness and pain when being handled. It may be red and inflamed-looking at first, but later it very frequently becomes bluish. After about 12 to 24 hours gangrene sets in; the swelling becomes cold and painless to the touch; the temperature falls sub-normal, and the animal becomes alarmingly weak. Death usually follows shortly after, unless the strangulation is relieved by operation and perhaps amputation of the strangulated portion of bowel. An obstructed hernia is usually merely the preliminary of strangulation.

Treatment.—Palliative treatment, such as is so very common in human beings consisting in the application of trusses, bandages, etc., is of no use whatever where animals are concerned. When an ordinary simple hernia appears in an animal an owner has, therefore, only one of two alternatives left if the life of the animal is to be protected; he must either satisfy himself that the condition is really a simple one and leave it alone, or he must call in advice and have a radical operation performed. With young animals of any species it is usual to leave herniæ alone provided they are not acute, for it very often happens that during the growth and development of the young creature the hernia disappears of its own accord, and the hole in the abdominal wall heals over. There is, however, always a danger that, as the result of some extra exertion, heavy feeding, boisterous playfulness, fighting, etc., strangulation may occur, and the condition may demand immediate attention.

The most rational method is one in which the animal is anæsthetised, the skin opened, the contents returned to the abdomen, the peritoneal sac obliterated if it is present, the edges of the ring carefully sutured so that they will form a strong union, and finally the skin wound closed.

Where strangulation has recently occurred it is possible by immediate operation to relieve the condition and save the animal, but where gangrene has set in nothing can be done with good chance of success; it is permissible to attempt operation, but in most cases humane destruction is the only procedure. The operation for a strangulated hernia differs from that for a simple one in that it is necessary to enlarge the tight ring, to allow restoration of the circulation. If the bowel is obviously gangrenous the dead portions may be removed and the ends united to each other, but the chances of recovery are small, for peritonitis will most probably have started within the abdomen.

With diaphragmatic herniæ, even where it can be diagnosed, operation is difficult and seldom successful. When a mare has developed a large ventral hernia during pregnancy nothing should be done until she has foaled, but after that, if the hernia is not too large, it should be operated upon before she is allowed to breed again.

A word of warning is perhaps advisable: an owner is very often much tempted to look upon what is actually a hernia with some contempt, and finding that it does not disappear within a few days, he decides to puncture it and 'evacuate the fluid'—with fatal consequences.

HERPES VIRUSES cause, for example, Aujesky's disease, equine rhinopneumonitis, equine arteritis, feline rhinotracheitis. (*See also* B. VIRUS and FADING.)

HERZTOD DISEASE.—A heart condition in pigs, which has similarities to 'Mulberry Heart.'

HETEROSIS.—Hybrid vigour.

HETEROZYGOUS (*see under* GENETICS, *page* 376).

HETP.—An organo-phosphorus insecticide used in agriculture and horticulture. Similar to TEPP (which see).

HEXACHLORETHANE.—A drug of value against the liver-fluke in cattle and sheep and also effective against *Hæmonchus* and *Trichostrongylus*. It is safer than carbon tetrachloride.

Poisoning does occasionally occur, however, and seems to be connected in some way with blood calcium imbalance. It is recommended that for several days before dosing with hexachlorethane, feeding-stuffs other than grass or hay should be withheld—roots and concentrates should not be given.

Symptoms of poisoning include: lowered temperature, coldness of the extremities, dullness which may develop into coma. Abdominal pain and blood-stained dung may also be in evidence.

HEXACHLOROBENZENE.—Used as a seed-dressing, it has given rise to a form of PORPHYRIA (which see) in children in Turkey, and might similarly affect livestock.

HEXACHLOROPHENE.—A drug used against liver flukes. It is stated to be safe for cows in milk and pregnant ewes.

In the ram, excessive doses can cause atrophy of the seminiferous epithelium of the testes.

HEXAMINE is a substance made by the action of ammonia upon formalin. It is excreted by the kidneys, and as it sets free formalin in an acid medium it has some antiseptic qualities when the urine is acid. As a consequence it is usually prescribed along with some acid salt, such as acid phosphate of sodium, unless the urine is naturally acid.

HEXAMITIASIS.—An intestinal disease of turkeys occurring in the U.S.A. and in Britain.

Cause.—*Hexamita meleagridis.*

Symptoms.—Day-old poults may be affected, but more commonly the disease attacks turkeys a few weeks old. The feathers become ruffled, the birds listless with drooping wings. The droppings become liquid and frothy. Birds stand silent and motionless with eyes closed. Loss of condition is rapid, with marked dehydration. In young birds mortality may reach 100 per cent. Recovered birds may act as carriers.

Treatment.—Tinostat has given some success. Antibiotics; furazolidone.

HEXYLRESORCINOL.—A urinary antiseptic, effective for alkaline as well as acid urine. It is not suitable for cats.

HEXŒSTROL.—The trade name for a synthetic œstrogen said to be more active than stilbœstrol. (*See* STILBŒSTROL, CAPONISING, etc.)

HIATUS HERNIA (*see under* HERNIA).

HIBITANE.—Chlorhexidine, a valuable disinfectant effective against some bacteria which cause mastitis in cattle.

HIGH HEELS, *i.e.* raised calkins, are sometimes put on to horses' shoes to relieve the strain upon the back tendons when these latter are sprained or injured. They do good in the early stages when the condition is acute, but if they are used too long there comes a time when the tendons shorten and the horse is unable to walk sound on a flat shoe. High heels are also put on to the heels of colts' shoes when they are being broken in, and when they show a tendency to the formation of bog spavins in their hocks. Very often when a bog spavin appears in a three-year-old colt, the addition of calkins to its shoes, and the application of a mild stimulating liniment to the swellings, will result in complete resolution, provided the animal is rested for two or three weeks.

HILUM, or (incorrectly) **HILUS,** is a term applied to the depression on organs such as the lung, kidney, and spleen, at which the vessels and nerves enter or leave, and round which the lymphatic glands cluster. The hilum of the lung is also known as its root.

HINNY.—The offspring of a stallion and a female ass.

HIP-JOINT is the joint formed between the head of the femur, or thigh-bone, and the depression on the side of the pelvis called the acetabulum. It is surrounded by a mass of very powerful muscle, which, assisted by ligaments, binds the two bones together so as to make dislocation uncommon. The joint is of the 'ball-and-socket' variety.

'HIP DYSPLASIA' IN DOGS.—This term, current among dog breeders, covers a number of abnormal conditions of the acetabulum and head of the femur.

Some of these conditions are hereditary.

They include: (1) *Subluxation,* in which the head of the femur is no longer firmly seated within the acetabulum. Deformity of the head of the femur gradually develops. The symptoms include: a reluctance to rise from the sitting position, and a sawing gait, observed when the puppy (most often an Alsatian, sometimes a Golden Retriever or Boxer) is 4 or 5 months old.

(2) *Osteochondritis dissecans* is seen in terriers with short legs, poodles, and Pekingese. It is possibly identical with Perthe's Disease. Muscular wasting and lameness is observed, usually in one limb.

(3) *Slipped Epiphysis.* This also causes pain and lameness at 4 to 6 months, but is difficult to distinguish from (2).

(4) *Congenital Dislocation,* in which the acetabula are too shallow to retain the heads of the femurs in position. Reported in the Black Labrador. A false joint forms in time. (*See also* PERTHE'S.)

HISTAMINE.—An amine occurring as a decomposition product of histidine (*see* AMINO-ACIDS) and prepared synthetically from it. Histamine is widely distributed in an inactive compound form in the body, particularly in the lungs, liver, and to a lesser extent in blood and muscle. As a result of trauma, burns, or infection, it may be liberated from the skin, lungs, and other tissues. Histamine dilates capillaries, reduces blood pressure, increases any tendency to œdema, stimulates visceral muscles and gastric and pancreatic secretions. Histamine toxicity is shown by engorgement of the liver, shock, and a tendency to urticaria-like skin lesions. (*See also* ANTIHISTAMINES, ALLERGY.)

HISTAMINASE.—An enzyme obtained from extracts of kidney and intestinal mucosa, capable of inactivating histamine and other diamines. It has been used in treating anaphylactic shock and other allergic conditions due to, or accompanied by, the liberation of histamine in the body.

HISTOPLASMA CAPSULATUM. — A fungus which causes disease, usually fatal, in dogs and man; also in cattle. The liver becomes involved, and there is also often dropsy. The disease, HISTOPLASMOSIS, is believed to be rare.

HISTOSTAB.—An antihistamine.

HOCK (*see* p. 114).

HODGKIN'S DISEASE (*see* PSEUDO-LEUKÆMIA).

HOG.—A male pig after being castrated.

HOG CHOLERA (*see* SWINE FEVER).

HOGG.—An uncastrated male pig. (*See also under* SHEEP.)

HOGGET (*see under* SHEEP).

HOLSTEIN-FRIESIAN.—This breed of cattle in the U.S.A. and Canada has its origin in animals imported from the Netherlands mostly between 1857–87. They are also known as American or Canadian Holsteins or Holsteins.

HOMATROPINE is an artificial alkaloid prepared from atropine. Its sole use is to dilate the pupil of the eye for careful examination of the deeper parts of that structure. It is more suitable than atropine, as it does not interfere with vision for such a length of time as does atropine.

HOMOGRAFT REACTION, THE.—The process by which an animal rejects grafts of another's tissue.

HOMOZYGOUS.—An animal is said to be homozygous for a given characteristic when all its germ cells transmit identical genes for that characteristic. (*See* GENETICS.)

HONEY is used in medicine mixed with various drugs as a soothing preparation for use in sore throat. Its price prevents its use in other than valuable animals.

If made by bees from plants treated with systemic insecticides, *e.g.* schradan, which persists in the nectar, the honey will contain schradan.

HOOF (*see* FOOT OF THE HORSE).

HOOF-PRINTS, and other places where the soil is exposed below the turf, are on wet pastures a common habitat of the snails which act as intermediate hosts of the liver fluke. Dressing with 28 lb. of finely powdered bluestone, mixed with 1 cwt. of dry sand, to the acre, will reduce the snail population if done each year in June and repeated in August.

HOOF REPAIR WITH PLASTICS.—Until recently it has been possible to alter the shape of a deformed hoof only by paring away horn; but a technique used in the U.S.A. enables a plastic material to be bonded with the horn, so that this can be built up. Cracks, deformities, and cavities can be repaired, using an acrylic substance in the form of a white powder, together with one of two types of fluid.* With one, the acrylic assumes in about 5 minutes the hardness of wall horn; with the other, that of the frog tissue. The former can be rasped and nailed; the latter rasped or trimmed with a knife. Large defects should be repaired with a series of layers in order to avoid damage from heat generated by the process. The latter is described in the *Journal of the American Veterinary Medical Association*, **147,** 1, 340.

HOOK WORMS.—These are voracious blood-suckers, and secrete *anticoagulins* in order to prevent the host's blood from clotting at the point abraded by their teeth. It is perhaps not widely enough known that skin disease and damage to the pads of the feet may result from hookworm infestation. The latter most commonly occurs in foxhounds, beagles, racing greyhounds, and other sporting dogs confined in kennels and runs. Sometimes it is a deterioration in the animal's performance which first draws the owner's or trainer's attention to foot abnormality.

Hookworm larvæ can penetrate the unbroken skin; their entry being facilitated by a substance which they secrete to soften or destroy the skin's outer layers. Where they have entered, there is redness; and this applies to areas of skin in contact with the ground when the dog is lying down, but especially to the skin between the pads of the feet. Redness here, with or without itching, which may be mild or intense, is often the first sign of foot abnormality. In severe cases, the pads become soft and spongy. Long-standing cases may be complicated by a secondary bacterial infection, giving rise to swelling of the pads and to deformity of the claws. (*See* PARASITES, p. 665.)

HOOSE (*see* HUSK).

HORDEOLUM (*hordeolum,* a barley-corn) is another name for stye (*see* EYE, DISEASES OF).

HORMONES (ὁρμάω, I stir up) are substances which upon absorption into the blood-stream influence the action of tissues or organs other than those in which they were produced. The internal secretions of the ovary, testicles, thyroid, parathyroid, adrenal, thymus, pituitary body, and the pancreas are examples of hormones. (*See* ENDOCRINE GLANDS.)

The inter-action of the hormones is far-reaching and complex. In health, a delicate balance—the 'endocrine balance'—is maintained. In ill health this balance may be disturbed by an insufficiency of one particular hormone or by excess of another. Some hormones are antagonistic to each other, so that an excess of one amounts to much the same thing as too little of another. In some conditions, such as 'milk fever' in the cow, a number of endocrine glands are believed to be involved; the imbalance being far from a simple one. The thyroid may be regarded as the 'master gland'; its secretion profoundly influencing growth, sexual development, immunity, and the rate of metabolism. Yet the thyroid is itself stimulated by a hormone secreted by the anterior pituitary gland—an example which illustrates the interdependence of the whole endocrine system.

* Hoof Repairing Material: H. D. Justi Division, Williams Gold Refining Co., Inc., Philadelphia, U.S.A.

An animal's disposition and its hormone secretions are closely linked. Fear or anger, for example, will cause an outpouring of adrenalin ; sex hormones may determine whether an animal chooses to fight or flee. And, probably, the animal's 'endocrine make-up' determines to some extent its capacity for, or tendency to, anger, fear, etc., as it does for sexual appetite.

Insulin (*see* PANCREAS, DIABETES, HORMONE THERAPY).

Thyroxine (*see under this heading and* THYROID GLAND).

Adrenalin (*see under this heading and* ADRENAL GLANDS).

Hormones of the anterior pituitary lobe stimulate the gonads (gonadotrophin), thyroid, adrenals, the skeleton, and milk secretion, etc.

Pituitary Gonadotrophin influences both the ovary and testis. In the latter it stimulates development of the sperm-secreting tissue and of actual sperm production, and of the interstitial tissue and the secretion of male sex hormones. In the ovary it stimulates growth of the ovarian follicles and development of corpora lutea. Pituitary Gonadotrophin is thus considered as having two parts or principles : F.S.H. (Follicle Stimulating Hormone) and L.H. (Luteinising Hormone).

Chorionic Gonadotrophin. This is a hormone resembling that of the anterior pituitary but formed in the placenta and excreted in the urine of pregnant women. The action of this hormone is predominantly luteinising.

Serum Gonadotrophin (P.M.S.) is a hormone similar to the above but predominantly follicle-stimulating, obtained from the serum of pregnant mares.

Pituitrin is the hormone from the posterior lobe of the pituitary, and comprises a pressor principle (*vasopressin*), which acts upon the heart and circulation, causing a rise in blood pressure, and an oxytocic principle (*oxytocin*) which stimulates involuntary muscles such as those of the intestines and of the uterus (when pregnant).

Natural œstrogens are hormones obtained from the follicles of the ovary and include *œstrin* and its chemical variants *œstrone*, *œstriol*, *œstradiol*, etc. At puberty œstrin brings about development of the teats, udder, vagina, etc. Œstrin is, to some extent, antagonistic to luteal hormone and the parathyroid secretion.

Synthetic œstrogens have a similar effect to the above. They include stilbœstrol, hexœstrol, and dienœstrol.

Progestin, *progesterone*, or the *luteal hormone* is produced by the corpus luteum. This hormone stimulates preparation of the lining of the uterus for pregnancy, and by counteracting other hormones ensures the undisturbed maintenance of the gravid uterus ; meanwhile suppressing œstrus, and—with the œstrogens—stimulates development of the udder and onset of lactation.

Androgen is the sex hormone secreted by the testes. A synthetic androgen, *e.g. testosterone, testosterone propionate*, is commonly used in hormone therapy. The male sex hormone is responsible for the development of secondary sexual characters, is capable of counteracting the female sex hormones, and apparently inhibits the deposition of fat.

HORMONE THERAPY is of great value in cases where a true endocrine failure or imbalance is at fault, but it is obviously not a panacea. Moreover, the indiscrimnate use of hormones is fraught with danger, and if persisted with may give rise to the production of ANTIHORMONES (which see). Therapy, as opposed to 'chemical caponisation', should be carried out by a veterinary surgeon only.

The uses of *insulin*, *thyroxine*, *adrenalin*, and *pituitrin* are described under these headings, and extracts of *thyroid* and *parathyroid* gland are similarly dealt with. Apart from these, considerable use is made in veterinary practice of the sex hormones. (*See* HORMONES *above*.)

Chorionic gonadotrophin is used in the treatment of nymphomania due to cystic ovaries, of cryptorchidism, and also of pyometra and of some cases of infertility due to a deficiency of luteinising hormone. In the mare and cow a single dose given intra-muscularly will usually correct nymphomania. Chronic gonadotrophin is obtained from the urine of pregnant women.

Serum Gonadotrophin (P.M.S.) is used in cases of anœstrus and infertility, and to obtain an extra crop of lambs.

Progesterone is used to prevent abortion or resorption of the fœtus occurring as a result of luteal deficiency. It is also used to treat cases of cystic ovaries, and may be tried to relieve uterine hæmorrhage. Luteal hormone preparations are given either intramuscularly (if in oil) or by implantation (if in tablet or pellet form).

Synthetic œstrogens, such as *stilbœstrol* and *hexœstrol*, are used for the 'chemical caponisation' of poultry. In other animals they are used in cases of retention of the afterbirth, in some cases of pyometra, uterine inertia and dystokia, and in order to cut short lactation. Some synthetic œstrogens can be given by the mouth. In the dog stilbœstrol is used in the treatment of enlarged prostate; in the bitch stilbœstrol diproprionate may be used by intra-muscular injection after mating to prevent conception.

Testosterone propionate is of use in sexually under-developed young males, and in adult males it may be given to improve fertility or to overcome impotence. In castrated or androgen-deficient males it may be of service in obesity, alopecia, and possibly eczema. In the female it may be used to cut short œstrus in racing bitches and mares, to suppress lactation, and in the treatment of pyometra. It has been used with success in the treatment of alopecia (baldness) in spayed cats and also in the bitch (non-spayed). (*See* CORTICOSTEROIDS, ENDOCRINE GLANDS, SYNCHRONISATION OF OESTRUS.)

HORMONES IN MEAT PRODUCTION.—The practice of implanting a pellet of hexœstrol into beef cattle and lambs in order to obtain a heavier carcase, has gained general acceptance in the U.S.A. In Britain, the practice came in for much criticism during 1957 and the early part of 1958, and largely fell into abeyance.

It has been suggested that there is a considerable risk of accumulation of hormone on pasture, with a risk to breeding animals subsequently grazing that pasture.

In Northern Ireland seven heifers aborted as a result of being given silage contaminated with hexœstrol. This case, reported by Mr. J. F. Rankin, B.Sc., M.R.C.V.S., Ministry of Agriculture, Belfast, deserves to be widely known.

It happened on a farm where some bullocks, receiving hexœstrol-impregnated cubes with home-mixed fattening meal, were housed. The litter, which the farmer had been told would be safe for spreading on the pasture, was used as a seal for a pit-silo. The hexœstrol evidently found its way from the manure into the silage, and the heifers eating it in due course aborted.

The leaner carcase—and especially the leaner brisket—is appreciated by the butcher buying implanted steers, but many butchers have complained of feminine sexual characteristics in carcases which would normally lead to their rejection.

In beef cattle, the treatment of two-year-old steers over a 100-day period appears to give the best results. Good feeding is essential.

In one small-scale Scottish trial, the gain in weight was approximately 42 per cent. In other trials, conducted at Nottingham University, increases in weight—over the non-treated control animals—have been reported as 63 per cent, in yarded cattle; and as 15½ per cent, 46 per cent, and 55 per cent on spring, summer, and autumn pasture, respectively. The extra weight of the treated steers could be worth anything up to £4 per head.

At Nottingham the majority of the treated steers were slaughtered first and reached a better degree of finish than the control steers. Carcases were leaner. In this respect the implanted steer differs from the capon, in which most of the extra weight is due to extra fat.

Over-dosage may result in a poorer quality carcase than that of the untreated steer, and must be avoided for this and other reasons.

The method of administration has been to implant a pellet of hexœstrol under the skin of the ear. Implantation is preferable to giving the hormone mixed in the food for the following reasons. It is not easy to be sure of giving the right dosage. Skilled mixing is required, and the workers who carry this out run a risk to their health. Mistakes might arise, and the hormone-containing food inadvertently be given to females or breeding stock or to animals other than cattle. An example of this occurred in the U.K.; 11 out of 14 ewes aborting after being fed cattle-fattening cake containing hexœstrol. Apart from these dangers, a much larger quantity of the hormone preparation is needed when it is to be given in the food, and that obviously multiplies the cost of the treatment.

The same remarks apply to sheep, the hand feeding of which may not be practicable. Implantation, using ordinary poultry caponising pellets, avoids these dangers, but not the possibility of side-effects. The worst side-effect was reported from America; lambs having a smaller urethra, which may lead to difficulty in passing water, blockage by 'stones' and other complications which can result in death. In one outbreak 2,000 out of 9,000 lambs died as a result of urethral obstruction after receiving 12 mg. stilbœstrol by injection.

In a Welsh experiment the implanted group was approximately 40 per cent heavier than that of the non-implanted control animals, and fetched an extra 9s. per head at December prices. In other experiments fattening hoggs have shown an added increase of 33 per cent over 30 days on turnips, and of 42 per cent over 150 days on turnips and concentrates. Lamb carcases are generally leaner. (*See also* TWINNING.)

HORN FLY.—*Lyperosia irritans* is a parasite of cattle in America, Hawaii, and Europe.

HORNS, INJURIES TO.—In the horned breeds of cattle, sheep, and goats, injuries to the horns are not uncommon. In spite of the great strength of the horns of cattle, fracture of the horn cores, from fighting, collision, etc., may arise with comparative ease when the force has been applied in a lateral or transverse manner. Very frequently the horn itself remains apparently intact, but the bony core is fractured, and the injury is not suspected until the animal is noticed bleeding profusely from one nostril, *i.e.* that on the same side as the injured horn. The explanation is that the blood finds its way into the hollow sinus in the core which communicates with the other sinuses to the head, and these in turn lead into the nasal passage of the same side, so thas the blood seeks an exit eventually through the nose. In other cases the tip of a horn may be broken clean off, and the external hæmorrhage is liable to be alarming.

Treatment.—It is firstly necessary to control the hæmorrhage. This may be effected by tying a cord round the bases of each horn in the manner of a figure-of-eight, first round one horn root and then round the other. A stick inserted in this loop and twisted like a tourniquet will tighten it sufficiently to control the bleeding. If the horn is still holding (*i.e.* if only the core is fractured) it will act as a natural splint, and a good recovery may be looked for; but if there is any degree of movement possible, it is necessary to fix a piece of board to the sound horn, to act as a splint, and to bandage the injured horn to it. Wounds of the horns, as a rule, are not serious once the bleeding has been arrested, but deformity is liable to result. (*See also* WOUNDS, ACCIDENTS, INJURIES.)

HORSE-MEAT.—Uncooked liver, lungs, etc., may be a source of the hydatid cysts of the tapeworm *Echinococcus granulosus* of the dog. (*See also under* MEAT STAINED GREEN.)

HORSE-POX (*see* VARIOLA).

HORSES, BREEDS OF

Horses will be considered as falling into the following groups for the purposes of this section:

(1) Heavy Draught Class:
- Shire.
- Clydesdale.
- Suffolk.
- Percheron.

(2) Light Draught Class:
- Cleveland Bay.

(3) Saddle and Harness Class:
- Thoroughbred.
- Hunter.
- Arab.
- Hackney.
- Hackney pony.

(4) Pony Class:
- New Forest.
- Dartmoor.
- Exmoor.
- Dales.
- Fell.
- Welsh cob.
- Western Islands.
- Connemara.
- Shetland ponies.

(*See also separate entries for* APPALOOSA, GARRON, AMERICAN QUARTER HORSE.)

The Shire Horse.—This is the largest, strongest, and heaviest of all the British breeds of draught horses, and has been in existence for many centuries. Records which go back to the Roman invasion show that a breed of horses was known in England then which was noted for its strength and activity. The origin of the breed is associated with the shires lying between the Humber and the Cam, *i.e.* the fenlands of Lincolnshire and Cambridgeshire, and extending westwards to the Severn valley.

Characteristics.—A stallion should stand at least 17 hands, and weigh one ton when adult. The legs should be big and massive, clean and flat in the bone, and plentifully provided with 'feather' at the back and sides. The hair on the legs should be silky though strong; it should not be wiry, woolly, or curly. The body should be large and massive, the muscles of the shoulders and thighs hard, well developed, and uniformly arranged, the gaskins and fore-arms strong and well clothed, and the head set upon a well-arched neck and thoroughly masculine. Mares are usually divided into two classes, over 16 hands and under 16 hands. Almost all colours are found, but chestnuts, roans, greys, and piebalds are not in favour. Dark rich browns are in most demand, and any white above the knees or hocks is not favoured in showyards.

The Clydesdale Horse.—This breed is generally accepted as being Scottish, but there is little doubt that it was originally a composite breed obtained by crossing native Scottish mares with Flemish stallions. Lanarkshire had always been associated with the breeding of Clydesdales in the past.

Characteristics.—Bays and browns are the commonest colours, although blacks, roans, and even chestnuts are sometimes met with. Of late years many animals show a few grey or white hairs scattered through the coat, and unseemly splashes of white have been noticed on the thighs, under part of the belly, and even on the quarters. Full-blaze faces are very common, and are often associated with 'wall eyes'. The height of a stallion is usually from 16 to 17 hands; a few of the biggest exceeding the latter figure. Mares are smaller, many of them only measuring 15·2 hh. As a breed Clydesdales are very active, possess clean, sound bones, good action at the trot and walk, and large, open, sound feet. Many show horses appear to have square feet, but this is due to artificial methods of shoeing, and in many cases it disguises an otherwise rather small foot. It is a practice which should not be encouraged. The 'feather' is confined to the back of the leg, and should be straight, fine, and silky. When trotting or walking away the hocks should be close together and the hind toes slightly thrown outward. The fore-arms and gaskins are much slimmer and less well muscled than in the Shire.

The Suffolk Horse.—This breed is named after its native county, where it has been regularly bred for over 500 years. The popular name 'Suffolk Punch' has arisen owing to the characteristic thick-set muscular body set upon short, stout legs. A good horse stands as high as a Clydesdale and weighs a ton. The breed is remarkable for the purity of its colour, which is always some shade of chestnut. Suffolks are noted for their gameness and docility. They are invaluable for slow, heavy work which would 'break the hearts' of Shires or Clydesdales, such as ploughing heavy clay lands.

Characteristics.—The Suffolk is an excellent mover at the trot and walk; the hoofs are well shaped at the present time, though formerly they were rather subject to certain foot diseases. The legs are clean and strong, but appear to be too small for such a large body, since they possess no 'feather', except a tuft at the back of the fetlock; this feature is entirely optical, for by actual measurement they compare well with Shire or Clydesdale. The body is massive and well developed, clothed with a powerful array of muscle, and covered with a fine silky close-fitting skin, which denotes purity of breed and quality. The quality is characteristic. Seven grades of colour are recognised, varying from a *dark chestnut* (almost brown-black), through *dull dark, light mealy, red, golden, lemon,* to a *bright chestnut,* which last is the most popular.

The British Percheron Horse.—The native heavy draught horse of France most nearly approaches to the type of the Suffolk so far as our own breeds are concerned, but it is a smaller and less 'top-heavy'-looking horse.

Characteristics.—Greys and blacks are the predominant colours, but roans, dark browns, and even bays are met with. The height is up to 16 hands for mares and to 16·2 hands or 17 hands for stallions, but many animals smaller than this are found. They weigh from 15 cwt. to 1 ton. A typical animal has clean sound legs, great activity for its weight, moving with a straight action, long deep bodies, and a very docile temperament.

The Cleveland Bay.—This is the oldest of the British breeds of clean-legged farm or large carriage horse, and has been in existence for about 200 years in the North and East Ridings of Yorkshire. The introduction of thoroughbred blood about a century ago probably endowed it with its attributes of courage and quality.

Characteristics.—A good horse should stand about 16·1 to 16·3 hands high, and should have good sloping shoulders, short legs and back, and be possessed of powerful loins and long quarters. The head is proudly carried, and there should be a general suggestion of strength and activity, with good clean action which is not at all exaggerated like that of the Hackney. The colour of the Cleveland is bay, either light or dark, with black points as a rule.

Black 'zebra-marks' across the back of the fore-arms and the front of the gaskins are supposed to denote purity of blood, but are not so common as formerly. White is not admissible except for a few white hairs forming a small star on the forehead, or a grey or white tuft on the heel. Blaze faces and white feet or legs indicate a recent or distant cross with another breed (often Hackney).

The Cleveland Bay is used for breeding heavy-weight hunters when crossed with a thoroughbred sire. It is also crossed with the Hackney for producing cross-bred carriage horses with some style about them. In coaching days the majority of the stage-coaches and mail-coaches were run with teams of Cleveland Bays.

The Highland Garron.—It is probable that the Garron is an offshoot from the Western Island ponies. They are heavy, strong, useful animals which have lost practically all pony character, and are admirably adapted for hill-farm work, such as on Highland crofts, and for carrying deer. There is little doubt that the Percheron has been used in the production of the Garron.

Characteristics.—Garrons stand up to 14·2 hands high, although a large number of smaller horses are met with. They have good, clean heads, bold eyes, often Roman noses, and strong muscular crested necks in both mares and stallions. The shoulders are rather heavy; the backs are long but strong; the quarters are good and powerful, though not always as well set as they might be; and the bone of the leg is apt to be rather round. The colours are black, brown, dun, piebald, black-and-white, brown-and-white, bay, mixed and dappled grey, and a number of red or blue roans.

The English Thoroughbred Horse.—This is a breed of mixed origin, horses of Arab, Turkish, and Spanish breeds having been utilised to form it. Charles II. imported a number of Eastern mares, and by crossing them with stallions also imported, there was founded a breed which, by careful selection for speed and stamina, has produced a horse superior to the Eastern breeds. During the last 200 years the height has also been considerably increased; as much as an inch every 45 years has been added, according to certain authorities. Long-distance races, the fashion formerly, have now given place to races of a shorter distance at a much faster pace, and the age at which horses are trained is now much less than originally; in fact, the majority of horses are at present in training before they are four years old. As a general rule the thoroughbred horse has not been subjected to as much in-breeding as have other breeds of animals, for stamina, speed, and courage are absolutely essential qualities in the race-horse, and these are only gained by outcrossing, and, once attained, are rapidly lost by intensive in-breeding.

Characteristics.—There is no height or weight which can be considered as typical of the thoroughbred, some good horses measuring under 16 hands, and quite a number being over 17 hands high. The commonest colours are bays and browns; chestnuts and greys are perhaps next commonest. Blacks are rare. The head should be of pleasing appearance, with fine, lean, distinct features, medium-sized ears, large, prominent, clear, intelligent eyes, fine nostrils, and a tightly fitting fine soft skin. The neck should be long, muscular, and arched, joining the chest smoothly without any 'collar-bed'. The chest should be deep and large, with high withers, and the shoulders should slope obliquely backwards to give freedom and elasticity in movement. The body should be short above and long below, with well-sprung ribs, back and loins level and well-balanced, and no slacknes in the coupling. The hind-quarters should be long and the thighs well clothed with muscle. The gaskins should be broad and prominent, and the hocks clean, deep and wide, and entirely free from thickening. The fore-arm should be firm and well muscled, long and tapered, leading to a broad, flat, clean knee, which is supported by a short, clean, wide cannon. The feet should be of medium size, wide, moderately upright, high at the heel and concave below. The whole appearance should suggest speed and vitality with very easy action at the gallop (which is the normal pace of the thoroughbred) and a low trotting action.

Hunters.—Hunters are not a distinct breed by themselves, but they are of such importance that they deserve some passing attention here. Almost without exception hunters are bred with a strain of thoroughbred blood in one of their immediate parents, and very often the sire is a pure thoroughbred. The type that is sought after is what might be described as a compact, stout, short-legged, well-balanced thoroughbred, true in action, moving freely at walk, trot, or gallop, and easily able to leap such obstacles as are encountered in an average hunting field. Consequently, since performance is more than appearance, it is very difficult, if not impossible, to judge a hunter's merits by his outward form. Many horses which would hardly appear to be likely to do credit to a cab are excellent performers in the field. In a way there are two types: the lady's hunter—an animal of a smaller, finer appearance; and the gentleman's hunter—a bigger, stronger animal able to carry a man of 12 stones weight. A lady's hunter usually stands about 15 to 15·3 hands high, and a gentleman's hunter may be up to 16·2 hands. It is not desirable to exceed this height, because the higher a horse the longer are his legs, and the less sure-footed will he generally be. Heavyweight hunters are bigger, stronger, thicker-set animals, which can carry up to 15 or 16 stones through a day's hunting.

A strong constitution is absolutely essential in a hunter, for it must be able to stand up to a hard day's galloping without food or water, and be able to recover without an unduly long rest.

The value of an Arab strain is very pronounced, for it is a matter of common knowledge that no horse is able to withstand hardship as does the Arab. There is some tendency for the first Arab cross to be small and rather light in the leg, but this is a matter which can be corrected in one or two generations. For cross-bred hunters a good plan is to start with a mare that has proved her worth in the hunting field, and to use a powerful thoroughbred stallion of a good riding type which has done well on the race-course. However, many useful animals are bred from a light cart-horse mare crossed with a thoroughbred stallion, or from a pony mare similarly crossed. Much depends upon the activity and conformation of the mare, and there is always a number of such crosses which prove very disappointing in the field.

The English Arab.—Records of the Arab go back a very long way, and the origin of the Arab pony in its native country is shrouded in the mists of antiquity. Some claim that it is descended from Barbary horses imported from North Africa into Arabia 2000 years ago. It is practically certain that it did much to originate the modern English thoroughbred.

Characteristics.—The Arab has the general conformation of a good saddle pony, and is more useful for carrying weights for long distances without undue fatigue than for short sprints. It shows great intelligence, and is noted for its stamina under adverse conditions. Greys are common, with bays, browns, and chestnuts occurring frequently. Many so-called Arabs are really crosses between Arabs and Egyptian or Turkish ponies, and are apt to be weedy. The pure-bred Arab is a very much better animal in appearance and performance. The Arab Horse Society has been started in Great Britain with the idea of promoting the breeding and importing of pure-bred Arabs from Arabia and other parts of the Near East, and there is little doubt that in time the influx of new blood will do much to put the breeding of light horses upon a better footing than it has been in the past.

The Hackney.—The foundation of the Hackney was most probably a cross between home-bred 'trotting mares' and an imported Arab horse called the Darley Arabian, but the greater influence was exerted by a horse called 'Shales' or the 'Schale's Horse', which was foaled in 1755 or about that time, and this animal is usually looked upon as the real founder of the modern Hackney. There is a good deal of Arabian and thoroughbred blood in the show Hackney of the present day, inherited from a cross that took place prior to the founding of the Hackney Horse Society in 1883. Lincolnshire and Cambridgeshire were at first associated with Hackneys, but the breeding spread from these counties to Norfolk and Yorkshire, and it became general in many parts of England, and in Scotland and Ireland as well.

Characteristics.—The height is usually from 15 to 15·2 hands high, but bigger horses than this are seen. At the walk and trot the Hackney has a jaunty, graceful, easy, springy movement, and a level action without any rolling. The head and tail are carried well up, and the knee flexion is pronounced. The limb should be lifted with the knee bent, and when the fore-arm is almost straight out the lower part of the limb below the knee is shot out straight in front of the animal, and the whole leg descends to the ground in a straight line from elbow to foot. The hind-legs are well and vigorously flexed, the feet being lifted clear and high, and the foot coming to the ground in a straight line with the fore-feet. The back and loins require to be strong and well muscled to enable the horse to carry himself with an absence of jar, and the back should be such as will suggest that it can keep a saddle in place. Records of performance show that a good horse was able to trot for 15 miles at a fast pace carrying 20 stone and not become unduly tired.

Chestnuts are very numerous, bays are common, and both blue and red roans are often seen, but blacks and greys are not in favour.

New Forest Pony.—Some Arab and thoroughbred blood has been introduced at various times. The height varies in different parts of the Forest, but it is usually between 12·2 and 13·2 hands in the wild state, although individuals reaching 14·1 hands may be reared under domestication. Flea-bitten grey is a common colour, probably due to Arab influence. The great characteristic of the New Forester is to be always gay and alert; and though they are extremely good-tempered when well-broken, they may be somewhat troublesome until mastered. They are never sulky. A number are used for children's hunters, but they make better driving ponies when of good size.

Dartmoor Ponies.—They are noted for hardiness. They are very intelligent, and their heads are square and clean-cut Dark bay and brown are the common colours, and the height is about 12·2. hands high. Their bone is hard and firm, the feet are unusually good, and the back is short and well ribbed. There is probably a close resemblance between the Dartmoor and the Exmoor ponies.

Exmoor Ponies.—This breed shows more quality as a rule than the Dartmoor, and is usually smaller and lighter, its height being between 11·2 and 12 hands high. Brown bay or dun with mealy noses are the prevailing colours, and the characteristic of the nose is nearly always present in pure Exmoor ponies. The head is typically of the pony type, clean-cut, with small ears and lively eyes, and the whole conformation suggests power and endurance. Crossed with suitable sires, both these two breeds (Dartmoor and Exmoor) are used for the rearing of small children's hunters and polo ponies. They are pre-eminently riding ponies.

Dales Ponies.—The breed known as Dales ponies are found in Yorkshire, Westmorland, and parts of Durham county. They are very often bred on small farms, where they are general workers, at home in the saddle, between shafts and in chains. They are also good pack ponies, and enthusiastic admirers enjoy some good hunts mounted on a Dales pony. In height they stand 14 to 14·2 hands, and the colour of the true-bred pony is black, dark brown, or occasionally grey. Other colours indicate crossing with Hackney, Shire, or Clydesdale.

Fell Ponies.—This is one of the largest and heaviest of the English breeds of ponies, and in some respects is like the Garron. Fell ponies are found in the highlands of Northumberland, Cumberland, Westmorland, Durham county, and Yorkshire. They stand up to 14 hands high, are of a thick, powerful build, possess deep chests and strong loins, have very well-developed fore-arms and thighs, and are much used for harness, draught, and weight-carrying purposes. The prevailing colours are black, dark brown, and a few greys are found.

Welsh Cobs and Ponies.—There is no doubt that both these breeds are descended from the same stock, and the difference between them is chiefly one of size. They are both noted for hardiness and endurance, and for being extremely sure-footed. Crossed with suitable sires they breed foals which very often turn out good polo ponies. They are good harness ponies, and as a rule are better between shafts than under the saddle, although many children's riding ponies are of this breed. Welsh ponies are supposed to measure from 12 to 12·2 hands, and cobs from 13·2 to 14·2 hands high. Other colours give rise to the suspicion that some previous crossing has taken place. Cobs are very often crossed with the Hackney, and some assert that this has been bad for the breed.

Highland Ponies are 13 to 14 hands high. Colours: dun, grey, black, brown; occasionally chestnut. No white markings. Shapely 'pony' heads, a good, prominent eye, short legs. They do all the work on the Western Islands crofts; they are good to ride on the hills, and make first-rate deer carriers.

Connemara Pony.—This breed has existed in the rough hilly districts of Connemara for centuries, and is still bred there. There is a good deal of variation in size and type. The colours are dun, grey, black, or bays, and the height is from 14 to 14·2 hands. The croup and the withers are the same height; the head is rather large; the neck strong and muscular; the shoulders are straight; the body is long and deep, and the legs are short.

Shetland Ponies.—As the name suggests, the home of this well-known little pony is the group of bleak, wind-swept islands lying north of Scotland, where it has existed for many hundreds of years. It is one of the oldest of British breeds. A Stud Book was started in 1889, and this was the first of the pony breeds to have one. The height varies, but from 38 to 40 inches at the shoulder is the usual, while animals measuring more than 42 inches when four years old are disqualified from registration.

In some cases full-grown ponies may only measure 30 or 32 inches. Black and dark browns are favourite colours, but practically all colours are met with, greys being least common. The head should be small and intelligent-looking, with short, sharp ears, nostrils wide and sensitive, and mane and forelock full and flowing. The body should be compact, the legs short.

HORSES, DISEASES OF,—These include: Acne, contagious; aneurism; anhidrosis; anthrax; asthma; azoturia; blouwildebeesoog; blue nose disease; borna; botriomycosis; 'broken wind'; brucellosis; chronic catarrhal enteritis; colic; Comeny's infectious paralysis; coronary thrombosis; dourine; entêquê seco; epizootic lymphangitis; equine biliary fever; equine contagious pleuropneumonia; equine Ehrlichiosis; equine encephalomyelitis; equine filariasis; equine infectious anæmia; equine infectious bronchitis; equine influenza; equine piroplasmosis; equine rhinopneumonitis; equine viral arteritis; fistulous withers; foals, diseases of; glanders; grass disease; grease; guttural pouch diphtheria; horse sickness, African; Japanese B. encephalitis; Kimberley horse disease; laminitis; mal de caderas; mal du coit; periodic ophthalmia; 'poll evil'; purpura; rabies; rhinosporidiosis; senkobo; strangles; stringhalt; summer sores; tetanus; tuberculosis; ulcerative lymphangitis; uterine infections; urticaria; variola. (*see under these headings*.)

HORSES, FEEDING OF.—Oats have become the staple food of horses in almost all countries. Other foods used are barley, maize, wheat, rice, rye, bran, beans, peas, and other legumes. These latter, when of good quality, can be substituted to some extent for oats, but the horse must always be allowed time to accommodate himself to a change of food, lest digestive disturbances occur. It has been found that the horse, owing to its peculiar digestive apparatus, requires a certain amount of coarse, bulky food, partly to act as a mechanical stimulant, and partly to reduce the concentration of the other foods, so that along with the oats or other grains hay or straw, either chopped into chaff or long, is fed. The following rules should be adhered to as far as the feeding of horses in Great Britain is concerned:

(1) Water before feeding, and allow the horse as much as it desires to drink.

(2) Feed in small amounts and as often as the nature of the work or other circumstances will allow.

(3) Do not work immediately after the horse finishes feeding. An hour should be given for a full feed.

(4) Give the first feed of the day early, and give the majority of the bulky food at the last feed of the day, so that the horse can eat it at its leisure.

(5) Always buy the best quality of food obtainable; it is false economy to use inferior food-stuffs.

(6) Inspect the teeth periodically, and have any errors corrected at once.

The quantity of food given naturally depends upon the size and type of the horse, upon the nature of its work, upon individual variations (some horses being able to exist upon more sparing diets than others), and upon the district and the climate, but the following rough summary may be taken as an example of the amounts that are given to horses of various types:

	Oats.	Bran.	Hay.
Heavy draught horse	15 lb.	4 lb.	18 lb.
Light draught horse	12 ,,	3 ,,	12 ,,
Carriage horse . .	10 ,,	3 ,,	10 ,,
Pony	8 ,,	2 ,,	10 ,,

HORSE-SICKNESS, AFRICAN.—This disease, which is also called AFRICAN HORSE-PLAGUE, PERREZIEKTE or PAARDENZIEKTE, etc., is a disease of horses, mules, and occasionally of donkeys, which is prevalent in summer and autumn, attaining its height about the end of the latter season. Nine days or so after the first frost of the winter, it suddenly ceases.

During 1960 the disease spread to the Near East, Turkey, and Cyprus. F.A.O. were concerned at the risk of its spread into Western Europe.

Cause.—A virus transmitted by biting insects, and which can perhaps live in some alternative host other than the horse. Dogs may die after eating infected horse-meat.

Symptoms.—There are four types of the disease that can be recognised clinically. In *the horse-sickness fever*, the temperature slowly rises—about one degree per day—until it reaches its maximum, which may be almost anything up to 106° F.

and then gradually returns to normal. Typically the duration of this rise and fall is from 12 to 14 days, and the actual obvious fevered condition is present for about eight days. The respirations and the colour of the visible membranes remain unaltered, however, and there is only slight general disturbance. In the *pulmonary form*, which is locally known as the ' dunkop ' (meaning ' thin head '), horse-sickness is at its worst. The temperature rises much more rapidly, reaching its maximum in three days. A sudden breathlessness and labour in breathing become apparent. The nostrils are fully distended, the head and neck are extended, the ears nod, patchy sweating occurs, and the rate of the respirations may be as much as 60 to 80 per minute. With each respiratory movement there is a kind of double action ; the thoracic muscles contract first, and immediately after them the abdominal walls contract. This double-breathing is considered by the farmers to be quite characteristic. Soon after this stage a harsh, dry, painful cough appears, accompanied by some slight discharge. As the cough increases so the discharge becomes more and more copious. The cough gets softer and is accompanied by a gurgling sound, and quantities of frothy yellow liquid are brought up. Should the horse or mule manage to bring up large amounts of this material (bucketfuls, literally), there is hope that it will recover, but far more often the horse chokes and drowns in its own serum.

The *œdematous* or *cardiac* form, locally known as ' dikkop ' (meaning ' thick head '), is characterised by a very striking swelling of the head and neck, which may extend to the body, and by the grave disturbance of the heart.

The *mixed form* of horse-sickness is rare when compared with ' dunkop ' and ' dikkop ', and consists of the symptoms of both of these superimposed upon each other. As a rule, pulmonary symptoms are the first to appear, and then local swellings suddenly arise, but at other times an animal showing mild ' dikkop ' will suddenly become breathless and commence to discharge frothy material from the nose, and dies in a very short while.

Certain complications are comparatively common in cases of horse-sickness, and of these paralysis of the œsophagus, which leads to an inability to feed and swallow properly, and blindness are common.

Treatment.—No success has followed treatment of actual cases. All that can be done is to treat the symptoms.

Prevention.—*Protection against night-flying insects* is of the greatest importance. A vaccine is used.

HORSES : Names given according to Age, Sex, etc.—In different parts of the country local names are given to horses at different periods of their life, and in the following list the most usual names have been selected and are given with the above reservation, *i.e.* that they may be local :

Foal : a young horse from birth to a year old ; if a male it is called a *colt* or *horse foal* ; if a female, a *filly* or *mare foal*.

Colt : a young male.

Filly : a young female.

Gelding : a castrated male.

Rig : a horse whose testicles have been retained in the abdominal cavity instead of descending into the scrotum ; the technical name is *cryptorchid*.

Yearling : a year-old horse of either sex.

Yearling filly.

Yearling colt.

Two-year-old colt or **filly.**

Three-year-old colt or **filly.**

Four-year-old, etc.

Stallion : an adult male uncastrated horse over 4 years old, also called an *Entire*.

Mare : an adult female over 4 years old.

Mule : the offspring from the male ass and the mare.

Hinny : the offspring from the stallion and the female ass.

Janet : a female mule.

Jenny or **Jenny ass :** a female ass.

HORSE-TAILS, POISONING BY.—In different localities and under different conditions there may be considerable variation in the chemical composition of species of *Equisetum*, with results accordingly. It would appear that on the continent of Europe and in great Britain *Equisetum palustre* and *E. sylvaticum* are the most dangerous, and that in America *E. arvense* is most to be feared, particularly when they are fed among hay.

For pathology, symptoms, and treatment, see BRACKEN POISONING.

HORSES, WORMS IN.—The following table shows those adult worms regarded as of most importance. (The list of small strongyles totals 11 and their names are omitted here.)

Adult Worms in the Intestines

Of considerable importance.

1. Large strongyles
Strongylus edentatus
Strongylus equinus
Strongylus vulgaris

2. Small strongyles

Adults mainly in Other Tissues

Echinococcus granulosus (larval stage)
Dracunculus medinensis
Draschia megastoma * (larval stages in the skin)
Dictyocaulus arnfieldi
Fasciola spp.
Habronema spp. (larval stages in the skin)

(With acknowledgements to M. C. Round, B.Sc., and the Animal Health Trust.)

HOST *(see* 'Parasitism' *on p.* 628 *and also* DEFINITIVE HOST).

HOUSING OF ANIMALS.—This is, obviously, a vast subject, and for detailed information reference should be made to up-to-date books on veterinary hygiene, to the Agricultural Research Council's series of bibliographies of farm buildings research, and to the Journal of the Farm Buildings Association.

Two things must be said at the outset. The first is that, generally speaking—given windbreaks, the possibility of shelter in inclement weather and of shade in summer, the avoidance of muddy conditions and of overstocking—animals kept out-of-doors are likely to be healthier than those which are housed for long periods. In the past, housing of animals has so often meant overcrowding in dark, damp, draughty or ill-ventilated buildings. Under such conditions disease is almost inevitable—rickets, pneumonia or scours in calves; infertility in the bull; agalactia in the sow; tuberculosis in the dairy cow.

The second thing is that, from a health point of view, not every 'development' is an advance. Commercial competition may dictate the overcrowding of chickens to the point where feather-picking has to be counteracted by red lighting or de-beaking; this may lead to short-term economic gains, but it is the antithesis of good animal husbandry, and the solving of the veterinary problems raised must be viewed accordingly. Intensivism can surely be pushed to a stage where not research, but only a return to good husbandry, will succeed in reducing the incidence of disease—and also, incidentally, the size of the drug bill.

On the other hand, the dairy cow has undoubtedly benefited from another dictate of economy—the change from cowshed to the yard-and-parlour system—for instead of being yoked or closely chained for long periods, she is free to move around; and such exercise is in itself important. (*See* CUBICLES FOR COWS.)

Cattle were housed on slatted floors in England in 1860—with straw; the current revival of the practice, without straw, may lead to hygromata, damaged teats or injured legs to an extent not readily admitted in the first flush of enthusiasm; and it is, of course, important that there should not be a draught blowing through the slats, or the money saved on straw will be lost in other ways.

Intensivism has led to development in forced-draught ventilation, and to the efficient insulation of walls and roof of animal houses by means of Polystyrene, Fibreglass, and other substances. (*See under* CONTROLLED ENVIRONMENT.)

It costs over 4 times as much to keep an animal warm by feeding concentrates—'an internal fuel'—as by warming the livestock house. Minimum economic temperatures are given below.

Housing has an important bearing upon the feeding of animals. Pigs, for instance, confined on concrete have no opportunity for the normal scavenging which can obviate mineral or vitamin deficiencies, and special rations accordingly become necessary for such housed animals. Vitamin A and B deficiencies are particularly likely to occur. In store cattle, lack of a vitamin A supplement causes blindness on many farms.

Residual infection is obviously important, and advice is given on this under SALMONELLOSIS and DISINFECTION. In a building used for calves and pigs, or pigs and turkeys, for example, a cross-infection between the species may arise with a particular strain of *E. coli*. On land surrounding buildings it is worth remembering that the worm *Trichostrongylus axei* is common to cattle, sheep, horses, and goats.

Cattle.—An adjustable open-ridge method of ventilation is still recommended as the best for cowsheds. In winter, the optimum temperature inside appears to be within 44–55° F. Milk yields are said to be depressed when the temperature

* Frequently, but incorrectly, called *Habronema megastoma.*

falls below freezing point. In summer, there is an upper limit of about 77°, at which point cattle begin showing distress. High humidity, at a temperature above 60°, appears to diminish milk yield.

For young calves, the temperature should not be allowed to fall below 60° F.

For covered yards, ventilators should be provided at the highest point, with a gap of 2 feet between the top of the walls and the eaves. Open-fronted covered yards should not have a gap.

Pigs.—Given adequate straw, the most primitive arks on range will yield better results than a cold, damp house. A warm environment will reduce the risk of overlaying by the sow. While different optimum temperatures have been given by different research workers, it seems that 70° is about the figure to aim at in the farrowing house. For artificial rearing, a temperature of 86° has been recommended for the first 4 days. Cold, damp floors result in liver disorders which do not appear in buildings where the pigs have a warm, dry bed. Pregnant sows are better not housed.

For fattening pigs, an optimum temperature would appear to be about 65°; and 60° should be the minimum. Humidity does not appear to have an adverse effect, though few authorities recommend it. Good ventilation is advocated.

Sheep.—In general, the disease problems associated with the housing of sheep have been less serious than might have been expected, and there is a credit side as well as a debit side. For example, if lambs are born and reared to market weight indoors, there is far less risk of worm infestation causing trouble. It is recommended that pens should not contain more than 15–25 ewes, grouped according to lambing dates.

Ewes and hoggs housed for the winter after grazing should be wormed during the first week. If it is a liver-fluke area, dosing against flukes is advisable six weeks after housing.

Lambs *must* be protected against lamb dysentery, and any from unvaccinated ewes should be given antiserum.

Infestation with lice may be aggravated by housing and spread more rapidly. Since it can cause serious loss of condition, dipping or spraying before housing is recommended.

E. coli infections are as much a threat to the housed lamb as to the housed calf. Overcrowding and dirty conditions at lambing predispose to coli septicæmia, which is usually a sequel to navel infection. In early weaned lambs, the quality of the milk substitute is important if scouring is to be avoided; and measures should be taken to minimise contact between housed sheep and their dung. Slatted floors, regular cleaning, copious use of bedding material, periodical disinfection—all help in this direction.

Good ventilation can go a long way towards reducing the risk of acute pneumonia. In lambs and older sheep this is often associated with Pasteurella infection, sometimes aggravated by lungworm infestation. Pasteurella pneumonia vaccine *may* be effective in prevention, but is useless against other forms of pneumonia—which can be caused by other bacteria, moulds, and viruses. With reference to the latter, parainfluenza 3 vaccine may well have a place, according to expert veterinary opinion.

Infections which give rise to abortion may prove more troublesome indoors than out, and vaccination against enzootic abortion, caused by a virus, seems worthwhile. (*See also* COPPER POISONING *and under* SHEEP BREEDING *and* INTENSIVE.)

Poultry.—Chickens probably do best at temperatures between 55° and 65° F. Egg-production declines at temperatures below 40° or above 75° F. A relative humidity of 50 per cent is considered the optimum for grown birds. A cold, dry house is better than a warm, wet one. Ventilation requirements vary; for example, a bird may need as much as 1 cubic foot per minute per lb. bodyweight in the hottest weather, but only one-sixth of this in the coldest weather. (*See also under* CHICKS, NIGHT LIGHTING.)

For other aspects of housing, *see under* CONCRETE, LEAD POISONING, WOOD PRESERVATIVES, CUBICLES, BULL HOUSING, LOOSE BOXES, DEEP LITTER, INTENSIVE LIVE-STOCK PRODUCTION.

HUCKLEBERRY POISONING (*see* GARDEN NIGHTSHADE POISONING).

HUMERUS is the bone of the arm, lying between the shoulder-joint and the elbow-joint. It has a rounded head which, with the corresponding depression of the scapula, forms the 'ball-and-socket' shoulder-joint. At the opposite extremity it forms with the radius and ulna the hinged elbow-joint.

HUMOUR (humor) is a term applied to any fluid or semifluid tissue of the body, *e.g.* the aqueous and vitreous humours in the eye.

HUNTING ACCIDENTS.—Varieties.— Perhaps one of the commonest accidents in the hunting field in ordinary country is a fall on to hard ground, with consequent bruising. The parts affected are the lips and lower jaws, the sides of the face, and the shoulders, when a horse has come down at a jump ; the knees and hocks, and the sides of the chest and abdomen, when it has fallen from a slip or stumble ; the knees, cannons, fetlocks, or coronets when it has struck the top of a gate or wall when jumping but has regained its feet ; and the quarters and region of the dock when it has turned a somersault at a bad jump. The bruising may be accompanied by tearing or laceration of the surface tissues if the weather is dry or if the ground is stony, but, usually, there is little to be seen at the time beyond a coating of mud or the loss of some hair. Sprains of the tendons, causing immediate lameness, or only making the horse go stiff at the time, are also common. The tendons of the fore-limbs are perhaps more frequently strained or sprained than those of the hind-limbs, but the accident may happen in either. They usually result from landing on to hard ground, a macadamised road, or on to a rock, in the fore-limbs, and from excessive effort before the jump in the hind-legs. Putting a foot into a rabbit hole or on to a rolling stone may also produce a strain in any leg. In a country where there are many 'bullfinch' hedges, or where there is much wire, tears of the skin or of skin and superficial muscles, and pricks by thorns or the barbs of wire, are common. They are generally worst about the fore-end of the horse, but they may occur behind. Where there are many low-made fences on top of a bank, containing stakes at short distances apart, penetrating injuries from stakes are not uncommon. Such hedges are usually easy to jump, and the horse does not make a sufficient effort, and perhaps slips as he takes off, consequently landing with his chest on to or with his belly across the fence. The stake very often penetrates a certain distance and then snaps off short, leaving one piece in the hedge and the point in the horse's chest, abdomen, or leg. Stake wounds are serious, because, firstly, when the stake is removed there is often an alarming rush of blood ; and secondly, it is not always possible to be certain that the point of the stake has not injured a large nerve or artery, or has not perhaps punctured the pleural or peritoneal cavity. In addition to these types of accident, such injuries as are inflicted by kicks from other horses must be considered ; over-reaches, treads, brushing and speedy-cutting, may occur ; but as these are liable to result in horses other than hunters they can hardly be considered as purely hunting accidents.

For the treatment of these conditions, reference should be made to BRUISING, WOUNDS, OVER-REACHING, etc.

HUSK is a disease of cattle, sheep, and goats characterised by bronchitis, which gives rise to a husky cough. Typically, husk is a verminous bronchitis (*see* PARASITES, p. 662), but it is possible that some atypical cases in adult cattle may be due to a virus. Husk was formerly regarded as an acute disease of young animals turned out to grass during their first summer, but of recent years the importance of husk in milking cows has been emphasised. Although husk in calves is of greater economic importance, nevertheless the cost of an outbreak in a milking herd may be very high—not as a result of death so much as of loss of milk and the need for extra feed.

Mild, wet weather enables the parasites to survive away from the animal body for a longer period, especially on marshy land, and these factors together with overstocking are contributory causes of the disease.

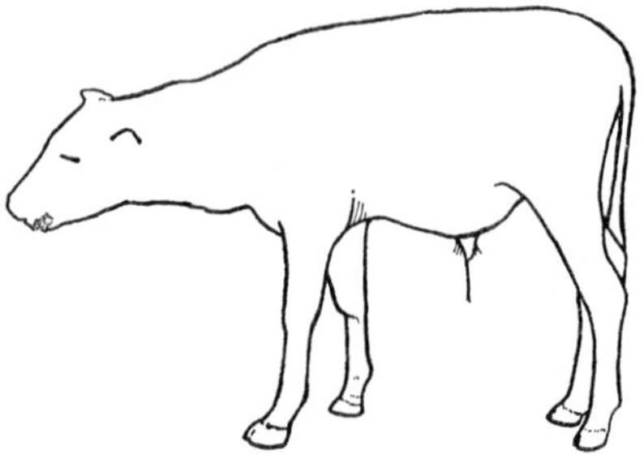

Husk—the neck is held extended and there may be continual coughing and/or distressed breathing.

Symptoms.—The disease takes its name from the husky cough which is present in nearly all cases of mild husk. In acute cases, however, the cough may be absent, and the outstanding symptom is distressed breathing. It is only necessary to add here that in adult cattle husk is generally less severe but lasts a longer time, though in some cases pregnancy is terminated a week or two before full time owing to the coughing.

In calves, death may occur from actual suffocation due to masses of worms in the air passages, or it may be brought about from progressive debility, or sometimes by pneumonia. In adult cattle, pneumonia, with *C. pyogenes* acting as secondary invaders, is more common. Œdema of the lungs and emphysema may be present as described in FOG FEVER.

Treatment.—In adult cattle especially, when fever suggests bacterial complications, sulpha drugs or antibiotics may save life. Anthelmintics have been introduced for the treatment of husk. These include diethylcarbamazine, methyridine, and tetramisole.

A drug cannot, of course, unblock the air spaces of the lungs or undo the damage caused by the parasites. Calves very severely affected usually die despite treatment. The administration of oxygen may save life in the Fog Fever type of husk.

Prevention.—As a preventative, which stimulates natural defence against the worm larvæ and renders them incapable of migrating to the lungs, a vaccine may be used on farms where husk is likely to be encountered each year. Two doses, at 4-week intervals, are necessary; one can be given when the calf is 2 months old or over. The vaccine must be given about eight weeks before the calves go out to grass.

The vaccine, which consists of lungworm larvæ subjected to X-rays, is given by mouth.

Vaccinated calves which have been out on contaminated pasture should not be regarded as free from infestation and mixed with unvaccinated stock—or the latter may become ill with Husk; some of the vaccinated calves acting as 'carriers'. Otherwise, prevention of Husk is largely a matter of good husbandry—the provision of sufficient nourishing food and the avoidance of overstocking or the grazing of heavily infested pastures—together with the routine dosing against parasitic worms in the intestines, enabling the animal to put up a higher degree of resistance to the husk worms. Other recommendations: (1) take a hay crop or make silage from pasture subjected to controlled close grazing before letting the cows return to it; (2) only use the chain harrow when the weather is dry and the herbage short; (3) and do not let cattle run back too far on to the parts they have already grazed. (*See under* MANURE HEAPS.)

HYALURONIDASE.—An enzyme which breaks down the hyaluronic acid forming part of the material in the interstices of tissue, and so facilitates the absorption of injected fluids. It assists the rapid distribution of drugs injected either subcutaneously or intramuscularly. It has been used in the treatment of urinary calculi.

HYBRID.—At one time this word meant a cross between two inbred lines; recently it has been used to describe a simple cross between two different breeds.

HYBRID VIGOUR (*see* GENETICS, p. 379).

HYDATID (ὑδατίς) is a cyst produced in various parts of the body by the growth of the immature forms of tapeworms. (*See* PARASITES, p. 646.) Hydatidosis is the name for the infestation. In man it is prevalent throughout S. America, and has as its source dogs, ruminants, pigs, foxes, and rodents.

HYDRAGOGUES (ὕδωρ, water; ἄγω, I move). (*See* PURGATIVES.)

HYDRARGYRUM is another name for mercury.

HYDROCELE (ὕδωρ, water; κήλη, tumour) means a collection of fluid present within the outer proper coat of the testicle (tunica vaginalis) or within the spermatic cord. It is not a common condition among domesticated animals, although a small amount of fluid is very often present in apparently normal animals.

HYDROCEPHALUS (ὕδωρ, water; κεφαλή, head) is a condition in which a large amount of fluid collects within the brain cavity of the skull. It may be present before birth (*congenital hydrocephalus*), in which case the large size of the head may present an obstruction to parturition, or it may arise during life (*acquired hydrocephalus*). In the congenital form which is met with in foals, calves, and puppies, there is a large prominent swelling over the forehead, and a rounded dome-like cranium. Animals born in this condition are usually dead, or if they are living they die soon after birth. The swelling is composed of fluid, which is probably derived from the normal cerebro-spinal fluid within the brain cavity. The bone of the cranium is thin and shell-like, and the brain substance is atrophied. It frequently becomes necessary to puncture the swollen skull and evacuate the fluid before delivery can be effected.

In the acquired form, which is chiefly met with in the horse and dog, the fluid collects in the ventricles of the brain, or under the meninges, as the result of some preceding inflammatory condition, such as meningitis, which has interfered with the free circulation of the cerebro-spinal fluid, or has produced an exudate from the engorged blood-vessels. When due to meningitis it is usually an acute condition, and its symptoms are masked by those of the meningitis ; when due to other causes in which there is obstruction to the flow of cerebro-spinal fluid it is usually chronic, and the symptoms are those of pressure on the brain. The animal becomes gradually dull, sleepy, insensitive to its surroundings, and stands in almost any position as if it could not be bothered standing properly. The gait is irregular and often staggering, and while the horse may be encouraged to walk forwards it is usually almost impossible to induce it to back. The general appearance is that of a 'dummy', without volition, intelligence, or interest in anything. As the condition slowly progresses, however, there usually comes a time when the 'dummy' suddenly becomes seized with a frenzy of excitement, when it will damage itself and those around without knowledge. Convulsions may occur, and during one of these death is liable to take place. (*See under* HELLEBORES.)

HYDROCHLORIC ACID is a gas which, when dissolved in water, forms a clear colourless fluid of sour taste and smell. It is normally found present in the gastric juice, to the extent of about 2 parts per 1000 (*see* DIGESTION). In the concentrated form it is like all other mineral acids, a corrosive and irritant poison.

Uses.—Its main use is as a stomach tonic in cases where the normal amount of acid in the gastric juice is diminished. It is useful in some cases of diarrhœa due to indigestion, and it has some stimulating action on the liver.

HYDROCYANIC ACID is the scientific name for prussic acid. (*See* PRUSSIC ACID.)

HYDROGEN BOMB EXPLOSIONS.—When a hydrogen bomb explodes 45 per cent of the energy is released in the form of a blast, which will destroy things for a distance of up to twenty miles ; 40 per cent of the energy is dissipated in the form of heat, dangerous for fifteen miles ; and the remainder of the energy is in the form of alpha, beta, and gamma rays (which will kill up to three miles).

Donkeys, used as test animals, appeared normal twenty-four hours after exposure to these gamma rays, then became dull and listless. Some pressed their heads against solid objects continually before dying ; others lay down. Some lived for nearly seven weeks, dying from internal hæmorrhage eventually. Some survived and after four years were breeding normally.

Cattle near the Nevada site were found to have 'highly radio-active' thyroids, containing $\frac{1}{10}$ of a microcurie per gram. (The radio-activity of the luminous dial of a watch may amount to 1 microcurie.)

From an American report two things emerge. One is that radiation intense enough to cause infertility will have other and far more immediately obvious effects upon the animal. Secondly, there appear to have been some remarkable survivals among cattle exposed not merely to fall-out but to direct radiation. Cows calved —and did not produce monsters ! (*See also* RADIO-ACTIVE FALL-OUT.)

HYDROGEN PEROXIDE is a colourless, odourless, syrupy fluid which only differs from water in that while it contains two atoms of oxygen, and has the formula H_2O_2, water only contains one atom and has the formula H_2O. It has the property of being able to give up this atom of oxygen in the presence of heat, pus, or decomposing organic matter. It is prepared in the form of a gas dissolved in water, so that the resulting solution will yield up ten times its own volume of oxygen. It is this oxygen in a fresh or *nascent* state that is the active antiseptic agent. It is either as this solution that it is used for application to wounds, or as a dilution of 1 part in 2, 4, or up to 10 of water, according to the condition.

HYDRONEPHROSIS (ὕδωρ, water; νεφρός, kidney) is a condition in which the capsule of the kidney, or even the kidney itself, becomes greatly distended with urine which is unable to pass along the ureter into the urinary bladder owing to some obstruction in that channel, such as calculus, a twist, or owing to the pressure of some organ near by. The kidney swells in size, and causes pressure upon the surrounding organs with pain over the lumbar region, and in severe cases a bulging of the muscles just behind the last rib. It is treated by either the removal of the whole kidney, provided the other one is healthy, or else by the removal of the obstruction.

HYDROPS (ὕδρωψ) is another name for dropsy or ascites.

HYDROPS AMNII (*see* UTERUS, DISEASES OF).

HYDROPS UTERI (*see* UTERUS, DISEASES OF).

HYDROSALPINX.—An accumulation of serous fluid in the Fallopian tube. It is stated to be a common cause of permanent sterility in gilts in America.

HYDROTHORAX (ὕδωρ, water; θώραξ, the chest) means a collection of water on the chest, *i.e.* in the pleural cavity. This is one of the results of certain forms of pleurisy.

HYGIENE (ὑγίεια, health) means the study of the various methods that should be taken to conserve the health, and to prevent preventable diseases. (*See* CLOTHING, EXERCISE, VENTILATION, SANITATION, WATER-SUPPLY, DIET AND DIETETICS, DISINFECTANTS, SLURRY, etc.)

HYGROMA (ὑγρός, moist; -ωμα, tumour) is the name applied to a swelling occurring in connection with a joint, usually the knee or hock, which is the result of repeated bruising against a hard surface (*See* CAPPED HOCK, etc.)

Hygroma in cattle may arise through an insufficiency of bedding, whereby the knee is bruised every time the animal lies and rises, or it may be brought about through too high a feeding-trough, in which case the cow strikes her knees against its front edge when she lies or rises. The result of this bruising is that the tendon sheaths lying in front of the knee become inflamed and their contained synovia increases. At first a diffuse thickening occurs over the knee, with but little pain (unless the condition is produced through a single violent blow, when heat and pain are marked); this gradually increases until a comparatively large, usually soft, fluctuating swelling is present. In time there is a gradual hardening, until in the course of two or three months the enlarged knee is almost as hard as bone, and very often covered over with a layer of horn (a process called 'keratinisation').

Sometimes the tendon sheaths are not involved, but the skin tissues are thickened. Treatment depends upon the stage to which it has progressed. In the early stages it may be opened and the fluid contents evacuated. When it has been in existence for a long time it should either be left alone, or if it is causing lameness it should be operated upon and dissected away. Occasionally a large welling which will eventually develop into a hygroma results from the presence of a thorn, stone, piece of glass, etc., embedded in the skin. This possibility should be remembered where a cow suddenly becomes affected with a swelling of a knee.

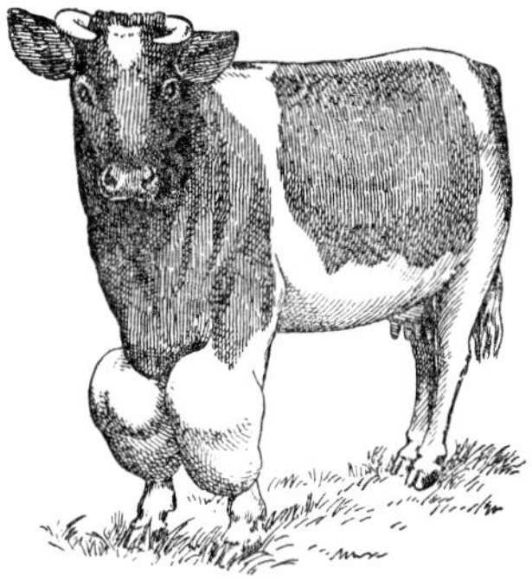

Severe bilateral hygroma in a cow. The swellings in this case were responsible for stiffness in walking, and difficulty in rising from the ground. They had been in existence for over 3 years when the photograph (from which this diagram was prepared) was taken. The cow was a Friesian kept in too short a stall, so that the knees came into contact with the trough when rising or lying.

HYGROMYCIN B.—An antibiotic used in the U.S.A. as an anthelmintic, and claimed to be effective against large roundworms and whipworms.

HYOID is the name of the bone which gives support to the root of the tongue and to the larynx. It has some similarity to the letter U.

HYOSCYAMUS (*see* HENBANE).

HYOSTRONGYLUS RUBIDUS. — A parasitic worm of pigs.

HYPER- (ὑπέρ, over) is a prefix indicating excess.

HYPERÆMIA (ὑπέρ, over; αἷμα, blood) means congestion, or the presence of an excessive amount of blood in a part.

HYPERÆSTHESIA (ὑπέρ, over; αἴσθησις, sensation) means over-sensitiveness of a part, as, for example, in tetanus there is hyperæsthesia of the skin, and in many eye diseases there is hyperæsthesia to light.

HYPERCHLORHYDRIA is a form of indigestion associated with excessive secretion of hydrochloric acid.

HYPERGLYCÆMIA (ὑπέρ, over; γλυκύς, sweet; αἷμα, blood) means excess of sugar in the blood, the condition preceding and accompanying diabetes mellitus.

HYPER-IMMUNE SERUM.—The serum of an animal which has been hyper-immunised by repeated injections of a toxin or vaccine. It is rich in antibodies, and is used for curative treatment of *e.g.* tetanus.

HYPERKERATOSIS.—This means an excess of horn or KERATIN (which see). The specific disease is also characterised by hardening of the skin. In the United States it was formerly known by the provisional name of 'X Disease'. A few cases have been reported in the United Kingdom. Mortality is often high.

Cause.—The disease is due to poisoning by minute quantities of chlorinated naphthalene compounds (and possibly other chemical substances also). These are found in many wood-preserving compounds, in insecticides, lubricants, and electrical insulation material. These substances apparently bring about a secondary vitamin A deficiency. In America the disease has followed the feeding of pellets prepared by machinery lubricated with grease or oil containing naphthalene compounds—an indication of the minute quantities sufficient to cause trouble. Usually, however, the disease is a sequel to housing stock in recently creosoted buildings.

Symptoms.—A thickening of the skin, sometimes with loss of hair, on neck and shoulders. In calves, stunted growth, a discharge from the eye (often with a corneal opacity), frothing at the mouth, weakness and emaciation occur, and death may precede any obvious skin changes.

Treatment.—Vitamin A will assist recovery.

HYPERMETROPIA (ὑπέρ, over; μέτρον, measure; ὤψ, eye). (*See* VISION.)

HYPERPLASIA (ὑπέρ, over; πλάσις, formation) is the term applied to abnormally great development of some tissue.

HYPERPOTASSÆMIA.—Too high a level of potassium in the blood-stream. This may be brought about artificially, with fatal results, by the mistaken use of potassium iodide intravenously instead of sodium iodide.

HYPERPYREXIA (ὑπέρ, over; πυρεξία, fever) means an excessive degree of fever. (*See* FEVER, TEMPERATURE.)

HYPERTENSION.—High arterial blood pressure.

HYPERTHYROIDISM.—Excessive activity of the thyroid gland. (*See* THYROID GLAND.)

HYPERTROPHY (ὑπέρ, over; τρέφω, I nourish) is the condition that results from an increase in the amount of work that an organ or member has to perform, from an increase in the amount of nourishment that it receives, or from some other alteration in the body economy, by which the particular organ or tissue increases in size and efficiency. Thus in certain valvular diseases of the heart when obstruction to the free flow of blood occurs, the muscle wall of the heart becomes increased in thickness and strength, and a compensation results. In the training of horses the trainer aims at getting the maximum efficiency from the skeletal muscles, which under the influence of judicious training and feeding become hypertrophied. After one organ of a pair has been removed, as, for instance, the kidney or the ovary, the remaining organ becomes increased in size so as to be able to perform practically the same amount of work as was previously done by the pair.

HYPERVITAMINOSIS.—Disease associated with an excess of a particular vitamin. For example, chronic hypervitaminosis A occurs in cats fed exclusively or virtually so, on an all-liver diet. (*See under* CAT FOODS.)

HYPNOTICS (ὕπνος, sleep) are measures which, strictly speaking, produce sleep.

Certain drugs possess the property of inducing sleep, and of these the chief are the barbiturates, chloral hydrate, morphia, and hyoscine. In general, hypnotics are employed when the pain or discomfort resulting from some disease will allow the suffering animal no rest. They are sometimes employed after operations, when the animal is restless and likely to disturb bandages, dressings, or when it is liable to induce hæmorrhage by movement. (*Compare* TRANQUILLISERS.)

HYPO- (ὑπό, under) is a prefix indicating a deficiency.

HYPOCALCÆMIA is the name under which those conditions are grouped which exhibit the uniform symptom of an acute deficiency in the amount of total calcium circulating in the blood-stream. The actual physiological causes of this drop are not well understood, but *see under* MILK FEVER.

Further details will be found under the headings of those conditions which are associated with a lowered blood calcium. (*See* MILK FEVER; TRANSIT TETANY; LAMBING SICKNESS IN EWES.)

HYPOCHLORITES.—These are widely used as disinfectants, being relatively non-toxic and non-irritant to the skin. Their efficacy depends upon the amount of available chlorine, which is more active against viruses than most disinfectants. Hypochlorites are unable to penetrate grease and are often combined with detergents. Sodium hypochlorite is useful for disinfecting premises after an outbreak of a virus disease. (*See also* TEAT-DIPPING.)

HYPOCUPRÆMIA.—A condition in which there is too little copper in the blood-stream. This occurs in SWAYBACK in lambs, and is also associated with serious ill health in cattle. On the Shropshire-Cheshire border, for example, hypocupræmia is accompanied by scouring and stunted growth. Two-year-old heifers have been mistaken for 8-month-old calves. In Caithness hypocupræmia is liable to occur on 75 per cent of the farms unless precautions are taken. Scouring is not a common symptom there but calves of the beef breeds show a stilted gait and progressive unthriftiness. The black hair around the eyes turns grey in some cases, giving the calves a 'spectacled' appearance. Copper salts by mouth or injection obviate the trouble, but the indiscriminate dressing of land with copper salts is likely to result in copper poisoning.

HYPODERMIC (ὑπό, under; δέρμα, the skin) administration of drugs. (*See* INJECTIONS.)

HYPOGLOSSAL NERVE (ὑπό, under; γλῶσσα, the tongue) is the 12th cranial nerve and supplies the muscles of the tongue, together with others nearby.

HYPOGLYCÆMIA (ὑπό, under; γλυκύς, sweet; αἷμα, blood) is the term applied to a deficiency of sugar in the blood. It may occur in states of starvation, but is of special importance in connection with the administration of insulin, which is injected to lower the blood sugar from an abnormal amount, and which, if given in too large doses, may produce too great reduction with symptoms of nervousness, breathlessness, and excitement. In human medicine hypoglycæmia may be a sequel to the use of sulphonamides, *e.g.* sulphadiazine. These symptoms are relieved by taking some food containing sugar and by an injection of adrenalin, which checks the action of insulin. (*See* BABY PIG DISEASE.)

HYPOMAGNESÆMIA.—A condition in which there is too little magnesium in the blood-stream.

Hypomagnesæmia is of particular importance in cattle, in which the condition is sometimes called 'Grass Tetany', or, formerly, 'Lactation Tetany'. It is experienced when a herd is turned on to lush spring grass after being stall fed during the winter, but an interval of a few days elapses before symptoms appear. Hypomagnesæmia occurs in bulls as well as in cows, and also in beef calves and sheep. It is encountered during the late autumn or winter in yarded animals receiving fodder crops in large amounts with little or no good hay, sometimes—but not invariably—after a snowfall or cold, wet spell.

Hypomagnesæmia is apparently far more common in the Ayrshire than in other British breeds of cattle. Cows which have had several calves are more prone to it than heifers.

Hypomagnesæmia is commonly seen in animals grazing pastures which have recently received a heavy dressing of nitrogenous or potash fertiliser.

Cause.—The exact cause is still unknown, but it appears to be associated with a high protein diet and too little fibre. Whole milk is not by itself an adequate source of magnesium for a rapidly growing young animal, and the condition may accordingly occur in calves.

Symptoms.—Sudden death or the finding of a dead cow. Intense excitement, convulsions, and paralysis may precede death. In a less acute form of Hypomagnesæmia the animals appear ' nervy ' —responding violently to sensations of touch or sound.

Treatment.—This must be prompt and consists in the intravenous injection of magnesium salts. Successful in perhaps 75 per cent of cases. Great care is necessary, however, in giving the injection and even approaching the animal—which may otherwise die at the prick of the needle.

Prevention.—The feeding of magnesium-rich supplements 3 weeks before early spring grazing and for 1 week or so afterwards; or, in sheep, the use of a magnesium lick, from a month after service till a month after lambing. (For adult cattle a daily dose of 2 oz. per head of calcined magnesite, mixed with damp sugar-beet pulp, is recommended.) A mixture of magnesium acetate solution and molasses may be offered *ad lib.* from ball feeders placed on pasture, as an alternative. Magnesium ' bullets ' are also used. Top-dressing pasture with calcined magnesites (about 10 cwt. per acre) is helpful. (*See* MAGNESIUM MILK FEVER.)

HYPOMYELINOGENESIS CONGENITA IN SHEEP.—A congenital disease of lambs, characterised by trembling or twitching, staggering, and sometimes shaking of the head.

HYPOPHOSPHATÆMIA.—A condition in which the level of blood phosphorus is too low. (*See* MILK FEVER.)

HYPOPHOSPHITES of lime, iron, etc., are often administered as tonics in cases of great depression and lack of energy resulting from disease or anæmia.

HYPOPHYSIS.—The pituitary gland.

HYPOPLASIA. — Under-development. Hypoplasia of the genital organs is one cause of sterility.

HYPOTENSION.—Low arterial blood pressure.

HYPOTENSIVE DRUGS are used to produce temporary hypotension in order to diminish hæmorrhage. In veterinary practice their use is still largely experimental. Methonium compounds are examples.

HYPOTHERMIA.—A technique used in human surgery for operations within the dry heart and based upon experimental work carried out upon dogs. The venous blood is cooled in a circuit outside the body (a method now preferred to the use of ice packs or refrigerated blankets) until a body temperature of 68°—77° F. is obtained, when the flow of blood to the heart can be stopped for several minutes to allow the operation to proceed

HYPOTHYROIDISM.—A condition associated in cattle with a high incidence of aborted, stillborn, or weakly calves. (*See* GOITRE.)

HYSTERECTOMY.—A surgical operation for removal of the uterus. Usually the ovaries are removed at the same time. (*See* OVARIO-HYSTERECTOMY.)

HYSTERIA (CANINE).—This is a disease of dogs of doubtful cause. It has become rare during recent years in the U.K. since the use of agenised flour was discontinued.

Symptoms.—Young dogs which appear to be normal in every way are liable to attack so soon as they are subjected to any degree of exertion or excitement. For example, greyhounds may suddenly exhibit symptoms during the first few yards of a race, and gun dogs may succumb to an attack so soon as work begins, or when the first shot is fired.

The dog suddenly appears to ' go mad '. It races around with a fixed stare in its eyes, yelling or howling. It pays no attention to words of command, and if on the leash continually struggles in a most violent manner to free itself. Enormous muscular energy is expended, and in 3 or 4 minutes, or less, the dog usually loses control of its movements and falls to the ground in convulsions. It may gradually become quiet and, after a somewhat dazed phase, recover its normal appearance and, apart from exhaustion, may seem little the worse. Attacks may pass in 2 or 3 minutes, or may last for 20 minutes or half an hour. Sometimes one attack succeeds another fo a whole day, the duration of lucid intervals being either short or long.

In a kennel, should one dog be seized with an attack, other dogs near may suddenly be affected almost immediately afterwards, especially so if they are running together in an exercising yard.

Prevention.—Many theories have from time to time been advanced to account for hysteria. It has been mainly attributed to the use of agenised flour. Flour containing spores of *Tilletia tritici* (a parasite of wheat), a diet deficient in vitamin B_1 and the presence of parasites in the external ear or of intestinal worms are other possible causes. A change of diet is always indicated, especially if the dog has been subsisting largely on dog-biscuits.

Treatment.—If possible, isolate the animal in a dark place away from noise. A sedative or tranquilliser is indicated. (*See* TRANQUILLISERS.)

I

I.B.K.—Infectious Bovine Keratitis (Infectious Ophthalmia of cattle, p. 325).

I.B.R.—Infectious Bovine Rhinotracheitis. (*See* RHINOTRACHEITIS.)

ICELANDIC PNEUMONIA (*see under* JAAGZIEKTE.)

ICE, ICEWATER.—Of use in cases of hæmorrhage from the stomach, as an aid to control bleeding from wounds, and as an application in cases of meningitis, paraphymosis.

ICHTHYOSIS (ἰχθύα, shark-skin) is a rare condition of the skin in the dog, especially over the elbows and hocks, in which large and irregular cracks appear and a general scaliness of the surface is seen. The fissures become filled with dirt, and suppuration results.

ICI 33828.—A chemical compound derived from hydrazine which has the property of inhibiting the output of pituitary gonadotrophins, and hence of suppressing œstrus. It is being extensively tested in pigs, and is expected to have an application in relating controlled breeding to artificial insemination. In poultry it may be used to induce rapid moulting in a pullet flock so that birds may be kept on for a second year without an unduly long non-productive period intervening. Another possible use is to delay the onset of laying in pullets.

ICTERUS (ἴκτις, a weasel) is another name for jaundice. (*See* JAUNDICE.)

IDENTICAL TWINS are those derived from the division of a single egg.

IDENTIFICATION OF CATTLE.—Nose prints, taken in the same manner as finger-prints, have been used in New Zealand. This may have value in black-skinned animals for which tattooing is of little value.

IDENTIFICATION OF HORSES.—In the U.S.A. thoroughbreds are identified, under a race-course system, by a set of four photographs—one of each chestnut.

IDIOPATHIC (ἴδιος, peculiar; πάθη, suffering) is a term applied to diseases to indicate that their cause is unknown.

IDIOSYNCRASY (ἴδιος, peculiar; σύγκρασις, mixture) means a peculiarity of constitution causing an animal to react differently from most animals to a drug or treatment.

ILE DE FRANCE.—A large French breed of sheep.

ILEOCÆCAL refers to the junction between ilium and cæcum, that is, between the end of the small intestine and the commencement of the large. The so-called ileocæcal valve is formed by the cæcum in such manner that while food material may readily travel from ilium into cæcum, it is difficult for it to pass in the opposite direction. The region around the ileocæcal valve is frequently the site of the ulcers, which are characteristic lesions of swine fever in pigs.

ILEUM (εἴλω, I twist about) is the last arbitrary division of the small intestine. (*See* INTESTINES.)

Inflammation of the ileum—which becomes thickened and stiff, almost like a piece of rubber hose—is a cause of death in piglets in two to four months old. It has been suggested that there is a hereditary predisposition to this condition, which often affects the whole litter. In many instances, the trouble is recognised only at the bacon factory, having caused no *apparent* illness in the pigs. Those that die, on the other hand, do so from perforating ulcers and peritonitis, after showing evidence of thirst, a bluish colour of the skin, and collapse.

ILIUM (*ilia*, the flank) is another name for the haunch-bone, the outer angle of which forms the 'point of the hip'. The ilium is the largest and most anteriorly situated bone of the pelvis. (*See* BONE.)

IMBALANCE.—A term used to describe, for example, a faulty calcium-phosphorus ratio in the food of an animal; or an excess of one hormone in the blood-stream, or a deficiency of another—with resulting disease. (*See* RICKETS, OSTEOFIBROSIS, INFERTILITY.)

IMMOBILON.—An analgesic and immobilising agent. (*See under* ETORPHINE.)

IMMUNE BODIES.—Antibodies.

IMMUNITY (*immunis*, exempt) is the power to resist infection, or the action of certain poisons. It is noticeable that in a herd of cattle, for example, there are some individuals that do not contract a disease no matter to what extent they may be exposed to the infection, and that there are others that will become affected on every possible occasion. The same is seen in other animals. This immunity to the attack of disease is either (1) inherited; (2) acquired naturally; or (3) acquired artificially.

Natural immunity.—There are some species of animals that are not affected by diseases or by poisons that are dangerous to others. The snake-killing mongoose of India possesses an immunity against cobra venom; the pigeon can withstand large doses of morphine without harm; fowls are resistant to tetanus and anthrax; the horse does not become affected with foot-and-mouth disease; rats are not attacked by tuberculosis; the ox is immune from glanders; man is not affected by swine fever and many other diseases that are fatal to the lower animals, while, with the exception of the monkey, animals are not susceptible to syphilis. It is probable that species immunity cannot be broken down even by massive inoculation of the causal agent, but when vital resistance is low an animal may be attacked by a disease to which it is otherwise immune.

It is probable that much of the ordinary resistance of an animal is transmitted to it by the medium of the colostrum in its mother's milk. It is well known as a principle of protection in some diseases. For example, lambs acquire a high degree of protection from lamb dysentery through colostrum from the ewe, which has been itself inoculated (*see* LAMB DYSENTERY).

Acquired immunity results from an attack of some disease from which the animal eventually recovers. It is probable that all, or at least most diseases confer a certain amount of immunity, but this varies greatly. It may be lifelong, or virtually so, as in sheep pox, swine erysipelas, or distemper. In most instances, however, its duration is less, and in some only temporary. *E.g.* cattle may be attacked by foot-and-mouth disease several times during their lives, and horses after recovery from one attack of tetanus may have a second natural attack. The immunity conferred by recovery is liable in many of the virus diseases (*e.g.* Bluetongue), and in some protozoal diseases to break down in the presence of massive infection subsequently. Recovery from a disease is actually a process of natural immunisation against that disease, the poisonous principles present in the body being destroyed by antagonistic substances which are elaborated by the body tissues, until the symptoms the poisons produce have all disappeared.

Artificially acquired immunity is of two varieties, either active or passive.

(*a*) *Active immunity* may be artificially produced by inoculating an animal with a vaccine (*i.e.* dead or attenuated bacteria or virus) or with a toxoid.

(*b*) *Passive immunity* is that form of artificial immunity obtained by injecting into the body of one animal blood-serum drawn from the body of another animal which has previously been rendered actively immune by injecting particular antigens. The serum contains antibodies or ' antitoxins ', which assist and amplify the antagonistic forces of the threatened animal, so that it is less liable to become affected with the disease, and if it does, the attack is milder than it would otherwise have been. The principle of the production of passive immunity, which never lasts for any great length of time, is made use of against tetanus, swine fever, anthrax, rinderpest, distemper, and a number of other common diseases in different parts of the world. The theory of the action is, that the antitoxic serum contains certain chemical substances (antitoxins) which have been produced by the cells of the animal from which it is prepared, and which combine with or neutralise the poisons (toxins) produced by the disease factor in the animal that is under treatment. (*See* SERUM THERAPY, GLOBULIN, COMPLEMENT.)

There are many complexities involved in immunity, which is far from being the simple subject it may here appear. Immunisation is not always attained without risk of side-effects. (*See under* CRYSTAL VIOLET VACCINE.) In human medicine, both serum shock and serum neuritis may occasionally follow the use of equine antitetanus serum or of antitoxin made from this. (*See Lancet*, November 27, 1965.)

IMMUNOFLUORESCENT MICROSCOPY.—This is a useful laboratory method of diagnosis, described as specific and very sensitive. It enables a virus to be identified during the course of an unknown infection. It can demonstrate the presence of swine fever virus, for example, even before the appearance of symptoms. Results can be obtained within a matter of hours.

The principle involved is that antigens in tissues are identified by using their ability to respond to, and fix, the homologous antibody previously labelled with a fluorescent tracer which does not affect its properties.

The method has demonstrated swine fever virus using impressions from lymph nodes taken from pigs killed during the first 60 hours after experimental infection. The virus is revealed first in the cytoplasm as a diffuse granular fluorescence; later bright, fluorescent particles become visible within the nucleus.

The term fluorescent antibody test is applied to this technique. (*See also under* RABIES.)

IMPACTION (*impactio*) is a term applied to a condition in which two things are firmly lodged together. For example, when after a fracture one piece of bone is driven within the other, this is known as an impacted fracture; when a temporary tooth is so firmly lodged in its socket that the eruption of the permanent one below is prevented, this is known as dental impaction. Impaction of rumen or of colon means that food materials or fæces have become tightly packed into these organs, generally owing to absence of proper muscular tone in the intestinal walls, or due to a paralysis of these from toxin absorption or nervous disturbance.

IMPERFORATE ANUS.—A congenital defect in which the rectum has no external opening.

IMPETIGO (from *impeto*, I attack) is a skin disease of dogs and cattle particularly, characterised by the formation of painless pustules, shallow, thin-walled, and usually projecting upwards above the level of the surface of the skin. It is seen in puppies affected with worms, distemper, and teething troubles, in bitches and cows after parturition, when the mammary glands are usually affected, and in other animals when the vitality is lowered. It is caused by a micrococcus.

Symptoms.—The areas appear as pustules varying in size from a millet seed to half an inch in diameter, yellow in colour, soft in consistence, slightly raised above the surface of the surrounding skin, and, although surrounded by a red ring of inflammation, painless to the touch. The pustule soon bursts, liberates a quantity of yellowish-white discharge, which dries into a scab, falls off, and rapidly disappears.

Treatment.—The general tone of the body should be raised by good food and tonics. The pustules should be dressed with some antiseptic such as acriflavin, a hypochlorite solution, or gentian violet. Sulphanilamide ointment is sometimes used and the scabs removed.

IMPLANTATION.—This term is used in connection with the application beneath the skin of pellets composed of, or containing, synthetic hormones. Thus, in chemical caponisation of poultry, pellets of hexœstrol or stilbœstrol are implanted; while for increased meat production they are likewise implanted in steers (and sometimes heifers, too) and in lambs.

Hormone treatment is sometimes carried out by this means rather than by intra-muscular injection. Strict asepsis is necessary.

IMPOTENCE is loss of the ability to copulate in a male animal. Causes include malformation of the genital organs, weakness, starvation, constrictions resulting from injuries or operations, or it may be only a temporary phase in the life of the animal from which it recovers with rest and good food. Stallions that are used excessively for the service of mares are apt to become impotent towards the end of the season. It is often difficult or impossible to arrive at the real cause, and when the animal is a valuable one, it must be remembered that a previous owner may have maliciously severed the spermatic cord without in any way altering the appearance of the genital organs, so that impotence results and the continuance of a particular strain or family is impossible. This is advantageous if the previous owner holds a monopoly of that strain. (*See also* INFERTILITY.)

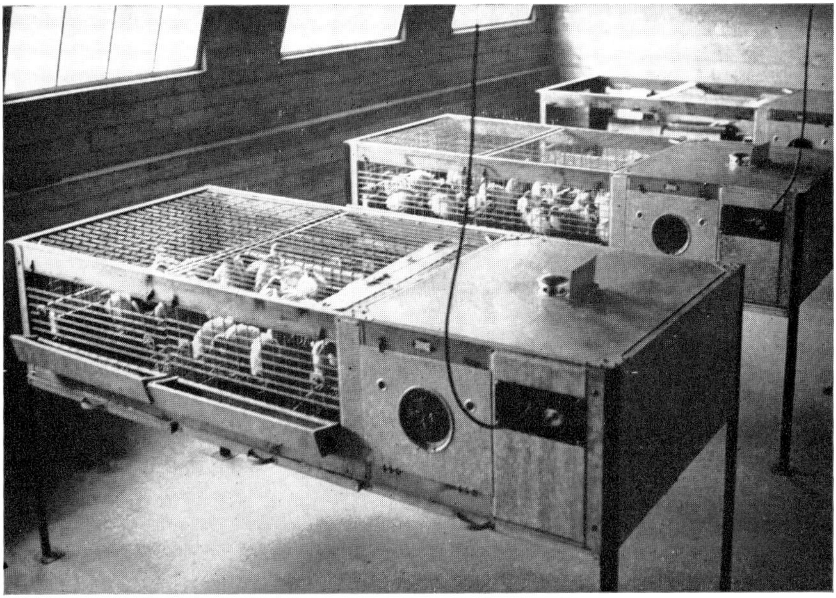

Turkey poults in a brooder with wire floor and thermostatic control.

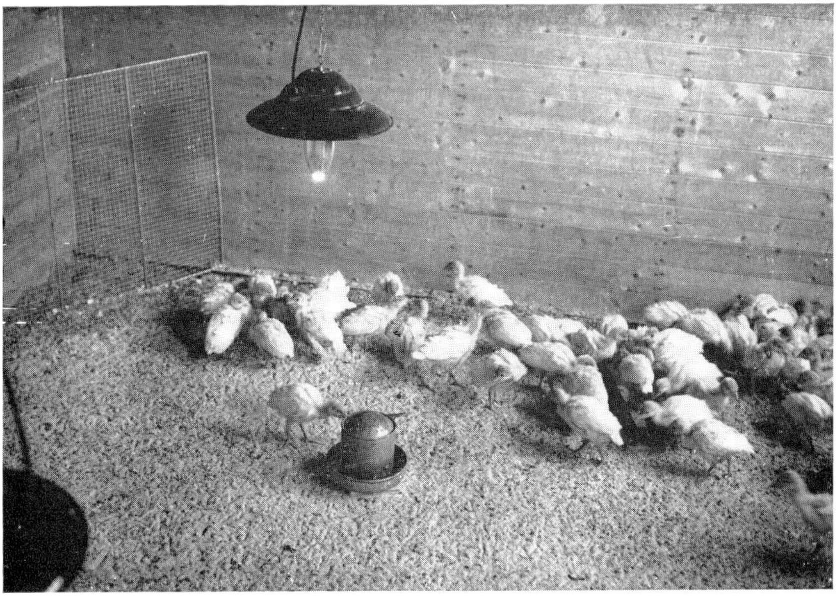

Brooding under lamps. The corner screen is to prevent crowding.

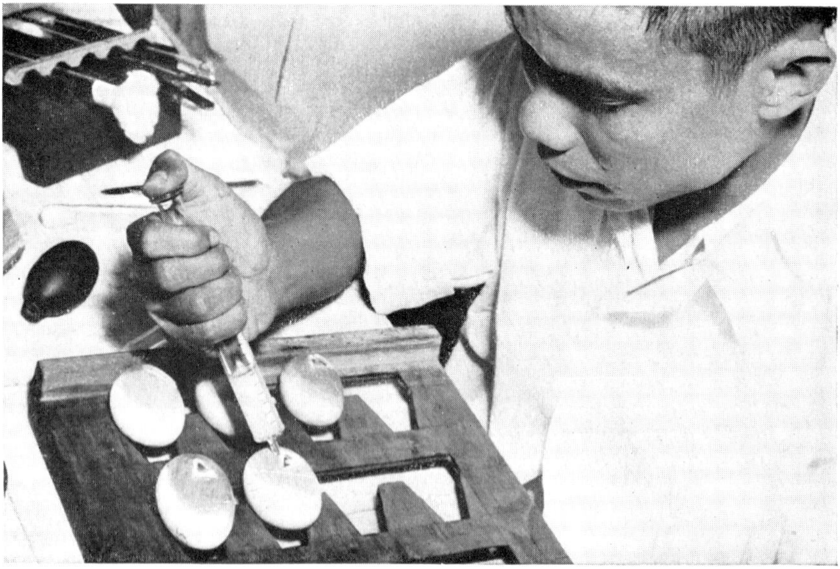

A Siamese technician, working under the auspices of the United Nations Organisation, inoculating chick embryos with cattle plague virus as a preliminary step to the production of 'avianised' vaccines used to immunise cattle and buffaloes against this dread disease.

See VACCINES.

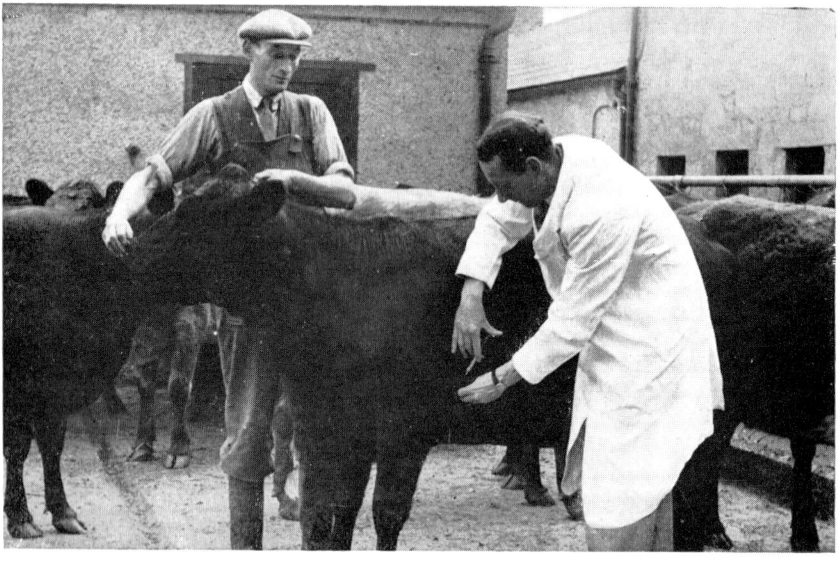

Preventive medicine is the keynote of modern veterinary practice. Here a veterinary surgeon is seen inoculating a heifer with vaccine against brucellosis.

See IMMUNITY, INFERTILITY *and* VACCINE.

IMPRINTING.—This is a mental process in which an inborn tendency in the animal causes it to attach itself to a set group of objects or a single object within a few hours after birth. It is a very important process if the young lamb or calf is to be properly suckled and cared for.

IN VITRO.—In the test-tube.

IN VIVO.—In the living body.

INCISOR is the name applied to the cutting teeth of each jaw. There are no upper incisor teeth in domesticated ruminants. (*See* TEETH.)

INCLUSION BODIES.—Round, oval, or irregular-shaped structures of a homogeneous or granular nature, found in cells during the course of virus infections. *E.g.*, Negri bodies in nerve cells in rabies, Bollinger bodies in epithelial cells in fowl pox.

INCOMPATIBILITY is a term applied to unsuitability in a prescription owing to the fact that its different contents either cannot be mixed, or that when mixed they undergo chemical changes, or that their pharmacological actions are antagonistic.

INCOMPETENCE (*in*, neg.; *competo*, I meet accurately) is a term applied to the valves of the heart when, as a result of disease in the valves or alterations in the size of the chambers of the heart, the valves are unable to close the orifices which they should protect. (*See* HEART DISEASES.)

INCONTINENCE (*in*, neg.; *contineo*, I hold) is a term applied to the inability to retain the contents of the urinary bladder or of the bowels, and occurs in diseases of these organs, in injuries and diseases of the spinal cord, and occasionally as the result of fear or other emotion. From the dog-owner's point of view, puddles on the floor mean incontinence—and this may be associated with a dog with an enlarged prostate gland relieving bladder pressure indoors.

INCO-ORDINATION is a term meaning irregularity in movement. Various muscles or, in some instances, portions of one muscle contract or fail to contract without relation to each other or to the whole. Deliberate purposive movements are no longer possible or are carried out imperfectly.

INCUBATION (*incubo*, I hatch) means the time that elapses between the actual time of the infection of an animal by a particular disease and the appearance of the first of the symptoms. Most of the acute infectious diseases have fairly definite intervals of incubation, and it is of great importance that owners of animals should be acquainted with these periods, since they are of the greatest value in coming to a decision in any particular case when an outbreak of a contagious disease occurs on a premises, and when other animals have been in contact with the diseased but themselves do not exhibit any symptoms. By isolating and carefully watching these 'contact' animals, and taking precautionary measures when symptoms do develop, many serious losses may be avoided. Generally speaking, contact animals, although themselves infected, do not infect other healthy animals during the incubative period.

The average incubation periods for the commoner infectious diseases are:

Contagious abortion	Up to 126 days.
Anthrax	12 to 24 hours or more.
Black-quarter	1 to 5 days.
Braxy	12 to 48 hours.
Distemper	3 days to 3 weeks.
Dourine	15 to 40 days.
East Coast fever	10 „ 20 „
Erysipelas (swine)	2 „ 3 „
Foot-and-mouth disease	12 hours to 12 days.
Glanders (*i.e.* including farcy).	1 to 6 weeks or more.
Heart-water	11 to 18 days.
Influenza	3 „ 10 „
Lymphangitis, epizoötic	8 days to 9 months.
Mediterranean fever	3 to 4 weeks.
Piroplasmosis, British bovine.	14 days at earliest.
Piroplasmosis, other forms	Up to 3 weeks.
Pleuro-pneumonia, contagious bovine.	3 weeks to 3 months.
Pleuro-pneumonia, contagious equine.	3 to 10 days.
Rabies	10 days to 5* months.
Rinderpest	4 to 5 days.
African horse-sickness	6 to 8 days.
Strangles	3 „ 8 „
Surra	5 „ 30 „
Swine fever	5 „ 15 „
Tetanus, horse	4 days to 3 weeks.
Tetanus, ox	5 to 8 days.
Texas fever	6 weeks.
Tuberculosis	2 weeks to 6 months.
Variola caprina (goat-pox)	1 to 7 days

(* but *see under* RABIES)

Variola equina (horse-pox)	6	,, 8	,,
Variola ovina (sheep-pox)	4	,, 20	,,
Variola vaccina (cow-pox)	6	,, 9	,,

All of these times are liable to some variation on different occasions and under different circumstances. The longer periods given usually apply to a mild attack, and the shorter to severe and acute attacks. For practical purposes it is wise to allow at least a week more than the longest incubation period given before an animal that has been in contact with an infection and has not developed the disease is allowed to resume its place with other healthy animals. (*See also* INFECTION, QUARANTINE.)

INDICATOR.—A substance used in chemistry, etc., to show by a colour change that a reaction has taken place. (*See also* COMPLEMENT FIXATION TEST.)

INDIGESTION (*see* DYSPEPSIA).

INDUCTOTHERM an electrical apparatus used in the treatment of sprained tendons, etc. (*See* DIATHERMY.)

INFARCTION (*infarcio*, I cram in) means the changes which take place in an organ when an artery becomes suddenly plugged up, leading to the formation of a dense wedge-shaped mass in the part of the organ that was originally supplied by that artery. (*See* EMBOLISM.)

INFECTION (*inficio*, I taint) is the name given to the process by which a disease is transmitted or communicated from one animal to another, and it is also applied to the invasion of the tissues by organisms capable of producing disease. All diseases transmissible from animal to animal are called *infectious*. The infective agent (*e.g.* a virus or bacterium), on being transmitted to a second animal in small amount, is capable of reproducing itself in larger quantity and renewing the particular disease.

The infective agent may be transmitted to a healthy animal by direct contact with a diseased creature, when the term 'contagious' is applied, a term that is, however, quite artificial; or it may be transmitted by indirect contact. Indirect contact is of the greatest importance among the lower animals, because there are so many different means by which it becomes established. Thus the following agents may act as carriers of contagion and spread disease by indirect contact: the attendant of a sick animal, eating or drinking utensils, grooming tools, animal clothing, the litter or bedding, harness, the walls and floors of buildings, railway loose-boxes, lairages at ports or markets, the soil and herbage of the open field; other animals, such as rats, rabbits, hares, foxes, or wild birds, that are not themselves liable to contract the disease; insects and other invertebrate creatures; running streams, drainage systems; and even strong currents of air may carry infection.

INFECTIOUS AVIAN NEPHROSIS.—A disease of chickens usually 4 to 9 weeks old, possibly caused by a variant of the infectious bronchitis virus. Symptoms include depression, and sometimes sneezing and coughing.

INFECTIOUS BOVINE RHINOTRACHEITIS.—(*See under* RHINOTRACHEITIS.)

INFECTIOUS BRONCHITIS OF POULTRY.—This was considered rare in Britain in 1960, but had previously assumed serious economic importance among broilers in the U.S.A. Coughing and sneezing may be detected only at night. Reduced egg yield may be the only symptom. Secondary infection may cause infectious bronchitis to resemble C.R.D. The laying of mis-shapen eggs may follow recovery. Now a serious disease in Britain, it is usually known as Infectious Bronchitis. Vaccines are available, including a combined one against both this disease and Newcastle disease. A live vaccine was introduced in the U.K. in 1970. Mortality is usually low, but intensively housed stock may die from secondary infections, *e.g.* E. coli, P.P.L.O. The cause of Infectious Bronchitis is a coronavirus.

INFECTIOUS NASAL GRANULOMATA IN CATTLE.—In certain parts of India cattle in restricted areas (sometimes in single herds only) may become affected with this condition. Large tumour-like masses develop in connection with the frontal sinus and the turbinated bones in the nasal passages.

The frontal sinuses appear to be the more usual site of origin of the growths, and from here they may spread either forwards into the nasal passages, backwards into the throat, or sideways when the pressure exerted may be sufficient to cause one or both eyeballs to bulge.

Some research workers have produced

evidence that a Rhinosporidium is responsible, while others state that a Schistosome is present.

Treatment.—Intravenous injection of tartar emetic repeated 5 or 6 times at weekly intervals. Lithium antimony thiomalate intra-muscularly has now replaced tartar emetic to some extent.

INFECTIOUS NECROTIC HEPATITIS (*see* BLACK DISEASE).

INFECTIOUS PUSTULAR VULVOVAGINITIS (*see under* VULVOVAGINITIS).

INFECTIVE DRUG RESISTANCE.—Resistant strains of bacteria may arise as a result of chromosomal mutation. In 1959 Japanese workers demonstrated another type of resistance transmissible from a resistant bacterial cell to a sensitive one merely by contact. (*See* ANTIBIOTIC RESISTANCE.)

INFERTILITY.—Insidious but great losses are directly due to failure to breed on the part of otherwise promising animals. The immediate loss to the individual owner of live-stock is not so apparent as with certain specific diseases, but it is infinitely greater than the loss accruing from any other single specific or non-specific disease. This loss is made up by the keep of the barren animals, the absence of offspring, reduction of the milk supply, and interference with breeding programmes.

Causes.—The most common and important causes of sterility or infertility can be grouped under several headings, as follows, but it must not be thought that the classification is perfect, or the list exhaustive. The causes are arranged in this way merely for convenience.

I. FEEDING AND CONDITION.—Underfeeding is a common cause of infertility in heifers. There must be adequate protein in the diet, and adequate vitamin A (and perhaps C), plus adequate copper, iodine, and other trace elements. These include manganese. A diet rich in calcium but poor in phosphorus may, in the in-calf cow, lead to resorption of the fœtus.

Excessive fat, on the other hand, may also lead to infertility or to inability on the part of the male to accomplish coitus.

In cows, temporary infertility may apparently be closely associated with the feeding at about the time of service. Cows losing weight are likely to be affected, especially if fed on poor-quality hay or silage. With *ad lib.* feeding systems, heifers and more timid cows may not be receiving enough roughage. Kale is sometimes responsible.

In ewes, infertility and fœtal death are always serious in many hill areas, the result—to quote Dr. John Stamp—'of keeping pregnant sheep under conditions of near-starvation during the winter months when weather conditions are atrocious'. (*See* DIET, FLUSHING OF EWES, STILL-BORN, REPRODUCTION, VITAMINS, KALE, SELENIUM.)

II. ENVIRONMENT AND MANAGEMENT.—A sudden change of environment, close confinement in dark quarters (the lot of many a bull), lack of exercise may all predispose to, or produce, infertility. Abnormal segregation of the sexes and the use of vasectomised males (for purposes of detecting œstrus) are other factors. A low level of nutrition may cause a quiescent or dormant state on the part of the ovaries. At the same time there are seasonal cycles of sexual activity, and a 'failure to breed' during the winter months may be natural enough, even if the farmer regards it as infertility. This 'winter infertility', as it is often called, may be influenced by temperature length of daylight, lack of pasture œstrogens, underfeeding, etc. At this season, heifers often have inactive ovaries, while

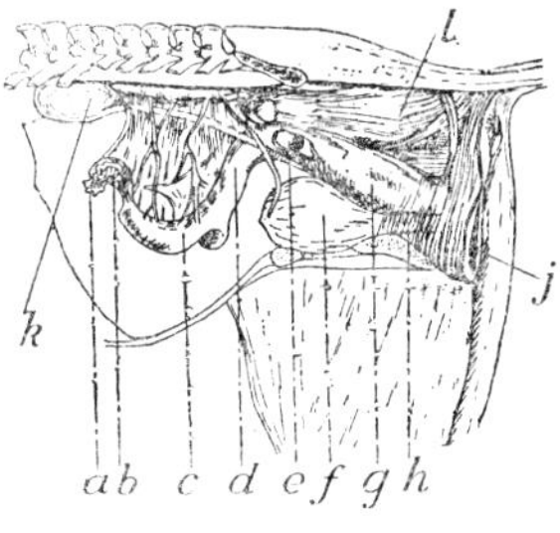

Diagram to illustrate the relative positions of the generative organs in the mare, as seen from a deep dissection of the side of the pelvis. *a*, Fimbriated end of oviduct; *b*, left ovary supported by its ligament; *c*, left horn of uterus; *d*, body of uterus; *e*, cervical canal of uterus; *f*, urinary bladder; *g*, vagina, into which is inserted the penis of the male during coition; *h*, urethra; *j*, external part of vulva; *k*, left kidney with the ureter leading from it; *l*, rectum.

in cows irregular and 'silent' heats give low conception rates.

III. DISEASES OF THE GENITAL ORGANS IN FEMALE.—This is a very long list, and includes some of the commonest and most important conditions which bring about infertility.

Inflammation or other disease of the

ovaries.—Ovaritis; the non-maturation of Graäfian follicles, from any cause, and the presence in the ovary of large or small, single, multiple, or multilocular cysts (which often form from a corpus luteum), are causes of infertility; another is blocked Fallopian tubes.

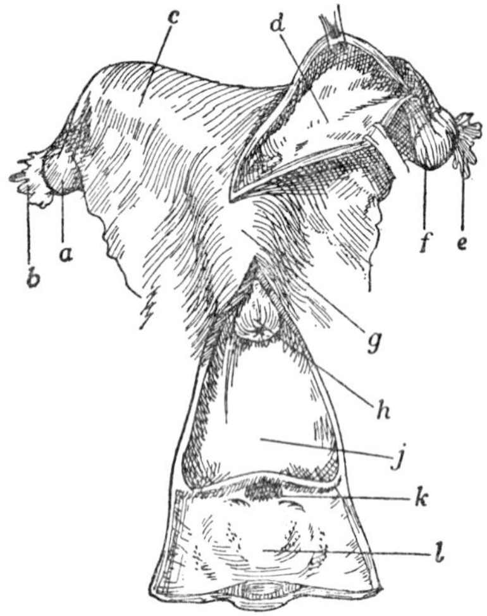

Generative organs of mare, seen from above. The vagina and vulva have been laid open by an incision along their upper parts, and the right horn of the uterus has been incised. *a*, Left ovary; *b*, fimbriated end of left oviduct; *c*, left horn; *d*, right horn of uterus laid open; *e*, end of right oviduct; *f*, right ovary; *g*, body of uterus; *h*, cervix; *j*, vaginal interior; *k*, opening of urethra from urinary bladder; *l*, interior of vulva.

Persistent corpora lutea.—Not only do they apparently predispose to uterine infection, but they inhibit the ripening of the next Graäfian follicles, and therefore ovulation cannot occur. Spurious œstrus may be shown, but service is always unsuccessful.

(*See under* Ovaries, Diseases of; Hormones *and* Hormone Therapy.)

Inflammation of the uterine mucous membrane.—A very large number of cases of infertility can be ascribed to infection of the uterus or the oviduct by organisms. **(For a list of the infections which cause infertility, see under ABORTION. For infections causing infertility in the mare, see under UTERINE INFECTIONS.)**

When the condition is mild, following a previous calving, it may disappear spontaneously, but in many instances it persists and becomes chronic. Associated with inflammation of the mucous membrane of the uterus or oviduct is often a persistent corpus luteum in the ovary. Carelessness during parturition, the use of unclean instruments or appliances, decomposition of retained membranes, and other similar factors, also bring about infection of the uterus. *Brucellosis* though not necessarily itself a cause of sterility, by lowering the vital resistance of the uterus, favours infection by a multitude of other organisms which normally may be non-pathogenic. The details of uterine infection, including salpingitis (inflammation of the oviduct), in the causation of sterility, are highly technical, but, generally speaking, it may be said that the presence of organisms in the uterus, or the presence of the products of their activity, either kills the male germ-cells, or renders the locality unsuitable for anchorage of the fertilised ovum (or ova), with the result that it perishes.

Abnormalities of the cervix may prevent conception—mechanically when the lumen is occluded or plugged by mucus of a thick tenacious nature, and pathologically when there is acute inflammation of the mucous membrane of the cervix, or even of the whole uterus. Scirrhous cervix—where much fibrous tissue is laid down in the cervix—when very advanced may cause sterility, but by itself is not usually of great importance. It is much more serious as a hindrance to parturition. (*See, for example,* Ring-womb of the ewe.) Cysts and fibrous bands in the os are seldom sufficiently extensive to occlude the passage through the cervical canal. Occlusion may, however, occur as the result of swelling and congestion of the mucous membrane, due to infection and inflammation. In such cases the sperms are unable to penetrate into the uterus, and fertilisation does not occur. In this connection it should be noted that acidity of the uterine or vaginal secretion—brought about as the result of a very mild infection—tends to coagulate the albumin in the cervical and vaginal mucus, rendering it thick, tenacious, and even semi-solid, and making it difficult, if not impossible, for the travelling sperms to penetrate. Syringing the vagina a short time before service with a weak alkaline solution (*e.g.* 5 per cent bicarbonate of potassium)—a well-known method of inducing successful service in many cases in mares and cows—acts by counteracting acidity, and dissolves a certain amount of coagulated mucus, thereby opening up the hitherto closed entrance through the cervix. To be successful the syringing should be carried out about half an hour before service, as there is then sufficient time given for the softening or solution of the mucus. (*See* 'WHITES,' 'EPIVAG').

Tumours, either malignant or benign, in connection with any part of the female tract, may act mechanically to prevent conception, may destroy vital structures —*e.g.* the ovary—or by the suppuration they induce may produce conditions in the uterus unsuitable for pregnancy.

Specific disease, such as tuberculosis in cattle, strangles, or glanders in mares, etc., may also give rise to sterility. When the genital tract is extensively diseased, from any specific cause, it is obvious that the intricate process of maternity cannot be accomplished. (*See* VULVO-VAGINITIS.)

IV. HEREDITY, CONGENITAL ABNORMALITIES IN THE FEMALE.—*Freemartin.* —A heifer calf born as a twin with a bull calf is sexually impotent in at least 80 per cent of cases, and probably in more than this. Freemartins are only met with in animals of the ox tribe, for sheep and goats frequently produce twins which are both sexually potent.

Hypoplasia or under-development, may occur as an inherited condition in the female. It may involve one or both ovaries, causing either infertility or complete sterility. The uterus, also, may be hypoplastic. (*See also under* GENETICS.)

Endocrine failure.—Heredity may be involved.

Hermaphrodism.

'White heifer disease' (*see under this heading*).

It was stated in 1967 that 10 per cent of female pigs are sterile. Group studies have shown that 25 to 50 per cent of infertile gilts had abnormalities of the genital tract sufficient to cause sterility, and two-thirds of these were regarded as hereditary.

V. DISEASE OF THE GENITAL ORGANS IN MALE.—*Orchitis*, or inflammation of the testicle, and *Epididymitis*, inflammation of the epididymis, due to injury from kicks, or to infection from external wounds, or from specific infection, such as *brucellosis* or *trichomoniasis* in the bull, strangles in the stallion, etc., disturb the spermatogenic functions. In addition there may be such accompanying pain that sexual desire is in abeyance. Chronic inflammation, which may be due to tuberculosis in bulls, or to continual mild injury from excessive pendulousness in any animal, by stimulating the formation of much new fibrous tissue which crushes the spermatic tubules, may reduce the total amount of sperms formed, but only when it is advanced does it cause complete absence of spermatozoa. When acute inflammation subsides the tissues may return to normal and spermatogenesis recommence, but in some cases the sperm-producing tissues suffer permanent damage. Occasionally, also, adhesions in testicle or epididymis may occlude the passages or block the vasa deferentia, and produce sterility.

Tumours of the testicles may destroy the tubules or prevent spermatogenesis, and on the penis, or in connection with the prepuce, may act as purely mechanical agents, which prevent coitus by the male.

Adhesions between penis and prepuce, the result of acute or chronic balanitis, though rare, may cause mechanical inability to protrude the penis and fertilise the female.

Inflammation in the secondary sexual glands—*i.e.* in prostate, seminal vesicles, or other glands—may occlude the vasa deferentia or ejaculatory ducts, and cause inability to pass semen, while in other cases the semen may be so altered as to cause death of the sperms in the female passages.

Affections of the prepuce, such as balanitis, and injuries accompanied by laceration or severe bruising, may cause temporary sterility, but when recovery occurs fertility returns.

Specific diseases, such as tuberculosis, strangles, influenza, and many others, may cause sterility in certain cases.

VI. HEREDITY, AND CONGENITAL ABNORMALITIES IN THE MALE.—*Cryptorchidism*, in which one or both testes do not descend into the scrotum, is a well-known cause of infertility in the male. When one testis properly descends, and is fully developed, conc ption may follow service, and a sire suffering from this disability has upon some occasions been regularly used in a flock or herd; but when the rig animal has both organs retained, although sexual desire may be emphatic, service is usually unsuccessful. The condition unfits a male animal for use as a breeding sire, since there is evidence that it is a hereditary unsoundness. (*See* HORMONE THERAPY.)

Hypoplasia or under-development of the male sex organs, particularly of the testis, is an important cause of sterility. It may involve both testicles or only one.

Endocrine Failure may arise as a result of an inherited predisposition. In bulls this may occur in later life, rendering them sterile *after* they have produced a number of progeny which, in their turn may perpetuate this form of infertility.

Hermaphrodism, or *Hermaphroditism*, in which an animal possesses both male and female organs, but is without a full complement of either, is usually, but not always, associated with sterility.

Malformations of the urethra, in which there is a fistula in the wall of the tube, and sometimes no external urethral aperture, the urine escaping by a side exit, may render a male animal mechanically unable to fertilise the female. (*See also* GENETICS.)

VII. PHYSICAL OR PSYCHICAL INABILITY OR DISTURBANCE. — Under this heading are grouped a number of conditions which are difficult to classify elsewhere. Some occur in the male, some in the female, and some are common to both sexes.

Incompatibility between the blood of sire and dam may be responsible for some cases of abortion in cattle, etc. (*See* HÆMOLYTIC DISEASE.)

Old age.—When an animal reaches a certain age reproduction becomes impossible. The periods of œstrus cease, and fat is usually laid down in considerable quantities, so long as the teeth and digestion remain normal. Breeding ceases earlier in the females than in the male.

Discrepancies in size between male and female may result in failure to breed. The penis may be too short, or too large; the vagina may be too long or too small; the female may not have the strength to carry a heavy male; or the male may not be tall enough to reach the female.

Stunted growth in the female may result in a backwardness of development of the genital organs and sterility.

Masturbation, or sexual self-abuse, may lead to temporary infertility.

Injuries to the back, hips, hind legs, or feet of the male, and sometimes to the same regions of the female, may be severe enough to prevent successful coition, and temporary or permanent sterility results. Recovery may occur later, and breeding then again becomes possible.

Treatment.—Much of the infertility among farm animals could be prevented by exercising more care before, during, and after parturition upon previous occasions (*see* PARTURITION), and by rational methods of feeding, exercise, and a restrained use of breeding-sires, limiting the number of females served to a reasonable maximum. When disease is in existence, professional advice should be sought, and measures should be taken early to cure or eliminate it. To discover the cause of sterility necessitates a careful clinical examination, and often a microscopical examination of the semen, and sometimes a search through breed records. (*See also* articles on BREEDING OF ANIMALS; REPRODUCTION; EMBRYOLOGY; UTERUS, DISEASES OF; HORMONE THERAPY; GENETICS; ELECTROPHORESIS; etc.)

INFESTATION is a term used to indicate the presence of parasites upon or within an animal. The word is used in the same way as infection, but the latter is restricted to include only single-celled parasites, such as bacteria, protozoa, or fungi, while infestation implies the presence of parasites which are composed of many cells, such as worms, lice, fleas, mange-mites, etc.

INFLAMMATION (*inflammo*, I set on fire) may be briefly defined as the reaction of the tissues to any injury, short of one sufficiently severe to cause death. There are four cardinal symptoms of inflammation, viz. heat, pain, redness, and swelling, to which may be added interference with function. The swelling is usually the most pronounced and noticeable among animals when the surface tissues of the body are affected.

The first sign of inflammation consists in a dilatation of the arteries and veins of the affected part, so that the blood circulates in it more quickly and in larger amounts than before, thus causing heat and redness. Very soon, however, and apparently as the result of some change in the walls of the veins, the circulation becomes gradually slower, and white cells of the blood push their way in great numbers through the walls of the capillaries, migrating into the surrounding tissues along with large quantities of the fluid material of the blood and a few red cells. Hence the swelling, which is the most characteristic feature of inflammation. The white cells attack the bacteria which have invaded the tissues. They also remove tissues that are dead or useless. Others of them, at a later stage, when the source of irritation has been removed, play a part in assisting the new tissues to repair the damage that has been done, though the greater part of this reparative process is carried out by the cells of the part themselves.

One of two results may follow inflammation. Either *re-solution* may take place, or else *abscess-formation* occurs.

Symptoms.—As mentioned before, heat, pain, redness, and swelling, with interference with function, are the classical signs of inflammation, and there are general symptoms, such as high temperature, feverishness, etc., varying with the severity of the inflammation. Certain definite symptoms are set up in special localities; for example, inflammation of the mucous membranes of the stomach and intestines leads to a copious excretion of mucus, and is known as 'catarrh'.

For the inflammations of special organs *see under* PNEUMONIA, PLEURISY, PERITONITIS, MAMMARY GLAND; etc.

INFLUENZA (Italian word meaning 'influence'). Scientifically, this term is now applied only to diseases caused by a myxovirus.

The World Health Organisation was much exercised as to what happens to the virus of human influenza between epidemics. It has long been known that there is a relationship between this disease and swine influenza. The human influenza virus (Type A) was isolated from the parasitic pig lungworm. Larvæ of these lungworms are harboured by earthworms—the only known intermediate hosts—which live for as long as ten years.

In 1957 W.H.O. stated: 'In the inter-epidemic periods, the virus is not found in the tissues of the pigs. However, earthworms taken from infected pig farms seem to carry inapparent viruses, and these can develop, in pigs eating the worms, into normal viruses capable of being isolated from the respiratory system. The question, therefore, arises whether the pigs are, in fact, the virus reservoirs, rather than being secondarily infected by the human virus, as some have maintained.' (*See also* SWINE INFLUENZA.)

Influenza in the horse—(*see under* EQUINE INFLUENZA)—and in the cat are different and distinct diseases. Pneumonia in calves may be caused by a virus of influenza-type.

Avian strains of type A influenza virus cause a number of diseases in hens, ducks, turkeys, etc. Fowl plague is an example.

INFLUENZA, CAT (*see* FELINE INFLUENZA).

INFRA-RED lamps are used in the creeps of piggeries and in poultry brooders. Either 'bright' or 'dull' emitters are available; the latter being preferred for chick-rearing. They have many advantages, but a power-cut can cause severe losses. (*See also under* LIGHT TREATMENT; TOES, TWISTED.)

INFUSIONS are preparations of vegetable drugs made by steeping them for some time in water and then straining. In order that an infusion may keep well it is usually concentrated and mixed with spirit, being diluted again just before it is dispensed.

INGUINAL CANAL is the passage from the abdominal cavity to the outside down which pass the spermatic cords and their associated structures in the male, while in the female the vessels of the mammary gland pass through the canal to the udder. It is a slit-like opening, about 5 inches long in the horse, and is directed downwards, inwards, and forwards. It is bounded behind by a strong band called the inguinal or *Poupart's* ligament. The canal is important, because if it is dilated from any cause some part of the small intestines may pass through it, resulting in inguinal hernia. (*See* HERNIAS.) It serves as the opening through which retained testicles are removed in the 'rig' or cryptorchid animal.

INGUINAL REGION is the region of the inguinal canal, that is, that part of the posterior and uppermost division of the abdominal wall which lies in below the brim of the pelvis. The scrotum, penis, and their vessels, etc., are situated in the inguinal region in the male horse, and in the female the mammary glands with the vessels that supply them. In some animals, such as the dog and boar, the scrotum is farther back, *i.e.* in the perineal region, while in the bull and ram the penis is farther forwards.

I.N.H. is the abbreviation for isonicotylhydrazile, a drug used in the treatment of tuberculosis.

INJECTIONS.—May be hypodermic or subcutaneous, intradermal, intra-muscular, intravenous (into a vein), intraperitoneal (into the abdominal cavity), epidural. Precautions must be taken against the introduction of bacteria, dirt, etc. The hair should be clipped away at the site of injection, and the skin cleaned with spirit or an antiseptic. Needles and syringes should be sterilised before use, unless of the disposable type intended for once-only use and already sterilised and in a sealed wrapper.

Where the material to be injected is already fluid, this is generally guaranteed sterile by the manufacturers, and is put up in sealed vials. In cases where the drug has to be dissolved in water first, only water that has been recently boiled and allowed to cool should be used, and solution of the drug should take place in a perfectly clean vessel. Neglect of these precautions is likely to be followed by the formation of an abscess at the point of injection or even by septicæmia.

The syringe having been filled with the drug in solution, a fold of the skin is picked up between the thumb and forefinger of the left hand, and the needle is inserted into the middle of this fold. The nozzle of the syringe is slipped into the head of the needle and the piston is slowly but firmly pressed home so as to expel the contents into the loose tissues under the skin. Care should be taken that all air-bubbles are excluded from the barrel of the syringe, as it is unwise to introduce them.

Cautions.—When using powerful and dangerous agents, such as strychnine, atropine, or arecoline, the dose given should always be smaller than when these are administered by the mouth, and care should be taken not to inject the drug into a large vein, for the consequences may be immediately fatal. Restless animals should always be secured so that they will not make a sudden plunge when the needle is introduced, and break the stem of the needle. Abscesses in hams are common in pigs, and doubtless result from anti-anæmia intra-muscular injections made without due precautions as to cleanliness and to broken-off needles.

Inoculations should not be carried out in a dusty shed. (*See* ANTHRAX.)

With stable compounds the route of administration has little influence on the end result; not so, however, with unstable ones. 1000 mg. per kg. of thalidomide produces no central depression in mice when given subcutaneously. The same dose given intraperitoneally gives rapid and profound sedation. Clearly, if one pharmacological action can depend on the route of administration, another may. (K. Hellman, *Lancet*, February 19, 1966.) (*See also* DETERGENT RESIDUE *and* ENEMA.)

INJURIES FROM SHOEING.—The fitting of an iron shoe on to horses' feet is so purely artificial that injuries often result from it. These are not always the fault of the smith. There are some horses with such bad feet that it may be quite impossible to shoe them without running the risk of injuring the sensitive structures in the process. The nails, toe-clips, or even the shoe, may inflict damage.

(1) **The nails** may produce lameness either by actually penetrating the sensitive laminæ—a condition called 'pricking'; or, by being driven too close to the laminæ, they may press upon the sensitive structures—a condition known as 'binding'.

Pricking may be only slight when the farrier knows that the nail has stabbed the quick and immediately withdraws it, or if he is unaware of the misdirection, it may become a very serious condition. All nail injuries should receive attention at once, for they are usually easily amenable to treatment in the early stages; but if neglected they rapidly suppurate, and the pus burrows until it finds an escape, causing the horse great pain and often permanent damage. The shoe should be removed if the horse becomes lame when returning from the blacksmith's shop, and the track of each nail tested by pressing upon it with pincers. If the horse flinches, the nail-hole in the foot should be pared out and a small pledget of tow covered with Stockholm tar pressed into the cavity and the shoe replaced, with the exception of the nail, at that particular place. In more severe cases the foot will require immersion in an antiseptic foot-bath for some hours, and perhaps the application of a poultice. Should much pus be found when the nail-hole is pared out, it will be necessary to strip off the covering horn and thoroughly cleanse the track.

Binding is not so serious. Generally it suffices to remove the shoe, allow the horse to remain barefooted for a day or so, and then to replace the shoe, taking special care that the nails are not driven too coarsely upon the second occasion. The lameness in this case very often only appears two or three days after the horse has been shod, and is attributed to some other cause.

(2) **The clip** may produce lameness by being driven too coarsely, and either burning the sensitive structures when being fitted, or pressing upon them unduly when hammered into position afterwards. When side-clips are used, *i.e.* one on each

side of the foot, if they are forced home too far the foot is jammed in between two rigid structures which will not allow it to expand and contract with each movement of the foot, and lameness results. In each instance the trouble is easily detected by either pressing on the horn over the clip when the horse flinches, or by tapping the wall near the clip when he again objects. The shoe should be removed, the horse given a day or two's rest, the clips altered, and the shoe reapplied, when he will usually go sound. If burning is suspected, the same procedure may be adopted, but if the lameness persists, it is probable that some pus has formed which will require evacuating before the horse will cease to walk lame. It sometimes happens that if the clip is very high and sharp, and if the shoe loosens till it is only holding by one nail, or if the shoe is partially torn off, the horse may tread on the clip which penetrates the sole of the foot and inflict a very severe wound. This is treated as for pricking, the area being pared out and the foot immersed in a hot foot-bath, etc.

(3) **The shoe** may cause injury if it has an uneven surface and pressed upon one part too much. This is particularly liable to happen when the horn of the foot is weak and thin. Horses with flat feet, or those with dropped sole, may develop bruises of the sole if the web of the shoe presses upon the outer circumference of the sole, where it joins the white line. In such cases the shoe should be removed and the unevenness corrected, orthe bearing surface of the foot should be eased. Some horses may require to be shod with a bar-shoe, so that the frog may take some of the weight off the affected part, and others need a run at grass and a blister over their coronets to stimulate the growth of new horn. Burning of the sensitive parts of the foot may occur through the carelessness of the smith, not by making the shoe too hot, but by holding it in position on the foot for too long a time, so that it may 'bed itself in'. This is a most reprehensible practice and should not be tolerated. The injury usually results in a separation of the horn from the sensitive tissues below, and some weeks pass before the horse can resume his work again. (*See* CORNS, BRUISED SOLE.)

INJURIES (*see* ACCIDENTS, HUNTING ACCIDENTS, WOUNDS, FRACTURES, BLEEDING, SHOCK).

INNOMINATE (*in*, neg.; *nomen*, a name, is a term applied to the bone of the pelvis and to structures associated with it. The pelvis is composed of six separate bones, three on either side, viz. ilium, pubis, and ischium.

INOCULATION (*in*, into ; *oculus*, a bud) is the process by which infective material is brought into the body through a small wound in the skin or in mucous membrane. Many contagious diseases are contracted by the accidental inoculation with germs. Inoculation may also be carried out as a preventitive against certain diseases. (*See* INJECTIONS *and* IMMUNITY.)

INSECTICIDES.—The use of unsuitable insecticides can lead to fatal poisoning in cattle, etc. (*See* TEPP.) Poisoning may occur following absorption of an insecticide spray through the skin. This, or inhalation of spray droplets, may lead to dangerously contaminated milk. In the U.S.A. the following insecticides are *not* recommended for dairy and cowshed use on account of this risk: DDT, aldrin, dieldrin, chlordane, lindane, methoxychlor, toxaphene, and heptachlor. (*See* CHLORINATED HYDROCARBONS.)

Some insecticides may be safe for one species of animal but fatal to another. For example, on a farm in New York State an insecticide spray containing thiophosphate had no effect on 50 chickens, but killed over 7,000 ducklings.

Dieldrin, used as a seed dressing, has caused fatal poisoning in wood-pigeons and other wild birds. Lambs have been killed by ALDRIN (which see). (*See* BHC, DDT, DIELDRIN, DERRIS, TEPP, PARATHION, PYRETHRUM, SYSTEMIC, NANKOR, GAME-BIRDS, etc.)

INSECTS.—For a general description of these, *see page* 668.

INSPISSATION (*inspissatio*) is a term applied to the process of drying or thickening of fluids or excretions by evaporation. Inspissated abscesses are characteristically found in old-standing tuberculosis of lymph glands.

INSUFFLATION (*insufflatio*, a blowing-in).—The blowing of powder or vapour into a cavity, especially through the air passages or into the eye, for the treatment of disease. It is the word also used to indicate that pus or other fluid from nose or throat has been drawn down into the lungs by gasping respirations. Fatal results usually follow the insufflation of purulent material, regurgitated food, etc.

INSULATION OF BUILDINGS, FLOORS (*see under* HOUSING OF ANIMALS).

INSULIN is the active principle prepared from the pancreas, where it is produced by the cell-islets of Langerhans. It can also be prepared synthetically. Insulin is now greatly used in the treatment of human diabetes, but less so in dogs and cats because it is seldom or never justifiable to keep diabetic animals alive. It is given by hypodermic injection.

Insulin is sometimes used in acetonæmia in sheep and cattle, when it is given with large doses of sugar or glucose to overcome the acidosis, and for indolent wounds.

INSURANCE.—Comprehensive policies are now issued by Lloyds covering veterinary fees for dogs, the life of the dog, third-party risks, etc. Disease-risk policies for other animals are available in Britain ; *e.g.* for foot-and-mouth disease, brucellosis.

INTENSIVE LIVESTOCK PRODUCTION.—This means, generally speaking, having farm animals indoors to a greater extent, and also having them within a smaller space inside a building.

The tendency in the latter direction is illustrated by Dr. D .W. B. Sainsbury's comparison of figures:

	1950s	1960s
Beef cattle (in yards)	70 sq. ft.	15 to 25
Bacon pig	10	6
Broilers	1·0	0·6

The economic *advantages* claimed for intensive livestock production are the economies of scale through reducing costs of labour and equipment per animal housed ; lower feed costs through bulk buying and home mixing ; the ability to afford skilled management and labour ; also a saving in acres of valuable land.

The *disadvantages* are the effect on stocks of large concentration, disease, cannibalism and all the problems of stress, and intensive feeding methods.

Intensive livestock production was the subject of a government enquiry. (*See under* BRAMBELL.)

The following describes potential hazards and health problems, and should not be regarded as condemnation of all current farming methods !

Poultry.—De-beaking, badly done, can reduce resistance to infection. Birds debeaked and unable to take a dust bath are prone to severe infestation with lice and mites, both now commonly resistant to the commonly used parasiticides ; and infestation is a problem in battery houses. Lack of exercise is conducive to fatty degeneration of the liver in battery birds. Among birds crowded together on deep litter coccidiosis and worm infestations are apt to be serious. Faulty ventilation often gives rise to a harmful concentration of ammonia in houses where there is litter, and also predisposes to C.R.D., infectious bronchitis, and other respiratory infections. The greater the concentration of birds, the greater the stress, it seems ; and the more chance of an increasing proportion both of susceptible birds and of ' carriers ' of various infections.

Beef cattle.—In calf-rearing units, salmonella infections cause a high proportion of the deaths of bought-in calves. Bronchitis is also an important cause of losses, which often amount to 7 per cent.

In units taking in 12-week-old calves, respiratory disease, principally virus, infections, are important. Other conditions encountered include : foul-in-the-foot, infectious bovine keratitis, and bloat.

If trough space is too limited, inflammation of the eyes may be caused by cattle flicking their ears into their neighbours' eyes—simulating the effects of infectious bovine keratitis.

Among veal calves, pneumonia and a peracute coliform septicæmia are major causes of losses. Anæmia, parasites, and a form of anaphylactic shock are also among the hazards of rearing.

Pigs.—These animals are particularly prone to the effects of stress (discussed under that heading), and of confinement in poorly ventilated buildings which favours respiratory infections such as enzoötic pneumonia.

Dr. D. W. B. Sainsburg has strongly advocated the use of farrow-to-finish pens which accommodate pigs from birth to slaughter day, and obviate four or five moves to strange surroundings with its accompanying stress.

Sheep.—Respiratory troubles, including various forms of pneumonia, are a danger in buildings where ventilation is poor. There are some very successful flock houses, with one end virtually open, where disease problems have been minimal; foot-rot being controlled by regular use of a foot-bath. In such buildings, the ewes lamb indoors, to the great advantage of the shepherd. Straw is used for bedding. Yorkshire boarding assists ventilation. (*See also* HOUSING OF ANIMALS.)

INTERCOSTAL (*inter*, between; *costa*, a rib) is the term applied to the muscles nerves, and blood-vessels that lie between the ribs, as well as to diseases affecting these structures.

INTERCURRENT (*intercurrens*, running between) is a term applied to one disease which occurs during the course of another disease already present, and modifies its course or increases its severity.

INTERDIGITAL CYST, or INTERDIGITAL ABSCESS, is a condition commonly affecting the feet of dogs, in which abscesses about the size of a pea or larger appear in the spaces between the digits of the paws. It most often affects Spaniels, Airedales, Scots terriers, Sealyhams, Dandie Dinmonts.

Cause.—Germs usually found are the bacillus coli communis, streptococci, and staphylococci, but how these obtain access is not always quite clear. Some hold that the condition is an infection of the hair follicles found between the toes; others believe that the condition is caused by the entrance of sand and grit into the skin between the toes when the dog is outside at exercise; while some believe that the condition is in the nature of a general disturbance. In some instances, the lesion may be a true retention cyst.

Symptoms.—The dog is first noticed to lick at his foot when lying, but upon examination there is nothing to be seen. Later on he begins to go lame when he puts the paw to the ground, and in a short while will carry it altogether. A hard, painful swelling is found occupying the upper part of an interdigital space in the foot affected. This comes to a head in the course of a day or two and finally bursts, discharging a small amount of blood-stained purulent material. After bursting, the dog gets relief, and if there are no complications the small wound heals up and the trouble disappears. As a rule, however, it is not long before a second abscess forms and bursts in the same way. This may be repeated for some time at more or less regular intervals till, instead of a single abscess, a crop of them form. In such a case the dog may have them on two or more of his feet at the same time, and be quite unable to walk. At the place where each abscess formed there is left a scar and some thickening of the skin, while in dogs that have been badly affected there is a hard and irregular lumpy thickening. After the abscesses have been forming for some time they suddenly cease, and the dog has a rest for perhaps months at a time. Sooner or later, however, they are almost certain to recur at varying intervals.

Treatment.—The first-aid treatment consists in the hot fomentation of the paw. In addition, with a view to preventing a recurrence, many veterinary surgeons cauterise the lining of the cyst under anæsthesia. The foot is bandaged to keep the wound clean, dressed daily until the pus ceases to discharge and the wound has healed. This does not prevent other abscesses from forming, however; in fact, it seems almost impossible to effect this. Whatever treatment is adopted there are always some cases in which it fails.

INTERFERING is another term for what is generally called 'brushing'. (*See* BRUSHING.)

INTERFERON.—A recently isolated substance which inhibits the multiplication of viruses within living cells.

INTERMITTENT (*intermitto*, I leave off) is a term applied generally to fevers or other diseases which continue for a time, subside, and then recur. Intermittent pulse is a symptom of a weak heart, when the pulsation in an artery cannot be felt for one or two beats, and then becomes full and strong for a number of succeeding beats.

INTERNAL HÆMORRHAGE may result from rupture of some large blood-vessel; or it may be the result of an injury to some organ that is richly supplied with blood, such as the liver or spleen. In either case the bleeding occurs into one of the body cavities and the blood is lost to the tissues of the animal. (*See also* ANTICOAGULANTS, WARFARIN POISONING.) Unfortunately internal hæmorrhage is generally such that little or nothing can be done to check it, and the animal dies from 'shock'. It is shown by a paling of the mucous membranes of the eyes and mouth, by an increase in the rate of the respirations, which sometimes assume the character of a series of gasps, by an acceleration of the pulse at first, followed by a diminution in its strength and frequency, and terminating in beats so weak and slow that they are imperceptible. When death is approaching, the animal is usually heard to give one or two long and deep sighs, and there are often a few short convulsions. In cases where hæmorrhage is less severe, the animal should be kept quiet, recumbent, and warm. Water (containing a teaspoonful of salt to a pint) should be offered. Adrenalin may also be given by injection. (*See* SHOCK, BLOOD TRANSFUSION, DEXTRAN, VITAMIN K.)

INTERNAL HÆMORRHAGE OF FOWLS.—This is a condition described *under* 'HÆMORRHAGIC DISEASE'.

INTERNAL SECRETIONS (*see* ENDOCRINE GLANDS).

INTERVERTEBRAL DISC PROTRUSION (*see under* SPINE *and* NANDROLONE).

INTERSTITIAL (*interstitiaiis*) is a term applied to cells of different tissue set amongst the active tissue cells of an organ. It is generally of a supporting character and formed of fibrous tissue, but the interstitial cells of the testis are actively secretory. The term is also applied to diseases which specially affect this tissue, as interstitial nephritis.

INTESTINE (*intestinus*, that which is within) is that part of the alimentary canal that is situated beyond the stomach. In it the greater part of the digestion and absorption of the food-stuffs take place. (*See* DIGESTION.) The size of the intestine varies both in length and calibre in the different animals, and is best considered under the heading of each animal separately, but in all animals the bowel is divided into a *small intestine*, immediately following the stomach, and a *large intestine*, between the end of the small intestine and the outside opening—the anus.

Horse.—(1) Small Intestine.—The first part of the intestinal system in the horse measures about 70 feet, and is divided into a fixed portion—*duodenum*, and a more or less free portion—*jejunum* and *ileum*. Its diameter varies from 1½ to 3 inches when moderately distended, and its capacity is about 12 gallons. The duodenum is the first part succeeding the stomach, measuring about 3½ to 4 feet, and is shaped like a horseshoe. It receives the bile and pancreatic ducts at a point about 5 or 6 inches from its origin at the pylorus of the stomach, and ends by becoming the jejunum just under the left kidney. The jejunum and ileum are free

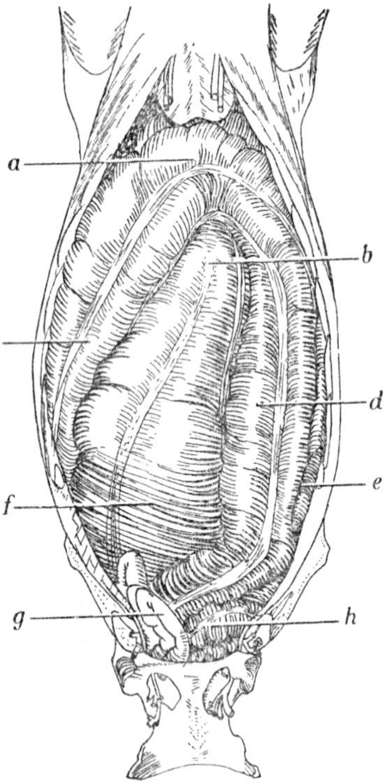

Diagram of the abdominal organs of the horse, viewed from below with the animal upon its back. *a*, Ventral diaphragmatic flexure; *b*, apex of cæcum; *c*, right ventral colon; *d*, left ventral colon; *e*, portions of small intestine; *f*, cæcum; *g*, small intestine; *h*, small colon. (After Bradley's *Anatomy*.)

in the abdominal cavity except for the mesentery which suspends them to the roof of the abdomen, and by which they receive their blood, lymph, and nerve supply. Their position varies according to the other organs of the abdomen and the state of their contents, but they lie mainly in the upper left section of the abdomen mixed up with the coils of the small colon. The ileum ends at the *ileo-cæcal* valve, where it joins the cæcum—the first part of the large intestine.

(2) Large Intestine.—This extends from the end of the ileum to the anus, and

measures about 25 feet in length. Its diameter varies in different parts from about 3 inches in the small colon to nearly 20 inches across the widest part of the cæcum. It is divided into *cæcum*, *large colon*, *small colon*, and *rectum*. The cæcum is a large blind sac lying on the right side of the abdomen and extending downwards and forwards to within a hand's-breadth from the sternum. It is shaped somewhat like a reversed comma, having both its entrance and exit near the base, and has a capacity of about 8 gallons Food-stuff

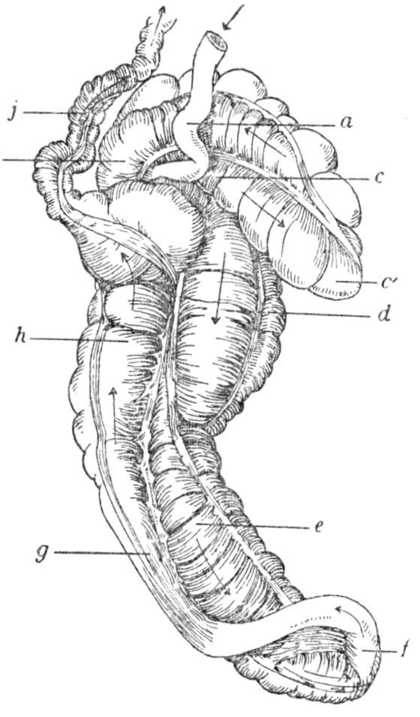

Diagram to show the arrangement of large intestines of horse. *a*, ileum; *b*, base of cæcum; *c* and *c′*, cæcum and its apex; *d*, right ventral colon; *e*, left ventral colon; *f*, pelvic flexure; *g*, left dorsal colon; *h*, right dorsal colon; *j*, commencement of small colon. The arrows show the directions in which the food passes through this part of the alimentary system. (After Bradley's *Anatomy*.)

enters it by the ileo-cæcal valve, and leaves by the *cæco-colic valve*, whence commences the large colon. The large colon has a particular shape and position; it lies in the form of four parts, designated by the numbers 1 to 4. First part, the right ventral colon, lies along the lower part of the right side of the abdomen, beginning at the cæco-colic valve and ending by crossing over to the left side of the body just in front of the apex of the cæcum, to become the second part, the left ventral colon. This runs back to the entrance to the pelvis and turns upwards and forwards to become the left dorsal part, the third part. From this point the colon retracts its position back to the right side of the body immediately above the previous parts. That is, the left dorsal part runs forwards to the anterior region of the abdomen, crosses over to the right side to become the right dorsal colon, and ends near where it began. The small colon continues the direction backwards, lying loosely in the space in the middle of the abdomen, and ends by joining the rectum lying in the pelvis. This latter is simply the short fixed tube in which the motions accumulate before being discharged to the outside. It is often dilated in a bottle-shaped manner.

Ox.—The intestines lie entirely to the right side of the middle line of the abdomen. (1) Small intestine, measuring 130 feet in length, lies in the lower part of the right side of the abdomen, filling in the spaces left between more fixed organs. (2) Large intestine is much smaller than in the horse, and not so complicated. The cæcum lies in the upper posterior part of the abdomen, with its blind sac posteriorly in or near the pelvic inlet. The cæcum is about 2½ feet long and is followed by the colon (there is no small colon in the ox), which has a length of about 35 feet. The colon is arranged like the coils of a watch-spring, with each coil double, consisting of one part running towards the centre—*centripetal*, and a corresponding part running from the centre—*centrifugal*. It lies in the right flank of the abdomen, about half-way between spine and abdominal floor. The last centrifugal fold runs straight back to become the rectum.

Sheep.—With certain slight modifications the intestines of the sheep are similar to those of the ox.

Pig.—(1) Small Intestine.—This varies from 50 to 65 feet in length, and mainly lies on the left side and floor of the abdomen, with some coils pushed across on to the right side of the body. (2) Large intestine is about 15 feet long and considerably wider than the small bowel. The cæcum lies in the upper part of the right flank, with its blind extremity close to the entrance to the pelvis. The colon is arranged in three double spiral folds between the small intestines on its left face and the right flank on its right face. The spiral is not all in the same plane as in the ox, its centre being, so to speak, pulled out away from the rest. Its commencement is of considerable diameter, but it becomes narrower as it nears the rectum.

Dog.—The intestines are short in this animal, only reaching a length of about 15 or 16 feet, of which the small intestine measures 12 to 14 feet. The small intestine occupies the right side of the abdomen and part of the floor. It is attached by the mesentery to the region under the lumbar vertebræ. The large intestine has a course somewhat like that of man. It commences at the cæcum, a small, snail-like piece of bowel, which does not seem to have the same valve-action that is met with in other animals, lying on the right side of the body fairly far forward. From here the colon has a short course upwards towards the head, turns across to the left side of the body, and then runs backwards to end in the rectum.

Structure.—In all animals the intestines, both small and large, are constructed of four main coats. These vary to some extent in the different animals, and in different parts, but they all consist of an inner mucous membrane lining, a submucous coat, a middle muscular coat, and an outer peritoneal covering. The thickness of the bowel wall measures from less than an eighth of an inch in the smaller dogs, up to half of an inch in the thickest parts of the colon of the horse.

Mucous membrane coat.—This is the soft, moist, velvety lining which is found in all parts of the intestine. It consists of a layer of pillar-like cells, placed side by side, with their lower ends resting upon a fine, smooth membrane, below which is a loose network of connective-tissue fibres bounded by a layer of muscle fibres called the 'muscularis mucosæ'. Throughout the whole of this system there are the multitudinous ramifications of blood and lymph vessels which supply the region with nutritive substances, and which are instrumental in the absorption of the food materials resulting from the process of digestion. In the small intestine the surface of the mucous membrane is studded with very fine hair-like projections called 'villi'. These are supplied with both a central lymph system, the lacteal, and a network of capillaries, and are the agents of absorption in this part. Lying between these villi are numerous intestinal glands which pour out a secretion of mucous and digestive juices, known as the 'succus entericus'. At various areas there are what are called 'Peyer's lymphoid patches', which are concentrations of lymphoid tissue somewhat similar to what are found in lymph glands. Scattered here and there in the small intestine, and much more thickly in the large intestine, are special cells that pour out a lubricating

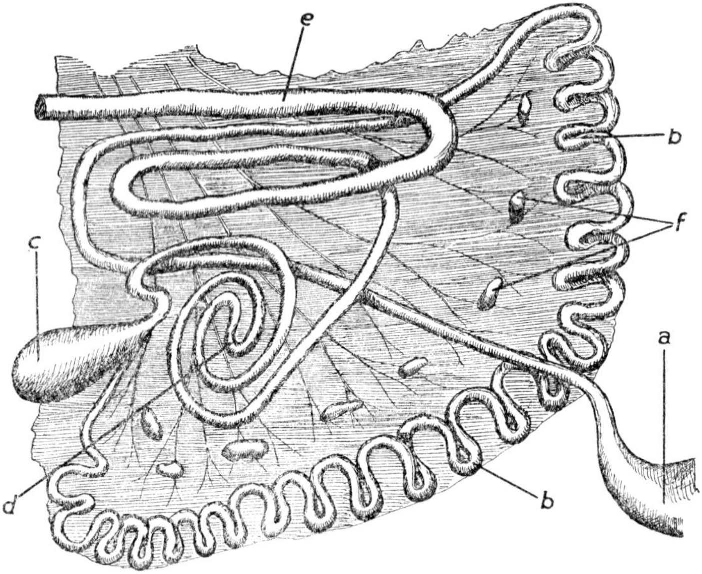

Diagram of the arrangement of the intestines of the ox. *a*, Fourth stomach; *b*, coils of small intestine; *c*, cæcum; *d*, spiral colon; *e*, rectum; *f*, lymph glands.

mucus; owing to their shape they are called 'goblet cells'. The large intestine in all animals does not possess villi, and the ridges seen in the small intestine are not so marked.

Submucous coat.—Lying between the muscularis mucosæ of the previous coat and the true muscular coat there is a large amount of loose connective tissue, which allows the mucous membrane to move freely under the action of the muscles of the bowel. This possesses a large and copious supply of blood and lymph vessels which communicate with the smaller vessels in the mucous membrane.

Muscular coat.—There are two definite layers of muscle fibres in the wall of the bowel. The innermost of these has its fibres all running in a circular manner round the submucous coat, and the outer layer has fibres running lengthwise. In the large intestine some of these longitudinal fibres are collected into distinct bands called 'tænia', which being somewhat shorter than the other fibres cause a certain amount of puckering of the bowels. The muscular arrangement of the intestines is very important, as it is owing to it that all the movement of the bowels occurs. In health it is continually contracting and expanding, shortening and lengthening, and moving the food either onwards or backwards. During the process the food is squeezed and churned and most thoroughly mixed with the digestive juices. The movement is called 'peristalsis' when it tends to move the food towards the anus, and 'anti-peristalsis' when it is in the opposite direction.

Peritoneal coat forms the outermost covering of the bowel. It is continuous for the whole length of the canal from the pylorus to the anus, except for certain comparatively small regions where, for example, the duodenum and the cæcum are bound directly to the roof of the abdomen or to other organs by fibrous tissue. It is a tough membrane with a layer of smooth glistening cells on its outer surface which rub against similar cells on the surfaces of adjacent organs and reduce friction to a minimum. (*See* PERITONEUM.)

Attachments.—The intestines are hung or held in position by folds of peritoneum which bind them, directly or indirectly, to some part of the abdominal wall. The fold in which the free part of the small intestine hangs is called the 'mesentery of the small intestine', and it is through this that the blood and lymph vessels and the nerves enter and leave the bowel. It is composed of two layers, in the middle of which pass the vessels. The arrangement allows of the freest possible movement for the intestine, and at the same time tends to hold it just as much in position as is necessary to prevent the gut from becoming twisted around other structures.

INTESTINE, DISEASES OF.—The intestinal system of animals is probably the seat of more diseases than any other system in the body. It will, therefore, not be possible to include more than a brief description of the conditions here, and for details the reader must refer to sections such as: ACTINOBACILLOSIS, ANTHRAX, CALCULI, CONSTIPATION, COLIC, DIARRHŒA, DYSENTERY, HERNIA, INTUSSUSCEPTION, JOHNE'S DISEASE, ŒDEMA OF THE BOWEL, PARASITES, PERITONITIS; RECTUM, DISEASES OF; SWINE FEVER, SCOURS; etc.

PERFORATION OF THE BOWEL may occur at almost any time either as the result of injury or disease. Stabbing injuries, such as the goring of other animals by bulls and boars, war injuries to horses, accidents with agricultural implements, etc., crushing injuries, especially when the bowels are full, such as run-over accidents to dogs; ulceration of the bowel, such as sometimes happens during swine fever, distemper, collections of concretions, and penetrating injuries from the swallowing of sharp objects, are all possible causes of the condition.

Symptoms.—Interference with the continuity of the bowel wall allows amounts of the food materials to escape into the peritoneal cavity, and a general peritonitis results. In certain cases where the damage has been small a localised inflammation occurs which limits the activities of the escaped organisms, an abscess forms, becomes closed round with fibrous tissue, and recovery follows. In more severe cases the abdomen becomes extremely painful to the touch, the walls of the cavity become tense and hard, the back is arched, the animal shows signs of great distress, the temperature rises, the pulse becomes fast and hard and gets gradually weaker, and sweating and laboured breathing are manifested. In some cases small quantities of blood- or mucus-containing motions are passed with straining. After a few hours, or perhaps one or two days, the animal collapses, becomes unconscious, and death rapidly follows.

Treatment.—All food should be withheld, and only very small mouthfuls of water should be allowed whenever the condition is suspected. In the case of the commercial food animals immediate slaughter is best, both from the humane and from the economic aspect. In other animals if the injury is small there is a chance that recovery may take place, but if the temperature rises and great distress is shown this is not likely, and humane destruction is the only course failing immediate veterinary aid. If conditions are suitable an immediate operation, in which the abdomen is opened, the perforation sought, and the hole in the bowel wall stitched up, is the best course. Sometimes it is necessary to remove a small piece of bowel and sew the divided ends together. Penicillin and/or sulpha drugs are used to overcome the infection.

INFLAMMATION, of the intestines, or enteritis, is a common disease of animals.

Causes.—In the great majority of instances there has been some error in the feeding which has resulted in an irritation—the first stage of inflammation. Excessive amounts of any food material may be a cause; some hard foreign body, which is not sharp enough to produce perforation, may have been eaten with the food; substances of chemical or vegetable origin such as arsenic, strychnine, castor oil, croton seeds, etc., may result in inflammation; parasitic worms in any animal may be the cause; and it appears during the course of certain specific diseases, such as anthrax, hæmorrhagic septicæmia, swine fever, distemper, etc. In the case of the carnivora it is often brought about by the eating of partially decomposed flesh or fish. (For inflammation of the ileum in pigs, *see under* ILEUM.)

Symptoms.—In the mildest cases there may not be very much general disturbance, especially in the early stages. The animal is disinclined for food, has shivering fits, passes motions that are usually coated with mucus, and develops a thirst. The bowels may be heard to rumble, flatus or gas is frequently passed, and there may be some straining. The temperature may be normal or only slightly raised and the pulse and respirations are not appreciably altered. Later the condition may pass off, or it may become intensified, with a high temperature, frequent and painful straining, often causing the animal to call out in pain. The back is arched, the larger animals do not lie down, the smaller ones object to having their abdomen handled, and prostration gradually sets in.

In chronic enteritis the animal partially recovers, but has periodic attacks of foul-smelling diarrhœa, in which strands of mucus may be seen. The appetite is never fully restored, and there is always a tendency to drink larger amounts of water than usual. The abdomen becomes permanently 'tucked up', the animal ceases to thrive, gradually gets weaker, and finally dies from exhaustion.

Treatment.—This depends totally upon the cause of the inflammation. When it is due to large amounts of irritant food, a purgative which will not increase the inflammation is necessary. If poisoning has been the cause, the appropriate antidote must be given. (*See* ANTIDOTES *and* POISONING.) If parasites are responsible they must be expelled. Otherwise, it is treated by administration of soothing and demulcent food-stuffs, such as linseed-, barley-, or oatmeal-gruels, milk containing flour, arrowroot, cornflour, etc., white of egg, soda-water, and so on, according to the animal affected; intestinal antiseptics; intestinal astringents. (*See also* DIARRHŒA, NURSING OF SICK ANIMALS.)

OBSTRUCTION OF THE BOWELS is a common cause of colic in the horse, and is considered under that heading. In cattle, sheep, pigs, and carnivores, it may be produced by constipation.

Causes.—In the first place it may be due to the thrusting of a portion of the bowel through some hole in the wall of the abdomen, when the condition is known as hernia. (*See* HERNIA.) On the other hand, it may be brought about by something that interferes with the normal movement of the food along the intestinal tube, such as the presence of a tumour projecting into the lumen of the bowel, the thickening and constriction that results from an ulcer, the twisting of one portion of intestine round another, producing a kink, the pressure of diseased or damaged organs on a loop of bowel, or that curious condition known as 'intussusception' (*see* INTUSSUSCEPTION), and lastly some body, such as a concretion or calculus, or a piece of bone may have become lodged in a na row part of the bowel and prevent the food materials from travelling along it.

Symptoms.—In the early stages there are frequent attempts to defæcate, but only small amounts of dry motion are evacuated. Later, the attempts become painful and unsuccessful. The animal assumes the characteristic position of defæcation, and strains violently in a vain endeavour to get rid of the accumulated matter. It may grunt or moan, and frequently looks round at its hind-quarters. Cattle and sheep generally grind their teeth and paddle with their hind feet; they separate themselves from their mates when at pasture, and become dull and depressed. Pigs lie much between the attempts at defæcation, and become lethargic and annoyed, giving vent to their feelings in short, irritated grunts or squeals when made to move. Dogs and cats are noticed to assume a crouched position for long periods at a time and to strain continually. They may drag themselves along the ground and lick at their hind parts. The abdomen becomes hard and tucked up in all animals unless gas is formed, when it swells. There is usually a fœtid smell from the body of an animal suffering from obstruction of the bowels. If the condition is not relieved in the course of a day or so, signs of toxæmia appear. The temperature rises. The mucous membrane of the eyelids assumes a dirty yellow colour, denoting that the bile is not being evacuated into the bowels but is being absorbed into the general circulation. Animals that are able to vomit, do so. In the last stages the vomit consists of the material that has passed far down the intestinal system, is fæcal in character, and has a very objectionable putrid smell.

Treatment.—Purgatives simply increase the symptoms and the seriousness of a strangulated hernia, while no amount of purging will clear a passage past a large tumour, or straighten out a piece of twisted or kinked bowel. In these cases the rational treatment is a surgical operation, in which the abdomen is opened, the obstruction sought, and an endeavour made either to reduce it by massage, or else to remove it by opening up the bowel. Dogs and cats may be given a dose of liquid paraffin, from 2 drams to an ounce, according to the size of the dog. The cat takes about half the dose for the dog. If an enema of hot soapy water can be given, it has most beneficial and stimulating effects in all animals; in fact, there are many cases in which, if an enema is given and repeated in an hour or so, no further treatment is necessary, as the obstructed material is able to be evacuated by its influence. Massage to the abdomen, the application of hot packs, and gentle exercise are helpful.

INTOXICATION is a state of poisoning. The poison may be some chemical substance introduced from outside, *e.g.* alcohol, or it may be due to the products of bacterial action. The term 'auto-intoxication' is applied to the absorption of waste products.

INTRACRANIAL (*intra*, within; *cranium*, the skull) is the term applied to structures, diseases, or operations associated with the contents of the cranium Intracranial inoculation means inoculation through the parietal or occipital bone into the brain.

INTRADERMAL.—Means into the thickness of the skin. *See* TUBERCULIN TESTING for an example of intradermal injections.

INTRAMEDULLARY.—Within the marrow cavity of long bones. Thus, intramedullary pins—used in the treatment of fractures.

INTRAMUSCULAR.—Within a muscle; *e.g.* intramuscular injection.

INTRA-PERITONEAL INJECTIONS are those made direct into the abdominal cavity.

INTRATHECAL.—Into a sheath; intraspinal.

INTRATRACHEAL—Into the 'windpipe'. (*See also* ENDOTRACHEAL ANÆSTHESIA.)

INTRAVENOUS INJECTION.—An injection direct into a vein, a technique employed in anæsthesia and where much fluid has to be injected.

INTUBATION is a simple process consisting in the introduction of a tube into the windpipe by way of the mouth. It is resorted to during the administration of anæsthetics to lessen the risk of asphyxia (*see* ENDOTRACHEAL ANÆSTHESIA) or to facilitate operations on the mouth, nasal passages, larynx, or head.

INTUSSUSCEPTION (*intus*, within; *suscipio*, I receive) is a form of obstruction of the bowels in which a part of the intestine enters within that part immediately above or below itself. It is an extremely serious condition, and attended by intense pain. It occurs in the horse and in puppies chiefly. It may be due to the griping action of a severe purge to the overloading of one part of the bowel, while other cases occur without any apparent cause. If the condition is not relieved it leads to the stopping of the blood-supply in that part of the bowel which is enclosed within the other. Acute swelling and inflammation supervene, absorption of harmful products of digestion results, and the animal dies rapidly. The symptoms include loss of appetite, uneasiness due to abdominal pain, straining, and blood in the fæces. In the dog a sausage-like swelling may be palpated in the abdomen, or there may be protrusion from the anus of a turgid, cylindrical mass having four thicknesses of bowel wall. Treatment involves manipulation under anæsthesia (after laparatomy in most cases), and sometimes the surgical removal of the innermost portion of the bowel and the stitching of the remaining ends to each other.

INUNCTION (*in*, into ; *inguo*, I anoint) is the method of administering drugs by rubbing them into the skin mixed with oils or fats.

INVOLUTION.—A change back to its normal condition which an organ undergoes after fulfilling its normal function, *e.g.* involution of the uterus following pregnancy.

IODIDES are salts of iodine.

Actions.—They are rapidly excreted from the body, and in the process stimulate the kidneys, skin, mucous surfaces, and the glands generally, to increased activity. Iodides hasten the process of repair and so aid in the absorption of diseased or damaged tissues. Taken in excess they cause a condition known as 'iodism' or iodine poisoning. The symptoms of this are diarrhœa, loss of appetite, emaciation, total refusal of water, a dry, scurfy condition of the skin with a loss of hair, and in some cases catarrh of the nasal mucous membranes.

Uses.—In dropsical conditions of the pleura and peritoneum, and in the secondary stages of pneumonia, iodides are given to hasten the absorption of the exudate. Potassium iodide is given with good results in purpura hæmorrhagica, actinomycosis, 'scirrhous cord', lymphangitis, to stimulate the absorption of the thickenings that often remain after an attack, and in 'periodic ophthalmia'. It is an antidote to lead and mercury poisoning when chronic, disengaging them from the tissues and allowing of their excretion. Sodium iodide has similar actions, but is less depressant to the heart, **and can safely be given by intravenous injection which the potassium salt cannot.**

Externally the red iodide of mercury is used mixed with lard in the proportion of 1 : 8 or 10, as the familiar 'red blister'. (*See* BLISTERS.)

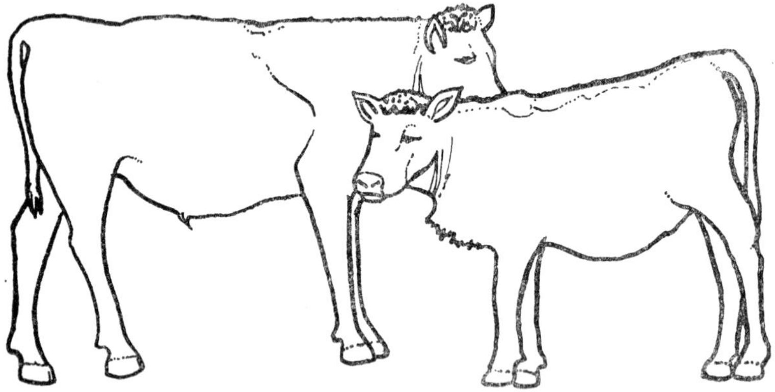

Iodine deficiency—comparison of body size between the normal and deficient animal.

IODINE is a non-metallic element which is found largely in seaweed. It is prepared in the form of dark violet-brown scales, which are soluble in alcohol and ether. It has a pleasant but pungent smell and a burning taste. If applied to the skin either as flakes or in strong solution, it causes staining of the skin and leads to its peeling off. Internally it is a violent irritant poison. (*See also under* RADIO-ACTIVE IODINE.)

Uses.—Pure iodine in the form of scales is never used. The ordinary tincture of iodine that is a common household remedy contains 2½ per cent of iodine. This is used to clean the skin prior to surgical operation, to paint on to swollen glands, as a mild counter-irritant in small bursal or synovial enlargements, and is often applied to the surface of an abscess which is slow in 'coming to a head'.

A mild IODOPHOR, *e.g.* Iosan CCT, is used for teat-dipping in modern dairy hygiene for the prevention of mastitis.

IODINE DEFICIENCY ON THE FARM.—Iodine is required by the body for the formation of thyroxin, the hormone produced by the thyroid gland, and the common sign of iodine deficiency is goitre. Acute iodine deficiency occurs in fourteen of the United States. In Britain, typical iodine deficiency is not common in farm stock, although in some areas the question of iodine intake below the optimum for health and fertility is of economic importance. The remedy is to provide salt licks or mineral mixtures containing traces of iodine. This is particularly important when large quantities of kale, cabbage, or turnips are being fed.

IODO-CASEIN.—An artificially prepared thyroid active protein sometimes used instead of thyroxine.

IODOFORM is a saffron-coloured crystalline substance made by the action of iodine upon a mixture of alcohol and potash. It has a most penetrating and rather pleasant smell, and a strong taste. It is insoluble in water, but dissolves in alcohol, ether, and oils. It acts as a powerful antiseptic when brought into contact with discharges from a wound. If applied in large amounts to a raw surface it is apt to be absorbed and cause poisoning.

Uses.—The commonest use of iodoform is in the treatment of wounds, when it is applied as a dry dusting powder mixed with several times its own amount of starch, zinc oxide, etc. A deodorant as well as a strong antiseptic, it keeps wounds clean and sweet. Made into a paste with bismuth and liquid paraffin it forms the well-known 'Bipp', used in wounds that have been neglected and are purulent or very dirty; and since it can be left in position for several days before it has exerted all its antiseptic powers, it is most useful for animal administration. Since the advent of sulpha drugs iodoform is less used.

IODOPHOR.—An 'iodine-bearer'. (*See under* IODINE.)

IODOPHTHALEIN is the sodium salt of tetra-iodophenol-phthalein, a bluish-violet crystalline powder. As it is excreted quickly by the liver, collects in the gall-bladder, and casts a shadow with X-rays, it is administered by the mouth or by intravenous injection for the diagnosis of disease of the gall-bladder by means of radiography.

IONIC MEDICATION, or **MEDICAL IONISATION,** means the use of an electric current to cause substances to pass through the skin and subcutaneous tissues for curative purposes. The substances used must be soluble in water. A continuous current is necessary. The most commonly used electrolytes are sodium chloride, magnesium sulphate, copper sulphate, cocaine hydrochloride, quinine sulphate, and adrenalin. These are made into solutions in which pads of felt or lint are soaked, and the pads are applied to the area to be treated. One large electrode of brass or aluminium is laid over the pad, and another applied to some suitable part of the body, and the current is applied. This causes a disintegration of the electrolyte into its constituent ions, which are driven through the skin and exert their curative action on the body cells and tissues of the area.

Uses.—Ionisation is used to stimulate sluggish ulcers to heal, in the treatment of diseases, to soften scars, to exert powerful local antiseptic or germicidal actions, to allay pain, and to induce local constriction of vessels in treating inflammatory changes.

IPECACUANHA, IPECAC, or HIPPO, is the root of *Cephælis ipecacuanha*, a Brazilian shrub. It contains an alkaloid 'emetine' which acts as an irritant when brought into contact with the mucous membrane of the stomach, and induces vomiting. After absorption into the bloodstream the same effect is observed owing to the action on the central nervous system. In small doses it acts as a gentle stimulant to the mucous membrane of the air passages. In bronchitis it is given as an expectorant.

IRIDECTOMY (ἶρις, ἐκ, out; τέμνω, I cut) means an operation by which a part or the whole of the iris is removed from the eye, and the size of the pupil is thereby increased.

IRIS (ἶρις, a halo) is the muscular and fibrous curtain which hangs behind the cornea of the eye and serves to regulate the amount of light that is allowed to reach the inner parts of the eye. It possesses radiating and circular fibres which, when they contract under the influence of light, enlarge and decrease the size of the pupil respectively. (*See* EYE.)

In the horse there are often projecting growths seen on the edges of the iris, to which the name 'nigroid bodies' is applied. The function of these is not understood, but when they are of large size it is affirmed that they are liable to cause the animal to shy. It may be necessary to perform iridectomy and remove the bodies.

IRITIS (ἶρις, a halo; *itis*, termination meaning inflammation) means an inflammation of the iris. (*See* EYE.)

IRON is a metal which is not only necessary in small amounts in the bloodstream, in the red blood corpuscles, and in various organs, but is used as a drug as well. All salts of iron have a powerful astringent action on the bowels, and in some cases on wounds and bleeding surfaces.

Uses.—Internally iron compounds are of value in microcytic anæmia, that resulting from hæmorrhage, nutritional anæmia in young animals, anæmia occurring during pregnancy, and chronic wasting diseases. Alone it is of no value in the treatment of pernicious anæmia in man, but is used as a supplement to liver therapy. Iron salts are frequently given together with arsenic, quinine, strychnine. Excessive doses of iron have caused fatal poisoning in children, and may occur in young domestic animals. The freshly prepared or moist oxide of iron is a fairly satisfactory antidote to arsenical poisoning. The sulphate is employed in worm powders. The phosphate of iron is much used as a tonic. (*See* PARRISH'S FOOD, EASTON'S SYRUP.) Iron salts are given to prevent piglet anæmia. Externally, iron is used as an astringent dressing for grease, canker, and cracked heels in horses.

IRON POISONING.—As stated above, this may occur from overdosage, or from the eating of an iron preparation left within reach. (*See also under* FLOOR FEEDING OF PIGS, for the danger of concrete made with sand rich in iron.)

Piglets have been poisoned by iron-dextran preparations given to prevent anæmia. A diet rich in vitamin E, for the sows before farrowing, may help to reduce losses.

In the dog, ferrous sulphate or ferrous gluconate in doses as low as 0·3 to 0·75 gramme respectively of ferrous iron per kg. bodyweight, have caused severe illness with diarrhœa, vomiting and ulceration of stomach and intestine.

IRRADIATION is the term applied to treatment by various forms of light and radiant activity. (*See* LIGHT TREATMENT.) Husk (lungworm) larvae have been irradiated for vaccine purposes. (*See* HUSK.) (*See also* 'RADIATION SICKNESS').

IRRADIATED ERGOSTEROL.—Vitamin D_2.

IRRIGATIONS is the name given to the washing out of wounds or cavities of the body by means of large amounts of hot or cold water containing some antiseptic in solution. The method is employed in the treatment of inflammations of the uterus, bladder, and in certain forms of colic, when the irrigation is applied by the rectum. (*See* ENEMA.)

Easily improvised apparatus may consist of a length of ordinary ½- or ¾-inch hose-pipe, to one end of which a funnel or petrol-filler is attached, while the other is either used as it is, or has a nozzle inserted. The nozzle is introduced after lubrication with vaseline or soap if necessary, and fluid is poured into the funnel held at a higher level than the rest. It is important to allow a small quantity of the fluid to escape before introduction, so that all the air is excluded from the tube. In this way two or three pailfuls of fluid may be conveniently given as a uterine douche. No efforts should be made to prevent the overflow from escaping in douching the uterus, as septic material is mechanically carried to the outside.

As antiseptics for use in irrigation many drugs are used. For the uterus in any animal a weak solution (1:1000) of permanganate of potash is very suitable.

Coal-tar products are not suitable.

Many of the acridine products are useful, such as acriflavine, proflavine, brilliant green, etc. (*See also* DETTOL.)

Various solutions are employed for the irrigation of wounds. (*See* ANTISEPTICS.)

ISCHÆMIA.—Local anæmia.

ISCHÆMIC CONTRACTURE (*see under* MUSCLES, DISEASES OF).

ISCHIUM (ἰσχίον, the hip-joint) is the bone which forms the most posterior part of the pelvis, and forms the point of the buttock.

ISCHURIA (ἴσχω, I check; οὖρον, urine) means insufficiency in the amount of urine passed, due either to suppression of excretion in the kidneys or retention in the bladder.

ISOLATION is an important procedure in the control of the spread of infectious disease, and is applied to the animals themselves, to the attendants, and to the premises.

Isolation of individual animals affected with some mildly contagious disease is generally carried out by their removal to a loose-box, away from other healthy stock. They are attended to by the same attendants who feed, water, groom, and look after the healthy, but they are not touched until last, after the others have been attended to.

In more contagious diseases, affected animals should not only be isolated themselves, but separate attendants should be provided whenever possible.

In very serious outbreaks of contagious diseases, such as foot-and-mouth disease, glanders, contagious pleuro-pneumonia, and swine fever, the premises are isolated. No animals may enter or leave that are liable to contract the particular disease, unless for purposes of immediate slaughter. All persons are prohibited from entering such premises unless on particular duty, and these are made to take precautions with regard to disinfection. (*See* INCUBATION, INFECTION, QUARANTINE.)

ISONIAZID.—A drug used in the treatment of tuberculosis.

ISOQUINOLINIUM chloride lotion has been used in the treatment of ringworm in cattle.

ISOTONIC is a term applied to solutions which have the same power of diffusion as one another. An isotonic solution used in medicine is one which can be mixed with body fluids without causing any disturbance. An isotonic saline solution for injection into the blood, so that it may possess the same osmotic pressure as the blood serum, is one of 0·9 per cent strength or containing 80 grains of chloride of sodium to the pint of water. This is also known as normal or physiological salt solution. An isotonic solution of glucose for injection into the blood is one of 5 per cent strength in water. Solutions, which are weaker than or stronger than the fluids of the body with which they are intended to be mixed, are known as hypotonic and hypertonic respectively.

'ITCH, THE' (*see* MANGE).—'Sweet Itch' is an old name for eczema.

ITCHINESS (*see* PRURITIS).

-ITIS is a suffix added to the name of an organ to signify inflammation of that organ.

IXODES is the generic name of one of the varieties of ticks that infest animals. (*See* PARASITES.)

J

JAAGSIEKTE.—A disease of adult sheep, first recognised in South Africa but occurring also in the United Kingdom, Iceland, the U.S.A. It is characterised by pneumonia. The cause is unknown, but is probably a virus. Death occurs within a few weeks or a few months. Affected animals should be slaughtered.

In Britain, one East Anglian farmer lost 50 out of 200 half-bred ewes from jaagziekte during 1958. The disease is probably widespread but subclinical in hill sheep in Scotland. The disease is likely to assume considerable economic importance in intensively managed sheep.

JABORANDI, or PILOCARPUS, is the leaf of a South American plant, *Pilocarpus pennatifolius*. It contains an alkaloid, pilocarpine, upon which its action depends. When given internally it causes an increase in the secretion from the various glands of the body, but it does not cause sweating in animals in the same way that it does in man. The stimulation of the intestinal glands leads to a pouring out of fluid into the intestines and a consequent fluid condition of the fæces. The drug stimulates and tones up the involuntary muscles of the body, and an increase in the peristalsis of the intestines results. The heart-beat is increased in ordinary doses given by the mouth or subcutaneously, but large doses decrease its action, especially when given intravenously.

Uses.—The chief use is in the treatment of impaction or stoppage of the intestines. It is also the antidote to atropine poisoning. Pilocarpine constricts the pupil and is used to reduce intra-ocular pressure in cases of glaucoma.

JALAP is the tuber of *Ipomea jalapa*, a Mexican plant, which contains two resins with irritating properties.

Uses.—Powdered jalap was used as a powerful purge for swine, especially when combined with calomel. It is not suitable for horses or cattle.

JANET.—A female mule.

JAPANESE B ENCEPHALITIS.—This disease of man, caused by a virus, is transmissible to horses especially; experimentally also to cattle, sheep, goats, and pigs. In the latter, it may result in abortion and stillbirths. Horses' eyesight is affected and they later become drowsy. Recovery is seldom complete; many die.

JAUNDICE (Fr. *jaunisse*) is the name given to a yellowish discoloration of the visible mucous membranes of the body (eye, nose, mouth, and genital organs).

The symptom of jaundice, or icterus may be associated with a great variety of diseases. Thus, its appearance may indicate the destruction of red-blood corpuscles due to parasites, such as may occur in cases of Biliary Fever and Surra in the horse; Red-water in cattle; Malignant Jaundice (canine babesiosis), Canine Yellow Fever, and Leptospiral Jaundice in the dog. It may indicate an incompatibility between the blood of sire and dam-causing hæmolytic jaundice of the new, born foal or piglet. Or it may indicate an obstruction to the flow of bile or one of several other pathological conditions.

When bile cannot escape into the small intestine by the bile-duct from the liver in the usual way, it becomes dammed back, is absorbed by the lymphatics and the blood-vessels, carried into the general circulation, and some of its constituents are deposited in the tissues of the body. It may be caused, therefore, by some condition which interferes with free evacuation of the bile; this may either be in the bile-ducts themselves, such as a gall-stone, or a swelling of the lining mucous membrane produced by acute inflammation; in the intestines; or there may be some disorganisation of the liver. (*See also* CANINE VIRUS HEPATITIS.)

The causes responsible for the appearance of jaundice include: liver flukes and round worms in the bile-ducts (these, however, do not always cause jaundice), gall-stones, and collections of dried bile in the gall-bladder (*see* GALL-STONES, *also under* GALL-BLADDER, DISEASES OF), cysts or tumours in the liver substance or in such position that they press upon the ducts; cirrhosis, tuberculosis, bacterial necrosis, and various degenerations of the liver; it may also arise during the course of digestive disturbances, influenza, distemper, strangles, azoturia, etc. In addition to these causes, jaundice may appear when there is nothing obvious to account for it; for instance, it sometimes appears during pregnancy, œstrum, old age, and after eating large amounts of lucerne or sainfoin for the first time. It may be seen during poisoning with copper, mercury, phosphorus, chloroform, or lead, and after some snake-bites.

The condition may be either acute or chronic. In the acute form the yellow discoloration of the membranes suddenly appears; the temperature may rise to an alarming height; the animal becomes very dull and depressed; marked weakness in movement is observed; and there is a foul smell from the breath. If the condition is not soon relieved it is rapidly fatal. In the chronic type the yellow tinge gradually appears in the membranes and in the white of the eye, the temperature rises slowly, and dullness is not observed at once. The fæces become clay-coloured; the urine becomes bright yellow or even green in colour, and contains much bile pigments and salts. Constipation almost always supervenes. In the dog and cat, the acute type is often accompanied by convulsions and fits, and vomiting is excessive. In the chronic form the animal loses condition, becomes anæmic, often develops a dropsical condition of the abdomen, and gradually becomes weaker.

Treatment.—The treatment depends entirely upon the cause. In cases where there is some mechanical obstruction it is obvious that it is first necessary to remove this if at all possible. Where other disease exists it needs appropriate attention. (*See also* JAUNDICE, LEPTOSPIRAL; JAUNDICE OF THE NEW-BORN *under* FOAL DISEASES; *and* BILIARY FEVER.)

JAUNDICE, LEPTOSPIRAL, OF DOGS also called INFECTIOUS JAUNDICE, is a serious condition which appears to be indigenous in certain districts in Great Britain, and is characterised by a high mortality and a tendency to inflammatory or other bowel complications.

Cause.—The cause of the disease is a spirochæte, *Leptospira icterohæmorrhagiæ*, which also causes Weil's disease in man. It is present in about 40 per cent of apparently healthy rats. Contamination of food by rat urine, and eating rats which have been killed, are probably responsible for cases in dogs. Young sporting dogs are commonly affected. The organism is present in the urine of affected animals and man, and cases may occur from contamination of the unbroken skin by infective urine. The spirochæte gains a more ready access if the skin is injured, or through the minute lesions made by an insect bite.

Symptoms.—In most cases the first symptoms are those of jaundice; the dog goes off its food, may vomit, becomes very dull and depressed, and a yellowish tinge appears in the mucous membranes of the eyes and mouth. This becomes gradually worse, and in two days or so the eyes and mouth may be tinged a canary yellow. The dog rapidly loses condition, and its abdomen becomes tucked up and painful on pressure. There is at first a certain amount of constipation, and what fæces are passed are either clay-coloured or may be dark, in which case latter they contain blood. They always have a foul, fœtid odour. Diarrhœa with great straining may occur. In acute cases there may be general collapse; the temperature is high at first, then falls, the pulse is weak and rapid, spasmodic contractions of certain groups of muscles occur, and convulsive seizures may be exhibited just before death occurs.

In other cases of *L. icterohæmorrhagiæ* infection jaundice does not occur, the symptoms resembling more those of *L. canicola* infection. There is inappetence, occasional vomiting, acute depression, brownish discoloration of the tongue, a uræmic odour from the mouth, and a slight degree of fever. (*See* LEPTOSPIROSIS.)

Prevention.—Vaccination is recommended, and can be combined with distemper inoculation. (*See also under* DISTEMPER.) By frequent disinfection of kennels where large numbers of puppies are reared, the eradication of rats and mice, and also fleas and lice, and by a sufficiency of exercise in the open air, enzoötic jaundice has been practically stamped out of certain kennels where formerly it was difficult to rear even half the number of puppies born in a year.

Treatment.—This consists essentially in the early administration of anti-serum and/or penicillin. Physiological saline should be given by injection daily, when food and water may be withheld (apart, perhaps, from a little barley water). Good nursing is essential. (*See also* LEPTOSPIROSIS.)

JAUNDICE, LEPTOSPIRAL, OF OTHER ANIMALS (*see under* LEPTOSPIROSIS).

JAVA BEAN POISONING.—The 'Java' beans, *Phaseolus lunatus*, though not native to Great Britain, have been imported in large amounts, owing to the mistaken idea that they form a valuable food-stuff when not eaten in large quantities at a time. The beans are of varying origin, and differ in colour, thus: *Java* beans are as a rule reddish-brown, but they may be almost black; *Rangoon* or *Burmah* beans are smaller, plumper, and lighter in colour (so-called '*red Rangoons*' are pinkish with small purple splashes, and the '*white Rangoons*' are a pale cream colour); *Lima* beans are large cream-coloured beans somewhat like the 'butter beans' that are used for human consumption. As a general rule it may be taken that the coloured beans are the most dangerous for stock feeding; the white beans being usually safe, although it would always be advisable to obtain a written guarantee that they are safe for feeding when purchasing. Wild grown beans are always richer in poisonous principles than the cultivated varieties. The active poisonous agent in the beans is a substance called *Phaseolunatin*, which is a member of a group of glucosides that are capable of producing hydrocyanic acid (prussic acid) when there are suitable conditions of heat, moisture, etc., such as are found in the stomachs of animals; these glucosides are called in consequence *cyanogenetic glucosides*.

Symptoms.—These are exactly the same as those given under PRUSSIC ACID, which see.

JAW is the name of each of the bones that carry the teeth. The upper jaw-bones are two in number and are firmly united to the other bones of the face. The lower jaw—or mandible—is composed of a single bone in horse, pig, dog, and cat, but in the ruminants the fusion between the right and left sides does not occur until old age. Each of the jaws presents a number of deep sockets or 'alveoli' which contain the teeth. With regard to the licensing of bulls, 'a bull shall be considered abnormal if the four central incisors protrude to the extent of preventing contact between the upper part of these teeth and the dental pad'. (*See* DISLOCATIONS, FRACTURES, MOUTH, TEETH; *also* ATROPHIC MYOSITIS *and* EOSINOPHILIC MYOSITIS—both given in the Section headed MUSCLES, DISEASES OF.)

JEJUNUM (*jejunus*, empty of food) is the name of the central portion of the small intestine which has rather irregular divisions. (*See* INTESTINE.)

JENNY.—A female ass.

JERSIAN.—Also known as a F-J hybrid, this is a beef cross obtained from a Jersey bull on a Friesian cow. (In New Zealand, the reverse cross is used.)

JETTING.—This term is applied to a technique developed in Australia, involving the application of insecticide under pressure by means of a jetting gun—a handpiece with four needle jets for combing through the wool. The pressure used is 60 to 80 lb. per square inch, which can be achieved by an ordinary medium/high-volume agricultural sprayer.

In Britain, jetting was demonstrated at the 1965 Royal Show, and the following advantages were claimed for it:

1. Clean wash of constant insecticidal concentration is used, none of which is recirculated.

2. There is no wastage of wash as in dipping and spraying as the gun is only actuated while being used; there is virtually no run off and none has to be disposed of as in dipping. Jetting is therefore the most economical means of applying insecticide.

3. Insecticide is thoroughly applied to those areas of the sheep most susceptible to fly strike and individual sheep can be given special attention, *e.g.* if they are especially dirty.

4. The duration of protection against maggot fly strike is comparable with that given by dipping and longer than that provided through a spray race.

5. No equipment other than that normally present on a farm except a relatively inexpensive jetting gun is necessary.

6. Jetting can be carried out anywhere on the farm.

7. Sheep do not have to be lifted and so injury or distress is kept to a minimum.

8. Less labour is required than for dipping.

9. Jetting with one gun even for an inexperienced operator is as fast as dipping (about 100 sheep per hour), with two or more guns in operation correspondingly faster.

JEYES' FLUID.—A saponaceous solution of cresols, etc., a non-corrosive disinfectant, about six times as efficient as carbolic acid.

JIBBING IN HORSES.—There is no doubt that there is a good deal of misunderstanding concerning jibbing among people connected with horses. It is very often the case that the horse gets blamed when no blame is due.

Causes.—A very few horses, usually old and lazy creatures, jib when given a task heavier than usual. What began as pure laziness becomes a vice and a habit, and in such horses a little stimulation from the whip is excellent. The greater number of jibbers, however, commence the trick because of fear or nervousness. They may have been frightened when they first experienced some unusual sight or sound, and they learn to associate like occasions with unpleasant sensations. They refuse to pass a particular vehicle or object on the roads because they do not understand it, and from jibbing they soon proceed to the next stage, which is shying and bolting. (*See* BOLTING OF HORSES.) In other instances when a horse wears harness that does not fit comfortably, *e.g.* the collar may be too tight, or the breechings too loose, and is put to a heavier load than usual, he becomes afraid to try his hardest, since he knows from previous experience that ' something may happen '. This is especially the case with horses that have been ' piped ', *i.e.* have temporarily fainted through an obstruction to the circulation caused by too tight a collar. Rather than suffer again in the same way the horse will not try. In addition to these there are some horses which may be suffering from some physical disability which does not allow them to exert their whole pulling power on a load, or when going up a hill; when examined carefully they are found to be suffering perhaps from heart or circulatory trouble, such as incompetence of the valves, or sclerosis of the arteries (the latter a legacy from a previous infestation with round worms in the mesenteric arteries), or in a few cases some brain trouble. There are, however, other cases in which a horse that has hitherto worked in an honest and satisfactory manner suddenly becomes a ' rogue ', and refuses to pull.

Remedies.—It should be the aim of the owner of the nervous horse to overcome by intelligent kindness the harm which has been wrought by abuse, to gain the confidence of the horse by never asking it to do anything that is beyond its power or comprehension, and to give it every opportunity to become acquainted with unfamiliar objects. The fit of the harness should at all times receive the greatest attention, for while badly fitting harness may directly be the cause of injury, it may also indirectly result in trouble, as mentioned previously.

JOHNE'S DISEASE, CHRONIC BACILLARY DIARRHŒA, or PSEUDO-TUBERCULAR ENTERITIS, is a chronic infectious inflammation of the small and large intestines, affecting cattle particularly, but sometimes sheep, goats, and deer, characterised by the appearance of a persistent diarrhœa, gradual emaciation, and great weakness. The infection has been set up experimentally in the rabbit. It may occur naturally in the pig, and *post-mortem* findings may at first suggest tuberculosis.

Cause.—It is caused by *Mycobacterium paratuberculosis*, which is in many respects very like the tubercle bacillus. Like the latter, it belongs to the c ass of ' acid-fast ' bacilli, is similar to it in shape and size, and to some extent in its cultural characteristics. Infection takes place by way of the mouth through food-stuffs contaminated with excreta from other infected animals. Pastures, stagnant water, ponds, and animal buildings, may harbour the germs for long periods. The organism can survive for 17 to 19 months in tap-water. A case in a 9-month-old steer has been reported.

Symptoms.—The disease is very slow in its onset. Cattle that have become infected may not show any symptoms for as long as two years after the last case occurred on a premises, and not all infected animals actually develop symptoms. The first signs of the disease are loss of condition, general unthriftiness, a harsh, staring coat, and a laxness of the bowels, in spite of good food and a well-balanced ration. Milk cows, goats, and ewes, give less milk, and if suckling their young these may show similar symptoms. After a period of wasting, the symptoms become exaggerated. The temperature fluctuates a degree or two above the normal, the animal refuses food some days, but eats ravenously on others. It is about this time that emaciation begins to become very marked. The flesh wastes away, leaving the bones sticking up from the skin in a remarkably prominent fashion.

JOHNE'S DISEASE

Weakness and general debility become more and more pronounced, till some day the animal lies down and is unable to rise. It lies for a few hours making occasional

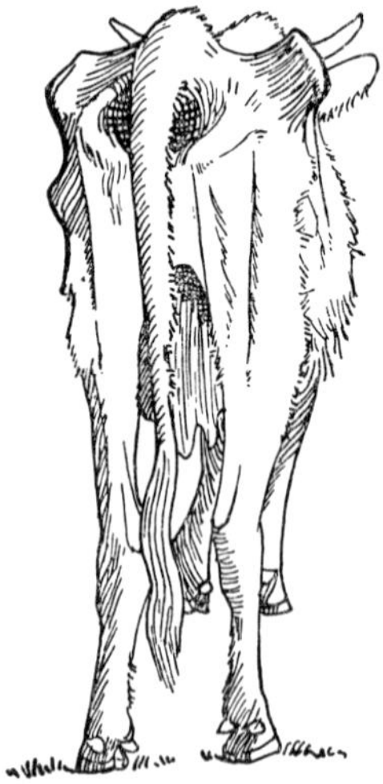

Drawing of a cow in an advanced stage of Johne's disease. The animal is extremely emaciated, and the bones stand out prominently.

struggles to regain its feet, until becoming weaker and weaker, death supervenes. In the ewe and the goat the symptoms are the same, except that diarrhœa is not so continuous. There are periods when the evacuations are formed and almost normal, but the wasting is none the less marked. It is often noticed that before parturition a pregnant female shows irregular symptoms that cannot be considered definite, but after the act of calving or lambing she manifests the disease in an acute form and dies in the course of a few weeks.

Prevention.—Much of the loss, both direct and indirect, can be avoided by the early diagnosis and the slaughter of affected cattle. There is no cure for the condition when once well established; the disease is invariably fatal sooner or later.

Great attention should always be paid to the prevention of infection to other animals, especially calves. Pastures that are suspected of being heavily infected should be left without stock for 4 or 5 months and may receive a top-dressing of lime or chalk. All infected litter should be stored in a dung-pit which is not accessible to other animals, and should be used for cultivated land. Loose-boxes, sheds, etc., that have housed a case should be carefully disinfected, and diseased animals should be fed after healthy ones. Ponds and water-courses should be fenced to prevent fouling by fæces, water for drinking being pumped out.

Diagnosis, Tests.—Rapid diagnosis is of great importance, and a material similar to tuberculin (called '*Johnin*') has been prepared. Suspected cattle can be tested, and reactors may thereby by identified and eliminated. The Johnin test is useful but not infallible—remarks which apply even more to the Complement Fixation test and the avian tuberculin test, which both suffer from being non-specific. (*See* NURSE COWS.)

From the export point of view the B.V.A. has stated: 'While these tests may have some merit in countries with a low level of non-specific infection or of Johne's disease, their use condemns many normal animals in Britain, where reaction to avian tuberculin and, therefore, to Johnin is common. Moreover, cattle which have passed the test in Britain sometimes fail when they are re-tested during quarantine in the importing country.'

It is emphasised that the fact that the tests are sometimes carried out in Britain before export does not imply official recognition either of their accuracy or usefulness. Every effort is made, however, to follow the same testing techniques as are employed in the importing countries. For example, Canadian Johnin has been used on animals going to Canada.

The non-specific infection eferred to above includes that with bacilli like tubercle bacilli but harmless, avian tuberculosis, and 'skin tuberculosis'. It is considered possible that normal tuberculin testing may provoke a temporary reaction to the Johne's disease Complement Fixation test. 'Although there is little practical value in C.F. testing an animal less than one year old, this is sometimes required for export purposes. It is, therefore, important to appreciate that calves may develop a temporary reaction following colostrum feeding by a reacting cow.'

Bacteriological examination of scrapings from the rectal mucous membrane reveal clumped masses of the acid-fast organism in most positive cases.

A vaccine became available to U.K. veterinary surgeons in May 1964. It is intended for use in calves up to a month old in problem herds. Care has to be taken to minimise its interference with interpretation of the tuberculin test. Vaccination is being practised in Iceland, Holland, Belgium, and France.

JOHNIN.—A diagnostic. (*See* JOHNE'S DISEASE.)

JOINT-ILL. NAVEL-ILL or POLYARTHRITIS is a disease of foals, lambs, and calves, in which abscesses form at the umbilicus and in some of the joints of the limbs, due, in the majority of cases, to the entrance of organisms into the body by way of the unclosed navel. There are numerous organisms associated with the disease, the commonest of which are streptococci, staphylococci, Pasteurella, *E. coli*, the necrosis bacillus, and *see under* FOALS, DISEASES OF.

Symptoms.—It is seldom that two cases present similar symptoms. There is a great variability in the severity of the attack. In a few cases the joints have been found swollen at birth; or the disease may arise at any time up to six months; but in the majority the symptoms do not appear till about 5 or 6 days after foaling. The young animal becomes dull, takes no interest in its dam, refuses to suckle; the breathing is hurried; the temperature rises from 2° to 4° F. above normal; the foal prefers to lie stretched out on its side, and may have attacks of either diarrhœa or constipation. If the navel is examined it is found to be wet and oozing with blood-stained serous material, or it may be dry, swollen, painful to the touch, and hard, owing to abscess formation within. In cases that appear later in life there may be no umbilical symptoms. In the course of a day or so, one or more of the joints swells up. The joints most commonly attacked are the stifle, hip, knee, hock, shoulder, and elbow, but it may be seen in any of the others. The swelling is tense, painful, hot, and œdematous, and the surrounding muscular tissues are also affected. A day or two later the joint bursts and discharges a quantity of blood-stained serous fluid, containing shreds of fibrinous clot. True pus is not often met with in the foal, but it is seen in the lamb and calf. The young creature gets progressively weaker, and loses condition very rapidly, till finally death occurs. When the internal organs are affected death takes place more rapidly, and there are local disturbances according to the seat of the lesion. Some cases recover, but it is seldom that a severe case ever develops into a thrifty and healthy animal afterwards. The mortality is about 50 per cent to 60 per cent of the affected, but it is much worse in some seasons and districts than others.

Prevention.—In the first place, it cannot be too strongly impressed upon the owner of stock that the eradication of joint-ill from his flocks, herds, and studs lies chiefly in his own hands. The most scrupulous attention must be paid to the cleanliness of the foaling-box, the calving-box, and the lambing-pen. Where climatic and other conditions are favourable the pregnant females should be allowed to give birth to their young out of doors. For mares, an open, or a partly open, shed should be provided in a sheltered corner of the paddock, and the mare may be encouraged to sleep there by being fed inside. The same principle should be followed with cattle on a farm that is badly affected. Lambing-pens should without fail be changed to a fresh site every year.

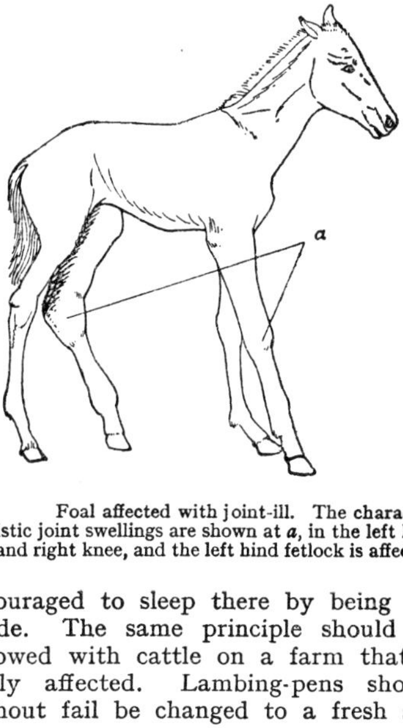

Foal affected with joint-ill. The characteristic joint swellings are shown at *a*, in the left hock and right knee, and the left hind fetlock is affected.

Recent investigations undertaken by the Animal Health Trust suggest that thoroughbred foals in the U.K. suffer severe illness as a result of being deprived of a not inconsiderable volume of blood when the navel cord is ruptured by human agency prematurely. Severance of the cord, it seems, is always best left to the mare. The use of strong disinfectants applied to the stump of the navel cord is likewise deprecated.

With calves, it is probably wiser to ensure clean surroundings, and to attempt to prevent navel-sucking by other calves, than to cut the cord and dress it with some strong disinfectant as a routine. Where joint-ill is a problem, an application of a sulphanilamide dry dressing may be safer than 10 per cent iodine solution.

When cutting the cord, it is necessary to maintain the strictest personal cleanliness if the disease is to be prevented. The hands and arms of the attendant should be first washed in a suitable disinfectant, and the finger-nails ought to be kept short. Scissors should be sterilised, and tape scrupulously clean.

It is necessary to ensure that the external genitals of the mother are as clean as possible. Where very valuable animals are concerned the young is sometimes caught upon antiseptic rubber sheeting, or on towelling, and retained there until the cord has been dressed.

Treatment.—Sulphonamides and antiserum are indicated. Abscesses are opened, and the contained material is washed out by syringing with suitable antiseptics, such as acriflavine; the umbilicus is opened up, evacuated, and disinfected. Great care should always be taken that the contents of abscesses are never allowed to become spilled over the floor, as they are liable to be carried on the boots of attendants to other hitherto healthy animals and infect them.

Calves that are living with others in calf-houses should be isolated as soon as they show symptoms, and should be attended to by the attendant after he has finished with the healthy. All pails, and other feeding utensils that are liable to get infected, should be washed out with boiling water or steamed before future use, and the pen or box that houses a case should be occasionally washed out with disinfectant.

In this connection the wisdom of housing animals in well-built, hygienic premises, provided with impervious floors and walls, and possessing the minimum of internal fittings, is very obvious. (*See also* FOALS, DISEASES OF.)

JOINTS.—A joint, or articulation, is formed by the union of two or more bones or cartilages by other tissues. Bone is the chief component of most joints, but in some cases a bone and a cartilage, or two cartilages, form a joint.

Structure.—Joints fall into two great divisions, namely, (*a*) movable joints, and (*b*) fixed joints. In a *movable joint* there are four main structures. Firstly, there are the two bones whose junction forms the joint; secondly, there is a layer of smooth cartilage covering the ends of these bones where they meet, which is called 'articular' cartilage; thirdly, there is a sheath of fibrous tissue known as the 'joint capsule', which is thickened into bands or 'ligaments' which hold the bones together at various points; and finally, there is a closed bladder of membrane, known as the 'synovial membrane', which lines the capsule and produces a synovial fluid to lubricate the movements of the joint. Further, the bones are kept in position at the joints by the various muscles passing over them and by the atmospheric pressure. This type of joint is known as a *diarthrodial joint.*

Some joints possess subsidiary structures such as discs of fibro-cartilate, which adapt the bones more perfectly to one another where they do not quite correspond, and allow of slightly freer movement, *e.g.* the stifle-joint. In others, movable pads of fat under the synovial membrane fill up larger cavities and afford additional protection to the joint, *e.g.* the hock-joint. In some the edge of one bone is amplified by a margin f cartilage which makes dislocation less possible than otherwise, *e.g.* the hip and the shoulderj joints.

In the *fixed joints* a layer of cartilage or of fibrous tissue intervenes between the bones and binds them firmly together (*synarthrodial joint*). This type of joint is exemplified by the 'sutures' between the bones that make up the skull. Classified among these fixed oints are the *amphiarthrodial joints*, in which there is a thick disc of fibro-cartilage between the bones, so that, although the individual joint is really capable of but limited movement, a series of these, like the joints between the bodies of the vertebræ, gives the column, as a whole, a very flexible character. In this connection it is noticeable that the movement in the region of the neck may be much more free than in some of the true movable joints, such as between the small bones of the hock or carpus.

Varieties.—Apart from the division into fixed and movable joints, those that are movable are further classified. *Gliding joints* are those in which the bones have flat surfaces capable only of a limited amount of movement, such as the bones of the carpus and tarsus. In *hinge-joints* like the elbow, fetlock, and pastern, movement can take place around one axis only, and is called flexion and extension. In the *ball-and-socket joints*, such as the shoulder and hip-joints, free movement can occur in any direction. There are other subsidiary varieties, named according to the shape of the bones which enter into the joint.

JOINTS, DISEASES OF.—The larger joints, on account of their exposed position in the body, are subject to frequent injury, and this, together with the wear they have to withstand, and the peculiarity of their blood-supply, renders them liable to a number of serious diseases. The joints that are most often affected are the stifle, hock, knee, and fetlocks, but the shoulder, hip, elbow, and the lower joints of the digit are not infrequently the seat of disease as well. Even minor injuries, in which the skin is broken and the joint cavities exposed, are liable to be followed by serious results from infection of the joint (a condition which is only second in seriousness to injury to the internal organs) ; while what appear to be very severe injuries often clear up with little or no bad after-effects, provided the skin over the joint remains intact. Among diseases that are associated with joints, and which are treated in separate sections, there are : RING-BONES, BONE SPAVIN, NAVICULAR DISEASE, THOROUGHPIN, CURB, WIND - GALLS, BOG SPAVIN, SLIPPED SHOULDER, SLIPPED STIFLE, HYGROMA OF THE KNEE, CAPPED ELBOW, CAPPED HOCK, KNUCKLING OF THE FETLOCK, and JOINT-ILL ; *see also* ARTHRITIS, BURSITIS, ANKYLOSIS, FRACTURES, DISLOCATIONS, GLASSER'S DISEASE, 'HIP DYSPLASIA', TUBERCULOSIS ; SWINE ERYSIPELAS, etc.

SYNOVITIS is the name given to any inflammation of the membrane lining a joint cavity. It may be acute, sub-acute, or chronic.

Causes.—Generally this is not a separate condition but occurs during the course of such specific fevers as glanders, joint-ill, strangles, distemper, or influenza, when it is due to the invasion of the delicate synovial membrane of the joint by some particular type of organism. It also occurs during rheumatism, rickets, gout (in poultry), severe sprains and bruises, and in a variety of other diseased conditions. Tuberculous joint disease often produces a chronic synovitis in the neck bones of the horse, which leads to an arthritis later. Conditions such as wind-galls, curb, bog spavin, etc., are really only synovitis that have become chronic, or are complicated with other pathological conditions. (*See* BRUCELLOSIS.)

Symptoms.—The synovial membrane becomes inflamed, thickened, and secretes an excessive amount of fluid into the joint. As a result the joint becomes hot, swollen, and painful. The animal goes lame in greater or lesser degree according to the extent of the inflammation. When at rest, the joint is usually kept flexed with the toe of the affected leg just resting on the ground. If it is a simple condition, such as a mild sprain, these symptoms last for a few days and then gradually pass off. In more severe cases, such as in joint-ill, there may be pus formation, septicæmia, and death. In the chronic type the swelling persists. The animal is able to use its limb as usual, but the blemish of the accumulated fluid in the cavity does not disappear (*e.g.* bog spavin, wind-galls, etc.).

Treatment.—Treatment depends upon the cause. In the simplest cases a short rest, with either cold or hot fomentations to affected part, generally results in a complete recovery. Other cases require to be tapped, and the fluid that has collected is removed, the joint being flushed out with some astringent solution afterwards. In those instances when the synovitis is only a localisation of some general fever, the treatment of the general condition is of greater importance than the local attention to the joint. In severe cases in the smaller animals it may be advisable to amputate the limb above the affected joint if the life of the creature is to be saved.

OPEN JOINT, which is also called 'open arthritis' or 'punctured joint', is a condition in which a direct communication has been formed between the inside of the joint and the outside. A small wound, which upon a muscular region of the body would be considered a very trivial affair, is likely to have serious or even fatal results if it is so situated that it involves an opening into a joint cavity. As compared with other domesticated animals, open joint in the horse is the most serious, but it is a condition that must be considered grave in any animal.

These serious changes which result from an open joint are not so much due to the initial injury as to the organisms that enter the joint, either at the time of the injury or afterwards. They cause a disintegration of the essential structures of the joint, invade the general circulation, and set up severe constitutional disturbances.

Notwithstanding all this, it does sometimes happen that an open joint in any animal may escape infection, and may heal up in quite a satisfactory manner; and with modern methods of treatment, more and more cases recover completely.

Causes.—Stabbing wounds, such as arise from falling on to sharp objects, stones, pavements, etc., from wounding with agricutural implements or tools, from kicks when a horse is shod with frost cogs, from barbed wire, from rusty nails, etc., are the most common; as well as from a blood-borne infection that attacks the joint from the inside, and causes it to burst to the outside.

Symptoms.—The most striking signs of open joint are, in the first place, the excessive degree of pain that seems out of all proportion to the visible amount of damage that has been inflicted; secondly, the great amount of swelling that is usually seen, not only on the side of the joint where the injury exists, but also on the opposite side; and thirdly, the discharge of a thin, straw-coloured or blood-stained sticky synovia which has a tendency to coagulate around the skin opening. After one or two days, general symptoms appear. The animal becomes fevered, goes off its food, may break out in a profuse perspiration, has shivering fits, and may show muscular tremors or quiverings. The temperature rises; the pulse becomes hard and fast; and the breathing is accelerated. The pain in the joint causes the animal alternately to move the limb backwards and forwards a short distance; no weight is put upon the affected limb, and any handling of the joint gives rise to obvious signs of great tenderness in the part. In the most severe cases, complications are common. After a course of from 6 to 7 days to about a fortnight, the animal generally dies from exhaustion or general infection. In those cases that recover, some improvement is usually seen by the 4th or 5th day. There may be some stiffness in the joint for a considerable time afterwards.

Treatment.—The horse should be placed in slings and made comfortable. Skilled assistance should be sought at once, as the condition is always most serious. Treatment includes the use of penicillin or the sulphonamides.

EPIPHYSITIS is the name given to inflammation situated at the end of a long bone just beyond the joint. In the commonest form among animals, it is due to rickets, and occurs in young puppies and little pigs. (*See* RICKETS.) The condition is also sometimes met with in adult oxen, when it is caused by tuberculous disease in the marrow cavity of the bone. It is accompanied by a swelling of the bone just clear of the joint, and is accompanied by much pain and lameness. The skin over the part may burst and discharge tuberculous pus, after it has been in evidence for some time. (*See* TUBERCULOSIS.) In another form, associated with excessively rich feeding and undue confinement in young animals, the uppermost extremities of the bones forming the points of the hocks separate from the shafts, and the condition becomes virtually one of 'hamstrung'. There is an acute epiphysitis, which is believed to be of a rheumatic nature.

STIFFNESS OF JOINTS may be due to various causes. It may result from bony disease of the edges of the bones that form the joint, which interferes with the freedom of movement of that joint, such as in ring-bone (*see* RING-BONE). It may be due to a sprain of the ligaments or tendons that pass rom one of the component bones to the other, which results in a shortening of these structures and consequent impediment to free flexion. Often a severe injury to the joint itself, such as a dislocation, or fracture of one of the bones, results in a stiffening of the movement of the joint. A very large number of comparatively slight, though continuous, injuries, set up a slow inflammation, which produces adhesions of fibrous tissue between the parts of the joint and limits future movement. In many cases of adhesions, lime salts are eventually deposited in the fibrous bands and the condition of 'ankylosis' results; this fuses one joint surface to its fellow in bony union. These cases are, of course, unable to be relieved.

LOOSE BODIES IN JOINTS result from inflammation of various types, the bodies being developed as projections on the synovial membrane or on the cartilage of the joint, and are later pulled off by its movement. They bring on repeated attacks of synovitis, and often cause sudden locking of the joint, so that for a time it is immovable. They are commonest among sporting dogs, and are sometimes removed by operation.

DISLOCATIONS (*see* DISLOCATIONS).

ARTHRITIS means inflammation which involves all the structures of the joint, viz. synovial membrane, capsular ligaments, cartilages, and the ends of the bones that take part in the formation of the joint. In almost every case it commences by a synovitis (*see* SYNOVITIS, under this section), but the degree of inflammation is severe enough to extend to the structures around the synovial membrane. Its causes, symptoms, and treatment are similar to those given for synovitis, but it commonly leads to ankylosis and fixation of the joint, if the affected animal survives. (*See* CORTISONE.)

BURSITIS, an inflammation of a bursa, commonly occurs in the region of a joint. The prominences of the hock, elbow, knee, stifle, etc., are protected by bursa, which are lined on their insides by synovial membrane. These sometimes become inflamed and lead to the formation of fluctuating swellings which have a tendency to become chronic. Capped elbow, capped hock, and hygroma of the knee, are of this nature.

JUGULAR (*jugulum*, the collar-bone) is the name of the large veins (one on either side of the neck) which carry the blood back to the chest from the head and anterior parts of the neck. The *jugular furrow* is the name of the groove between the windpipe and the muscles of the neck, in the depths of which lies the jugular vein.

K

K VALUE.—This is used as a measure of the insulating value of building materials such as glass fibre, wood.

KALA-AZAR, or DUMDUM FEVER, is a disease of human beings caused by a small protozoön parasite called the *Leishmania donovani*, which is met with in India, the Mediterranean countries, and in South America. A similar disease, called CANINE LEISHMANIASIS, is found in dogs in some of the same regions, and the parasite in them is indistinguishable from that found in human cases. The symptoms are similar. The principal, and often the only symptom, is wasting, with sometimes paralysis of the hind-quarters. The parasites are found in cells of the spleen, liver, and bone marrow. Affected dogs often suffer also from mange, and skin parasites (especially the sand flea) are blamed for transmitting the parasite. (*See* p. 634.)

KALE.—This contains a factor which gives rise to goitre if fed in large amounts, without other foods, over a long period. Hæmoglobinuria sometimes follows the grazing of frosted kale by cattle, which may suffer anæmia without showing this symptom. The illness can be serious, resembling POST-PARTURIENT HÆMOGLOBINURIA, and may result in sudden death. The frothy type of bloat may also occur in cattle eating excessive quantities of kale—especially, it seems, during wet weather, and when no hay is fed as well. There is some evidence to suggest that the feeding of large quantities of kale may lead to low conception rates, and to mastitis.

KAOLIN, or CHINESE CLAY, is a native aluminium silicate, which is used as a protective and astringent dry dusting powder. Kaolin is sometimes given internally as an adsorbent in intestinal disorders. Mixed into a paste with glycerine and some antiseptic, it is applied to acute sprains of tendons, to acutely inflamed tender organs such as the mammary gland and the testicle, and has superseded the old-fashioned linseed-poultice. 'Antiphlogistine' is the name of a proprietary kaolin poultice.

'KEBBING'.—Another name for Enzoötic Abortion of Sheep.

KED.—A parasite of sheep (*see under* PARASITES).

KEMPS.—Coarse hairs, the presence of which reduces the value of a fleece.

KENNEL LAMENESS.—A colloquial term for lameness arising from a nutritional deficiency, such as may occur in a dog fed entirely on dog-biscuits. (*See* RICKETS.)

KERATIN (κέρας, horn) is the substance of which horn and the surface layers of the skin are composed. It is a modified form of skin which has undergone compression and toughening. It is present in the hoof of the feet of animals, in claws, horns, and nails. (*See* FOOT OF HORSE.)

KERATITIS (κέρας, horn) means inflammation of the cornea, the clear part of the front of the eye. (*See* EYE, DISEASES OF.)

KERATOCELE.—A hernia through the cornea. (*See* EYE, DISEASES OF.)

KERATOMA (κέρας, horn, *-oma*, termination meaning tumour) is a horn tumour affecting the inner aspect of the wall of the hoof of the horse. It is a condition that may be present for a considerable period of time without causing any symptoms. It grows from the sensitive laminæ, and is often situated at the front of the hoof. It may be caused by pressure from a closely driven nail or from the toe-clip, but some cases appear to arise without any history of irritation. Sooner or later it will appear at the lower part of the wall on the inside of its circumference, in a position that is covered by the shoe. It may form a sinus leading up the wall, or the surface may be intact. In severe cases a keratoma will produce a groove by causing pressure and absorption along the outer surface of the pedal bone and render that latter liable to fracture. It is treated by surgical removal, but is likely to recur afterwards.

KETONE BODIES.—These arise from acteyl osenzyme A. They are not normal intermediates in the degradation of fatty acids, but are formed by special reactions to serve, together with free fatty acids, as a readily oxidizable fuel of oxidation in various tissues when the supply of glucose is restricted. The mild forms of ketosis, *e.g.* of starvation or of low carbohydrate diets, or of mild diaebtes, are physiological processes. 'The severe forms of ketosis of the diabetic coma or of the lactating cow are connected with the high rates of gluconeogenesis which occur under these conditions. Oxaloacetate, which is an intermediate in gluconeogenesis, is diverted from the tricarboxylic acid cycle to gluconeogenesis, owing to the high activity of the enzyme converting it to phosphopyruvate. The liver compensates the loss of energy from a reduced rate of the tricarboxylic acid cycle by an increased rate of oxidations outside the cycle. The main reaction of this type is the oxidation of fatty acids to ketone bodies. These arise grossly in excess of needs, as a by-product of reactions which satisfy the requirements for energy.'—(Prof. Sir Hans Krebs.)

Ketonuria is the term applied to the presence of these bodies in the urine.

KETOSIS (*see* ACETONÆMIA).

KICKING.—A great deal of misunderstanding exists concerning kicking in the horse. Many horse-owners look upon it as a vice only, but, while there are undoubtedly cases of vicious kickers, it is not too much to say that the *majority of horses do not kick because of viciousness.* Generally speaking, the horse prefers to depend upon his powers of speed for his safety, rather than upon his powers of self-defence, and it is most often under either immediate or remote provocation that the domestic horse will resort to kicking. In this connection it must be remembered that horses possess exceptionally long memories, and what they once learn they seldom forget. Authentic records of horses having 'savaged' unkind grooms long after the original cruelty occurred bear this out. Kicking in the horse can be looked upon as due to: (1) viciousness; (2) playfulness; and (3) disease.

(1) *Vicious horses* must be considered with the greatest amount of respect at all times, and every opportunity taken to teach the horse to associate the act of kicking with the infliction of some bodily punishment administered in a rational manner. This is by no means always easy. The horse has probably learnt that his show of physical superiority has overawed his 'master', and he therefore resorts to it whenever possible.

(2) *Playfulness* in a horse is often the result of either an insufficiency of exercise or work, or is induced by the attendants teasing the horse for the 'fun of seeing it kick'. As the consequences of a playful kick may be quite as serious as those of a vicious kick, both the above irregularities must be carefully guarded against. The teasing of a horse by a groom or stable-boy should be dealt with by the utmost severity, for it is by this most unfair treatment that many otherwise good horses are spoiled.

(3) *Disease* of the ovaries in the mare is responsible for those exhibitions of kicking, squealing, and the passage of urine often seen in the female. Cysts, multiple and small, or few and large, develop in the ovarian tissues, and, by their pressure, exercise an irritant effect on the nerve-endings in the organ, which appears to react throughout the whole system, producing either a condition of almost continuous season, or else an extreme irritability, which shows itself as a desire to kick upon the slightest provocation. The animal is diseased, and the disease needs to be dealt with. In extreme cases it is necessary to have a surgical operation performed, in which one or both ovaries are removed, or the cysts present are punctured.

KICKS (*see under* WOUNDS).

'**KIDNEY-DROPPING**', or 'JINKED BACK', are names that are loosely applied to various symptoms of weakness in the horse's back. Sometimes the terms refer to azoturia (*see* AZOTURIA), and at other times they are applied to that weakness that a horse will show when there is some obstruction in the arterial circulation of the hind-quarters of the body, such as thrombosis of the iliac arteries. When such a horse is being made to perform some very exacting work he will become weaker and weaker in the hind legs, and finally may sink to the ground into a sitting position. After remaining thus for a few seconds he will rise and continue as though nothing had occurred, but the process is repeated if the work continues to be severe. The condition is beyond cure. All that can be done is to ensure that the horse will get light, easy, slow work. In some parts of the country 'jinked back' is used to mean ankylosis of the spine.

KIDNEY WORM (*see* p. 665).

KIDNEYS are paired organs situated high up against the roof of the abdomen, and in most animals lying one on either side of the spinal column. Their function is the removal of certain waste products and water from the blood-stream, the excretion being called the 'urine'. The urine is carried away by the ureters—one from each kidney—and enters the urinary bladder, where it is stored until time and circumstances are convenient for its passage to the outside of the body by means of the urethra.

Horse.—The kidneys of the horse differ from each other both in shape and position. The right has the outline of a playing-card heart, and lies under the last two or three ribs and the transverse process of the 1st lumbar vertebra, while the left is roughly bean-shaped and lies under the last rib and the first two or three lumbar transverse processes. They are held in place by the surrounding organs and by fibrous tissue, called the renal fascia. Each of them moves slightly backwards and forwards during the respiratory movements of the animal.

Ox.—In the ox the kidneys are lobulated, each possessing from 20 to 25 lobes separated by fissures filled with fat in the living animal. The right kidney lies below the last rib and the first two or three lumbar transverse processes, and is somewhat elliptical in outline. The left occupies a variable position. When the rumen is full it pushes the left kidney over to the right side of the body into a position slightly below and behind the right organ, but when it is empty the left kidney lies underneath the vertebral column about the level of the 3rd to the 5th lumbar vertebra. It may lie partly on the left side of the body in this position in some cases.

Sheep.—In the sheep the kidneys are bean-shaped and smooth. In position they resemble those of the ox, except that the right is usually a little farther back.

Pig.—In this animal the kidneys are shaped like elongated beans, and they are placed almost symmetrically on either side of the bodies of the first four lumbar vertebræ. They sometimes vary in position.

Dog and Cat.—In these animals the kidneys are again bean-shaped, but they are thicker than in other animals, and relatively larger. As in most animals, the right kidney is placed farther forward than the left, the latter varying in position according to the degree of fullness of the digestive organs. In the cat the left kidney is very loosely attached and can usually be felt as a rounded mass which is quite movable in the anterior part of the abdominal cavity.

Structure.—The size of the kidneys varies in individuals according to their habit of life, and in different breeds according to the size of the adult. Typically the organ is enveloped in a fibrous coat continuous with the rest of the peritoneal membrane, and attached to the kidney capsule. This capsule does not permit of much swelling or enlargement of the organ, and consequently any inflammation of the kidney is attended with much pain. On the innermost border (*i.e.* that looking towards the spinal column) there is an indentation called the *hilus*, which acts as a place of entrance and exit for vessels, nerves, etc. Entering each kidney at its hilus are a renal artery and renal nerves; leaving the kidney are renal vein or veins, lymphatics, and the ureter. If the kidney be cut across there are two distinct areas seen in its substance. Lying outermost is the reddish-brown granular *cortex*, which contains small dark spots known as *glomeruli* or *Malpighian corpuscles*. Within the cortex is the *medulla*, an area presenting a radiated appearance, whose periphery is of a deep red colour. In this periphery there are seen the cut ends of the arciform vessels. If the kidney be compound, as in the ox, the medulla is seen raised into short blunt *papillæ*, which project into the funnel-shaped *pelvis*, from which the ureter takes its origin. In other animals these papillæ are not always distinct. Opening into the pelvis are the *papillary ducts*—the ends of collecting tubules that carry small amounts of urine to the pelvis. If one of these collecting tubules be traced upwards into the substance of the kidney it is found to split into a number of smaller tubules that pass right up through the medulla to the outer region of the cortex. Here each branches again into what are called *convoluted tubules*, and each of these after a very tortuous course ends in a glomerulus. In each glomerulus is a network of capillaries supplied by the terminations of the branches from the renal artery, and carrying blood to be relieved of its waste contents. Surrounding each of these bunches of capillaries are capsules (known as *Bowman's capsules*) which form the ends of the uriniferous tubules already described. The blood after circulating in the glomerulus is collected into a small vein which again splits up into a second set of capillaries that encircle the convoluted tubules. Once again it is collected into veins, and after these reunite many times, it finally leaves the kidney by the large renal vein at the hilus. By means of this double circulation, first through the glomerulus and then around the tube, it happens that a large amount of fluid is removed from the blood in the glomerulus, and then the concentrated blood passes on to the uriniferous tubule for removal of the waste part of its contents. The mixture of fluid and solid flows down the tubule and is collected in the pelvis, as the urine. The cells that form the tubules, etc., are nourished, not by the blood that is being purified, but by blood contained in other branches from the arciform arteries at the junction of

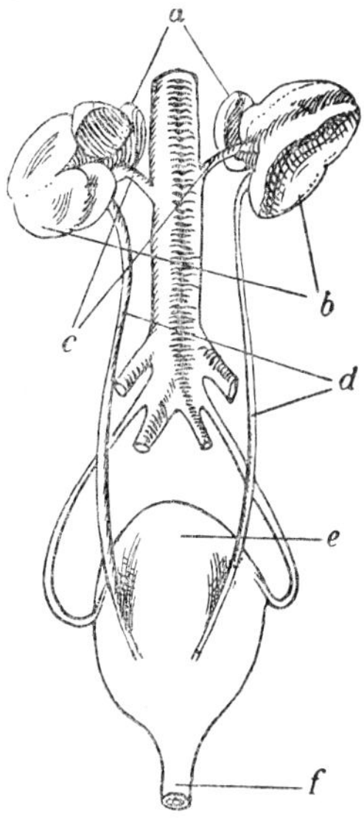

Diagram of the urinary apparatus of the horse. *a*, Adrenal glands; *b*, kidneys; *c*, renal arteries; *d*, ureters; *e*, bladder; *f*, urethra. The termination of the aorta is also shown lying between the ureters.

the cortex and medulla. After passing through a set of capillaries this blood is also collected and passed into the renal vein. In all animals, but especially in those of the cat tribe, there are arteries in the capsule of the kidney that assist in the circulation, and it is by dilatation of these that congestion or inflammation can be partly relieved by the application of hot packs to the region of the loins.

Function.—The chief function of the kidneys is to secrete or, more correctly, to excrete, urine from the blood-stream. In this process, solids which have been produced by the liver or by the activity of the tissues from the used-up material of the body are excreted. To keep these in solution a large amount of water is also excreted, and these two processes are, to a large extent, carried out by the different parts of the kidney. The watery part of the urine, as already mentioned, passes through the walls of the capillaries forming the glomerulus, into the interior of Bowman's capsule, by a process that may be roughly described as filtration, the cells forming the capillary walls exercising a selective action and allowing water to pass through, though in health they keep back the albumin, sugar, and other important constituents of the blood. It has been shown by Nussbaum, from experiments upon the kidney of the newt, which has separate blood-vessels for the glomeruli and for the tubules, that various salts and peptones are also extracted from the blood by the glomeruli. The fluid passed into Bowman's capsule runs from it down the much convoluted uriniferous tubule. The tubule, on the other hand, upon whose walls run capillaries containing highly concentrated blood, excretes the urea, uric acid, and other solids of the urine, and these solids are washed out and down into the pelvis by the water passing down the tubule from the glomerulus. That solids are excreted by the cells lining these tubules has been proved by Heidenhain, who experimented by injecting indigo into the blood-vessels of animals, and finding after death that these cells and the interior of the tubules contained quantities of the blue pigment.

When the kidneys fail to act, these solid waste substances accumulate in the blood, producing a condition of urine poisoning called 'uræmia', which, if not speedily relieved, soon causes death. The condition receives its name from urea, which is the chief waste product excreted by the kidneys, though in all probability it is not the substance mainly responsible for the poisoning.

KIDNEYS, DISEASES OF.—Owing to the large amount of tissue around the kidneys it is usually very difficult to examine the kidneys other than indirectly, and upon this account many diseases of these organs are not noticed when the animals are alive; it is only in the post-mortem room that the conditions are discovered. Moreover, partly by reason of their deep position in the body, and partly because of the inability of an animal to communicate to man the exact seat of pain or discomfort, symptoms of kidney disease are very often referred to other abdominal organs or to the muscles of the back. Exact diagnosis is based almost entirely upon macroscopic, microscopic, and chemical examinations of the urine in a laboratory.

Horse.—ACUTE NEPHRITIS is an inflammation of the kidney tissues as a whole, or of the glomerulæ and the secreting tubules only. The latter is much the more common among all animals. Since the diagnosis and symptoms of each are clinically the same, and as their differentiation is only possible by microscopic examination after death, it will suffice to describe the commoner type only.

Causes.—An acute attack generally arises from injuries to the tissues around the kidney which involve the kidneys themselves to a greater or lesser extent, depending upon the severity and the amount of damage done. Among these may be noted falls, contusions, blows, sudden reining-in when the horse is travelling at full speed, and sometimes injuries at foaling. Exposure to cold, chills, and draughts, by lowering the vitality of the kidneys and rendering them an easy prey to organisms, is a common cause. Poisonous agents, such as turpentine, cantharides, carbolic acid, and phosphorus, are to blame for some cases, and the products given off by fodder that is mouldy or damaged account for others. In addition to the above, certain infectious diseases, such as influenza, contagious pneumonia, and others, are sometimes complicated by acute inflammation of the kidneys.

Symptoms.—The symptoms shown by a horse suffering from this condition are obscure, but dull colicky pains, the passage of small amounts of highly-coloured urine at frequent intervals, arching of back, a stiff, awkward gait, and pain over the loins with difficulty in turning sharply round, suggest kidney trouble. There is always a certain degree of fever, but this depends on the case. In some cases food is refused, no urine is passed for several days, and the horse periodically breaks out in a sweat. The urine, when passed, usually has a high reddish or brownish colour in the early stages, and later it may become milky and curdled-looking. Collections of dropsical fluid often appear along the under parts of the abdomen, around the sheath, legs, and sometimes in the eyelids and throat. Abdominal dropsy may be seen, and water may form on the chest.

Treatment.—It is necessary to give the kidneys rest. No exercise may be allowed, no nitrogenous foods, such as oats, beans, peas, or feeding-cakes, should be given; the horse should be allowed plenty of water to drink, and the food should consist of gruels, linseed tea, sloppy bran mashes, milk, etc., with small quantities of alkaline substances, such as bicarbonate of soda or potash, and small amounts of salt should be allowed daily. The bowels must be kept moving by oily laxatives, and the horse should be provided with a warm rug over the loins. If the pain in the loins is great it is advisable to apply a hot pack of salt, or a wet pack (made by wringing a blanket out of hot water and applying it direct to the region, and covering with a dry rug). All drugs that have an irritating effect on the kidneys, such as nitre, turpentine, caffeine, and those that interfere with urinary secretion, such as the opiates, must be avoided. Should the secretion of the urine cease and the animal evince a distinct sour, urine-like smell from its breath, it is not likely to recover. Antibiotics are used.

Preventative measures should be taken by avoiding chills, etc., during the course of fevers and infectious diseases, by care in the use of the drugs above mentioned as causes, by continual supervision of the food and rejection of such as is not sound; and during convalescence from an attack the animal should not be given large quantities of nitrogenous foods in a vain endeavour rapidly to rebuild its lost strength, for serious and often fatal relapses attend such conduct.

CHRONIC NEPHRITIS is rare in the horse.

Causes.—Chronic inflammation may be a sequel to the acute form, or it may be due to the ingestion of harmful substances. such as lead in herbage, bad food, etc.

Symptoms.—The chief signs are similar to those of the acute type, but less severe. The temperature does not rise, food is taken; sometimes the horse passes considerable amounts of urine and at other times hardly any at all he shows slight pains at times when at work or exercise, may arch his back occasionally, becomes fatigued on slight exertion, and ceases to thrive in spite of good food and proper attention. The coat stares and is scurfy to excess, and a faint smell of urine is perceptible from the breath and often from the fæces.

Ox.—ACUTE NEPHRITIS is often produced during the course of infectious diseases, such as pneumonia, malignant catarrh, mastitis, and tuberculosis; it may occur as the result of large doses of the substances mentioned as blameworthy in the case of the horse; it has been produced through feeding on acorns; and colds, chills, and infection with *Corynebacterium renale*. (*See also* PYELONEPHRITIS, LEPTOSPIROSIS.)

Symptoms.—The ox stands in a rigid position, with its back arched; the amount of the urine is small; it is passed often, it may be blood-stained, and is absent in some cases. The appetite is lost, rumination ceases, tympany of the rumen may occur, temperature is elevated, and the pulse and respiration rates are increased. Convulsions and unconsciousness, denoting retention of urine in the blood-stream, may be seen, and are usually indicative of approaching death. The course is rapid, and either death or recovery takes place in from 2 to 5 days as a rule.

Treatment.—The principles of treatment given for the horse are equally applicable to the ox.

CHRONIC NEPHRITIS is but seldom noted before death in the ox, but is occasionally found in slaughterhouses and during the making of post-mortem examinations. (*See also* LEPTOSPIROSIS.)

Sheep and Pig.—NEPHRITIS in these animals generally arises during the course of specific diseases, such as hæmorrhagic septicæmia in sheep, and swine fever and swine erysipelas in the pig; in the pig it also occurs as a result of infection with *Corynebacterium suis*. (*See* PYELONEPHRITIS.)

Dog.—ACUTE NEPHRITIS.—This is common in the dog, and was formerly often diagnosed as gastritis on account of the vomiting. Many cases are associated with LEPTOSPIROSIS.

Symptoms.—In the early stages little or no urine may be passed; sometimes the urine is blood-stained. Vomiting is frequent, there is excessive thirst, fever, straining, and often arching of the back, together with stiffness. Ulceration of the mouth may occur. In very severe cases a condition of uræmia may be set up, indicated by convulsions. A test for albumen assists or confirms the diagnosis.

Treatment.—The animal should be warmly clothed and allowed to rest and fed upon easily digested, demulcent, laxative foods, such as broths made weak, gruels, barley-water, milk, Allenbury's, Mellin's, or Benger's foods. Water in limited amounts may be given to drink, but the patient must never be allowed to drink *ad lib*. After the excessive excretion of urine has passed off, gentle exercise is allowed, and the animal is gradually brought back on to its normal diet. Antibiotic drugs may be used.

CHRONIC NEPHRITIS (sometimes still referred to as Bright's Disease). This may be a sequel to an acute attack or it may occur insidiously without any acute inflammation having previously taken place. It is common in old or middle-aged dogs. (*See* RUBBER JAW.)

Symptoms.—The animal becomes thin, vaguely unwell, occasionally vomits, and often shows stiffness and periodic loss of appetite.

Treatment.—It is important to reduce the amount of exercise and to prevent, as far as possible, chills—which may lead to an acute attack of nephritis, often with fatal results. Put the animal on to barley water for a week or two, avoid giving fish, meat in quantity, but instead for a time try Benger's, milk puddings, brown bread, cod-liver oil and malt. Heart tonics are often indicated.

PURULENT NEPHRITIS, or 'suppurative nephritis', is a condition in which one or both kidneys show abscess formation. All species may be affected. It is caused by pus-producing (pyogenic) organisms, which may gain access to the kidneys either by the blood-stream—when the term *pyæmic nephritis* is used, or by the ureters from the bladder—when the condition is *pyelonephritis*. *Pyelitis*, meaning pus in the pelvis of the kidney, is used to indicate abscess formation in the pelvis only, and generally precedes the more severe form of pyelonephritis. It may be associated with stone formation (renal calculus).

Symptoms.—Pyæmic nephritis is always difficult to diagnose, and it is often only on post-mortem that the condition is revealed. It is usually associated with, or follows soon after, some general purulent infection, such as distemper complications, the organisms settling in the kidney cortex and forming many small abscesses. These may burst and pus will be discharged in the urine, but the condition often proves fatal before this happens. The symptoms shown by the animal are unsteady gait, weakness of the hind-limbs, pain on pressure over the loins, an irregular temperature, sometimes high and sometimes low, and death occurring after only a short illness.

Pyelonephritis is generally preceded by an attack of inflammation of the bladder, vagina, or uterus. It is commonest in cows and mares after parturition when the genital tract has become septic, but it is seen in all females under similar circumstances. It is not so common in male animals. Generally only one kidney is affected, and the animal exhibits pain when turned sharply to the affected side, and tenderness when that side is handled.

Pyelitis shows symptoms that are practically the same as those of pyelonephritis, except when due to renal calculus. In such cases it causes an obscure form of colic, and small amounts of blood-stained urine are passed at frequent intervals.

The differentiation of these varying forms is based upon the microscopic examination of the urine. In all cases pus in some form or another may be found. The organisms responsible can be isolated from the urine by culturing, and when a stone is present tiny crystals, or epithelium casts of the pelvis, may be passed and recovered from the urine.

Treatment.—In the smaller animals, when the condition only involves one kidney, excision of the affected organ may be followed by recovery—the remaining healthy organ enlarging and undertaking the functions of both—but this is impossible in horses and cattle, or where both kidneys are affected. In such cases but little can be done. Slaughter of the animal is recommended, either upon humane or economic grounds.

STONE IN THE KIDNEY.—A calculus or stone may sometimes form in the pelvis of the kidney as the result of the gradual deposition of salts from the urine around some particle of matter that acts as a nucleus. The diet of the animal has a considerable influence upon the formation of stone; foods rich in phosphates and calcium salts are at least predisposing causes. Among these commonly blamed in this respect are bran, pea, and bean straw, lucerne, bones, meat, fish, etc., given in excess, and excessively hard water, but it is not probable that food alone will produce a calculus.

Symptoms.—The symptoms are very vague, and resemble those seen in pyelonephritis. The urine is often blood-stained, and contains albumin. That voided at the end of micturition often shows a certain amount of greyish-yellow sandy or gritty deposit. This can sometimes be noticed on a concrete stable floor immediately after urine is passed, but care must be taken not to confuse it with the sand that is sometimes used for preventing slipping in the stable. In many cases the animal becomes seized with an intense spasmodic pain to which the name 'renal colic' is applied. These spasms last for an hour or more and then usually pass off. They recur at irregular intervals. Usually the condition affects only one kidney and the other one enlarges to fulfil the functions of both.

Treatment.—It is impossible to administer any drugs that exert a solvent action upon a stone already present, but by a well-balanced diet and the giving of common salt to induce a thirst and the subsequent large amount of water that flushes through the kidneys, a great deal may be done to keep a stone from growing larger at a rapid rate. Soft water should be supplied to all animals. Urinary sedatives and antiseptics should be given, such as hyoscyamus and hexamine.

PARASITES OF THE KIDNEY include LEPTOSPIRA in the dog, and occasionally *Eustrongylus gigas* in horses, dogs, and cattle, the larvæ of *Strongylus vulgaris* in colts, *Stephanurus dentatus* in pigs, and the cystic stages of certain tapeworms in the ruminants, are of most importance. (*See* PARASITES *and* LEPTOSPIROSIS).

TUMOURS OF THE KIDNEY are not common in animals.

CYSTS OF THE KIDNEY.—Under certain circumstances not well understood, but probably as the result of a localised inflammation, retention cysts occur in the kidneys. They appear as swellings containing fluid under the capsule. As a rule they do not cause any trouble unless they burst, when they may set up a uræmic peritonitis which ends fatally. The condition is technically known as 'hydronephrosis'.

INJURIES OF THE KIDNEY are not common, owing to the great protection that the lumbar muscles provide. They may be lacerated or bruised as the result of run-over accidents in the dog. Slips or falls in the hunting field may cause similar injuries. The kidney may be shattered and death from internal hæmorrhage occurs, or in less severe cases the hæmorrhage takes place below the capsule and blood is passed in the urine. If only one kidney is affected, and provided the bleeding is not great, the other hypertrophies and acts for both. The animal should be kept quiet, and as a first-aid measure hot applications should be applied over the loins.

KIMBERLEY HORSE DISEASE, or WALK-ABOUT DISEASE.—This was first described by Murnane and Ewart in 1928. It occurs in the Kimberley district of W Australia, and has a seasonal incidence—January to April (*i.e.* 'wet season'). Horses of all ages are susceptible.

Cause.—Whitewood (*Atalaya hemiglauca*) taken voluntarily or fed when food is scarce.

Symptoms.—Anorexia, dullness, wasting, irritability, biting other horses, and gnawing at posts. Yawning is a marked and almost constant sign Then muscular spasms lead to a phase of mad galloping in which the horse has no sense of direction and is uncontrollable. Gallops become more frequent but less violent, and gradually merge into the walking stage—slow, staggering gait, with low, stiff carriage of the head. The horse may walk about for hours, with a mouthful of unchewed grass protruding from its lips. (*See also* BIRDSVILLE DISEASE.)

'KINKY-BACK.'—The colloquial name for a condition in broiler chickens involving distortion of the sixth thoracic vertabra. It is the cause of lameness and sometimes paraplegia. It appears to be of hereditary origin, perhaps influenced by growth-rate.

KIRSCHNER-EHMER SPLINT.—Used in treating fractures in the dog and cat. It has transverse pins which are driven into parts of a long bone on either side of the fracture, and which are then held in position by an external clamp.

KLEBSIELLA.—It was suggested that *Klebsiella pneumoniæ* was an important cause of infertility in the Thoroughbred mare, and that this infection constitutes a venereal disease in the horse. The latter point was *not* substantiated by Lord Porchester's Commission (*see under* UTERINE INFECTIONS), but '*Klebsiella* may be passed on mechanically by a stallion from one mare to another'. The infection is not regarded as an incurable one, though its control may be difficult once it has become established in a mare.

In the dog.—Klebsiella infection may cause illness clinically indistinguishable from distemper, and may therefore account for some of the suspected 'breakdowns' following the use of distemper vaccines.

In the sow.—The infection may result in acute mastitis. Both piglets and sow may die.

KLEIN'S DISEASE (*see* FOWL TYPHOID).

KNEE is the name, wrongly applied, to the carpus of the horse, ox, sheep, and pig. This joint really corresponds to the human wrist and should not be called 'knee', but custom has ordained otherwise. (*See* JOINTS.)

KNEE-GALL, or KNEE THOROUGHPIN, is a distension of the carpal sheath at the back of the joint in the horse. It is sometimes a serious condition, especially when it is associated with some general infectious disease such as strangles, influenza, pneumonia, etc., or with a wound that has become infected. A sausage-shaped swelling appears at the back of the knee-joint, extending from an inch or two above the carpus down to the middle of the cannon. It may be tense and painful if it is acute and has appeared suddenly, or if chronic it is soft, fluctuating, and generally painless. The most common causes are overwork, strains, etc., involving over-extension of the joint and consequent damage to the tendon sheath.

Treatment.—In acute forms, cold applications by means of the hose-pipe, followed by bandaging with cotton-wool and an elastic rubber or flannel bandage on the outside, give the best results. In more chronic cases, where the contents of the swelling are solid, it is not always possible to reduce the galls. They may be treated by surgical removal.

KNEE SPAVIN, or CHRONIC INFLAMMATION OF THE KNEE-JOINT, is a diseased condition of the small bones of the carpus, which in many respects resembles bone spavin in the hock. Its causes are to a great extent the same, its symptoms are similar, and its treatment follows the same lines. It is, however, a more serious condition than spavin in the hind-limb, because when fixation or fusion of the small bones of the knee takes place there is likely to be some interference in the freedom of flexion of the joint, since in the knee there is not a single main joint as there is in the hock. In the knee each small joint between the bones of both rows takes an almost equal part in the flexion of the whole joint, and any impediment in one reacts upon the flexion of the joint as a whole. (*See* BONE SPAVIN.)

KNEE SPLINT is the name applied to a splint in the fore-limb of the horse when it occurs high up near to the knee-joint. It usually involves the head of one of the small metacarpal or splint bones, and may lead to an exostosis which impedes the movement of the knee-joint. As a rule the higher a splint is situated the more serious it is. (*See* SPLINTS IN HORSES.)

KNOCKED-UP SHOE is one in which the inner branch is hammered laterally so as to increase its height but decrease its width. There is one nail-hole at the inside toe, and four or five along the outside branch. The shoe generally has a clip at the toe and the outside quarter, and may have a small calkin on the outside heel.

It is used for horses given to brushing, cutting, or interfering with their hind-feet.

KNOCKED-UP TOE.—A term used in racing greyhound circles to describe a type of lameness associated with the digits. It sometimes yields to rest but may require surgical treatment (even amputation of the third phalanx).

KNUCKLING OF FETLOCK or OVER-SHOT FETLOCKS. The phrase simply means that the fetlock joints are kept slightly flexed forwards above the hoof, instead of remaining extended.

Knuckling of the fetlocks in calves of the Jersey, Ayrshire, and Friesian breeds is an inherited defect which can sometimes be corrected by a minor surgical operation.

Occasionally foals are born with their fetlocks knuckled, but, like many other deformities of a similar nature, the condition gradually disappears as the muscles of the young animal obtain their proper control of the joints which they actuate. In older horses the two chief conditions that are responsible for knuckling are: (1) Thickening and contraction of the tendons or ligaments behind the cannon; and (2) chronic foot lameness, such as is produced by ring-bones, navicular disease, chronic corns, etc. The horse assumes the position of partial flexion of the fetlock apparently in order to ease the pain he feels in one or other of these structures, and as the result of the relaxation of the tendons, shortening occurs, and it finally becomes impossible to straighten out the joint.

Symptoms.—By itself the condition is not a painful one, but some one or other of the causes which produce it may be associated with pain, so that it is wrong to conclude that all horses that show knuckling are quite fit for work. As a rule the degree of knuckling is no indication of the actual cause, nor yet of its seriousness. A chronic thickened flexor tendon may produce excessive flexion of the joint although the horse feels no pain. On the other hand, a ring-bone may only cause a slight amount of knuckling, and yet be painful enough to make the horse go very lame. Generally, horses with fetlocks that are knuckled over are only fitted for easy work at slow paces, and if called upon to exceed their usual pace they begin to stumble and may fall.

Treatment.—This depends upon the cause of the flexion. In many cases little can be done beyond shoeing in such a way that the horse may be able to obtain as much ease as possible, *i.e.* by the application of calkins to the heels, and by rolling the toes. This advice applies particularly to those cases in which the tendons are the seat of chronic inflammation. In other cases where there is no inflammatory process at work, and where the tendons have become shortened through enforced inaction, it is necessary to elongate the toes of the shoe and to reduce the heels, so that the tendons are subjected to a certain amount of stretch each time the foot comes to the ground. Surgical division of the contracted tendons sometimes gives good results, but it is an operation requiring that other conditions, such as age, conformation, etc., shall be favourable, and necessitating the greatest care in the after-treatment.

(*Note.*—For descriptive purposes the word 'flexion' in this article means a bending backwards of the lower section of the limb from the fetlock joint—the cannon remaining stationary. Otherwise confusion between 'flexion' and 'extension' of the fetlock might occur.)

KYASANUR FOREST FEVER.—This is a disease of man and monkeys, occurring in Mysore, and resembling Omsk Fever. The causal virus is transmitted by the tick *Hæmaphysalis spinigera*, and believed to have been brought by birds from the Soviet Union.

KYPHOSIS (κυφός, bent) is the term applied to a curvature of the spine when the concavity of the curve is directed downwards. It is sometimes seen in tetanus, rabies, etc., and is a symptom of abdominal pain in the dog.

L

L-FORMS OF BACTERIA.—Those which can survive without a true cell wall. L-forms of staphylococci and streptococci have been recovered from cases of mastitis, and they are completely resistant to antibiotics such as penicillin which interferes with bacterial cell-wall formation.

LABIAL.—Relating to the lips.

LABILE.—Unstable. Thermo-labile—unstable in the presence of heat.

LABIUM is the Latin word for lip or lip-shaped organ.

LABOUR (*see* PARTURITION).

LABURNUM POISONING.—All parts of the plant, whose botanical name is *Cytisus laburnum*—root, wood, bark, leaves, flowers, and particularly the seeds in their pods—are poisonous, and all the domestic animals and birds are susceptible.

Symptoms.—The toxic agent is an alkaloid called *cytisine*, which produces firstly excitement, then unconsciousness with inco-ordination of movement, and finally convulsions and death.

In the horse, when small amounts have been taken, there is little to be seen beyond a staggering gait, yawning, and a general abnormality in the behaviour of the animal. With larger doses the horse shows, in addition to the above symptoms, sexual excitement, sweating, muscular tremors, rapidity and noisiness of breathing, and later falls to the ground. In this position it cannot rise; the breathing becomes slow; heart-action is irregular; the temperature falls; and the animal becomes unconscious or dies in great agony.

In cattle and sheep, which are more resistant than the horse, the stomach becomes filled with gas, the limbs become paralysed, the pupils are dilated, the animal becomes sleepy, and later, salivation, coma, and convulsive movements follow each other. Fatal cases in these animals are not common; the symptoms may last for several days and then gradually pass off.

In the dog and pig, which vomit easily, the irritant and acrid nature of the plant causes free vomiting, and usually the animal is enabled to get rid of what has been eaten before the symptoms become acute. In other cases there is a similarity to what is seen in the horse.

Treatment.—There is no known specific antidote. Any treatment must aim at the elimination of the plant from the body, either by the stomach tube, by operation, or by the free use of non-irritant purgatives such as oils, treacle, and salts, etc.; and by giving heart stimulants. Tannic acid combines with the alkaloid to form an insoluble tannate. Very strong black tea or coffee that has been *boiled* instead of infused may be given as a drench.

LACOMBE.—A lop-eared pig from Alberta, Canada. Breeding: Danish Landrace 51 per cent, Chester White 25 per cent, Berkshire 24 per cent. (The Chester White comes from Pennsylvania, and originates from 18th-century imports.) The import of Lacombes was sanctioned in 1966.

LACRIMAL, or LACHRYMAL (*lacrima*, a tear) apparatus is the arrangement connected with the eye, for the moistening and cleansing of this organ. (*See* EYE.)

LACTATION (*lac*, milk) is the period during which the female animal is actively producing milk. It depends directly upon the fact that if the milk is not regularly removed the secretion will cease. It reaches its maximum duration in the cow and goat, which are milked by human agency for the production of milk for consumption. By this artificial method the duration of lactation and the quantities of milk have been enormously increased.

The definition of a lactation is now 305 days, commencing from calving and ending when the cow ceases to be milked at least twice a day and this is in line with other European records. The period for butterfat sampling continues to be from the fourth day after calving.

To produce 2000 gallons of milk the cow must secrete over $9\frac{1}{2}$ tons of milk from the mammary gland, *e.g.* roughly about twelve or fourteen times the weight of her whole body. That remarkable British Friesian cow, Manningford Faith Jan Graceful, which died at the age of $17\frac{1}{2}$, gave a lifetime yield of 145 tons, 14 cwt., 85 lbs.; and her highest 365-day yield—with her third calf—was 3829·5 gallons. A Jersey has, in 361 days, given over 2666 gallons

(1157·46 lbs. butterfat). An Ayrshire, Theale Maude 12th, established a world breed record in giving 20·1119 gallons milk (7371 lbs. butterfat) in 12 lactations, and was still milking. Another Ayrshire has produced over 3295 gallons at 3·73 per cent butterfat in 365 days. (*See* MILK YIELD, MAMMARY GLAND, MILK, WEANING; *also* section on Dairy Breeds of Cattle, *under* CATTLE, BREEDS OF.)

LACTATION, ARTIFICIAL.—The artificial induction of lactation may be brought about by means of hormones. For example, barren, anœstrus ewes have been rendered good foster-mothers to lambs by a single dose of 40 mg. stilbœstrol diproprionate in oil. (*See also under* SPAYING.)

LACTATION TETANY (*see* HYPOMAGNESÆMIA *and* HYPOCALCÆMIA).

LACTIC ACID (*see* MILK).—Excessive production of lactic acid in the rumen—such as occurs after cattle have gorged themselves with grain—is a serious condition, and is followed by absorption of fluid from the general circulation (with consequent dehydration), ruminal stasis, and often death.

LACTOSE.—Sugar of milk. (*See* SUGAR.)

LAKES (*see* ALGÆ POISONING, LEECHES).

LAMB DYSENTERY is an infectious ulcerative inflammation of the small and large intestine of young lambs, usually under ten days old, and characterised by a high mortality and an alarming tendency to spread and to attack larger and larger number of lambs year by year. It is a disease which has become a very serious menace to sheep farmers, particularly in the north of England and the south of Scotland. During recent years it has spread to Wales, and it appears to be spreading farther and farther each year.

When a farm becomes infected there are certain almost uniform features of the disease seen during the first few years until it becomes established. In the first year, only about a dozen lambs or so are lost towards the end of the lambing season; in the second year, perhaps 25 to 40 lambs die; in the third year, 50 to 60; in the fourth anything from 40 per cent to 60 per cent of the total number born.

When the disease first appears upon a farm it almost always attacks the lambs born towards the end of the lambing season, especially those dropped by late lambing ewes which have been drawn out from the rest of the flock, and are 'shed in' into a paddock or park near to the shepherd's cottage or the farm steading. In this way the ground of such enclosures becomes fouled, and as the sheep are frequently brought into these places for washing, hoof-trimming, dipping, clipping, drafting, and sorting, opportunity for contamination of the sheep is freely given.

Cause.—*Clostridium welchii*, type B. This organism is one of the gas gangrene group. After birth the lamb runs every risk of getting infection from its mother's udder, from the soiled wool of the hind-quarters, or from the soil itself. In other cases infection seems to occur through healthy living lambs smelling or nibbling at dead or moribund lambs which are infected with the disease. It should be noted that the first 24 hours of life are the most critical, the susceptibility then being greatest, and it is during this period that the newly born lamb can be protected by serum, as will be explained later.

Symptoms.—In the acute type nothing seems to be wrong with the lambs at night, but in the morning two or three are found dead. If symptoms appear during the day, lambs are seen to become suddenly dull and listless; they stop sucking and lie about half-asleep; their mother's bleat passes unregarded; if made to move they do so stiffly and painfully. When they attempt to pass dung there is difficulty and pain, but the dung at first is not altered in any way. Later, the fæces become brownish-red in colour (sometimes yellow), semi-liquid, and are often tinged with bright red blood. After a few hours in this state, the lamb becomes unconscious and dies. In less acute forms, the lamb may live for two or three days; it shows the same symptoms, but they are not so severe. In those cases occurring on farms which have been infected for a number of years, and those in older lambs, the first suspicious symptom is that the lamb lags behind its mother; she waits for it, and both get left behind the rest of the flock when they are being driven or when the sheep are shifting over a hill. The ewe's udder fills with milk, and the lamb only sucks in a half-hearted manner, or not at all. Its back is arched, its abdomen appears empty, and clinging to the short wool around the tail there is a mass of brownish or yellowish-red diarrhœic material, which has an extremely foul odour. The lamb becomes weaker and weaker, prefers lying in almost any posture and in almost any position, no matter how cold or exposed, and it soon passes into a state of unconsciousness, terminating in death in 1 to 4 hours.

Post-mortem examination.—When a dead lamb is opened and the contents of its abdomen examined, the bowels are usually found to be intensely inflamed. The peritoneal cavity may be full of fluid, or there may be only a small amount of thick gluey material which causes the gut to adhere to other organs. If a piece of the inflamed bowel is examined it is seen to be studded with small ulcers, usually best seen from the outside. Bowel contents are liquid and blood-tinged, and possess a very objectionable odour. The liver is larger and paler than normal, but otherwise there are no well-marked changes.

Prevention.—Two methods: The newly born lamb is injected as soon after birth as possible, and not later than 12 hours, with lamb dysentery antiserum. This gives it a passive immunity enduring long enough to protect throughout the dangerous period—generally about 3 weeks. A dual-purpose vaccine to give protection against both lamb dysentery and pulpy kidney disease is now available. An extra dose of this vaccine in the autumn will protect the ewes against enterotoxæmia (as pulpy kidney disease in the adult is usually called). (*See also under* VACCINATION.)

LAMBING, LAMBS (*see under* SHEEP BREEDING).

LAMBING DIFFICULTIES.—Abnormality of the fœtus, or its malpresentation, accounts for a high proportion of 'difficult lambings'. The failure of the cervix to dilate is another frequent cause of difficulty, which can usually be overcome by a veterinary surgeon. (*See* 'RINGWOMB'; *also* VAGINA, RUPTURE OF)

LAMBING SICKNESS IN EWES, which is also called parturient hypocalcæmia, or milk fever in ewes, is a condition similar to milk fever in cows. The symptoms and treatment are the same. It may be mistaken for Pregnancy Toxæmia or Louping Ill. (*See* 'MOSS ILL'.)

LAMELLA is a small disc of glycerin jelly containing an active drug for application to the eye. It is applied by inserting within the lower lid. The four official lamellæ are those containing atropine, cocaine, homatropine, and physostigmine.

LAMENESS.—It is proverbially difficult to define lameness, but since the majority of people understand what is meant by the term, a definition is not important. It consists of a departure from the normal gait, occasioned by disease or injury situated in some part of the limbs or trunk, and is usually accompanied by pain. It has been described as 'the language of pain in the limbs', but this is not correct, for there are certain forms of lameness which are definitely not associated with pain or tenderness; such are usually called 'mechanical lamenesses'. (*See also* RICKETS.) In simple cases lameness is not difficult to diagnose; but in obscure cases, and in those instances where more than one limb is affected, it may be extremely difficult for any one, professional or otherwise, to determine where the lameness is, and to what it is due.

It is important to remember that lameness in cattle, sheep, and pigs may be the first symptom of **foot-and-mouth disease.**

Causes of lameness also include: in **cattle:** foul-in-the-foot, fluorosis, laminitis, and 'milk lameness'

sheep: footrot, erysipelas infection. (*See under* SWINE ERYSIPELAS *and* DIPS AND DIPPING)

pigs: Bush foot, foot-rot, swine erysipelas.

In all species fracture of a bone may be the cause; or injuries to joints, ligaments, tendons or muscles.

The following remarks refer especially to the horse, but they are to a great extent applicable to the other four-footed animals

Signs of lameness.—The most characteristic and easily seen feature of practically all forms of lameness is some unusuality in the manner of nodding the head, either at the walk or the trot. Normally, the horse's head rises and falls to the same extent at each step, and, in lesser measure, the point of the croup (i.e. the highest part of the hind-quarters) follows the same course. If a horse be made to walk alongside a blank wall, the head is seen to describe a wavy line against the wall, the undulations of which are equal, provided the rate of the gait is uniform. In a lame horse these undulations become unequal. For purposes of description, the four-footed animal will be considered as being formed of two bipeds which are united together by a more or less rigid bar (the spinal column), which projects forward farther than the anterior pair of limbs, and has a weight (the head) hung on to its anterior extremity. When a biped animal, such as a man, is lame on one limb to such an extent that it cannot be placed upon the ground, progression, if it takes place at all, must consist of a succession of hops from the sound leg back on to it again. During this time the lame member swings through the air. The head in such cases *rises* when the *sound leg is off the ground*, and *falls* when the *sound leg is on the ground.* In less severe cases the affected member may rest upon the ground for a short period during the stride, but the greater part of the work of propelling the body forward falls upon the sound leg. In other words, the sound leg still makes a succession of hops, and the head rises and falls as before, in spite of the fact that the lame leg is coming to the ground. This principle holds good in the two separate bipeds of the horse, just as it does in man. The withers of a horse which is lame in one of its two fore-legs, rise when the lame leg is on the ground, and fall when the sound leg comes to earth. And this rising and falling is transferred along the rigid bar of the neck to the head. Accordingly, when a horse is lame in this way, its head is said to nod heavy on the sound leg, and to rise on the lame leg.

When this explanation is applied to the hind pair of limbs, every fact fits except so far as the rise and fall of the head are concerned. The croup rises when the lame leg is on the ground, and falls when the sound limb is there. But the croup is connected by a rigid bar, passing over a fulcrum (the withers), with the head. It will be seen, therefore, that any rising of the croup will cause a lowering of the head, since the spinal column acts as a lever working over a fulcrum. In the horse which is lame on one of its hind limbs, therefore, the head falls when the croup rises, that is, when the lame leg is on the ground ; it rises when the sound leg is on the ground. In other words, it behaves in a manner opposite to its behaviour when the lame limb is situated in front ; the diagonally opposite hind-leg is indicated.

Apart from the nodding of the head there are other very important signs of lameness in the four-footed animal. In the first place the length of the stride may be increased or decreased. It does not follow that a limb which makes a short stride is that which is lame, for in lamenesses that are situated at the toe of the foot the stride taken by the lame limb is almost invariably lengthened, and the foot is snatched up rapidly almost as soon as the sound foot has passed it in the stride. This fact has a human as well as animal application. The noise made by the lame limb falling to the ground is always less than the noise made by the sound limb, for obvious reasons. The lame limb may be lifted higher than the sound one during the walk, as in cases of sand-crack at the toe (often called 'symptomatic stringhalt' when affecting a hind limb), or, more often, it is not lifted so high (in most cases of pain in joints or in flexor tendons). On soft ground the footprint made by the lame leg is never so deep as that made by the sound leg, although this fact is not of great practical importance. In most lamenesses of the hindmost pair of limbs, the point of the haunch (external angle of the ilium) is carried higher on the same side as the lameness exists. This is most pronounced in lamenesses which involve the joints in greater pain when they are flexed. The raising of the pelvis on the same side as the lameness enables the foot to clear the ground during the stride with a lessened amount of flexion than would otherwise be the case. Finally, there may be some peculiarity of the swing of the lame limb through the air. It may be carried outward away from the normal straight line of flight (abducted), or it may be carried too near to the other limb (adducted). Some of these variations can be best determined by holding before the observer's eyes a piece of paper, or an envelope, etc., which can be used to cut off from view the whole of the upper part of the horse, and only allow the limbs to be seen, and to have the horse walked or trotted past.

Determining the lame limb.—The observer should see the horse walked away from him, towards him, and then past him at right angles. The horse should then be trotted in the same way. If he watches the head carefully, he will see how it is nodding, and as soon as he gets the rhythm of the nods he should immediately commence nodding his own head at the same rate. When he is sure that he is nodding in time with the horse's head, he should at once drop his eyes to the horse's fore-feet, and determine which fore-foot comes to the ground when the nod of his head is downwards. Having decided which fore-leg corresponds with a downward nod of the horse's head, he can state that the horse is lame either on the opposite fore-leg, or else the hind-leg of the same side. He should now attempt to decide whether the lameness is in the anterior pair of limbs or in the posterior pair. To do this it is necessary to observe carefully, with the aid of an envelope if necessary (see previously), in which pair of limbs there is some discrepancy in movement, either a long or short step, a lighter noise, adduction or abduction (see from in front and behind only), increased or diminished flexion, etc. By the aid of these rules practically all simple single-leg lamenesses can be determined. Where there are two or more limbs affected it is very much more difficult. The services of a veterinary surgeon should be obtained to diagnose the situation of the lesions and their extent and nature.

Determining the seat of the lameness.—The affected limb should be examined in a systematic manner, and a careful search made for injuries signs of disease, etc. The hand should be passed down the front and back of the limb, manipulating the bones in the first place. These can best be felt below the knee or hock, and it is below this region that the great majority of lamenesses due to bony conditions are situated. Search should be made for spavins, splints, ring-bones, side-bones, etc. Subsequently, the observer should feel the softer structures, tendons, ligaments, and should feel over the course of tendon sheaths, joint capsules, for signs of pain, swelling, or heat. Muscles should be manipulated fairly firmly, and heat, pain, or swelling in them looked for. The foot should be picked up afterwards, and, since more than half of all lamenesses are situated in the foot, it should be carefully examined. The shoe may have to be removed, and the foot should always be cleansed from soil, dung, etc. Pressure from pincers around the lower part of the wall, tapping with a hammer, both on the wall and on the sole, and passive manipulation of the joints, may elicit signs of pain from the animal.

For further information, the various sections upon diseases which are associated with characteristic lameness, such as RICKETS, SPAVIN, RING-BONE, LAMINITIS, BRUCELLOSIS, etc., should be consulted.

LAMINITIS.—Consists of inflammation, either acute or chronic, of the sensitive laminæ which lie immediately below the outer horny wall of the foot.

The disease should always be considered serious owing to the fact that the sensitive parts of the foot are enclosed in a comparatively rigid box which does not allow of the swelling that is one of the characteristic symptoms of inflammation. The inflamed parts do swell as much as they are able, but the process entails great pressure upon the sensitive nerve-endings, great pain, usually some separation between the horn and the parts below, and very often leads to deformity of the hoof.

Cause.—Is not yet thoroughly understood, but appears to be an allergic reaction to a surfeit of grain, or to breakdown products of a retained afterbirth (in the mare), or to bacteria in the uterus, etc.

LAMINITIS IN CATTLE

Laminitis has been encountered in both adult and young cattle. For over 50 years, overfeeding with barley has been regarded as a likely cause, and more recently the disease has been described among cattle 4½ to 6 months old in barley beef ' units.

Symptoms.—These consisted of arching of the back, awkward movements, and paddling of the feet. Heat in the feet and pulsation of the digital arteries may be detected. The head is held low and extended. Much time is spent lying down, and occasionally animals lie flat on their sides with all four legs fully extended. Muscular tremors are usually present, especially behind the shoulder and in the fold of the flank. No deformity of the hooves is visible, as a rule, for 8 or 9 days.

Differential diagnosis.—The symptoms may be suggestive of early meningitis, encephalitis, or tetanus; also of peritonitis or bloat. Local changes in feet and legs helps diagnosis.

Treatment.—Antihistamines, corticosteroids, and phlebotomy all proved unsuccessful. (*See Veterinary Record* for Feb. 12, 1966.)

LAMINITIS IN HORSES

Predisposing causes.—Any condition which puts undue weight upon the feet for ong periods, with insufficient exercise, is probably the most common cause. Among these may be mentioned: heavy body weight in fat stallions, ponies, pregnant mares, and pack-horses; unfit condition, as in horses left idle for long periods, and

LAMINITIS

in young horses being broken in; and overwork. (*See* AZOTURIA.)

Symptoms.—These are both general, affecting the whole body, and local, affecting the feet only. Of the general symptoms perhaps the most striking are the expression of acute pain in the face and the attitude assumed. The horse usually stands still, and refuses to move when asked. It may attempt a step, but groans or grunts, and ends by remaining in the same position. When lying on the ground it is almost impossible to make it rise, the pain being more acute when standing than when lying. The pupils are widely dilated, and the membranes of the eyes are a deep red colour. Respiration is distressed and rapid, and the pulse is very fast and strong in the early stages, but becomes weaker as exhaustion advances. The temperature is raised from 2 to 5 degrees above normal, and remains high till the termination of the case. In a typical case the nostrils are trumpet-shaped, the muscles of the face are contracted into an expression of agony, the body trembles with the pain, and sweat may run down the legs literallv in streams. The attitude assumed by the horse is almost characteristic. One, two, or four feet may be attacked. When only one member is affected there is usually some painful condition present in the opposite leg of the same pair, which has induced the horse to rest all or nearly all of the body weight upon the hitherto sound limb, with the result that it becomes overworked and is consequently attacked with laminitis. In such a case it is usually the fore-limbs which are involved, and the horse alternately shifts his weight from one leg to the other. Each time the foot with laminitis is lifted from the ground, it is snatched up and held for a few moments as if contact with the ground was painful; later it may be rested out in front of the horse with the heel only on the ground. In a short time the other leg tires and must be rested; a considerable amount of shuffling takes place before the affected foot can be safely posed, and the duration of the weight-bearing is generally shorter than with the other foot. When two feet are affected it is always either the fore pair or the hind pair; diagonal feet are never attacked. If the fore-feet are involved the horse stands with these thrust out well in front of him, resting on the heels as much as possible, while the hind-feet are brought up under the belly in order to bear as much of the body weight as possible. This leads to a definite crouch in the horse's appearance, and when considered along with the reluctance to move into a new position, may appear to indicate that the back has been injured. Moreover, an owner may fall into this error by observing the tenseness of the powerfully contracted muscles along the spine, and these facts have occasionally led to blistering or rubbing the back with liniments—a procedure which, needless to say, is futile. When all four feet are affected the position assumed by the horse is similar to what is seen when the fore-feet only are affected, but the horse does not tend to pivot round on his fore-feet when asked to move, as he may when the hind-feet are sound. When only the hind-feet are affected they are brought well under the abdomen so as to rest mainly upon their heels, while the fore-feet are placed as far back as possible to carry the majority of the body weight. The four legs are thus bunched together, the head is lowered, and the back is even more arched than in the previous instance, so that by the uninitiated injury to the back may be more easily suspected than when only the fore or all four feet are diseased.

If the feet themselves are examined, no matter which ones are affected, they are found to be hot to the touch, the arteries at the coronet are bounding with pulsations, pressure cannot be tolerated, and if the feet are tapped even gently with a hammer the horse groans or grunts with the pain, or snatches his foot from the ground. In all cases the toes of the feet are more severely affected than the heels, and the horse endeavours to rest his weight upon the heels rather than upon the toes. It is this fact which leads to the postures described.

In from 4 to 12 or 14 days the symptoms slowly subside and the horse regains its normal attitude and condition. Sometimes the disease becomes rapidly worse after the first few hours, owing to hæmorrhage having occurred between the horny and the sensitive walls. In the worst type of case the blood may actually burst out around the coronets. Death usually terminates such cases in from 12 to 24 hours.

In the chronic form, which often follows the acute, laminitis presents a slowly progressive change in the shape of the foot. The toe becomes more and more elongated, the heels and the pasterns become vertical, rings appear around the coronet and move slowly downwards as the horn grows, and a bulge appears in the concavity of the sole. This latter is produced by the tilting of the third phalanx of the foot, occasioned by the separation of the horny from the sensitive wall by the unorganised collection of exudate that results from the inflammation. The third phalanx (*as pedis*) has its anterior part pulled backwards and downwards by the action of the flexor tendon, presses upon the horn of the sole just behind the toe, causes it to bulge downward, and in very bad cases may actually pass through it. The degree of lameness varies according to the severity of the deformity, but in all cases there is a shortened step by the affected feet, difficulty in turning at a fast pace, and a stiffness and rigidity quite foreign to the normal gait of the horse. In other cases the lameness is very distinct.

Treatment.—An antihistamine has been used with success in some cases. Success has also been reported with ACTH.

Otherwise, treatment aims at reduction of fever and inflammation. Local applications of cold, alternated with heat to the feet, are efficacious. The horse should have its shoes removed in the first place, and its feet, if overgrown, must be reduced to their normal proportions. This is sometimes very difficult, and may necessitate casting. It may then have its cannons hosed, be made to stand in a running stream of water, or some other measure may be adopted to ensure that moist cold is applied for from 2 to 4 hours *continuously*. After that, warm, and finally hot water should be poured over the fetlocks for a period of about twenty minutes to half an hour. The cold applications are then resumed.

While the horse is suffering great pain, the exercise allowed should be only such as it will take voluntarily in a loose-box, but when the inflammation begins to subside it should be taken out of the box for fifteen minutes three or four times a day, and made to walk, very slowly, upon some convenient strip of soft ground near by. As healing proceeds, the exercise may be proportionately increased. Feeding should be of the lightest and most easily digested nature, and should be sufficiently laxative to keep the bowels moving. All substances rich in protein, such as oats, beans, etc., must be avoided.

Green food in small amounts is good, and a little hay should be supplied.

In chronic cases the shoeing is of great importance. As much of the overgrown horn at the toe as possible should be rasped away, and the overgrown heels should be pared. If the sole is very thin and the horse flinches upon pressure over the bulge, a leather sole packed with a small amount of tow soaked in Stockholm tar should be applied. The shoe should be wide in the web, seated out so as not to press upon the projecting sole, and made upon the 'rocker' or the 'rocker-bar' principle. In the 'rocker shoe' the iron is made thin at the toe, thick at the quarters, and thin again at the heels. In the 'rocker-bar shoe' there is a bar across the heels added. In either case the foot is enabled to roll from the time it is put down until it is lifted, instead of remaining stationary. In some cases, especially where the horse appears to 'feel with his heel' before placing the foot, it is advisable to leave long heels on the shoe, and it is sometimes necessary to relieve pressure from the wall at the toe by cutting or rasping the lower border, so that the shoe does not press upon it. (*See also* HOOF REPAIR.)

LAMPAS.—A swelling of the mucous membrane of the hard palate of the horse immediately behind the arch of the incisor teeth in the upper jaw. It is often seen about the time when the permanent teeth are cutting through the gums, *i.e.* at 2½, 3½, and 4½ years, and for a short time afterwards. It is erroneously thought that it is the *cause* of a falling off in condition which naturally occurs when the teeth are cutting; it is really rather an *effect*. It was the custom to lance 'lampas' in many parts of the country; this occasions unnecessary pain and discomfort to the horse, and if the incision is made towards one side instead of in the middle line there is a serious risk of wounding the palatine artery on that side.

LAMZIEKTE is a disease of cattle in South Africa which occurs as an enzoötic in animals on phosphorus-deficient areas of the veldt. The *Clostridium botulinus* is the actual cause of death. During spring the herbage usually contains adequate supplies of phosphorus and no cases occur, but during winter the lack of phosphorus leads grazing cattle to chew the bones of animals (often cattle) that have died, in an endeavour to take phosphorus into the body to make good the deficiency. This condition of bone-eating (osteophagia) is actually only the result of a craving for minerals; it is not cannibalism. Where the animals whose skeletons are left on the veldt, harboured in their alimentary canals, the *Clostridium botu-*

linus, this organism invades the carcase, and both it and its toxin are present in the decomposing remains. Both organism and toxin are capable of setting up botulism in cattle when taken in by the mouth.

Symptoms.—Death may occur only a few hours after eating the bones, or it may be postponed for 1 or 2 days. Recovery is rare, and only occurs after long convalescence. There is paralysis of the jaws, tongue, and throat; great muscular weakness; often prostration without unconsciousness, and other more vague symptoms. The severity of the symptoms varies with the amount of toxin taken in or liberated in the body. Recovery gives no immunity.

Prevention.—The researches of Sir Arnold Theiler and the workers at Onderstepoort showed that the best means of preventing lamziekte is to feed sterilised bone meal to cattle during the winter months in areas which are naturally deficient in phosphorus. In conveniently situated enclosed parts, artificial manuring with phosphatic compounds is also useful. Where possible, the carcases of animals which have died from lamziekte should be burned or buried before other cattle gain access to them or to skeletons.

Treatment is useless once symptoms have developed.

LANOLINE is a fat derived from the wool of sheep. It is used extensively for the making of ointments, because it does not become rancid with keeping, and because it is supposed to penetrate the skin more than other substances.

LAPAROTOMY (λαπάρα, the flank; τομή, an operation) is a general term which is applied to the opening of the abdominal cavity. The incision is either made in the middle line of the abdomen, or through one or other of the flanks. It is performed when diseased conditions of the organs in the abdomen or pelvis require surgical treatment, or for the removal of structures such as the ovaries in the female.

LAPINISED.—This term is applied to a virus which has been attenuated by passage through rabbits. An example is afforded by lapinised swine fever vaccine.

LARGACTIL.—A valuable sedative. (*See* CHLORPROMAZINE; *also under* ARTIFICIAL HIBERNATION.)

LARKSPUR POISONING.—Of the several varieties of Larkspur, most of which occur in America in the ranges of the West, where they cause great loss to cattle owners, only one species is commonly found in Great Britain—*Delphinium ajacis*, which grows mainly in cornfields in Cambridgeshire, Essex, and Suffolk. The seeds are the most dangerous parts of the plant, although the leaves have proved fatal when fed experimentally. Horses and sheep are not so susceptible as cattle. The active principles are four in number, viz. *Delphine*, *Delphisine*, *Delphinoidine*, and *Staphisagrine*, and of these the first three are highly poisonous. It is not certain whether they all occur in the British plant, but they have been isolated from foreign species.

Symptoms.—In general the symptoms are similar to those produced by aconite. There is salivation, vomiting, colicky pains, convulsions, and general paralysis. No specific treatment is known, but atropine by hypodermic injection has been recommended; also permanganate of potash dissolved in water and given in the form of a drench.

LARYNGITIS (λάρυγξ, the windpipe) means inflammation of the larynx. (*See* LARYNX, DISEASES OF.)

LARYNGOSCOPE (λάρυγξ, the windpipe; σκοπέω, I examine) is an instrument by means of which the throat and the back of the mouth may be examined. Strictly speaking, the name indicates that it is for the examination of the larynx, but it is only in dogs that this is feasible. In the larger animals, control is difficult, and in the horse the soft palate is so long that vision is obstructed.

LARYNGOTRACHEITIS, INFECTIOUS.—This is a disease of poultry caused by a Herpes virus, prevalent in N.W. England. Loss of appetite, sneezing and coughing, a discharge from the eyes, difficulty in breathing are the main symptoms. Birds of all ages are susceptible. Mortality averages about 15 per cent. No treatment is of value. Control is best achieved by depopulation and fumigation. A vaccine has been used.

LARYNX (λάρυγξ) is the organ of voice, and also forms one of the parts of the air passage. It is placed just between, and slightly behind, the angles of the lower jaw. Externally it is covered by the skin, by a small amount of fibrous tissue, and by the sterno-thyro-hyoid muscles; on either side of it lie the lowermost parts of the parotid glands when the neck is arched; above it, and to some extent on either side of its anterior part, lies the origin of the œsophagus (gullet), and it projects into the pharynx. Attached to its posterior part is the first ring of the trachea or windpipe. It is a complicated valve which regulates the volume of air in respiration, prevents foreign bodies from being insufflated into the trachea, and is the chief organ of voice-production.

Structure.—The larynx is formed of a framework of cartilages united by joints and ligaments, lined on the inside by mucous membrane similar to that of the trachea generally, and covered on the outside by both intrinsic and extrinsic muscles. There are three single cartilages—the cricoid, thyroid, and epiglottis; and one pair—the arytenoids. The *cricoid* cartilage is shaped somewhat like a signet ring and connects the rest of the larynx with the first ring of the trachea. To its upper part are attached the arytenoids and the posterior horns of the thyroids. A crico-tracheal membrane unites it to the trachea, and a crico-thyroid membrane unites it to the thyroid cartilage. The *thyroid* cartilage possesses a body which in man forms the protuberance known as 'Adam's apple', and two lateral wings which sweep outwards and upwards to end in horns which join the cricoid. At the upper anterior extremities of the wings are the anterior horns, one on each side, which are attached to the hyoid bone. To its body are attached the epiglottis and the vocal ligaments, which latter form the foundation for the vocal cords. The *epiglottis* lies in front of the body of the thyroid and curves forwards towards the root of the tongue; it is shaped somewhat like a pointed ovate leaf. The *arytenoids* are situated one on either side of the upper part of the cricoid to which they are attached. They are somewhat pyramidal in shape, and to them are attached the upper ends of the vocal ligaments. The spaces between the cartilages are filled by fibrous membranes, which bind them together, and the whole is lined by mucous membrane. The movable parts are actuated by muscles, the chief movements being those in which the vocal ligaments, and consequently the vocal cords, whose basis they form, are stretched tight or slackened, or are carried away from each other or made to approach. Air issuing from the trachea under pressure causes the vocal cords to vibrate, and according to the volume of air passing and to the tenseness or slackness of the vocal cords, so are the volume of sound and the pitch of the note varied. The larynx described is essentially that of the horse; in the other domestic animals there are minor differences. (For functions, *see under* VOICE.)

LARYNX, DISEASES OF (*see also* ROARING, WHISTLING, *and under* BRONCHITIS). The affections of the larynx are not numerous if we except such conditions as roaring, whistling, pneumonia, strangles, common colds, bronchitis, etc., which, while not specifically diseases of the larynx, may involve that structure.

Coughing is a symptom of irritation in the larynx or upper parts of the trachea. It may be brought about by a great variety of diverse conditions, such as the presence of a foreign body, inflammation, pain, compression, inhalation of noxious gases, etc. In the process of coughing, the larynx first closes by approximation of the vocal folds, the muscles of expiration—especially the abdominal walls—begin to contract and exert pressure upon the contained air in the chest cavity, the head is lowered, and then the pent-up air is suddenly released by the wide opening of the larynx. Any particles of irritating matter become caught in the rush of air and are carried up into the nasal passages and forced out through the nostrils, or, in some animals, are blown up into the pharynx and mouth.

A more or less continuous chronic cough is one of the common symptoms of tuberculosis in the ox, of broken wind in the horse, and of chronic bronchitis in the dog.

LARYNGITIS is an inflammation of the larynx, but particularly of the mucous membrane which lines its interior. It is often associated with pharyngitis or with bronchitis and tracheitis, when it is usually due to the spreading of inflammation from one of these neighbouring structures. It is a common symptom of influenza in the horse, and in many cases is one of the only definite symptoms in addition to those of fever.

Causes.—In ordinary acute laryngitis not complicated with other diseases there is usually the history of a chill, or exposure to damp, to draughts, or to the influence of sudden changes from a well-ventilated to a badly ventilated stable. Long journeys by rail, standing for long periods in sale-yards, shows, etc., are other contributory factors. It is probable that in all such instances the actual cause is invasion with organisms, made possible by the lowering of vitality occasioned by adverse conditions. In other cases exposure to the infections of strangles and influenza may result in an attack of laryngitis.

Symptoms.—In ordinary cases there is a cough, difficulty in swallowing, pain on pressure over the larynx, extension of the head to relieve pressure on the throat (a condition that is aptly described in popular terms as 'star-gazing'), and some amount of nasal discharge. In more severe cases food is refused although liquids can be taken; the discharge is copious, and a wheezing or roaring sound accompanies breathing. This may develop into œdema of the larynx, in which the membranes become so swollen as to interfere with respiration, and unless the condition is relieved by the use of a tracheotomy tube, the animal may become slowly suffocated. A slight rise in temperature and pulse-rate accompanies the milder forms, but when influenza is present, or if other specific diseases arise, the signs of fever are more distinct. Uncomplicated laryngitis usually lasts from a week to about a fortnight. Occasionally complications, such as roaring or whistling, follow recovery from the initial disease.

Treatment.—It is advisable to isolate all cases of laryngitis in a loose-box or other building, especially those arising in newly purchased animals, on account of the risk of contagious disease developing. The strictest attention must be paid to ventilation, and to the maintenance of body heat, to ward off pneumonia. Food should be soft, easily swallowed, and easily digested, such as mashes of bran, linseed, barley, or oatmeal gruels, teas, and finely chopped or chaffed green food. Clean cold water should always be available for drinking purposes. 'Antiphlogistine', smeared upon a piece of cotton or flannel, which is tied over the horse's poll, gives good results. In the drinking water the horse should receive some simple laxative such as Epsom or Glauber's salts twice daily, and small doses of electuary should be administered by smearing on the teeth or tongue several times each day. As convalescence is reached, walking exercise should be given, and after a time the horse may be turned out for an hour to grass in the sunny part of the day if the weather will allow. It is important to remember that even when the symptoms have subsided relapses are common, and the condition should not be considered to have subsided until the lapse of a week after the symptoms disappear.

TUMOURS may affect the cavity of the larynx and give rise to a chronic cough and distressed breathing at times, but they are not common.

TUBERCULOSIS may affect the larynx of the ox.

WOUNDS of the larynx are not common, owing to its comparatively sheltered position in the body. The objectionable habit of giving a ball to horses or other animals by placing it upon the sharpened end of a stick and poking it back into the throat is often responsible for injury to the larynx. *See also under* DRENCHING for a danger associated with the use of a drenching gun in pigs.

FOREIGN BODIES may gain entrance into the larynx from careless drenching or wrong administration of balls, from hastiness in swallowing, from a fright while feeding, or in the case of dogs and cattle, from playing with some small object which lodges in the back of the throat and finds its way into the larynx. The respirations are at once upset, and if the object is large and not soon dislodged the animal quickly becomes seriously distressed. The treatment is to remove the foreign body by some means or other. The hand may be passed into the back of the throat in the case of large animals and the obstruction removed, or forceps may be necessary to grasp the object.

LATERAL CARTILAGES are rhomboid plates of cartilage which are attached, one on either side, to angles of the third

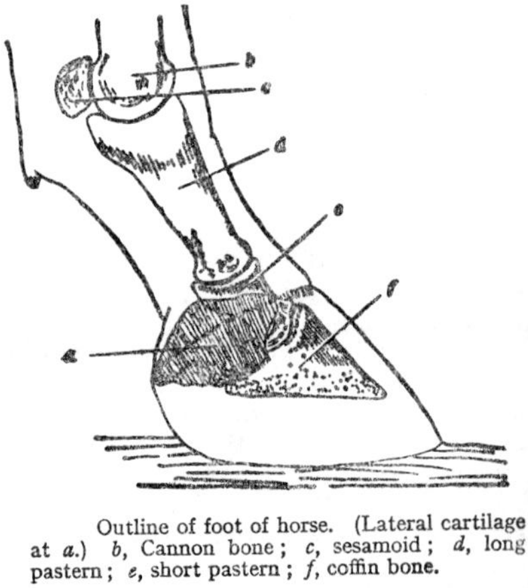

Outline of foot of horse. (Lateral cartilage at *a*.) *b*, Cannon bone; *c*, sesamoid; *d*, long pastern; *e*, short pastern; *f*, coffin bone.

phalanx (*os pedis*) of the foot of the horse. They extend above the coronet sufficiently to be felt distinctly at the heels and for a certain distance in front of this. In old age they often become ossified in their lower parts. When they ossify in their upper palpable margins the name 'side-bone' is applied to the condition. In certain cases they may become injured from treads or tramps by neighbouring horses or from the other foot, and the cartilage, being poorly supplied with blood, undergoes necrosis. This is accompanied by a greater or lesser amount of suppuration, and the pus eventually bursts out through the coronet and constitutes what is known as a 'quittor'. (*See* SIDE-BONES, QUITTOR, FOOT OF HORSE.)

LATHYRISM, or LATHYRUS POISONING, is a form of poisoning caused by feeding upon one or other of the various peas that are included under the general name of 'Mutter peas'. The peas which are usually understood to be included under this name are *Lathyrus sativus* principally, and *L. cicera* and *L. clymenum*, less frequently. The latter are found in samples of field peas grown in South Europe and North Africa, while *L. sativus* is imported from India mainly. They are poisonous to all the domesticated animals, but seem specially dangerous for horses. Many outbreaks have been recorded, and in most the percentage of deaths has been high, sometimes as much as 50 per cent of the affected.

Symptoms of poisoning may not appear until the lapse of as much as fifty days after the peas cease to be used as a food-stuff. The cause of lathyrism was shown in 1952 or thereabouts to be the high selenium content of the plants. (*See* SELENIUM.)

Symptoms.—Usually become visible when the animal is put to work or exercised. Typically, the chief symptoms are those of paralysis of some part of the body—usually the hind-limbs and the recurrent laryngeal nerve. This latter gives rise to the condition known as 'roaring', and unless quickly relieved the horse will die from asphyxia. In some instances the symptoms are so sudden in their onset that the horse drops while in harness and is unable to rise. In less severe cases there is staggering and swaying of the hind-quarters, great difficulty in breathing, dilated nostrils, a widely opened mouth, a fast and very weak pulse, and convulsive seizures. The paroxysms may pass off in a few minutes, or the horse may collapse and die.

Treatment.—Tracheotomy gives immediate relief in the majority of cases, but the tube must be left in position for some days. The removal of the cause is of course a *sine qua non*.

The antidote is ascorbic acid, added to the diet.

LAUDANUM is the popular name for tincture of opium. (*See* OPIUM.)

LAUREL POISONING.—The exceedingly common ornamental shrub *Prunus laurocerasus* has caused poisoning among cattle and sheep on the continent of Europe, but it would appear that the British varieties are not so toxic. Cases are occasionally recorded in which animals, chiefly cattle and sheep, have died from eating quantities of the plant, but they are not common. The plant possesses a rather characteristic odour and a bitter taste when its leaves are bruised and tasted. This is due to the cyanogenetic glucoside *Prulaurasin*, which is contained in the parenchyma of the leaves. There is also a certain amount of an enzyme-emulsion, and the interaction between these two substances results in the formation of hydrocyanic (or prussic) acid, which is the actual cause of the poisoning.

Symptoms.—Prussic acid is one of the most rapid of the known poisons, and produces its effects within a very short space of time after the leaves have been eaten. The animal staggers and falls; it may attempt to rise, but fails; the stomach becomes distended with gas; respirations are laboured and slow; convulsions, in which the limbs are repeatedly stretched out to their fullest extent and then moved spasmodically as if galloping, take place; the pupils are fully dilated, and unless the animal receives attention, death rapidly occurs. The respirations are the first to cease, and in from 1 to 4 minutes afterwards the heart stops beating.

Treatment.—*See* PRUSSIC ACID POISONING.

LAVAGE.—The process of washing out the stomach or the intestines. In gastric lavage a double-way tube is passed down into the stomach either through the mouth or by way of the nose, and water or some medicinal solution is poured or pumped through one channel in the tube, and after a time escapes by the other, carrying with it the contents of the stomach in small amounts. (*See also* ENEMA.)

LAW, THE, relating to animals in the United Kingdom is frequently added to or amended, and consequently it is advisable to consult the Ministry of Agriculture for the latest information on any particular subject. Recent legislation is referred to under ANÆSTHETICS, ANIMAL BOARDING ESTABLISHMENTS, MARKETS, TRANSIT OF CALVES, VETERINARY SURGEONS ACT, DISEASES OF ANIMALS ACTS, PET ANIMALS ACT, DOCKING AND NICKING ACT. Other relevant Acts are: the Riding Establishments Act, 1939; Coal Mines Act, 1911; Protection of Animals Act, 1911; Slaughter of Animals Acts, 1933 and 1954; Dogs Act, 1906; Injured Animals Act 1907; Cruelty to Animals Act, 1876. (*See also under* ANTIBIOTICS, ADDITIVES.)

LAXATIVES are mild purgatives. (*See* PURGATIVES.)

LEAD is one of the heavy metals which have little or no action upon the system when taken as the metal, but the salts of which are medicinal substances.

Varieties.—Externally, the acetate, the strong and the dilute solution of the subacetate of lead (Goulard's Extract and Goulard's Water), the oxide, carbonate, and iodide are now seldom employed.

LEAD POISONING in the acute form is extremely common in cattle which have eaten paint, licked out discarded paint tins, or licked newly painted railings, etc., or eaten tarpaulins. It is frequently fatal and many cattle are unnecessarily lost each year from this cause. Dogs and cats are prone to lick lead dressings from their skins, and cases have been recorded where paints (white-lead paint) have been licked from the floor when painters were at work. Lead poisoning in the chronic form is called *plumbism*. This results from the gradual accumulation of the metal in the body, taken in small doses, but in greater quantities than it is excreted. The effects are due to the irritation of the lead salt on the voluntary and involuntary muscles. Water which contains small amounts of lead is the cause of some cases; herbage near to smelting works which becomes saturated with lead salts, the repeated application of dressings containing lead and the absorption of these through the skin as well as by licking, are other factors responsible for chronic lead poisoning.

Experimental work in the U.S.A. (1966) showed that pigs can consume, without showing any symptoms at all, a daily dose of lead which would rapidly kill a cow.

Ten lead pellets can kill a goose; 25 pellets have caused death within 10 days.

Symptoms.—These vary in the different animals. In the horse, convulsions, partial paralysis, colicky pains, roaring and respiratory distress, thirst, and an increase in the amount of urine, have been seen. In cattle, brain symptoms, denoted by a staggering gait, impaired vision, and the assumption of unusual postures, are noted. In the dog and cat there are exhibited salivation, chronic diarrhœa, paralysis of the carpi or 'knees' in the fore-legs, loss of condition, sometimes convulsions, and sometimes a blue line along the gums. This blue line is seen in other animals in which the amount of lead taken has been small, but over a considerable length of time.

Treatment.—The 'first-aid' antidote is large doses of sulphate of magnesium (Epsom salts) for the sudden or acute cases, given in some oily or demulcent fluid, such as gruel, milk, and olive oil, etc.

The treatment of lead poisoning has been revolutionised by the introduction of the chelating agent, calcium di-sodium adetate, which converts inorganic lead in the tissues into a harmless lead chelate which is excreted by the kidneys. The drug must be given intravenously. In chronic cases, potassium iodide is given three or four times daily to hasten the elimination of the lead salt from the system. (*See also* CHELATING AGENTS.)

LEATHER SOLES are applied to horses' feet under the shoe for the purpose of protecting the sole of the foot from injury, to retain dressings in position, to minimise concussion, and to serve as an attachment for bar-pads and frog-pads. The leather is cut larger than the circumference of the foot, laid upon the prepared foot, the shoe is then nailed on so that the nails pass through the leather, and finally, the projecting edges of the leather are cut off close round the foot. It is advisable in all cases where leather soles are worn, that the space between the sole of the foot and the leather sole should be filled up with tow soaked in Stockholm tar to keep the sole moist, to preserve the leather, and to prevent small stones, etc., from working in between the leather and the horn.

LEECHES are invertebrate animals belonging to the class Vermes, provided with suckers and leading a semi-parasitic life. They suck blood from animals and are generally found about streams and ponds. They sometimes cause trouble by fastening on the throats or mouths of animals including domestic waterfowl.

Limnatis nilotica has been reported as causing extensive damage in North Africa and Europe, especially in Bulgaria, where cattle, buffaloes, horses, sheep, dogs, pigs, and men may become infected. *L. africana* and species of *Hæmadipsa* are active in West Africa and in the tropical forests of Asia and South America, respectively.

Two cases of infestation of dogs with *Diestecostoma mexicanum* have been reported from Honduras. In the non-fatal case, a catheter was passed through the inferior nasal meatus and a 50-ml. capacity syringe containing chloroform water attached. The solution was injected slowly while the catheter was revolved. Over seventy leeches emerged after the treatment. (*See also under* PARASITES.)

LEISHMANIASIS is the general name applied to diseases of the blood caused by minute protozoan parasites. They are of considerable importance in man, but not in animals other than the dog. Cutaneous leishmaniasis, or ' oriental sore ' is seen in Persia, India, parts of Africa, and South America, and is caused by *Leishmania tropica*. Visceral leishmaniasis, called also kala-zaar or ' dum-dum fever ', occurs in the coastal countries of the Mediterranean, and is caused by *Leishmania donovani*. There is evidence that they are both transmitted by the sand flea. Both forms are diagnosed by laboratory examination, and are treated successfully by intravenous injection of 10 c.c. of a 1 per cent solution of tartar emetic, which is a specific. (*See also under* PARASITES.)

LENS OF THE EYE is one of the refractive media through which the light passes before it reaches the retina of the eye. It is by the bulging and flattening of the lens, brought about by the automatic action of the ciliary muscles, that divergent or parallel rays of light coming from objects that are near at hand or far away, are focussed upon the retina. This property of being able to alter in curvature is lessened as age advances, and consequently in old animals there is not the same acuteness of vision as in young ones. The lens is the seat of the opacity that is called cataract. (*See* EYE, CATARACT, etc.)

LENS, DISLOCATION OF (*see under* EYE, INJURIES).

LEPTAZOL.—An antidote to barbiturate poisoning.

LEPTOMENINGITIS (λεπτός, thin; μῆνιγξ, membrane) means inflammation of the inner and more delicate membranes of the brain and spinal cord.

LEPTOSPIROSIS.—Infection with *Leptospira*. (*See under* SPIROCHÆTAE.) In 1958, 34 distinct pathogenic serotypes of leptospira were recognised. Eight of these were of public health or veterinary significance in the U.S.A. Cattle, horses, sheep, pigs, and dogs are susceptible to infection. Leptospirosis occurs in the U.K. and in many other parts of the world.

LEPTOSPIROSIS IN DOGS.—Jaundice in dogs caused by *Leptospira icterohæmorrhagiæ* is dealt with under JAUNDICE, LEPTOSPIRAL, OF DOGS. This organism also causes jaundice (Weil's disease) in man, and illness (with or without jaundice) in a number of domestic animals, including pigs and calves. Monlux showed in 1948 in the U.S.A. that of 100 rats used in a survey, 55 had leptospira in the kidneys, and that 23·07 per cent of the farm rats and 49, or 66·2 per cent, of the dump rats harboured leptospira in those organs. (The incidence of the leptospira in the rat varied with the location of the dump. Nearly all the rats obtained in one area were positive. If there is plenty of food, rats will migrate very little.) Similar surveys in the United Kingdom have shown 37·6 per cent rats infected.

In a Glasgow survey it was found that 40 per cent of dogs had at some time been infected with *Leptospira canicola* (the cause of Canicola Fever in man), which is two or three times more common as a parasite in dogs than *L. icterohæmorrhagiæ*. The parasite is the cause of much of the acute and sub-acute nephritis in younger dogs, especially between November and April.

Symptoms of infection with *L. canicola* are very variable. There may be loss of appetite, depression, and fever alone, or together with *marked thirst* and *vomiting*, loss of weight, and sometimes a foul odour from the mouth. In a few cases there is jaundice. Ulceration of the tongue may occur. Collapse, coma, and death may supervene. (*See* ' STUTTGART DISEASE '.)

The symptoms first described above are related to leptospiral invasion of the blood-stream. This may be followed by invasion of, and damage to, the kidneys. This primary nephritis may be followed later by chronic interstitial nephritis, kidney failure, uræmia, and death.

Treatment.—Penicillin has been used with considerable success in the early stages of *L. canicola* infection. Once the kidneys have been damaged, however, treatment is as for nephritis. In severe cases—where the ' Stuttgart ' syndrome or symptoms of uræmia are evident, the animal dies, as a rule, despite all treatment. (*See* KIDNEYS, DISEASES OF; URÆMIA, NURSING.)

Prevention.—A vaccine is available, the makers recommending that one should wait until the puppy is five months old before the first inoculation.

Most of the dogs which recover from leptospirosis excrete the organisms in the urine for long periods (sometimes 4 to 18 months). This obviously makes control of the disease difficult in the absence of vaccine.

LEPTOSPIROSIS OF CATTLE.—Some confusion has been caused by widespread statements that this does not occur in the United Kingdom. Such statements are incorrect. The confusion arose over *Leptospira grippotyphosa*, isolated from imported Charolais bulls in quarantine in 1961 and again in 1965. This particular infection had indeed never been reported in the U.K. before, but other forms of leptospirosis in cattle do occur; notably infection with *L. icterohæmorrhagiæ*.

Leptospiræ have been obtained from cows with symptoms of illness, secreting milk having a blood-tinged or thickened yellow appearance. Artificial infection led to variable symptoms—fever, albuminuria, and hæmoglobinuria, and sometimes death. A generalised infection occurs with localisation in the kidneys. Abnormal milk is a dominant symptom.

" A total of 406 cattle sera collected at the Edinburgh abattoir from animals of 63 different herds in various parts of Scotland, the north of England and Northern Ireland were tested against the following Leptospira serotypes: *icterohæmorrhagiæ, canicola, pomona, bratislava, ballum, sejroe, grippotyphosa,* and *bataviæ*; *saxkœbing* and *hardjo* were included when testing the last 80 cattle sera. The results of these tests revealed that 260 (64 per cent of the total) sera had agglutinins to one or more of these 10 serotypes." (*Vet. Record*, June 3, 1967.)

Leptospirosis of calves has been seen both in the United Kingdom (due to *L. icterohæmorrhagiæ*) and overseas (due to other *leptospiræ*). In Queensland an acute fever with jaundice and hæmoglobinuria has been known in calves for many years. It is rapid in onset and death occurs within a few hours to 4 days after the appearance of symptoms; dullness, temperature 104° to 107°, dark red urine, pale and yellow visible mucous membranes. *L. pomona* was demonstrated in kidney sections on post-mortem examinations. Recovered calves continue to excrete *leptospiræ* for up to three months. Infection may occur through inhalation of droplets of infected urine splashing on concrete, or as a result of insect bites. After an outbreak of abortion associated with *Leptospiræ* in Scottish cattle, wild mammals were examined. *Leptospiræ* were isolated from 22/108 rats, 3/49 mice and 1/3 hedgehogs; voles, mice and shrews were found to be infected on the farm where the leptospiral abortion had been diagnosed. Contamination of pastures by the urine of wild mammals may play a part in the spread of leptospirosis in cattle.

In the U.S.A., where the important species are *L. pomona, L. grippotyphosa,* and *L. sejroe*, abortion is reported to be the main symptom of leptospirosis in cows. In Illinois, a survey covering over 23,000 animals showed 14 per cent to be affected.

In Kenya, outbreaks of acute illness due to infection with *L. gryppotyphosa* have been reported in cattle, sheep, and goats. Jaundice is a symptom in some 30 per cent of cases, and death has followed within 12 hours of symptoms being observed. Snuffling, coughing, and holding down of the head are other symptoms. In cows, milk yield is reduced and is red in colour or otherwise abnormal. Urine varies from red to black. Temperature may rise to 105 degrees Fahrenheit.

In Europe, the above, *L. pomona* and *L. canicola* have been isolated.

LEPTOSPIROSIS OF PIGS.—Cases of

leptospiral jaundice in piglets due to *L. icterohæmorrhagiæ* and also to *L. canicola* have been reported in the United Kingdom, but overseas *L. pomona* is of more importance in the pig (and also from the public health aspect). In 1958 a U.K. survey showed the presence of antibodies to *L. pomona* in 287 out of 755 serum samples but "pomona cross-agglutinins are not uncommon in animals infected by other leptospiral serotypes '. (*Vet. Record,* June 3 1967.)

Symptoms in pigs include loss of appetite, fever, jaundice, and—in some cases—death. Pigs which have recovered excrete *leptospiræ* for some time afterwards. Indeed, infection in a herd may persist for years, with risk to human health. Sows may abort.

L. canicola can survive for 12 days in naturally infected pig kidneys kept in a refrigerator. (*See* CANICOLA FEVER, which pigmen may contract from pigs.)

LESION (*laedo,* I hurt) meant originally an injury, but is now applied to all diseased changes in organs or tissues.

LET-DOWN OF MILK (*see* MILKING).

LETHAL FACTORS (*see* GENETICS, p. 387).

LEUCIN (λευκός, white) is a crystalline substance which is found in most of the glands of the body as a result of the decomposition of proteins. It is found in the urine in quantity when the liver is diseased.

LEUCOCYTES (λευκός, white; κύτος, a cell) is the name given to the white cells found in the blood and lymph. (*See* BLOOD, INFLAMMATION, PHAGOCYTOSIS, LEUCOCYTOSIS, WOUNDS.)

LEUCOCYTOSIS (λευκός, white; κύτος, cell) is a temporary increase in the number of white cells in the blood. It occurs after a feed, during pregnancy, after exertion, and when the temperature is elevated. It is seen during certain specific diseases, when it is due to the action of the toxins and poisons produced by the organisms that cause the disease, when malignant tumours are present in the body, and in poisoning with chlorate of potassium, phenacetin, etc. (*See* LEUKÆMIA.)

LEUCODERMA (λευκός, white; δέρμα, skin) means a condition of the skin and hair when areas become white as a result of injury or disease. It is seen on the backs of horses that have worn badly fitting saddles and collars, when it is called 'saddle-mark' and 'collar-mark', and after ringworm.

LEUCOMA.—The presence of an opaque patch or spots on the surface of the cornea. (*See* EYE.)

LEUCOPENIA.—A condition in which the white blood cells are less numerous than normal. It occurs during the course of several diseases, *e.g.* swine fever, leptospirosis of cattle. (*See* FELINE ENTERITIS.)

LEUCORRHŒA (λευκός, white; ῥέω, I flow).—A chronic vaginal discharge, generally of a whitish or greyish colour. It is a symptom of vaginitis or of metritis. (*See* UTERUS, DISEASES OF, 'WHITES'.)

LEUCOSIS, BOVINE.—A notifiable disease in Denmark, where it is endemic on 70 farms and has an annual average incidence of 4·1 cases per 100,000 head of cattle. A symptomless, latent leukæmic state may persist throughout life or change to the overt, 'cancer' type of leukæmia, which is fatal within days or months and usually seen in cows 4–8 years old. A skin type of leucosis is seen occasionally in 2- and 3-year-olds and this clears up after a few months, but is liable to recur and end fatally. Calves and yearlings are sometimes the subject of sporadic cases of leucosis, but this is chronic and characterised by lymphadenitis.

Strict control measures—aided by laboratory diagnosis — are enforced. Leucosis-herds are supervised—no animals from them may be sold except for direct slaughter.

The name leucosis is a synonym for lymphosarcoma and LEUKÆMIA (which see).

LEUCOSIS COMPLEX OF FOWLS.—This group of diseases, which includes FOWL PARALYSIS (or neural lymphomatosis) and LEUCOSIS, has been known since 1907. Viruses may account for all forms, but this is not yet certain. The following refers to leucosis, which occurs mainly in birds 6 months old or over, often soon after they have begun laying.

Experimentally, the incubation period appears to be 2 to 8 weeks. A few sporadic cases occur, and even in laying tests, where a number of birds are penned up for a year in a relatively small space, it is exceedingly rare to have more than one case in any one pen. The affected birds show no definite symptoms during life, but are dull, cease laying, stand with feathers ruffled, and die in from four days to a week or ten days. The disease has been described as occurring in several forms, *e.g.* :

(1) Lymphoid leucosis.
(2) Myeloid leucosis.
(3) Erythroleucosis.
(4) Nodular form.
(5) Osteopetrosis.

In the first type the lesions seen at *post-mortem* examination are very typical. The liver and/or spleen may be enormously increased in size, has a pink and white mottled appearance, and is soft and pulpy. The spleen may on occasion reach the size of a small orange. In this type the blood picture is not materially changed. In myeloid leukæmia, liver and spleen enlargement also occurs, but there is a great increase in the number of white cells in the circulating blood and a decrease in the red blood cell content. The ratio of white to red corpuscles from being (normally) 1–100 or thereby may be increased to 1 to 2, and in some cases they may even outnumber the red cells. In the third type a severe anæmia is seen, the comb and wattles often having a yellowish appearance. There is an increase of the basophils in the circulating blood. In the nodular form, tumours with a chalky or cheesy appearance may occur in the chest or on or near the pelvis. Osteopetrosis is described under that heading. The presence of a sarcoma or carcinoma may be included in the term avian leucosis.

LEUKÆMIA (or **LYMPHOSARCOMA**) is a malignant disease—a form of cancer—involving lymphoid tissue especially. It occurs in all the domestic animals in which, as opposed to man, there is commonly but not invariably no increase in the number of lymphocytes in the bloodstream (an 'aleukæmic leukæmia'). Accordingly, lymphosarcoma is the better name.

In one form there may be a large tumour mass at the site of the thymus. Usually, many lymph nodes are involved, with enlargement of the spleen and infiltration of the liver. Tumours may occur in almost any organ.

In the dog, death commonly follows after 3 weeks, but the duration of illness varies from 1 to over 60 weeks. Most cats die, or have to be destroyed, within 8 weeks.

Leukæmia is the commonest malignant disease in the cat in Britain, and is caused by a virus, which can spread from cat to cat and can also produce the disease in dogs.

Symptoms.—Enlargement of superficial or of mesenteric lymph nodes, depression, emaciation, often diarrhœa. (For the disease in cattle, *see also under* LEUCOSIS.)

Treatment.—All attempts at treatment have been unsuccessful.

LEYS, NEW.—Cattle grazing these are, generally speaking, more prone to Hypomagnesæmia than when on permanent pasture. Clover-rich leys are also conducive to Bloat, unless precautions are taken.

LICE (*see* PARASITES).

'LICKED BEEF' is that which shows greenish or yellowish tracks made by the larvæ of warble-flies, with the formation of 'butcher's jelly'. This is of importance in food inspection.

LIEN is the Latin name for the spleen.

LIGAMENTS are strong bands of fibrous tissue that serve to bind together the bones forming a joint. They are cord-like in some instances, flat bands in others, and sheets in the case of the joint-capsule which surrounds a joint. (*See* JOINTS.)

LIGHT, INFLUENCE OF.—Adequate light is necessary for maximum fertility. This applies to poultry (*see under* NIGHT-LIGHTING), to bulls—too often kept in dark places—and sheep, etc. (*See also* RICKETS, VITAMIN D.)

LIGHT SENSITISATION.—This term is used to describe something more than mere sunburn and the 'peeling' so painfully experienced by holiday-makers. It implies a predisposing factor, such as the eating of a particular plant, which has the effect of making certain cells in the animal's body *abnormally* sensitive—for the time being—to light. Strong sunlight is then capable of causing serious and extensive damage, with a good deal of distress.

In Australia this trouble is frequently caused, in cattle, sheep, and pigs, through eating St. John's wort. Elsewhere overseas, clover and buckwheat are often responsible. Occasional cases of light sensitisation occur even in the United Kingdom. To give an example, a British Friesian heifer was discovered in obvious distress. Over nearly all the white parts the skin was dead and had partly sloughed off. Appropriate treatment, which included temporary confinement in a darkened loose-box, was followed by a rapid recovery. Bog Asphodel is believed to cause light sensitisation in sheep in Britain, where pigs have also been affected (probably by St. John's wort). In New Zealand, where the condition is called Facial Eczema, moulds have been incriminated.

It is always the white, pigment-free skin which suffers. Thus, some breeds of livestock are never troubled with light sensitisation, while white or partly white cattle are susceptible. Similarly, grey and piebald horses in the U.S.A. and elsewhere are sometimes affected.

Light sensitisation is associated with disfunction of the liver, and the presence of porphyrins in the bloodstream. It also occurs in some cases of PORPHYRIA.

Less uncommon is the inflammation of the eyes, occasionally seen in young cattle, during sunny weather, following a dose of phenothiazine. A greyish film forms on the surface of the eyeball (in bad cases there is ulceration), and there is weeping from the swollen lids. Prevention is simple. Keep young stock indoors for a day or two after treatment with phenothiazine if the weather is bright and sunny, especially if they are in rather poor condition. (*See also under* PHYLLOERYTHRIN.)

LIGHT TREATMENT.—The visible spectrum consists of the rays of light which lie between the red rays on the one hand and the violet on the other. The radiations below (that is of less frequency than) the red rays of the spectrum are known as *infra-red* or heat rays ; those immediately above the violet rays are called *ultra-violet* rays. Beyond these latter are many other varieties such as X-rays and the gamma rays which characterise radio-active substances.

Radiant heat.—Calorfic (heat) rays, luminous rays, and actinic rays, the calorific and heat rays predominating. Piggeries, and poultry establishments where winter-hatching is carried out, are equipped with artificial sunlight lamps. The rays penetrate a considerable distance into the tissues, but their chief effect is to promote warmth and induce dilation of superficial blood-vessels. Radiant heat is useful after surgical operations.

Ultra-violet light is much more effective and powerful than radiant heat, in that it is much more active chemically and induces certain changes in body cells which heat alone cannot effect, while ultra-violet rays are also definitely bactericidal.

Various special forms of lamp can be had for irradiation of cavities such as mouth and throat, vagina, uterus, etc., and others give variable degrees of radiant heat and ultra-violet irradiation, which are probably more beneficial than either can be alone.

In ultra-violet irradiation, the object is to concentrate the rays upon tissues near the lamp, especially the skin, since the rays are unable to penetrate any great distance. They act by destroying bacterial and fungus life in skin diseases such as eczema, certain cases of follicular mange (with gross secondary infection), ringworm, ulcerations of lips, ears, and skin, infected wounds, ringworm, etc.

During the course of rickets, after the diet has been corrected, ultra-violet irradiation is of great importance in converting the cholesterol stored in skin cells into ergosterol, and during convalescence from pneumonia, distemper, and other debilitating diseases, ultra-violet rays are effective in toning up the system.

In the horse, in addition to various skin diseases such as acne and ringworm, benefit often follows a course of irradiation in cases of localised grease and psoriasis.

LIGHTING OF ANIMAL BUILDINGS.—Recently, various kinds of glass substitutes have been put on the market, which are reputed to allow the ultra-violet rays of natural sunlight to pass through without appreciable absorption.

Adequate light is necessary to prevent rickets, and to ensure maximum fertility in poultry and other animals.

Artificial lighting of poultry houses is now a common practice. (*See* NIGHT LIGHTING.) Red light is used in many broiler houses and in some laying houses in order to reduce cannibalism.

LIGHTNING STROKE.—Cattle, sheep, and horses, are most often affected. Similar results are seen from contact with powerful electric currents, such as a high-tension wire falling on to horses in the streets, etc. The severity and intensity of the results depend on the current; some animals are killed outright, others are temporarily stunned and recover rapidly.

Symptoms.—Strong currents produce death instantaneously from paralysis and shock of the nervous system. In such cases the animal is often found with a bunch of grass between its teeth, and perhaps a mouthful of the same material. There is generally some amount of scorching, especially about the bases of the horns, and at the coronets. There may be an irregular 'lightning mark' connecting these places. On removal of the skin there is generally a streak of bruised subcutaneous tissue seen under the scorched areas. Wounds or fractures are sometimes met with, and in other cases there may be no visible signs of the electric shock. Decomposition of the carcase is rapid, the blood is not coagulated, *rigor mortis* is incomplete, and the veins are distended with blood. In less severe cases the animal may be found lying apparently asleep, but efforts at its awakening are unsuccessful. The stupor passes off in a variable time, and the animal rapidly recovers. In other cases recovery is not complete. An ear may be permanently paralysed, one or both hind-limbs may be useless, vision may be destroyed, or the muscles of the mouth may be incapable of function.

LIMBERNECK IN POULTRY.—This is a form of botulism which is occasionally seen in fowls in this country but appears to be more common abroad. The ingestion of carrion or of flies or their maggots infected with *Clostridium botulinus* may give rise to the trouble. The cardinal symptoms are a loss of power of the muscles of the neck, wings, and legs, affected birds first being dull and inactive.

LIME (*see* CALCIUM).

LIMING OF PASTURES.—If this be carried out *to excess* it can, according to André Voisin, lead to a deficiency in copper in the grazing animal and so bring about infertility (which see). Manganese deficiency is likewise a sequel when the soil becomes too alkaline.

LIMOUSIN.—A pure beef breed noted for high liveweight gains, high killing-out percentages, and freedom from calving difficulties. Its import from France was sanctioned in 1970.

LINDANE is an insecticide containing not less than 99 per cent of gamma BHC.

LINER, TEAT-CUP.—In selecting milking machinery equipment, one should avoid any liner with a hard mouthpiece.

LINGUAFULA SERRATA.—A 'tongue worm' parasitic in the nose of dogs, etc. (*See* p. 693).

LINIMENTS, or EMBROCATIONS (*linio*, I anoint), are preparations intended for external application, generally applied by rubbing. They are usually of an oily nature, poisonous, and should never be kept with medicines that are used for internal administration.

Varieties.—'A.B.C. liniment' consists of aconite, belladonna, and chloroform, mixed together to form a liniment. It is useful for painful muscular conditions, such as sprains, ruptures, and bruises, for acutely inflamed glands, and for painful rheumatic conditions in joints.

Turpentine liniment, ammonia liniment, and soap liniment, are preparations that are used for sprains, bruises, or tendinous or ligamentous swellings, when a reduction of the inflammation and absorption of the swelling is desirable. They are also used for rheumatism either in joints or muscles.

LINSEED is used either as the seeds, meal, or oil. The seeds, from the flax plant *Linum usitatissimum*, are sometimes given to stock, bruised so as to render the rich oily central parts open to the influence of the digestive juices, but more often they are ground to form linseed meal. The oil is obtained by expression from the seeds, and is subsequently purified. The residue is made into linseed cake and used for feeding to cattle, horses, and sheep.

Uses.—Linseed, taken internally, is a demulcent and nutritive substance which is of especial use in inflamed or irritable conditions of the throat, alimentary canal, and bladder. In the form of linseed tea or as boiled linseed, it is a valuable food for horses and cattle when recovering from the after-effects of severe illnesses. It is often taken when other forms of food are refused. Linseed tea is made by pouring 15 or 20 parts of boiling water on one of the seeds, or on four of the meal, and allowing the mixture to stand for one hour in a hot place where it will not boil, and for a subsequent hour in a moderately cool place. It is ready for offering to the animal when cool enough. Linseed oil is a gentle laxative in small doses, and a purgative in full doses. It is not to be recommended as a purgative agent for the horse, as it is nauseating and uncertain. It is often used as the vehicle in which irritating substances such as ether, turpentine, or ammonia preparations are given. For the dog it is not suitable. It is important to remember that *boiled linseed oil*, which often contains a poisonous substance called litharge, should never be substituted for the raw expressed oil.

LINSEED POISONING.—The flax plant contains small amounts of a cyanogenetic glucoside which, under conditions of dampness, may attain considerable proportions, and has occasionally proved harmful to animals eating it. When manufactured into cake, linseed has occasionally caused poisoning, when, during the process of manufacture, the temperature to which the cake is submitted is not sufficiently high to destroy the glucoside. The symptoms are similar to those seen in laurel poisoning, since they are also due to the production of prussic acid.

LIPASE.—A fat-splitting enzyme found in the pancreatic juice, blood plasma, and many plants.

LIPOMA (λίπος, fat; *-oma*, meaning tumour) is the name given to a tumour that is mainly composed of fat. These are liable to arise almost anywhere in the body where there is fibrous connective tissue, but are especially common below loose skin. They are occasionally seen in the abdominal cavity, where they develop in connection with the peritoneum, and sometimes encase the bowel and obstruct its function. (*See* TUMOUR.)

LIPS are musculo-membranous folds which act as curtains guarding the entrance to the mouth. In the horse they are covered on the outside with fine hairs, among which are longer, stouter tactile hairs, while some heavy draught horses have a ' moustache ' on their upper lips; on the inside the lips are covered by mucous membrane which is continuous with that of the mouth generally. In the horse they are extremely mobile, and the upper lip especially contains a very dense plexus of sensory nerves which serve tactile purposes. In the ox the lips are thick and comparatively immobile. The middle part of the upper lip between the nostrils is bare of hair and is termed the muzzle. It is provided with a large number of tiny glands which secrete a clear fluid in health, which keeps the part cool and moist. Within the lower lip are numbers of horny papillæ; its free margin is bare, but the under part of it is covered with ordinary and tactile hairs. The sheep possesses no hairless muzzle, but has a distinct ' philtrum ' instead. The lips are thin and mobile. In the pig the upper lip is thick and short and is blended with the snout or nasal disc, while the lower is thin and pointed. The angles of the mouth extend farther back than in the horse or ox. The lips of the dog vary with different breeds; in most they are thin and mobile, and capable of being retracted from the teeth. They are covered on their outsides with tactile hairs all over except for a small groove in the upper lip (philtrum) which blends with the muzzle above. In the bulldog this may be so deep as to give the appearance of ' hare-lip ', a malformation to which this breed is susceptible. (*See* HARE-LIP.) The lateral borders of the lower lip are provided with a number of projections which are usually pigmented a dark colour.

The lips are liable, from their situation, to injury from falling (horses and cattle), when fighting (dogs and cattle), and in other circumstances. The nature of the injury varies from a severe contusion or tear to the smallest abrasion. Owing to the very copious blood supply, healing is rapid and usually uneventful. A number of specific diseased conditions may involve the lips, and characteristic lesions may be produced upon them in some cases; thus in foot-and-mouth disease the vesicles which are found in that disease are sometimes situated within the margins of the lips. In ' calf diphtheria ' ulcerated areas may be found on the lips. Ringworm may attack their outer surfaces. Cancer may involve the lips.

LIQUOR is a solution of a drug in water.

LIQUORICE is the powdered root of *Glycyrrhiza glabra*, a plant of South Europe and Asia. It possesses demulcent and mild laxative actions, and is used in the preparation of many electuaries, cough powders, and as a coating for the outsides of pills and balls which have a nasty taste. (*See also* GLYCYRRHETINIC ACID.)

LISTERELLOSIS (*see* LISTERIOSIS).

LISTERIOSIS.—A disease caused by *Listeria monocytogenes* which attacks rodents, poultry, ruminants, pigs, horses, dogs, and man. It causes encephalitis and abortion in cattle and sheep, meningitis in man.

From studies carried out in Michigan, it appears that the infection in cattle and sheep occurs primarily in winter and early spring. Its duration is short in some cases, but as long as 10 days in others; generally much less in sheep than in cattle. The disease in sheep 'could easily be confused with ketosis or with the effects of over-eating'. In cattle, the infection may be confused with rabies or poisoning. The affected animal is seen to keep aloof from the rest of the herd, and is later unable to stand without support. If walked, it usually moves in a circle. The head may be held back to one side, with salivation and a nasal discharge. Some cows become violent in the terminal stages.

In one English outbreak, 12 out of 15 calves died between April and August, at 3 to 7 days old, from septicæmia. There was severe keratitis and conjunctivitis, extreme dejection, and distressed breathing.

Abortion is a common result of Listeriosis. There is also a septicæmic form, rare in adult cattle and sheep, which shows itself by depression, fever, weakness, and emaciation. Pigs may have swelling of the eyelids, encephalitis, paralysis, or occasionally septicæmia.

Infection may be spread by urine, milk, fæces, an aborted fœtus, and vaginal discharges.

Terramycin has given good results in treatment in a few reported cases which were not too advanced. No vaccines are effective. (*See also* AVIAN LISTERELLOSIS.)

LITHIASIS (λίθος, stone) is a general name applied to the formation of calculi and concretions in tissues or organs, *e.g.* cholelithiasis means the formation of calculi in)the gall-bladder. (*See also under* CALCULI.)

LITHIUM is a metal of which the carbonate and citrate were sometimes used in attempts to prevent or dissolve urinary calculi. Their action is not reliable. Lithium antimony thiomalate is used by injection to remove multiple warts.

LITHONTRIPTICS (λίθος, stone; τρίβω, I rub down) are substances which are reputed to have the power of dissolving stones in the urinary system. (*See* HYALURONIDASE.)

LITHOTOMY (λίθος, stone; τέμνω, I cut) is the term applied to the operation of opening the bladder for the removal of a stone.

LITHOTRITY, or LITHOLAPAXY (λίθος, stone; τρίβω, I rub down; λάπαξις, evacuation) is the name of an operation in which a stone in the bladder is broken into small fragments and removed by washing out the bladder with a catheter.

LITTER (*see* DEEP LITTER *and* BEDDING).

LITTER, OLD.—Broiler chicks reared on previously-used litter may, as a result of the ammonia fumes, develop a severe inflammation of eye-surfaces and eyelids. In one house, 3,000 broilers were affected. The birds cannot bear to open their eyes, and appear obviously dejected. Mortality is generally low, but the trouble is a serious one for all that.

LITTER SIZE (PIGS).—In Britain, the average is 10·7 pigs born alive and 0·6 pigs per litter born dead. An average of 2·2 pigs die between birth and 8 weeks old. (P.I.D.A. figures, 1959.) A litter of 34 has been recorded.

LIVER.—The liver is a solid glandular organ lying in the anteriormost part of the abdomen close up against the diaphragm. Its colour varies from a dark red-brown in the horse to a bluish-purple in the ox and pig; it is soft to the touch though it is rather friable in consistency, and it constitutes the largest gland in the body. Its functions are numerous, and even at present are not all perfectly understood, but they include the excretion of bile, the storage of glycogen, the breaking-down of old and worn-out red blood corpuscles, and the formation of waste substances from the broken-down tissues of the body, especially urea and uric acid, which find their way into the blood-stream and are excreted from the body in the urine by the kidneys. In all animals except those of the horse tribe, the bile is collected into a kind of reservoir, called the *gall-bladder*, from whence it may be poured out into the bile-duct to pass to the small intestine, where it assists the pancreatic juice in the digestion of food after a meal.

Shape.—There are probably few organs which vary so much in shape as the liver, not only in different animals, but in different individuals of the same species. Its general outlines only will be given here. *In the horse* it lies obliquely across the abdominal surface of the diaphragm, its highest and most posterior part being at the level of the right kidney. It possesses a strongly convex diaphragmatic surface which is moulded into the concavity of the diaphragm, and a posterior or abdominal surface which lies in contact with the stomach, duodenum, and right kidney, each of which organs forms a depression in the liver substance. It is only incompletely divided into three lobes in the horse; viz. a right, the largest; a middle, of small size; and a left, of medium size. Lying mainly in the right lobe and on its abdominal surface is the 'porta' of the liver, where the portal vein and hepatic artery enter and from whence the hepatic duct (bile-duct) emerges. Part of the posterior vena cava passes through the liver substance, whose blood it eventually drains. The liver is held in position by the pressure of other organs and by six ligaments. These are: the coronary, which attaches it to the diaphragm; the falciform, from the middle lobe to the diaphragm and abdominal floor; the round, to the umbilicus; the right lateral, to the costal part of the diaphragm; the left lateral, to the tendinous part of the diaphragm; and the hepato-renal or caudate, to the right kidney. *In the ox* it lies almost entirely to the right of the middle line through the body, and its long axis is directed downward and forward. It is thicker than in the horse. Its diaphragmatic surface fits into the concavity of the right part of the diaphragm, and its posterior surface is very irregular. It presents impressions of the two main organs with which it comes into contact—the omasum and reticulum. There is only one distinct lobe—the caudate. There is no left lateral ligament, and the round ligament is only found in the calf. A gall-bladder is present; it is situated partly in a slight depression on the posterior surface of the liver, and partly on the abdominal wall. It is pear-shaped in outline, has a cystic duct which comes off from the bile-duct, and it acts as a reservoir for the bile. *In the sheep* the liver presents small variations, but in the main is similar to that of the ox. The bile-duct joins the pancreatic to form a common duct instead of opening separately as in other animals. *In the pig* the liver is large, very thick, and very much curved. It lies in the anterior part of the abdominal cavity, occupying the whole of the anterior hollow of the diaphragm and more to the right than to the left side of the body, but it extends behind the level of the rib-cage on either side. It possesses four main lobes —right lateral, right central, left central, and left lateral, and on the upper part of the first of these is a small caudate process. The gall-bladder lies in a special little fossa on the right central lobe. *In the dog* the liver is very large, being about 5 per cent of the whole body-weight, and possesses six or seven lobes. The gall-bladder is buried almost completely in the space between the two parts of the right central lobe, only a very small portion of it being visible from the outside.

Blood supply.—The blood supplied to the organ is from two distinct sources, for the liver is peculiar in that the blood collected from the stomach and bowels into the portal vein does not pass directly to the heart, but is distributed to the liver, in the substance of which the portal vein breaks up into capillary vessels. The effects of this are that many harmful substances, absorbed from the food in the stomach and intestines, are abstracted from the blood-stream, altered in the liver into harmless products, and excreted again in the bile in an unabsorbable form, and that various constituents of the food are stored up in the liver for gradual use. The second supply is by a large hepatic artery from the cœliac artery, which also sends branches to the stomach and pancreas, etc. The blood from this artery nourishes the liver cells. After the blood from each source has circulated in the liver it is collected into hepatic veins which open directly into the vena cava, where it passes through the substance of the organ.

Minute structure.—The liver is enveloped in an outer capsule of fibrous tissue with which is blended the hepatic peritoneum, and from which strands run in along with the vessels, and, penetrating into the deepest recesses of the organ, bind its whole structure together. The hepatic artery, portal vein, and bile-duct divide and subdivide, the various branches of each lying alongside corresponding branches from the other two, till their finest divisions, known as interlobular vessels, lie between the lobules of which the whole gland is built up. These lobules, which vary in size in the different animals, form, each in itself, a complete secreting structure, and the liver is made up of many hundreds of thousands of such, exactly similar, lobules.

A single lobule has the following structure. From the small vessels lying around its margin, capillaries or 'sinusoids' are given off, which run in towards the centre of the lobule, where they empty into a small 'central vein'. These central veins from adjacent lobules collect together, and ultimately the blood passes into the hepatic veins, and so leaves the liver. Between the capillaries inside a lobule lie rows of large liver cells, forming the essential elements of the organ upon which its activity depends, Between the rows of liver cells also lie fine bile capillaries which collect the bile discharged by the cells and pass it into the bile-ducts lying around the margins of the lobules. The liver cells are amongst the largest cells of the body, and each contains one large nucleus. With careful special staining methods there can also be seen tiny passages or canals, passing into the cells themselves; some of these communicate with the bile-duct, and others with the ultimate branches of the portal vein. After a mixed meal many of the liver cells can be seen to contain droplets of fat, and granules of glycogen (animal starch) can also be determined. In addition to the cells above described, there occur at intervals along the walls of the sinusoids in a lobule stellate cells which represent the remains of the endothelium from which the capillary-like sinusoids are developed. They are known as 'Kupfer's cells'.

Functions.—As already noted, the liver has numerous functions, of which at least three have been discovered. The best known of these is that of the formation of bile, which constantly trickles from the bile-duct into the intestine, and is passed out in large quantities when a meal has been recently taken. In some animals it has a slight action on fats and starch, but its main function appears to be one of assistance to the activity of the pancreatic juice in the digestion of fats, starches, and to a lesser extent of proteins. Bile consists mainly of salts of two complex acids —glycocholic and taurocholic acids; the former is more abundant in the bile from human beings and herbivorous animals, and the latter is found in carnivorous bile and contains sulphur, which is absent from glycocholic acid. In addition there are bile pigments, mucus, water, and small amounts of fats, soaps, cholesterin, and mineral salts. Bile pigments—bilirubin and biliverdin—are derived from broken-down red blood corpuscles but do not contain any of the iron of the hæmoglobin, which appears to be stored up in the liver. Cholestrin is normally present in only small amounts, but when in excess it becomes deposited in the gall-bladder or bile-ducts as gall-stones. (*See* BILE.) The second function of the liver is the removal from the circulation of the waste products of muscular and other activities, their alteration into urea or uric acid, and their distribution into the circulation again, from whence they are excreted by the kidneys. In addition to the above functions the liver controls the amount of sugars circulating in the blood. When large quantities of sugar and starch are eaten, digested, and absorbed, instead of passing at once into the general circulation, which would throw a surplus of nutriment upon the tissues a short time after feeding and leave them destitute in the intervals, the sugar formed from the food is carried by the portal vein to the liver, and there deposited for future use. It is not stored as the soluble sugar, but as the animal starch called 'glycogen'. If an animal be killed a short time after eating a feed containing starch, and if its liver be examined, the liver cells are found crowded with granules of glycogen. This glycogen is either converted once more, as it is needed, into sugar and passed into the general circulation, or else it is altered into another form, in which it combines with materials in the blood, and is carried away to the muscles and other active organs. In this way the supply of sugars circulating in the blood is kept more or less definite, and usually measures about 0·6 per cent strength in the blood leaving the liver.

LIVER, DISEASES OF.—The liver is one of the passive organs of the body, and may be very extensively diseased without giving any outward sign of discomfort or disturbance, unless the circulation is hindered or the discharge of bile is interfered with or upset. One of the commonly known signs of liver disturbance is jaundice—a yellow coloration of the visible membranes, which is considered under JAUNDICE. Dropsy, which may arise through interference with the circulation of blood through the portal vein, as well as by other causes, is also considered separately. The presence of gall-stones, which is a complication of some liver diseases, is treated under GALL-BLADDER, DISEASES OF. Waxy degeneration is described under AMYLOID DISEASE OF THE LIVER. Under PARASITES are described those diseases, such as hydatid cysts, coccidiosis, fluke disease, or 'liver rot', etc., which are due to parasites living in the liver or in connection with it.

INFLAMMATION OF THE LIVER may be either acute, suppurative (in which abscesses are formed), or chronic. In acute inflammations the parts essentially affected are the liver cells themselves. In chronic inflammation the most marked changes are found in the fibrous tissue which forms the framework of the gland; it is called 'cirrhosis' of the liver.

Acute inflammation is usually a stage farther than acute congestion, which precedes it. It is produced by the absorption of poisons, either of bacterial, vegetable, animal, or mineral origin from the intestines, and it is sometimes caused by the migration of parasites through the liver. The symptoms are pain on pressure over the abdomen, an elevation of temperature, suppression of the appetite, a disinclination to move, and often diarrhœa or constipation in the later stages. (*See also* CANINE VIRUS HEPATITIS.)

Chronic inflammation accompanies very many diseased conditions among animals, the commonest probably being infestation with liver flukes, but it may also be present as a result of tuberculosis, feeding upon mouldy or damaged foods, large amounts of brewers' grains, distillers' offals, poisonous plants in small amounts for considerable periods of time, and in other cases the cause is obscure. It may be produced by feeding cattle upon the plant, ***Senecio jacobea***, a ragwort, and occurs in naturally occurring cases of ragwort poisoning.

Symptoms include a gradual loss of condition, irregular appetite, a staring coat, and a general unthriftiness. Indigestion is shown by irregularity in the passage and consistence of the fæces, listlessness, and pendulousness of the abdomen, as well as other more direct symptoms. Dropsy, due to interference with the abdominal circulation, is seen, especially in sheep with liver flukes, and in dogs and cats. In other cases the liver may be very much altered in appearance and size, but no symptoms are shown, and the condition is only found after death.

Suppurative inflammation is due to the entrance into the liver of pus-forming organisms, and is usually secondary to some other diseased centre in the body where pus is being manufactured. The lesions consist of abscesses in the substance of the liver. Symptoms are vague and diagnosis is often impossible.

FATTY DEGENERATION OF THE LIVER.—The disease is a slowly progressive one; no treatment is possible, even though accurate diagnosis were possible.

TUMOURS.—When small and placed deeply in the substance of the gland they may cause no symptoms whatsoever, but when large and pressing upon vessels or bile-ducts they may give rise to passive congestion, biliary obstruction with jaundice, or they may cause degeneration. The animal presents symptoms accordingly. In the case of large or rapidly growing tumours giving off metastatic or secondary growths, the symptoms are those of excessive tumour growth in any part of the body, with special manifestations connected with the liver. (*See under* TUMOURS.)

TUMOUR-LIKE GROWTHS are seen in large numbers in the livers of beef cattle and dairy cows in abattoirs; they are not true tumours, as a rule, but when cut into are found to be either actinomycotic, tuberculous, or necrotic abscesses, or perhaps cystic swellings due to the intermediate stage of some tapeworm. (These are dealt with under their appropriate headings.)

RUPTURE OF THE LIVER is an accident of comparatively common occurrence among old animals, especially dogs and cats. It may result from a blow, kick, run-over accident, or fall; from violent struggling, fractured ribs, swallowing a sharp-pointed foreign body; or it may arise from very simple exertion when the liver is diseased. It is serious, owing to the hæmorrhage which follows even a small wound in such a vascular organ as the liver, and an animal injured in this way often dies from internal hæmorrhage.

Symptoms.—When the injury has been small there are no marked symptoms beyond the initial pain of the injury. In cases where a larger tear has been sustained but where the capsule has remained intact, as from severe crushes, there is evidence of abdominal pain. The animal is dull, disinclined to move, exhibits pain when the area is handled, and often shows rigors or patchy sweating. Its pulse is weak; its membranes are pale in colour; the ears, feet, etc., are cold; and breathing is usually laboured. This condition may last from 12 to 36 hours, when it either gradually begins to pass off during the next few days and the animal recovers, or, more frequently, the capsule of the liver gives way and the animal dies from internal hæmorrhage. In other cases where the rupture of the liver has been complete (*i.e.* where the capsule is torn), death occurs in a few hours, or in the worst cases almost at once.

LIVER FLUKES are parasitic flat worms which infest the livers of various animals, especially sheep and cattle. They may cause severe illness and even death. Control measures include regular dosing, and destruction—so far as practicable—of the intermediate host snails. (*See* PARASITES.)

To be effective, control measures require a planned campaign rather than a single battle or weapon. In the sheep, infestation does not lead to subsequent immunity, and this fact gives very little hope of an effective vaccine (similar to the irradiated huskworm larvæ vaccine) ever being produced. Nor until 1971 was there any drug to kill all young, immature flukes within the body, and it is these which on their mass migrations through the liver can damage it so severely that sudden death inevitably follows.

However, it is claimed that diamphenethide kills all stages of the liver fluke, including those three days old and upwards. A single dose is given as soon as the outbreak is detected, and a further dose four weeks later. It is claimed to be safe for lambs and pregnant/in-milk ewes.

A vaccine against Black Disease—in which spores of one of the gas-gangrene group of organisms are stimulated into activity by young flukes in the liver—can prevent deaths from the resulting toxæmia. Against the liver flukes themselves, routine dosing is essential on all farms where they are likely to occur. Dr. C. B. Ollerenshaw, of Agriculture, has pointed out that, in the light of Australian experience, there is a tendency in this country to under-dose with carbon tetrachloride, and that consequently results have not been as good as they might have been. With the newer drugs, too, which are especially useful in tackling acute fluke disease problems, he suggests that dose-rates may have to be well above the minimum to obtain a high percentage of fluke kills. (*See* histogram, p. 513.)

Land drainage is still high on the list of control measures.

The use of snail killers is a recommended part of the campaign against fluke disease, but not a snag-free method. It is so easy to miss small areas inhabited by snails, and this applies even when using a knapsack sprayer—the only possible method of spraying if the land is too wet, as it often is, to take a tractor. Snail killers can be unpleasant to work with. The cheapest is sodium pentachlorophenate. N-trityemorpholine costs about 45s. per acre but has the advantages of being relatively harmless to stock, so that grazing need not be delayed for a fortnight as after copper sulphate dressings or pentachlorophenate. All are poisonous to fish.

Running ducks over snaily land is not among the official recommendations but it might prove of some value. A few farmers have tried it in the past. In Zambia two years ago a large-scale duck-rearing scheme was introduced in areas flooded by the River Zambesi as a method of fluke disease and bilharzia control. Hoof-prints, where the soil is exposed, are favourite habitats of the snails.

In man, water-cress is the chief source of infestation. Illness is most marked during migration of immature flukes. Eosinophilia is a pointer to aid diagnosis; eggs may not appear in the fæces for 12 weeks. (*See also under* ANTS.)

LIVER/KIDNEY SYNDROME OF CATS.—This illness resembles leptospirosis in the dog, but this infection has not been proved to be the cause.

LIVER/KIDNEY SYNDROME OF POULTRY.—This affects birds usually 2 to 3 weeks old. Symptoms may not be observed—or there may be depression for a day or two; occasionally trembling or paralysis of legs. Mortality: 1 to 5 per cent. The whole carcase may have a pink tinge. The liver is pale, swollen, and fatty. The kidneys may be very swollen. The cause is unknown.

The syndrome has to be differentiated from Toxic Fat disease, Gumboro disease, and Infectious avian nephrosis.

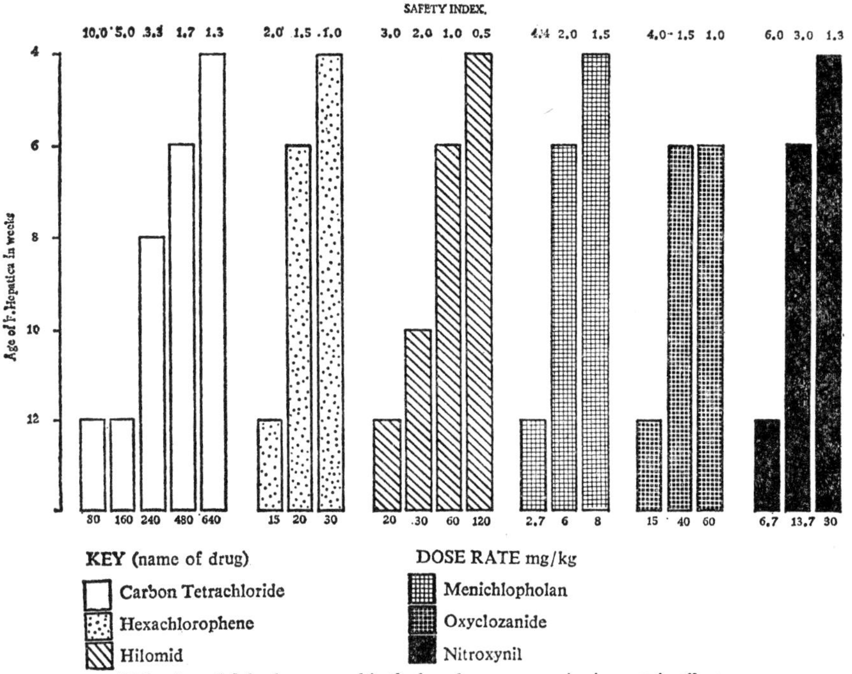

All the six anti-fluke drugs named in the key show a progressive increase in efficacy against immature flukes as the dose rate and size of the fluke increase.

LIVER ROT is the popular name for the condition resulting from mass migration of immature liver flukes. (*See* PARASITES *and* LIVER FLUKES.)

LIVER, RUPTURE OF (IN FOWLS) (*see* HÆMORRHAGIC DISEASE).

'LIZARD POISONING' IN CATS.—This term is applied to infestation with the liver-fluke *Platynosomum concinnum*, which has been reported from South America, the Caribbean Islands, Malaysia, the U.S.A. and, more recently, Nigeria. The life cycle of the parasite involves a large land snail, a crustacean, and lizards, frogs, and probably other amphibians and reptiles. Symptoms in the cat include listlessness, fever, jaundice, diarrhœa, vomiting, and emaciation; but sub-clinical infestations also occur.

LOBE (λοβός) is the term applied to the larger divisions of various organs, such as the lungs, liver, and brain. The term *lobar* is applied to structures which are connected with lobes of organs, or to diseases which have a tendency to be limited to one lobe only, such as 'lobar pneumonia'.

LOBULE (*lobulus*, a little lobe) is the term applied to the division of an organ which are smaller than a lobe; for example, the lobules of the lungs are about the size of a millet seed, and those of the liver a little larger. The term *lobular* is applied to disease which occurs in a scattered irregular manner affecting lobules here and there, such as 'lobular pneumonia'.

LOCK-JAW is a popular name for tetanus. (*See* TETANUS.)

'LOCO WEED.'—Legumes oxytropis and astragalus in the U.S.A. produce a chronic contracted front-leg condition in lambs born to ewes which ate just insufficient of the plant to cause abortion.

LOCUST BEANS are the broken-down pods of the carob tree, *Ceratonia siliqua*. The pods are fleshy, flat and pulpy, dark purple and glossy on the outside, and contain a number of small, extremely hard, polished seeds. The beans are rich in digestible carbohydrates, contain a proportion of proteins, and are consequently used for finishing off fat stock and for the feeding of working horses. The food is sweet, and usually readily eaten by stock. Occasionally the hard seeds, which are seldom chewed, collect in the stomach of the horse or in the abomasum of the ox, and give rise to indigestion. They sometimes serve as nuclei for calculi.

LOOSE-BOXES.—The best type has well-built brick or stone walls lined on the inside to the roof with cement-plaster finished off smooth. The floor is of cement-concrete, grooved to facilitate the draining away of fluids and to provide a foothold, and the corners are rounded off with fillets of cement. The only fittings inside are hay-rack, water-bowl, and manger, of iron, and rather larger than in the stall of a stable, so that cattle as well as horses may use them; in some cases one or two rings, to which animals may be tied, are provided. It is very useful to have a strong angle-iron beam running across the roof of the box, which will serve to support the block and tackle if it becomes necessary to use the box for slinging horses. One or more windows, high up out of reach of the animals' heads, should be included, and the door should always be made in two halves, so that horses with respiratory diseases may be able to stand with their heads out of the box, and so obtain a plentiful supply of fresh air. Wherever possible, loose-boxes should be built with a southerly aspect, so that the very important germicidal action of sunlight may be taken full advantage of, whenever sick animals are housed in the box.

LORDOSIS (λόρδωσις) means an unnatural curvature of the spine, so that the concavity of the spine is directed upwards. It is seen in tetanus, and sometimes in rabies.

LOTION (*lotio*, a fluid application) means a fluid preparation intended to be brought into direct contact with the skin, and used for washing a part. Lotions are generally of a watery nature, though some are alcoholic, and many are known as 'liquors'. External applications of an oily or a soapy nature are known as 'liniments'.

Varieties and Uses.—*Antiseptic lotions.* (*See* ANTISEPTICS.)

Astringent lotions are used to check discharges from inflamed mucous membranes, and to stimulate sluggish wounds or ulcers on the surface of the body. Sulphate of zinc in varying strength in water is an example. Calamine lotion, containing carbonate of zinc, is used in cases of wet eczema to stop the discharge and soothe irritation.

LOUPING-ILL, which is also called TREMBLES, TREMBLINGS, TWITCH, DIZZY STAGGERS, THE JUMPS, and a number of other names indicative of the above conditions, is an infective paralytic disease of sheep, transmitted by *Ixodes ricinus*, the tick commonly present on hill pastures. It occurs in western Scotland, the North of England, and the North-west of Ireland. It has a definite seasonal incidence, most cases occurring between March and June, and between September and October, and only few sporadic cases are met with at other times of the year. All breeds of sheep are susceptible. It has been recorded as affecting pigs, but is not generally recognised as a disease causing much loss among these animals. It is also transmissible to man, producing fever and muscular pain.

On upland grazings where ticks abound, louping-ill has, of recent years, become of economic importance **in cattle.** The animals become dull and uninterested in food, walk in an unnatural way, sometimes with their heads down, and occasionally become excited.

Cause.—A virus, introduced into the general circulation by the bites of infected ticks (adult or nymphal). The virus primarily multiplies in the blood, and in certain cases invades the central nervous system at a later stage in the infection. This invasion is responsible for the typical symptoms of the disease. It would appear that accessory conditions favour such invasion, *e.g.* tick-borne fever, a disease also transmitted by the *I. ricinus*. The periods when outbreaks of the disease are commonest correspond with the first and second tick crops during the year.

The ticks can survive, in the absence of sheep and cattle, on deer, rabbits, hares, voles, field mice, grouse, etc., and these animals may act as host of the virus.

Symptoms.—Two forms of the disease are recognised: viz. an acute and a subacute form. In the *acute form* the symptoms may appear in from 4 to 6 days after the sheep are infested with the carrier ticks. The sheep becomes uneasy, lies down and rises frequently during the day. Its temperature ranges between 104° and 107° F. during the next week or ten days, and it develops nervous symptoms. At first, it is merely more timid and more easily frightened than usual; later, the muscles of the jaws and neck begin to twitch and quiver, and there may be frothing at the mouth. It staggers when made to move rapidly or turn suddenly, and as the disease becomes firmly established it may be seen taking short spasmodic jumps, rising apparently from all four feet at the same time, and landing upon all four feet again. In this way an affected sheep can usually be easily noticed among a flock when the sheep are being driven or collected by a dog. In more advanced stages the animal becomes paralysed, unable to stand, and often has its head drawn round over its fore flank. Unconsciousness quickly appears, and the animal dies a short time afterwards.

In the *sub-acute type* the first symptoms are slight. Later, the sheep is seen taking very high steps with its fore-legs; it holds its head very high, and sometimes carries it to one side (often the left); the pupils are dilated, and the expression of the sheep is one of extreme fear when caught. It may attempt to feed, but actually eats very little. Tremblings of the muscles, staggering and falling, and sometimes paralysis of one or more groups of muscles, are seen, but it is not common for convulsive seizures and elevation of the temperature to be present in this type. As time goes on the sheep loses condition, at first very slowly, but later very rapidly. If not attended and fed by hand it dies from starvation in the course of two or three weeks, but if fed by hand it may live for two months.

A number of sheep recover from each type of the disease even when left to themselves, but it is common for such to retain some legacy from louping-ill which shows in the carriage of their heads, either a greater elevation than usual, or a twisting to one side, or their mode of progression may change. Recovery from one attack confers a definite degree of immunity, which may last for life. As far as is known, recovered sheep are not carriers of infection.

Treatment.—There is no known curative treatment. Affected sheep, if not numerous, should be slaughtered. Prevention should aim at the eradication of the infecting ticks from grazing lands. This is not easy, as the tick can live under rough herbage without access to the living sheep for as long as one year. Under PARASITES a description is given of the life-history of the tick.

A vaccine against louping-ill, developed at Moredun, had to be withdrawn in 1966 because of the infection of laboratory staff engaged in its commercial production. An improved vaccine, also developed at Moredun in 1969, gives a degree of immunity equal to that resulting from a natural infection within 7 to 10 days of injection. Vaccination of ewes confers protection in their lambs. Inoculations are carried out in spring prior to the season when ticks become active.

LUBRICANTS.—The type of lubricant used in pellet mills and other forms of machinery for processing animal feeding-stuffs may be of the greatest importance. Lubricants containing chlorinated naphthalene compounds and used on such machines may give rise to Hyperkeratosis in cattle eating the food so contaminated by the minutest quantity of lubricant.

LUGOL'S SOLUTION.—A solution of 50 gm. iodine and 100 gm. potassium iodide in distilled water to 1000 c.c.

LUING.—A beef breed evolved by Messrs. Cadzow from Beef Shorthorn and Highland cattle, and named after the island. Colour: red with a touch of gold; or roan; or white. There are a breed society and herd book. Recognised by Secretary of State, Scotland, 1965.

LUMBAR (*lumbi*, the loins) is a term used to denote either the structures in or disease affecting the loins, that is, the region lying between the last rib and the point of the hip, from one side of the body to the other. There are lumbar vertebræ, lumbar muscles, etc.

LUMBAR ANÆSTHESIA (*see* EPIDURAL ANÆSTHESIA).

LUMEN.—The space inside a tubular structure, such as an artery or intestine.

LUMINAL, or **PHENOBARBITAL,** is a sedative drug used particularly in canine hysteria, but also in other nervous conditions. It is given in doses of ½ to 2 grains. Luminal sodium is a soluble preparation given in similar doses for the same purposes.

'LUMPY SKIN DISEASE'.—A highly infectious and important disease of cattle in Africa. The cause is a virus. A discharge from the eyes and nose, lameness, and salivation may be observed—

depending upon the site of nodules which sometimes involve mucous membrane as well as skin. No specific treatment is available.

Permanent sterility may follow this disease ; likewise death.

The disease is a pox, and a modified sheep-pox vaccine is used.

'False lumpy skin disease' is a name for an African disease caused by a virus similar to (or identical with) that of bovine mammillitis. (*See* VIRUS INFECTIONS OF COWS' TEATS.)

LUMPY WITHERS is a condition in the working horse in which small lumps, about the size of a walnut or more, appear on either side of the withers where the collar lies. There may be several, but one on each side is the common number. They are produced by irritation of the synovial bursa which lies under the skin along the spines of the withers, resulting in the production of an excessive amount of synovial secretion. Unless they receive attention they often lead to the production of fistulous withers. (*See* FISTULOUS WITHERS.)

LUMPY WOOL, or wool rot, is a condition caused by a fungus which attacks the sheep's skin during wet weather, causing irritation and the formation of a hard yellowish-white scab about ⅛ inch thick. Healing soon occurs and the wool continues to grow, carrying the hard material away from the skin as a buff or brownish zone in the wool. Severe infection may lead to loss of wool.

The fungus causing this mycotic dermatitis—as Lumpy Wool is technically known—is *Dermatophilus dermatonomus*. (*See also under* STREPTOTHRICOSIS.)

LUNGING (from *allonger*, to lengthen) is a method of exercising horses whereby the horse is made to travel in a circle round a man who stands at its centre holding a long rope. The circle is at first small in diameter, but as the horse learns what is required the rope is lengthened, and the circle becomes larger. By this means a horse may be given half an hour's trotting exercise in small enclosures without the necessity of carrying a man or pulling a vehicle.

LUNGS.—The lungs are a pair of organs situated in the thoracic (chest) cavity, in which exchange of gases between the blood and the air takes place. The air enters by the nostrils, passes through the nasal passages, pharynx, larynx, trachea, and bronchi, and finally enters the air cells in the lungs themselves. (*See* AIR PASSAGES.) The blood is carried to the lungs by the pulmonary artery, which divides and subdivides into tiny capillaries which lie around the walls of the air cells.

Lung is composed of very highly elastic tissue which consists of multitudes of tiny sacs arranged at the terminal parts of the smallest of the bronchioles, and which collapse when the balance of pressure between the air in the sacs and on the outside of the lung surface is disturbed. Thus a lung shrinks to about one-third of its normal size when removed from the chest cavity.

Horse.—The lungs occupy the greater part of the thoracic cavity, and are accurately moulded to the walls of the chest and to the other organs contained within it. The right is considerably larger than the left, owing to the presence of the heart, which lies mostly to the left side of the middle plane of the cavity. In the equidæ the lung is not divided into lobes as it is in some of the other animals. The apex is that portion which occupies the most anterior part of the chest cavity, and just immediately behind it is the deep impression for the heart. Behind this again, and a little above it, is the 'root' of the lung, which consists of the blood-vessels entering and leaving the lung, lymph vessels, nerves, the bronchus, and here also are situated the bronchial lymph glands. In cross-section each lung is somewhat triangular in shape, with one of the angles rounded. The rounded angle lies in the uppermost part of the chest, alongside the bodies of the thoracic vertebræ, and the more acute of the remaining angles lies along the floor of the chest.

Ox.—In the ox the lungs are thicker and shorter than in the horse, and there is a greater disproportion in size—the right weighing about half as much again as the left. They are divided into lobes by deep fissures. The left has three lobes, and the right four or five. The root in each case is almost immediately above the impression for the heart. The apical lobe (*i.e.* the most anterior of the right lung) receives a special small bronchus from the trachea direct. In the sheep the lungs are like those of the horse—the lobation being at best very incomplete.

Pig.—The left lung is like that of the ox, but the right lung has its apical lobe very often divided into two parts. Otherwise there are no great differences. Three bronchi are present, as in the ox.

Dog.—The lungs are thicker than in either the horse or ox in conformity with the more barrel-like shape of the chest. There is no cardiac impression in the left lung. Each has three large lobes, but the right has a small extra mediastinal lobe, and there may be one or more accessory lobes in either lung.

Colour.—In the perfectly fresh lung from a young unbled animal the colour of the lung is a bright rose-pink, with a glistening surface, the pleural membrane, but in the lungs of older animals there is usually a certain amount of deposit of soot, dust, etc., which has been inhaled with the air and collected in the lymph spaces between the air cells. In an animal which has been bled the lung is of a pale pink, owing to the lesser blood content. In the case of pit ponies, town dogs, and other animals which have breathed a comparatively impure atmosphere, the lungs show a greater or lesser degree of pigmentation, so that the colour of the normal lung may vary from a slate-blue to a jet black, and yet be quite healthy.

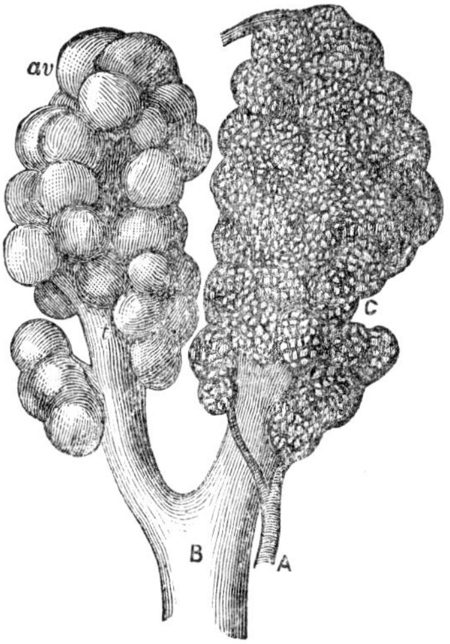

The outer surface of two infundibula in a lobule of the lung. *A*, branch of the pulmonary artery ramifying over the air alveoli; *B*, the small bronchial tube of the lobule; *C*, capillaries; *av*, air vesicles or alveoli; *t*, air terminal bronchiole.

Changes at birth.—Before the birth of a young animal the lungs are collapsed and look not unlike cooked liver, being pale grey in colour, dense in consistence, and firm to the touch. They are smaller in size, and sink in water. Immediately upon taking the first breath the tissue of the lungs expands, the colour suddenly changes to a bright red, the consistence becomes spongy, and if placed in water they will float. These changes are of use in determining whether a dead foal or calf, etc., has been born dead or has died after first breathing.

Connections.—The lungs are firmly anchored in position by their roots to the heart and trachea, and by the pleura to a longitudinal septum running vertically from front to back, called the 'mediastinum' (*see* PLEURA). The pulmonary artery, carrying impure blood to the lungs, divides into two large branches after only a very short course. Each of these branches enters into the formation of the root of the lung, and there begins to divide up into a very large number of smaller vessels. These subdivide many times until the final capillaries are given off around the walls of the air-sacs. From these the blood, after oxygenation, is carried by larger and larger veins, till it eventually leaves the lung by one of the several pulmonary veins. These number six or seven or more, and leave the lungs by the roots. In addition to the blood carried to the lung for aeration a small bronchial artery carries blood to the lung substance for nutritive purposes. This accompanies the bronchi and splits into branches corresponding to the small bronchi and bronchioles. The lymph vessels in the root of the lungs are very numerous, and are all connected with the large bronchial glands at this part. The glands are important, for when disease germs gain entrance into the lungs it is the duty of the lymph system to pick them up, carry them to the glands, and there destroy them. In certain cases, especially in tuberculosis, there comes a time when the lymph glands are unable to deal with the bacilli in an effective manner, and, not being destroyed, the organisms set up disease in the glands themselves. The lymph glands are therefore useful indicators of the healthiness or otherwise of the lung.

Minute structure.—The main bronchial tube, entering the lung at its root, divides into branches, which subdivide again and again, to be distributed all through the substance of the lung, till the finest tubes, known as 'bronchioles' or 'capillary bronchi', have a diameter of only about $\frac{1}{100}$th of an inch. In structure, all these tubes consist of a mucous membrane surrounded by a fibrous sheath. The trachea, as well as the larger and medium-sized bronchi, have in the fibrous layer pieces of cartilage which, in the trachea and largest bronchial tubes, form regular but incomplete rings, and in the smaller tubes are arranged as plates. These cartilages have the function of preventing the tubes from closing or being compressed, and so obstructing the passage of air. The larger and medium bronchi are richly supplied with glands secreting mucus, which is poured out on to the surface of the lining membrane and serves to keep it moist. The surface of this membrane is composed of columnar epithelial cells, provided with little whip-like processes known as 'cilia', which have the double function of moving any expectoration upwards towards the throat, and of warming the air as it passes over them. The walls of the bronchial tubes are rich in fibres of elastic tissue, and immediately below the mucous membrane of the small tubes is a layer of plain muscle fibres placed circularly. To this muscular layer belongs the function of altering the lumen of the tube, and, consequently, its air-carrying capacity. It is a spasmodic contraction of the muscular layer that produces the characteristic expiratory 'cough' of true asthma.

The smallest divisions of the bronchial tubes open out into a number of dilatations, known as 'infundibula', each of which measures about $\frac{1}{20}$th of an inch across, and these are covered with minute sacs, variously known as 'air-vesicles,' 'air-alveoli', or 'air cells'. An air cell consists of a delicate membrane composed of flattened plate-like cells, strengthened by a wide network of elastic fibres, to which the great elasticity of the lung is due; and it is in these thin-walled air cells that the respiratory exchange of gases takes place.

The branches of the pulmonary arteries accompany the bronchial tubes to the farthest recesses of the lung, dividing like the latter into finer and finer branches, and ending in a dense network of capillaries, which lies everywhere between the air vesicles, the capillaries being so closely placed that they occupy a much greater area than the spaces between them. The air in the air vesicles is separated from the blood only by two most delicate membranes, viz. the wall of the air cell and the wall of the capillary, and it is through these walls that the respiratory exchange takes place.

LUNGS, DISEASES OF.—The diseases of the lungs, on account of their great importance, are considered, to a large extent, separately under their respective headings. (*See under* BROKEN WIND, BRONCHITIS, CHILLS AND COLDS, GLANDERS, PLEURISY, PNEUMONIA, STRANGLES, TUBERCULOSIS, JAAGSIEKTE, etc.)

CONGESTION OF THE LUNGS is the condition which almost always ushers in an attack of true pneumonia, and is therefore often considered as the first stage of pneumonia. It is characterised by an abnormally large amount of blood in the lungs. It may be brought about by anything which induces an increase in the inflow without a corresponding increase in the outflow of blood, or anything which decreases the outflow without altering the inflow. The first of these results is an active congestion, and the second is a passive congestion. It is commonest in the horse.

Causes.—The commonest cause of congestion is an attack upon weakened tissues in the lung by numbers of the ever-present germs. Chemical irritants, smoke, medicines, exposure to chills and colds, lower the vitality of the delicate lung cells, and bacterial activity proceeds unchecked. The body attempts to counteract this activity by sending a larger amount of blood than usual to the area, and active congestion results. In passive congestion there is usually some obstruction to the return flow of blood to the heart, such as weakness or disease of the right heart, which does not supply sufficient driving power to effect the return of the blood to the left heart, or obstructions on the valves of the left side of the heart which is unable to deal with the blood as fast as it is returned from the lungs. These conditions are frequently seen in horses that are not in fit condition and are called upon to perform some particularly strenuous work or exercise. Pressure upon the pulmonary veins from a tumour or an inflammatory condition, such as pericarditis, also results in passive congestion. There is another form of congestion, known as 'hypostatic congestion', in which undue pressure is put upon the lungs through lying on one side for long periods at a time, and the lowermost part of the under lung becomes filled with blood in response to the laws of gravity. It is to prevent this that it is so necessary to turn over on to the other side animals that are unable to stand and have been lying for some time.

Symptoms.—In acute congestion the symptoms are severe, and the animal is in great distress. Its respirations are very rapid and difficult; it stands with head outstretched, nostrils dilated, eyes anxious-looking, and the breathing comes and goes in great sobs. If made to move it may lose balance and fall as if fainting. The membranes are deeply injected and may be bluish or even purple. The pulse is small and weak, and often cannot be felt. The temperature is only slightly elevated in the early stages, but rapidly rises to 106° F. or over. There may be some bleeding from the lungs which issues by the nostrils. In less acute cases the symptoms come on more slowly, and are less alarming. The condition may pass off in twelve hours or less, or may become complicated by pneumonia, laminitis, œdema of the lungs, etc., but in animals with a diseased heart a repetition is very likely at a future time.

Treatment.—The animal must be immediately released from all work or restraint, and placed where a free supply of fresh air is available. Immediate relief is obtained by bleeding from the jugular vein, which lessens the tension on the heart and enables it to regain its lost ground. The surface circulation should be stimulated by friction and the application of rugs, bandages, etc. Heart stimulants, such as caffeine, camphor, strychnine, or digitalis, may be administered hypodermically.

Afterwards, if complications do not ensue, the horse requires a long period of rest, careful building up, courses of heart tonics, regulated exercise, etc., before he is fit to be put to strenuous exertion again.

PULMONARY ŒDEMA, or œdema of the lungs ('Pulmonary Apoplexy'). It is usually very sudden in its onset, and after only a few hours of extremely laboured breathing the animal in most cases expires. The condition is brought about by a transudation of the blood serum (sometimes accompanied by corpuscles) from the engorged capillaries into the air cells, where the pressure is lower than in the vessels. It is due to the same causes as congestion, but it is very much more serious. It is seen in 'Fog Fever' and in animals which have breathed smoke from a burning building. Other causes include an allergy, certain poisons such as Antu, broncho-pneumonia, and occasionally nephritis or a nerve injury.

Symptoms.—The preliminary symptoms are the same as those in congestion, but become exaggerated with great rapidity. A considerable amount of serum and frothy discharge may be coughed out from mouth or nostrils, but no relief is obtained. In a short time signs of suffocation supervene, and the animal becomes virtually drowned in its own blood serum.

TUMOURS OF THE LUNG are not at all uncommon among the smaller animals, but they are usually of metastatic origin, *i.e.* they are secondary growths which have started from another centre in the body, being carried to the lung tissue either by the blood- or lymph-stream. The symptoms vary from only a slight breathlessness during exercise, to acute dyspnœa (difficulty in breathing) upon the slightest exertion. Treatment is impossible.

ABSCESS IN THE LUNG may follow pneumonia from ordinary causes or it may be specific, as in glanders, strangles, tuberculosis, pleuro-pneumonia of cattle, and other diseases. (*See* these headings.)

GANGRENE OF THE LUNG may be a complication of or a sequel to pneumonia, and is usually fatal. It is characterised by the presence of a foul-smelling, usually rusty-red, and almost always very copious discharge from both nostrils, in addition to the other symptoms of pneumonia. It is commonest in the horse as a sequel to ordinary pneumonia, and in other animals it may occur when the pneumonia has been produced through faulty drenching. (*See* Pneumonia.)

COLLAPSE OF THE LUNG occurs under several conditions. The lungs are so resilient, in consequence of the elastic fibres throughout their substance, that if air be admitted within the pleural cavities the lungs immediately collapse to about a third of their natural size. Accordingly, if the chest wall is wounded and air gains entrance through the wound (pneumothorax), the lung collapses. After the wound has healed, and provided no complications occur, the elasticity is restored as the air is absorbed. In the same way, when there is an effusion of fluid during pleurisy into the pleural cavities, the lung also collapses. This collapse is liable to be permanent if the fluid remains in position for any considerable length of time, and when adhesions form. When a foreign body or growth blocks up one of the bronchial tubes the air behind the block is absorbed and collapse of the lung again results. The lungs of a fœtus at birth are collapsed until the first breath has been taken, and any signs of expansion of the lungs in such is proof that the creature was not born dead. (*See* Lungs.)

WOUNDS OF THE LUNG are serious on account of the air admitted through the chest wall, which leads to collapse; on account of the damage they cause to the lung, as well as on account of the hæmorrhage, and the difficulty of checking it, they usually lead to local pneumonia. The lung may be wounded by the end of a fractured rib pointing inwards, by some sharp-pointed body which penetrates through the chest wall, or by some hard, sharp body passing down the gullet and tearing through its wall. The symptoms are not uniform, and the treatment of each case must be according to its nature and extent.

PARASITES OF THE LUNGS include the worms responsible for 'husk' (*i.e.* stronggyles, in each domestic animal), larval stages of *Ascarides*, as well as the cystic stage of *Tænia echinococcus*, one of the dog tapeworms, etc. Flukes are also sometimes found living in the lungs of cattle and sheep; lung flukes attack cats, dogs, pigs, and man in the Far East and the United States, and other parasites are met with more rarely. (*See section on* PARASITES.)

LUPINES, POISONING BY.—Lupines of different species have often been found to cause poisoning of sheep, but although horses, cattle, and goats may be affected, it is rare in other animals. In the United States of America great loss among sheep flocks has been occasioned by feeding on lupines animals not accustomed to them, although those which had eaten small amounts previously, and had probably gained some tolerance to the toxic agent, were not affected. In Europe the most dangerous species is the yellow lupine, *Lupinus luteus*, although both the blue lupine, *L. angustifolius*, and the white lupine, *L. albus*, may be poisonous when eaten in quantity. In addition to acquired tolerance, another factor which varies the toxicity of the plant is the nature of the soil upon which it is grown, and the stage of growth at which the plant has arrived when eaten. Thus lupines eaten before the seed pods have formed are almost harmless, while the ripe, or nearly ripe, seed-pods will kill a sheep in from a half to one hour if eaten in quantity. The nature of the poison is not yet fully understood, but it appears that there are two alkaloids and a substance called *lupinotoxin*, which possess poisonous properties. The alkaloids are *lupinine* and *lupinidine*.

Recent evidence from Australia confirms an old theory that lupine poisoning is due to a fungus which is parasitic or saphrophytic on the plant, and that when this fungus is absent the lupines are quite harmless. In Australia lupinosis causes losses after summer rainfall.

In the U.S.A., 'crooked calf disease', in which calves are born with twisted backs or necks, malaligned legs, or cleft palates, is a sequel to in-calf cows eating lupines, and is important in Idaho.

Symptoms.—In Europe, by far the greater number of cases are of a chronic type, which results in the production of a train of symptoms to which the name 'lupinosis' has been given. In America, however, the symptoms are of an acute type. The variation may be due to the amount of the plant eaten, and each form may be met with in either continent.

In the *acute type* the sheep become suddenly ill and die in from a few hours to six days, most deaths occurring between the fourth and the sixth day. The appetite is lost; breathing is very difficult; the temperature rises very high; blood is passed in the urine; and circulatory and digestive troubles arise. After a time the animals lose their balance, fall to the ground, may show convulsions, rapidly lose condition, collapse, and die. Jaundice and œdematous swellings of the lips, eyelids, and ears may be seen.

In the *chronic form*, *i.e.* lupinosis, the sheep show less severe symptoms and may live for 15 to 20 days before death or recovery takes place. The characteristic lesion in luprinosis is a great increase in the supportive framework of fibrous tissue in the liver, which leads to pressure upon the liver cells and consequent derangement of function. Gastric inflammation accompanies the liver disturbance and makes feeding impossible. The animal loses condition, becomes dropsical about the head and neck, lies about without interest in its surroundings, and finally, in the period stated, collapses and dies. A few animals recover, but they seldom thrive well afterwards.

LUPUS (*lupus*, a wolf) is a term sometimes used to indicate tuberculosis of the skin, in which the areas affected are of small size and in the form of intractable pimples or ulcers. The word is borrowed from human medicine, in which lupus is a recognised condition.

LUTEIN.—An internal secretion of the ovary.

LUXATION (*luxus*, a dislocation) is another name for dislocation. (*See* DISLOCATION.)

LYMPH (*lympha*, water, strictly speaking) is the fluid which circulates through the lymphatic spaces of the animal body. It is a colourless fluid, rather more watery than, but otherwise similar to, the blood-plasma. It contains salts similar to the blood-plasma, and the same kinds of proteins, viz. fibrinogen, serum-albumin, and serum-globulin. It also contains colourless lymph corpuscles, derived from the lymph glands, and similar to some of the white blood corpuscles. After meals, certain of the lymphatic vessels contain large amounts of fat globules in the form of a milky emulsion, and are therefore called ' lacteals '. These vessels are those which absorb fat from the food passing through the small intestine and convey it to the thoracic duct, from whence it passes direct into the blood-stream.

Lymph may be regarded as the material through whose agency the tissues are directly nourished, and by which waste materials are collected from the tissues and taken back into the blood-stream. There are certain tissues which are not provided with a blood-supply at all, *e.g.* the cornea of the eye, cartilage, horn, etc., and in them the lymph is the only nourishing medium.

The lymph is derived in the first place from the blood-stream, of which the watery constituents exude through the fine walls of the capillaries into the tissue spaces. This is partly the result of the higher blood-pressure in the capillaries, and partly due to the vital action of the cells composing their walls, which take up blood-plasma from the blood and pass it through themselves to the spaces in the tissues. At first, very incompletely, but later more regularly, these spaces are lined with an endothelium which eventually takes the form of tiny lymph vessels which permeate throughout the whole of the tissues of a part. The lymph capillaries consist of a single layer of cells similar to the smallest blood-capillaries, and like them they unite with each other eventually to form larger vessels which are called the ' lymphatics ', or ' absorbent vessels '. These ramify through the body, passing here and there through lymph glands, into which they discharge their contents, and from which they collect them again, until finally they open into veins at the root of the neck and the now purified lymph is restored to the blood-stream. Other lymph vessels commence as small spaces in the peritoneum and pleuræ, and act as drains for these otherwise closed cavities. It is in this way that fluid effusions of pleurisy and localised peritonitis are absorbed. (*See also under* GLANDS.)

The circulation of the lymph is effected by means of ' lymph-hearts ' in some of the lower forms of animal life, but in the higher animals there is no lymph-heart, the circulation depending upon the pressure at which it passes through the capillaries, and upon the squeezing action of muscular contraction during exercise. The lymph capillaries and vessels are copiously provided with valves, which prevent any back-flow of the lymph-stream, so that the pressure exerted by contraction of a muscle results in the driving of the fluid in one way only, and space is left behind for the exudation of more lymph. From this fact alone one can understand the great importance of muscular action in the economy of the body.

Lymph possesses, like blood, the power of clotting when exposed to the air or to surfaces that are roughened. When it does clot it forms a colourless or only faintly yellow coagulum, over the surface, and protects cells which are perhaps abraded, below. In small wounds and scratches, where the injury is so small that little or no hæmorrhage takes place, this film of coagulated lymph can be easily seen.

The term ' lymph ' is also applied to the material which collects in the vesicles of cow-pox (and other poxes) which is used for vaccination. (*See* VACCINATION, VARIOLA.)

LYMPHADENITIS (*lympha*, lymph; ἀδήν, a gland) means inflammation of lymphatic glands. (*See* GLANDS, DISEASES OF.)

LYMPHADENOMA (*lympha*, lymph; ἀδήν, a gland; *-oma*, meaning a tumour) is another name for Hodgkin's disease. (*See* HODGKIN'S DISEASE.)

LYMPHANGITIS (*lympha*, lymph; ἀγγεῖον, a vessel). This word essentially means an inflammation of the lymphatic vessels, but through custom it has come to be used for a particular condition among horses, in which the chief symptoms are associated with an inflammation of the lymph vessels of one or more limbs. This disease will be described here. (*See also* EPIZOÖTIC LYMPHANGITIS, ULCERATIVE CELLULITIS, which is often called 'ulcerous lymphangitis', *and under* GLANDERS.)

Other names by which this disease is popularly known are: 'weed'; 'Monday morning disease'; 'a shot o' grease'; 'water farcy'; 'big-leg', etc.

The disease is essentially a disease of horses, although a condition almost similar is seen in the dog and in cattle. It is met with in all breeds, sexes, and ages of horses kept under all conditions of management, and receiving almost any of the foods used for the feeding of horses. It may attack one or two hind- or fore-limbs, although it is certainly commonest in one or other of the hind-legs.

Causes.—Since it is most often seen in heavy draught horses of a sluggish temperament, which have thick 'greasy' or puffy legs, these factors are considered as at least predisposing causes. Moreover, since lymphangitis is more often seen in horses receiving full feeds rich in protein constituents and doing little or no work, it is further considered that these factors also may act as predisposing causes. It is due to this that the disease, seen so very often on a Monday morning, after the week-end's rest, is called 'Monday morning disease'. In other cases it frequently appears after horses come in from a run at grass and are put straight on to hard corn feeding, especially if this contains beans or peas in any quantity.

Symptoms.—The preliminary symptoms are not always seen, but they consist of attacks of shivering and fever, with sometimes cold sweats. The temperature rises 3° F. or more; the pulse is fast and bounding; the breathing is rapid; the eyes and nostrils are injected, and the animal stands apparently dejected. In a short while, acute lameness develops in one or more legs. One or other of the hind-limbs is most often attacked, but it is also seen in a fore-limb, and sometimes two limbs may be affected. The lymph glands on the inside of the thigh or armpit become swollen and extremely painful to the touch, and the leg is usually raised from the ground when they are handled. The distended lymph-vessels can be felt as cords running up the inside of the limb, and pressure upon them evinces signs of pain. About this time a diffuse swelling of the whole limb below the stifle or elbow commences. It spreads from above downwards, and is often clearly marked off from the healthy part above. The swellings are at first painful to the touch all the way down the limb, but after a time the pain decreases. Occasionally the swellings will pit upon pressure, like dough. This is the typical appearance of the horse in the morning when the condition is first noticed. The preliminary symptoms develop during the night and early morning, and are not often seen.

In the greater number of cases no dung will be found behind the horse, as constipation is almost always present, but small amounts of thick, heavy urine are passed. The appetite is lost for a day or two, but the horse is usually very thirsty. Under appropriate treatment, the severity of the symptoms abates in 2 or 3 days' time, or sooner; and although lameness still persists, perhaps for as long as a week, the general appearance of the horse rapidly improves. Some cases, where the horse lies down and is frightened to rise, become complicated with bed-sores and abscess formation, and extend into weeks before they recover, but the horse is usually able to resume work in from ten days to a fortnight.

Horses which have once been attacked are very liable to a recurrence, and each succeeding attack leaves the leg a little larger than it was before, until, when one leg has been affected three or four times, it becomes permanently thickened.

Prevention.—Horses of a sluggish or lymphatic temperament should be kept short of concentrated rations when standing idle in the stable at week-ends or holidays. A bran mash containing a handful of Glauber's salts with a little nitre (about a teaspoonful) and sulphur (3 drams) added, should be given at night as a routine when the horses are to be idle the next day. Hay in reasonable amounts may be allowed as bulky food, and the horse should receive as much water as it desires. It is sometimes a wise plan with horses that have been once attacked to give them half an hour's exercise, either by walking or lunging, during an idle day, or to turn them out for an hour or two into a grass paddock, where possible.

Treatment.—The horse should be taken to a loose-box, with as much care as possible. It will be found that a horse with lymphangitis has great difficulty in negotiating a doorstep, and it is useful to lay some short straw down on either side of a high step. It is necessary to rug up the horse, and make comfortable with plenty of bedding and a liberal supply of cold water. In very painful cases it is sometimes necessary to give some sedative. Laxatives are indicated. Hot fomentations are advisable over the affected leg, but they are not essential. If used, a blanket wrung out of hot water and applied to the limb for a minute or two, is better than bathing with very hot water. Afterwards the limb may be either gently rubbed with mild embrocation, or it may be massaged in an upward direction, covered with a piece of blanket (dry), and a straw- or hay-band may be applied fairly tightly. For food the horse should be given mashes, green food, a small amount of good, old hay, and all foods rich in protein should be avoided until the acute symptoms abate. As soon as the horse can bear weight upon the leg it should be given a few minutes' exercise three or four times daily, but there is some danger in over-exercising. The return to the normal hard feeding should be gradual; and as the horse recovers and becomes fit for work, it should commence with short easy journeys for the first week.

Antihistamines may be tried.

LYMPHATICS is the term generally applied to the vessels which convey the lymph through the body. (*See* LYMPH.)

LYMPHOCYTE (lymph, and κίτος, cell) is a variety of white blood-cell. (*see under* BLOOD.)

LYMPHOCYTIC CHORIOMENINGITIS.—A virus disease of mice transmissible to human beings. Dogs may act as symptomless carriers.

LYMPHOMA (*lympha*, lymph ; *-oma*, meaning tumour) is another name for lymphadenoma or Hodgkin's disease. For lymphomatosis of poultry, *see under* FOWL PARALYSIS and LEUCOSIS.

LYMPHOSARCOMA (*see* LEUKÆMIA).

LYSINE is an amino-acid.

LYSIS (λύσις, relief from sickness) means the gradual ending of a fever, and is opposed to 'crisis', which means the sudden termination of disease. The word is also used to signify the solution of bacteria in certain substances which are produced by the body in disease, and the process is called 'bacteriolysis'. (*See also* HÆMOLYSIS.)

LYSOFORM is a liquid soap containing formalin, by virtue of which it possesses great antiseptic powers.

LYSOL is a brown, oily fluid, with antiseptic properties, made from coal-tar by dissolving in fat and extraction with alcohol or by combining cresol with soap. When mixed with water in a 2½ per cent solution it forms a useful antiseptic soapy fluid for cleansing the hands. (*See* DISINFECTANTS.)

LYSSA (λύσσα, frenzy) is another name for rabies. (*See* RABIES.)

M

'M. & B. 693'.—Sulphapyridine, one of the sulphonamide drugs (which see).

MACROCYTE (μακρός, large; κύτος, cell) is the term applied to an unusually large red blood corpuscle especially characteristic of the blood in some forms of anæmia.

MACULES (*macula*, a spot) are spots or stained areas of the skin or of mucous membrane, which are either brownish, red, or purple in colour. They are due either to small hæmorrhages, to diseases of the internal organs, to eczema occurring previously, to pregnancy, or to burns.

'MAD ITCH'.—The colloquial name for Aujeszky's Disease (which see).

MADNESS IN DOGS (*see* RABIES, MENINGITIS).

MÆDI.—A chronic disease of sheep, probably caused by a virus, occurring in Iceland, and characterised by pneumonia. The disease also occurs in India, and is seen in goats. Incubation period: 2 years or more.

MAGGOTS IN SHEEP.—In many parts of the world certain dipterous flies may lay their eggs on the wool of sheep during summer, and the eggs hatch into maggots which either live on the surface of the skin or burrow down into the subcutaneous tissues. They cause great loss from wasting of flesh, destruction to fleeces, and sometimes result in the death of the affected sheep. The green-bottle flies (*Lucilla cæsar* and *L. sericata*, in Great Britain, and *L. macellaria*, in both North and South America) are those responsible for this condition. (*See under* MYIASIS *and* PARASITES, p. 671.)

MAGNESIUM is a light white metal which burns in air with the production of a brilliant white flame, leaving a white powder as a residue. The salts of magnesium used as drugs are the oxide, carbonate, and sulphate. There is a heavy oxide, known as 'magnesia ponderosa', a light oxide called 'magnesia levis', a heavy carbonate, and a light carbonate. Both the oxides and the carbonates are antacids and slightly laxative. The sulphate of magnesium is commonly called 'Epsom salts'. (For blood magnesium, (*see under* HYPOMAGNESÆMIA.)

Uses.—Magnesia, whether light or heavy, is usually prescribed for foals, calves, and dogs when these require a mild antacid and laxative. Mixed with the sulphate and dissolved in peppermint water it forms 'White Mixture', a valuable laxative medicine. The sulphate of magnesium, which has a dosage as follows: cattle, 1 to 1½ lb.; sheep, pigs, small calves, 2 to 4 ounces, is a saline purgative of very wide applicability. In smaller doses, about ⅙th to ⅛th of the above, it is very useful as a febrifuge, and can be given in the drinking water. In a weak concentration (less than 5 per cent solution) Epsom salts usually fail to produce any purgative results, so that when administered they should not be dissolved in too large quantities of water. In concentrated solution they have a somewhat bitter taste, and it is therefore usual to dissolve them in treacle-water made a little warmer than blood-heat. A quart of water is usually quite sufficient for a full dose for the ox. Magnesium sulphate is not the best purgative agent for the horse, and except for special occasions it is better to use other substances. (*See under* PURGATIVES.)

In treating tetanus, hypodermic injections are sometimes given to control the muscular spasms; in lead and carbolic acid poisoning it is the physiological and chemical antidote; in cases of conjunctivitis it was used as an eye lotion; and it is often used in saturated solution for external application to bruised and inflamed joints, tendons, etc.

Calcined magnesite is used as a top-dressing for pastures in an attempt to prevent hypomagnesæmia (about 10 cwt. per acre). For cattle, a daily dose of 2 oz. calcined magnesites is considered to be of great value in the prevention of hypomagnesæmia, but it should be fed only during the 'danger period'. This is because prolonged feeding of magnesium salts is apt to accentuate any latent phosphorus deficiency and may lead to 'milk lameness' or similar conditions.

A mixture of magnesium acetate solution and molasses has been used, being available on a free-choice basis to cattle from ball feeders placed in the field.

MAINE-ANJOU.—A French dual-purpose breed of cattle. Colour: red and white, and roan.

MAIZE (*see* PHYTIN).

MALACIA (μαλακία).—Softening of a part or tissue in disease, *e.g.* osteomalacia or softening of the bones.

MALAISE (*French word*) means a vague feeling of feverishness, listlessness, and languor, indicated by evidences of these feelings, by an absence of desire to feed, and often by shivering fits. It usually precedes the onset of acute diseases.

MALARIA OF BIRDS (*see under* PLASMODIUM).

MALATHION.—An organic phosphorus insecticide used for the control of external parasites in cattle. It is relatively safe since it is detoxified by the mammalian liver—unless another organic phosphorus compound, which destroys the relevant enzyme, is absorbed at the same time. (*See* POTENTIATION, INSECTICIDES.)

Malathion is also used on crops, and at least 24 hours should be allowed between spraying and grazing.

MAL DE CADERAS, or MALADIE DE CADERAS, is a trypanosome disease of the horse, occurring in Brazil, the Argentine, Bolivia, and Paraguay, being most serious in the latter country. It is caused by the *Trypanosoma equinum*. (*See* PROTOZOÖN PARASITES, p. 634).

MAL DE PLAYA.—A form of poisoning in cattle by a plant *Lantana camara*.

MAL DU COIT, or MALADIE DU COIT, is another name for the trypanosome disease which is more commonly known as 'Dourine', a disease of the horse, occurring on the continent of Europe, in many parts of Africa, in India, and in the United States of America, and caused by the *Trypanosoma equiperdum*. (*See* PROTOZOÖN PARASITES, p. 634).

MALE FERN.—The growing point of Male Fern may attract cattle on bare pasture, and lead to poisoning. In Scotland 61 out of 68 head of beef cattle were involved in this way, with 45 wholly blind, 10 partly blind, and 21 recumbent. All recovered within a week except for 4 cows and 4 calves, which remained completely blind. One cow was additionally recumbent and was destroyed. (*Vet. Record*, December 20, 1967.) (*See* EXTRACT OF MALE FERN.)

MALFORMATION (*see* DEFORMITIES).

MALIGNANT (*malignus*, of an evil nature) is a term applied in several ways to serious disorders. Tumours are called malignant when they grow rapidly, tend to infiltrate surrounding healthy tissues, break up easily and become carried to other parts of the body by blood- or lymph-streams, where they set up fresh growths, called *metastases*. (*See* TUMOURS.) The term is also applied to manifestations of disease which are much more severe than generally; thus there is malignant icterus, malignant œdema, etc.

MALIGNANT APHTHA OF SHEEP (*see* ORF).

MALIGNANT CATARRHAL FEVER OF CATTLE, or GANGRENOUS CORYZA, is an infectious fever of cattle, in which there are acute inflammatory changes in the mucous membranes, particularly those of the respiratory system. It occasionally occurs in the British Isles, the continent of Europe, Australasia, North America, but is most common in Africa. It is not contagious between cattle.

Cause.—A virus, which is carried by sheep and wildebeest, and causes illness in buffaloes and cattle.

Incubation period: 3 to 8 weeks.

Symptoms.—In the early stages, the visible mucous membranes show a deep red injection, which passes on to a stage of swelling, infiltration with pus, the production of false or croupous deposits, and finally, when these fall off, ulcer formation accompanied by purulent discharge. As stated, the mucous membranes of the respiratory system are the most frequently affected, but those of the digestive and other systems may also be affected. The animal shows all the classical symptoms of fever—an elevated temperature, a fast, full pulse, rapid respirations, absence of appetite, cessation of rumination, and a diminution in the milk supply. The muzzle is dry and hot; the coat stares; and the animal stands with its back arched and its head lowered. Loss of condition is very marked in fat cattle, and in severe cases there is great depression, the animal lying stretched out on the ground almost continually. An inflammation of the lining membranes of the eyelids usually accompanies the condition, and the animal's eyes are swollen and partly closed. As pus-production and the formation of the false membranes take place, a yellowish-green, purple, or merely blood-stained discharge appears at the nostrils, and, when the mouth is affected, dribbles from between the lips. If the sinuses of the head are attacked, as they may be from inflammation spreading from the nose, the horns may be shed, and the discharge, always foul-smelling, becomes intensely objectionable from decomposition within the enclosed cavities. The lesions may be present in the membranes of the stomach and intestines, when there are symptoms of gastritis, and diarrhœa. Sometimes the genital passages are attacked, when the same lesions are encountered. Occasionally hoofs are shed, and in such cases the skin is usually found affected around the coronets.

The mortality from catarrhal fever is high; usually one out of every two animals attacked dies in from 3 to 5 days. Where the symptoms are less severe the animal may be ill for 4 or 5 weeks and then recover.

Treatment.—No specific treatment is known. Internally, the administration of antibiotics is indicated.

MALIGNANT JAUNDICE OF DOGS (*see* Biliary Fever).

MALIGNANT ŒDEMA (*see* Gas Gangrene).

MALIGNANT PUSTULE (*see* Anthrax.

MALIGNANT STOMATITIS (*see* Calf Diphtheria).

MALIGNANT THEILEROSIS OF SHEEP and GOATS.—A tick-borne disease caused by the protozoan parasite *Theileria hirci*, and occurring in E. Europe, the Middle East, Egypt, and Sudan.

Symptoms include high fever, constipation, glandular enlargement, pale anæmic mucous membranes with later jaundice and death; but the disease may be very mild in animals with some locally acquired immunity.

MALLEIN TEST is a method of testing for the presence of glanders in a horse, somewhat similar to the tuberculin test for tuberculosis. A small quantity of a filtered extract of the bacilli of glanders, called 'Mallein', is injected either below or into the substance of the skin. After a variable period the temperature of the horse rises and there is some amount of local reaction shown by swelling at the point of injection, in a typical positive case, while in a negative case there is no result. The most satisfactory method of applying the test consists of the injection into the skin of the lower eyelid of a concentrated form of mallein in 2 minim doses; this causes a reaction in the form of a conjunctivitis, in positive cases. It is used to test horses that have been in contact with the disease, or that are suspected of being affected, and proved of great value in preventing outbreaks of glanders among Army horses during the 1914 and 1939 wars. (*See* Glanders.)

MALLENDERS and SALLENDERS are diseases of the horse affecting the skin in the flexures of the carpus or 'knee' (mallenders), and of the tarsus or 'hock' (sallenders), which are of the nature of psoriases, and may be hereditary.

The superficial layers of the skin in these situations become inflamed, excessive amounts of epithelium are formed from an almost raw surface, and the condition is aggravated by the continual bending of the joints, which does not allow of healing.

Symptoms.—In severe cases there may be extensive cracking of the skin and lameness, but more often the condition does not interfere with work.

Treatment.—It is necessary first of all to remove the shed cells from the area and expose the skin below, by washing with a hot solution of washing soda and hard soap. The hairs may need to be clipped from the back of the knee in horses with much feather, but usually this is not necessary. The area should be thoroughly dried with a towel afterwards, and an ointment applied daily for a week.

MALT is a substance derived from barley by allowing a certain amount of growth to take place in the germinated seed, and then suddenly raising the temperature to kill the growth, and grinding the grain. It contains an albuminoid ferment called 'diastase', together with a large amount of malt-sugar and dextrine, the latter constituents being still further developed from the starch of the barley by the action of the ferment, so long as the temperature is kept at about 104° F., and when moisture prevails. The ferment will convert a large amount of the starch in flour into sugar, if malt be mixed with the flour; this action is similar to what takes place in physiological digestion.

For these reasons malt is often given along with starchy foods for dogs that have an inadequate digestion, or those that will not thrive. A mixture of cod-liver oil and malt extract is often given to young puppies that are threatened or are actually suffering from rickets.

MALTA FEVER, also called UNDULANT FEVER, is a disease affecting goats and man particularly, but also sometimes other animals.

Causes.—*Brucella melitensis*, which is closely allied to *B. abortus*, which gains entrance into the body mainly through contamination of food. The germ can pass slowly through an unbroken mucous membrane, but it easily passes through an abrasion. Many cases of infection among laboratory workers are on record. The milk and the urine especially, and to a less extent the fæces, and saliva, of an infected animal are infective, and when these contamina tethe food-stuffs of other healthy animals, the disease is spread through them.

Symptoms.—One of the difficulties of the control of Malta fever is that infected goats and other animals may not show any perceptible signs of ill health for long periods, although they are discharging from their bodies the causal organism. They may appear in poor condition, and a chronic inflammation of the udder may be present, in severer cases, but it is not till late in the disease that the milk undergoes any noticeable change. A chronic cough is sometimes seen, and 50 to 90 per cent of pregnant females may abort.

Lameness may occur both in males and females, and vague inflammatory conditions, which usually disappear without treatment, may attack the testes and udder. The disease is very rarely fatal among animals, but its mportance lies in the possibility of its transmission to man, where the symptoms are much more serious. Accurate diagnosis demands the services of a skilled bacteriologist working in a laboratory.

Treatment.—A sensitised vaccine is used to treat the disease in man, and would be useful in countries where the disease is widespread among goats; but in other parts, where only a few animals are attacked, it is better to kill the infected, carry out careful disinfection of premises, avoid water-supplies which may be infected, adopt strict measures of personal cleanliness among human beings, and ensure hygienic surroundings and good feeding for the goats. Goat milk should be avoided, or pasteurised by heating to 145° F. for twenty minutes. (*See also under* BRUCELLOSIS, UNDULANT FEVER.)

MALUCIDIN.—A yeast extract which has been used in America for bringing about resorption of fœtuses in the bitch. It has no value as a contraceptive. If given during the last third of pregnancy, abortion will occur. A 3 per cent solution was used in appropriate dosage intravenously.

MAMMARY GLAND, or UDDER, is the name of the organ which secretes milk. Mammary glands are found in the most highly developed animals—the *Mammalia*, or mammals—for the purpose of suckling their young until such time as they are capable of supporting themselves by other foods. As a rule they are confined to the female sex, although males may at times possess functional glands. They are developed in the skin, and are, in fact, highly modified skin glands. Their form, situation, and number vary in the different domesticated animals, and deserve separate description.

Mare.—The mammary glands are two in number, situated in the inguinal region. Each is shaped like a compressed and inverted cone, with the teat as apex. They are independent of each other, being separated by a dense septum of fibrous tissue, which sends strands into each gland and acts, along with the remainder of the fibrous capsule, as a supportive structure. The tissue of the gland consists of lobes, each of which is split into lobules composed of many tiny tubules lined with a secretory epithelium, and leading into ducts. The gland tissue is supported by the strands of fibrous tissue already mentioned. The ducts from one gland all eventually lead into a milk sinus, at the upper part of the teat, and from the sinus three or four larger ducts, called ‘ lactiferous ducts ’, pass to the extremity of the nipple. The lactiferous ducts are closed by a ring of muscular tissue which acts as a sphincter preventing loss of milk.

Cow.—There are four glands in the cow normally, although Nature has made provision for six in most animals, but the two situated most posteriorly are non-functional except in rare cases. In reality, it would be more correct to consider the udder of the cow as composed of *two* glands only, each of which is provided with two teats, but it is customary to speak of four

MAMMARY GLAND

'quarters' of the udder, and they may be considered as four glands, since each teat drains its own particular area. A strong septum divides the two right-hand glands from the two on the left side, but there is no line of demarcation between fore- and hind-quarters on the same side of the body. The septum is important, for it prevents disease from readily spreading across the body, although there is no hindrance to inflammatory processes spreading from a fore- to a corresponding hind-quarter, or *vice versa*.

The structure of the gland is similar to what is seen in the mare, being composed of lobes and lobules, held in position by fibrous tissue, and sending ducts down into an irregular milk sinus. This latter is large, and partly divided into compartments by folds of mucous membrane. From it leads one large lactiferous duct down the teat to its apex, which possesses a sphincter muscle of almost $\frac{3}{8}$ths of an inch in width.

Ewe.—There are two mammary glands, each of which has a single teat. They are situated in the inguinal region, as in the mare and cow.

Sow.—The mammary glands number twelve in most sows (although a few have more), and are arranged in two rows reaching from just behind the level of the elbows along the abdomen to the inguinal region. As a rule, the glands which are situated towards the middle of the series are the best developed and secrete the most milk. Each teat has two ducts as a rule.

Bitch.—As in the sow there are two rows of glands along the lower line of the abdomen. They are known as 'pectoral', 'abdominal', and 'inguinal', according to their position. They are usually ten in number, but in the smaller breeds there may only be eight, and in the larger breeds there are sometimes twelve. The teats each possess from ten to twelve tiny lactiferous ducts.

Variations in size.—In the young virgin animal the mammary glands are small and undeveloped, although readily distinguishable, until the first period of heat or œstrum, when they become swollen and turgid. It is not until after the first pregnancy that they show any very remarkable change, however; towards the end of that period, as parturition approaches, the glands become actively enlarged as the result of an increase in the gland tissue they contain, until at or shortly after the birth of the young they contain milk. In the lactation period succeeding parturition they continue to increase for a time, under the influence of suckling or milking by hand; but as the young animal grows, starts feeding, and makes less demand upon its mother, once again they shrink. In subsequent lactation periods they again increase in size, until between the fourth and seventh or eighth parturition they attain their maximum functional activity. After this time, although the glands may appear to increase in size still more, less milk is secreted; the increase in size is due to the deposition of fat or fibrous tissue between and around the gland tissue. In the case of dairy cattle, a great alteration in the size of the udder has been effected by artificial selection and management. Actual size alone, however, is no certain indication that the cow is a good milker; in old animals there is a quantity of fat deposited in the udder, and in many animals the amount of the fibrous tissue framework also increases the size—giving rise to the term 'fleshy udder'. It is often difficult to distinguish whether a cow with a large udder is really a good milker or not, but cows with fleshy udders or those that are fat will show less variation in size between the full and the recently milked udder. As a general rule the udder should collapse after milking, and when handled should feel like silk enclosed within the skin, the skin hanging in folds when viewed from behind. If the udder is fleshy or fat, the decrease in size is not marked and the recently milked udder feels like a piece of muscle enclosed within the skin, which does not become wrinkled into folds.

Secretion of milk.—This is a continuous process, initiated at parturition or before by the hormones prolactin (from the pituitary gland) and thyroxine (from the thyroid). The milk accumulates in the alveoli, upper channels, and milk cisterns; the rate of secretion decreasing as internal udder pressure rises.

Milk 'let-down' in the cow, associated with the hormone oxytocin, is referred to under MILKING.

The stimulus to milk secretion, when once established, is sucking or milking. In the absence of these, the glands begin to atrophy in the course of a few days, and their secretion ceases. A cow can withhold her milk by the contraction of the sphincter muscles of the teat, but no animal is able to discharge the milk from her udder until it is distended. If the tension becomes considerable, milk may pour from the teats owing to the pressure exerted upon the sphincter by the contained milk; but after the pressure is somewhat lessened by the escape of a little milk, the muscle once more contracts and shuts the canal.

During the actual process of secretion two distinct proceedings are involved. In one, certain parts of cells lining the secreting tubules (alveoli) are shed to form the fat globules of the milk, and in the other, the water, salts, and other substances are elaborated from the lymph by a process similar to what occurs in other glands of the body. The first milk to be secreted by the udder after parturition, is found to contain large numbers of these cells, or parts of cells, while later in the lactation period they are few in number or absent. This is because the secretory alveoli are at first packed full with such cells, and, accordingly, the first milk contains the greater numbers. They are known as 'colostrum corpuscles', and serve important functions which will be considered later. It must not be thought that all the fat globules in the milk originate from the shedding of cells from the alveoli, for in the milk of carnivores, where the fat content is low, a process of fat secretion, like any other secretion, takes place, the droplets of fat being manufactured inside the living cells of the tubules originally, and then passed out through the cell-envelope into the lumina of the ducts and tubules. It is probable that a similar process accounts for much of the fat in the milk of cows and other animals also.

Colostrum is the name given to the first milk that is secreted by the udder.

(The importance of the newly born of any species of animal getting a supply of colostrum-containing first milk, soon after it is born, is explained under COLOSTRUM.)

(For other information concerning milk, *see* MILK.)

Conditions affecting the milk yield of cows.—(1) *Breed.*

(2) *Temperament.*—There is no doubt that a placid but not sluggish, alert but not highly nervous, cow makes the best milker.

(3) *Health.*—It is, of course, necessary that a cow should be in good general health if the best results are to be obtained from her. The importance of hygienic, well-lighted, well-ventilated, well-drained cow-byres, and of judiciously regulated exercise in summer and in winter, is very great, and most marked improvements are seen when cows with a previously ordinary milk yield in a badly managed herd are introduced into a well-run herd.

(4) *Age.*—A cow in good health improves in her milk-yield up to her 7th or 8th year, and remains at a high level until her 10th or 12th year. The milk of a young cow is much richer in fats and solids than that of an aged animal, so that the ideal position in a herd is to have enough young stock to counteract any possible deficiency in those substances from the milk of the old cows.

(5) *Lactation.*—A cow yields the greatest amount of milk between the 6th and 8th week after calving; thence she gives a smaller amount each day till about the 300th day, when she goes dry. Cows give best results when their lactation period does not exceed 8½ to 9 months, *i.e.* when they are dried off about six weeks before they are due to calve, having settled in-calf at the first or second service.

(6) *Period of year.*—In the spring and early summer when the grass is young and flush the cows at pasture give more milk than they do in dry, hot weather, when the fields are full of the woody stems of grasses that are past their flowering period. In summer weather there is an increase in the *olein* content of the butter-fat, and in winter an increase in the *stearin* content, so that butter in summer is more oily than in winter, irrespective of the temperature under which it is kept.

(7) *Œstrus or heat.*—In the majority of cases œstrus reduces the milk yield of cows, but there are cases where no diminution takes place. The butter-fat content, however, is always low (sometimes as little as 1 per cent for 2 or 3 days), and butter made exclusively from such milk is white in colour.

(8) *Food.*—The influence of the food upon milk production is of great importance. There may be no marked change in the actual composition of the milk, but quantity is decreased and the 'churnability' is lowered upon diets which are not sufficient or are badly balanced. (*See* FIBRE.)

(9) *Soils.*—The nature of the soil and of the geological formations of a farm influence the milk, probably through the quality of the pasture and the water. Limestone soils always yield milk richest in butter-fat, and of the best 'keeping quality'; clay soils are the exact converse in these respects, and gravelly or stony soils are intermediate.

(10) *Water-supply.*—A plentiful supply of good sound water is absolutely necessary both in summer and winter if the cows are to milk well. Cows require about 1 lb. of water for every 4 lb. dry food, or 1 lb. water for every 5 lb. of milk produced, but by far the best method is to allow the animals to satisfy their thirsts without restriction. This can best be effected by the provision of individual drinking bowls in the byre, and a self-filling trough at pasture.

(11) *Temperature.*—Cows appear to do best when they are kept in an even temperature of about 50° F. in the summer, and 40° to 50° F. in winter. There are occasions when these temperatures cannot be maintained, but by proper ventilation, avoidance of overcrowding, etc., in the byre the temperature should never be allowed to pass far beyond these limits. In any case, it is better to have a byre too cool than too hot.

(12) *Treatment.*—Gentle treatment is of the utmost importance in maintaining a dairy herd at the highest pitch of efficiency. Anything which upsets a cow's temper, whether occasioned by the attendants, by her neighbours, by dogs or other animals, etc., will cause her to hold up her milk, and will eventually decrease the daily yield. Quick, efficient, and clean milking stimulates extra secretion of milk, while slow, slovenly, careless work reduces the amount given. (The importance of udder stimulation in relation to 'let-down' of milk is referred to on p. 556.)

MAMMARY GLANDS, DISEASES OF.—When it is remembered that the udder of the cow has become extraordinarily highly specialised by selection and management, it is not surprising that it has also become liable to a large number of diseased conditions. Its situation in the animal body, moreover, is one which exposes it to injury and contamination from which it would be exempt were it placed at the other end of the cow. Nevertheless, with careful management, good hygiene, regular and efficient milking, the economic losses from diseases of the udder can be greatly reduced.

ABSCESS FORMATION may be the result of acute or chronic inflammation of the gland itself, or it may be due to entrance through the teat canal of foreign substances, etc. Other causes of abscess may be the larvæ of one or other of the blow-flies in summer. The eggs are laid around the teat orifice, are not wholly dislodged by milking, and the maggots, when they hatch, invade the teat canal, and by their presence and irritation set up local inflammatory changes which result in abscess formation.

Symptoms.—In instances where injury has been inflicted, there will be evidence of this in abrasions of the skin, wounds, etc., and the cow will resent milking operations. The milk may contain blood. When examined, the abscess may not be discovered until two or three days afterwards, before which an ordinary mild injury would be getting better. It will be perceptible as a hard mass of tissue, varying in size from a walnut to an orange or larger, and signs of pain will be shown when it is pressed. In more chronic abscess formation the symptoms appear more slowly; for a time there may be more tenseness than usual after milking, and the cow may be fidgety during the process. Her milk yield from the affected quarter may fall, and the milk often appears ropy or stringy.

Treatment.—As soon after diagnosis as possible the abscess must be opened by a veterinary surgeon and its contents eliminated. Sometimes it is necessary to encourage the abscess to 'point' by the use of hot fomentations, liniments, etc. After the pus has been eliminated the cavity must be irrigated with antiseptic and the wound left open for drainage. Penicillin or sulpha drugs are indicated. (*See* ABSCESS. Specific abscesses are considered under ACTINOMYCOSIS, TUBERCULOSIS, etc.)

MASTITIS, or inflammation of the udder, affects either the secreting cells or the fibrous tissue strands between them, and usually ends by affecting the whole of the tissues; which obviously alters the amount and quality of the milk, and often terminates by its total suppression; and which is almost always accompanied by severe general symptoms. All the domestic animals are liable to the disease, but it is commonest in the cow, ewe, and goat. (For mastitis in the cow, *see under* MASTITIS.)

Mare.—Mastitis is rare in the mare, but cases occasionally occur when the udder becomes the seat of inflammation as the result of strangles, purulent wounds, etc., in either the mare or her foal, and the contamination of the teats by the discharges from these conditions. In other cases it has been produced by the stings of wasps or hornets, by scratches and abrasions becoming contaminated with

MAMMARY GLANDS, DISEASES OF

flies, and through the mare continually kicking to ward off the attacks of flies, while some cases appear to arise through sudden changes in the food of the mare, *e.g.* when she leaves a poor bare pasture and is suddenly put on to a field of second-cut (*i.e.* aftermath) clover, rye-grass, lucerne, sainfoin, etc., where the growth is rank and flush. It is usually seen in nursing mares with large udders, but it may occur before foaling, and has been seen in virgin mares. It may also arise where the foal is weaned or dies when the udder is in full milk, and when no manual stripping is carried out.

Symptoms.—The general disturbance is not unlike what is seen in the cow, but the condition is almost always acute. Temperature is high, pulse is fast and full, breathing is faster than normal and usually shallow, the appetite is in abeyance, and shivering fits may occur. Sometimes colicky pains may be noticed. Locally, the mare shows great tenderness and pain in the udder. She walks with stiffness in the leg on the affected side when the condition attacks one side of the udder only, and with difficulty when both halves of the udder are attacked. The udder is swollen and tense. A varying amount of œdema accompanies the disease, and spreads along the belly in many cases. The milk is altered to a sticky serous thin fluid, and this soon turns blackish in colour, thickens, and finally becomes purulent. It possesses a disagreeable odour. Abscess formation may take place, or gangrene may set in. In either case, and in fact in most cases of mastitis in mares, the function of the affected part of the udder is destroyed. Death may occur when there is an extensive inflammation, and especially when the gangrenous area is large.

Treatment.—The mare should be brought in from pasture and isolated in a loose-box. If the foal can be induced to feed from the manger or from the pail, it may be left with its mother, provided she is not worried by it, but where the mare is seriously ill, and where the foal continually annoys her by trying to suck, it should be taken away from her and either put to a foster-mother, or, if possible, reared by hand. In some cases it may be left in the loose-box, but should be shut by itself in a partition in one corner. It must receive daily exercise when so treated. The local treatment of the diseased udder is essentially the same as that given for the cow.

Ewe.—Mastitis in the ewe may be either gangrenous, due to *Staphylococcus aureus*, or of the suppurative type, due to *C. pyogenes*. It is very common in some years and in some districts, and may be rapidly contagious or sporadic. It occurs in sheep under all types of management, but is usually most severe in low-ground flocks on intensively stocked land.

Symptoms.—The disease appears suddenly in animals that were apparently normal a few hours previously. The affected ewes separate themselves from the rest of the flock, move with difficulty and pain, disregard their lambs, and refuse to feed. The affected half of the udder is found to be swollen, hot, painful to the touch, and œdematous. It soon becomes gangrenous and commences to slough out. Violet patches of the skin surface indicate gangrene. The discharge from the teat is purulent and of a putrid odour. In the suppurative form, hard nodular abscesses can be felt below the skin, and deformity of the udder occurs in consequence. In either case death may occur in three days to one week, or sloughing of the affected areas may be followed by recovery. A subnormal temperature precedes death.

Treatment.—When cases appear among a flock the healthy should be immediately separated from the diseased, and should be taken with their lambs to a clean pasture and attended by a different shepherd if possible. They should be dipped first. The diseased ewes should be separated from their lambs, and enclosed in a sheltered pen. The lambs must be reared by hand. Antibiotic treatment is indicated. A toxoid is available for prevention.

Goats.—Two forms of mastitis are met with in the goat: (1) *Gangrenous*, and (2) *Purulent*. The former of these is almost identical with that of the ewe (see above), and in the latter there is a great tendency towards the formation of abscesses in the udder. These burst and give rise to discharging sores that persist for long periods. A considerable amount of destruction of the gland tissue follows, but ultimate recovery usually occurs.

Sow.—One, two, or more piglets out of a litter are often lost because the sow has mastitis. This may take the form of an acute infection within a few days of farrowing; the sow being obviously ill and some of the udders painful to the touch. Or the attack may be subacute, occurring when the piglets are a week or

 MAMMARY GLANDS, DISEASES OF

a fortnight or more old ; the sow seeming well enough in herself though a hardening of some of the udders can be felt, and the plight of the piglets is apparent. Several different germs are responsible for mastitis in the sow, *e.g. Streptococcus agalactiæ, S. dysgalactiæ, S. uberis, S. viridans, Staphylococcus aureus,* and *B. coli.* In cases where the veterinary surgeon has been called in and a bacteriological examination has incriminated *B. coli,* an anti-serum may prove a very useful preventive in herds where this is a recurring trouble. Actinomycosis may occur in sows on stubble fields.

Bitch.—Although by no means common, mastitis in the bitch is very liable to occur when conditions under which the udder may become contaminated prevail. Thus it is seen in kennels where the sanitary conditions are bad, where the puppies have sores about their mouths or feet, and where the bitch licks herself when fed upon a flesh diet. An insufficient number of puppies suckling a bitch in which the milk secretion is copious is also a contributory factor.

Symptoms.—The attack comes on suddenly as a rule, though some cases are sub-acute. The animal is very sick and feverish ; she lies stretched out on her side, moaning, and food is refused. The affected glands are swollen, tense, reddened, and tender on pressure. The secretion from them is mainly pus, and the puppies are clamorous for food. Abscesses develop and burst, and ulcerating wounds are left behind. Absorption of poisons frequently takes place and the animal dies from toxæmia. In non-fatal cases hard lumpy swellings are left behind, which may persist for weeks afterwards, and sometimes give rise to the ' mammary tumours ' which are so common in bitches.

Treatment.—The bitch should be given cascara or other gentle laxative and the glands may be fomented. Penicillin and/or sulpha drugs may be prescribed by the veterinary surgeon. When abscesses are present they should be opened and evacuated. The puppies must be removed and reared by hand or foster-mother, and stripping of the healthy glands is essential.

TUBERCULOSIS of the udder is an extremely common condition among cattle where no anti-tuberculous management exists. It is of great danger to human beings, for the milk from such an udder, although perhaps normal looking to the naked eye, almost always contains the bacilli of tuberculosis and is capable of infecting human beings. (*See* TUBERCULOSIS.)

TUMOURS, if we exclude warts, are not common in the mammary glands of animals with the exception of the bitch, in which growths composed of a mixture of tumour tissues (adenoma, fibroma, lipoma, chondroma, and even osteoma), are encountered. As a rule they are of slow growth, occasion no pain or inflammatory reaction, are usually enclosed in a capsule, and when totally removed, do not tend to reappear. Sometimes malignant tumours, which have their primary seat in some other part of the body, may invade the udder by metastatic spread, and, owing to the good blood-supply, grow very quickly. (*See* TUMOURS.)

WOUNDS AND INJURIES of the udder and teats are commonest in the cow and sow, owing to greater pendulousness than in other animals. The injuries inflicted vary from mere superficial scratches from thorns, stubble, etc., to large and deep bruised wounds, such as may be caused by horn-gores, kicks, stakes in hedges, barbed wire, bites from dogs, pitchforks, etc. All wounds of the udder and teats are serious on account of the danger of infection from even a tiny scratch, and the development of mastitis as a result. The larger the wound, and the deeper it penetrates, the more serious is the consequence. If the gland substance has been penetrated, or if the teat canal has been opened by the object causing the injury, blood-stained milk flows freely from the wound in lactating animals. At other times the injury presents the usual appearance of a wound. With deep wounds gangrene is liable to follow udder injuries, and a slough occurs some time later, the remaining cavity being easily made to bleed when the cow moves about. Wounds of the teat which open the milk canal are extremely difficult to induce to heal while the cow is in milk, partly because the milk flows out through the wound as soon as it collects, and partly because the operation of milking irritates the wound and retards healing by disturbing the granulation tissue as soon as it forms. In addition to this the teat has a more dense structure and a less copious blood-supply than other tissues. A wound from which milk continues to flow for some time after infliction, and which does not tend to heal, is known as a ' milk fistula '.

Treatment.—As a first-aid treatment wounds of the teats and udder should be washed with warm water and an antiseptic, dry sulphanilamide powder afterwards being applied.

When a teat has been torn or injured so that milk escapes from the canal it is usually difficult to get the fistula, so formed, to heal until the cow goes dry. It may be here noted that a fistula in a teat constitutes an unsoundness in a cow, which entitles the purchaser to return her if she is sold with a guarantee. An operation is usually necessary to obtain healing. This procedure necessitates the cow remaining dry for at least two months. In some cases a cow with a fistula is better turned out to grass at once, and made to rear calves until her milk flow ceases, when she can be taken in and undergo the operation.

ERUPTIONS ON TEATS may be either specific, such as are seen during outbreaks of foot-and-mouth disease, cow-pox, malignant catarrhal fever, rinderpest, etc., or they may be caused by infection of the teat with germs from the mouths of calves suffering from calf diphtheria, or from streptococcal infection, while in a few cases they may arise through contamination of the hands of the milkers with infection from sores or wounds occurring in the human being, or on animals with which they are in contact. The great majority of teat sores, however, are caused through ' chapping ', or ' cracking ' of the delicate skin of the teat. In cases of cows that suckle their calves the saliva and the milk leave the teat wet, and when drying takes place the skin cracks and ' chaps '. Turning cows out in cold weather in winter, when there is frost or snow, with their teats wet has the same effect. The cracks and sores may appear at any part of the teat, but they are more serious when at the tip than in other places, because the serous discharge collects there, and, becoming infected, serves as a means whereby germs can pass into the teat canal, and perhaps set up mastitis.

One other most important cause of sore teats is attack by biting flies. Apparently they are induced to settle on the teats by the odour of the film of milk left after milking, and thereafter bite through the skin and suck blood.

Treatment.—Prevention is better than cure, and endeavours should always be made to prevent the delicate teats of heifers from becoming cracked and attacked by sores. The observance of the measures of cleanliness mentioned under ' MASTITIS ' (in this section) will do much to prevent teat sores.

WARTS ON TEATS (*see* WARTS).

TEAT OBSTRUCTIONS.—Difficulty in milking may be caused by stricture of the sphincter, milk clots or (rarely) calculi in the teat canal, or by the presence of warty growths inside the canal. The latter condition is considered under WARTS. Stricture of the sphincter is the common cause of ' toughness ' in milking. It consists of an abnormally small opening at the tip of the teat. Almost all owners of cows are so familiar with the condition that no further description is necessary. It may be relieved by the use of teat bougies, which are left in position between milkings. A short length of red or blue thread should be left hanging to facilitate removal. Their use requires that they shall be aseptic when inserted to avoid the introduction of infection. Milk clots are usually the indication of chronic disease in the udder, and cows showing them should have their udders examined. Calculi, composed of lime salts, casein, etc., are occasionally present in the teats and give rise to difficulty in milking. They are recognised by the freedom with which they may be moved about in the teat, and are sometimes called ' peas ', owing to their resemblance to these legumes. They can be removed through the tip of the teat when small, but when large must be taken out through an incision when the cow is dry. (*See also* MASTITIS ; MILK.)

MAMMILLA is the Latin term for the nipple.

MAMMITIS.—Another name for mastitis.

MANDELIC ACID.—A urinary antiseptic, effective in *acid* urine.

MANDIBLE (*mandibulum*) is the bone of the lower jaw. (*See* JAW.)

MANDIBULAR DISEASE (*see* SHOVEL BEAK).

MANGANESE, which should not be confounded with magnesium, is a metal of which the oxides are abundantly found in Nature. The most common, and indeed the only, manganese salt that is used to any great extent, is the permanganate of potassium, which is used as a disinfectant, antiseptic, or oxidising agent.

At one time manganese butyrate and colloidal manganese injections were in vogue for the treatment of boils and other staphylococcal skin infections. Manganese is a trace element, and lack of sufficient in the pasture herbage may cause infertility in cattle, *e.g.* in Devon and Cornwall. (*See* POTASSIUM PERMANGANATE, TRACE ELEMENTS, *and* SLIPPED TENDON.)

MANGE (*see under* PARASITES, p. 688).

MANURE HEAPS.—It is important to prevent grass growing near these and to fence them, as such herbage tends to become heavily infested with Husk parasites and constitutes a menace to cattle. Pig manure can be a source of *trichomoniasis* in cattle.

MARASMUS (*μαραίνω*, I waste away) means a general wasting. (*See* ATROPHY.)

'MARBLE BONE' DISEASE (*see* OSTEOPETROSIS).

MARBURG DISEASE.—A virus disease of vervet (and perhaps other) monkeys which can prove fatal to man. (*See* MONKEYS.)

MAREK'S DISEASE.—This disease was first described in Austria-Hungary in 1907 but has only become generally prevalent within recent years. It was first recorded in America in 1914, and in Great Britain in 1929, and spread widely. It forms part of the still controversial 'Avian Leucosis Complex'. In Britain, Fowl Paralysis itself (Marek's disease) has of recent years become more common, and is occurring at an earlier age. It has caused a sudden and high mortality in several broiler flocks.

A vaccine is available.

Cause.—The cause is a Herpes virus. At the same time there is some evidence for believing that in natural outbreaks there is a hereditary basis for the disease. Perhaps both causes may operate in outbreaks, the virus only attacking those birds which have inherited some particular weakness from their parents.

Mortality.—The mortality varies, but in birds 6–8 weeks old may exceed 20 per cent. It is difficult actually to arrive at a satisfactory figure as this disease may co-exist with others, *e.g.* coccidiosis, tapeworm infestations, tuberculosis, vitamin deficiency, etc.

Symptoms.—Fowl-paralysis affects birds most commonly between the ages of three and eight months, but cases have been recorded in broilers a little over 3 weeks old, and also in birds over a year old. It is frequently noticed that certain strains of birds are affected, in-contact birds of a different parentage remaining healthy. Affected birds may show lameness of one or both legs. This lameness becomes progressively worse, and general paralysis results. A common attitude for an affected bird to adopt is to lie about with one limb extended in front and the other extended behind. In spite of this the bird appears alert and will feed if placed beside a supply. Paralysis at first is flaccid, but later appears to become spastic in nature, a peculiar bunching or clutching appearance of the claws being noted. Drooping of one or both wings may be noted, at first perhaps scarcely perceptible, but gradually becoming worse till in some cases the tip of the wing may touch the ground. Twisting of the head may also be noticed in some members of the flock, and sometimes a flaccid paralysis of the neck muscles is also met with. In certain birds, eye lesions may be seen. The iris tends to become a dull grey colour and encroaches on the pupil which, instead of being circular, is distorted, and may be oval, eliptical, slit-like, or even completely obliterated. Other birds may show digestive troubles, such as dilated and pendulous crops, or constipation followed by diarrhœa. In some affected flocks the above symptoms may be met with, whereas in other cases one set of symptoms predominate, *e.g.* most of the birds show blindness. On noticing such symptoms, several birds showing characteristic manifestations should be sent to a poultry laboratory for diagnosis.

Control Measures.—On the disease being diagnosed, all affected birds should be destroyed as soon as the first symptoms are observed, as these are usually in good condition and may be used for food purposes. If, however, this is not done at once, paralysis progresses and becomes general, condition is rapidly lost, and the bird becomes a total loss. There is no method of detecting the disease in apparently healthy birds. Blood examinations have been carried out, but these cannot be recommended as being of practical value. The disease is always introduced to a farm by the purchase of fresh stock, either in the form of eggs, day-old chicks, or adult birds.

Control measures consist in careful selection of the source of fresh stock.

A live attenuated vaccine can be used for prevention.

Both the fowl tick, *Argas persicus*, and the Darkling beetle, can harbour the virus of Marek's disease.

MARES, INFERTILITY IN (*see under* UTERINE INFECTIONS).

MARIE'S DISEASE.—This was first described in Man in 1890. It has been reported in the dog (*see under* ACROPACHIA) and in the horse. In the latter it has occurred in the absence of either tuberculosis or tumours. In Africa, the round-worm *Spirocerca lupi* has been reported as associated with the condition in the dog. The cause is not definitely known, but possibilities are a tumour toxin; a hormone imbalance; an autonomic vascular reflex.

Marie's Disease is also known as Hypertrophic Pulmonary Osteoarthropathy.

MARKETS.—A common source of infection. (*See under* SALMONELLOSIS.) In the U.K. covered accommodation must be provided for dairy cows in milk, calves, and pigs, in accordance with the Markets (Protection of Animals) (Amendment) Order, 1965.

'MARMITE DISEASE'.—A form of dermatitis encountered in piglets 3 days old and upwards. (*See* 'GREASY PIG' DISEASE.)

MARROW means the softer substance that is enclosed within the cavities of the bones It is of two kinds—*yellow marrow*, which is found in the tubular spaces in the centres of the long bones, especially the limb bones, and *red marrow*, which fills up the spaces found in the short bones such as the vertebræ and in the ribs, etc. In emergency, as for example after severe hæmorrhage, the yellow marrow may become red, and assist it in its function. There is no essential difference between the two, though yellow marrow owes its colour to the large amount of fat contained in it, while red marrow is of a highly cellular structure. The cells peculiar to the marrow known as 'myelocytes' are similar to the white blood corpuscles but larger. It is supposed that the red corpuscles of the blood-stream are formed from certain nucleated corpuscles of the bone marrow.

Red bone marrow is used medicinally for weak or delicate carnivorous animals, especially after debilitating diseases. It is either given on bread or is scraped from the centre of beef bones and given mixed with the food. The bone should not be broken up and given to the dog to 'pick'. (*See also under* BONES, DOGS'.)

MARSH MARIGOLD POISONING.—The Marsh Marigold, or 'King cup' (*Caltha palustris*), has occasionally been the cause of poisoning, but as a rule animals will not eat it unless there is a scarcity of other herbage. The plant is supposed to be harmless when young, and only poisonous at, and after, the time of flowering. Cattle are most often affected, and show symptoms of gastric disturbance, diarrhœa, loss of milk secretion, and sometimes bloating and blood in the urine. The treatment consists of the administration of stomach sedatives, demulcent drinks, plenty of water, and feeding on good hay for a few days. Fatal results are seldom met with.

MASHAM.—The cross resulting from a Blackface ewe × a Wensleydale ram.

MAST CELL is a type of connective tissue cell containing numerous granules which stain with basic dyes. Blood mast-cells are known as Basophils.

MASTITIS (μαστός, the breast).—Inflammation of the udder. (*See* MAMMARY GLAND, DISEASES OF, for mastitis in animals other than the cow.)

MASTITIS IN THE COW.—Inflammation of the udder, involving either the secreting cells of the mammary glands, or its connective tissue, or both. Mastitis may be unaccompanied by obvious symptoms. This **subclinical** mastitis commonly reduces milk yields by 10 per cent or so, and is consequently of great economic importance. A simple test can now be used to detect the presence of an abnormally high content of white cells in an ordinary-looking sample of milk, and so indicate the presence of mastitis. Once it is known that it exists, bacteriological tests can be used to identify the organisms responsible and to determine the best treatment. Sometimes an excess of white cells (over 500,000 per ml.) in the milk is the result of inflammation due to trauma and not to infection. Thus, the California or Whiteside Test may draw attention to

MASTITIS IN THE COW

a faulty milking machine or bad milking technique.

The mastitis situation in a herd can be monitored on a monthly basis by laboratories operating electronic cell counters. The table shows the ranges of white cell counts.

Cell Count Ranges (cells/c.c.)	Estimate of Mastitis Problem	Estimate of Milk Production Loss per cow per year
Below 250,000	Negligible	—
250,000—499,000	Slight	42 gallons
500,000—749,000	Average	74 gallons
750,000—999,000	Bad	169 gallons
1,000,000 and over	Very bad	197 gallons

(With acknowledgements to Beecham Laboratories Ltd.)

The graph, reproduced with acknowledgements to the Milk Marketing Board, shows the spread of mastitis in an autumn calving herd.

Seasonal variations in herd cell counts.—Due to the calving pattern of a herd and the fact that the cell count of a cow will rise towards the end of the lactation, it is best to take a series of monthly cell counts to obtain the most accurate estimate of mastitis in the herd. This is why the Board is making this a twelve-month contract.

Mastitis tends to rise as the winter progresses and falls when the cows first go out to grass. The cell counts rise again in July and August chiefly because of the high proportion of the cows nearing the end of their lactation. Cell counts and mastitis levels fall again in September when some of the older cows are being culled and first calf heifers are coming into the herd. Mastitis levels rise again through the winter period.

Clinical mastitis—in which the symptoms are observable—affects 3 per cent of our national dairy herd on any one day, according to Mr. C. D. Wilson, M.R.C.V.S., who adds: 'A cow with clinical mastitis will lose 20 per cent of its expected yield as the result of an attack.'

Mastitis should always be regarded as a hard problem and not as affecting only a single animal.

Mastitis may also be acute, sub-acute, or chronic. In general, adopting this classification, symptoms may be described as follows:

Acute.—Shivering may usher in the attack. Later, there is a rise in temperature, fast, full pulse, short, quick respirations, an uneasy appearance. The animal paddles with her feet, but is usually afraid to lie on account of the pain occasioned to the udder. She refuses food, and rumination is in abeyance. When the udder is examined it is found that one (or more) quarter is swollen, tense, reddened, and very painful to the touch; so painful may it be that the cow stands with her hind-legs straddled apart. In a short time the appearance may change to a deep purple or bluish colour, and the swelling increases. A little yellow serum may be drawn from the teat during the first few hours, but this later changes into flocculent material, containing blood and

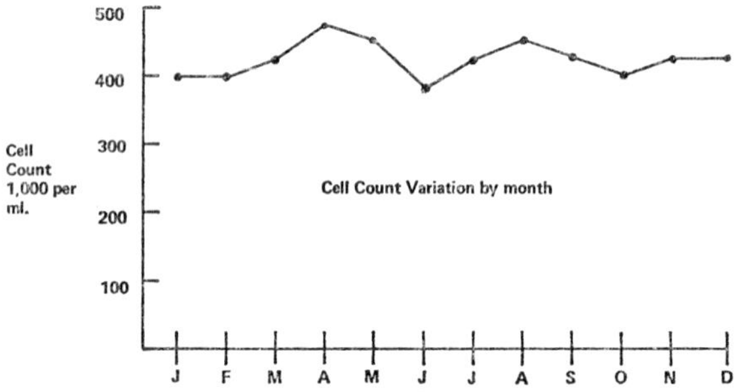

MASTITIS IN THE COW

pus cells, and in the later stages nothing but pus can be obtained. Occasionally it is impossible to draw any fluid at all from the teat, and in such cases the pain is intense. Gangrene of the lower part of the quarter around the base of the teat is frequent. It is shown by a change in colour to a greenish-purple, by stiffness, coldness, and a lessening in surface sensibility. There is an oozing of a blackish-green discharge which possesses a very objectionable odour. In a few days the area of gangrene will slough out and leave a raw cavity. If the gangrene affects a large part of the quarter, or when more than one quarter is attacked, the condition of the cow is serious in the extreme.

Sub-acute.—The disease runs a course not unlike that of the acute form, but the symptoms appear much more slowly. There is a greater difficulty in milking, the first drawn milk often containing little clots and always large numbers of shed epithelial cells, and later, as a gradually increasing pain and swelling in the affected quarter, accompanied by an alteration in the colour of the milk to yellowish, yellowish-grey. The amount of milk decreases. As a rule, appetite remains normal, pulse and breathing are unaltered, and if there is any rise in the temperature it is slight.

Chronic.—There is a minimum of general constitutional disturbance, and an almost complete absence of pain, a slowly progressing increase in the density of the gland, a diminution in the secretion of milk, and a gradual *increase* in the size of the affected quarter or quarters. Chronic mastitis with increase in size is one of the characteristics of tuberculosis of the udder.

MASTITIS AND ANTIBIOTICS.—When penicillin became available for veterinary use, it began to change the bacteriological picturenof mastitis in our dairy herds. The orga ism chiefly responsible for mastitis was then *Streptococcus agalactiæ*, and penicillin proved not only successful in treatment but has provided a means of eradicating this infection from entire herds.

Unfortunately, evidence suggests that antibiotics have not made mastitis a less common disease. Other bacteria have stepped into the breach, so to speak, left by *S. agalactiæ*, and now the one most commonly isolated from infected udders is *Staphyloccus pyogenes*. Strains of *Staphylococcus pyogenes* resistant to antibiotics have been increasing over the years as the table shows.

Antibiotic	*Percentage resistant strains*	
	1958	**1961**
Penicillin	62·0	70·6
Streptomycin	3·6	20·0
Oxytetracycline	0·4	6.0
Chlortetracycline	0·4	4·3
Novobiocin	0·0	3·3
Chloramphenicol	0·4	1·0

Mr. C. D. Wilson, M.R.C.V.S., Central Veterinary Laboratory, Weybridge, has emphasised the figures in the second column above—that of 500 strains of staphylococcus obtained from clinical cases of mastitis, over 70 per cent were resistant to penicillin G, 20 per cent to streptomycin, and over 5 per cent to the tetracyclines.

Several other kinds of bacteria, which at one time were regarded as of little or no significance in the production of mastitis, are now increasingly found, and some have shown themselves capable of causing serious damage to the udder.

Mastitis due to *E. coli* is more frequent now than it was in the 1960s.

An organism with the cultural characteristics of the pleuropneumonia group (*Mycoplasma*) was isolated from udders showing a painless swelling of the quarter in an outbreak of mastitis in Britain. Bedsonia have also been implicated, as well as ' true ' viruses, *e.g.* those causing Vesicular Stomatitis and Infectious Bovine Rhinotracheitis.

In a large dairy unit of 560 milking cows over 700 cases of clinical mastitis occurred in three months; 95 per cent of them being associated with *Streptococcus agalactiæ*—and it was found that L-forms of these were involved. (*See* L-Forms).

Corynebacterium bovis, an organism commonly found in the udder and for long regarded as non-pathogenic, may possibly be a cause of some cases of ' non-specific ' mastitis.

It is estimated that over 700 cases of tuberculoid mastitis occur in Britain each year, and are almost invariably caused by the introduction of antibiotics into the teats before cleaning them.

Pathological changes in the udder may render any antibiotic ineffectual, and it is on prevention—by hygiene—that one must pin one's main hope.

Antibiotics can more economically be used when the cow is in the dry period. Long-acting antibiotics can then be given

MASTITIS IN THE COW

without aggravating the problem of antibiotic residues in milk. (*See under* MILK.)

MYCOTIC MASTITIS.—It is now generally recognised that *sometimes* the use of antibiotics in the treatment of various diseases, in various species of animal, encourages the multiplication of fungi. These, perhaps having no longer to compete against antibiotic-sensitive bacteria, may become masterful and harmful to their host. This sort of thing has been experienced with dairy cows, and now—in addition to a not-so-short list of bacteria implicated in mastitis—over 25 species of fungi have been incriminated. The worst of these is called *Cryptococcus neoformans* and it can cause outbreaks of mastitis severe enough to lead to cows being slaughtered.

Not all the fungi are as bad as this one. With some, the mastitis may even clear up on its own, either quickly or after a period of months. Unfortunately, routine culture and staining methods used for the identification of bacteria leave the fungi undiscovered.

Man-to-Cow Infections. — Occasionally, mastitis in cattle arises from infection by human beings. The kind of streptococci which can give rise either to a severe sore throat or to scarlet fever

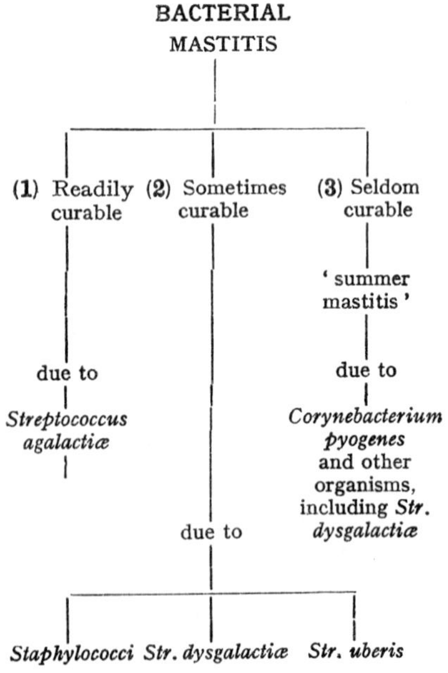

can result in an outbreak of mastitis in a dairy herd, and several such outbreaks have been reported in various countries. The pneumococcus, a cause of human pneumonia, has been isolated from the udders of cows with streptococcal mastitis in Essex, Bedfordshire, and other counties; the source being the cowman's throat.

Ignoring, for a moment, the fungi, perhaps the simplest and most helpful classification of mastitis is referred to in the table above.

1. Streptococcus agalactiæ infection.

Symptoms.—The disease is insidious and animals may harbour the germs for some time before signs of mastitis appear. The first indication is usually the presence of small flakes or clots in the fore-milk. These may disappear during a period of temporary improvement, or the signs of an acute mastitis may appear, namely: heat, pain, and swelling of the affected quarter. As the disease progresses, clots in the milk become more obvious and the quarter hardens.

The Spread of Infection.—Evidence has accrued that infection enters by way of the teat and that it can easily be spread from cow to cow by milker's hands or the cups of the machine, but apparently less easily by the latter method. Udder cloths and towels are also commonly infected. It has also now been shown that in an infected herd a large proportion of sores or chaps harbour the germ, and these may be a source of infection of the udder itself in the same cow or another. It has been shown also that the skin of the teats and the milker's hands may remain infected from one milking to another, and that in a heavily infected herd, the skin of the cow's body, milker's clothes, floor, partitions and, in fact, everything in the byre, become contaminated and may remain so for considerable periods.

There is also reason to believe that the udder of the calf occasionally becomes infected when it is sucked by another calf whose mouth has become contaminated by infected milk, and that this infection may persist until she calves. As far as is known, there is no reservoir of *Str. agalactiæ* in the cow's body, except the udder. There is some fairly recent evidence that older cows can be infected more easily than younger ones and that amongst cows of the same age there are differences in the ease with which they can be infected. As a result, some animals can overcome an infection, but in the majority persistent infection is the rule.

Treatment and Eradication.—Proper treatment depends upon a correct diagnosis and the use of penicillin in adequate dosage, introduced into the udder with aseptic precautions so as not to introduce further (and perhaps more virulent) infection. Adequate dosage is important as otherwise strains of penicillin-resistant *streptococci* may arise. In some cases sulphanilamide may be used.

Treatment of infected cows only may result in quick eradication if the numbers of infected cows in a herd are not large. If the incidence is high, however, better and quicker results can be obtained by treatment of all cows in milk or dry, infected or not, at the same time.

Results to date show that in herds so treated, clots or other signs of *Str. agalactiæ* mastitis disappear at once, that in over one-third of the herds eradication may be expected at once, and that in most of the remainder new infections or recrudescent infections are confined to a few cows. Some herds give more difficulty, usually because of persistent skin infections of the udder, the owner's reluctance to remove or isolate a res stant case, or bad sanitary conditions.

Infected cows which have been treated should be tested between one and two weeks afterwards. If still infected, they should be re-treated at once and re-tested. If a cow fails two treatments, her history and clinical state should be given weight and, if an old case, she should be disposed of unless of exceptional value. Cows remaining infected after the herd treatment must be isolated or every precaution taken to prevent spread to other cows, pending re-treatment and test.

If any infection was found at the first test, the whole herd should be re-tested every two months until two tests have been passed, covering four months from the date when the last infection was treated; then at twelve-monthly intervals. If no infection was found at the first herd test, another should be made after twelve months. Any *cow* purchased should be treated at once unless she has recently passed a bacteriological test. All the other additions (purchased heifers, cows re-calving and home-bred heifers) should be tested at once and handled with penicillin cream on hands and udders until proved clean—unless they have been proved clean in the previous lactation.

Another method of eradication which has given good results is treatment of all infected cows when they go dry. This has, however, the disadvantage that eradication must take at least one year and that clean cows are returned to an infected environment unless a separate herd is formed.

2. Infections other than S. agalactiæ. These infections also arise via the teat canal. They differ from *Str. agalactiæ*, however, in that they can be harboured in the tissues of the cow's body and, in the case of the staphylococci, are resident flora of the cow's skin as well as of human hands, forearms, and nose. Mastitis due to *Str. uberis* is mainly chronic, not easily distinguished from *Str. agalactiæ* mastitis, and often responds to penicillin treatment. Mastitis due to *Str. dysgalactiæ* and to *staphylococci* may likewise be chronic, but more often assumes an acute form, with considerable heat, pain, and swelling in the affected quarter. In some cases due to *staphylococci* there is a generalised illness with or without gangrene of the quarter and death. Treatment consists in the administration of antibiotics, or staphylococcal toxoid, or hibitane, together with formentations of the udder and sometimes the use of belladonna liniment to reduce pain. Eradication of these types of mastitis is not possible. (For treating infection with *Staphylococcus pyogenes*, *see under* Mastitis and Antibiotics, p. 537.)

3. 'Summer Mastitis' occurs most commonly in July, August, and September, usually in heifers and dry cows, occasionally just after calving. In such cases the uterus may act as a reservoir of infection.

Symptoms.—The affected animal may stand aloof from the rest of the herd, sometimes paddles with her hind feet, and is obviously in pain. On examination the trouble is soon located to the udder, where hardness—but not necessarily swelling—of a quarter is detected. Foul-smelling pus (grey, greenish-yellow, or blood-stained) is present.

Treatment.—As a first-aid measure, apply hot fomentations and gently strip out the quarter. This may already be irretrievably damaged, so far as future milk production is concerned, but no time should be lost in calling in the veterinary surgeon who may administer antiserum, toxoid and sulpha drugs, and succeed in saving the animal's life, though use of the quarter is usually lost.

Prevention.—The injection of long-acting penicillin prior to turning out, repeated every 3 weeks during the summer. Give such protection against flies as is practicable.

MASTITIS IN THE COW

The Control of Mastitis.—Dr. F. Dodd, of the NIRD, has emphasised that the present farm practice of treating clinical cases of mastitis with antibiotics cannot give adequate control, partly because many preparations are ineffective against staphylococci, but mainly because the level of infection is not much reduced—it remains in the untreated, subclinical cases. To detect all infected cows by means of laboratory techniques, and then treat them, would in his view be too expensive, and likely to be ineffective without some complementary means of preventing new infection. Moreover, it would aggravate the problem of antibiotic residues in milk.

His conclusion is that 'a satisfactory control can only be based on the prevention of new infection, and at the present time the only methods which show promise of being practical, economic, and effective are specific hygiene techniques'. This is also the long-held view of many veterinary authorities. The British Veterinary Association endorsed it in the early 1950s.

Among techniques recommended, teat-dipping now comes very high on the list. 'The teat-dip, first adopted by a veterinary surgeon in 1916, has proved to be the most important procedure in the hygiene system,' is the view of Mr. F. K. Neave of the NIRD. He compares the method favourably with the pasteurisation of teat-cups 'which does nothing to prevent infection of the teat canal'. The liquid mainly used for teat-dipping is an iodophor—a type of disinfectant containing iodine but extremely mild in its effect upon the tissues. (*See* TEAT DIPPING.)

A second recommendation is the wearing by the cowman of smooth rubber gloves, which can be dipped in disinfectant before the udder is washed. They represent a partial solution of the problem created by the fact that hands cannot be sterilised.

Warm water sprays may be used for udder washing, and disposable paper towels for drying. The latter obviate cross-infections from udder cloths.

If warm water sprays are not available, wash udder (if very dirty) with plain warm water first, then with, *e.g.* ICI Udder Wash.

It is significant that in herds with a low incidence of mastitis, udder washing is avoided in 40 per cent and practised only in 11 per cent.

Questions which the farmer must ask himself are as follows:

(1) Is the cowman capable of handling the cows properly, and keen to do so?

(2) Are the vacuum gauges and cup liners kept correctly adjusted?

(3) Is hand stripping avoided?

(4) If a disinfectant is used, is it used at the correct strength?

(5) Are there disposable paper towels?

(6) Are there any old, chronically infected cows in the herd which do not respond to treatment and would be better disposed of?

Rough inexpert milking and stripping predispose to mastitis. With machine milking the use of a badly designed teat-cup liner, for instance, or leaving the cups on an empty quarter may lead to trouble. (*See under* MILKING MACHINES for faulty use of these leading to mastitis.) Bruising is an important predisposing cause, and for this reason cows should never be hurried, especially before milking, as the udder may be injured. This applies particularly to older cows in which the udder is large and pendulous. Chilling must be avoided, and also chapped teats. The latter should be left dry after milking. Even the smallest injuries and sores on the teats should be carefully attended to, since the germs which gain entry to these so often gain entry to the udder later.

The routine use of the strip cup is helpful. If flecks or clots are seen in the milk, segregate the cow(s) if practicable, and—in any case—milk after the others. When a strip cup is used care should be taken to see that neither the handle nor the fingers become a source of infection to clean cows. Use the cup *before* the udder is washed.

Dry-cow therapy.—It has been shown in large-scale field experiments that the best time to treat cows to eliminate infection from the udders is during the dry period. Particularly with staphylococcal infection, there is a better chance (Mr. C. D. Wilson has stated) of removing infections at this time than during lactation, and better results are achieved when cows are treated in the subclinical phase of the disease rather than during a clinical attack. Treatment during the dry period not only eliminates most of the existing infection; it also prevents most of the new infections from occurring during the dry-period, including 'summer mastitis'. Another advantage is that there is no problem of milk being contaminated with antibiotic(s), provided that a cow is dry for six weeks or longer. It is advisable to treat *all* cows. Preparations containing cloxacillin have proved very effective.

MAXILLA (*maxilla*, a jaw) is the name applied to the upper jaw-bone which carries the cheek teeth. It forms part of the roof of the mouth, and the floor of the nasal passage.

MEADOW SAFFRON POISONING.—The Meadow Saffron, Autumn Crocus, or Naked Ladies (*Colchicum autumnale*), is a common inhabitant of meadows, hedge bottoms, and woodland areas in England and Wales, and is a serious cause of poisoning among horses and cattle. Pigs may sometimes eat the bulbous root (corm) and suffer, but sheep and goats are resistant. All parts of the plant are poisonous, both when green and when dried in hay, but the toxicity varies at different times of the year. Cases of poisoning are usually seen in the spring, when the leaves and seed-vessels are produced, and then again in summer and autumn (from August to October), when the flowers are formed.

The poisonous agent contained in the plant is present in largest amounts in the seeds and corms (' bulbs ') ; it is called *Colchicine*, and is cumulative in its action due to the fact that it is only slowly excreted by the kidneys.

Symptoms.—These do not usually appear until several hours after the plant is eaten, and if only small amounts have been taken daily for a long period the symptoms may develop very slowly. When only small quantities have been taken there is an absence of appetite, suppression of rumination, profuse dribbling of saliva, and diarrhœa. The excretion of acrid colchicine by the kidneys cause irritation in the urinary bladder, and induces the animal to pass urine in small amounts almost as soon as it is formed. Blood may be present in both the urine and the milk of dairy cows. When large amounts have been eaten the symptoms are more severe. The animal loses its balance, staggers about, and finally falls stupefied. Its pupils are dilated ; a profuse perspiration breaks out over the whole body ; signs of acute abdominal pain are evident, and blood-stained liquid fæces and urine are passed with considerable straining. Death takes place in about 16 to 24 hours in rapidly fatal cases, but when less of the plant has been eaten it may be delayed until the third or fourth day after the appearance of the symptoms. Recovery occurs when the amount taken has not been great, but it is always slow, and accompanied by much loss of flesh, and a serious falling off in milk secretion. As a rule, if the pulse is but little disturbed the animal will recover, but cases showing a small, weak, irregular pulse usually end fatally. Abortion is common in pregnant cows and heifers.

Treatment.—The antidotes to colchicine are tannic acid and gallic acid given in large doses when the alimentary canal still contains quantities of the plant, and the administration of demulcent drinks of barley-water, linseed tea, gruels, etc., to allay the irritation ; and the intravenous injection of potassium permanganate solution in physiological salt solution is calculated to neutralise toxic principles absorbed into the general circulation.

The plant should be eradicated from pastures in the autumn when its striking pale purple crocus-like flowers can be easily seen. The bulbs should be dug out or cut with a hoe, and the plant collected.

MEAL FEEDING IN PIGGERIES.—This can result in a very dusty atmosphere under some circumstances, causing coughing and a feeling of tightness in the chest in people working there, and to a sometimes false assumption that the pigs are coughing because of Virus Pneumonia.

MEASLES IN BEEF is due to the presence of the cyst stage (*Cysticercus bovis*) of the tapeworm *Tænia saginata*, which is a parasite of man. Oxen swallow the eggs of the adult tapeworm, and these hatch in the intestines, liberating young embryos, which burrow until they settle in muscle fibre or connective tissues. Here they appear as small oval spots, from $\frac{3}{16}$ths to $\frac{1}{4}$th of an inch long, containing fluid, and each possessing the head of a potential tapeworm. The disease causes no symptoms in cattle, but it is of great importance from the meat inspection point of view, since if the meat is not well cooked, a person eating it becomes infested with tapeworms. (*See* PARASITES, p. 652.)

MEASLES IN PORK is due to the presence of the cyst stage (*Cysticercus cellulosæ*) of the tapeworm of man—*Tænia solium*. It is extremely common among pigs in eastern lands, which have access to garbage and human ordure, from whence they pick up the eggs passed through the human intestines. The eggs undergo a development similar to those of the beef measles tapeworm. (*See* PARASITES, p. 652.) Man may also himself harbour the cystic stage.

MEASLES VACCINE.—An attenuated measles virus vaccine has been developed for use in the dog to give protection against distemper. The vaccine can be given to the puppy when 3 weeks old. Immunity is normally established within 72 hours and lasts at least 5 months. The measles virus is not excreted by the puppy. (*See also under* DISTEMPER.)

Forney, Bordt and Theodore (1967) reported a series of experiments which demonstrated a limitation on the use of measles vaccine. 'This limitation is due to the fact that puppies born of bitches vaccinated with measles virus may possess sufficient maternally acquired measles antibodies to interfere with their response to vaccination with measles virus. Such puppies would be expected to become susceptible to canine distemper in a manner similar to non-vaccinated puppies.'

MEAT INSPECTION (*see under* FOOD INSPECTION).

MEAT SCRAPS, BONES can be a source of foot-and-mouth disease or swine fever infections. (*See* SWILL.) (*See also last two paragraphs of section* TUBERCULOSIS.)

MEAT (STERILISATION) REGULATIONS, 1969.—These require all knacker meat to be sterilised before being supplied to owners of pets, kennels, etc.

MEATUS (*meatus*, passage) is a term applied to any passage or opening, *e.g.* external auditory meatus, the passage from the surface to the drum of the ear.

MECHANICAL STAGE.—A device fitted to a microscope for moving, horizontally, the glass slide on which is the preparation to be examined. It enables a careful search to be made of the 'field' of view.

MECKLE'S DIVERTICULUM, of human pathology, apparently has a veterinary equivalent—a finger-like projection from the small intestine, recorded as a congenital abnormality in the dog.

MECONIUM (*μηκώνιον*, poppy-juice) means the brown or blackish, viscid, semifluid or hard material which collects in the bowels of young animals prior to birth. It should in all cases be discharged soon after birth. In the first milk of the dam there is a natural purgative for this purpose.

MEDIASTINUM (*medius*, middle) is the name given to the space in the chest which lies between the two lungs. It contains the heart and the great vessels, the gullet, the extremity of the trachea, the thoracic duct, the phrenic nerves, as well as other structures of less importance.

MEDICINES ACT, 1968. (*See* VETERINARY PRODUCTS COMMITTEE and ADDITIVES.)

MEDITERRANEAN FEVER.—A tick-borne disease of cattle and the water-buffalo, occurring in S.E. Europe, Africa, and Asia, and caused by *Theileria annulata*,

Symptoms.—Fever, loss of appetite, a discharge from eyes and nose, anæmic pallor of mucous membranes, constipation followed by diarrhœa. Survivors recover very slowly.

MEDIUM.—In bacteriology this term is applied to a liquid (*e.g.* broth) or a solid (*e.g.* agar) in which bacteria are grown in the laboratory.

MEDULLA (*medulla*) is another word for marrow. The word is generally restricted to the marrow of bones, or to designate a part of the brain, but it occasionally means the spinal cord, which is called the spinal medulla.

MEDULLA OBLONGATA (*medulla*, marrow; *oblongus*, long), or BULB, is the hindermost part of the brain, which is continued backwards as the spinal cord. It contains the centres which govern many of the vital functions of the body, such as that controlling the heart, respiration, etc. (*See* BRAIN.)

MEGA- and **MEGALO-** (*μέγας*, great) are prefixes denoting largeness.

MEIBOMIAN GLANDS are minute glands situated in the eyelids, which under certain circumstances become the seat of abscesses; these are often called 'styes' or 'eye-cysts'.

MELÆNA (μελαίνω, I blacken) means a condition of the fæces in which dark tarry masses are passed. It is due to hæmorrhage from the anterior parts of the alimentary canal, such as the stomach, or small intestines. The blood undergoes chemical changes as the result of the action of the digestive juices, which produce large amounts of sulphide of iron.

MELANOTIC μέλας, black) is a term applied to certain tumours which become infiltrated with a black pigment called 'melanin', which is derived from the colouring matter of hair, etc. Such tumours are commonest in old horses that have been grey and are turning whiter; they are frequently, but not always, of a malignant nature. (*See* TUMOURS.)

MELIOIDOSIS.—A disease resembling glanders, caused by *Pfeifferella pseudomallei*, and occurring in rodents—occasionally in human beings and farm animals—in the tropics. Diagnosis: 'whitmorin' test. In man, chloromycetin is used in treatment. Cases have occurred in Germany.

MELOPHAGUS OVINUS.—Sheep ked.

MEMBRANA NICTITANS (*see* end of section headed EYELIDS).

MEMBRANES (*see* AFTERBIRTH, BRAIN, MENINGES, MUCOUS MEMBRANES, SEROUS MEMBRANES, etc.).

MENAPHTHONE (*see* VITAMIN K).

MENINGES (μῆνιγξ, a membrane) are the membranes surrounding the brain and spinal cord. These membranes carry the blood-vessels which nourish the brain substance and the inner layer of the skull. Hæmorrhages from these vessels, and consequent pressure from blood-clots, form the great dangers of fractures of the skull, or concussion of the spinal cord. (*See* BRAIN, SPINAL CORD.)

MENINGITIS (from μῆνιγξ, a membrane) is a term applied to inflammation affecting the membranes covering the brain (cerebral meningitis), spinal cord (spinal meningitis), or both (cerebro-spinal meningitis). When the outer membrane is affected the condition is called 'Pachymeningitis', and when the inner membrane it is known as 'Leptomeningitis', although clinically it is not often that these distinctions can be determined, for inflammation readily spreads from one to the other, passing along the strands of the middle (arachnoid) membrane. Owing to the very close association between the inner membrane (pia mater) and the surface of the brain, it is hardly possible for leptomeningitis to be present without the brain substance also becoming inflamed (encephalitis), so that whenever the pia mater is involved the animal's condition is extremely serious.

Causes.—Meningitis frequently develops in association with virus or bacterial diseases of animals, such as strangles, glanders, tuberculosis, swine erysipelas, distemper, and Borna disease. It may be caused through the presence of the bladder stage of *Tænia cœnurus* in the sheep or ox (gid or sturdy), or of strongyle larvæ in the horse. It may be produced through an external injury which fractures the skull and allows entrance to organisms, or it may appear during the course of other head injuries in which there is no fracture. It accompanies most cases of encephalitis caused by viruses.

Symptoms.—As a rule the first signs are those of restlessness and excitement. The animal moves about in a semi-dazed fashion, and stumbles into or against fixed objects. At times, fits of delirium are seen, and the animal may do itself serious damage. The pulse, respiration rate, and almost all natural movements, are faster than usual. The temperature is high, and the pupils are dilated. Neighing, bellowing, squealing, and barking, apparently at nothing, may be noticed, and at times the animal exhibits a wild frenzy. After an attack of delirium or frenzy the animal becomes dull and quiet; the head hangs, the eyes stare, the expression is vacant, and the animal may either stand still or lie down. As the disease develops a period of lessened activity supervenes. Dullness and depression are continually present; food is only taken when it is placed near; fæces and urine are retained; and the animal remains in one position for hours unless vigorously roused. Other symptoms, such as touring in circles, rolling over and over along the ground, turning forward and backward somersaults, resting the head upon any convenient fixed object, such as a loose-box door, lying curled up in an unusual attitude, etc., may be seen in some cases. Paralysis of one side of the body (hemiplegia), of both hind-limbs (paraplegia), or of a group of muscles, is not infrequent in the smaller animals. In the dog a form of chronic meningitis occurs in which bony tissue is laid down in the spinal canal towards the posterior part of the vertebral column. It is called 'chronic ossifying pachymeningitis' as a consequence. It mainly affects old dogs, and only causes inconvenience when severe. It may be suspected in an animal that becomes frequently affected with constipation, and that takes long periods to evacuate the rectum. In such the hind quarters are sometimes held high in the air, the dog balancing itself upon its fore feet for seconds at a time, immediately after the act of defecation. It may lead to complete paralysis of the hind limbs, accompanied by incontinence of urine and fæces.

Treatment.—In the larger animals death almost always follows severe cases of meningitis, and it is questionable whether immediate destruction would not always be the most rational method of dealing with such cases, especially if the carcase has a food value. In valuable animals, treatment, if undertaken, must be according to the symptoms. Absolute quiet in a darkened loose-box is essential. The nervous irritability requires the use of a sedative, and antibiotics or sulpha drugs may be tried.

Treatment must depend upon a professional diagnosis.

In all animals in which meningitis follows injury, the skull should be examined for fractures.

***MENINGOENCEPHALITIS EOSINOPHILICA* OF PIGS.**—This is characterised by death of the cells in the grey matter of the brain in front of the *corpora quadrigemina*, and by thickening of the blood vessels around which are found considerable numbers of eosinophils.

Symptoms include: walking in circles, pressing the head against a wall, champing of the jaws, convulsions.

The cause, or a cause, is considered to be salt poisoning.

MENISCUS (μηνίσκος, crescent) is the term applied to a crescentic fibro-cartilage in a joint.

MEPACRINE HYDROCHLORIDE.—An antimalarial drug which has been used in the treatment of coccidiosis in cattle.

MEPYRAMINE MALEATE.—An antihistamine which is given by the mouth, by intra-muscular injection, or applied to the skin as a cream. Used in the treatment of laminitis, azoturia, urticaria, etc. (*See* ANTIHISTAMINES.)

MERCUROCHROME.—An antiseptic, and a stain for spermatozoa.

MERCURY, also known as QUICKSILVER, and HYDRARGYRUM, is a heavy silver-coloured liquid metal. The metal has been used in a state of fine subdivision in the form of an ointment, with chalk as a grey powder, and as blue pill. The metal itself, however, is inert, and its effect upon the system is probably the result of the action of body fluids upon it, which convert it into one or another of its powerful salts.

Actions.—The salts of mercury are of two varieties: mercur*ic* salts, which are very soluble and powerful in action; and mercur*ous* salts, which are less soluble and act more slowly and mildly. Mercuric salts are all highly poisonous to animal and bacterial life, so that they act as strong antiseptics. In strong solution they may be caustic, and in weaker solutions are irritant, the biniodide being used as a blister in consequence.

Internally, the mercuric, and to a less extent the mercurous salts are purgative, and clear bile away from the intestines. They are absorbed into the body only slowly as a compound with albumin, or along with the chlorides of the blood and lymph, and their excretion is also slow. When given in single large doses, or in repeated small doses, they are poisonous. (*See* MERCURY POISONING.)

Uses.—Preparations of mercury are less used than formerly. Mercury ointment was a former dressing for ringworm. It must be used with care in dogs on account of the danger of poisoning through the dog licking the dressing. Yellow oxide of mercury is also the active agent in 'golden ointment'. Calomel, the subchloride of mercury, is used internally as a stimulant cathartic, clearing away bile from the intestines, and promoting a greater secretion from the intestinal glands. It is usual to administer a saline purge 6 or 8 hours after giving calomel, so that there is little absorption of the drug into the system. Corrosive sublimate, the perchloride of mercury, is a powerful antiseptic, and an irritant and corrosive poison. It is not now used in the treatment of wounds, many alternative and less poisonous drugs being available.

Biniodide of mercury, or red iodide of mercury, made up into an ointment, forms the base of the common 'red blister'.

With all these preparations it is essential that care be taken, for the drug may enter the system by absorption from the skin, or by the animal licking itself.

MERCURY POISONING cases have occurred where herbage near chemical works has become impregnated with mercury or mercury compounds, and cattle have died from eating it. In the smaller animals frequently, and in the larger animals sometimes, toxic results follow the use of mercuric dressings applied to the skin. Mercury can readily be absorbed through the unbroken skin, and more rapidly through wounded areas, so that use of mercury compounds on the skin requires care. In animals that are given to licking themselves (especially cattle and dogs) poisoning may result when mercury dressings are used. Feeding dressed seed corn has led to the death of pigs, and might well do so in other animals.

Acute poisoning results when large amounts of the drug have been taken into the system. The animal becomes suddenly ill, vomiting and severe purgation occur in the smaller animals, and there is a profuse watery or blood-stained diarrhœa and excessive salivation in horses and cattle. Acute abdominal pain is evident; the animal is very restless, and in a few hours collapse and death occur. In milder cases the symptoms are similar but less severe; the pulse becomes weak, breathing is irregular, the temperature falls below normal, and death occurs in two or three days, usually from exhaustion.

Chronic poisoning, or *mercurialism* takes place when smaller amounts have been taken into the system frequently for a considerable time. The drug may be absorbed comparatively rapidly, but is only slowly excreted from the body, so that it accumulates in the tissues. There is an excessive amount of salivation, blanching of the mucous membranes of the mouth, and loosening of the teeth. (It should be remembered that the incisor teeth of the ox are movable *normally*.) The coat stares and the skin becomes scurfy and dry; the hair may fall out in patches. The skin and surface muscles lose their elasticity, and loss of condition takes place. Mercury is said to be excreted in the milk.

Antidotes.—In acute cases no time should be lost in giving a drench composed of the whites of from two to eight or ten eggs (the smaller number for the smaller animals) mixed up with about half their volume of ordinary flowers of sulphur, and made thin enough to swallow with warm water. The whites of egg precipitate the albuminate of mercury, and the sulphur combines with the metal to form the insoluble sulphide of mercury. In chronic cases the same treatment should be adopted three or four times a day, and doses of potassium iodide may be given to hasten elimination of the drug.

Where poisoning has occurred through the skin, the mercury dressings should be washed off with soap and warm water to which has been added a little ordinary washing soda. (*See* CHELATING AGENTS.)

MERCURY, POISONING BY DOG'S.—Both Dog's Mercury (*Mercurialis perennis*) and Annual Mercury (*Mercurialis annua*), which closely resemble each other except that the former is perennial and the latter annual, are poisonous when eaten in quantity by live-stock. The objectionable odour possessed by the plants, however, causes animals to avoid them unless there is a shortage of green food. Cows are most often affected. The poisonous principles are variously stated as being either *Mercurialine* or else *Trimethylamine*, but, in any case, they are cumulative, since animals may not show any symptoms until from 7 to 10 days after the plants are first eaten.

Symptoms.—The mercury plants are emetic and purgative, the purging action being very severe and frequently fatal. It is stated that the first effects are constipation and colic, and that diarrhœa does not follow till later. In some cases the diarrhœa gives place again to constipation later still. The plant is irritant and causes inflammation of both the digestive and urinary systems. Urine is passed frequently, accompanied by painful straining, and is of a blackish or blood-red colour, as is the diarrhœa. The animal rapidly becomes weak and depressed. Pulse-beats continue strong, though fast; there is no change in the breathing, but the temperature is high. Milk secretion is almost completely stopped in the case of dog's mercury, and is often of a bluish or blood-red colour when annual mercury has been eaten. The milk may cause digestive disturbances to animals consuming it. Recovery is very slow owing to the gradual elimination of the toxic principle from the system, and paralysis of a muscle, or of a group of muscles, may remain after the other symptoms disappear. Deaths have occurred.

Treatment.—The animal should be given strong black tea or coffee, along with demulcent drinks of gruels, linseed tea, whites of eggs, etc. Plenty of water should be provided for drinking purposes to flush out the kidneys. Diarrhœa or constipation should receive appropriate attention.

MESENCEPHALON is the mid-brain connecting the cerebral hemispheres with the pons and cerebellum.

MESENTERY (μέσον, middle; ἔντερον, the intestine) is the name given to the double layer of peritoneal membrane which supports the intestine. The mesentery supports the small intestine, the colic mesentery supports the colon, and the other organs of the abdominal cavity are held in position by various folds of peritoneum which are sometimes called mesenteries.

MESOCOLON (μέσος, middle; κόλον, colon) is the name of the fold of peritoneum by which the large intestine is suspended from the roof of the abdomen.

MESOMETRIUM is the name of the fold of peritoneum running from the roof of the abdomen to the uterus. It consists of two layers, between which run the blood and lymph vessels, and the nerves to the uterus, and it acts as an elastic suspensory ligament supporting the uterus in position. During pregnancy it gradually stretches under the weight of the fœtal contents, but retracts again after parturition under normal conditions.

MESOSALPINX is the suspensory ligament of the oviduct.

MESOVARIUM is the suspensory ligament of the ovary.

MESULPHEN.—A parasiticide which allays itching, used in cases of sarcoptic mange.

METABOLIC.—Relating to metabolism

METABOLIC PROFILE TESTS.—To quote a paper by Dr. J. M. Payne, M.R.C.V.S. and colleagues at the Institute for Research on Animal Diseases, Compton, 'modern farming imposes severe strains on the metabolism of dairy cows. Every effort is made to secure high yields at minimum cost. This is likely to increase, because high yielding cows are advantageous both in terms of financial return and in efficiency of protein conversion. New types of feed and unconventional methods of husbandry are also likely to be employed, thus adding to the strain and possibly introducing hidden dangers to the metabolic health of the animals. The metabolic profile test was devised to help meet this situation.'

The method depends on the fact that *imbalances between feed input and production output are reflected in abnormal concentrations of key metabolites in the blood.* The test appears to be of most value in (a) monitoring optimum input/output balances in apparently normal dairy herds; and (b) as an aid in diagnosing basic nutritional inadequacies in herds suffering from production disease problems.

As a first step in devising the test it was necessary to establish 'normal' values, and this was provisionally achieved by analysing 2,400 blood samples from 13 dairy herds. The second step involved carrying out routine metabolic profile tests in 50 dairy herds. In many of these, abnormalities were detected which could be associated with actual or potential production disease problems. If necessary, a change of diet was recommended, and the effects of this monitored by repeated tests.

Haemoglobin levels were low in herds sampled at the end of the winter indoor period, but rose steeply when cows were turned out to pasture in the spring. 'This was so marked as to suggest that in some herds animals were saved from clinical anaemia only by the spring grass!'

Low blood sugar levels were associated in one herd with a severe and unexplained ketosis (acetonæmia) outbreak; but the effects of somewhat ham-handed over-correction in another herd led to secondary ketosis, following supplementation with a mixture of brewer's grains, sugar beet pulp and rolled barley. Two herds with low blood sugar showed few clinical problems, but many cows failed to come on normal heat in winter—a situation remedied by supplements.

Serum urea concentrations tended to be low on conventional indoor winter rations, but high in herds grazing highly fertilised pastures. The latter gave rise also to high concentrations of inorganic phosphate and potassium in the blood.

A dramatic example of low serum magnesium was shown in one herd where the farmer thought that his cows were dying from calving injuries. Magnesium supplements in the diet overcame the trouble. The detection of low serum magnesium levels may, of course, be valuable in the prediction of impending outbreaks of clinical hypomagnesæmia. Indeed, in one herd—apparently clinically normal—two animals died of grass tetany before the supplementation recommended after testing could become effective.

The dietary intake of sodium may be too low. For example, in an experiment 30 cows grazing known sodium-deficient herbage licked surrounding objects, each others' coats and even urine. This craving disappeared when sodium supplements were given.

Too little blood albumin was a feature in some herds on low-cost, low-protein diets. Cows on highly fertilised pastures tended to have high blood albumin levels.

Until recently, the number of blood samples involved would have been far too great for the metabolic profile tests to be applied on anything but a small, laboratory scale; but now new automatic analytical equipment together with a computer allow a rapid and large-scale analysis and interpretation of data.

As time goes on, the 'normal' values may need revision, and trace elements and other metabolites may be included in the test which, it is hoped, will 'be of value in providing a link between the veterinary surgeon and the dairy farmer in the application of modern preventive medicine'.

But the test must be carried out in a carefully planned and standardised manner, under veterinary supervision. In other words, it is not a 'do-it-yourself' procedure, with a few samples at random taken from a dairy herd and sent through the post for testing.

METABOLISM (*μεταβολή*, change) means tissue change, and includes all the physical and chemical processes by which the living body is maintained, and also those by which the energy is made available for various forms of work or production. The constructive, chemical, and physical processes by which food materials are adapted for the use of the body are collectively known as *anabolism*. The destructive processes by which energy is produced with the breaking down of tissues into waste products is known as *catabolism*. Basal metabolism is the term applied to the amount of energy which is necessary for carrying on the processes essential to life, such as the beating of the heart, movements of the chest in breathing, chemical activities of sereting glands, and maintenance of bodycwarmth. This can be estimated when an animal is placed in a state of complete rest, either by observing for a certain period the amount of heat given out from the body or by estimating the amount of oxygen which is taken in during the act of breathing and retained.

METABOLITES.—Any product of metabolism, but especially of catabolism.

METACARPAL (*μετά*, beyond; *καρπός*, the wrist) region is the part of the limb lying between the carpus or wrist, and the phalanges or digits. This region in the horse is commonly called the region of the 'cannon' on account of the comparatively straight tubular form of the large or 3rd metacarpal bone. The bones in the metacarpal region of the horse are three in number, of which the central or third is the largest, and the inner (2nd) and outer (4th) are rudimentary. In the ox there are two large metacarpals fused together; the sheep is similar; the pig has four separate from each other, and the dog possesses five bones in this region.

METAL DETECTOR (*see under* Mine Detector).

METALDEHYDE POISONING has been encountered in the dog and cat following the eating of 'Meta' tablets used for killing garden slugs. Symptoms may include: excitement, vomiting, muscular tetany, nystagmus in the cat, partial paralysis, and stupor. The animal should be kept quiet in the dark pending veterinary aid, when anæsthesia may be required.

METAPHYSIS (*μετά*, beyond; *φύειν*, to grow) is the name applied to the vascular active extremity of the diaphysis, or central portion, of a young bone. The metaphysis lies immediately below the epiphyseal cartilage where growth in length of a bone takes place.

METAPLASIA is described as 'the change of one kind of tissue into another; also the production of tissue by cells which normally produce tissue of another sort.'

METASTASIS (μετάστασις, a change of place) and 'metastatic' are terms applied to the process by which a malignant tumour spreads to distant parts of the body, and gives rise to secondary tumours similar to the primary. Thus sarcoma in some part of the abdomen may spread to the thorax by pieces of tumour or clusters of cells breaking away from the parent growth, and being carried by the blood-stream to the lungs, etc., and setting up new sarcomatous growths there.

METATARSAL (μετά, beyond; ταρσός, the instep) is the name given to the bones and structures lying between the tarsus or hock and the digit of the hind limb. It corresponds to the metacarpal region in the fore limb, and has a somewhat similar arrangement of bones.

METHÆMOGLOBIN is a modification of hæmoglobin, the pigment of blood, which is found in blood, and sometimes in urine after administering large doses of certain drugs, such as acetanilid, and also in some diseases. Chemically, methæmoglobin is the same as oxyhæmoglobin, except that it cannot part with its oxygen so readily as the latter.

METHALLIBURE is a non-steroidal pituitary inhibitor, which causes artificial anœstrus. On termination of treatment, follicular activity rebounds with synchronisation of œstrus. It has been used for the synchronisation of œstrus in gilts.

METHANE (MARSH GAS) has the chemical formula CH_4. Large quantities may be formed in the rumen in cases of tympanitis in the cow. The gas is inflammable. (*See* SLURRY.)

METHIOCARB.—A snail-killer used in agriculture. Poultry and other animals must be kept away from treated areas for at least a week.

METHONIUM COMPOUNDS block impulses in sympathetic ganglia and are employed in arterial hypertension, *e.g.* Hexamethonium.

METHYL is the name of an organic radicle whose chemical formulæ is CH_3, and which forms the centre of a wide group of substances known as the methyl group. For example, methyl alcohol is obtained as a by-product in the manufacture of beet-sugar, or by the distillation of wood; methyl salicylate is the active constituent of oil of wintergreen; methyl hydride is better known as marsh gas.

METHYLATED SPIRIT is a mixture of rectified spirit with 10 per cent by volume of wood naphtha, which renders the spirit dangerous for internal administration. (*See* ALCOHOL.)

METHYRIDINE.—An anthelmintic, for use in cattle and sheep, introduced in 1961. A colourless, sweet-smelling liquid, readily miscible with water, methyridine in solution is given by subcutaneous injection.

The drug is claimed to be very effective against *Trichostrongylus* species in the abomasum; *Ostertagia*, *Cooperia*, and *Nematodirus* in the small intestine; and *Trichuris* species in the cæcum and large intestine. 'The drug also has exceptional activity against *Bunostomum*, *Chabertia*, and *Œsophagostomum* species. Variable results,' say the makers, 'are occasionally experienced against *Hæmonchus* and *Ostertagia* species in the abomasum, although in the majority of animals a high percentage of the worms are eliminated.'

An outstanding advantage claimed for Methyridine is the efficient removal of immature stages of all these species.

The drug has appreciable activity against adult lungworms. (*Dictyocaulus* species.)

Dosage.—One ml. of solution per 10 lb. bodyweight, with a maximum dose for cattle of 60 ml.

Mode of action.—After injection the drug is rapidly absorbed and distributed throughout the tissues. Appreciable amounts diffuse into the alimentary canal where they remain until metabolism of Methyridine in the tissues causes the blood concentration to fall. When this happens re-absorption takes place. This is because the drug passes from blood to intestine and *vice versa* according to the concentration gradient. However, while the concentration of Methyridine along the entire length of the intestine always closely matches that present in the blood, the levels in the abomasum are higher and more persistent. It is believed that this is because the acidic contents of the abomasum attract Methyridine in the same way as they attract other basic substances.

Toxicity.—Twice the therapeutic dose

may cause death from respiratory failure. Dullness and ataxia may be observed with lesser over-dosage. There is no antidote.

Side-effects.—Occasionally dullness may be observed for 24 hours after dosing. In cattle, especially, a swelling may occur at the site of injection, and sometimes proves troublesome.

Precautions.—The liquid will de-fat the skin if the hands come into contact too much with Methyridine. Absorption through the unbroken skin can occur. The drug will attack rubber, paintwork, etc.

METRIC SYSTEM (*see under* EQUIVALENTS, TABLES OF).

METRITIS (μήτρα, the womb) means inflammation of the uterus. (*See* UTERUS, DISEASES OF.)

MEUSE-RHINE-IJSSEL (M.R.I.).—A dual-purpose breed of cattle from Holland, with good milk yields and high butterfat. Its import was sanctioned for the Shorthorn Society in 1970.

MICE (*see* LYMPHOCYTIC CHORIOMENINGITIS *and* RODENTS).

MICRO- (μικρός, small) is a prefix meaning small.

MICROCEPHALY (μικρός, small; κεφαλή, head) is a term applied to abnormal smallness of the head.

MICROCYTE (μικρός, small; κύτος, cell) means a small red blood corpuscle.

MICRON.—0·001 mm., the unit of measurement in microscopical and bacteriological work. Its symbol is μ.

MICRO-ORGANISMS are organisms so small as to require the high powers of the microscope for their demonstration. (*See* BACTERIOLOGY.)

MICROPHTHALMIA.—An abnormal smallness of the eyes, accompanied by blindness. In piglets it is believed to be associated with a Vitamin A deficiency.

MICROSCOPE.—The ordinary microscope with oil-immersion lens gives magnification up to 1500 diameters. (*See also* ELECTRON MICROSCOPE.)

MICROSPORUM.—A group of fungi responsible for ringworm. (Formerly called MICROSPORON.)

MICTURITION (*micturio*, I make water) means the act of passing water.

MIDDLINGS (*see* WEATINGS).

MIGRAM.—A disease of sheep on the Romney Marsh. The cause is unknown.

MIL is a contraction for millilitre, equal to one cubic centimetre of fluid.

MILIARY (*milium*, a millet seed) is a term, expressive of size, applied to various disease products which are about the size of a millet seed, *e.g.* miliary tuberculosis.

MILK.—Composition.—Cow's milk is a very valuable food substance as it contains all the essential food constituents, viz. proteins, carbohydrates, fats, and vitamins, in addition to a considerable percentage of mineral matter. The most important protein in milk is casein; it is present in a state of partial solution Carbohydrates are represented by the milk-sugar or lactose which is dissolved in the liquid portion of the milk. They, along with the fat which occurs as spherical globules, are heat and energy-producing substances. The mineral matter consists, to a very large extent, of compounds of lime and phosphorus. These substances are the essential constituents of bone.

The percentages of the main constituents of milk vary considerably, particularly as regards the percentage of fat, which alters most; the following are average figures:

	Per cent
Protein	3·40
Milk-sugar	4·75
Fat	3·75
Mineral matter	·75
Water	87·35
	100·00

In the young growing animal muscle and bone are being formed rapidly. Hence the food of the young must be adequately provided with protein and mineral matter in particular. Milk, since it contains considerable quantities of both of these constituents, and vitamins, is an excellent food for growing animals; but not a complete one—it will not provide adequate iron in the piglet or adequate magnesium in the calf.

APPROXIMATE COMPOSITION OF THE ASH OF COW'S MILK

	Per cent
Potash	29·0
Lime	20·0
Soda	7·0
Magnesia	3·0
Iron oxide	0·5
Phosphoric acid	29·0
Chlorine	14·0

Legal Standards.—In Great Britain, under the 'Sale of Food and Drugs Act', milk containing less than 3 per cent of butter fat, or less than 8·5 per cent of non-fatty solids (*i.e.* proteins, sugar, and ash), is deemed to be not genuine (until or unless the contrary is proved) by reason of either the addition of water or the abstraction of some of the fatty or non-fatty solids. (*See* SOLIDS-NOT-FAT.)

The specific gravity of cow's milk varies between 1·028 and 1·032. The greater the fat content the lower the specific gravity because fat is lighter than water and solids, bulk for bulk.

The reaction of the milk of the herbivorous animals is generally approximately neutral, while that of the carnivorous animals is acid.

APPROXIMATE COMPOSITION OF MILK PRODUCTS

	Water.	Proteins.	Fats.	Sugar.	Ash
Separated milk	90·0	3·7	0·2	4·9	0·8
Skimmed milk	90·0	3·6	0·8	4·6	0·8
Butter milk	91·0	3·3	0·5	3·4	0·6
Cream (thin)	64·0	2·8	30·0	3·5	0·5
Cream (thick)	39·0	1·6	56·0	2·3	0·4
Whey	93·0	0·9	0·2	4·8	0·5

APPROXIMATE COMPOSITION OF MILK OF DIFFERENT ANIMALS

	Water.	Proteins.	Fats.	Sugar.	Ash.
Mare	90·5	2·0	1·2	5·8	0·4
Cow	97·4	3·4	3·8	4·8	0·8
Ewe	81·9	5·8	6·5	4·8	0·9
Goat	84·1	4·0	6·0	5·0	0·8
Sow	84·6	6·3	4·8	3·4	0·9
(Human)	(87·4)	(2·1)	(3·8)	(6·3)	(0·3)

Germ content.—Cow's milk by the time it reaches the consumer also contains a variable and frequently large number of bacteria (*but see* PASTEURISATION). The number present in a particular sample of milk depends on:

(1) Whether the milk was produced under hygienic conditions;

(2) The length of time the milk has been kept since milking;

(3) The temperature of keeping.

All the bacteria present in milk are by no means harmful forms from the point of view of the consumer. The great majority are quite harmless or even useful. The microbe occurring in largest numbers (sometimes 99 per cent of the total) is one which causes the milk to turn sour and curdle. Sour milk, however, is not at all injurious to the consumer provided it is clean sour milk; under certain conditions it may be quite a valuable article of diet.

If milk is produced under dirty conditions it is liable to contain a microbe which can bring about a form of souring which is of a highly undesirable nature.

Germs in milk may include those of tuberculosis, mastitis, brucellosis, anthrax, and Q Fever, and cow-pox, and they (*see* UNDULANT FEVER) can be conveyed to man by the drinking of infected milk. The germs of tuberculosis, contagious abortion, and anthrax as a rule infect the milk of the cow while it is still in the udder. The viruses of foot-and-mouth disease and cow-pox are added to the milk during the operation of milking, as a result of the rupture of vesicles on the teats. (*See also* Q FEVER.)

Milk may also be infected with disease germs after it has left the cow. The main disease microbes which enter milk after it is drawn are those of typhoid, dysentery, diphtheria, scarlet fever, septic sore throat, and sometimes tuberculosis. Such infection is brought about by the handling of milk by persons suffering from or who have recently suffered from the disease or who have been in contact with infected individuals, *e.g.* milkers, dairymen, milk dealers, etc.

There is another disease which is believed to be conveyed by milk, viz., infantile diarrhœa, or 'Summer complaint'. This disease is considered by many to be due to consumption by infants of milk highly contaminated with organisms fro manure—the abnormal milk-souring organisms already referred to. These organisms often multiply with great rapidity in dirty milk in hot summer weather.

'Fore milk' is more highly contaminated than that drawn last (called the 'strippings') as the following figures indicate:

Bacteria per c.c. in:

Fore milk . .	55,000 to 97,000
Strippings . .	0 to 500

Frequently large numbers of bacteria find their way into milk during milking, especially if the udder and flanks of the cow are dirty.

The byre should be cleaned preferably twice a day, and the animals provided with clean bedding. It is important, however, that the removal of the manure and the foddering or littering of the byre should not be carried out during the two hours that precede milking. During these operations the air is filled with clouds of dust and bacteria, and if the cows are milked soon afterwards large numbers of these germs settle into the milk pails.

In order to minimise bacterial contamination of milk during milking, the cow's udder should be wiped with a disposable towel wrung out of water containing a disinfectant, and the hands of the milker should be thoroughly washed before the milking of each cow (preferably in water containing a disinfectant). (*See* p. 540 for recommended procedure.)

The numbers of bacteria present in milk after milking do not remain constant. They, as a rule, show a slight fall during the first few hours, followed by a very rapid and relatively enormous increase. The higher the temperature up to a point the more rapid is the multiplication as a rule. This is well illustrated in the following table:

BACTERIA PER C.C. IN MILK

Temperature at which Milk was kept.	Fresh.	After 24 hours.	After 48 hours.
40° Fahr. .	4295	4138	4566
50° " .	4295	13,900	127,700
60° " .	4295	1,587,300	33,011,100

It will be noted that at 40° F. there is practically no increase in numbers. Lower temperatures are still more effective.

The bacterial numbers in milk may also increase after milking as a result of dirty utensils. Cleaning of the milk utensils must, therefore, be thorough, and a sufficiently high temperature must be used to destroy most of the bacteria present.

Normal changes produced by bacteria.—Souring is due to the action of the normal milk-souring organism. This germ attacks the milk-sugar and converts it into a substance called lactic acid. One must, however, distinguish souring from curdling. The sour taste is due to lactic acid and is sometimes noticed before the milk actually curdles. Curdling is also due to lactic acid but indirectly. The casein of milk is normally present in a state of partial solution from which it is precipitated by acids. As soon as the acidity due to lactic acid reaches a certain level the casein is thrown out of solution and appears as an insoluble mass—the curd. Curdling is therefore due to the activity of the lactic acid bacteria. Anything which retards the activity of the organisms will prolong the period during which milk can be kept 'sweet'.

Abnormal changes produced by bacteria.—One of the most frequent is a change in consistency as the result of which 'ropiness' is produced. If a spoon is dipped into ropy milk and removed, the milk becomes drawn out into slimy threads of varying lengths. This condition may be found in milk when it is drawn from the udder, where it is generally due to an inflammation of the gland tissue. More often, however, it is not present immediately after milking, but develops on keeping. In such cases the cause is bacterial. Ropy milk of this nature is quite wholesome, although it does not sour normally. Milk which shows ropiness on being drawn from the udder is not only unwholesome, but may be positively dangerous, and should on no account be used for human consumption.

White blood-cells in milk.—'A cow with a healthy udder should not be producing milk with a white cell count regularly in excess of 500,000 per ml.' (L. H. Aynsley and J. M. Buol, *Vet. Record* April 3, 1965.) An excess of white cells, as indicated by the California Milk Test, for example, makes the milk undesirable for human consumption. The cause is subclinical mastitis due to (*a*) trauma, defective milking machine or technique; or (*b*) infection; (*c*) or both.

Plant	Change in Milk.	Change in Butter.
Autumn Crocus (*Colchicum autumnale*). *See* Meadow Saffron.		
Bog asphodel (*Narthecium ossifragum*) *	Poisonous, causes diarrhœa.	
Buttercups (*Ranunculus* sp.) :		
R. acris *	Bitter taste.	
R. scleratus *	Lessened secretion, reddish coloration.	
R. repens *	Strong unpleasant flavour.	Distinctly bitter taste and high colour.
Butterwort (*Pinguicula vulgaris*)	Disagreeable taste, stringiness.	Disagreeable flavour.
Camomiles :		
(1) Corn Camomile (*Anthemis arvensis*)	Disagreeable flavour.	
(2) Stinking Camomile (*A. Cotula*)	Lessened secretion and disagreeable taste and flavour.	
(3) Wild Camomile (*Matricaria Chamomilla*)	Disagreeable flavour.	
Cowbane (*Cicuta virosa*) *	Lessened secretion and acridness.	
Cow-wheat (*Melampyrum arvense*)	Supposed to increase secretion.	
Fool's Parsley (*Aethusa Cynapium*) *	Unusual odour.	
Garlics (*Allium* sp.)	Strong 'oniony' flavour and smell.	'Oniony' flavour.
Hellebores :		
(1) Green Hellebore (*Helleborus viridis*) *	Bitter milk having purgative effect on calves.	
(2) Stinking Hellebore (*H. fœtidus*) *	Bitter milk and unusual odour.	Unusual odour.
(3) Black Hellebore or Christmas rose (*H. niger*) *	As above (No. 1).	
Hemlock (*Conium maculatum*) *	Unpleasant flavour.	
Henbane (*Hyocyamus niger*) *	Greatly lessened secretion and unpleasant taste.	
Hogweed (*Polygonum aviculare*)	Bitter taste.	
Horsetails (*Equisetum* sp.) *	Lessened secretion of watery milk poor in fat.	Greasiness and unappetising odour.
Ivy (*Hedera Helix*)	Bitter taste.	
Kingcups (*see* Marsh Marigold)		
Lesser Wartcress (*Senebiera didyma*)	Unusual taste.	
Lesser Sium (*Sium angustifolium*)	Disagreeable flavour.	
Marsh Marigolds (*Caltha palustris*) *	Loss of milk secretion.	
Meadow Saffron (*Colchicum autumnale*) *	Suppression of milk or a bluish coloration; poisonous to calves and infants.	
Mercury Plants :		
(1) Dog's Mercury (*Mercurialis perennis*) *	Often entire stoppage of secretion.	
(2) Annual Mercury (*M. annua*) *	Thin watery milk poor in fat; sometimes a bluish or reddish tinge.	

* Those plants marked with a star are also poisonous.

Plant.	Change in Milk.	Change in Butter.
Mints (*Mentha* sp.)	Minty odour and taste; rennet action prevented.	
Monkshood (*Aconitum Napellus*) *	Lessened secretion.	
Oak (*Quercus* sp.) * :		
Acorns	Changes in milk.	Cheeses develop a sharp acid flavour in about one month after making.
Leaves	Reduction or entire cessation of secretion.	Bad flavour.
Ox-eye Daisy (*Chrysanthemum Leucanthemum*)		Disagreeable flavour.
Pennycress (*Thlaspi arvense*)	Disagreeable flavour.	
Pepper saxifrage (*Silaus pratensis*)	Cream frothy and contains gas.	
Rhododendron (*Rhododendron* sp.) *	Bitterness, reduced secretion, reddish colour.	
Runch (*Raphanus Raphanistrum*)	Bitter flavour.	
Stinking Mayweed (*see* Camomiles)		
St. John's Wort (*Hypericum perforatum*)	Diminution in secretion.	
Spurges (*Daphne* sp.)	Diminution in secretion.	
Tansy (*Tanacetum vulgare*) *	Bitter taste.	Bitter taste.
Tormentil (*Potentilla Tormentilla*)	Stringiness in milk.	
Turnips (*Brassica* sp.)	' Turnip taint '.	Strong ' turnip taint '.
Water Parsnip (*Sium* latifolium)	Objectionable flavour.	Objectionable flavour.
Wood Anemone (*Anemone* sp.)*	Disagreeable acid flavour.	
Wood Sorrel (*Oxalis Acetosella*) *	Difficulty in churning.	
Wormwood (*Artemisia Absinthium*)	Disagreeable flavour.	Disagreeable flavour.
Yarrow (*Achillea Millefolium*)	Characteristic bitter taste and strong odour.	Bitter taste and strong odour.
Yew (*Taxus baccata*) *	Diminution in milk supply during convalescence when plant has not caused death.	

* Those plants marked with a star are also poisonous.

Antibiotics in milk.—A 1961 survey showed that in Great Britain 11 per cent of the supplies of milk which were tested contained antibiotics. The most common one (90 per cent) was penicillin. Fortunately, results of tests carried out by M.M.B. creameries in 1964 indicated that the incidence of antibiotic residues in milk approximately halved during the intervening period.

For a number of years concern over the presence of antibiotic residues in milk has been expressed by the medical profession, as well as by the manufacturers of cheese and yoghourt. Some people are allergic to antibiotics, and if they drink milk containing them they may suffer severe effects, *e.g.* a troublesome rash and a period off work. It has also been feared that the continual consumption of small quantites of antibiotic may result in people becoming sensitised, later undergoing a severe reaction when given that antibiotic by their doctor. A third danger is the development of organisms resistant to antibiotics, which could possibly give rise to illness not responding to antibiotic treatment. In 1963 a report issued by the World Health Organisation stated that the undesirable effects of the presence of penicillin in milk were solely of an allergic nature, and that the danger of sensitisation had not been proved. That, however, is not to say that it does not exist.

The sale conditions for the Milk Marketing Board stipulate that 'a producer shall not deliver any milk produced from a cow that shows any symptom of disease of the udder, or is undergoing treatment of the udder by chemotherapy including the use of antibiotics, or produced from a cow which has undergone any such treatment unless he believes that sufficient time has elapsed since such treatment to avoid the presence of antibiotics in milk'.

Originally, an antibiotic was defined as 'a chemical compound produced by micro-organisms and in minute concentrations capable of inhibiting the growth of other micro-organisms'. Not all the preparations used in the treatment of mastitis fall within this category, since they are not produced by micro-organisms; but, for all that, they count in the penalty scheme.

Abnormal changes in colour are not infrequent. A red colour in milk may be due to blood, if it is present when the milk is drawn from the udder and does not increase on keeping. Red, blue, and yellow colours may develop in milk on keeping, and are due to certain forms of bacterial activity. Very often abnormal odours or flavours, such as the flavour of turnips, are due to other types of bacterial action.

The germs producing these changes may be derived from the cow's udder or from the skin, from the food, fæces, water supply, or from the air of the byre, or from dust in the byre or milk-house, etc. (*See* TUBERCULOSIS; MAMMARY GLAND; MAMMARY GLAND, DISEASES OF; MASTITIS.)

Plants affecting the milk.—A large number of plants affect milk or milk secretion in animals eating them, and very often the real cause of unusual tastes or odours in the milk is some common wild plant, when the blame for this is laid upon the udder. Some plants give the milk a characteristic taint or odour (such as garlics), and others alter its colour; some decrease the total secretion and others lessen the fat content; a few alter the colour and character of butter made from the milk, and one or two, whose poisonous principles are excreted by the mammary gland, render the milk actually poisonous. These are considered in tabular form, as shown on p. 552.

MILK, ABSENCE OF, in the mammary glands following parturition, is discussed under AGALACTIA.

'MILK FEVER', which is also called PARTURIENT FEVER, is a complex condition—mainly hypocalcæmia of milk cows, milk goats, and sometimes of ewes, bitches, and cats in which there is a partial or complete loss of consciousness, paralysis of the hind-quarters, and sometimes paralysis of other parts. The disease is not a fever; in fact, the temperature is usually found to be subnormal.

In the hill ewe the condition is colloquially known as MOSS-ILL (which see). Hypocalcæmia also occurs in lowland ewes.

'Milk fever' would appear to be one of the diseases that is to some extent traceable to artificial methods of management, for it is not known among wild animals, nor yet among those whose existence most nearly approximates to the wild state. It is most frequently, though not exclusively, met with in heavy milking cows, of the essentially dairy breeds. Animals in good condition, liberally fed, and getting only a minimum of exercise, are more often affected than are those under opposite conditions of management. It is commonest between the third and fifth calving, and animals having had an attack are liable to a repetition when they next calve. A few cases occur some hours before calving, but the majority take place within three days subsequent to parturition. 'Milk fever' may not arise until as long as four weeks after calving, but, as a rule, delayed cases are mild, though they take longer to recover. It is more common after easy parturition than after a difficult one, though this rule has many exceptions.

Causes.—As previously mentioned, 'milk fever' is a hypocalcæmia (fall in the level of blood calcium), but what exactly brings this about is not yet fully known. The condition is not a mineral deficiency in the accepted sense of the term. If it were, it could possibly be averted by liming of the pastures or by the addition of calcium salts to the feed, but neither of these procedures is effective. The level of the calcium in the blood falls even though the amount taken in by the mouth remains constant. Research has shown that as cows grow older they assimilate less calcium from their food.

Experimental work has shown that a cow in full lactation not infrequently secretes daily in her milk about twelve times the amount of calcium present in her blood. As all the calcium salts in the milk have to come from the blood-stream, it follows that the blood calcium must be replaced about twelve times a day. Should anything go wrong with the 'mechanism' controlling the calcium supply for the blood, then symptoms of hypocalcæmia or 'milk fever' begin to appear.

Recent research suggests that the calcium-controlling 'mechanism' is a very complex one, involving all the internal-secreting glands and both the sympathetic and parasympathetic nervous systems. One theory is that the exaggerated development of the cow as a milk-producer brings about over-activity of the pituitary gland, which secretes hormones to such an extent that the delicate balance—if one may use these mechanical similes by way of explanation—of the calcium-regulating mechanism is upset. It then only requires the birth of a calf to put things right out of gear. The level of blood calcium falls. Symptoms of illness appear.

It must be added that blood samples have shown that as well as a shortage of calcium in the blood, there may be too little phosphorus and either too much or too little magnesium. This accounts for the differing symptoms in what is collectively called 'milk fever'.

Symptoms.—The animal at first shows a certain amount of excitement. She paddles with her hind-feet, stares around her in a somewhat affrighted manner, may bellow, and if tied attempts to break loose. The pupils are dilated, and the iris muscles twitch. After a time she staggers on her feet, loses balance, and falls to the ground. When down she may make one or two efforts to rise, but after struggling for a time she gives it up and remains quiet. In very many cases a characteristic position is assumed. The cow lies on her brisket, but with her hind-feet splayed out almost at right angles to the rest of her body. The head is turned round over one shoulder (often the left), and the muzzle points to the stifle. In this position she may snore or moan for a time, but later becomes unconscious. If the head be straightened out (often a difficult procedure) it almost immediately swings round into the original position as soon as released, and apparently automatically. Other positions may be assumed such as lying stretched out on the side at full length, in which there is a great tendency to gas collection in the stomach, difficulty in breathing, and perhaps death from suffocation, or the cow may lie with her head and neck along the ground in front of her, or resting on the edge of the manger or food trough. The breathing becomes deep and slow, pulse is fast but weak, the extremities of the body—horns, ears, and feet—grow cold, the temperature falls to 4 or 5 degrees below normal.

Whereas formerly the mortality was 90 per cent or so, it has been reduced to less than 5 per cent in cases that are treated.

It is necessary to emphasise here that in well-marked cases with symptoms such as the above, the muscles of swallowing are paralysed, and if drenches be forced over the cow's throat, a proportion is sure to find its way into the trachea, and thence into the lungs, where it sets up a septic pneumonia, from which cattle seldom or never recover.

It should also be emphasised that not every cow showing symptoms of partial paralysis is suffering from 'Milk Fever'.

Treatment.—The intravenous or subcutaneous injection of calcium borogluconate solution with or without magnesium. (*See also* UDDER INFLATION.)

When a deficiency of blood phosphorus complicates 'milk fever', and this does not completely respond to calcium treatment, phosphorus in the form of 3 oz. of sodium acid phosphate may be given by mouth twice daily.

Prevention.—Recent research has demonstrated the efficacy of suitable doses of Vitamin D, which enables the body to increase the absorption of calcium and phosphorus. The owners of otherwise excellent oldish or middle-aged cows prone to milk fever would be well advised to discuss Vitamin D with their veterinary surgeon. The dose has to be large, given night and morning for between 3 and 7 days prior to the expected calving date. Other preventive measures are at present being investigated.

'MILK LAMENESS'.—This is a translation of the Swedish name for a condition encountered in high-yielding dairy cattle, and characterised by hip lameness During one stage they assume a characteristic posture.

Some unthriftiness and sluggishness of movement may be observed in the herd. Animals stop frequently to rest.

The cause of 'milk lameness' is a deficiency of phosphorus in the blood-stream, and—since hip lameness may have several causes—blood tests are necessary in order to confirm a diagnosis.

In a Scottish outbreak, recovery soon followed the feeding of sterilised bone-flour in small amounts. It seemed that

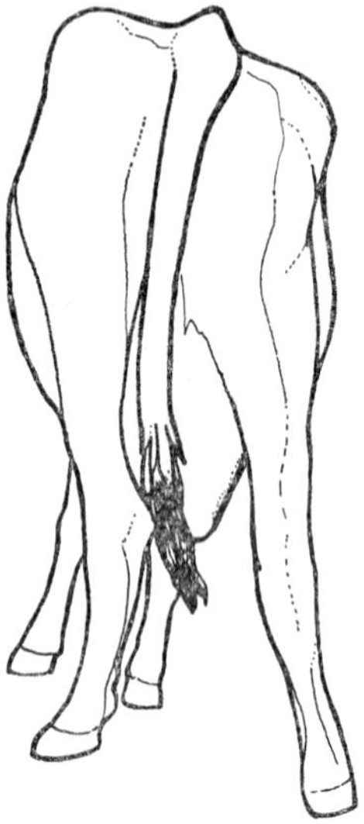

'Milk lameness'—the characteristic posture.

the cows had been unable to acquire sufficient phosphorus from unsupplemented grazing, although the phosphorus-content of the herbage was probably normal.

Lameness associated with a blood-phosphorus deficiency is, of course, well known in many parts of the world—subjected either to drought or to high rainfall—where the soil or herbage are deficient in phosphorus.

MILK RING TEST, THE, for brucellosis, is a valuable, method of detecting infected herds of dairy cattle. It has been recommended that a sample of milk for ring-testing should be from not less than 15 or more than 150 cows. The test is of no value in detecting the disease in individual animals.

Occasionally, as with most biological tests, false positives or false negatives are given. Colostrum, or milk from a cow with mastitis, will sometimes affect the accuracy of the test adversely.

The test is used in many countries to assist in disease-eradication programmes.

'MILK SCALD' around the mouths of pail-fed calves may be a mycotic dermatitis caused by the fungus which produces Lumpy Wool or Wool-Rot in sheep.

MILK SINUS is the chamber situated at the base of each of the teats in the cow (and in other animals), into which the milk tubules discharge their milk, and from which the teat canal leads to the tip of the teat. (*See* MAMMARY GLAND.)

'MILKSPOT LIVER'.—This is a name given to pigs' livers showing whitish spots or streaks of fibrous tissue, the result of chronic inflammation caused by the larvæ of the roundworm *Ascaris lumbricoides*.

MILK TEETH are the temporary or deciduous teeth of young animals. For the time of their appearance, *see* DENTITION.

MILK YIELD.—Before the 1939–45 war, the average yield of dairy cows in Britain was about 560 gallons, and total production in England and Wales was about 1,000 million gallons. The average yield in 1960 was in the region of 750 gallons per cow, with nearly 1,900 million gallons total production in England and Wales. In recorded herds, cows averaged 926 gallons in 1960–61, heifers 792 gallons. National average for 1969 was about 815 gallons.

Daily milk yield: at Olympia during the 1960 Dairy Show, an Ayrshire cow gave over 13½ gallons in the 24 hours. Expressed in pints, the yield of the 1962 supreme champion (British Friesian) was 91 in 24 hours. (For other figures *see under* LACTATION.) (*See also* STRESS.)

Butterfat: In 1969 a Guernsey cow gave 16,371 lb. milk at 10.16 per cent butterfat in 305 days.

MILKER'S NODULE.—Human infection with pseudo-cowpox. (*See under* TEATS, COWS', INFECTIONS OF.)

MILKING (*see* p. 540 *and also under* MILKING MACHINES).—At milking time the 'milk let-down' mechanism begins to operate; it is actuated by the hormone 'oxytocin' which is secreted in the posterior pituitary gland and which is released into the blood-stream on the receipt of a nervous stimulus. This stimulus may be caused by the rattling of milk pails, the placing of food in the manger, the washing of the udder, etc.

The hormone causes a contraction of the cells which surround the alveoli and milk channels, and milk is squeezed downwards into the milk cisterns and from these it is driven into the milk pail by the squeezing action of the milker's hand or the squeezing-suction action of the teat cup of the milking machine or the mouth of the sucking calf. The let-down action of the hormone seems to last about 7 to 10 minutes after which time it is more difficult to extract milk from the udder.

MILKING MACHINES.—The action of milking machines simulates that of the sucking calf. The teat orifice is opened and milk withdrawn by means of a partial vacuum applied to the outside of the teat. As continuous vacuum would restrict circulation of the blood in the teat, cause pain, and inhibit milk ejection, the vacuum is applied intermittently by means of a pulsator.

The basic principles of machine milking are, in fact, vacuum and pulsation, and the way in which these are applied to the teat in the teat-cup assembly.

For maintenance of a healthy udder, what is required is, first, a strong stimulus to 'let-down', followed by rapid milking. As soon as the machine ceases to milk, the udder should be stripped and the machine removed. In practice, attention to this involves the cowman not having too many units to cope with, or other tasks to perform.

Milking machines can be made to milk faster by increasing the degree of vacuum, increasing the pulsator rate, or by widening the pulsator ratio. If, however, the cowman already has more to do than he can manage, a faster milking can result only in prolonged attachment. The milking routine must be re-organised to avoid this—or mastitis will follow.

A liner with a hard mouthpiece is likely to cause trouble. One of the best, and also the cheapest, types consists of a straight rubber tube with a metal ring inserted to form one end into a mouthpiece.

In one herd badly affected with mastitis, a change from slack, wide-bore liners to the narrow-bore stretched type resulted in a spectacular improvement.

Mr. C. D. Wilson, of Weybridge, has pointed out: 'A fallacy which has died hard is that leaving milk in a cow predisposes to mastitis. More harm is done to a cow by pulling on four quarters for milk contained in only one, than by leaving a pound of milk in the udder.'

Investigation has shown that the slow milker is almost invariably the cow with a small teat orifice. If it is not practicable to cull such an animal, the milking machine pulsation ratio may, with advantage, be altered. At 60 pulsations per minute, and at 15 inches of mercury, a ratio of 4 : 1 (*i.e.* the liner being open for four times as long as it is closed) will reduce milking time—*especially with slow milkers*—without hurting her, or adversely affecting the stripping yield.

Common faults in milking machines are: incorrect vacuum level, or vacuum fluctuations, blocked air bleeds, unsuitable pulsation rate, and faulty liners. Such faults can lead to MASTITIS. Regular, skilled maintenance of milking machines is therefore all important.

During a survey among 71 farms participating in a mastitis control scheme, 95 per cent of the milking machines were found to be faulty. The importance of this is shown by another survey, of a small number of herds with a serious mastitis problem, in which cell counts were carried out before and after machine testing and adjustment. It was found that cell counts fell by about 25 per cent following the first annual test, and by about 15 per cent following the second annual test. **This shows that the correction of milking machine faults really can achieve something worthwhile, whether measured in cow health or farmers' profits.**

MILKING PARLOURS (*see under* DAIRY HERD MANAGEMENT).

MILLERS' DISEASE (*see* OSTEOFIBROSIS).

MINE-DETECTOR.—This instrument has been put to veterinary use in the confirmation of a diagnosis of a (metal) foreign body in the reticulum of cattle.

MINERALS (*see under* PHOSPHORUS, CALCIUM, TRACE ELEMENTS).

MINIMAL DISEASE PIGS.—Those reared free from certain infections. (*See also* S.P.F.)

MINK, DISEASES OF.—These include distemper (caused by the virus of canine distemper), botulism, salmonellosis, tuberculosis, paralysis due to a vitamin B deficiency, mastitis, metritis, and paragonimiasis. A vaccine against botulism is available. (*See* ALEUTIAN DISEASE.)

MISCARRIAGE (*see* ABORTION *and* CONTAGIOUS ABORTION).

MITES, PARASITIC.—These include the 'red mite' of poultry, the northern fowl mite, the tropical fowl mite, the 'itch-mite' of sheep, the harvest mite, and the mites associated with mange in all animals. (*See under* PARASITES.)

MITOSIS.—The usual process of cell reproduction. Hence, MITOTIC RATE.

MITRAL VALVE is the left atrio-ventricular valve of the heart, which is so-called because of its supposed likeness to a bishop's mitre. Disease of the mitral valve is a common condition in the dog. (*See* HEART.)

MIXTURE is the name given to any compound of drugs in the form of a liquid, for internal administration.

MOLAR TEETH (*molaris*, a millstone) are, strictly speaking, the last few cheek teeth on either side top and bottom in the horse or any animal, which are not represented in the temporary dentition. 'Molar' is often applied indiscriminately to all or any of the cheek teeth. (*See* DENTITION.)

MOLLITIES OSSIUM (*mollities*, softness; *ossium*, of the bones) is another name for osteomalacia. (*See* OSTEOMALACIA.)

MOLYBDENUM.—This trace element is commonly present in soil and pasture grasses, and is beneficial except when it occurs in excessive amounts—such as in the 'teart soils' of central Somerset, and of small areas of Gloucestershire and Warwickshire. Here 'molybdenosis' causes scouring in ruminants, especially cattle. The scouring is worse from May until October when the grass contains most water-soluble molybdenum. Staring coats, marked loss of condition and evil-smelling fæces are observed in affected cattle. A daily dose of copper sulphate (2 grammes for adults and half this for young stock) obviates or remedies the trouble.

Molybdenosis may occur also as the result of aerial contamination of pasture in the vicinity of aluminium-alloy and other factories, and of oil refineries. In an outbreak in 1960 near the Esso Refinery at Fawley, younger cattle showed a marked stiffness of back and legs, with great difficulty in getting to their feet and reluctance to move—in addition to diarrhœa.

If an animal is receiving extra molybdenum in its diet, it is likely to need extra copper. Levels of molybdenum which interfere with copper metabolism also inhibit the synthesis of B_{12}, the cobalt-containing vitamin, by the rumen microflora.

MONILIA.—A group of yeast-like organisms.

MONILIASIS.—This is a disease due to the yeast-like organism *Candida albicans*. In humans it follows, in some cases, the use of certain antibiotics.

The disease occurs in turkeys and fowls, in other domestic animals, including dogs and cattle, and it must be borne in mind when using antibiotics. A high temperature, loss of weight, and œdema of the lungs may result.

Nystatin has been used—successfully, it is claimed—in the treatment of turkeys with moniliasis.

MONKEYS, DISEASES OF.—These include:

(1) Infection with B virus. This is easily transmitted to people who are bitten by monkeys (or perhaps to people merely handling monkeys with B virus lesions), and is of the greatest importance, as an encephalitis or encephalomyelitis is produced in man, with death as the usual outcome. This infection should be suspected in monkeys showing vesicles on the lips, tongue, inside of the cheeks, or on the body. The vesicles burst and give rise to ulcers and scab formation. Occasionally, affected monkeys have conjunctivitis and a thick discharge from the nose.

(2) Tuberculosis. This is generally the miliary form, due to the human type of tubercle bacillus. Symptoms include: loss of weight, of appetite, dullness; sometimes cough and rapid breathing.

(3) Pneumonia (unconnected with tuberculosis). A monkey that is coughing and sneezing can be assumed to be seriously ill. Death from pneumonia can occur within 24 hours, and affect a high proportion of any group of monkeys.

(4) Dysentery due to *Shigella* organisms.

(5) Phycomycosis.
(6) Marburg disease, which can be fatal both in monkeys and man, has been seen in laboratory workers in contact with blood and tissues of Vervet monkeys. (See *Lancet*, November 25, 1967.)
(7) Rabies.
(8) Ringworm.
(*See also* KYASANUR FOREST FEVER).

MONKSHOOD POISONING (*see* ACONITE).

MONOPLEGIA (μόνος, single; πληγή madness) means paralysis of a single limb, or part. (*See* PARALYSIS.)

MONORCHID.—This term is commonly used by dog-breeders to mean an animal in which only one testicle has descended into the scrotum. Such an animal is correctly called a unilateral cryptorchid; the term Monorchid being reserved for the animal with a single testicle (a far rarer condition).

Under Kennel Club rules, a dog which has not both testicles in the scrotum cannot be entered for Shows; but there is as yet no ban on the registration of dogs sired by a cryptorchid.

Cryptorchidism is an inherited condition (though it has been claimed that feeding rats on a biotin-deficient diet caused their testicles to return to the abdomen after two or three weeks), but the precise mechanism of inheritance has not yet been determined.

MONOSACCHARID is the term applied to a sugar having six carbon atoms in the molecule. Among monosaccharids are glucose, galactose, levulose, etc.

MONSTERS or grossly deformed young are occasionally born to all species. Hæmolytic disease, for example, is responsible for abnormal piglets. (*See also under* BULL-DOG CALVES, GENETICS.)

MORBID (*morbus*, disease) means 'diseased'. Morbidity, as distinct from mortality, refers to the proportion of animals which become infected with a given disease: *e.g.* 'morbidity is 60 per cent

MOREL'S DISEASE.—This affects sheep and is caused by a Gram-positive micrococcus. The disease bears some resemblance to caseous lymphadenitis, with abscesses in subcutaneous tissue and intra-muscular fascia, and has been reported in France and Kenya.

MORLAM.—A strain of sheep bred at Beltsville, U.S.A. The best ewes have given 6 lambs in 2 years; lambs being born in September, January, and May—an 8-month breeding cycle.

MORNING GLORY.—The pink or reddish flowered *Ipomœa muelleri* is said to have caused losses of up to 7000 sheep on some sheep stations in Western Australia. There is a loss of condition, and after a time forced exercise gives rise to a swaying, inco-ordinated gait, and knuckling of the hind feet, with panting when the animal is driven a few yards.

MORPHIA (Μορφεύς, the god of sleep), or MORPHINE, is the name of the chief active principle of opium. It is of an alkaloidal nature. (*See* OPIUM.)

MORPHOLOGY.—The study of shape, *e.g.* of bacteria.

MORTAR-EATING by cattle may be regarded as an indication of a mineral-deficient diet—probably it is calcium and magnesium which the animals are seeking.

MOSAICISM (*see under* ERYTHROCYTE MOSAICISM).

'MOSS-ILL.'—A colloquial name for hypocalcæmia (*see under* MILK FEVER) in hill ewes. It is seen mainly in the mature ewe, and during the weeks preceding and following lambing. It often follows within 12 to 48 hours of a move to fresh pasture.

Symptoms.—Stilted gait, abnormally high carriage of the head, muscular tremors—particularly of the lips in the early stages—recumbency, coma.

Treatment.—Calcium borogluconate by subcutaneous injection.

MOTH BALLS (*see* NAPHTHALENE POISONING).

MOTOR is a term applied to those nerves and tracts in the brain and spinal cord that have to do with the impulses which pass from the higher nerve centres to the muscles causing movement. (*See* NERVES.)

MOULDY FOOD (*See* DIET *under* PALATABILITY, *and* FOXY OATS, *also*

GROUNDNUT MEAL). Mouldy hay or straw can lead to farmers' lung, and to abortion in cattle.

'MOUNTAIN SICKNESS'.—A disease of cattle kept at high altitudes in N. and S. America. Local cattle are affected to an extent of only 1 per cent or so; recovery is unusual. Death occurs from congestive heart failure, after symptoms of depression, dropsy of the brisket, and distressed breathing on slight exertion.

MOUTH is the cavity into which the food is first received, and where it is prepared by chewing and admixture with saliva for the other stages of digestion. It possesses an opening, small in herbovores and large in carnivores, bounded by lips, which vary in thickness and mobility, a floor, formed mainly by the tongue and its associated structures, a roof, made up of hard and soft palates, and walls formed by the cheeks. Posteriorly, an opening leads into the pharynx or throat. Projecting into the cavity of the mouth are the upper and lower teeth and the tongue. The interior of the cavity, except for the teeth, is lined by mucous membrane, which is thickest on the hard palate, and thinnest at the tip of the tongue in most animals. Scattered throughout this membrane are the openings of many glands, and localised in certain places are the specialised 'taste-buds'. The ducts which carry saliva secreted by the salivary glands also open into the mouth. The tongue is a mass of intricately arranged muscle, which governs the food in its passage through the mouth, and has other functions, such as that of licking the surface of the skin in some animals. (*See* TONGUE.) The teeth serve the purpose of triturating the food into smaller particles, to allow of easy swallowing, and in certain animals are used as weapons of offence or defence. (*See* TEETH.)

MOUTH, DISEASES OF.—The mouth being one of the few internal cavities which can be examined by direct vision, its examination affords valuable, even if sometimes uncertain, evidence in cases of disease. The state of the mucous membrane lining the mouth as regards pallor, pigmentation, and other conditions, gives a general idea of the extent to which other mucous membranes in the interior of the animal body are affected in anæmia, jaundice, etc. It is therefore advisable to have a good general idea of the appearance of the mouth of an animal in health, and to have some knowledge of the commoner diseased conditions to which it is liable.

Conditions of the tongue.—The tongue of any animal in health should be of a pink glistening appearance, soft and moist to the touch in the horse, sheep, pig, and dog, and rough in the ox and cat. (There are a few breeds of dogs, such as the chow, in which the tongue is normally black or bluish.) When handled the tongue should possess a considerable power of retraction; a weak flabby tongue usually indicates general muscular weakness. When at rest the tongue should touch the inner edges of all the lower teeth. When it becomes greatly swollen it presses against the teeth and these leave indentations around its margin. Swelling of the tongue may result from inflammation, a dropsical condition of its membrane, or may be produced by a cystic swelling underneath it to which the name 'ranula' is given. In cattle there is a raised part or 'dorsum', behind the free tip, which is instrumental in forming the food into boli for swallowing, and this should be regular and free from ulcerated areas or tumorous swellings, which often indicate actinomycosis. Digestive troubles, especially gastritis, usually cause alteration in the appearance of the tongue: a soapy-white appearance indicates indigestion, especially when accompanied by a foul odour acute gastritis in dogs and cats produces a fiery red or copper-coloured tongue; in leptospirosis there are very often patches of necrosis around the free tip, and an odour of decomposing flesh. In foot-and-mouth disease the typical vesicles which affect other parts of the mouth may also be present on the tongue, usually towards its tip. Ulcers along the free edges of the tongue may be produced by diseased teeth, and, in such cases, the ulcers correspond in position with the affected teeth. In the disease called 'calf diphtheria', which is not due to the diphtheria bacillus of man, the tongue may be the seat of raised areas of false membrane which will also be seen in other parts of the mouth. The tongue may be injured or wounded from too severe a bit in the horse, or from carelessness in breaking in a young colt. In such cases there is usually a distinct mark across the tongue's upper surface, behind which the organ appears normal, and in front of which it is reddened and swollen. Foreign bodies, such as pins, needles, nails, wire, splinters of bone, etc., may become fixed in the tongue, and lead to protrusion of the organ, difficulty in swallowing, salivation, and a disinclination on the part of the animal to allow of the mouth being handled or examined. (*See also* TONGUE, 'BLACK TONGUE'.)

Conditions of the mouth.—As a rule the symptoms that lead one to suspect that the mouth is diseased are as follows: salivation and difficulty in feeding in all animals; 'cudding' or 'quidding' the food in the horse (the food is taken into the mouth, but, instead of being swallowed, is chewed time and time again, until it collects and is finally dropped out of the mouth into the manger); smacking of the lips, in the ox particularly; rubbing the mouth along the edge of the trough, floor, etc., or pawing at it with the front feet; holding the head to one side; frequent yawning, and much working of the jaws. Dogs may occasionally hold their mouths open, especially when a piece of bone or other substance becomes fixed between the teeth, but this symptom is not commonly seen among the other domestic animals. Indigestion often has its origin in bad teeth, and the passage of whole oats by horses in poor condition nearly always points to the teeth not functioning properly.

All young animals are liable to go off their food very suddenly about the time when they are changing their teeth. The two periods when this is most marked in the horse are at 2½ years, when the first two permanent molars on either side top and bottom are replacing the corresponding temporaries, and at 3½ years, when the third permanent molars do likewise. In the ox and other animals, owing to greater variations in feeding and development, there are not such precise periods, but whenever a young immature animal begins to feed indifferently its teeth should be examined. (*See also* 'BROWN MOUTH'.)

ACTINOMYCOSIS affects the mouth cavities of cattle, forming irregular tumorous swellings which interfere with feeding and cause salivation. (*See* ACTINOMYCOSIS, ACTINOBACILLOSIS.)

APHTHA is the name applied to a condition in which numbers of vesicles, containing a clear fluid, appear in the mouth, and after a time burst and liberate their contents. Sometimes the blisters contain pus and are numerous, but generally they are not serious. They are treated by syringing out the mouth with a solution of chlorate of potash, or Milton, etc. In severe cases they may require touching with a strong astringent, such as copper sulphate crystals.

BLEEDING FROM THE MOUTH occurs when some injury has been inflicted. Hæmorrhage is apt to be very profuse, as the mucous membrane is well supplied with blood-vessels. Animals may bite their own tongues when fighting, or if they fall with their tongues between their teeth, and sometimes the bit inflicts an injury to the gums which bleed to an alarming extent. A drink of cold water, or douching out the mouth with strong salt and water solution, will stop hæmorrhage from small vessels, and when large arteries have been injured it is necessary to apply compression, torsion, or ligature to the cut end. (*See* BLEEDING, THE ARREST OF.) A serious bleeding sometimes accompanies the operation of lancing the gums for the relief of 'lampas', when the palatine artery is accidentally severed. (*See* LAMPAS.)

CALF DIPHTHERIA occurs as areas of a whitish deposit of membrane raised above the level of the surrounding mucous membrane, either on the gums, insides of the cheeks, or upon the tongue. The areas are the centres of activity of the *Actinomyces necrophorus*. (*See* CALF DIPHTHERIA.)

CRIB-BITING causes an alteration in the apposition of the incisor teeth of the horse, and may prevent him from grazing since he is unable to bite off the grass. It is shown by an irregular wearing of the tables of the teeth. (*See* CRIB-BITING.)

DEFORMITIES OF THE MOUTH occasionally occur in all animals, but they are commonest in sheep. Two varieties are very common: 'parrot mouth', in which the upper jaw bones are longer than the lower, and the upper incisor teeth, or the dental pad in ruminants, project farther forward than the lower; and 'hog mouth', or 'sow mouth', in which the lower jaw is longer than the upper. In either case the animal has difficulty in feeding, and may never thrive. (*See* HARE-LIP.)

FOOT - AND - MOUTH DISEASE lesions are characteristic in that they are irregular, eroded, very painful, accompanied by great salivation and smacking of the lips, and tend to spread throughout a herd with amazing rapidity. They commence as blebs or blisters, which burst and leave a raw shallow reddened area, which is commonly referred to as the 'ulcer' of this disease. (*See* FOOT-AND-MOUTH DISEASE.)

MUCOSAL DISEASE (*see under this heading*).

ORF, or **OOF**, is a disease of young sheep and lambs in which irregular scabby areas appear about the lips and face, and sometimes within the mouth cavity. It is a contagious disease, and very liable to spread through a flock of lambs about weaning time. (*See* ORF.)

LAMPAS is a swollen condition of the gums behind the upper incisor teeth of the horse, which may be due to dietetic errors, indigestion, or to the cutting of the permanent teeth in young animals. (*See* LAMPAS.)

SALIVATION accompanies most, if not all, of the diseased conditions of the mouth which are accompanied by pain. It may originate from diseased teeth, injuries or wounds of the mucous membrane or of the bones, from various forms of poisoning, especially those in which the poison is irritant or corrosive, or it may be produced in certain specific diseases, such as foot-and-mouth disease. It is well to understand that there are some drugs which produce salivation when given in ordinary doses, *e.g.* arecoline or eserine.

In the cat (especially under one year old), salivation may be a symptom of ulcerative glossitis, believed to be caused by a virus, possibly that of feline enteritis. Water is refused.

SALIVARY CALCULI and **SALIVARY FISTULÆ.** (*See under* SALIVARY GLANDS.)

STOMATITIS means inflammation of the mouth. It may arise from such drugs as Lysol, ammonia, chloral hydrate, carbolic acid, turpentine, etc., administered in too strong solution, it may result from animals licking blister from areas that have been blistered, or it may arise from causes already mentioned or from a lack of riboflavin (vitamin B_2) in the diet. In some cases the inflammation is diffuse, involving all the superficial structures of the mouth, while in other cases it remains localised to the gums, the cheeks, or the tongue, and usually forms vesicles. The first of these varieties is often called *catarrhal stomatitis*, and the second, *vesicular stomatitis*. The severity of the symptoms is according to the extent of the inflammation, but in most cases the animal refuses its food, resents the examination of the mouth, and discharges quantities of saliva from its mouth. The treatment consists in giving mouth washes of mild astringent and sedative antiseptics. Plenty of water should be allowed, and a handful of common salt added to each pailful will keep the cavity from becoming further inflamed from discharges, etc. In severe cases of stomatitis there is also some pharyngitis usually present. This necessitates the use of an antiseptic elecutary.

LEPTOSPIROSIS in the dog presents lesions in the mouth in which the edges of the tongue become necrotic and small cr large areas slough out. In very bad cases almost the whole of the tip of the tongue may separate from the rest and become thrown off. There is always great pain, refusal of solid food, though liquids may be taken, great thirst for water, an excessively foul odour from the breath, and often dribbling of blood-stained saliva. (*See* LEPTOSPIROSIS.)

TUMOURS in the mouth are not very common in the larger animals, if tumour-like conditions such as actinomycosis are excluded, but they are sometimes seen in dogs. In these latter, cancerous growths similar to those occurring in almost any part of the body, sometimes affect the mucous membrane of the inside of the mouth, occasionally the muscles of the tongue or cheeks, and more rarely the bones of the jaws. Multiple small white warty growths, scattered over the mucous membrane of the whole of the cavity of the mouth, varying in size from a millet seed to a large pea, and sometimes possessed of a considerable stalk, are comparatively common in young adult dogs and are seen also in puppies.

WOUNDS AND INJURIES of the mouth may result from a very large variety of causes, among which may be mentioned the following : badly fitting bits ; stones, pieces of wire, nails, or other hard foreign bodies in the food ; 'run-away' and 'run-over' accidents ; kicks, blows, falls, etc., which may produce fracture of the jaws or laceration of the cheeks, lips, etc. ; carelessness in drenching or balling ; irregularities, deformities, or diseases of the teeth ; the lancing or burning of the swellings of lampas by ignorant people, etc. The injuries resulting may be slight abrasions of the membrane, contusions of the deeper structures, wounds of the tongue, lips, gums, etc., penetrating wounds through the cheeks, palate, or floor of the mouth, and combinations of these. The symptoms depend upon the cause and the extent of the damage done. In the majority of cases mouth wounds do not prove serious after any foreign bodies have been removed, for the whole cavity is so well supplied with blood-vessels that healing is always rapid. Hæmorrhage may be alarming at first.

but, unless a large artery has been severed, it soon ceases. Large tears in the mucous membrane or in the skin of the lips or cheeks, should be sutured. Antiseptic mouth washes should be applied afterwards. When the wounding has been severe an animal will often refuse to eat solid food, and may require to be fed on liquids for a few days. Plenty of water should always be provided for drinking purposes. It keeps the wound clean, and if a little salt is added, not only will the beneficial action of the salt be evident, but it will create a thirst.

MUCILAGE is prepared from acacia or tragacanth gum, and is used as an ingredient of mixtures containing solid particles in order to keep the latter from settling as a deposit. It is also a demulcent. (*See* DEMULCENTS.)

MUCORMYCOSIS.—Infection with *Rhizopus microsporus* is a cause of death of piglets under a fortnight old. The organism has been isolated from stomach ulcers in piglets which, before death, showed symptoms of vomiting and scouring. In many cases Moniliasis was also present. Abortion in cattle has been attributed to mucormycosis.

MUCOSAL DISEASE.—One of a group —perhaps identical, perhaps due to different types of the same virus—of which Virus Diarrhœa was first described in New York State in 1946.

Most cases in Britain are mild—so mild as often to escape detection by stockmen. A few ulcers in the mouth, perhaps also in the nostrils, may be the sole indication of the disease. Often, though, the animal is feverish, with a temperature of 104° or 105°. Loss of appetite, scouring, and a drop in milk yield may be observed. The feet may be involved, with ulceration in the cleft, but not invariably lameness.

Severe cases have been seen in many parts of England and Scotland, among both housed and grazing stock. On one farm 21 out of 50 calves died, and in other outbreaks mortality has been high. Symptoms are as described above.

Chronic outbreaks may involve a farm for months on end, with adult cattle becoming ill and miserable one after the other, and showing marked loss of condition, fever, scouring, mouth and foot ulceration ; all this being reflected in the milk yield.

Treatment has to be symptomatic. There is no specific treatment for Mucosal Disease—no antiserum, no drug which will destroy the virus. Sulpha drugs or antibiotics can be used to overcome secondary infection by bacteria, tonics can be given to assist recovery.

The virus which causes Mucosal Disease can survive storage at a temperature of 4° C. for at least sixteen months ; also repeated freezing and thawing.

Mucosal Disease has to be differentiated not only from foot-and-mouth disease, and the diseases mentioned above, but also from Johne's disease, Cattle Plague, and other conditions.

There is an immunological relationship between the mucosal disease virus and that causing swine fever.

MUCOUS MEMBRANE is the general name given to the membrane which lines many of the hollow organs of the body. These membranes vary widely in structure in different sites, but all have the common character of being lubricated by mucus, derived in some cases from isolated cells upon the surface of the membrane, but more generally from definite mucous glands situated beneath the membrane, and opening here and there through it by ducts. The air passages, the whole of the alimentary canal and the ducts of the glands which open into it, the urinary passages, and the genital passages, are lined by mucous membranes.

In structure a mucous membrane consists of a basis of fibrous tissue not unlike the true skin, though looser and lighter in texture, in which the blood-vessels, nerves, and mucous glands lie. This is covered on its surface by a layer of epithelium resem-

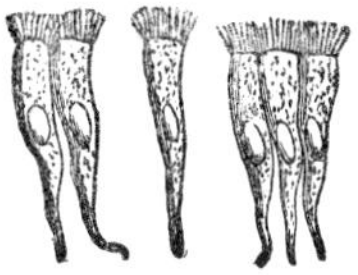

Ciliated columnar epithelial cells from the mucous membrane of the respiratory passages. (Turner's *Anatomy*.)

bling the epithelium of the skin, but possessing softer, moister, and more delicate cells than those of the outer skin, and it is in this epithelial layer that variations in the arrangement, shape, size, and function of the cells occur in the different mucous membranes of the body. In the air passages they are, almost everywhere except over the vocal cords, of a pillar-like shape, provided with thread-like processes, and called ' ciliated cells '. Over the vocal folds the cells resemble those of the skin, except that they possess no hairs. In the digestive system generally the cells are like simple pillars, and are known as 'columnar cells'. They are arranged side by side in an upright position as a whole, but differ in various parts. In the mouth and gullet the cells are very densely arranged and are called 'stratified'; in the stomach and intestines they lie more loosely, and amongst them there are the mouths of the specialised digestive glands, or the ducts from these glands. In some parts large clear cells, known as 'goblet cells' from their shape, are met with. In the urinary passages the epithelial cells are thickly and densely arranged some-

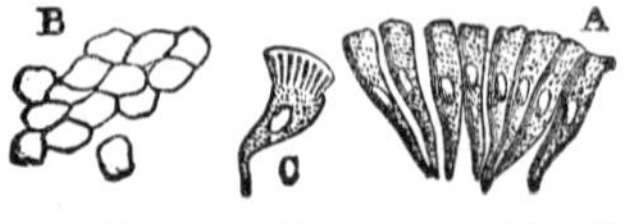

Columnar epithelium. *A*, Side view of a group of cells; *B*, surface view of the ends of a group of cells; *C*, a columnar cell from the mucous membrane of the small intestine. (Turner's *Anatomy*.)

what like Roman paving, and are called 'stratified squamous' or 'transitional squamous'. Their dense arrangement is to prevent damage to the nerves and

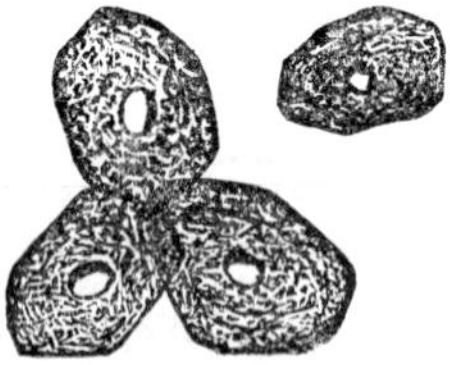

Scaly epithelium from the roof of the mouth. (Turner's *Anatomy*.)

delicate structures below them by the strong urine.

Lying close beneath the epithelium there is, in most mucous membranes, a thin layer of involuntary muscle fibres called the 'muscularis mucosæ', and to this, as well as to the extremely loose attachment of mucous membranes to the hollow organs which they line, is due the great pliability and elasticity of these membranes.

MUCUS (*mucus*, the discharge from the nose) is the general term for the slimy secretion derived from mucous membranes, such as those lining the nose, air passages, stomach, intestines, etc. Mucus is mainly composed of a substance called *mucin*, which varies according to the particular mucous membrane from which it is derived, and it contains other substances such as cells cast off from the surface of the membrane, ferments, particles of dust, soot, and various germs. All mucin has the following characters. It is viscid, clear, and tenacious; when dissolved in watery secretions it can be precipitated by the addition of acetic acid; and when not in solution already, it can be dissolved by weak alkalies such as lime-water. It is a compound of protein (albuminous material) with carbohydrate (starchy material), and can be partially transformed into sugar.

Under normal circumstances the surface of a mucous membrane is lubricated by only a small quantity of mucus, and the appearance of large amounts of mucus upon its surface is a sign of inflammation of the membrane. This is seen especially well during a cold or catarrh of the nasal passages, when the excess discharge of mucus comes away from the nostrils. Use can be made of the flow properties of cervical mucus for pregnancy diagnosis; a simple apparatus being used to measure the way in which a tiny 'blob' of mucus flows in a narrow tube. A correct result is given in about 96 per cent of cases.

MUCUS AGGLUTINATION TEST.—This is used in the diagnosis of VIBRIC FŒTUS INFECTION in cattle (which see).

MUD FEVER is the popular name for a variety of erythema that attacks the heels and coronets of horses' feet when these parts are subjected to long-continued irritation. It may arise during the winter time from frost, during muddy weather (especially if the horses' feet are not kept clean), from the irritation of the mud which cakes on to the skin and prevents free aeration and circulation, and from other causes. The skin surface becomes reddened and slightly swollen, and the area is painful to the touch. It may be itchy, and the horse may damage the skin surface by rubbing or biting. It is usually easily controlled by washing all the mud etc., away from the feet, especially in long-feathered horses, and applying some simple astringent lotion. Better management, and more careful attention to horses' feet in bad weather, will usually prevent the condition.

'MULBERRY HEART'.—A cause of death in pigs from about 10 weeks of age upwards. There is œdema (dropsy) of the pericardium and epicardial hæmorrhages. The cause is not known, but usually Mulberry Heart is seen in pigs which were in good bodily condition and it has been suggested that there may be some connection between this and œdema of the bowel, or that rancid fats in the diet may be responsible.

Experimentally, the syndrome has been produced by a variety of diets containing high levels of unsaturated fatty acids. Vitamin E and a selenium salt were shown to be effective in preventing Mulberry Heart.

The condition is most common in animals 2–4 months old.

Landrace pigs appear especially susceptible.

Symptoms include lack of appetite, shivering—especially of shoulders and hindquarters. The forelegs may be splayed in an effort to maintain balance, and the snout may be rested on the ground. A sitting-dog posture may be assumed. Black spots on buttocks, ears, etc., may be seen on many pigs in the herd. Temperature is subnormal. Distressed breathing may be observed. Death usually follows within 12 hours of the onset of symptoms. Occasional survivors are usually blind and unsteady on their legs. (*See also under* HEART, DISEASES OF.)

MULE.—The offspring of a male ass and a mare; also a Blackface × Border Leicester crossbred sheep.

MULES'S OPERATION.—This involves the removal of a fold of skin from the crutch of Merino sheep and is carried out by Australian sheepmen for the control of blowfly strike. Mulesing is a synonym.

MULTIPLE SUCKLING (*see under* NURSE COWS).

MULTIPLE VACCINES (*see under* VACCINATION).

MUMMIFICATION OF FŒTUS.—This sometimes occurs after resorption of fluid from the placenta and fœtus following the death of the latter. It is not uncommon in dairy cattle. In sows, it has been reported following Aujesky's disease. In ewes, it may be associated with toxoplasmosis and ovine virus abortion.

MUMPS is another name for parotiditis or inflammation of the parotid glands at the base of the ears and at the back of the angle of the lower jaw. (*See* PAROTIDITIS.) According to American reports, antibodies against the human mumps virus have been detected in the blood-serum of dogs.

'MUNGA'.—The African name for the grain of the bulrush millet, *Pennisetum typhoides*. The grain, when parasiticised with ergot, has in Rhodesia caused agalactia in sows without other symptoms A heavy piglet mortality resulted.

MURMUR is the name given to a prolonged sound heard by auscultation over the heart, lungs, and certain of the large blood-vessels in abnormal conditions. The so-called 'vesicular murmur' is heard when the air enters and leaves the vesicles or air alveoli of the lungs in the normal condition, but owing to the thickness of the chest walls and to the covering of hair or fur in animals, its keen appreciation is often very difficult or impossible.

MURREY GREY.—An Australian beef breed, originating from a roan Shorthorn cow and an Angus bull.

MUSCLE (*musculus*, a muscle), popularly known as FLESH, is the tissue by which, in virtue of its power of contraction, all movements are made in the higher animals. Muscular tissue is divided into three great classes, *Voluntary muscle, Involuntary muscle*, and *Cardiac muscle*, and of these the former only is under the control of the will, the two latter working automatically. Voluntary muscle is often called 'Striped' or 'Striated', because under the microscope each muscle fibre shows very distinct cross striping, while involuntary muscle does not, and is consequently often called 'Unstriped', 'Non-striated', or 'Plain'. Cardiac muscle is striated in an imperfect manner, is not under the control of the will, and has a specialised arrangement of its fibres.

Structure of muscle.—*Voluntary muscle* forms the chief clothing of the skeleton, and is the red flesh forming beef, mutton, pork, etc., of the food animals. The voluntary muscles are arranged in a definite manner over the body, the majority of them being attached to some part of the bony or cartilaginous skeleton, and are hence called 'skeletal muscles'. Each has an *origin*, from the stable part of the skeleton to which it is attached, which is succeeded by a *fleshy belly*, the motive part, and an *insertion* into the part of the skeleton which it moves. When contraction occurs, the insertion is brought closer to the origin, and this is known as the *action* of the muscle. In some muscles, such as the brachiocephalic running from the shoulder to the base of the skull, either attachment may be alternately origin or insertion, depending upon which part of the skeleton is fixed at the time.

Each muscle is enclosed in a sheath of fibrous tissue, known as the 'fascia' or 'epimysium', and from this partitions of fibrous tissue, known as 'perimysium', run into the substance of the muscle, dividing it into small bundles of 'fibres'. A muscle fibre is about 1/500th of an inch thick, and of varying length. If the fibre be cut across and examined by the microscope, it is seen to be further divided into 'fibrils', the cut ends of which are known as 'Cohnheim's areas'; but as all fibrils of a fibre act in unison, this is needless subdivision. Each fibre is enclosed in an elastic sheath of its own, which allows of lengthening and shortening, and is known as the 'sarcolemma' σάρξ, flesh; and λέμμα, a husk). Within

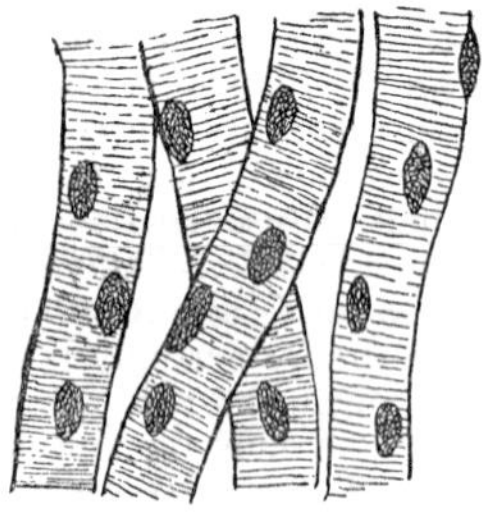

Diagram of the fibres composing voluntary muscle. The nuclei are found immediately below the sarcolemma or sheath, and are quite large. The cross striation of the fibres can be seen.

the sarcolemma lie numerous nuclei belonging to the muscle fibre, which was originally developed from a single cell. To the sarcolemma, at either end, is attached a minute bundle of fibrous tissue fibres, which unites the muscle fibre to its neighbour or to one of the connective tissue partitions in the muscle, and by means of these connections the fibre produces its effect upon contracting. The sarcolemma is pierced by a nerve fibre, which breaks up upon the surface of the muscle fibre into a complicated 'end-plate', and by this means each muscle fibre is brought under the guidance of the central nervous system, and the discharge of energy which produces muscular contraction is controlled. When the muscle fibre within the sarcolemma is examined by a high-power microscope, it is found to show alternate light and dark transverse stripes, with a fine dotted line (called 'Dobie's line' or 'Krause's membrane') running across the middle of each light stripe. In some cases an ill-defined clear line is seen running across the fibre in the middle of each dark band, and is known as 'Hensen's line'. By a careful study of these minutiæ it has been found out that the fibre is really made up of a number of superimposed discs of different material, some connective and some contractile, which are the active agents in bringing about contraction of the whole.

Between the pillar-like muscle fibres run many capillary blood-vessels. They are so placed that the contractions of the muscle fibres empty them of blood, and

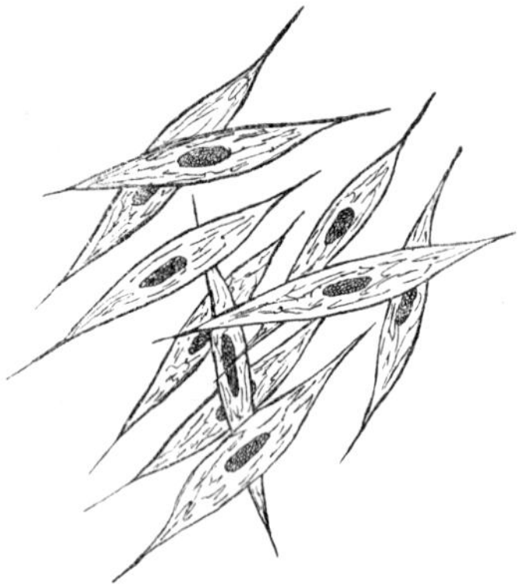

Diagram of involuntary muscle fibres from a teased-out portion of the wall of the small intestine. The nuclei are central in each fibre.

thus the active muscle is ensured of a continually changing blood-supply. None of these capillaries, however, pierce the sarcolemma surrounding the fibres, so that the blood does not come into direct contact with the fibrils themselves. They are nourished by the lymph which exudes from the capillaries and bathes the outside of the sarcolemma, passing into the fibrils by a process of osmosis. The lymph circulation is also automatically varied, as required, by the muscular contractions. Between the muscle fibres, and enveloped in a sheath of connective tissue, lie here and there special structures known as 'muscle spindles'. They appear to be the organs of sensation by which the brain is made aware of the state of contractions of any one particular muscle.

Involuntary muscle is that which composes the greater part of the walls of the hollow organs of the body, such as stomach, intestines, bladder, etc., and the walls of the blood-vessels, ducts from glands, the uterus and Fallopian tubes, the urethra, ureters, the iris and ciliary muscle of the eye, the 'dartos' tunic o the scrotum, and is associated with various glands of the body, like the prostate, and with the skin and hair follicles. The fibres are very much smaller than those of voluntary muscle, though they vary greatly in size. Each is pointed at the ends, has usually one oval nucleus in the centre, and a delicate sheath of sarcolemma enveloping it. The fibres are grouped in bundles, much as are the striped fibres, but they adhere to one another by a cementing material, not by tendon bundles found in voluntary muscle.

Cardiac muscle is a specialised form of involuntary muscle in which the fibres are provided with numbers of projections, each of which is united to a similar projection from an adjacent cell, so that the whole forms an intricate network or meshwork of fibres instead of an arrangement

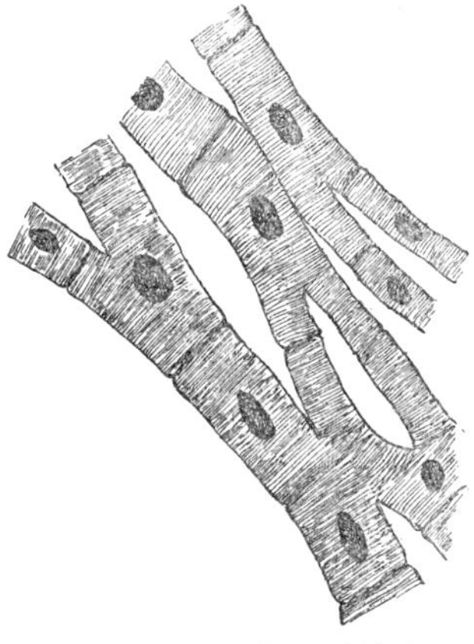

Diagram of the fibres which form cardiac muscle. Each fibre has processes which unite with processes from other fibres to form a highly intricate network or 'syncytium'.

of bundles. Each fibre possesses a large nucleus which is more or less central in position.

Development of muscle.—All the muscles of the developing animal arise from the central layer (mesoblast) of the embryo, each fibre taking origin from a single cell. Later on in life muscles have the power both of increasing in size, as the result of use, for example in race-horses and greyhounds and other animals that are trained to be fit, and also of healing themselves after parts of them have been destroyed by injury or removed surgically. This occurs by development of certain cells called 'myoblasts' in the same way as muscle is formed in the growing embryo, and it was once thought that it might occur by proliferation from the existing fibres. Unstriped muscle as well as striped muscle can take part in this increase in size, as witness the development of the muscular wall of the uterus during pregnancy. In this case not only do the numbers of muscle fibres increase, but each becomes three or four times its previous size. The fully pregnant uterus increases its weight about 20 times what it is when empty, and in the course of a month to six weeks after parturition decreases again in weight and size.

Chemistry of muscle.—Each muscle, as already stated, is composed of muscle tissue and fibrous tissue; the latter does not differ in essentials from fibrous tissue in other parts of the body, but the muscle tissue, or 'sarcoplasm', falls into a class by itself. In the living animal it is of a semi-fluid nature, and in the very recently killed animal it can be squeezed out from the cut ends of the fibres. It clots on standing, just as blood clots, the substances formed being muscle serum and myosin (the clot), produced from myosinogen, just as fibrin forms from fibrinogen. A dead muscle does not possess the same composition as a living muscle, and living muscle cannot be analysed, so that while the following figures of the composition of voluntary muscle are usually given as applying to living muscle, they must be accepted with reservation:

	Per cent
Water	75
Proteins (myosinogen, etc.)	20
Fat	3
Carbohydrates . . .	0·4 to 1
Nitrogenous waste products	0·2
Salts (mainly complex compounds of phosphorus)	1 to 1·5

When a muscle is made to contract for some time the glycogen (animal starch) stored up in it becomes transformed into sugar, destined probably to act as fuel to supply the energy of contraction. At the same time carbon dioxide and sarcolactic acid are produced by this combustion, and there is a certain amount of waste produced by the wear and tear of the permanent tissues. All these waste products are removed by the lymph and the blood, to be eliminated from the body by the lungs, kidneys, and other organs of excretion. In certain cases the rate of production of these waste substances is greater than the rate of their elimination, with the result that they collect in the body, and by their action on nerve-endings and other parts, they are responsible for the production of fatigue (*see later*).

Action of muscles.—It is impossible to attempt to explain fully the various processes that take part in the production of a voluntary muscular contraction in such a work as this, but briefly they may be stated as follows: A nerve impulse originates in some part of the brain or spinal cord, either as the result of volition or as a reflex, passes down the fibres of the motor nerve to the muscle, and is distributed throughout the muscle substance by the terminal nerves. Each of these ends by splitting into a number of tiny fibrils which pass into the sarcolemma and break up into the complicated end-plate already mentioned. The impulse reaches the end-plate and by some means activates the muscle fibrils, which give a twitch. If a series of stimuli pass into a muscle at the rate of about ten per second, a succession of twitches occurs, but complete relaxation does not take place between them. If the rate of the impulses is increased to about twenty-five or thirty per second, no appreciable relaxation occurs between one twitch and the next; in other words, the contraction is sustained as long as the impulses arrive at the same rate. When they cease, the contraction ceases and relaxation occurs. During contraction each fibril swells in diameter and decreases in length, very much as does a strip of solid elastic rubber when it returns to its normal state after being stretched. When not actively contracting the fibres are relaxed, but still retain their elasticity and a certain amount of tenseness. This elastic tension ensures that no time is lost when a muscle comes into action, as there is no slack to take up. Electrical changes occur in a muscle when it contracts, but their full significance is not yet well understood. A still more important change accompanying contraction is the development of heat, the smallest twitch of a muscle giving an appreciable rise in its temperature. Muscle in this respect is a very economical machine for doing work, for while a locomotive steam engine only converts about 4 per cent of the available energy of its fuel into work, the remaining 96 per cent being lost as heat, a muscle, according to Fick, transforms about 25 per cent of the available energy into work, and there is some probability that the perfectly fit muscles of a trained race-horse may be even more economical. As is well known, the heat obtained from muscular action is employed for the maintenance of body heat generally, but there are occasions when the amount of heat produced is in excess of requirements, especially when muscular exertion is violent. On account of this it is more economical for the animal to perform its work by making a large number of small efforts than by making fewer more intense and powerful efforts. Thus it is less tiring to proceed to a height by a gentle slope than to arrive by one that is steeper, although both involve the same amount of work. This principle is of the greatest importance in the training of horses for hunting or racing purposes.

In involuntary muscle slow, steady, deliberate movements occur instead of the twitches seen in the voluntary muscles. The process of contraction is wave-like, spreading from certain areas outwards from one muscle fibre to another. The nerves are arranged in an intricate network or 'plexus', and scattered throughout the muscle are concentrations of nerve cells known as 'ganglia'. These are able to control the actions of the plain muscles without any assistance from the brain or spinal cord, as can be shown if the abdomen of a newly killed animal be opened and the intestines removed. Until the absence of blood and the chilling of the outside air kill the muscles in their walls, the various parts of the intestinal system can be seen rhythmically contracting and expanding in the way they do during life. This has led some authorities to maintain that the nerve ganglia and plexuses present in plain muscle are capable of carrying on movement, and governing action, independent of the rest of the nervous system. It is as if each tiny area of muscle had its own little brain, with its own little set of nerves. That the brain and spinal cord do exert some control, however, can be readily demonstrated when some of the central nerves are cut, or are specially stimulated. By studying the results of such operations, it has been found that while primary movement probably does originate in the ganglia, the central nervous system, through its 'sympathetic' fibres, governs the actions of the involuntary muscles by two sets of nerve fibres; one set *tsimulates* action, and the other set *inhibits* it. Excitation of the stimulating fibres results in increased action, and of the inhibitory fibres in a slowing or cessation of movement. *Muscle tonus* is the state of partial contraction of a muscle by virtue of which it is ready for work at all times. Tonus is specially evident in the plain muscle fibres present in the walls of the arteries, and it is owing to it that such striking and rapid changes in the amount of the blood in a part can occur. If the inhibitory fibres (called 'vasodilators') in the arteries are activated an immediate increase of blood takes place, while if the stimulating fibres (called 'vasoconstrictors') are acted upon, the muscle fibres in the walls contract, the calibre of the vessels is decreased, and the blood-supply is lessened.

One more form of activity of the plain muscular system must be mentioned, viz. that known as 'peristalsis'. This is the process by which food-stuffs are moved along the lumen of the bowel. The presence of food in the intestine causes first a wave of dilatation to travel along the gut, and immediately behind it a wave of contraction or constriction follows. The constriction forces the food into the slightly dilated part of the bowel just in front of it, and the sum total of many peristaltic waves is responsible for the passage of the food through the whole of the alimentary system. In the small intestines a reverse movement, in which the waves proceed towards the stomach instead of away from it, alternates with the regular peristalsis, so that the food becomes well mixed before passing into the large bowel. This reverse wave is called 'anti-peristalsis'. During peristalsis the portion of bowel alternately becomes shorter and longer by virtue of the contraction and relaxation of the longitudinal fibre in its wall, and by this means food material is assisted in passing round flexures of the bowel. Given ordinary conditions, these movements are sufficient to prevent the collection of too much food at any one part of the bowel, but when through overloading, or through the action of some harmful substance in the food, one section of the bowel does not perform its function as thoroughly as the rest, it becomes full of food, dilated and inert, and a 'stoppage' or 'impaction' results. This is frequently encountered in colic.

Heart muscle, although somewhat similar to skeletal muscle in appearance, is involuntary, and possesses a characteristic action of its own. The heart is governed by sets of nerve fibres which are 'motor' (stimulating contraction) and 'inhibitory' from the central nervous system. In some animals there are ganglia present, but they have not yet been demonstrated in all. The original impulse for contraction may either arise in the muscle fibres themselves, or may be controlled by the ganglia. That it is not the central nervous system that is responsible for the initiation and maintenance of heart action is proved by the fact that the mammalian heart can continue to beat for days after removal from all nerve connections if it be kept in an even body temperature, supplied with certain chemical salts in solution, and kept well supplied with oxygen. The accelerator motor and inhibitory nerves are responsible for alterations in the pulse rate and force.

Fatigue of muscle is caused by the using up of the contractile substances in the fibres and by the concentration of waste chemical products in the sarcoplasm. The chief material responsible for fatigue seems to be sarcolactic acid, in fact if sarcolactic acid be artificially injected into a muscle its power of contraction is lessened. It affects the end-plates of the nerves and probably also the muscle spindles, lowering the conductivity of the former, and irritating the latter in such a way that messages of fatigue are passed to the brain, and the animal becomes 'tired'. When only a slight muscular action is undertaken, the waste products are swept away by the circulating blood and eliminated from the system, but when muscle action is sustained for any length of time, the excretion is slower than the formation, and the percentage of waste substances present in the muscles and in the blood rises. They may have a clogging action upon the nerves of the central system as well, but this has not been established.

During the period of rest which normally follows excessive muscular activity the excretion of the waste substances continues through the kidneys, lungs, etc., and after a time the muscles and the blood are freed from them and the animal is ready for further maximum muscular effort. The importance of a sufficient period of rest for animals that have been called upon to perform some great exertion, such as hunting or racing, is obvious. It is also on this account that the flesh of hunted animals does not keep well, and that authorities insist upon a period of rest before slaughter in the case of the food animals, when they have been travelled by road to abattoirs.

Rigor mortis, or the 'stiffness of death', is a condition which comes on in the muscles after death. They become firm and solid, lose their elasticity, and no longer respond to electrical stimuli. The muscle substance (sarcoplasm) clots, just as does the blood, and some muscle serum is expressed into the spaces around the fibres. In animals that have been hunted to death, or in those that have died when fatigued, rigor mortis sets in very rapidly, but passes off quickly. The 'setting of the flesh' in animals slaughtered for human food is simply another name for rigor mortis. In certain cases where there has been violent injury causing immediate death, rigor mortis appears instantaneously; animals killed thus are found rigidly fixed in the attitude in which death occurred.

Condition is that remarkable state into which horses and other animals can be brought by care in feeding, general management, and carefully regulated work, which is the highest pitch of perfection to which muscles can attain. It is a potential quality not possessed by all animals, and, even when attained, does not last for long periods. In the process of training it is possible by overmuch enthusiasm to produce a condition of 'staleness', in which speed or staying power diminishes, but recovery from which follows a period of rest. Condition consists in a gradual education of the muscles of the skeleton, of the heart and respiratory organs particularly, as well as of the body generally, so that they will sustain fatigue with greater and greater facility. All superfluous fat and watery tissues are removed from the body, the volume of the muscles is increased, their elasticity, tone, responsiveness to stimuli, power of contraction, and blood-supply are heightened; the respiratory system is made to accommodate itself to the oxygenation of vastly greater amounts of blood in a shorter space of time than normally; the heart muscle, the main pump of the circulation, hypertrophies, and the walls of the smaller arteries, the secondary pumps of the circulatory system, are keyed up to the highest state of responsiveness to local requirements. In the production of all this lies the art of the trainer, an art requiring a long education. Rough tests of the state of condition of a horse consist in taking the pulse and respiration rates when at rest, and then again at varying periods after exercise, and noting the time it takes for each of these functions to settle down to the normal. For purposes of illustration, but not for practical reference, the following table compiled by Wadley and quoted by Smith may be given; in this fit and unfit horses were made to perform the same work for the same time, and the times taken for subsidence of pulse and respiration rates to normal are noted.

	Fit horses.	Unfit horses.
Pulse Rates:	per min.	per min.
Before work . .	40	39
At cessation . .	88	113
2 mins. later . .	55	66
5 ,, ,, . .	46	56
Respiration Rates:		
Before work . .	10	12
At cessation . .	41	48
2 mins. later . .	21	28
5 ,, ,, . .	16	19

MUSCLES, which are collectively and popularly known as the 'flesh' of an animal, comprise the voluntary muscles, and amount to over one-third the weight of the whole body in an average animal of ordinary condition. The total number of voluntary muscles is over 700 in the horse, and more than this in some of the other domesticated animals, so that they each one cannot be described in detail here. Each voluntary muscle is named, its blood- and nerve-supplies are mentioned, and its shape, relations, and actions are considered in works on Comparative Anatomy, to which reference must be made for further details.

Generally speaking, muscles which cause a joint to bend are called 'flexors', those which straighten a bent joint are 'extensors', one which carries a limb farther away from the middle line of the body than previously is an 'abductor', one which has the opposite action is an 'adductor', and one which causes a segment of a limb to revolve is a 'rotator', or 'supinator', or a 'pronator', according to its position. A sphincter is usually involuntary, but a few are voluntary; they cause a contraction of the ring-like opening which they circumscribe. Many muscles have an insertion distant from their fleshy part (called the 'fleshy belly') by means of a tendon which is composed of fibrous tissue strands. Tendons may be long or short, and are usually attached to some eminence or roughness on a bone. They are so constituted that they are usually able to withstand more than the maximum tensile strain that the muscle can exert, and consequently do not readily rupture. (*See* TENDON.) Some of the more important muscles of the horse will be considered.

Fore-limb.—*Connecting the limb with the rest of the body* are the following: trapezius, rhomboideus, and latissimus dorsi, outside; and the brachiocephalic, superficial and deep pectorals (each of which is double), and the ventral serratus, also in two parts, inside. *In the shoulder region* lie the deltoid, supraspinatus, infraspinatus, teres minor, subscapularis, teres major, coracobrachialis, and capsularis; of these the last four lie on the inside of the region of the shoulder-blade. *The muscles of the arm, i.e.* around the humerus, are the biceps brachii, brachialis, tensor of the antibrachial fascia, triceps brachii (with three parts), and the anconeus. The triceps forms the great mass of muscle which is inserted into the elbow point, and extends the elbow in locomotion. *In the fore-arm,* the muscles which extend the limb below the carpus ('knee') are the radial carpal extensor, common digital extensor, lateral digital extensor (or extensor digiti quinti), and the oblique extensor of the carpus. Behind the bones lie the muscles which flex the carpus; these are the radial carpal flexor, the ulnar carpal flexor, the ulnar carpal extensor (which is really a flexor), the superficial digital flexor, and the deep digital flexor. The tendons of these last two muscles form the 'back tendons', at the back of the cannon. There are five small muscles below the carpus.

Hind-limb.—*The hip muscles* are the main muscles of propulsion. Most of them are attached to and act on the femur, but two—the psoas minor and the quadratus lumborum—flex the pelvis or the loins. The psoas major and iliacus flex the hip and rotate the thigh outward, being instrumental in carrying the limb forwards during locomotion. The muscles which extend the hip and propel the body forward are the middle gluteal, one of the largest muscles, biceps femoris, semitendinosus, and semimembranosus. The tensor fascia lata flexes the hip and extends the stifle, the superficial gluteal flexes the hip and abducts the limb, and the deep gluteal abducts the thigh and rotates it inward. *The muscles of the thigh* are sartorius, gracilis, pectineus, adductor, quadratus femoris, external and internal obturators, and gemelli, which adduct the limb and rotate it, and the quadriceps femoris (in four parts) and small capsularis, the former of which raises the patella and so extends the stifle-joint. *In the leg* on the anterior aspect are those muscles which extend the lower segment of the limb; these are the long digital extensor, peroneus longus, peroneus tertius, and anterior tibial. On the posterior aspect are the flexors, viz. gastrocnemius, soleus, superficial and deep digital flexors (whose tendons form the 'back tendons' of the hind-limb), and the popliteus.

Head and Face.—*The muscles of the ears* are divided into two sets: the intrinsic and the extrinsic. The former of these run between the cartilages of the ear and assist the more important extrinsic muscles. They are three in number. The extrinsic muscles are attached from some part of the head or neck near the ears into the cartilages. They are 7 in number, of which one muscle has four parts, two have three parts, two have two parts, and the remaining two have a single part, so that there are really 16 muscles altogether. This is not surprising when the extreme mobility of the ears of horses is remembered. *The eyelids* have four small muscles which close and open them. *The muscles of mastication* are six in number. The masseter forms the large dense mass of the cheek; its action is to close the jaws or to twist the lower jaw to one side. The temporal lies in the depression behind the eye and serves to assist the closure of the jaws. The two pterygoids lie on the inside of the lower jaw opposite to the masseter, and have actions like the latter. The other two muscles are the jugulo-mandibular and the digastric. *Attached to the hyoid bone* are 8 muscles only one of which is single. Their actions are to raise the floor of the mouth, tongue, and hyoid bone, to draw the base of the tongue and the larynx upward and backward, to draw these parts forward, or to assist other muscles in bending the neck. *The muscles of the lips, nostrils, and cheeks* assist in gathering food for the teeth to crop, manipulate the food during chewing, dilate or contract the nostrils, elevate or depress the lips, and give a certain amount of expressiveness to the lower part of the face. They are thirteen in number.

Ventral part of neck.—Just above the jugular groove, and reaching from close behind the ear down to the shoulder, can be easily seen the large brachiocephalic muscle, which may either swing the head round or advance the shoulder. Lying below this and covering the trachea in the lower part of the neck is the sternocephalic, while beneath this latter, and covering the trachea in the upper part of the neck, where the sternocephalic diverges laterally, are the sterno-thyro-hyoids and the omohyoids. The scalenus, the greater and lesser straight capiti, the lateral straight capitus, the long and the intertransverse neck muscles all lie deeply. They either flex the head or neck downwards or laterally.

Dorsal part of neck.—Lying in the dorsal part of the neck there are 12 muscles which serve to lift the head and neck upwards, to turn them laterally, or to rotate the head and cervical vertebræ to one side or the other. They are arranged in pairs separated down the middle line by the 'ligamentum nuchæ', a very powerful ligament which is elastic enough to allow the horse to depress the head, but of sufficient tenseness to take the greater part of the strain of supporting the head in an upright position off the muscles of the neck.

Trunk.—In addition to the muscles of the fore-limb, which attach it to the trunk, there are two dorsal serratus muscles, attached to the rib-cage, clothing the anterior part of the chest, a long transversalis costarum, and the longissimus dorsi, which lie external to the bony chest cavity. The last two of these along with the multifidus dorsi muscle lie along on either side of the spines of the vertebræ, and give the back its form and outline. When these muscles are weak and underdeveloped the spines of the horse stand out prominently from the contour of the back, and the horse is said to be 'razor-backed'. *In the tail* there are five muscles which are responsible for the extreme mobility of this part. *The thorax* has seven sets of muscles which are attached to the thoracic vertebræ, to the ribs and their cartilages, and to the sternum. They take part in the movements of respiration. The levatores costarum draw the ribs forward during inspiration, and are assisted by the external intercostals, a layer of muscle between each rib and the next. In expiration the following muscles take part: internal intercostals, the retractor costæ, the transverse thoracic, and the abdominal muscles. *The muscles of the abdomen* form the lower and side walls of the cavity, and consist of thick muscular layers between which lie strong sheets of fibrous tissue. In the horse the muscles are assisted in carrying the weight of the abdominal organs by a special layer of fascia called the 'yellow abdominal tunic'. Three muscles form the side walls: (1) the external oblique, the largest, which runs from the outer surfaces of the last 14 ribs and from the lumbar fascia, in a downward and backward direction, to end in a strong sheet (or aponeurosis) which passes to the middle line of the abdomen, where it meets its fellow aponeurosis of the opposite side; (2) the internal oblique, which lies under the external, and which arises from the angle of the haunch bone and runs downward and forward to end in an aponeurosis similar to that of the external; and (3) the transverse abdominal, whose fibres run in a transverse direction arising from the rib cartilages and the lumbar transverse processes, and end in an aponeurosis which joins those of the oblique muscles. Running down the middle line of the abdomen is a 'white line', called the *linea alba*, which is formed where the aponeuroses of the three above-mentioned muscles meet. It extends from the xiphoid cartilage of the sternum back to the brim of the pelvis. Lying on either side of this line are the straight abdominal muscles. These run from the cartilages of the fifth to the ninth ribs, and are inserted into the pubis by the prepubic tendon. All these abdominal muscles have a more or less common action; they raise the floor of the abdomen, compress its contents, and cause arching of the back. They are employed in expiration, urination, defecation, and during foaling. They are also used in galloping, to bring the pelvis forward after the stretch, especially the straight muscles, and to a less extent in drawing or backing loads. *The inguinal canal* is a passage through the posterior part of the abdominal wall through which pass the spermatic cord and its associated structures in the male, and the mammary blood-vessels and nerves in the female.

The Diaphragm, or 'Skirt', is the muscular and tendinous dividing structure between the chest and abdominal cavities. It bulges forward in a dome-like manner, so that the thoracic surface is markedly convex and the abdominal surface concave. It is attached to the cartilages of the ninth to the fifteenth ribs, and to the last three ribs themselves, to the upper surface of the xiphoid cartilage, and to the lower parts of the first five lumbar vertebræ. When it contracts, its domed part, which is mainly tendinous, becomes flattened, so that the longitudinal diameter of the chest is increased. It is accordingly the main structure effecting inspiration. In addition to this action it assists in circulation by carrying the abdominal contents backwards and increasing the intra-abdominal pressure, and thus tending to squeeze blood from the veins of the abdomen into those of the chest. It is pierced by three openings: the first of these, called the *hiatus aorticus*, contains the abdominal aorta, the vena azygos, and the cisterna chyli; the second—*hiatus œsophageus*—allows passage for the œsophagus, the vagus nerves, and small arteries; and the third—*foramen vena cava*—allows the vena cava to pass into the chest.

Cutaneous muscles.—Lying immediately under the skin and in some cases embedded in the subcutaneous tissue, there are numerous arrangements of cutaneous muscles, which pass from a comparatively rigid part of the underlying muscles or their tendons, to be inserted by thin fibrous sheets into the skin itself. These muscles are very highly developed in the horse, and serve the purpose of causing the skin to quiver and dislodge any particles of offending matter, flies, etc.

MUSCLES, DISEASES OF.—Atrophy of muscles may occur as the result of inaction, diminished blood-supply, or nerve injuries, as well as from malnutrition.

INFLAMMATION of muscle, or MYOSITIS, may arise as the result of injury through kicks, blows, falls, etc., which produce immediate consequences, or it may follow the irritation produced by badly fitting collars, breechings, or other harness. It frequently arises as the result of a sprain or strain in the limbs of animals, and it may be associated with partial or complete rupture. Horses that are called upon to perform some violent exertion when out of condition may suddenly go lame the day following from inflammation of the flexor muscles of the fore- or hind-limbs. As a rule, a bad bruise of the surface of the body is the complement of inflammation of the underlying muscles when external injury has led to myositis.

Symptoms.—The part affected usually becomes swollen and is painful on manipulation. The muscles affected are held relaxed, and if in a limb the foot is rested. When handled, they contract and become hard to the touch, and upon occasion they may crackle or be œdematous. When resulting from external injury there is usually some sign of this on the covering skin, but when due to strain no external lesions may be seen. Occasionally, after injury, an abscess may develop in the affected muscle, but much more frequently there is a pouring out of serum under the skin, and a 'blood-blister', or *hæmatoma*, forms below the skin. This feels soft to the touch, gives the impression of containing fluid, and after a short time loses its tenseness and fluctuates when the animal moves. After the acute stage of myositis passes off, some amount of atrophy and degeneration persists for a time. In severe cases the atrophy may be noticeable for the rest of the animal's life, but usually it disappears after a few months. When a complete rupture has occurred there may be fixation of some part of the limb, through the unrestrained action of the antagonistic muscles on the opposite side of the joints.

Treatment.—As soon after injury as possible the animal should be placed by itself, and complete rest ensured. It may be necessary to sling a horse or an ox where the damage is extensive, or where important supportive muscles are affected. The affected parts should then be gently bathed with hot water for half an hour two or three times daily, or hot moist compresses may be applied. A cooling, astringent, stimulating liniment is rubbed in during intervals between the fomentations. Later, exercise and hand rubbing are beneficial.

ATROPHIC MYOSITIS.—This has been described in the dog. The cause is unknown, but possibly damage to the fifth nerve due to over-extension of the tempero-mandibular joint.

Symptoms.—Inability to eat solid food or to lap, atrophy of the jaw muscles, very little voluntary movement of the jaws, and any attempt to force the jaws apart is resisted.

With careful nursing, recovery takes place naturally in a high proportion of cases after 3 to 6 months. (*See also* 'STIFF-LIMBED LAMBS'.)

EOSINOPHILIC MYOSITIS.—A disease of dogs, especially Alsatians, in which there is hardening of the muscles of mastication and of the temporal muscles. The dog assumes a foxy appearance. The nictitating membrane is in evidence. There may be tonsillitis. The cause is unknown; the outlook grave. Diagnosis may be confirmed by blood smear.

ISCHÆMIC CONTRACTURE.—A disease of muscles due to failure of their arterial supply. There is necrosis and the muscle is replaced by fibrous tissue which contracts or shortens. The condition has been reported in the dog.

MUSCULAR DYSTROPHY.—This is most common in beef cattle, but is occasionally seen in dairy cattle also. In calves and lambs it is often called 'White Muscle disease'. Muscular dystrophy also occurs in foals. It may prove fatal.

In human medicine the concept that it is an abnormality of muscle-fibre has been challenged, and the idea put forward that this may be primarily a disease of nerves.

Cause.—This appears to be complex and may include a vitamin E deficiency. This may be brought about by giving cod-liver oil in conjunction with rations low in vitamin E, such as dried skim milk powder, for research has shown that the inclusion of cod-liver oil in the diet leads to a striking increase in their requirements of vitamin E. The disease may also be associated with poor quality food, such as the mainly turnip and oat straw diet fed to pregnant cows during the winter in Scotland. Deterioration of food in storage, and especially of those containing unsaturated fatty acids may be associated with the condition.

Symptoms.—Stiffness and a peculiar gait. Some calves die due to the heart muscles and the diaphragm being affected.

Prevention.—Give the cow and calf vitamin E, or alternatively plenty of good quality silage.

'Small amounts of selenium will prevent the muscular dystrophy of cattle in north Scotland, a disease which is also prevented by relatively large amounts of α-tocopherol. The farms concerned were on soils derived from arenaceous sands of old red sandstone origin, which suggests that on comparable soils dietary deficiency of selenium might also occur. Such deficiency might well be masked by an adequate tocopherol intake as instanced by the absence of the disease on farms in the Moray Firth area, which feed rations containing silage and green fodder and its limitation to those feeding turnips and straw, a ration which provides about one-tenth of the tocopherol of silage rations.' (See *Veterinary Record*, Aug. 15, 1959.)

MUSCULAR RHEUMATISM is a form of myositis which attacks dogs and pigs especially, although horses and cattle are also affected. Certain animals seem to have a susceptibility to this trouble.

Causes.—Exposure to cold, draughts, and dampness, insufficient protection against changes in the weather, standing for long periods in rainy weather, and insufficiency of bedding (especially in piggeries and kennels). It is stated that an excess of damaged hay, barley, or maize will produce a train of symptoms that are not distinguishable from those of rheumatism.

Symptoms.—The affected muscles are found tense and quivering, and manipulation of them causes such excruciating agony that the smaller animals often scream with the pain when the parts are handled, and the larger animals may grunt or moan. Sometimes voluntary movements in the part of the animal itself excites the same distress. The muscles of the neck, shoulders, and abdominal wall are those most often affected in all animals; the muscles of the lower jaw are frequently affected in dogs; and the condition may attack almost any of the muscles of the body. When the loins are affected the condition is called *lumbago*, and when the croup and thigh are involved it is known as *sciatica*.

Treatment.—Massage of the affected muscles with some mild liniment, such as soap liniment, hot applications, exercise, and warmth are necessary outwardly, and internally salicylates should be given. For this purpose aspirin in the dog and salicylate of soda in the larger animals are useful. In all cases the bowels must be kept open.

CRAMP of the muscles is common in animals that are not in a fit condition when they are worked or exercised. (*See under* CRAMP, *and also* SCOTTIE CRAMP.)

PARASITES are sometimes met with in the muscles of pigs and cattle, giving rise to the terms 'measly pork' and 'measly beef', but they generally cause no appreciable external symptoms. The muscles of sheep may contain numbers of bodies known as '*sarcosporidia*', but their full significance is not yet known. They also occur in other animals.

TUMOURS are occasionally met with, the most common being fibroid, fatty, and sarcomatous growths, although tumour-like swellings are associated with botriomycosis in the horse, which is probably more common than those mentioned. (*See* BOTRIOMYCOSIS.)

SHIVERING, STRINGHALT. For these two muscular diseases of horses, *see under* those headings.

(*See also* MYASTHENIA.)

MUSCULAR DYSTROPHY.—*See* MUSCLES DISEASES OF.)

MUSCULAR RELAXANTS are drugs, other than anæsthetics, which produce relaxation or paralysis in voluntary muscle, such as does curare. They are sometimes used in conjunction with a general anæsthetic, since a larger dose of the latter is usually required to obtain muscular relaxation than to abolish pain; and large doses of some anæsthetics can give rise to poisoning. Muscular relaxants can, however, only too easily be misused, and should be reserved for the specialist anæsthetist.

'MUSHY CHICK' DISEASE.—Omphalitis. (*See under this* heading.)

MUSTARD is a yellowish powder, consisting of the dried ripe seeds of *Brassica nigra* and *Brassica alba* ground together. The former contains an active principle called 'sinigrin', the latter contains one named 'sinalbin', while both contain a quantity of a ferment named 'myrosin' which, in the presence of cold or lukewarm water, converts the two active principles into the volatile oil to which the action of the mustard is due. This oil is extremely irritating to the skin and to mucous surfaces with which it or its vapour comes into contact.

Uses.—Externally, mustard was used as an irritant to the skin, to produce a local superficial inflammation of a transitory nature.

Internally, it is sometimes used as an emetic for dogs when other and more suitable substances are not at hand. For this purpose, from a dessertspoonful to a tablespoonful is mixed into a thin paste with water and given by the mouth. Vomiting occurs in from 1 to 5 minutes after administration.

Poisoning.—Cattle have died as a result of white mustard seed being swept off the floor of a barn on to pasture. Symptoms included: walking backwards and in circles, profuse salivation, and curvature of the spine.

MUSTY FOOD.—This should not be used for animal food. It is very unpalatable; and a small quantity can spoil a large amount of food. It is not easily digested, and may lead to serious digestive upsets. There is also a risk of ASPERGILLOSIS.

MUTATION.—A permanent change in the characteristics of bacteria or viruses. This is the usually implied, though not exact, meaning. (*See also* GENETICS.)

MUTING OF DOGS.—This involves a surgical operation under general anæsthesia, when the vocal cords are completely excised. It was performed during the 1939–45 war on Army dogs.

MUTTER-PEA POISONING (*see* LATHYRISM).

MUTUALISM (*see* PARASITES, p. 628).

MUZZLE, TAPE (*see under* RESTRAINT, DOG).

MYALGIA (μῦς, a muscle; ἄλγος, pain) means pain in a muscle.

MYASTHENIA GRAVIS.—A disease which affects chiefly the muscles of the skeleton, but occasionally also the muscles involved in breathing. It is characterised by fatigue. A difficulty in swallowing may be noticed. The condition is believed to be due to some difficulty in the transmission of impulses across the neuromuscular junctions. It has been reported in the dog as well as in man. (*See Vet. Record*, April 28, 1962.) Diagnosis can be made with the aid of prostigmin, which gives relief within the hour. Relapse may follow treatment with prostigmin.

MYCOBACTERIUM.—One of a group of organisms which include the causes of tuberculosis and Johne's disease.

MYCOPLASMA.—An infective agent distinct from bacteria as well as from viruses. In size they resemble a large virus and they are filterable, but they can be cultivated on artificial media. They are also known as the Pleuro-pneumonia-like organisms (P.P.L.O.).

Mycoplasma mycoides was isolated from cattle with pleuro-pneumonia in 1898; *M. agalacticæ* from goats in 1923. Since then other species of mycoplasma have been found in man, dogs, pigs, fowls, turkeys, rats, and mice. The species most commonly associated with disease in the turkey and chicken are *Mycoplasma gallisepticum*, *M. meleagridis* and *M. synoviæ*. Several other species such as Iowa 695 and W.R.1 have also been found associated with disease in these birds while *M. anatis* has been isolated from an outbreak of sinusitis in ducks.

MYCOPLASMOSIS.—A mycoplasma infection. (*See under* CONTAGIOUS BOVINE PLEURO-PNEUMONIA, VULVO-VAGINITIS, ENZOÖTIC PNEUMONIA OF PIGS, SINUSITIS, INFECTIOUS of turkey.)

MYCOSIS (μύκης, a fungus) is the general term applied to diseases due to the growth of fungi in the body. Among the commonest are actinomycosis, ringworm, sporotrichosis, aspergillosis, etc.

MYCOTIC INFECTIONS are those caused by a fungus. Mycotic dermatitis in sheep is described under the heading LUMPY WOOL. Mycotic mastitis is of importance in dairy cattle, and 26 or more species of fungi are involved. (*See also* RHINOSPORIDIOSIS, FUNGOUS DISEASES, SPORIDESMIN.)

MYCOTOXICOSIS.—Poisoning by toxins produced by fungi.

MYDRIASIS (μυδρίασις) means an unusual state of dilatation of the pupil of the eye. Drugs which cause mydriasis, such as belladonna and cocaine, are called ' mydriatics '

MYELIN (μυελός, marrow) is the name given to the white fat-like substance forming a sheath round medulated or myelinated nerve-fibres in the nerves and in the central nervous system.

MYELITIS (μυελός, marrow) is a disease, or rather a diseased condition, in which destructive changes occur in the spinal cord. It usually follows upon viral infections. Paralysis of a muscle or of groups of muscles may occur; there may be twitchings or spasms of muscles; the penis may hang from the prepuce; the bladder and rectum become unable to retain their contents, and finally a form of paraplegia often occurs. The paralysis may gradually pass forwards; the sensation is lost in the skin of the loins, then of the back, and later the fore-legs become unable to support the weight of the body. Occasionally the condition disappears spontaneously, but the majority of cases end fatally in from 7 to 10 days. (*See also* OSTEOMYELITIS.)

MYELOCYTE (μυελός, marrow; κύτος, cell).—Red bone-marrow cell, from which the granular white corpuscles of the blood are produced. They are found in the blood also in certain forms of leukæmia.

MYELOGRAPHY.—The introduction of contrast media to outline the spinal cord for radiography. It has been used to demonstrate protrusion of the intervertebral disc in the dog, but is a technique not free from risk.

MYELOID (μτελός, marrow; εἶδος, form) is a term applied to sarcomatous tumours which present cells similar to those found in bone-marrow. (*See* LEUCOSIS COMPLEX.)

MYIASIS (μυῖα, a fly).—The presence of larvæ of dipterous flies in tissues and organs of the living animal, and the tissue destruction and disorders resulting therefrom. In sheep blow-fly myiasis is commonly known as ' strike '. The condition may occur in cats. (*See* PARASITES *and* ' STRIKE ', *also* UITPEULOOG.)

MYOCARDITIS (μῦς, muscle; καρδία, the heart) means inflammation of the muscular wall of the heart. (*See* HEART, DISEASES OF.)

MYOCLONIA CONGENITA (*see* TREMBLING of pigs).

MYODYSTROPHIA OF LAMBS (*see* ' STIFF-LIMBED LAMBS ').

MYOGLOBINURIA.—The presence of muscle pigment in urine. It occurs in azoturia. In humans, it occurs during muscular dystrophy. (*See* AZOTURIA.)

MYOMA (μῦς, muscle; *-oma*, meaning tumour) is the term applied to a tumour which consists almost totally of muscular tissue. They are rare in animals, and when encountered are generally found in the wall of the uterus.

MYOPATHY.—Non-inflammatory degeneration of muscles, such as may occur in muscular dystrophy.

MYOPIA (μύωψ, blinking ; from μύω, I close ; ὤψ, the eye), or SHORT SIGHT, is a condition in which, owing to the lens of the eye being too convex or the ball of the eye too long, rays of light are brought to a focus before they reach the retina. It is the opposite of hypermetropia. (*See* VISION.)

MYOSIS (μύω, I close) means an unusual narrowing of the pupil.

MYOSITIS (μύς, muscle) means inflam mation of a muscle. (*For* EOSINOPHILIC MYOSITIS *and* ATROPHIC MYOSITIS *see also under* MUSCLES, DISEASES OF.)

MYOTICS (μύω, I close) is the term applied to drugs which contract the pupil of the eye, such as eserine and opium.

MYSOLINE.—An anti-convulsant drug used in the treatment of epilepsy.

MYXŒDEMA (μύξα, mucus ; οἴδημα, a swelling) is a disease due to an insufficiency of the internal secretion of the thyroid gland, in which certain changes occur in the body. It is not common among animals, but a condition similar to myxœdema is seen in some of the calves of the Dexter breed of cattle. It has also been seen in piglets. (*See* THYROID, DISEASES OF.)

MYXOMA (μύξα, mucus ; *-oma*, meaning tumour) is the name applied to a tumour consisting of imperfect connective tissue, among the fibres of which there is a peculiar mucus-like juice. (*See* TUMOURS.)

MYXOMATOSIS, INFECTIOUS.—A disease of rabbits caused by a virus. Hares are occasionally affected also, but not domestic animals. The disease has a very high mortality rate when introduced into a country, but later the virus may become less potent or the survivors more resistant. Myxomatosis appeared in wild rabbits in Kent and Sussex in October 1953, and spread rapidly throughout most of Britain. Symptoms include: conjunctivitis, 'gummed' eyelids, swellings of the nose and muzzle, and of the mucous membrane of the vulva and anus. Orchitis is caused in the male. Emaciation, fever, and death follow. The disease is transmitted by the rabbit flea and, mechanically, by thistles.

MYXOVIRUS.—This is a group of viruses which includes those causing mumps, para-influenza, influenza A, swine influenza, fowl plague, and influenza B.

N

NÆVUS (*nævus*, a mole) is the term applied to tumours consisting of a mass of dilated blood-vessels. They occur in man chiefly, but cavernous hæmangioma of the liver in cattle is of the same nature.

NAGANA is a disease of cattle and other domesticated animals occurring in various parts of Africa, due to the presence of trypanosomes in the blood-stream. These parasites may be of several varieties, but *Trypanosoma brucei* is the one usually associated with the disease. The koodoo, hyena, and bush-buck, as well as other wild animals, act as reservoirs of the disease, which is transmitted to stock by the bites of flies. (*See* Parasites, p. 633.)

NAIL BINDING is the condition produced by driving a nail too close to the sensitive parts of the foot, but without actually puncturing them. Pain is caused by the pressure of the nail on the hoof matrix. (*See* Injuries from Shoeing.)

NAILING AND NAIL-HOLES.—In shoeing horses' feet it is of considerable importance to ensure that the nails used are of suitable size, shape, and strength, and that the nail-holes are sufficiently large, neither too fine nor too coarse, and of the correct pitch. Machine-made nails are almost exclusively used at present, and, although perhaps not superior to the hand-made kinds, they are very reliable. They are made in graded sizes from 2 to 16. A horseshoe nail is made with one of its sides flat from tip to head. When the nail is being driven through the hoof, instead of following a straight course it tends to veer *towards* the flat side, and is driven so as to come out through the wall by keeping the flat side to the outside of the foot. The nail-hole in the shoe is slanted or ' pitched ' in such a direction as will assist this outward tendency. If the pitch is too steep the nail (especially at the toe) will come out through the wall too low down and may split the horn; while if the pitch is sloped too much the nail will pass too close to the sensitive parts, or may penetrate them. When the series of nail-holes in a shoe is too close to the outer circumference of the web of the shoe, it is spoken of as ' fine nailing '; and when the holes are too near the inner circumference they are called ' coarse '. In fine nailing the nails leave the wall too soon, the clenches are too low and do not obtain a good grip of the horn, and the shoe is easily pulled off; in coarse nailing the nails are too close to the sensitive parts, which they may enter, and the clenches are high. The distance between the outer edge of the shoe and the nail-holes always depends upon the size of the horse's foot and the thickness of the wall, as well as upon whether the shoe is to be fitted so as to project beyond the wall, or to lie inside its outer circumference. (The former is called fitting ' full ', and the latter fitting is ' close '.)

In all cases the nails should enter the foot by passing through the ' white line ', which is found at the junction between the wall and sole of the foot. Passing through the white line they then enter the wall, and after a short course through it they come to the outside. The tip of the nail is broken off, and a piece of the stem is turned down to form the ' clench '. Clenches should be higher at the toe than at the quarters, as the wall is thickest at the toe, should lie flat in their grooves or ' beds ', and should be turned down for a distance about equal to the width of the nail, so that the clenches are square when finished off.

In driving the nails one of those at the toe is usually driven first, and as the shoe often shifts during the driving of the first nail, it should be tapped back into position before the second, usually the opposite heel nail, is driven. Afterwards the nails are driven alternately: an outside, then an inside nail. The heads should be well buried in the nail-hole, for otherwise they project, rapidly wear away, and the shoe easily loosens. (*See also* Injuries from Shoeing, Shoeing, *and* Foot of Horse.)

NAILS, or Claws, are composed of modified skin substance which has become horny or *keratinised*. They serve as weapons of offence or defence in the carnivora, and as hard dense resistant structures in the ruminants, protecting the softer parts of the foot from wear; while in the horse and other one-toed animals (*solipeds*) they have become modified into very elaborate structures called ' hoofs '. A nail is a curved conical horny process possessing a matrix with blood-vessels, nerves, etc., from which it grows and is nourished. Lying within the matrix is the bone of the terminal phalanx of the digit, which gives the nail its characteristic form in the different animals. When not in use in the carnivora they are retracted by ligaments in an upward direction; this is more marked in animals of the cat tribe, where the nail may almost disappear, than in those of the dog tribe.

NAILS, DISEASES OF.—The nails of cats and dogs sometimes become torn or broken through fighting or violent contact with hard objects. As a rule the matrix is damaged, and the nail often sloughs off afterwards, a new nail ultimately taking the place of the first. Sometimes only the tip is injured, and the matrix higher up is undamaged; in such cases a fine pellicle of horn covers the tip until such a time as the horn has grown down from above, and the whole nail is not shed. In other cases germs gain entrance under the horn, suppuration with great tenderness occurs, and the pus burrows up and bursts out at the root of the nail. In yet other instances germs enter under the fold of skin that overlaps the root of the claw, cause swelling and painfulness, and there is production of pus and shedding of the nail. Occasionally several claws, perhaps on different feet, are attacked, and the animal becomes quite crippled.

Treatment.—Injured ragged portions should be cut off with a strong pair of scissors, taking care not to injure the matrix more than necessary, and the whole foot should be cleansed and soaked for a few minutes in an antiseptic bath. An antiseptic dressing should be applied afterwards, and cotton-wool and a bandage fixed over all. Where suppuration is very severe it is necessary to have the terminal part of the digit amputated under a local or general anæsthetic.

INGROWING NAILS occur upon the ' dew claws ', on the insides of the paws of dogs. These more or less rudimentary digits do not touch the ground, and are consequently not subjected to wear from friction. The nails grow, and owing to their curve eventually penetrate the soft pad behind them. The condition usually causes the dog to lick the part persistently for some days before the nail actually enters the skin. In such cases the nail should be clipped short or filed off, and no harm results. Where actual penetration has occurred the nail should be cut short and an antiseptic dressing applied. It is customary for owners of sporting and other dogs to have the dew claws removed during puppyhood to avoid future trouble of this nature. Where this has not been done and trouble is experienced, amputation of dew claws can be carried out in the adult under anæsthesia.

ONYCHOMYCOSIS, or a fungus infection of the claws, is a not uncommon condition in cats, and is of public health importance as a reservoir of ringworm transmissible to children. (*See* Plate 14.)

NAIROBI SHEEP DISEASE is an acute infectious fever of sheep and goats, caused by a virus, which is reported from the area around Nairobi in Kenya, and possibly occurs in other parts of Eastern Africa. The virus is transmitted by ticks. Adults, the larvæ, and nymphal stages are capable of transmitting the virus, and it is only possible for a tick to retain the virus in an infective form from one stage to the next immediately succeeding. The virus may, however, be carried from adult female ticks through the egg stage to the larvæ.

Symptoms.—Affected sheep usually show an acute febrile disturbance within 5 or 6 days after being infected by the ticks. This lasts for up to 9 days and then a fall in temperature occurs and other clinical symptoms appear. Death may take place a day or two later, or a second rise in temperature may be shown, death or recovery following. There is rapidity and difficulty in breathing, a mucopurulent nasal discharge and green watery diarrhœa, which may contain mucus or blood. The genital organs of ewes are swollen and congested and abortion may occur in pregnant ewes.

Immunity.—In the great majority of cases, recovery confers a strong and lasting immunity.

NANDROLONE.—A hormone used in relieving pain from intervertebral disc protrusion and in orthopædics generally.

NANKOR.—The proprietary name of an organic phosphorus insecticide intended, after dilution with oil, for use on cattle. It is applied to sacking, wrapped round a length of chain, etc., used as a back-rubber by the cattle. It is a useful means of fly control on pasture land, and is officially approved for use on dairy cattle as well as on stores. Loops of string may be soaked in it and hung up in poultry houses and other buildings. It may also be sprayed on to cattle.

NAPHTHALENE POISONING might arise from the ingestion of moth-balls. In the dog, it has been shown experimentally to give rise to hæmolytic anæmia. (In children, poisoning from moth-balls gives rise to 'port-wine coloured' urine.) Another symptom is cataract. Chlorinated naphthalenes have been identified as one cause of HYPERKERATOSIS in cattle.

NAPHTHOL is a coal-tar derivative produced during the manufacture of coal gas. Two forms are recognised: Alpha-naphthol (*α-naphthol*) and Beta-naphthol (*β-naphthol*). Both forms are sometimes used as parasiticides externally.

NARCOSIS (νάρκωσις, a benumbing) is a condition of profound insensibility usually induced by drugs, which resembles sleep in that the narcotised animal can be roused temporarily and is not quite indifferent to severe external stimulation. It is produced by drugs, such as opium, by plants, such as darnel and poppy, and it occurs in some diseases, such as milk fever.

NARCOTICS (ναρκωτικός, making numb) are substances which produce narcosis. (*See* HYPNOTICS.)

NARES is the Latin word for the nostrils.

NASAL DISORDERS (*see* NOSE, DISEASES OF).

NASAL GLEET is another name for chronic nasal catarrh. (*See* NOSE, DISEASES OF.)

NASO-PHARYNX is the name given to the upper part of the throat lying posterior to the nasal cavity. (*See* NOSE.)

'NATURE' (*see under* DROPSY).

NAVEL-ILL (*see* JOINT-ILL).

NAVICULAR BONE (*naviculus*, a little ship) is the popular name for the sesamoid of the third phalanx of the horse. It is a little boat-shaped bone, developed just above the deep flexor tendon, and serves, as do all sesamoid bones, to minimise friction where the tendon passes round a corner of another bone. It enters into the formation of the 'coffin-joint', between the 2nd and 3rd phalanges of the digit. It is of great importance in deep punctured wounds of the foot when these are situated towards the heels, for, when damaged, its

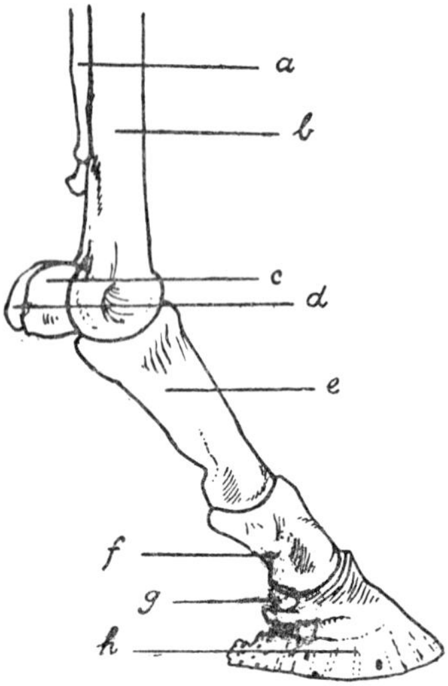

Diagram of the bones of the lower part of the horse's leg. *a*, Small metacarpal or splint bone; *b*, large or third metacarpal or cannon bone; *c* and *d*, sesamoids of first phalanx; *e*, long pastern bone; *f*, short pastern bone; *g*, navicular bone, or sesamoid of third phalanx; *h*, coffin or pedal bone.

surface becomes inflamed, the inflammation spreads to the coffin-joint and may produce incurable lameness. In the disease known as 'navicular disease' it is the chief structure affected.

NAVICULAR DISEASE is a chronic bony inflammation affecting the navicular bone and its associated structures. The fore-feet are usually both attacked, though the condition may arise in only one of these, or in the hind-feet (rarely). Externally, there are usually few definite symptoms to be noticed, but the condition after death shows as an ulceration of the cartilage first and later of the bone on the surface over which the deep flexor tendon plays.

Causes.—The direct exciting causes of navicular disease are not yet fully known, but the factors which predispose to its development may be briefly mentioned as follows:—(1) Irregularity in work, especially standing idle for long periods and then being put to fast or severe work; (2) Allowing the feet to become narrow, upright, and contracted at the heels, through bad shoeing; (3) Absence of frog pressure, such as when high calkins or very thick heels are worn; (4) Allowing the toe to grow very long and so throw undue strain upon the back tendons; (5) Excessive concussion upon hard ground, such as that to which the feet of cab-horses are constantly exposed; and (6) Hereditary influences probably act by lowering the vital resistance of the bones of the feet.

The condition is commonest in horses of the carriage type, although it is very often seen in ponies, hackneys, and other light breeds. It is very seldom seen in heavy draught animals, and when it does occur it is generally in those that have to work at the trot in towns.

It is thought that absorption of toxins by the system, during or following influenza or strangles, or perhaps after unnoticed attacks of rheumatism, may act as the actual cause by altering the density of the bone and rendering it less able to withstand the stress to which it is normally subjected.

Symptoms.—Navicular disease usually develops so slowly that the owner has considerable difficulty in remembering exactly when the first symptoms were noticed. In fact, little or no importance may be attached to the almost characteristic 'pointing' of one or both fore-feet, because 'he has *always* done that'. This indicates the first marked symptom: viz. 'pointing', which consists of the horse resting the affected foot (or feet) by placing it a short distance in advance of the other when standing in harness or in the stable. When both feet are affected, each is alternately pointed. Later, the horse may go lame or be tender on his feet at times, but with a rest he generally becomes sound again. As the disease advances, he may either start off in the mornings stiff and become better with exercise as he warms to his work, or he may commence sound but become lame as the day goes on. It depends upon the situation and extent of the ulceration. Sooner or later, however, there comes a time when he will go permanently 'pottery', or 'groggy'. The length of the stride decreases and there is difficulty in advancing the feet, as to suggest that the shoulder is the seat of the lesion. When made to turn, the horse pivots round on the fore-feet instead of lifting them, and when made to back, drags the toes. If the wearing shoe of such a horse is examined it is usually found to be more worn at the toe than at the heels. In fact a 'groggy' horse may wear his shoes quite thin at the toes before the heels show much sign of wear at all. In the final stages the horse becomes distinctly lame and unfit for work. When observed in the stable it is noticed to be continually shifting from one foot on to the other, and the resting foot is placed well out in front. In this state, if made to perform some violent exertion, the navicular bone sometimes fractures, and the foot cannot be placed upon the ground, or the tendon ruptures with equally severe results.

Treatment.—Old methods, for which good results were claimed, have proved useless in extensive modern trials. Good results sometimes follow any line of treatment, not because of any specificity of the treatment, but because adhesion has accidentally occurred between the tendon and the bone, thereby eliminating the friction which causes the pain.

In order to make the animal workable, it is customary to perform the operation of neurectomy (un-nerving), which consists of section of the plantar or median nerve of the limb. In a favourable case, following operation, the horse becomes apparently sound, although the diseased condition is still at work in the bone. No pain is felt, and the horse is fit for light work at slow paces. The feet require constant attention to ensure that no stones, nails, etc., lodge in the hoof, for even when these inflict serious damage the horse still goes sound, not feeling the pain.

More recently, success has been claimed for injections of hydrocortisone. (*See Vet. Record*, Dec. 16, 1961.)

NEAR EAST ENCEPHALITIS.—A tick-borne virus infection of horses, donkeys; less frequently of cattle and sheep. Convulsions/paralysis may follow fever and precede death.

NECK is that portion of the body which extends from the anterior limit of the chest to the base of the skull. Its main function is to support the head, for which special provision is made by the strong '*ligamentum nuchæ*', a powerful ligamentous sheet stretching from the spines of the withers to the posterior part of the occipital bone. This, being very elastic, takes the strain off the muscles running along the top of the neck, and enables an animal to carry its head without undue fatigue. In the lower part of the neck lie the trachea and the gullet—passages for the air and food. In all mammalian animals, whether the giraffe or the mouse, there are seven cervical vertebræ; down through the bony rings of these runs the cervical portion of the spinal cord, from which proceed the nerves that control the movements of the neck and to some extent the fore-limbs.

On the under surface of the neck can be felt the larynx, close behind the level of the angles of the lower jaw, and extending downward from it is the trachea or windpipe. Lying at first immediately above the trachea, but later inclined to the left side (usually), is the œsophagus or gullet, whose situation can be well seen when a horse is drinking water. Running along on either side in the groove just above the trachea (called the 'jugular groove') there is the jugular vein and, deeper in, the carotid artery—blood-vessels of the head and upper neck. Lying in connection with the first ring of the trachea are the lobes of the thyroid gland, while situated at various places down the neck are the cervical lymph glands. (*See also* MUSCLES, LARYNX, AIR PASSAGES, BONES, etc.)

NECROPSY (νεκρός, a dead body; ὄψις, a view) is another name for autopsy or *post-mortem* examination. (*See* AUTOPSY.)

NECROSIS (νέκρωσις, a state of death) means death of a limited portion of tissue. (*See also* NECROSIS (BACILLARY).)

NECROSIS (BACILLARY), or NECROBACILLOSIS, is the name given to infection with *Fusiformis necrophorus*. The organism is very widespread through Nature, and is found as a normal harmless inhabitant of the alimentary system in health. When it gains entrance to the body it generally produces sporadic effects in one particular animal, but upon occasion its passage through an animal so enhances its virulence that it becomes capable of spreading disease to other healthy animals which are ordinarily immune. In all cases it gains entrance into the tissues through a breach in their continuity; scratches, bruises, wounds, ulcers, burns, or other injuries to the skin afford a place of entrance for the germs, and when once established they are difficult to eliminate. In the intestinal canal the organisms enter through minute scratches or ulcers in the epithelial covering of the mucous membrane, or through larger lesions in some cases, and set up their effects locally. Sometimes the bacilli get into the blood-stream, are carried to distant parts of the body such as liver or lungs, and form disseminated abscesses in these parts. The typical result is the death of the cells of the area and their partial or complete adherence to the living cells around. A crust of dead cells forms, and under this the germs multiply and produce further cell death by the elaboration of a toxin which kills living tissue with which it comes into contact. In this way the diseased (or necrotic) process spreads deeper and deeper, the germs penetrating further and further into the body and spreading over gradually enlarging areas of the surface. A characteristic odour (which is said to resemble a mixture of old cheese and glue) is associated with the process of bacillary necrosis, but it is not always in evidence.

A very large number of diseased conditions among animals are due to the *F. necrophorus*, either alone, or associated with filterable virus, streptococci, staphylococci, or pyogenic bacilli, and the slow healing of comparatively slight wounds is often due to its activity. Among the more important particular conditions for which it is partly or wholly responsible are the following:

Horses: Cracked heels and Necrosis of the coronet;
Fistulous withers (*see* FISTULOUS WITHERS);
Abscesses in lungs and liver;
Poll evil;
Quittor (*see* QUITTOR);
Ulceration of intestines;
Joint-ill (*see* JOINT-ILL);

Cattle: Foul-in-the-foot (*see* FOUL-IN-THE-FOOT);
Calf diphtheria (*see* CALF DIPHTHERIA);
Multiple abscess formation in the liver;
Joint-ill;
Necrotic pneumonia of calves associated with white scour (*see* WHITE SCOUR IN CALVES);

Sheep: Orf or Oof (*see* ORF);
Necrosis of the skin of the head;

Pigs : Ulcers of swine fever (*see* SWINE FEVER) ;
Foot-rot, or Foot-foul ;

Dogs : Necrotic dermatitis ;
Pyorrhœa (*see* PYORRHŒA) ;

Fowls : Avian diphtheria, or Roup (*see* AVIAN DIPHTHERIA) ;

Rabbits : Schmorl's disease, or Necrobacillosis :

and in addition to these, it is very often found in diseased conditions of bones, tendons, ligaments, cartilage, or other varieties of connective tissue.

In a general way, among the above conditions those that affect the skin or surface tissues of the body are not immediately dangerous to life, while those that affect the mucous membranes, or some part of the internal organs of the body, very often end fatally.

The conditions mentioned (where reference is not made to other sections) will be briefly considered here.

CRACKED HEELS and **NECROSIS OF THE CORONET** are two conditions in which the lesions are of the same nature but situated in different parts of the foot. They are very common in the horse, usually sporadic but sometimes spreading from one horse to others in the same stable, occur during the winter time especially, and may cause death of the horse through infection spreading to the lungs. In muddy, wet, or frosty weather, when horses have to stand out-of-doors for long periods, the skin of the coronet or in the hollow of the heel becomes softened or damaged, the necrosis bacilli gain entrance, and a lesion appears. In some cases treads, bruises, injuries from calkins or frost studs, and punctured wounds of the feet become infected with dung or soil containing the necrosis germs, with the same result. The horse becomes very lame, and if the feet are examined an area varying in size from a shilling to a five-shilling piece is seen, usually affecting the skin of some part of the coronet. It is painful on pressure, cold to the touch, of a bluish or greenish colour, and when pressed a little foul-smelling pus can be forced from under the necrotic surface. With prompt treatment, which consists of the removal of the dead surface of skin and the application of strong antiseptics such as iodine, healing commences and the case recovers. When neglected, however, large areas of the skin may slough off, leaving purulent discharging sores and perhaps exposing the tendons or other structures below, or the infection may gain the general circulation and set up severe symptoms of ' blood-poisoning '. In the latter case the horse stands holding the affected limb off the ground ; the temperature is high ; breathing and pulse-rate are fast ; the appetite is lost ; the appearance is indicative of great suffering, and the animal is often bathed in perspiration. Death may follow in a few days, or the condition may become chronic, when there is much loss of flesh, great weakness, and finally death from exhaustion. In some of the acute cases restlessness and even delirium may be observed. In other cases general symptoms are not seen, but the process of necrosis penetrates deeper and deeper into tissues about the coronet, until the lateral cartilages or the fibrous tissue around them becomes invaded, and a quittor results.

ABSCESS FORMATION in the lungs or the liver of the horse may result from cracked heels or may originate through spreading of infection from the intestines. In either case, numerous small abscesses form throughout these organs, and death usually follows in a few days from pneumonia or acute hepatitis. As in practically all conditions of necrosis of the internal organs, treatment is hopeless. (*See* PNEUMONIA.)

ULCERATION OF THE INTESTINES may follow when an animal has received a dose of some irritant poison which is not sufficient to cause immediate death, although enough to destroy the vitality of the mucous membrane. The symptoms are those of enteritis, and usually consist of acute blood-stained diarrhœa, severe straining, and signs of per-acute fever.

MULTIPLE ABSCESS FORMATION in the liver in the ox is often due to infection of that organ with necrosis bacilli which have invaded the blood-stream from the intestines, and have been carried to the liver by the portal vein. The condition is often found in abattoirs in animals which showed no characteristic symptoms before death. The condition, even when it can be diagnosed before death, is untreatable.

NECROSIS OF THE SKIN OF THE HEAD of sheep is a condition which is common in some seasons and in some districts. It is somewhat like orf, but it attacks sheep of all ages, and those belonging to hill as well as lowland flocks. It is said to be commonest in wet seasons, and in areas where the land is badly drained or heavily manured. It is caused by the necrosis bacillus, and becomes infectious in a flock.

Symptoms.—The first signs are usually

those of dullness and depression. One or two sheep separate themselves from the rest, or lag behind when the flock is being driven. When examined they are found to be salivating freely at the mouth ; eyes and nostrils show a discharge, and the eyelids are often so swollen that the eyes are closed. The appetite is lost ; the respiration is panting ; temperature is high ; the pulse is fast ; and the skin and fleece become harsh and dry. In a short while patches of skin on the face, cheeks, forehead, or on other parts of the head, become swollen and purple in colour. A day later these patches are scabby or scaly on the surface, and a small amount of pus exudes from under them. In the course of time the skin from the patches falls or is rubbed off, and a raw, red, angry-looking sore results. Contiguous sores become confluent, and large areas of the head are exposed. The feet are not affected in typical cases. Complications such as pneumonia, or mammitis in suckling ewes, often arise, and result in a fatal termination.

Treatment.—As the disease spreads from one sheep to another, the affected members of the flock should be isolated as soon as the symptoms are seen. Folds, lambing pens, and troughs, which they have used, should be disinfected before healthy sheep are allowed to use them. The healthy flock should be taken on to fresh clean pastures, and each sheep should be examined once daily. As new cases are found they also are eliminated from the healthy. If the time of the year and the local circumstances are favourable, it is wise to dip all the healthy sheep, paying some attention to the head.

Affected sheep should be caught one by one, and the scabs should be removed by a piece of wood shaped like a knife-blade, in such a way that as little damage is sustained by the underlying tissues as possible. Each area is then painted with crystal violet.

FOUL-IN-THE-FOOT, or FOOT-FOUL, or FOOT-ROT, sometimes affects the feet of pigs that have been driven for long distances over hard roads and then have been housed in dirty badly littered piggeries. It also occasionally affects pigs that have been bought through the open store market, where it is probably contracted from similar causes. It is due to the bacillus of necrosis, if not wholly, at least in part. Its symptoms and treatment are essentially the same as those of 'Foul-in-the-foot of cattle', which see.

NECROTIC DERMATITIS in the dog's skin is characterised by the formation of numerous small abscesses in the skin, which on bursting discharge a small amount of blood-tinged thin pus, and leave fistulæ. The discharge contains the bacillus of necrosis and sometimes other organisms. It is often seen about the anus, the tail, the feet, hocks, elbows, outer surfaces of the stifles, and the tips of the ears, but it may arise upon almost any part of the body. It is commonest in old sporting dogs that are past the most vigorous period of their lives, have become fat, and lie about on hard floors for the greater part of the day. The most satisfactory method of treatment is to excise the whole area of the affected skin if this is not too large. Otherwise the fistulæ must be opened and their internal passages, cavities, etc., curetted or cauterised. The use of sulpha drugs and autogenous vaccines are other methods of dealing with this condition. When the areas affected are very large, it is more humane to destroy the animal.

SCHMORL'S DISEASE, or NECRO-BACILLOSIS OF RABBITS, is a condition which attacks both tame and wild rabbits, and also occurs in rats and a number of other wild animals, from any of which it may be contracted by dogs or cats. It is due to the necrosis bacillus, but is usually associated with the presence of large numbers of round worms in the stomach and intestines. It manifests itself either by the formation of necrotic patches about the lips, nostrils, eyelids, throat, and front of the chest, or else by abscess formation in various parts of the body. In the case of tame rabbits, the stock should be separated into apparently healthy in-contacts and healthy non-contacts, while every affected animal should be killed and the hutches thoroughly disinfected. In warrens, when the disease appears the rabbits may be eradicated by shooting or poison, but dogs or ferrets should not be employed. No dogs should have access to infected warrens, and all destroyed rabbits should be burned.

(See also sections to which reference has been made above.)

NECROTIC ENTERITIS.—A condition of unweaned and older pigs, characterised by scouring. It may closely resemble Paratyphoid.

The lesions are in the cæcum and ileum. (*See also under* ILEUM.)

Cause.—Probably a vitamin B deficiency, often associated with a chronic infection. Cold, damp, dirty surroundings appear to predispose to Necrotic Enteritis.

Research in Canada has demonstrated an apparent relationship between necrotic enteritis and infestation with Œsophagostomum worms, which stimulate pathogenic bacteria.

The following table is reproduced with acknowledgements to Mr. M. G. Pay.

A SUMMARY OF DIAGNOSTIC DIFFERENCES BETWEEN *Salmonella choleræ-suis* INFECTION AND NECROTIC ENTERITIS

Necrotic enteritis	*S. choleræ-suis*
Diarrhœa prominent feature	Diarrhœa occasional
Chronic wasting	Per-acute septicæmic deaths
No discoloration of extremities	Purple discoloration of extremities
S. choleræ-suis rarely found in organs	*S. choleræ-suis* easily found in organs
Lesions in small intestine consistent	Small intestine lesions uncommon
No prevention with *S. choleræ-suis* vaccine	Prevented with vaccine
Arsanilic acid and oxytetracycline in feed useful as medication	Oral medicaments useless
Larger pigs more resistant	Larger pigs more prone to

NECROTIC ENTERITIS IN CHICKENS.—This has been reported in Australia, among broilers, associated with *Clostridium perfringens* and probably some defect in nutrition.

NECROTIC STOMATITIS (*see* CALF DIPHTHERIA).

NEGRI BODIES are comparatively large rounded bodies which stain by special methods found in nerve cells in the brains of dogs and other animals which have died of rabies contracted under natural conditions. They are not present in cases affected with 'fixed virus'. The diagnosis of rabies once depended upon their demonstration in the affected animal. Negri Bodies are one form of Inclusion Bodies. (*See* RABIES.)

NEMATODE (*νῆμα*, thread) is a general term applied to the parasitic *Nemathelminthes*, which include the round worms, as distinct from the *Platyhelminthes*, or flat worms. (*See* PARASITES.)

'NEMATODE POISONING.'—In the U.S.A. larvæ of *Anguina agrostis* on Chewing's fescue in immature hay has caused an outbreak of poisoning in cattle. Symptoms included knuckling of the fetlocks, head tucked between the forelegs, recumbency, convulsions, and death.

NEMATODIRUS.—Parasitic worms of sheep (and calves in the case of *N. battus*). (*See* PARASITES, p. 660.)

NEMBUTAL (PENTOBARBITONE) (Sodium ethyl/methylbutyl barbiturate).—A white crystalline powder, soluble in water, and used for its narcotic and anæsthetic effects.

First used as a general anæsthetic in veterinary surgery in America in 1931, nembutal was brought to the notice of the veterinary profession in the United Kingdom by Professor J. G. Wright, who studied and improved the technique of its administration.

Nembutal has been used to produce anæsthesia in all the domestic animals including the fowl, but it is not recommended for horses,* calves, or sheep. For anæsthesia in the dog and cat, however, nembutal is very extensively employed, and is usually given by the intravenous route—a method which permits of varying depths of anæsthesia being obtained and the avoidance of overdosage. The drug may also be given by intra-peritoneal injection or by mouth; narcosis being then slower in onset (8 to 20 minutes), and occasionally preceded by some degree of excitement, while the dose has to be an estimate calculated on the basis of bodyweight.

Deep anæsthesia with nembutal may last for an hour, being followed by 2 to 7 hours of narcosis.

* 'In my opinion the place of the barbiturates in equine anæsthesia is as continuation or deepening anæsthetics and in these connections I use them widely. For abdominal operations such as ovariectomy or cryptorchidectomy, it is my practice, having induced light anæsthesia with chloral hydrate, to deepen and maintain it by the intravenous injection of pentobarbitone sodium. In a horse of 11 cwt., to which chloral hydrate in a dosage of 6·5 g. per cwt. has already been given, an initial dose of 20 gr. of nembuta is injected in a time of about 1½ minutes. Should sluggish response to stimuli persist or return

an additional 10 gr. is injected as required. In prolonged operations such as supraspinous bursitis as much as 60 gr. has been given during its course. The action of the two drugs is summative, each will be detoxicated or excreted separately and the total recumbency period will not be significantly greater than would have been the case with chloral hydrate alone.' (Professor J. G. Wright, 1958.)

NEOARSPHENAMINE.—A drug effective against Blackhead in turkeys.

NEOMYCIN.—An antibiotic obtained from *Streptomyces fradiæ*. It must not be given by injection, owing to resulting kidney damage.

NEOPLASM (νέος, new; πλάσσω, I mould) means literally ' a new formation ', and is applied to tumours in general.

NEPHRECTOMY (νεφρός, kidney ἐκ, out ; τέμνω, I cut) is the name given to the operation by which one of the kidneys is removed. (*See* KIDNEY, DISEASES OF.)

NEPHRITIS (νεφρός, kidney) means inflammation of the kidneys. (*See* KIDNEY, DISEASES OF ; LEPTOSPIROSIS.)

NEPHROLITHIASIS (νεφρός, kidney ; λιθος, stone) is the term applied to the condition where a stone is present in the plevis of the kidney.

NEPHROPTOSIS (νεφρός, kidney ; πτῶσις, falling) means the condition in which a kidney is movable or ' floating '. (*See* KIDNEY, DISEASES OF.)

NEPHROSIS, INFECTIOUS AVIAN.—Possibly caused by a variant of the infectious bronchitis virus, this is a disease of chickens mainly 4 to 9 weeks old, and gives rise to a mortality of up to 15 per cent. The carcase is found to be dehydrated ; the kidneys swollen and the tubules and ureters often distended with urates. In some outbreaks depression may be observed ; in others mild respiratory symptoms.

NEPHROTOMY (νεφρός, kidney ; τέμνω, I cut) means the operation of cutting into the kidney, in search of calculi, or for some other reason.

NERVES (*nervus*, a nerve).—The nervous system consists partly of fibres and partly of cells. The fibres can be looked upon as long processes extending from nerve-cells, which transmit impulses originating in the cell to some distant part of the body. The nerve-cells are situated mainly in the grey matter of the brain and spinal cord, while the white matter of these parts, as well as the nerve trunks which run through the body, are made up of nerve-fibres. The brain and spinal cord are often spoken of together as the ' central nervous system ' ; the nerves which proceed from them are named the ' cerebro-spinal nerves ' or the ' peripheral nerves ' ; while the system composed of ganglia and intricate nerve plexuses, which controls the action of involuntary organs such as stomach, intestines, variouss ecretory glands, the blood-vessels, heart, and others, and which is situated mainly in the neck, thorax, and abdomen, is known as the ' sympathetic nervous system '.

The nerve-cells originate, or receive, impulses and impressions of various kinds, which are conveyed from them to muscles, blood-vessels, etc., by ' efferent nerves ', or are received by them through ' afferent nerves ', coming from the skin, organs of sense, joints, muscles, etc. The sympathetic system is mainliy concerned with the movements and other functions of the internal organs, secreting glands, etc., whose activities proceed independently of, though related with, the central nervous system. It is very important to realise that nerve-fibres, whatever their situation, are only able to transmit impulses *in one direction*, viz. either towards the central system or away from it, and that nerve trunks, which consist of collections of nerve-fibres, may be composed of both afferent and efferent fibres.

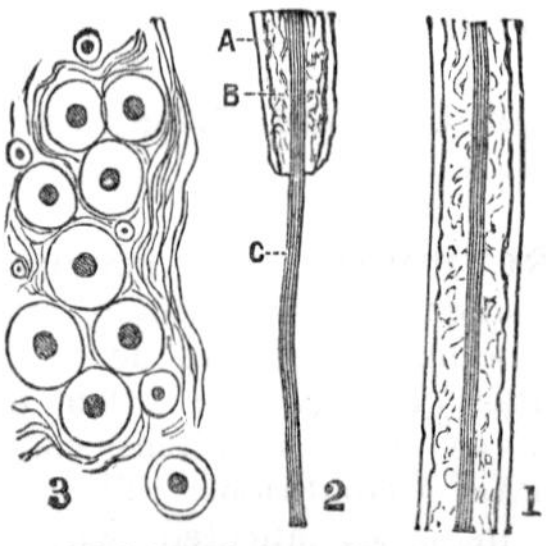

1, Medullated nerve-fibre ; 2, similar fibre in which *A* points to the neurolemma, *B* to the medullary sheath, *C* to the axis-cylinder ; 3, transverse section through part of a nerve, showing the varying sizes of the nerve-fibres. Magnified × 400. (Turner's *Anatomy*.)

Structure.—(1) *Nerve-fibres.*—The nerves of the body vary in size from the sciatic, which in the horse is almost as thick as a man's finger somewhat flattened, to the smallest twigs of nerve which are distributed to tiny areas of the body, and may consist of only one or two fibres. A large nerve consists of an outer strong fibrous sheath which connects the nerve to the structures through which it runs, and which is called the *epineurium*, within which lie bundles of nerve-fibres separated from one another by partitions of fibrous tissue in which run tiny capillaries which nourish the nerve. Each of these bundles is surrounded by a sheath of its own, known as the *perineurium*, while the delicate fibrous tissue that lies between the nerve-fibres themselves is known as the *endoneurium*. Running throughout the trunk there are blood-vessels and lymph-vessels, some of which pass into the spaces between the fibres lying in the fibrous tissue, and the large nerves have small sensory nerves ramifying in the epineurium. The finest subdivisions of the nerves are called nerve-fibres, and are of two kinds—*medullated* and *non-medullated*.

Medullated fibres, or white fibres, are characterised by the presence of a ' medullary sheath '. This is a layer of fatty substance which encircles the essential part of the nerve, the ' axis-cylinder ', and is itself encircled by an outer membranous sheath known as the ' neurolemma ' or ' nucleated sheath '. The medullary sheath is composed of soft, white, fatty substance, and to it is due the white colour of such nerves as are medullated. In the peripheral nerve-fibres it is interrupted at intervals of about 1/12th of an inch by short gaps, known as the ' nodes of Ranvier ', but across these gaps the axis-cylinder and the neurolemma are continuous. They bear some resemblance to the nodes seen in a cane of bamboo. The medullary sheath is usually regarded as fulfilling the purpose of an insulating investment of the axis-cylinder, preventing nerve impulses passing along one nerve-fibre from influencing other fibres in the vicinity. The axis-cylinder is the conducting part of the fibre ; it appears to be longitudinally striated, almost as if it were composed of fibrils. Non-medullated fibres are much thinner than the average medullated fibres, and differ from the latter in that they possess no medullary sheath. They are greyish in colour, frequently branch (medullated fibres seldom branch), and possess numerous nuclei. They are found most plentifully in the nerves of the sympathetic system just before they reach their destinations, although they are present in small numbers in practically all nerves.

(2) *Nerve-cells*, from one of which springs each nerve-fibre, are found in the grey matter of the brain and spinal cord, and in little groups on the course of some of the peripheral nerves, where they often form nodular swellings which are called ' ganglia '. Specialised nerve-cells are also found in connection with the organs of the special senses. They vary much in shape and size, some being amongst the largest cells in the body. The most common appearance is that of a large granular cell containing an oval nucleus, and running out at various points into long, usually branched processes. In a typical nerve-cell all of these processes except one, called the ' axon ', ' axis-cylinder ', ' neuron ', or ' nerve-fibre process ', branch again and again like the limbs of a tree, and are brought in apposition to similar processes from other cells to form what is known as a ' synapse '. These branching processes are known as ' dendrites ', ' dendrons ', or ' dendritic processes '. It is by means of synapses that communicating messages, or impulses, are conveyed from one nerve-cell to another. The axon is the long fibrillated structure which may either become a non-medullated nerve-fibre or becomes clothed with a medullary sheath and forms the axis-cylinder of a medullated fibre. The body of a nerve-cell, or more correctly the cell-body or ' cyton ', contains peculiar angular masses called *Nissl's granules*, which vary in size and shape in different cells and according to the activity of the cell ; thus in fatigued nerve-cells, and in those in which the axon has been cut, the granules become disintegrated or may be almost completely absent. Running through the nerve-cell there are extremely fine canals through which flows lymph which nourishes the cell, and in certain enormously large cells there are tiny blood-vessels penetrating into the nerve-cell.

In the cerebrum the cells are distinctly pyramidal in shape, the axon is extremely long, and there are usually many dendritic processes ; such cells are usually called ' multipolar '. Other cells are ' bipolar ', *i.e.* they possess only two processes, one of which is the axon ; while there are also ' unipolar cells ', possessing one process only, *e.g.* the cells in the ganglia on the dorsal roots of the spinal nerves, where each single process divides in a T-shaped manner. Lying here and there in amongst the important nerve-cells in the grey matter there are other cells, known as 'neuroglia cells', which are provided with innumerable processes running in all directions and forming a dense interlocking feltwork which acts as a supporting structure for the nerve-cells and fibres. They are of two kinds; some have branched processes, and others have processes which do not divide.

(3) *Nerve-endings.* — Each nerve-fibre proceeds from a nerve-cell to end in a definite organ, to or from which it carries a special kind of nerve impulse. The manner of ending of a nerve-fibre varies in different cases. The medullated nerve-fibres upon reaching the involuntary muscles, of the intestines, for example, end by forming an intricate network, or plexus, between the layers of muscle-fibres. In some instances they may pass into the fibres, but as a rule the network lies around the muscle-fibres which it actuates. In the heart muscle the arrangement is similar. In the voluntary muscles each motor nerve-fibre splits into smaller branches which pass to adjacent muscle-fibres. Each of these branches penetrates a muscle-fibre, the medullary sheath ceasing at the level of the sarcolemma, and the axis-cylinder spreads out into an end-plate composed of granular material and possessing what appear to be nuclei. The sensory nerves of muscle are distributed to the muscle-spindles, which are large fusiform bodies possessing a connective tissue sheath externally and ramifications of nerve filaments within. The function of these muscle-spindles seems to be one of acquainting the higher centres of the state of contraction of the muscle, and they also probably receive messages of pain when the muscle is injured. The ending of the sensory nerve-fibres in the skin is more complex. Most of these end not on the surface but in the true skin below the cuticle. Each nerve-fibre here forms a little bulb, called a tactile corpuscle, which lies within a capsule of connective or other tissue. Inside some of these tactile corpuscles the nerve-fibre may form a complicated network, while in others it ends abruptly. In the snout of the pig the sensory nerves end in discs; in the cornea of the eye they form a plexus in the deeper layers with little tendrils of nerve passing between the surface cells and ending amongst them; in the conjunctiva of most animals the endings are oblong or cylindrical bulb-like swellings; in the skin covering the bills of some birds and in the tongue of the duck the endings are called *corpuscles of Grundy*, and are arranged as three or more cells lying superimposed with tactile discs between them; and in other places there are other kinds of terminations, such as *genital corpuscles* in the external organs of both sexes, *articular corpuscles* in connection with joints, in the lips there are end-bulbs, and so on. In some parts specialised large bodies, known as *Pacinian corpuscles*, are found. In these there is an outer coating of connective tissue within which are layers arranged like the coats of an onion. A single medullated nerve-fibre passes to each and appears as its stalk, penetrates the outer coat, and the axis-cylinder either spreads into an arborisation or ends as a bulbous swelling. These corpuscles are particularly numerous in the mesentery of the cat, and are also found in the deeper layers of the skin, in the periosteum of bones near tendons and ligaments, and in connective tissue in other parts of the body. It is probable that Grundy corpuscles are either degenerate or imperfect forms of Pacinian corpuscles.

Development and repair.—The whole nervous system is developed from the epiblast or outer layer of the embryo, the brain and spinal cord arising from an infolding of the surface along the back to form a tube, and all the nerves are budded out directly or indirectly from this primary neural tube, increasing in length until they reach the skin, muscle, glands, or other tissues to which they are distributed. Each nerve-fibre, as already stated, is the process of a nerve-cell, and if the nerve be cut that portion of its fibres which is separated from the cells immediately starts to degenerate. The degeneration is first seen in the medullary sheath, if that be present, but later involves the whole nerve-fibre. Eventually the fibre shows as an outer sheath containing numerous droplets of a fatty substance. Within a few weeks or days, however, from the cut end of the nerve each severed fibre begins to sprout out new delicate fibres, sometimes as many as three new axis-cylinders growing from what was originally one. Each axis-cylinder becomes clothed with a new medullary sheath, and grows down through the old nerve-sheath, through any scar tissue that is not too dense, and eventually down to the organs or tissues which the original nerve supplied before section. The process is hastened when the cut ends of a nerve trunk have been brought together by careful suturing, so that no scar tissue has to be pierced, and there have been cases where, when the suturing has been performed before degeneration has had a chance to become established, immediate action has been restored to the muscles supplied by the nerve. It is on this principle that attempts have been made to restore the function of the vocal cords in the horse affected with roaring, but so far they have not been successful in cases occurring naturally.

Functions of nerves.—The greater part of the bodily activity originates in nerve-cells, either in the brain, spinal cord, or in ganglia, and during the process food materials are used up in considerable amounts. Consequent upon the activity in nerve-cells impulses are transmitted down the nerve-fibres to muscles, glands, blood-vessels, etc., and the tissue cells in these parts perform their appropriate work. These impulses are transmitted from the nerve centres to the tissues by the 'efferent' set of nerves (*e*, short form of *ex*, from; *fero*, I carry), *i.e.* by the motor nerves. At the same time the various kinds of sensory nerve-endings, whether these be situated in the organs of the senses, in Pacinian or other corpuscles, in end-bulbs, or in other receptive structures, are being stimulated by changing local or general, external or internal conditions, and 'afferent' (*ad*, to; *fero*, I carry) nerve-fibres transmit impulses of sensation (whether perceptible to the mind or not) towards the cells from which they spring, and so onwards to the higher nerve centres. The efferent nerves carrying outgoing impulses can be compared to the electric wires that explode a mine, for the nerve impulse produces a sudden chemical change in the tissues to which it passes; while the afferent nerve impulses are not unlike the electric current which travels along a telephone wire to affect the receiver at the other end. Nevertheless, it must not be understood that the impulse passing along a nerve is a form of motion similar to an electric current in all respects, for nerve impulses only travel at the comparatively slow rate of about 100 feet per second; they are probably more like the motion of air particles which produce sound.

In many cases muscular activity results from a train of events somewhat as follows: sensory nerve-endings on some part of the skin receive a sensation of pain; afferent impulses pass by the sensory nerves to the spinal cord, and after rearrangement are sent to the brain. During the change in the spinal cord, motor cells in the vicinity have been activated and efferent motor impulses are flashed down the motor nerves to the muscles of the area, and the injured part is violently moved away from the situation of danger. Meanwhile the brain has received the sensation, the mind becomes aware of the injury through the familiar unpleasant sensation of pain, and, if necessary, measures are taken which may involve the movement of all the skeletal muscles, and the animal struggles or runs away. The process is actually much more complicated than this, and will be further explained later.

The important fact that the ventral and dorsal roots of each spinal nerve differs in function was discovered in 1822 by Sir Charles Bell. He found that when the ventral roots were cut the power of movement in a part of the body was destroyed; while division of the dorsal roots abolished sensation in the parts concerned. Therefore he concluded that the ventral roots consist of motor fibres going to muscles, and the dorsal roots of sensory fibres from the skin. Actually, the ventral roots consist of efferent fibres passing to muscles, blood-vessels, secreting glands, etc., and the dorsal roots of afferent fibres bringing impulses from skin, muscles, tendons, bones, joints, and other organs.

Sensation in man is popularly supposed to be derived through the five senses—sight, smell, hearing, taste, and touch, but in addition to these, impulses are carried by special nerve-fibres and are converted in the brain into sensations which furnish impressions of movement, locality, proximity to danger, a sense of pain, and a sense of heat and cold, and it is very probable that in wild animals especially, and in domestic animals to a great extent, these secondary sensations and the apparatus by which they are received, are very much more acute and highly organised than in man. What is commonly spoken of as 'instinct' may ultimately prove to be a greater power of the appreciation of external conditions, rather than an inborn hereditary 'something' which advises the animal to perform, or not to perform, certain acts.

The connection between the sensory and motor systems of nerves, already briefly referred to, is important. The simplest form of nerve action is that known as *automatic action*, which is carried out by the *autonomic nerves*. In this a part of the nervous system, controlling, for example, the lungs, goes on rhythmically discharging from its motor cells sufficient impulses to keep the muscles of respiration in regular action, influenced only by occasional impressions from various sources, which increase or diminish its activity according to the needs of the body. The motions of the stomach and intestines, the contractions and dilatations of the blood-vessels, the beating of the heart, the control of the secretions from all glands, the action of ureters, uterus, the pulsation of the liver and spleen, and many other functions which are not normally under the control of the will, are carried out through the agency of the autonomic system.

In *reflex action* the parts engaged are a sensory nerve ending, say, in the skin of the horse's lower fore-limb ; a sensory nerve leading from it to the spinal cord in the region of the withers and base of neck, where it ends by splitting up into processes near the nerve-cells ; a nerve-cell, or a series of nerve-cells, stimulated by the sensory impulse, and motor nerves leading from the region of the spinal cord concerned down to the muscles of the upper part of the fore-limb, shoulder, etc. Imagine the part smartly struck with a light stick ; almost before the stick has left the spot the horse has snatched up its foot and replaced it. In fact, sometimes the events happen so suddenly that the horse is actually startled, not so much by the stick as by the fact that it has moved its foot. The spinal cord has carried out a definite action without any assistance or control by the brain. Reflex action is very much more highly developed in animals than it is in man ; the movements of wild animals, lightning-like in their rapidity, are made possible only by reflex action. The movements of man, even those of the perfectly trained athlete, are slow and very deliberate when compared with the swift suddenness of the falcon hawk swooping to strike at its prey, or to the 60-miles-an-hour speed of the charging lion, or to the agility of the startled antelope.

Voluntary action is much more complicated than reflex. The same mechanism is involved, but, in addition, the controlling power of the brain is brought into play. This exerts first of all an ' inhibitory ' or blocking effect which prevents immediate reflex action, and then the impulse, passing up to the cerebral hemispheres, sets up a secondary rearrangement of impulses in a series of cells there, the complexity of which depends upon the intellectual processes involved. Finally, the inhibition is removed and an impulse passes down to the motor cells of the spinal cord, and a muscle (or a set of muscles) is brought into play through the motor nerves.

The *trophic function* of nerves is another most important part of their activity, for it appears as if the constant passage of nerve impulses down the nerves of any part were necessary for proper nutrition. Thus, if sensory nerves be diseased or injured, ulceration of the skin, shedding of the hoofs, and other changes are liable to occur, while if the motor nerves to muscles are destroyed atrophy of the muscles, and finally almost complete disappearance of the muscle tissues, may be seen. This constitutes one of the dangers of the operation of neurectomy in the horse. For certain forms of lameness where pain may be present, but where there is no great structural change, it is sometimes advisable to cut the sensory nerves (neurectomy) of the limb ; as a rule the animal goes sound afterwards, since it does not feel the pain. But untoward sequelæ may arise through section of the trophic nerves which cannot be separated from the sensory nerves concerned, and the horse may shed its hoof, or an ulcerating sore which may appear will not heal. In the mule, this operation cannot be satisfactorily performed because the animal almost always commences to chew at the coronet, producing a large ugly wound which incapacitates it for further work. The cause of this behaviour has not been determined.

Nervous system.—The brain and the twelve pairs of cranial nerves are dealt with under BRAIN, the spinal cord and the origins of its nerves are treated under SPINAL CORD.

Each of the spinal nerves arises by two roots, a dorsal and a ventral, the dorsal being the larger and possessing a ganglion beyond which it joins the ventral root. The junction occurs before the nerve passes out of the bony canal or ' intervertebral foramen ', but it is outside the dura mater in all regions except the coccygeal. The size of the spinal nerves varies greatly; in the cervical and lumbar regions they are large, for in these places the nerve trunks which supply the limbs have their origins, and in the coccygeal (tail) region they are small, since they only supply a few fibres to the muscles and skin of the tail. Each spinal nerve divides into two main divisions either just within, or immediately after it leaves, the intervertebral foramen ; one of these, the dorsal branch, is small

NERVES

and is distributed to the muscles and skin of the back, the ventral branch is larger and supplies the muscles and skin of the lower parts of the body including the limbs. Each nerve is connected by a small communicating branch with one or more adjacent ganglia of the sympathetic system, and some ganglia, especially in the abdomen, are connected with two or even three spinal nerves. As already stated the dorsal root is sensory or afferent, and the ventral root motor or efferent. This arrangement obtains with variations in all animals; for illustration, the distribution of the nerves in the horse will be considered in some detail.

The ventral branches of spinal nerves do not run straight to the parts which they supply, but first enter into the formation of plexuses with other nerves. They are arranged in regions according to the parts of the spine from which they take origin; *i.e.* cervical, thoracic, lumbar, sacral, and coccygeal.

The *cervical nerves* at the beginning of the series, *i.e.* the first six, have dorsal branches distributed to the muscles and skin of the upper crest of the neck from the poll to the withers. The ventral branches form an irregular cervical plexus, which supplies muscles and skin, etc., in the lower part of the neck. The sixth has a large ventral root, one part of which enters into the formation of the brachial plexus, and another furnishes a radicle to the *phrenic nerve* which supplies the diaphragm, while the remainder of the ventral root of this nerve supplies muscular and skin branches. The dorsal roots of the seventh and eighth nerves are distributed to the skin and muscles of the withers and shoulders. Their very large ventral roots, along with the ventral roots of the first two thoracic nerves, form the *brachial plexus*, while the seventh adds the posterior radicle of the phrenic nerve. This latter runs through the chest cavity, following a different course on either side of the body, and ends by dividing into several large branches which are distributed to different parts of the diaphragm. The brachial plexus is formed by the union of the last two cervical and the first two thoracic ventral branches, and usually also receives small twigs from the sixth cervical, and, in addition to furnishing branches which supply some of the muscles of the root of the neck and shoulder and the skin of the front of the chest and arm, it gives off the following large nerves: suprascapular, musculocutaneous, median, ulnar, and radial. The suprascapular supplies the muscles lying on the outer aspect of the shoulder-blade. The musculo-cutaneous supplies the biceps and other muscles of the arm, and sends a large branch to the median. The median is the largest of the plexus as a rule, and descends the limb in company with the brachial artery. It is the chief nerve of sensation of the fore-limb, and is severed in the operation of median neurectomy. Its branches are distributed to the skin of the carpus, metacarpus, fetlock, and foot, but before reaching the level of the carpus it divides into a medial volar, and a branch which joins the ulnar to form the lateral volar nerve. Muscular branches are given off before it reaches the shoulder or soon after. The ulnar is the other sensory nerve of the limb. It runs down to the elbow and then is joined by the ulnar vessels, passes down the outside of the forearm to end by dividing into a superficial branch to the skin, and a deep branch to join the outer division of the median in the formation of the lateral volar nerve. At the level of the elbow it gives off a muscular branch to supply some of the muscles of the forearm. The radial nerve is a very large branch from the brachial plexus which winds round the shaft of the humerus to gain the flexor aspect of the elbow-joint. It is distributed to the muscles which maintain the limb in an upright position; *i.e.* the triceps, and the extensors of the carpus and digit. Injury to this nerve results in paralysis of these muscles, and constitutes what is known as 'radial paralysis', or 'dropped elbow'.

The *thoracic nerves* are 18 in number on either side of the horse. Each has a dorsal branch which supplies the skin and muscles of the back lying above the spinal column, and a ventral branch which runs down between a pair of ribs and is distributed to the intercostal muscles, to some of the muscles of the chest, to the diaphragm in the case of those towards the end of the series, and sensory branches pass to the skin of the chest and abdomen. The ventral roots of the first two thoracics concur with the cervicals in the formation of the brachial plexus as already noted.

The *lumbar nerves*, Nos. 1 and 2, are about the same size as the thoracics and are distributed in a similar manner, but the last four are much larger and help to form the lumbo-sacral plexus, as well as sending muscular branches to the muscles of the loins, etc.

The *sacral nerves*, five in number on each

side have small dorsal branches distributed to the skin and muscles of the croup, and large ventral branches, the first two of which unite with the last four lumbars to form the lumbo-sacral plexus, while the third and fourth, after first having united with each other, form the nerves that supply bladder, rectum, genital organs, and other structures in the vicinity. The fifth unites with the first coccygeal.

The *lumbo-sacral plexus* gives off the branches which supply the pelvic limb and the greater part of the pelvis. The nerves arising from the plexus are as follows :— femoral, obturator, cranial and caudal gluteals, and the great sciatic. The femoral passes outward and backward and ends by supplying the mass of muscle above the stifle known as the quadriceps. The obturator passes down the inside of the pelvis to the obturator foramen, runs through it along with the artery and vein of the same name, and is distributed to the muscles on the inside of the thigh. The cranial gluteal curves up through the sacro-sciatic foramen round the shaft of the ilium, and is distributed to the three gluteal muscles, tensor fascia lata, and the piriformis muscle. The caudal gluteal emerges from the pelvis along with the sciatic but nearer to the centre of the sacrum, and divides into two parts, one of which ends in the biceps of the leg, while the lower branch becomes the lateral cutaneous femoral which ends in the skin of the hip and thigh. The sciatic, or great sciatic, is the largest nerve in the body, and appears in company with the caudal gluteal, as a broad flat band often thicker than a man's finger. It passes downward and backward behind the hip joint and descends the thigh. In its descent it lies below the biceps femoris and above the semimembranosus and semitendinosus muscles. At the level of the heads of the gastrocnemius it becomes the tibial nerve, which divides about a hand's breadth from the point of the hock into the medial and lateral plantar nerves. These run down the limb, at first together but diverging at the hock, and supply the skin and other structures below this level. The sciatic nerve supplies practically the whole of the mass of muscle below the level of the stifle, and a good deal of that in the leg above this joint.

The *sympathetic system* is joined by a pair of small branches given off from each spinal nerve, quite close to the spine. The system consists of two parts. There is firstly, a pair of knotted cords running down the length of the vertebral column, and situated near the bodies of the vertebræ if not actually upon them, and containing three pairs of ganglia in the head region, two pairs in the neck, and after that one pair opposite each vertebra. From these two ganglionated cords innumerable branches are given off, and these unite, in the second place, to form complicated plexuses connected with the internal organs. In certain regions there are other large and small ganglia associated with various organs, and from these twigs pass off in all directions to other ganglia or plexuses near by. The chief plexuses of the body are as follows, the name indicating the situation in each case :— carotid and pharyngeal plexuses, in the neck ; aortic, cardiac, œsophageal, pulmonary, and coronary plexuses in the chest ; solar, cœliac, gastric, hepatic, splenic, cranial and caudal mesenteric, renal and adrenal, spermatic, utero-ovarian, and hypogastric or pelvic plexuses in the abdomen ; while there are other smaller peripheral plexuses in connection with the bladder, prostate, and vagina.

In the other domestic animals the general arrangement of the nervous system is somewhat similar to that of the horse, with modifications according to the variation in the size, shape, and arrangement of the various organs and tissues.

NERVES, INJURIES TO.—Owing to their protected situation in the body nerves are not so frequently injured as other structures, but they are liable to be involved particularly in large and deep wounds of the limbs of animals. Continued or repeated severe pressure upon a nerve trunk may be sufficient to damage it and result in paralysis ; severe bruising in which a nerve is driven against a bone with considerable force may produce paralysis or inflammation of the nerve ; a nerve may be severed along with other tissues in a deep wound ; fracture of a bone, such as the first rib, may produce rupture of any nerves that lie upon or near to it ; and other accidents may also involve the nerves of the part. A nerve may sometimes be injured at its origin before it leaves the brain or spinal cord by hæmorrhage or apoplexy. (*See also under* IMMUNISATION.)

Symptoms.—Usually, it is not until after a wound has healed that the injury to the nerve becomes obvious. In ' radial paralysis ', or in other cases where large and important motor nerves have been damaged, the resulting paralysis of the muscles they supply is seen at once. (*See* RADIAL PARALYSIS.) When a sensory nerve is injured, sensation is more or less destroyed in the part of the body supplied by the nerve. The extent of the paralysis depends upon the degree of injury. When a motor nerve is injured, and especially when it is severed, the muscles which it supplies lose their power of contracting, waste, and may eventually so degenerate that they almost disappear. If this occurs in a limb the animal is unable to bear full weight upon that limb, and goes lame as a consequence. In the case of unilateral ' facial paralysis ', which very often follows accidents in which the side of the face has been badly bruised, the muscles on one side become paralysed but those on the opposite side are unaffected. This absence of antagonism between the two sides results in the upper and lower lips, and the muscles around the nostrils, becoming drawn over towards the unaffected side, and the animal presents an altered facial expression. The ear on the injured side of the head very often hangs loosely and flaps back and forward with every movement of the head, and the eyelids on the same side are held half shut. Other results that sometimes follow nerve injury are :—an alteration in the appearance of the skin, the hair falls out, the surface becomes cold, glossy, and may ulcerate, due to an interference with the trophic functions ; permanent deformity of a limb, or other appendage, through removal of the antagonistic action of the paralysed muscles, as indicated above ; difficulty in swallowing, when the pharynx is affected ; permanent protrusion of the penis in paraphymosis ; paralysis and sloughing of the tail ; an intolerable itch in the parts originally supplied by the nerve, which induces the animal to chew persistently at a paw, foot, or other part ; and sometimes hyperæsthesia of an area of apparently quite healthy skin.

NEUROMA. (*See* NEUROMA.)

NEURITIS, or inflammation of a nerve may accompany injuries, or it may arise as the result of some general specific disease, such as strangles, distemper, or tuberculosis, and some cases occur without any assignable cause. There are cases, however (*e.g.*, when a large or important nerve is situated near to a developing abscess in which the nerve sheath becomes involved, causing paralysis of muscles, or excessive pain perhaps with lameness in a distant part of a limb), when definite nerve symptoms are seen, and diagnosis is possible. Persistent shaking of the head, with no obvious cause, is thought to be due to neuritis of the maxillary (sensory) nerve. (*Note.*— ' Sciatica ' in the horse (a neuritis affecting the great sciatic nerve) has been recorded as the cause of certain obscure forms of lameness of the hind limbs, but is of academic rather than of practical interest.)

NERVOUS DISEASE.—For information under this heading *see* sections, such as APOPLEXY ; BRAIN, DISEASES OF ; CHOREA ; EPILEPSY ; HYSTERIA ; NERVE INJURIES ; AUJESKY'S DISEASE ; PARALYSIS ; SPINAL CORD, DISEASES OF ; RABIES ; TETANUS ; DISTEMPER, etc.

NETTLE-RASH is another name for urticaria. (*See* URTICARIA.)

NEURECTOMY (νεῦρον, nerve ; ἐκτομή, excision) is the term applied to an operation in which part of a nerve is excised. The operation is sometimes performed to give relief from incurable lameness in the horse.

NEURILEMMA (νεῦρον, nerve ; λέμμα, sheath) is the thin membranous covering which surrounds every nerve-fibre.

NEURITIS (νεῦρον, a nerve) means inflammation affecting nerves or their sheaths. It is often followed by paralysis of the part supplied by the nerve, or by a local lack of sensation of a part of the skin, according to whether a motor or a sensory nerve has been involved. (*See* NERVES, INJURIES TO, *and under* IMMUNISATION.)

NEUROGLIA (νεῦρον, nerve ; γλία, glue).—A fine web of tissue and branching cells which supports the nerve-fibres and cells of the nervous system.

NEUROMA (νεῦρον, a nerve ; *-oma*, meaning tumour), means a tumour connected with a nerve, generally of a fibrous nature and very painful.

NEURONE (νεῦρον, nerve) is a modern name applied to a single unit of the nervous system, consisting of one nerve-cell, with all its processes, and the nerve-fibre or axon springing from it. (*See* NERVES.)

NEUROTROPIC VIRUS (νεῦρον, nerve ; τροπος from τρέπειν, to turn) is a virus, which shows a predilection for becoming localised in, and fixing itself to, nerve tissues. The best known of these is that of rabies, which, though present in saliva, is absent from blood and other body fluids. Rabies virus enters the body through torn nerve-fibres at the seat of an injury, such as a bite, and, growing along them, eventually reaches the spinal cord and brain. Other neurotropic viruses are those of louping-ill sheep, and Borna disease in horses and cattle.

NEWCASTLE DISEASE (Fowl Pest).—This is an acute febrile infectious disease of fowls, somewhat resembling fowl plague but caused by a separate and immunologically distinct virus. It was given this name because it was first recorded near Newcastle in 1926. It re-appeared in 1933, and was reintroduced into Britain in 1947 when frozen table poultry was—contrary to veterinary advice—imported from Poland and Hungary. Few species of birds can withstand a massive dose of virus, but except in the fowl the disease is usually mild. The domestic fowl is subject to the peracute 'Asiatic' form encountered in Britain in 1947. This, however, was eradicated in the early 1950s, leaving the acute form and a mild form in which symptoms can be so slight as to escape notice. The disease may be transmitted to humans and gives rise to a conjunctivitis. The incubation period varies from 4 to 11 days.

The high incidence of Newcastle disease has been associated with intensive rearing and particularly with broiler plants. The best of these are well run, with buildings suitably spaced, and facilities for safe disposal of carcases. In others the reverse has been true. Overcrowding of birds increases risk.

Since the compulsory slaughter policy was replaced in 1963 by one of voluntary vaccination, the number of confirmed outbreaks fell steadily from over 2,000 to under 100 in 1968, and to only 36 in 1969. An epidemic in Essex in 1970 was followed by outbreaks in 33 other counties in the same year, and the disease continued to cause heavy losses in 1971.

Symptoms.—Direct contact between a healthy bird and a diseased bird invariably results in infection. A marked drop in egg yield is often the first symptom, and the eggs may be misshapen and soft-shelled. Inappetance followed by somnolence, and later paralysis is noticed. A long, gasping inhalation through the opened beak is a characteristic symptom, and there is frequently a discharge of mucus from the nostrils. This is often accompanied by a yellowish white evil-smelling diarrhœa. Nervous twitching of the head and neck may be seen. A high death-rate among young birds is to be expected.

Treatment.—No curative treatment has proved of value, and in naturally affected flocks the mortality may reach 100 per cent. The disease is notifiable in the U.K. and suspected cases must be reported to the police. The bodies should be carefully disposed off by burning or burying in quicklime, and thorough disinfection carried out. If the disease is suspected overseas, several fowls should be sent to a laboratory for diagnosis. The H.I., or Hæmagglutination-Inhibition Test, is of great value.

Differential Diagnosis.—The disease must be distinguished from fowl plague, fowl cholera, and fowl pox. In cholera, the causative organism, *Pasteurella aviseptica*, is demonstrable in the blood. Pigeons are generally not susceptible to fowl plague but are readily affected with Newcastle disease. There is generally no well-marked period of illness in plague, but to differentiate accurately, laboratory tests must be carried out. The presence of Newcastle disease in flocks of turkeys and ducks may go unsuspected for some time, as symptoms may be very slight.

Control.—In Britain, vaccination was not permitted until 1962, but then the use of approved dead vaccine became official policy. This must be given by injection (as described below). In 1971 two live vaccines were licensed for use: the Hitchner B1 and La Sota. These vaccines are *not* administered by injection, but as described later. La Sota is not recommended for birds under 28 days old, except under veterinary advice.

Inoculation Technique *.—First of all, there is the vaccine itself to be considered—this *must* be one approved by the Ministry of Agriculture. Secondly, needles and hypodermic syringes must be sterilised. Thirdly, there is the development of a good inoculation technique so that birds are not injured.

With young stock, 10 to 20 days old, the greatest care is necessary because the amount of muscle is small. There are two sites of injection to consider:

* With acknowledgements to *Farm & Country* and to Glaxo Laboratories Ltd.

NEWCASTLE DISEASE

(a) *Breast muscle.* This is a relatively safe site for injection of the small bird. The needle must be introduced from the head end of the bird into the breast muscle about ½ inch to the side of the point of the breast bone as shown in Diagram 1. The vaccinator must locate the point of the breast bone with the thumb of his left hand and use it as a guide. It is important to make sure that the thrust of the needle is always parallel to the line of the breast bone so that no damage is done to the chest of the bird. (Diagram 2.) The bird must be held with the breast region uppermost so that the vaccinator can approach the bird with plenty of room.

(b) *Leg muscle.* Injection is best carried out into the back of the chick's leg in the mid line above the point where the feathers begin. (Diagram 3.) The vaccinator should grasp the leg himself while the bird is held upside down with the legs towards him. It is important to introduce the needle carefully and parallel to the bone; otherwise damage may again be brought about since important nerves and blood vessels pass in this region.

Adult birds may be injected at any one of three sites: (a) Breast muscle; (b) Leg muscle; (c) Behind the head. In these older birds there is a larger mass of muscle to inject into, but care is still very necessary. Birds in batteries are best injected into the leg muscle simply by carefully pulling the leg through the feeding gap. Adult turkeys are normally vaccinated behind the head.

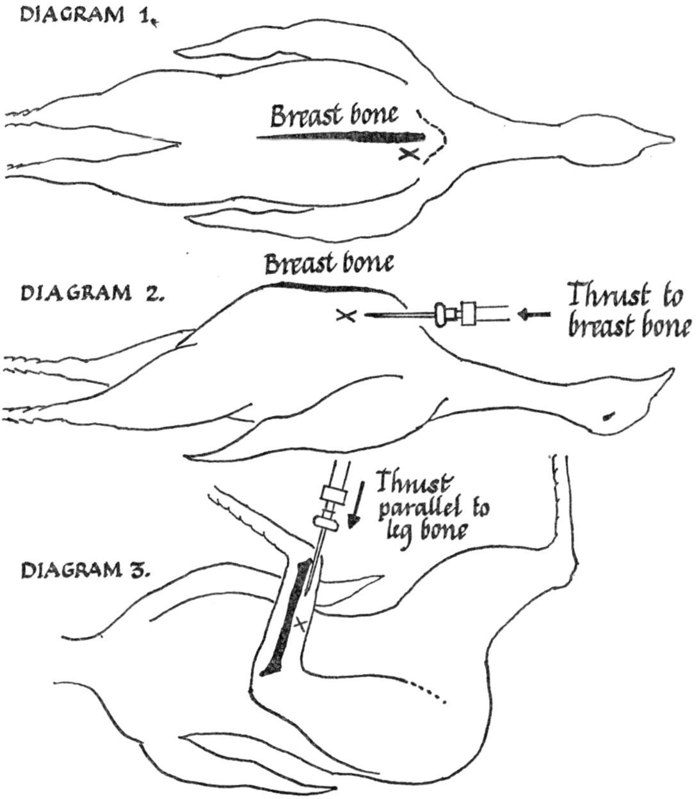

Inoculation technique.

Where the actual vaccination is being carried out by a visiting contractor or teams of vaccinators, the farmer should insist upon the highest standards of hygiene for their clothes, their persons, and their instruments.

The Ministry has pointed out that it

will sometimes happen that vaccination will be carried out in a flock in which, unknown to the owner, some of the birds are in the incubation stage of the disease. In other words, although no symptoms of illness will be shown by those birds, people handling them can become heavily contaminated with the virus of Newcastle disease—on their hands, face, clothes, boots, vaccine bottles, and cartons. It follows, of course, that unless they begin the next day's work with fresh bottles of vaccine, with boiled syringes and needles, with freshly laundered overalls, caps, and Wellington boots disinfected, a vaccinating team can carry such infection on to the next farm. This is important because it takes birds 10 to 14 days to acquire immunity following inoculation. (At least 2 inoculations needed.)

It is preferable for farm staff to carry out vaccination, if practicable, rather than rely on outside help.

In the human being, Newcastle disease virus may cause conjunctivitis and an influenza-like illness.

Administration of live vaccines.— These vaccines are in a freeze-dried form and have to be dissolved in water before use. They can cause stress and therefore should be given only to healthy, vigorous birds. Administration can be by individual dosing or by mass methods :—

(1) eye dropping—suitable all ages including day-old
(2) beak dipping—suitable day-olds only
(3) spraying—suitable day-olds only*
(4) in drinking water†—suitable over 3 days old

(* Operators must wear a face mask and goggles.)

(† adequate trough space essential—additional temporary drinkers needed—deprive of water 1 or 2 hrs beforehand.)

The Ministry has issued detailed schedules for vaccination of broilers, layers, turkeys, pheasants, quail and partridges suitable for (1) emergency use ; (2) where the disease is not already occurring.

'NEW FOREST DISEASE' (Infectious Bovine Keratitis) A painful eye condition which can lead to blindness if neglected (*see* p. 325.)

NEW FOREST FLY.—A blood-sucking fly, found in many parts of Britain. *Hippobosca equinus* attacks horses and cattle. It deposits larvæ (not eggs) in the soil. When disturbed, it makes a characteristic sideways movement.

'NEWMARKET COUGH' (*see* EQUINE INFLUENZA).

NICKING.—This is defined in the Docking and Nicking of Horses Act, 1949, as 'the deliberate severing of any tendon or muscle in the tail of a horse'. The practice is illegal.

NICOTINE is the active principle, of a fluid nature, upon which the action of tobacco depends. It should not be used as a warbles dressing in cattle owing to the risk of fatal poisoning. Nicotine poisoning may also arise from the old practice by shepherds of dosing with tobacco against parasitic worms.

NICOTINIC ACID.—A component of vitamin B_2, present in yeast, meat, eggs, milk, etc. Deficiency causes Black Tongue.

NICTITATING MEMBRANE is the 'third eyelid'. (*See* p. 319.)

'NIGHT BLINDNESS' in Irish setters is a condition of atrophy of the retina. (*See* PROGRESSIVE RETINAL ATROPHY *under* EYE, DISEASES OF, *and also under* NYCTALOPIA.)

NIGHTSHADE POISONING. (*See* GARDEN NIGHTSHADE, also DEADLY NIGHTSHADE.)

NIGROID BODIES (*niger*, black) are black or brown irregular outgrowths from the edges of the iris of the horse's eye. (*See* IRIS.)

NIGHT LIGHTING is now commonly practised in poultry houses, using 40-watt lamps to give a 14-hour day, or 1,500-watt lamps for three 20-second exposures a night. The object is increased egg production during the winter months, and the effect is due not merely to the provision of extra feeding-time, but also to the influence of light indirectly on the ovaries.

NIKETHAMIDE (*see* CORAMINE).

NIPPLES.—Infection and necrosis of sows' nipples is not uncommonly caused by *Fusiformis necrophorus*, and may lead to the death of piglets from starvation.

NISIN.—An antibiotic, prepared from *Streptococcus lactis*, which has been used experimentally in the treatment of mastitis.

NIT.—Egg of louse or other parasitic insect.

NITRATE OF POTASSIUM, or NITRE, also known as ' saltpetre ', and when in the form of sticks or balls as ' sal prunelle ', is a crystalline substance with a sharp saline taste.

Actions.—It is eliminated from the body by the kidneys, sweat glands of the skin, and by the mucous membrane of the bronchial tubes. In its passages through these structures it increases the various secretions, and helps in the removal of waste products from the blood.

Uses.—It is used during fevers, catarrhal conditions, and in other cases where toxins are produced in the body. It is usually prescribed with Epsom salts and given in the food or drinking water to all animals. If well diluted it is not objected to, but when given concentrated an animal will often refuse to eat or drink. As a diuretic it is given in œdematous conditions of the limbs and body generally, but it must be used with care in disease of the kidneys.

NITRATE OF SILVER, also called Lunar Caustic, is a heavy crystalline salt of silver, very soluble in water, and generally prepared in sticks along with potassium nitrate, called ' indurated caustic '.

Silver nitrate is caustic, astringent, and antiseptic. Its chief use is in eye lotions in conjunctivitis, ophthalmia, and corneal opacities, and as a caustic for the removal of small warts, for repressing exuberant granulations, and in solution for painting on to sluggish ulcers or wounded areas that have little tendency to heal. For the eye, it is used as an 0·1 per cent to a 2½ per cent solution and is instilled or painted on to the affected surface ; for caustic uses the sticks of ' indurated caustic ' are most useful ; for painting on to diseased areas of the skin or mucous membrane it is dissolved in distilled water to the strength of 8 to 12 grains to the ounce. In all cases when silver nitrate is being dissolved, distilled water should be used as the salts in ordinary tap-water are apt to throw the silver out of solution and precipitate it as the inert chloride of silver.

NITRATE POISONING (*see* NITRITE POISONING).

NITRE (*see* NITRATE OF POTASSIUM).

NITRITES are salts which have a powerful effect in paralysing the action of involuntary muscle. They dilate blood-vessels, check spasms, and relieve distressed respiration resulting from constriction of the smaller arterioles, as well as tending to lower pressure in the right side of the heart in certain conditions when this part is excessively dilated. The most common are amyl, ethyl, and sodium nitrites. Erythrol-tetranitrite and nitroglycerine have similar actions.

NITRITE POISONING.—Poisoning as a result of eating plants with a high potassium nitrate content is common in some of the western parts of the U.S.A. The nitrate is reduced to nitrite by substances within the plant under certain climatic conditions, and when such a plant is eaten the nitrite is rapidly absorbed from the digestive system and converts hæmoglobin into methæmoglobin. This is incapable of giving up its oxygen to the tissues and as a result the animal dies.

Sodium nitrite is used for curing meat and has found its way into swill, causing fatal poisoning in pigs. The main symptoms observed were vomiting, squealing, and distressed breathing. Nitrite poisoning has also occurred, in piggeries with poor ventilation, from condensation dripping down. It may arise, too, in grazing animals where nitrogenous fertilisers have been spread during dry weather, or before rain has had time to wash it all in. This could be called nitrate poisoning, but the nitrate itself has a fairly low toxicity, being converted into the poisonous nitrite. The nitrate content of heavily fertilised plants may increase the animal's intake of nitrates.

NITROFURANS.—A group of drugs developed in the U.S.A. during the 1940s, and including Nitrofurazone, Furazolidone, and Nitrofurantoin (for urinary tract infections). They are effective against a wide range of bacteria ; some against protozoa and fungi. It is thought that they interfere with the carbohydrate metabolism of micro-organisms.

NITROFURAZONE.—A drug of value in the control of coccidiosis. It can be given in mash to poultry. It may, however, be associated with rupture of the aorta in turkeys.

It has also been used in the treatment of Paratyphoid in pigs.

NITROPHENIDE POISONING, characterised by paralysis, has occurred in pigs fed medicated meal intended for poultry and containing nitrophenide as a treatment for coccidiosis.

NITROSAMINES.—These are very powerful chemical carcinogens. They cause cancer of specific organs irrespective of the route of administration.

NITROTHIAZOLE.—The drug 2-amino-5-nitrothiazole is effective in controlling Blackhead in turkeys (by preventive medication).

NITROUS OXIDE GAS is used as an anæsthetic in human medicine and is sometimes employed for small animals. (*See* ANÆSTHETICS.)

NITROVIN.—A growth promoter for pigs, sold under the brand name Payzone. (*See* ADDITIVES.)

NOCARDIOSIS.—Infection with *Nocardia asteroides* in cattle, dogs, cats, and man. It resembles actinomycosis but may affect the brain. The fungus has occasionally been isolated from the udders of cows affected with mastitis, and has been reported as the cause of ' incurable mastitis ' in an outbreak on a Texas farm. Involvement of the liver and mesentery, with marked loss of condition, thirst, and some diarrhœa—calling for euthanasia—has been recorded in the dog in Britain.

NODE (*nodus*, a swelling) means a localised swelling generally upon a bone or nerve fibre, in the latter case being only detectable by the microscope, and occurring normally. When affecting a bone, nodes are usually due to localised irritation, or to a fracture which has healed and left a thickening.

The term is also used with reference to the lymphatic system and lymphatic glands in particular.

NORMAL SALINE, or **PHYSIOLOGICAL SALINE,** is a solution of sodium chloride in sterile distilled water, which is isotonic with the strength of this salt in the bloodstream, that is about 0·9 per cent for mammals. For practical purposes this is usually reckoned as 90 grains per pint of water.

Normal saline has very valuable uses if injected subcutaneously at body heat in cases of dehydration during severe disease. It also has at least a temporarily good effect in the treatment of surgical shock, whether due to loss of blood or otherwise. Normal saline is also useful for diluting solutions of powerful drugs, hormones, etc., so that a larger amount of actual injection can be used; more accurate dosage and better and more rapid absorption are ensured than if strong compounds are used.

To be effective, large amounts of normal saline solution may have to be used. Thus, for dogs, from $\frac{1}{4}$ to 2 pints may be needed; for horses or cattle, up to 1 gallon, and these amounts may have to be repeated.

(*See also* DEHYDRATION, DEXTRAN.)

NORMOBLAST (*norma*, rule, and *βλαστός*, germ) is the term applied to a red blood corpuscle which still contains the remnant of a nucleus.

NOSE AND NASAL PASSAGES.—The ' nose ' of an animal, which is more often termed the ' muzzle ', or ' snout ', according to the species, serves two important functions. It forms the outermost end of the respiratory passage, and it lodges some of the end-organs of the sense of touch.

Horse.—*Externally*, the rims of the nostrils are built up on a basis of cartilages covered over by a fold of delicate skin possessing long tactile hairs. The cartilages are not complete laterally, thereby allowing the nostrils to become greatly distended during occasions of emergency. Situated at the upper and outer part of each nostril there is a pouch-like sac which opens into the nostril at one end, but is blind at the other. This is often called the ' false nostril '. Lying just within the entrance to the nasal passages about an inch or so inside each nostril is the lowermost opening of the lacrimal duct carrying tears secreted by the lacrimal gland of the eye. *Internally*, each nostril, and the nasal passage to which it gives access, is completely divided from the other by the *septum* of the nose and its associated structures. This is composed partly by the vomer bone, and partly by a wall of cartilage which is continuous with the cartilages of the nostrils. The walls of each passage are lined by mucous membrane which is reflected on to the two turbinated scroll-like bones that are found in the passage, and this membrane, being well supplied with blood, and being continually moist from the secretion of its mucin glands, serves to warm and moisten the incoming air before it passes to the lungs, and to extract the larger particles of dust, soot, etc., that the air picks up, by causing them to adhere to its sticky surface. The entrance to the air sinuses of the skull leads out from the posterior part of each passage, the mucous membrane lining the sinuses being continuous with that of the nose. (*See* SINUSES OF SKULL.) The end-organs of the sense of smell are scattered throughout the nasal mucous membrane in the upper parts particularly. The olfactory nerves from the brain, which pass out of the cranial cavity into that of the nose by way of the ethmoid bone, are distributed to these end-organs. Posteriorly, the nasal passages lead into the pharynx through the 'posterior nostrils'.

Ox.—The nostrils, situated one on either side of the broad expanse of moist hairless muzzle, are smaller and thicker than in the horse. No false nostril is present, and the opening of the lacrimal duct is not visible. The nasal cavities are short and wide anteriorly, and are narrow and incompletely divided by the septum posteriorly.

Sheep.—The nostrils are narrow and long, and the space between their inner extremities is small. There is no hairless muzzle.

Pig.—The nostrils are small, rounded in outline, and situated on the flat surface of the almost vertical and hairless snout. The skin of the snout is thin and possessed of large numbers of tactile corpuscles, and has a sparse covering of very fine hairs. The nasal cavities are long and narrow, and each is divided into an upper and a lower part posteriorly. The septum of the nose is partly membranous.

Dog.—The nostrils are situated on the muzzle with which the upper lip blends, and are somewhat comma-shaped in outline. Their appearance varies with the breed of the dog; *i.e.* whether of the bulldog or fox-terrier type, and the colour depends to some extent upon the marking of the rest of the face. In most breeds white nostrils are not considered to be good show points. The nasal cavities are also dependent upon the shape of the face, but generally speaking, they are of large size, possess well-developed turbinated bones with many folds and grooves, and are divided into an upper and a lower part posteriorly. The olfactory areas are entirely situated far back.

NOSE AND NASAL PASSAGES, DISEASES OF.—Diseases and disorders of the nasal apparatus are common in all animals, and are often misleading in their significance. For instance, a discharge from one nostril only very often originates from the root of a diseased tooth, the pus collecting in the maxillary sinus, escaping through the naso-maxillary opening, and trickling from the nostril; and the nasal passages themselves are, in reality, not the seat of disease at all. In other cases parasites may lodge in the upper parts of the nasal cavities and cause discharges, but by far the most common cause of a mucoid or purulent running at the nose is acute or chronic inflammation of the mucous membrane. (*See* GUTTURAL POUCH.)

INFLAMMATION or **RHINITIS**, which is also called 'Nasal catarrh', 'Coryza', 'Nasal gleet', and 'Ozœna', may be either acute or chronic. *Acute catarrh* is very often the preliminary or an accompanying symptom of such diseases as strangles, glanders, influenza, pneumonia, bronchitis, or pharyngitis, in the horse, or of distemper and other diseases in the dog. It may also occur without any other symptom, when the mucous membrane has become inflamed through local causes, such as the inhalation of irritant vapours, the entrance of foreign bodies into the nasal chambers, and it is seen when the larvæ of the nostril fly (*Œstrus ovis*) have invaded the nasal cavities of the sheep, or when *Linguatulæ* are present in the dog or cat. In most cases the direct cause of the inflammation is the infection of the lining mucous membrane with organisms. They are able to produce their effects when the general vitality of the body, or when the local vitality of the membrane itself, is lowered through some predisposing cause. Among such may be mentioned exposure to draughts, cold, etc. (*See also* RHINITIS, ATROPHIC of pigs.)

Symptoms.—Nasal irritation is first evidenced by snorting and shaking of the head in horses and cattle, and by sneezing in dogs. In a few hours there is an excessive secretion of nasal fluid of a clear nature, which soon changes to a thick white, and forms a definite discharge, soiling the muzzle and, in the dog, drying into scales. At the same time the mucous membrane will be found swollen and reddened in colour if the nostrils are examined. The eyes appear heavy, the conjunctivæ are injected, and tears may overflow from the eyes and run down the face. This latter symptom is due to occlusion of the lacrimal duct through inflammation and swelling of its lining. The temperature often rises one or two degrees in severe cases. In *chronic catarrh* there is a persistent or intermittent discharge of glairy, mucoid, purulent, or blood-stained material from both nostrils as a rule, but sometimes from one only. Where the discharge has a fœtid odour, diseased turbinated bones or tooth roots are usually found to be the cause. Ulceration of the mucous membrane may occur, the ulcers in some cases being visible when the nostrils are gently everted in horses. If the ulcers are about the size of a threepenny piece, and have a 'punched-out' discrete appearance, glanders should be suspected. (*See* GLANDERS.)

Treatment.—All cases of nasal catarrh should be considered contagious, for most of the contagious respiratory diseases of the horse and dog commence with nasal catarrh, and at this very early stage they are probably most contagious. The animal should be isolated accordingly, and attention paid to comfort, ventilation, and suitability of food, as discussed under NURSING OF SICK ANIMALS. Symptoms of other diseases must be looked for, especially when the temperature is high, and a professional diagnosis should be obtained. Penicillin may be indicated. The nostrils should be kept moist and pliable by rubbing small quantities of Vaseline around their rims daily, after sponging away discharges.

Diseased conditions of the turbinated bones or of the molar teeth call for surgical measures for their correction; parasites in the nasal cavities must be expelled (*see* PARASITES); and if other foreign bodies are present they must be removed.

CYSTS may sometimes form in the false nostril through partial or complete occlusion of its normally open lower end. When present they may cause some interference with breathing if large, but small cysts are unimportant. The condition is technically known as *Atheroma*. They are treated by incision or excision according to circumstances.

HÆMORRHAGE from the nostrils may occur under a variety of conditions. It may be due to injuries which cause tearing or laceration of the mucous membrane; it may occur during violent exertion, such as racing or hunting with horses not in maximum condition; it may be produced by particles of dust (especially irritant dust such as is found in lime-kilns, etc.) being inhaled for long periods and inducing sneezing fits; it may be associated with ulceration, congestion, tumour formation, or other diseased condition of the nasal mucous membrane; it may be due to fracture of a horn core in cattle and sheep, the blood entering the nose from the sinuses of the skull; in horses it may be seen in GUTTURAL POUCH DIPHTHERIA.

Treatment.—When the hæmorrhage is only slight, little more than keeping the animal quiet, and applying douches of cold water to the bridge of the nose, will be required. A thin trickle of blood coming from one nostril only can be disregarded, as it will generally cease of its own accord. When the bleeding is very profuse, and there may be danger of collapse more drastic measures are needed. Where only one nostril is affected it should be plugged with swabs of cotton-wool enclosed in gauze, and o arranged that some of the gauze is left outside the nostril to allow of removal some hours afterwards. In other cases, where both nostrils are affected, injections of normal saline containing adrenalin, into each nostril may be carried out; or both nostrils may need to be plugged after first having performed tracheotomy. These measures must be undertaken by a veterinary surgeon.

TUMOURS occasionally affect the nasal passages, and by their presence give rise to obstruction in the breathing, discharges from the affected side, and sometimes bulging of the side of the face. They require surgical measures for their removal.

Among other conditions in which the nose or the nasal passages are affected may be mentioned: mucosal disease, malignant catarrh, glanders, urticaria, purpura hæmorrhagica, strangles, and influenza (*see* these headings, *also* INFECTIOUS GRANULOMA).

NOSTRIL (*see* NOSE).

NOSTRIL FLIES, or the *Œstridæ*, are members of the class of two-winged flies, whose larvæ are parasitic in the nasal cavities, and in the air sinuses of the skull, of sheep. (*See* PARASITES.)

NOTIFIABLE DISEASES are those which, when they break out upon farm premises, must be notified to the police or government department concerned. In Great Britain these diseases are:

Group I—Still occurring (late 1971)

Anthrax
Fowl pest
Bovine tuberculosis (but virtually eradicated from cattle herds)

Group II—No longer occurring (late 1971)

Cattle plague
Epizoötic lymphangitis (in horses)
Glanders and farcy (in horses)
Parasitic mange (in horses)
Pleuro-pneumonia (in cattle)
Rabies
Sheep pox
Foot-and-mouth disease
Sheep scab
Swine fever

(*See under* DISEASES OF ANIMALS ACT, for duties and responsibilities of animal-owners.)

NOVOCAIN, or **KEROCAIN,** is a synthetic substitute for cocaine identical with PROCAINE HYDROCHLORIDE (which see).

NUCLEAR WEAPONS (*see under* HYDROGEN BOMB *and* RADIO-ACTIVE FALL-OUT).

NUCLEIN is a protein substance containing phosphorus derived from the nuclei of cells.

NUCLEUS (*nux*, a nut) means the central body in a cell which controls its activities. (*See* CELLS.)

NURSE COWS.—As a precaution it is wise to have these tested for Johne's disease, which some of them transmit to calves. The complement fixation test is useful for the purpose.

NURSING OF SICK ANIMALS.—In former times it was customary to ascribe all good results to the administration of drugs often severe in their actions, rather than to the healing powers of Nature. Very frequently animals recovered *in spite of*, rather than as the result of, the pills and potions they received. Nowadays, the belief is that the best that man can hope to do is but to *assist* Nature's reparative processes in so far as he is able. And to say this is not to discount the value and importance of anti-sera, penicillin, and the sulpha drugs—or, indeed, any drugs—which *assist*.

The aim of the attendant upon a sick animal should be that of one who tries to help Nature, fully realising, however, that while he may not be able to do much to assist, he at least should do nothing to hinder.

The competent nurse will realise his, or her, own limitations, and will not attempt diagnosis or treatment of any but minor ailments, leaving these tasks to the veterinary surgeon.

Cleanliness.—It is necessary to ensure cleanliness of the patient and his attendant, cleanliness of the loose-box, bedding, air, food, water, and of everything which comes into direct or indirect contact with the animal. The fact that a sick animal is discharging quantities of purulent infective material is no excuse for a disregard of simple methods of cleanliness. It entails but little trouble to take a small quantity of water containing a weak antiseptic, and to sponge out eyes, nostrils, or the external genital organs, once or twice daily, and the freshening effect of water alone about the head is of importance.

Where possible, a separate attendant should be provided to nurse sick animals, but if not practicable the healthy animals should be attended to first, and the hands and arms should always be washed in antiseptic after dealing with the sick. The sick-box or pen that houses the patient should not be in close proximity to healthy stock. It should be well ventilated, free from draughts, and is best lined with concrete to facilitate easy cleansing and disinfection. A plentiful supply of long, clean, dry wheat straw makes the best bedding material for the larger animals, and hay for dogs and cats. Pillows, rugs, blankets, or towels, etc., are sometimes useful for these latter animals, but when once soiled they require washing and boiling before use again.

Comfort.—A seriously ill animal requires all its resources to enable it to fight against the disease, and every little source of irritation acts unfavourably. Comfort should be assured by the provision of a plentiful supply of bedding, by the maintenance of bodily warmth effected by the application of suitable clothing, such as a horse-rug, hood, bandages for large animals, and of a coat, chest-protector, or piece of flannel for dogs and cats. Pigs can usually keep themselves warm if well littered, and the sheep, by its fleece, has an adequate protection against cold. In this connection it is well to avoid the application of too much heavy clothing; it is seldom that more than two rugs are needed by horses and cattle even in the coldest climate. Adequate ventilation should always be provided, especially in respiratory disease, but the animal should not be exposed to chilling draughts.

Whenever possible, windows or doors that face towards the sunlight should be left open, for not only do animals naturally enjoy basking in the sunlight, but it is a very efficient germicide, and the rays all play a part in hastening metabolism generally. In certain cases, however, such as tetanus, and in diseases of the eye, it is sometimes necessary to provide partial or complete darkness, for, in these, light may be injurious.

Grooming is of mportance, not only because it effects the removal of waste products from the skin, but also because it acts as a surface massage, stimulating the circulation, and rendering the skin more able to eliminate the poisons that are constantly being produced in the system. Where the chest is affected, and in cold weather, one side of the rug should be raised while that side of the body is being groomed, and replaced while the other side is being dealt with. In the same way an attendant should never omit to wipe away the discharges from the eyes and nose of an animal suffering from catarrhal condition.

Suitability of food.—The diet of sick animals is of the greatest importance, for, as a rule, so long as food is being taken there is no immediate danger, and animals are more fastidious when sick than when well. The food should be offered in small quantities at frequent intervals and, if refused, the manger should be cleaned out before more is given. A sour bran mash, stale feed, decomposing meat, or curdled milky food, left before an animal is sufficient to strangle any yearnings for food, and when the appetite is capricious the patient will often starve rather than eat unpalatable food.

Variety is important in feeding the sick. The food selected should be such as is easily digested, fairly nutritious, laxative, easily swallowed, and if specially prepared by heating or cooking it should not be offered until cool enough to take. During fevers all highly nitrogenous foods should be avoided; in stomachic disorders fluids are better tolerated than solids; in affections of the mouth and throat the food should be made thin and semi-fluid so as to ensure easy swallowing; in diarrhœa from simple causes the food should be such as will exert a demulcent and slightly astringent effect upon the bowels, and in other diseases the food should be equally suitable. In convalescence give gradually increasing amounts of concentrated food, allowing exercise proportionally.

The following is a list of the commoner sick-foods, with brief instructions for their preparation:

Bran mashes are laxative, easily swallowed, though of little nutritive value. They are prepared by scalding about half-a-pailful of good clean broad bran in a clean pail for half an hour. Boiling water is poured over the bran, the whole is well stirred, covered with a sack, and allowed to stand. When cool it is given after again stirring. The addition of a tablespoonful or two of common salt, and a little treacle, increases the palatability. If allowed to stand for long, until cold, the mash turns sour, and is not readily eaten. Sometimes a handful of oats, a little pulped turnip, freshly cut carrots, potatoes, apples, or mangels spread on the top of the mash will induce horses to eat it; while a handful of freshly picked and bruised ivy leaves stirred through will increase its palatability for the ox. Tonic, laxative, and stimulating drugs are often given in mashes.

Bran and linseed mash is prepared by boiling about a pound of whole or two pounds of ground linseed in 3 quarts of water for 3 hours, and adding 2 lb. of bran and 1 oz. of common salt, thoroughly stirring, and allowing to cool. It is more nutritious than a plain bran mash.

Oatmeal porridge is made by boiling 1 lb. of oatmeal in 1 gallon of water for 1 minute, and then allowing it to simmer over a slow fire until it becomes thick. Constant stirring is necessary. It may be given thinned down with milk or water when cool. A little salt should be added.

Oatmeal gruel.—Mix 1 lb. of oatmeal with a little cold water to make a paste; add 2 gallons of boiling water to scald, stirring the while; set aside for a few minutes; add cold water and a little salt, and give with the chill off. This is the same as 'oatmeal drink'.

Linseed tea is made by boiling 1 lb. of linseed in 2 gallons of water until the grains are soft.

Hay tea.—Fill a bucket with good hay; scald with boiling water; cover and allow to stand until cool; remove the hay and give as a chilled drink. Hay seeds, provided they are free from grit and dirt, may be used instead of the hay.

Scalded oats are made by pouring boiling water over 2 or 3 lb. of (preferably crushed) oats in a pail, and allowing to stand for 15 minutes. A little salt should be added. They are useful during convalescence for animals with a poor appetite.

Boiled barley, made by boiling 2 lb. of whole barley in a gallon of water until the grains are burst, and then adding a little bran and allowing to stand till cool, is useful in building up strength after a debilitating illness, but if given to excess may cause digestive disturbance. It should only be given once daily, and is best when mixed with hay chaff.

Milk is a food of great nutritive value, easily digested, and generally readily taken when a little salt is added, by all animals. It is of most use for dogs and cats, and the young of other animals, but adult horses and cattle can often be induced to drink it, and benefit by it. A beaten up egg may be added to it, or the white only. It is especially necessary to ensure that utensils in which milk is given are rinsed out with cold water and scalded after use.

Barley-water (*see* BARLEY-WATER).

Other foods that have their uses during sickness are as follows :—Green clover, lucerne, rye grass, etc. ; malted barley and malt coombs ; various cereal meals ; peptonised milk and beef-tea ; rabbit jelly, brains boiled in milk, sweetbreads, minced steak or liver, both cooked and raw ; milk puddings, especially arrowroot, cornflour, ground rice, and boiled rice ; as well as many proprietary foods, such as Benger's, Mellin's, and Allenbury's Food, Glaxo, etc. (*See also* HYDROLISED PROTEIN.)

Isolation.—It is a matter of common experience that whenever an animal is ill it always does better under treatment when it can be isolated away from association with other animals; and with contagious diseases isolation is essential.

Nursing of horses.—The affected horse should be removed from its stall in the stable and placed in isolation by itself. It should have plenty of bedding, be provided with clean water, and if the weather is cold and it is suffering from a fevered condition it should be clothed with a rug. In cases where the horse is unable to stand, a specially thick straw bed should be given, and one or two bags filled with straw, or bales of hay, are useful to prop it up in an upright position on the breast. Horses that are down must be turned over onto the other side twice or thrice daily. The rectum and bladder may require evacuation artificially, if it does not occur naturally. If bed-sores appear, they should be dressed twice daily with tincture of iodine, and more bedding should be supplied. In respiratory diseases the most important factor in nursing is the adequate provision of fresh air. Small feeds should be offered several times daily, and when a horse refuses one type of food it should be offered another. In all fevered conditions with elevated temperature, oats, beans, peas, cereals, and other foods rich in nitrogen, should be sparsely fed or avoided altogether. They load the blood with acids, and throw extra labour on the excretory organs. Accordingly, during kidney, liver, and most of the intestinal diseases, large amounts of demulcent drinks should be allowed if the animal has any thirst. Whenever the breathing is faster than normal drenching should be avoided. It is better to give medicines in ball form, or as hypodermic injections, in respiratory troubles.

During convalescence the horse should be given some exercise. The amount depends upon its strength, the duration of its illness, and the state of the weather. As a general rule, 10 minutes' walking exercise should be sufficient for the first day. This is given twice on the second day, and each succeeding day it is kept out longer, until when able to withstand an hour's walk every day for a week it may either be put out to grass for a few hours during the middle of the day, or may be given a short period of light work. A word of warning is necessary with regard to work ; after all severe diseases a too early return to work is very liable to be followed by a relapse, or by the development of further symptoms. It is better to lose a few more days' work and have the horse quite better, than to work it too soon and perhaps lose it altogether later. Finally, the attitude of the attendant should be one of kindness and extreme patience ; the horse is a very responsive animal both to kindness and to ill-treatment ; any extra trouble expended upon it, either in health or disease, is amply repaid ; any neglect to which it is subjected results in a lowering of its utility, whether as a beast of burden or as a companion of man.

Nursing of cattle.—Bulls are usually kept in a bull-box, and this is removed from the rest of the buildings. If it is unoccupied when illness occurs it will make quite a good sick-box, provided no better exists. Cows and bullocks should be removed from the byre or feeding-yard and isolated. Store cattle should be taken in from grass and housed in a box or calf-pen. Calves should be shut alone in a pen. The same conditions as to bedding, clothing, water, ventilation, etc., apply to cattle as well as to horses. In the case of food, however, it is essential to realise that sick cattle do not usually require the coaxing and encouragement that is lavished upon the horse. Very often, especially with fat well-fed cows suffering from stomach disorders, actual starving must be resorted to, and in other cases the supply of food must be cut down. Patient kindly treatment, the avoidance of all unnecessary fuss and haste, and a gentle firmness are essential.

Nursing of cows with mastitis forms a special branch of the cowman's duties. With such the frequent stripping of milk or pus from the udder, the hand massage of that organ, and the application of anti-inflammatory dressings in such a way that as little pain is inflicted as possible, and so that the animals shall be comfortable afterwards, are matters of great importance. In the case of digestive disturbances, cattle must be given a certain amount of coarse fibre before the functions of the stomach (*i.e.* rumination, etc.) are fully re-established. Fluids and semi-fluid foods do not form complete foods for cattle, on physiological grounds, since they pass to a great extent through into the later stomachs and only a small amount finds its way into the rumen. A little hay, oat straw, or chaff in the food should always be given, even when fluids must form the greater part of the nourishment. Salt should be added to all mashes, gruels, or fluids, for cattle, and if it is desired to increase their thirst for water, salt should be given both in food and water.

Nursing of dogs and cats.—With these small animals greater care and attention are often given than in the farm animals, and they frequently respond better. Conditions of cleanliness, ventilation, warmth, and comfort, can be provided to approximate to what prevails in human hospitals, and a greater variety in the food is possible. There is a greater tendency, however, for the owner of the dog to dabble in patent and quack medicines, and many amateur canine nurses are liable to become so impressed with their own curative powers, or with the supposed specific qualities of ' somebody's something ', that a word of warning is needful. A dog should not be ' dosed for worms ' whenever it becomes ill, nor should it be given such drugs as castor-oil indiscriminately. Very often the patient requires nothing further than a rest from food for a time. Far more harm is done by over-feeding than by under-feeding ; the preponderance of cases of indigestion over all other kinds of canine ailments very conclusively substantiates this fact.

Fondling, handling, and too much interference with the patient are harmful. In sickness, an animal desires peace just as much as does a human being. After food has been offered it should not be allowed to remain beside the animal until it has begun to decompose. Some animals are shy feeders and will only eat when alone, so that a reasonable opportunity should always be given for feeding. Generally speaking, the principles of human invalid diet apply here. If nausea or a tendency to vomit is apparent, rely upon glucose, with perhaps a little Benger's Food as improvement occurs. In fevers, try milk, Benger's or Allenbury's Food, and fish. The large bones should be removed. Both dogs and cats will be less likely to suffer from withholding their excreta if a metal tray containing damped ashes or clean earth is placed in a sick-room in an accessible position. Such a procedure materially helps to keep down objectionable odours in the house, and allows of great ease in disposal. In contagious diseases all dressings, swabs, cotton-wool, etc., that have been used for the sick animal should be burnt in the fire, or may be wrapped up in an old newspaper and disposed of in the kitchen grate. Care should be taken that other dogs or cats are not allowed to enter a sick-room where a case of contagious disease is being treated, and the attendant should always wash his hands before handling a healthy animal and after coming out from the sick-room.

For further details connected with nursing, reference should be made to what is given under the heading of **Treatment** under each disease, and also to such sections as: ANTISEPTICS, BEDSORES, DISINFECTION, ENEMA, MASSAGE, DEHYDRATION, BARLEY-WATER, VOMITING, FOMENTATIONS, VENTILATION, R.A.N.A.

NUTRITIONAL ROUP.—This is a condition noticed in fowls under restricted conditions which have been fed for a long time (a month or two) on a diet deficient in vitamins, especially vitamin A. They appear pale in the comb and wattles.

Egg production falls, and a loss of flesh and general unthriftiness may be noted. Birds fall ready victims to coccidiosis, fowl pox, or any disease to which they may be exposed. Diarrhœa may be present, and a whitish discharge is often noticed from the eyes. On examination of the mouth, characteristic whitish areas are seen.

NUTTALIA is the name given to a genus of piroplasms which cause biliary fever in horses in many parts of the world. There are two forms involved—*Babesia* (*Nuttallia*) *equi*, which is the smaller and more important, and *B.* (*Nuttallia*) *caballi*. Each is transmitted by one or more ticks. (*See* PARASITES.)

NUX VOMICA is the seed of the *Strychnos nux-vomica*, an East Indian tree. It has an intensely bitter taste. The medicinal properties are due to two alkaloids—*strychnine* and *brucine*, which the plant contains. Brucine has an action similar to, though much weaker than, strychnine. (*See* STRYCHNINE.)

NYCTALOPIA (*νύξ*, night, *ἀλαός*, blind, *ὤψ*, the eye), or night-blindness, is a condition that sometimes affects horses and mules in countries where the glare of the sunlight is very intense during the day. At night such animals are quite unable to see, and will stumble into objects that are easily discernible to human beings. It is recommended that cavalry horses and mules in foreign countries should be provided with cloth masks when at work or exercise in glaring sun during the day, if there is little or no shade. Camels are seldom affected, owing to the effective protection afforded to the retina by the overhanging eyelids and deeply placed eyeballs. (For the condition in the dog, *see under* 'NIGHT BLINDNESS'.)

NYLON is a convenient suture material which has largely replaced silk for skin sutures.

NYMPHOMANIA (*νυμφή*, a bride; *μανία*, madness) is the name given to an exhibition of uncontrollable sexual desire by mares especially, although the females of any species may be affected. The condition is associated with pathological changes, often of a cystic nature, in the ovaries. Hormone treatment may be tried under veterinary advice; or removing the ovaries by surgical measures, as early as possible after the erotic symptoms have made their appearance. (*See* OVARIES, DISEASES OF; HORMONE THERAPY.)

NYSTAGMUS (*νυσταγμός*, drowsiness, nodding) is a condition in which the eyeballs show constant fine jerky movements of an involuntary nature. The condition prevents the eyeball from coming to rest when it is directed towards a particular object; it moves rapidly to and fro in a lateral direction before becoming fixed upon the object. It is due to diseased conditions of the internal ear, of the cerebellar hemispheres, of the muscles of the eyeballs, or to intoxication with the products of bacterial activity which affect the nervous system. The condition may pass off when the principal disease clears up. No treatment is possible where it persists, and the animal may be but little inconvenienced if it is not called upon to perform some rapid or violent exertion.

O

OAK POISONING.—Both the acorns and the leaves of the oak (*Quercus* sp.) may be dangerous when eaten by stock, but the leaves are usually harmless unless eaten in large quantities. In a Northumberland outbreak, however, in a herd of 40 Galloways, 6 cows died and 4 aborted. A taste for oak buds was acquired early in the year when trees were felled and keep was scarce. Felling went on until September, when symptoms (fever and scouring with blood-stained fæces) were first shown after one cow had aborted and died. Colic and hæmaturia was reported (1961) in horses that ate the leaves.

Acorns comparatively often produce acute poisoning Pigs, sheep, and horses appear to possess a greater degree of immunity than do cattle, especially those under two years of age. It is when there is a scarcity of food in pastures towards the end of very dry summers that symptoms of poisoning occur. The animals most affected are young store cattle.

It is well known that both pigs and sheep can eat acorns to the extent of a peck per head per day so long as some laxative, such as bran, is fed along with them, and so long as the acorns are gradually introduced into the ration. For feeding purposes they should be ripe, dry, of a rich brown colour, and fresh when gathered, should be stored upon a boarded floor, spread out into a layer of about 6 inches thickness, and should be given at the rate of about a pound per day, gradually increased to about ten pounds. It is unwise to feed the maximum of one peck per head per day except when the acorns have been fed for long periods previously.

Symptoms.—Animals that have eaten acorns in quantity become dull, cease feeding, lie groaning, and appear to be in considerable pain. At first, there is severe constipation accompanied by straining and colicky pains, cessation of rumination, weakness of the pulse, and a temperature below normal. Later, small amounts of inky-black fæces are passed, and a blood-stained diarrhœa sets in. There may be a blood-tinged discharge of mucus from the eyes and nose, and the eyes sink in their sockets. Great prostration is seen, and the animals die in from 3 to 7 days when large amounts have been eaten. In chronic cases there is always great loss of flesh, and death does not take place till two weeks or more after the beginning of the symptoms.

The symptoms that are recorded as occurring when large amounts of oak leaves have been eaten are as follows :

' Loss of appetite ; less (and more difficult) rumination ; constipation which increases ; animals lie down, gaze at the flank as in colic, rise and attempt to urinate, which results in the passing of rosy-coloured liquid in jets ; loss of milk-production, which may drop to nothing ; fever, trembling, enfeebled condition.' Usually the course of the illness is not rapid, but death may occur in as short a time as 24 hours after the first signs are seen. (*See also above*.)

Treatment.—Cattle should be given long hay. The animals should be made comfortable, plenty of bedding being provided, and water being available. During convalescence, the animals require liberal feeding to make up the loss of flesh they have sustained.

OAT HAIR BALLS.—In some cases, in horses that are fed upon the sweepings from mills where oatmeal is made, or where oats are rolled or crushed, or even sometimes in those that receive ordinary crushed oats, the very fine hairs that are seen within the outer husk of the oat grain collect into masses in the stomach or intestines. These fine hairs, swept up along with other cereal refuse from mill floors, are sometimes sold cheaply for feeding purposes under the name of ' scree-dust '. They cohere together and are moulded into a more or less spherical ball by the movements of the bowel. When present in large numbers, or when of large size, they may be responsible for periodically recurring attacks of colic. They are often passed when about the size of a cricket ball, and can be seen in the fæces. They are commonly called ' dust balls '.

OATMEAL is made from oats by grinding, screening, and blowing off the greater part of the husks and the dust of the oat grains subsequently. Varying degrees of fineness are given by different types of mills. For animals, it is better to use oatmeal which has a considerable proportion of the husk left in the meal, since this has a very valuable stimulating effect on the intestines—providing 'roughage' and aiding in maintaining bowel movement.

Oatmeal may be fed either as dry meal (to pigs and poultry) or as a constituent of wet mash (cattle), or it may be used as gruel or porridge for sick or convalescent animals of all species.

Oatmeal porridge or brose should not form the main permanent diet of sheep-dogs which often suffer from 'BLACK TONGUE' as a result.

For poultry, 'Sussex-ground oats', also called 'Sussex-ground oatmeal', consists of oats ground coarsely so that the whole of the grain, including husk, is incorporated in the meal. (*See* PHYTIN.)

OBSTETRICS (*obstetrix*, a midwife) is the art of the delivery of the young, and the study of the abnormalities and diseases incidental thereto. (*See* PARTURITION.)

OBSTRUCTION OF BOWELS (*see* INTESTINES, DISEASES OF).

OBSTRUCTION TO RESPIRATION may be caused by a very large number of abnormal conditions.

Nearly all the more severe respiratory diseases are accompanied by, or associated with, a greater or lesser degree of respiratory obstruction. (*See* LARYNX, DISEASES OF; BRONCHITIS; PNEUMONIA.)

Irritation or inflammation is caused by parasites; for example, in the dog—*Linguatulæ*; in the sheep—*Œstrus* larvæ, and the worms causing verminous bronchitis; in the pig and ox—the worm parasites of the bronchial tubes; and in the fowl—*Syngamus trachealis*. (*See* PARASITES.)

Pressure from surrounding organs or tissues may cause narrowing of the air passages and lead to distressed respiration; *e.g.* inflammation of the parotid gland; abscess development in some of the glands about the throat during the course of strangles, actinomycosis, tuberculosis or glanders; atheroma of the false nostril; urticaria; malignant œdema; obstruction of the gullet with food or foreign bodies; or pus formation in the guttural pouch. Tumours may form either in organs or tissues lying around the air passages, or actually within them, and cause obstruction to the passage of air to and from the lungs. In the disease of the horse known as 'roaring', the vocal cord on one or both sides, instead of being held on one side out of the way of the stream of air, is allowed to hang loosely, almost half-way across the glottis, through paralysis of the muscles which should actuate it; while in 'spasm of the glottis' the laryngeal muscles become suddenly tensed to their fullest extent, and air may be entirely prevented from entering or leaving the thorax for seconds at a time. Sometimes when animals are being put under the influence of a general anæsthetic the tongue lolls back into the pharynx, gets drawn into the glottis by the in-going air, and obstructs the passage. The same thing may happen when the tongue is paralysed and the animal's head is held high. A condition known as 'stenosis of the larynx', in which the whole of the larynx shrinks and the calibre decreases, may follow operations upon the larynx or injuries to the laryngeal cartilages. A throat-lash that is too tightly fastened may compress the throat and obstruct breathing when the horse is put to violent exercise, although it does not usually cause distress when the horse is doing slow light work. This is often found to be the cause of horses becoming very easilv 'puffed' when they are over-keen and have to be held with a tight rein. The horse arches its neck in obedience to the pull on the reins, and in the process the throat expands and fills the throat-lash.

Overfeeding, by increasing the volume of the abdominal cavity and pressing the diaphragm forward, may produce difficulty in respiration, and collections of gas in the rumen of the ox may produce the same result. In fact, great distress and sometimes death from suffocation may be occasioned by extensive gas formation.

Pleurisy, in which there are adhesions formed between the lung surface and the chest wall, or in which there are quantities of fluid produced in the pleural space, may cause impediment to the breathing of a temporary or permanent nature.

Foreign bodies, which have been inadvertently taken into the pharynx, and, instead of being swallowed, are passed into the larynx, give rise to the most sudden and often very alarming difficulty in breathing. Puppies playing with small objects sometimes get them lodged in their larynges with disastrous results. Among the large animals, careless drenching is a very common cause of true 'choking'.

This may occur when some ordinary dose of medicine is being given to the horse, ox, or pig, but is more likely to happen when bitter, irritating medicines are being given, or when there is some diseased condition of the throat, such as laryngitis or pharyngitis, when the respiration is upset as in pneumonia, bronchitis, etc., or when the throat is paralysed, as in milk fever, or spasmodically contracted, as in tetanus. Small animals may be held up by their hind feet and slapped smartly on the back, when small objects can be dislodged from the larynx, and the larger animals should always have their heads released when they show the slightest tendency to cough when being drenched.

Fracture of the nasal bones, or of the turbinated bones, in which the nasal passages are blocked either by the fractured bone or by the hæmorrhage which accompanies the condition, are other possible causes of respiratory distress. (*See also* AIR PASSAGES.)

OCCIPUT (*occipitium*, the back of the head) is the name given to the uppermost posterior part of the head where it meets the neck. The occipital bone lies in the part of the skull which forms the occiput, and can be felt as a hard bony plate in most animals. Some of the neck muscles are attached to the occipital bone, and the powerful ligamentum nuchæ, which is the main supporting structure of the head and neck, is inserted into the prominence that can be felt between the ears. Within this part of the skull, the centres that are concerned with co-ordination of muscular movements are situated, and consequently injuries to the bone are attended with serious results, and often a lack of balance.

ODONTOMA is a tumour arising in tissues which normally produce teeth. They are encountered in horses and cattle in association with the roots (usually) of teeth, where they may appear either as rounded or irregular masses attached to an otherwise normal tooth (sometimes making extraction extremely difficult), or they may occur as large, irregular, solid masses replacing the greater part of a normal tooth and causing a swelling on the side of the jaw. They are usually extremely dense and difficult to cut, presenting an ivory-like appearance on section.

A so-called 'temporal odontoma' is a tumour, not uncommon in horses, about the size of a bantam's egg occurring in connection with the temporal bones. These tumours generally have an opening to the surface of the skin just below, or just in front of, the base of the ear. They contain one or two large, or many (sometimes over 100) small, imperfectly formed teeth enclosed in a single fibrous capsule. They may cause brain disturbances, shown by giddiness, loss of sense of perfect balance, a tendency always to swerve to right or left when walking or trotting, or difficulty in galloping or turning sharply. They are successfully treated by a radical operation in which they are dissected carefully away from the surrounding tissues and removed intact.

ŒDEMA (οἴδημα, swelling) means a dropsical swelling due to the passage of fluid through the walls of the blood- or lymph-vessels, into the spaces of the connective tissues below the skin, into the submucus region of a part, or into the substance of an internal organ. (*See* DROPSY *and* BOWEL ŒDEMA.) Œdema of the lungs occurs in an animal exposed to smoke in a burning building, during the course of HUSK, and as the result of an allergy.

ŒDEMA, MALIGNANT (*see* GAS GANGRENE).

ŒSOPHAGEAL GROOVE (*see* p. 877). Reflex closure of this groove is desirable when administering drugs such as Tetrachlorethylene (which see) as otherwise they pass into the rumen instead of the abomasum. Copper sulphate solution is used as a closure stimulant.

ŒSOPHAGOSTOMIASIS. — Infestation with *Oesophagostomum* worms. In calves, there is a reduced intake of food for several weeks; anæmia, and diarrhœa. In goats, peritonitis has been recorded in India. In pigs, these worms may be important in the causation of necrotic enteritis and paratyphoid. Third-stage larvæ of these (and also *Ostertagia*) worms have been found clinging to psychodid flies cultured from pig fæces. Larvæ have also been recovered from flies caught near a field in which pigs were grazing. It is possible that rats may also transmit larvæ from farm to farm.

(*See also* 'THIN SOW SYNDROME' *and under* PARASITES.)

ŒSOPHAGOTOMY.—A surgical operation involving incision of the œsophagus for removal of a foreign body, etc.

ŒSOPHAGUS (οἰσοφάγος), or Gullet, is the tube which conveys the food and drink down to the stomach from the mouth. It commences about the level of the last cartilage of the larynx, and first lies in the middle line of the neck. At the level of the 4th vertebra of the neck in the horse it inclines over to the left side, and runs down in this position till it reaches the entrance to the chest, where it assumes a middle position once more. From there it lies between the right and left lungs, passes over the base of the heart, and reaches the abdominal cavity by passing through the diaphragm, after which it terminates by opening into the stomach at about the level of the 14th thoracic vertebra. These relations are somewhat important in view of the comparative frequency of ' choking '.

The œsophagus is composed of a thick muscular wall, covered on the outside by loose fibrous tissue, and lined by mucous membrane. Food passes down from the mouth by a process of ' peristalsis '. (*See* Peristalsis.) Obstruction of the œsophagus is not uncommon. In the tropics, stricture of the œsophagus in the dog may be caused by *Spirocerca lupi* larvæ. (*See under* Choking.)

ŒSTRIN, or, more correctly, *ŒSTRONE*, is the name given to one of the hormones produced by the ovary. Its chief function is to promote those changes in the uterus and vagina which are associated with the phenomena of œstrus or heat. Œstrin also forms the basis for the biological test for pregnancy. (*See* Pregnancy Diagnosis Tests.)

ŒSTROGENS.—Substances, either of natural origin or prepared synthetically, which have the effect of inducing œstrus. (*See under* Hormones.) Pasture œstrogens may cause abortion.

ŒSTRUS, ' Season ', or ' Heat ', are names applied to the period during which the female exhibits a desire for the company of the male. It coincides with the ripening of an ovum, or ova, in the ovary. It is characterised by a peculiar systemic excitement that usually lasts for a definite period and then passes off. Females of each species behave in a slightly different manner, but their behaviour has, in each case, the following points of similarity: the genital organs become swollen and congested with blood, and there is a discharge of mucus from the vulva. The anima is feverish and irritable, and its appetite becomes irregular, though thirst is usually increased. It becomes restless, and shows an uncontrollable tendency to seek the society of the opposite sex. Some individuals change their temperament; becoming docile if they were refractory before, or vicious if they were previously of a gentle disposition.

The œstrous cycles in animals vary in different species and in different breeds, and to some extent in different individuals. Probably in the wild state œstrus only occurs once a year, and then at such a time as will allow the young animals to arrive when climatic, dietetic, and other conditions are most suitable for their survival. Artificial methods of domestication have so altered the conditions of life that in the domestic animals œstrus is much more frequent. It occurs for the first time much earlier, reappears during a part of the year, or throughout the whole year, at more or less definite intervals, and subsides later in life. In all animals it normally ceases during pregnancy and reappears a variable time after parturition, and it is always more regular in animals that are habitually used for breeding purposes than in those that are not used for these purposes. In some animals, such as the cow, it may only last 4 to 12 hours, and in others, such as the bitch, it may persist for from 14 to 16 days, or even for longer. (*See* Œstrus, Suppression of.)

Mare.—During the œstral period the mare behaves unusually. She may become irritable or sluggish, and is easily tired. Her appetite is capricious and she may lean against the stall partition when in the stable. If her flanks are accidentally touched she may squeal or kick. The clitoris is frequently raised and there is usually a discharge of some amount of slimy mucus from the vulva. Urine may be passed at frequent intervals. She shows a strong desire for the society of the male —even occasionally for that of the usually scorned gelding. Occasionally hysteria may be seen when the animal becomes quite unmanageable.

Cow.—A great deal of demonstration usually accompanies œstrus in the cow and heifer. The animal frequently bellows and gallops about the pasture with her tail raised. She mounts her fellows or stands to be mounted by them. Very often a cow in œstrus will break out from her pasture and wander away in search of the bull. Both cows and heifers in milk usually give less milk during the œstral period than in the intervals.

Sheep.—The ewe (and goat) is less excited, but a certain amount of playfulness and desire for the ram is shown. Very often there is a small amount of blood-tinged discharge from the vulva which stains the wool of the hind parts a rusty-red colour.

Sow.—The sow becomes torpid and lazy, and when asked to move often grunts in a peculiar whining manner. If housed with others she behaves like the cow—mounting or being mounted. The vulva is usually distinctly swollen, and there is sometimes a blood-stained discharge.

Bitch.—She wanders away from home accompanied by a crowd of male followers attracted to her by the strong odour of the blood-stained vaginal discharge, and may remain away for days at a time. Generally it is only during the last seven days of œstrus that the 'wander-lust' is most marked, and that she will allow service by the male.

Cat.—There may be evidence of pain and/or a strong desire to have her back and flanks rubbed or scratched. She will roll over and over on carpet or floor, rub herself against furniture, etc., and emit little pleased mews. If allowed her freedom she will probably remain out of doors all night, and take part in one of those nocturnal concerts which so annoy the lieges in cities and large towns.

In all animals there is a greater or lesser degree of swelling of the external genitals and a more or less profuse discharge of mucus, which has a powerful odour and attracts the attention of the male, arousing procreational instincts in him.

In the males of some species there is an œstrous cycle in which there are exhibited somewhat similar signs to those seen in females. This applies to the deer, camel, and the elephant in particular. The condition is spoken of as 'rutting' in the deer and camel, and as 'must', 'mast', or 'love-madness' in the elephant.

ŒSTRUS, SUPPRESSION OF.—The **bitch and cat** may be prevented from coming 'on heat' by oral dosing with the synthetic equivalent of a naturally occurring hormone. Various forms of 'The Pill' are available for animal use, but some have been withdrawn and veterinary advice should be sought concerning proprietary brands currently available.

ŒSTROUS TABLE.

Animal.	Time of Year.	Periodicity of Œstrus.	Duration.	First Occurrence after Parturition.
Mare . .	Feb. to July	21 days (14 to 28 days or more)	2 to 6 days	3 to 12 days; service on 9th day often successful.
Cow . .	All year; most intense midsummer	20 days (16 to 24 days or more)	4 to 24 hours	30 to 60 days (see below).*
Ewe . .	End of Aug. till Jan., depending on breed and district.	16 to 17 days (10 to 21 days)	1 to 2 days	(See below).†
Sow . .	Oct. to Nov. and Apr. to June	21 days (15 to 30 days)	1 to 3 days	8 weeks after farrowing, or 1 week after weaning of litter.
Bitch . .	Usually Dec. to Feb., and in spring	Once only during each period	9 to 18 days	(See below).‡
Cat . .	Jan. and Feb., and again often in late spring and autumn	Once during each period	7 to 10 days	As the dog.

* In the cow that is suckling a calf it is seldom that œstrus occurs until after weaning, when its appearance is somewhat variable, but often on 3rd to 12th day.

† With the exception of ewes of the Dorset Horn breed, which comes into season twice a year, and can rear two crops of lambs per year, sheep only show season in the autumn. It depends upon the breed as to how soon the rams may be put out with the flock. Generally speaking, the more low-lying the district and the milder the climate the earlier the ewes come into season; thus Suffolks are served from August till the end of September, and lamb from January till March. Mountain breeds are served from November till January, and lamb in April, May, and June.

‡ The bitch and the cat usually come in season twice a year, but great variation takes place with the smaller toy breeds and with those living a very artificial life: these may show œstrus as often as four times in the twelve months.

For a technique in **ewes,** *see under* SYNCRO-MATE *and* ARTIFICIAL INSEMINATION; likewise for **sows.**

OFFALS (*see* WEATINGS).

OILS are divided into *fixed oils*, which are of the nature of liquid fats, and are derived by expression from nuts, seeds, etc., and *volatile* or *essential oils*, which are obtained by distillation. The fixed oils are used as food-stuffs, and in large quantities as mild laxatives; *e.g.* linseed oil, olive oil, cod-liver oil; and several have special properties owing to active principles that they contain, *e.g* castor oil and croton oil. The volatile oils have actions similar to each other; all are antispasmodics in small doses; they dull pain, have a stimulant action on the heart, and possess powerful antiseptic or disinfectant actions. Examples of volatile oils are the oils of aniseed, cajaput, eucalyptus, peppermint, and turpentine. (*See also* PARAFFIN.)

OINTMENTS are mixtures of medicated substances with lard, benzoated lard, paraffin or petroleum jelly, or lanoline, intended for external application to the surface of the skin or to mucous membrane. Those that have lanoline as a base are more rapidly absorbed than others.

OLDENBURG.—A breed of sheep native to the Hamburg Marshes, West Germany. Fleece weights up to 14 lb. and lambing percentages of 170–180 are claimed.

OLFACTORY NERVE, or the NERVE OF SMELL, is the first of the cranial nerves.

OMASUM, or 'Many-plies', is the name given to the third stomach of ruminants. It is situated on the right side of the abdomen at a higher level than the fourth stomach and between this latter and the second stomach, with both of which it communicates. From its inner surface project large numbers of leaves or *folia*, each of which possesses roughened surfaces. In the centre of each folium is a band of muscle fibres which produces a rasping movement of the leaf when it contracts. One leaf rubs against those on either side of it, and large particles of food material are ground down between the rough surfaces, preparatory to further digestion in the succeeding parts of the alimentary canal.

OMENTUM is a fold of peritoneum which passes from the stomach to some other organ. There are several such folds, but the most important is that which passes to the terminal part of the large colon and the beginning of the small colon, and which is called the **great omentum.** This does not run direct to the colon from the stomach, but forms a loose sac occupying the spaces between other organs in the abdomen. In health, there is always a considerable amount of fat deposited in the folds of the great omentum, and this, in the ox, sheep, and pig, forms part of the suet of commerce.

In the dog the great omentum lies between the abdominal organs and the lower abdominal wall, and acts as a kind of protective bed which supports the intestines, etc.

OMPHALITIS.—'Navel ill.'

OMPHALITIS OF BIRDS.—Infection of the yolk sack, by bacteria found in the alimentary canal and on the skin of the hen, leads to the death of embryos and chicks. These bacteria may be relatively non-pathogenic elsewhere than in the yolk. The disease occurs where hygiene is bad, and takes two forms: 'Mushy Chick' disease (with deaths occurring up to 10 days after hatching), and a true omphalitis or 'navel ill'.

OMPHALO-PHLEBITIS (ὀμφαλός, navel; φλέψ, a vein) means inflammation of the umbilical vein. It occurs in young animals and is commonly present in the early stages of navel ill.

OMSK FEVER.—The cause of this is related to the Russian Spring-Summer Virus (which see), but is more serious in its effects and is spread by the tick *Dermacentor pictus*.

ONCHOCERCOSIS is the name applied to infection with worms belonging to the class *Onchocerca*. (*See* PARASITES, p. 662.)

ONCOGENIC.—Giving rise to tumour formation.

ONDIRI DISEASE (*see* BOVINE INFECTIOUS PETECHIAL FEVER).

'ONTARIO ENCEPHALITIS.'—A disease of piglets, as young as 4–7 days.

ending in a fatal encephalitis, and caused by the H.E.V. virus. (*See* VOMITING AND WASTING SYNDROME which may be identical.)

ONYCHIA (ὄνυξ, the nail) means an inflammation affecting the nails or claws of animals. (*See* NAILS, DISEASES OF.)

ONYCHOMYCOSIS.—Infection of the claw with a fungus. In cats, *Microsporum canis* Bodin infection is not uncommon. (*See* RINGWORM *and* Plate 14.)

OOPHORECTOMY (ᾠόν, egg; φέρω, I carry; ἐκ, out; τέμνω, I cut) is a term applied to removal, by operation, of a healthy ovary. When the ovary is removed because of some diseased condition, the term 'ovariotomy' is usually employed. (*See* SPAYING.)

OOPHORITIS is another name for ovaritis or inflammation of an ovary.

OPENING THE HEELS means the cutting away of the horn at the angles of the heels of the horse's foot, by which the continuity between the horn of the wall and of the bar on either side of the foot is destroyed. It is performed by some blacksmiths and owners in the hope that it will allow the heels to expand and so produce a 'fine open foot'. Actually, the operation results in an interference with the shock absorptive mechanism of the foot, and eventually produces *contraction* of the heels. It is by no means to be recommended. (*See* FOOT OF HORSE.)

OPEN JOINTS (*see* JOINTS, DISEASES OF).

OPHTHALMIA (ὀφθαλμία) means inflammation of the whole of the structures of the eye, but is sometimes restricted to mean keratitis. Contagious Ophthalmia is caused by *Rickettsia conjunctivæ* in sheep, and by *Moraxella bovis* in cattle. Verminous ophthalmia also occurs in cattle. (*See* EYES, DISEASES OF.)

OPHTHALMIC TESTS.—Tests in which a drop of mallein or tuberculin is instilled into the pouch of the lower eyelid. A positive reaction, indicating that the animal is affected is shown by a whitish or greyish-yellow copious discharge. The ophthalmic test is now seldom used.

OPHTHALMOSCOPE (ὀφθαλμός, the eye; σκοπέω, I look at) is an instrument used for the examination of the back of the eye and for the detection of defects in its transparent contents.

OPISTHOTONOS (ὀπισθότονος, drawn backwards) is the name given to the position assumed by the back-bone during one of the convulsive seizures of tetanus, and also sometimes seen during epileptiform convulsions and strychnine poisoning. The spinal column is markedly arched with the concavity facing upwards away from the lower parts of the body, so that the head is drawn backwards, and the tail and hind parts of the body are pulled forwards. The condition is due to the spasmodic contraction of the powerful muscles lying above the vertebral column. (*See also* 'BERENIL' poisoning.)

OPIUM (ὄπιον) is the dried milky juice of the unripe seed-capsules of the White Indian Poppy—*Papaver somniferum.* The juice obtained from poppies of this variety, when grown in temperate regions, is almost useless for medicinal purposes. It is obtained by cutting the green seed-capsules before they are ripe, and collecting the exuded, sticky, white juice on the next day. This is carefully dried, kneaded, and tested. Good opium should contain about 10 per cent of *morphine*, the chief alkaloid and active principle. It also contains other alkaloids in variable amounts, the most important of which are *codeine, narcotine, thebaine, papaverine, apomorphine*, etc.

The preparations of opium used in veterinary medicine are now less numerous, but have included the following: (1) Powdered opium, which is the dried juice powdered, contains about 9·5 per cent to 10·5 per cent morphine. (2) Tincture of opium, or 'laudanum', consists of the powder treated with distilled water and alcohol, and contains about 1 per cent of morphine. (3) Opium extracts, one dry of 20 per cent morphine, and one liquid of 3 per cent morphine, as well as a fluid extract which contains about 5 per cent morphine. (4) Compound tincture of camphor, or 'Paregoric', containing 2 grains of opium in every ounce; doses are double those of the tincture. (5) Compound ipecacuanha powder, or 'Dover's Powder', contains 10 per cent of opium, and is given to the horse in doses of 1 to 4 drams, and to the dog in 5 to 25 grain doses. (6) Gall and opium ointment, containing 7·5 per cent of opium, is used as an astringent ointment for piles and prolapsed rectum. (7) Compound tincture of morphine and chloroform, which contains $\frac{1}{11}$ grain of morphine, $\frac{3}{4}$ minim of chloroform, $\frac{1}{2}$ minim of dilute prussic acid, as well as Indian hemp and capsicum, is similar to the proprietary mixtures which are called 'Chlorodyne'. Morphine, codeine, apomorphine, heroin, and dionin are also preparations from or derivatives of opium that are used either pure in salt form or dissolved in some fluid such as glycerine. They are often given as hypodermic injections.

Actions.—Externally, the action of the preparations of opium is not reliable. Internally, medicinal doses produce a diminution in the secretion of the saliva, causing dryness of the mouth, and when long continued a difficulty in swallowing from absence of the lubrication which the saliva provides for the food. The peristaltic motions of the bowels are slowed or checked altogether in all animals. On the nervous system the effects vary according to the animal. In the horse, the sedative and hypnotic effects so well marked in man are not seen to the same extent. The administration of moderate doses will often soothe the animal, but sleep is seldom induced. Large doses cause delirium, shown by restlessness, symptoms of excitement, pawing at the ground, walking in a circular direction, and later a staggering gait, drowsiness, and extreme nausea. In cattle, the action of the drug is even less certain. Large doses produce excitement, and dangerous doses must be given before the sedative effects of the opium are marked. In the majority of cattle more or less delirium is exhibited, and as a natural consequence the drug is not used for these animals. In the dog, the action is more nearly like that in man. Narcosis can be induced by giving of large doses, especially if morphine be used hypodermically, but there is always a primary stage of excitement, during which vomiting often takes place. The sensory nerves are first stimulated and later are paralysed. The result of this is that pain in almost any organ of the body is diminished. Opium has little effect on the heart or blood-vessels, except a mild dilating action on the latter. Respiration is slowed down, and reflex acts, such as coughing, are less liable to occur. The bronchial secretion is lessened in quantity, and this action is made use of in some forms of bronchitis, when the discharge is too profuse. Ordinary doses cause no skin action, but large doses induce profuse sweating. The kidneys are unaffected, but the administration of large amounts may remove the desire for micturition, and a fully distended bladder sometimes results. In the horse the pupil of the eye is generally dilated, but in the dog it is more often contracted. Opium is excreted by the alimentary canal, no matter how it is given, and this elimination begins very soon after the drug has been given ; large doses may take several days before they are completely got rid of, and to this is probably due the great nausea that attends the use of the drug in all animals.

Uses.—As mentioned, the drug is uncertain in its effects when given externally, and is little used. Internally, preparations of opium are used as sedatives in inflammations of the internal organs, such as the bowels, bladder, bronchi, uterus, etc. ; to check profuse secretions from the various glands of the mouth, intestines, bronchi, etc. To prevent straining or pressing when the rectum or uterus is everted, either opium or morphine was used to quieten the spasms and relieve the pain. Morphine is one of the antidotes to strychnine poisoning, and is generally given in large hypodermic doses in these cases.

OPIUM POISONING is not of common occurrence. Some animals, especially dogs, have an individual idiosyncrasy or a particular susceptibility to opium, and will only tolerate small doses.

Symptoms.—Large doses in the horse induce violent delirium ; the animals become partially blind, rush against surrounding objects, stagger and fall, but rise again, sweating and blowing. After these exciting happenings the animals become depressed, stand immovable, and are extremely nauseated. Constipation is present, and just before death supervenes convulsions are seen. In the dog, large doses cause vomiting, delirium, and laboured respiration.

Treatment.—The antidotes are potassium permanganate and vinegar or acetic acid, given by the mouth. In the dog, if the drug has been taken by the mouth an emetic should be given first, and for this purpose the hypodermic injection of apomorphine is recommended. Hot and cold douches to the head and neck are useful to ward off the depression that always follows. Artificial respiration is necessary in some cases, and the injection of atropine is desirable. Strychnine and enemata of strong coffee are also useful.

OPSONINS (ὀψωνέω, I get food) are substances present in the serum of the blood which act upon bacteria, so as to prepare them for destruction by the white blood cells of the blood.

OPTIC NERVE is the second cranial nerve running from the eye to the base of the brain. It conveys the sensations of light that are received by the retina, and registers them in the optic centres of the brain. (*See* EYE, VISION.)

ORBIT (*orbita*, a track) is the bony cavity on either side of the skull in which the eye and some of its muscles, etc., are contained.

ORBITAL GLAND.—(*See* HARDERIAN GLAND *and* EYE, DISEASES OF.)

ORCHARDS.—Animals grazing in orchards may run the risk of poisoning if fruit-trees have recently been sprayed with copper or lead-arsenate insecticides or fungicides. Orchards, like paddocks, sometimes become a reservoir of parasitic worm larvæ. (*See* PADDOCKS; *also* ALCOHOL POISONING.)

ORCHITIS (ὄρχις, a testicle) means inflammation of the testicle. (*See* TESTICLE.)

ORF.—A disease of sheep, cattle, and goats which has a very wide distribution and many names. Among its numerous designations are the following: 'Ulcerative stomatitis'; 'Contagious pustular dermatitis'; 'Contagious ecthyma'; 'Necrobacillosis of sheep'; etc.

It is enzoötic in the Border counties of England and Scotland, but outbreaks may arise in any county in Great Britain, as well as in Germany, France, Austria, the United States of America, and other sheep countries. It was described as long ago as 1745.

The disease attacks sheep of all ages, sexes, and breeds; and kept under all conditions of management. It very frequently attacks lambs just before or after weaning, or after docking or castration, and from them it may spread to the teats of the ewes. In other cases it is common among gimmers until they are one year old.

Causes.—The essential cause of orf is a virus, but secondarily the *Fusiformis necrophorus* is very important. This organism is of almost universal distribution, but the virus is required to produce pox-like lesions first, which the necrosis organism then invades. The virus cannot be transmitted experimentally to rabbits, which distinguishes it from the poxes. *F. necrophorus* produces a toxic substance which kills surrounding cells; these form a scab under which the activity of the germ increases. A small amount of foul-smelling discharge is produced, which contains numbers of the bacilli of necrosis whose virulence and pathogenicity are greatly enhanced. Once orf has become established in a flock it usually spreads with rapidity so that several cases are first noticed simultaneously, and on subsequent days almost 50 per cent of the sheep may become affected.

Symptoms.—In the benign form of the disease vesicles, followed by ulcers, appear on the lips—especially at the corners of the mouth. Sometimes healing takes place uneventfully; in other cases verrucose masses form and persist. The animal loses weight.

In the malignant form the inside of the mouth becomes involved in most cases, and in addition other parts of the body such as the vulva and the skin of the face, legs, tail, etc. A greyish-black crust often appears which, if removed, leaves a raw, angry-looking surface. When there is much swelling around the nostrils breathing may be laboured, if the eyelids are severely attacked the swelling may close one or both eyes, and if the mouth is affected there is usually a good deal of salivation and the animal becomes shy of feeding. In some cases mastication only takes place on one side of the mouth, or it may be extremely slow and obviously painful. Sheep with such lesions on the head frequently rub their muzzles on their fore-feet, or scratch at their heads with their hind-feet. In this way the feet and legs often become affected. On the hair-bearing parts of the legs the crust-like scales appear and develop in much the same way as they do upon the head, but when the region of the coronet is affected a form of 'foot-rot' appears. In this the pustules are large—giving rise to the term 'carbuncle of the coronary band'—and abscesses form in the region of the coronet. The sheep becomes extremely lame, so much so that it is frequently unable to put the affected leg to the ground, and hobbles about on three legs. If both fore-feet are affected—which is commonly the case—the animal may be observed feeding from a kneeling position. In severe cases the horn separates from the sensitive structures below, large quantities of foul-smelling thick pus are produced, and the hoof may be shed. The space between the claws, and the parts around the front and sides of the coronets, are the commonest situations of the lesions. In the variety of the disease known as 'red foot', which occurs in Germany and the United States of America, the feet are almost exclusively affected, and the disease attacks the deeper structures, so that large irregular, penetrating sores, which discharge quantities of pus, are common.

Less commonly the external genitals of both male and female are affected. When it is seen there are usually typical lesions on some of the sheep in a flock. The lesions in this form appear as small pale spots on the mucous membrane of the vulva or prepuce, each of which has a yellow centre. These form ulcers which gradually extend, become confluent, and the whole area may ultimately become affected. A sticky putrid discharge appears, and if coition occurs the disease is spread to other sheep. As already mentioned, when sucking lambs suffer from orf they are liable to infect the udders of their dams. The disease in the udder appears as a painful swelling of the gland in the early stages, the ewes walk stiffly and refuse to allow their lambs to suck. Acute inflammation and suppuration follow, and parts of the udder are sloughed out. The ewes become useless for further breeding, although the mortality is not usually great among them.

Treatment.—As soon as a case of orf appears among a flock of sheep it should be isolated at once, and the remaining healthy sheep should be dipped. Many sheep farmers consider that such drastic measures are unnecessary, since cases of death from orf are not common, but if much indirect loss is to be avoided they should not be neglected. The loss of condition among growing lambs especially, and also among fat adult sheep, is very marked—as would naturally be supposed when it is remembered that feeding is rendered difficult or impossible, and that pain alone will cause wasting of flesh.

The isolated sheep that are already affected usually do best when they can be shut up indoors, given hand feeding, and provided with clean dry litter. A dressing is applied over the raw ulcerated area and around its margin. Crystal violet is very suitable as a dressing, and antibiotics are useful in treatment.

When dealing with the feet it is essential to open up any enclosed areas where abscesses have formed, and to evacuate the pus and discharges. Overgrown horn should be reduced, and all diseased horn should be carefully pared away. The foot should then be dressed with the crystal violet.

Bad foot cases should always be kept indoors in a fold, shed, etc., until healing is well advanced, for otherwise fresh supplies of germs enter from the soil, and the condition takes a much longer time to resolve.

On farms previously heavily infected, and where orf was very common on the feet, passing the whole of the sheep through a foot-bath at 3-weekly intervals has resulted in a complete disappearance of the disease. (*See* FOOT-BATHS FOR SHEEP.)

When lesions are present on the genital organs in either sex, strict isolation is absolutely essential. In the male the sheath, and in the female the vagina, should be syringed out with a solution of 1 in 500 potassium permanganate in water, or 1 in 25 of hydrogen peroxide, while in very severe cases chinosol in glycerine, 3 grs. per ounce, is to be advised.

Infected sheep after recovery should not be put out with the healthy flock until 2 weeks after the lesions have healed, and it is always advisable to dip them first.

The shepherd, or the attendant who treats the affected sheep, should ensure that he does not carry infection from one sheep to another by contamination of his clothes or hands. He ought always to wash in some disinfectant immediately after attending to cases of orf, since his hands and arms may become affected with orf. Indeed, orf is well recognised a an occupational hazard of shepherds.

Sheep may be immunised against the virus by means of a vaccine.

ORF IN THE DOG.—An outbreak of orf in a pack of hounds was reported in 1970 (*Vet. Rec.*, **87**, 766), and was characterised by circular areas of acute inflammation, with a moist appearance, ulceration and scab formation.

ORGANIC DISEASES, as distinct from 'functional diseases', are those in which some actual alteration in structure takes place, as the direct result of which faulty action of the organ or tissue concerned, follows. (*See* FUNCTIONAL DISEASES.)

ORGANIC SUBSTANCES are those that are obtained from either animal or vegetable sources, or which resemble in chemical composition those derived from such origins. They are peculiar in that they all contain carbon.

ORGANO-PHOSPHORUS POISONING.—This may arise from contamination of crops, or other food material, with organic-phosphorus insecticides such as dimethoate, schradan, parathion, or dimefox.

Treatment.—Atropine sulphate given intravenously or intramuscularly, and repeated in 30 minutes. Barbiturates may be needed to control excitement. Oxygen for distressed breathing and gastric lavage are recommended in the human subject. In the latter, P.A.M. has been recommended as an antidote to parathion and other insecticides in this group—in conjunction with atropine.

ORNITHOSIS.—The name now given to diseases of the psittacosis group other than that specifically affecting parrots. Pigeons, petrels, fowls, mice, ferrets, and man may be affected. In Britain, the disease is probably most common in pigeons. It occurs in ducks, and in the U.S.A. in turkeys. Budgerigars are sometimes a source of infection.

In one Edinburgh outbreak, 100 out of about 300 budgerigars in an aviary died. Human cases followed, and a dog was found to be excreting the organisms and to have a lung infection due to, or associated with, these. (*See also* PSITTACOSIS.)

OSSIFICATION (*os*, bone; *facio*, I make) means the formation of bone tissue. In early life the bones are represented by cartilage or fibrous tissue, and in these, centres appear in which the cells undergo a change and lime salts are deposited. This process proceeds until the areas or centres meet each other, and the tissue is wholly converted into bone. When a fracture occurs, the bone unites by ossification of the blood-clot which forms between the broken ends of the bone. (*See* FRACTURES.) In old age, ossification takes place in parts where normally there are cartilages found, such as in the larynx, in the rib-cartilages, in the scapular cartilages, etc., and these parts lose their normal elasticity and become easily broken. (*See* SIDE-BONES.)

OSTEITIS (ὀστέον, bone), or **OSTITIS,** means inflammation in the substance of a bone. (*See* BONE, DISEASES OF.)

OSTEOARTHRITIS (ὀστέον, bone; ἄρθρον, joint) is a term applied to a chronic inflammation of the bones composing a joint, and leading to deformity.

OSTEOCHONDROSIS.—A condition in which there is destruction of bone and cartilage; associated with degeneration of an intervertebral disc. (*See* 'RUNNERS'.)

OSTEODYSTROPHIC diseases (*see* p. 117).

OSTEOFIBROSIS (*Osteodystrophia fibrosa*).—A condition seen chiefly in the horse, but not uncommonly in pigs, goats, and dogs. There is a loss of calcium salts from the bones, which become fragile. Osteofibrosis makes its appearance within 12 months in a horse fed exclusively on bran, which contains much phosphorus but little calcium. Miller's disease', 'bran disease', and 'big head' are colloquial names for the condition.

OSTEOMALACIA (ὀστέον, bone; μαλακός, soft), is the equivalent of rickets occurring in the adult animal. The bones become softened as the result of the absorption of the salts they contain. The cause of the disease is obscure, but it appears to be more common in pregnant females than in other animals, and it may be associated with a deficiency of vitamin D. (*See* VITAMINS.)

The most serious feature is the deformity which occurs in the softened bones, owing either to the weight of the body or to the pull of the muscles upon them. When the deformity is located in the pelvis of the dam, great difficulty is often experienced at the birth of the young animal, and fractures of this part are not unknown. So far as treatment is concerned it is necessary to give cod-liver oil, good nourishing food, which contains an abundance of phosphates, and well regulated exercise; bone-marrow in the raw form and thyroid extracts have been recommended. It is not wise to breed from females of any species which have ever shown signs of this disease, even although they have quite recovered. It may be influenced by heredity.

OSTEOMYELITIS (ὀστέον, bone; μυελός, marrow) means an inflammation of the bone-marrow. It may follow wounds, and occurs during atrophic rhinitis of pigs, and actinomycosis in cattle. (*See* BONE, DISEASES OF.)

OSTEOPETROSIS, or MARBLE BONE DISEASE, forms part of the 'Avian Leucosis Complex'. It is characterised by thickening of the legs of poultry.

OSTEOPHAGIA (ὀστέον, bone; φαγεῖν, to eat) means bone eating, and is a symptom shown by sheep and cattle in certain parts of South Africa which are deficient in phosphorus and sometimes in calcium in soil and herbage. (*See* LAMZIEKTE.)

Deer living wild in forests where there is a similar deficiency, as in many parts of the Scottish Highlands, exhibit osteophagia by chewing and actually eating portions of shed antlers. Sheep exhibit similar tendencies in the same areas.

OSTEOPOROSIS is a rarefying condition of bones which lose much of their mineral matter and become fragile and often deformed. It occurs in OSTEOMALACIA and OSTEOFIBROSIS.

OSTERTAGIASIS.—Infestation with species of Ostertagia worms, which produce gastro-enteritis. It is seen in calves and lambs. This is an important disease in Ireland. (*See* PARASITES.)

OTITIS (οὖς, the ear) means inflammation of the ear. (*See* EAR, DISEASES OF.)

OTORRHŒA (οὖς, the ear; ῥέω, I flow) means a discharge from the ear. (*See* EAR, DISEASES OF.)

'OULOU FATO.'—A form of rabies occurring among dogs in parts of Africa, and probably Asia also. People are rarely bitten, epidemics are uncommon, infected dogs may show either no symptoms, or transient symptoms followed by recovery. Repeated attacks prove fatal, however.

OVARIES are the essential organs of generation in the female. They vary in size according to the size and age of the animal, but are about the size of a small hen's egg in the mare and cow, and smaller in other animals. They are suspended in a fold of peritoneum from the roof of the abdomen, called the 'mesovarium'. In the *mare* they are situated in the abdomen, lying a little below and behind the kidneys, usually in contact with the muscles of the lumbar region. Each possesses a groove which gives the organ a shape not unlike a bean, and which is called the *ovulation fossa*. It is into this groove that the ripe ova escape from the ovary, and it is the only part covered by germinal epithelium in the mare. In the *cow* the ovaries are oval in outline and possess no fossa. Each is situated about half-way up the shaft of the ilium of the corresponding side of the body. The ovaries of the *sow* are usually situated in a position similar to those of the cow, but their position changes somewhat after breeding has occurred. They are studded upon the surface with

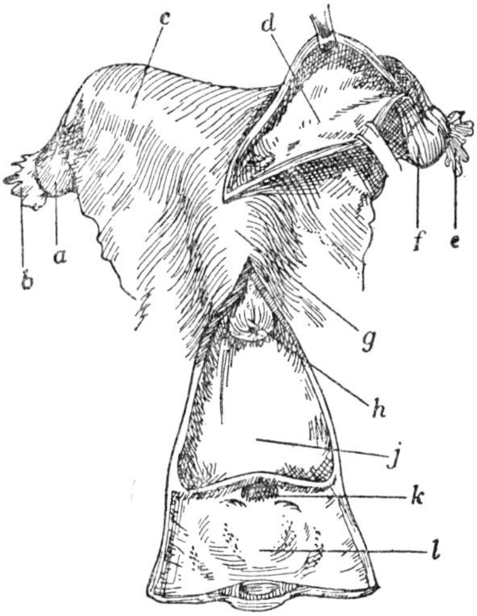

Generative organs of mare, seen from above. The vagina and vulva have been laid open by an incision along their upper parts, and the right horn of the uterus has been incised.

a, Left ovary; *b*, fimbriated end of left oviduct; *c*, left horn; *d*, right horn of uterus laid open; *e*, end of right oviduct; *f*, right ovary; *g*, body of uterus; *h*, cervix; *j*, vaginal interior; *k*, opening of urethra from urinary bladder; *l*, vulva.

irregular prominences, so that the organs present a mulberry-like appearance, and are enclosed in a 'purse' of peritoneum. In the *bitch* the ovaries are situated in close proximity to, if not in actual contact with, the kidneys of the respective sides.

Structure.—Each ovary is composed of a stroma of dense fibrous tissue in whose spaces are numerous blood-vessels, especially towards the centre. On the surface of the organ is a layer of *germinal epithelium* from whose activity result the *Graäfian follicles.* The follicles vary very much in size: when young they are microscopic, and lie immediately under the outer surface, but as they grow older they become more and more deeply situated, and finally, as ripening occurs, they once more come to the surface. In a ripening Graäfian follicle there is one (rarely two) of the essential female germ cells, called an *ovum.* This is situated at the pinnacle of a mass of cells which project inwards from the inner surface of the follicle, and which is known as the *cumulus.* When the follicle is ripe, a process known as *ovulation* occurs, in which the outer surface wall of the follicle ruptures and liberates the contained ovum, which escapes from the ovary. The ovum is caught by the oviduct, and either fertilised or passed on through the female system to the outside. The cavity of the Graäfian follicle fills up afterwards with spindle-shaped cells, and the structure is called the *Corpus luteum.* It possesses some not well understood influence over milk secretion, and is related to the development of the fœtus in the uterus. (*See* EMBRYOLOGY, REPRODUCTION, etc.)

OVARIES, DISEASES OF.—In cystic degeneration large cavernous cysts appear in the substance of the organ, and fill with fluid. For a time there are no definite symptoms shown, but after the cysts attain considerable size the animal begins to exhibit signs of fretfulness and excitability. As time goes on these symptoms increase in violence until in the mare, in which the condition is quite common, it usually becomes dangerous to work her. Upon the slightest provocation, and often with no provocation at all, the mare starts to kick. After her bout of kicking is over she resumes her normal behaviour, but another attack may come on at any time afterwards.

Cysts are also met with in cows where they may be associated with sterility, and in bitches where they are frequently present along with tumour formation in the mammary glands. They are recognised in America as a common cause of sterility in gilts; heat periods being irregular and the clitoris becoming enlarged. Hypoplasia of the ovaries may also occur.

Treatment.—The only treatment that has proved of any benefit is the removal of the ovaries by surgical measures, or the rupture of the cysts by pressure, and even where this is done there are cases where no good results follow. Probably the longer the condition has been in existence the less likely will benefit follow these procedures. (*See also under* INFERTILITY.)

OVARIO-HYSTERECTOMY.—Surgical operation for removal of the uterus and ovaries. This is carried out in the dog and cat in cases of pyometra, and following dystokia where a recurrence is feared. (*See also* SPAYING.)

OVARIOTOMY.—Surgical operation for removal of a diseased ovary.

OVERGROWN FOOT is one in which the horn of the wall all the way round has continued to grow downwards and outwards, without any compensatory wear along its lower edge. A horse with overgrown feet, which may arise either from too long periods between successive shoeings, or from living on marshy land where the unshod foot gets no wear, is unable to walk correctly. The frog does not reach the ground, the toe is too long, and the heels are too high, so that the normal anti-concussion mechanism of the foot is thrown out of action. The condition predisposes to the occurrence of sprains

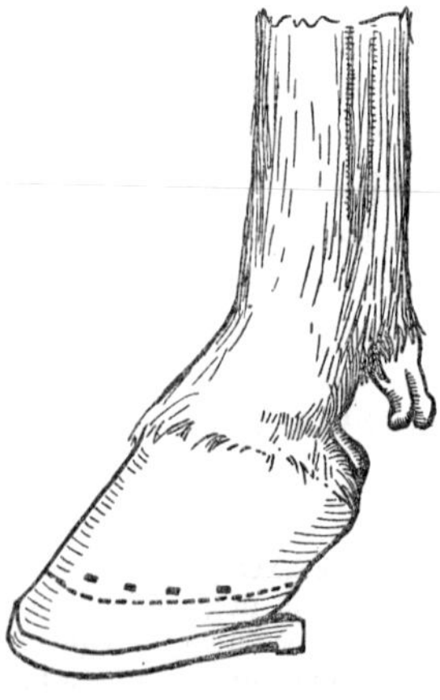

Overgrown hoof, showing how much should be cut away at the next shoeing.

and contractions of tendons, upright pasterns, and splitting of the horn, with the production of sandcracks as a consequence. Horses' feet that are shod should have the shoes removed at least once a month, and the growth since the last shoeing should be removed by rasping the lower edge of the wall. Young colts, running out at grass, should have their feet properly reduced at least once during every two months or so. Overgrown foot is of importance in cattle and sheep, and in animals confined in ' zoos '.

OVERLYING by the sow is one cause of PIGLET MORTALITY (which see) and can be prevented by the use of farrowing crates, rails, and the roundhouse. It should be remembered, however, that an ill piglet is more likely to be crushed by the sow than a healthy one ; and it has been shown that after one hour in an environmental temperature of 35° to 40° a piglet becomes comatose. (*See under* ROUNDHOUSE for an effective means of preventing overlying.)

OVER-REACHING, and ' Forging ' or ' Clacking ', are imperfections in the gait of horses in which one of the hind toes strikes against some part of one of the fore feet or a fore shoe. When the toe of the hind foot strikes the sole of a fore foot, or the iron of the shoe, with a resultant click, the condition is called ' Forging ', or ' Clacking '. When the toe of a hind foot strikes the heel of the fore foot, and wounds it, the condition is then ' Over-reaching '.

When a horse forges, not only is the noise produced objectionable to the owner, but the blow from the hind foot may throw the stride of the fore foot out of balance and cause stumbling. It is commoner at the trot than at other paces, but it may also occur at the walk, canter, or gallop. It may be caused through bad shoeing—*e.g.* when the toes are left too long ; it may arise through an imperfection in the gait—*e.g.* when the hind feet take too long a stride, and the fore feet too short a stride ; and it may occur in any horse that is tired. The explanation of its occurrence in the tired horse is probably that the fore feet, carrying almost 66 per cent of the body weight, tire out a little sooner than the hind feet, and are a little slower in leaving the ground.

Over-reaching is much more serious, since although there is no noise it is as likely to cause stumbling as is forging, and it entails the infliction of an injury. The analysis of the events resulting in an over-reaching injury is as follows : (1) the hind foot is carried forward in the stride to a point level with, or a little in front of, the position occupied by the fore foot which is just about to leave the ground (in ordinary normal progression the fore foot is lifted clear a fraction of a second before the hind foot comes to rest) ; (2) the fore foot has not left the ground, and the hind foot comes into collision with it ; (3) the toe of the hind foot enters into the hollow above the heels of the fore foot, just as the latter is leaving the ground ; and (4) a strip of skin is torn away from the bulbs of the fore heels by the sharp inner lower edge of the shoe of the hind foot. The typical injury from an over-reach is characteristic in that the flap of skin is usually attached by its posterior margin to the bulb of the heel.

Treatment.—In many cases the amelioration of these conditions primarily consists in better general management. Unfit horses that are easily tired should be brought into hard condition by exercise and good feeding, and should not be over-worked. Young colts being broken should not be schooled for too long periods at a time, especially after being newly shod.

Otherwise the shoeing should receive attention. The toes of all four feet should be shortened, and the hind shoes should be set back on the feet. The iron at the toes of all the feet should be bevelled along its lower inner edge (concaved), or rounded off, so that there is no sharp edge on the hind feet to cut the heels of the fore, and so that there is less iron to be struck on the fore feet.

With horses that easily tire it is usually advisable to roll the toes of the fore feet so that the foot is encouraged to leave the ground faster, and not obstruct the placing of the hind feet on the ground.

In advanced cases of forging, where the wall at the toe of the hind foot becomes worn, it is sometimes advisable to shoe with a piece of sheet iron covering the damaged portion of the wall of the hind foot. This guard or shield is welded or riveted on to the shoe.

OVERSTOCKING.—This term refers both to the cruel practice of exposing in a market cattle in urgent need of milking (with the object of obtaining better prices for animals with impressive udders) ; and also to an excess of grazing animals on a given acreage of pasture. (*See* STOCKING RATES.)

OVIDUCT (*see* FALLOPIAN TUBES, SALPINGITIS, EGG-BOUND, PROLAPSE OF OVIDUCT).

OVINE ENCEPHALOMYELITIS.—Louping Ill.

OVINE EPIDIDIMYTIS.—Brucellosis of sheep, important in Australia and New Zealand, and caused by *Brucella melitensis var. ovis.* (*See* BRUCELLOSIS.)

OVINE INTERDIGITAL DERMATITIS (O.I.D.).—This has been described in foot-rot free flocks in Australia, and is caused by *Fusiformis necrophorus.* (See also ' SCALD ' and ' SCAD.')

OVULATION (*see under* OVARIES *and* REPRODUCTION).

OVUM (*ovum*, an egg) is the cell derived from the female, out of which, after fertilisation, a future individual arises. (*See* EMBRYOLOGY, OVARY.)

OXALIC ACID is a rapid irritant poison, and generally a fatal termination precludes any possibility of treatment. If it has been given inadvertently, a large drench of lime-water, chalk and water, whitening, bicarbonate of soda, or other common alkali should be administered immediately in large quantities of water. This neutralises the acid and forms a salt which should be hastened out of the system by a subsequent demulcent purge, such as castor and olive or rape oil

Salts of oxalic acid occur in rhubarb, sorrel, mangolds, and other plants.

OXYCLOZANIDE (**' Zanil '**).—A drug for use in sheep and cattle against liver flukes. It has a very low toxicity and can be given to pregnant animals and those in poor condition.

OXYGEN (ὀξύς, acid; γεννάω, I produce) is a colourless gas, devoid of smell, and slightly heavier than common air. It forms about one-fifth of the atmosphere by volume.

Action.—When inhaled by animals in the pure state it causes an acceleration of all the body functions, and soon leads to death from over-stimulation of all the nerve centres. If given mixed with air to animals that are suffering from partial asphyxia, due to any cause, it gives almost immediate relief, but it is not always available for this purpose. It provides a means for supplying the essentials of respiration when, owing to pneumonia, bronchitis, or other disease of the lung, a sufficiency of oxygen cannot be obtained from the air. Cylinders of oxygen are used in connection with anæsthesia for the smaller animals, *e.g.* a combination of ether and oxygen, and for relief of œdema of the lungs. In the form of potassium permanganate, or hydrogen peroxide, both of which are salts which readily give up their oxygen content, it is sometimes used as a disinfectant or antiseptic for wounds.

OXYTETRACYCLINE.—An antibiotic (*see* TERRAMYCIN which is a brand name).

OXYTOCIN.—A hormone, secreted by the posterior pituitary gland, which actuates the ' milk let-down ' mechanism.

OXYURIS (ὀξύς, sharp; οὐρά, tail) is another name for the thread worm, which possesses a long finely tapered tail. (*See* PARASITES, p. 658.)

OZÆNA (ὄζαινα, a fœtid polypus in the nose) is a chronic inflammatory disease of the nasal passages. (*See* NOSE, DISEASES OF.)

P

PACHYMENINGITIS (παχύς, thick; μῆνιγξ, a membrane) means inflammation of the dura mater of the brain and spinal cord. (*See* MENINGITIS.)

PACINIAN CORPUSCLES are minute bulbs at the ends of the nerves scattered through skin, subcutaneous and other tissues, and forming the end-organs of sensation. They are abundant in the mesentery of the cat and in subcutaneous tissues of the penis and muzzle of most animals.

PADDOCKS.—These often become reservoirs of parasitic worm larvæ—a point for animal owners to bear in mind. Paddocks need 'resting' for 12 months or grazing by a different species of animal periodically.

Paddock grazing is a system of grassland management in which a given area of land is divided into a number of paddocks by fences and used for what André Voisin described as 'Rational Grazing'.

In Britain, on farms costed by ICI, paddock grazing of dairy cows has given very good financial results. The system should be set up on an area of grassland as near to the farm buildings as possible, allowing one acre for every two cows; *e.g.* 21 acres for a 42-cow herd. This area is then divided into 21 paddocks each of one acre, over which the herd should circulate in about three-weekly intervals; one day's grazing per paddock being ideal. Paddocks should be squarish rather than long and narrow, and well supplied with water. Fencing need cost no more than 30s. per acre or 3s. per cow per annum. A 21-acre cutting block should yield the bulk fodder for the winter, and each acre must therefore produce enough silage for two cows, *i.e.* 14 tons.

Fertiliser, especially nitrogen, is the key to the success of this system, and must be applied regularly throughout the grazing season. After the first graze, grass growth may be such that the farmer may have to take full silage cuts from a number of paddocks without grazing, so that the cows could circulate in a shorter cycle over a fewer number of paddocks. The cut paddocks would come back into the grazing system at a time when grass is slightly less abundant. Topping will be needed at least once in the early part of the season, and should be done without delay after the cows have left the paddock. (*See also under* PASTURE MANAGEMENT.)

The two-sward system involves the use of paddocks for grazing and of separate areas of grassland for conservation.

In order to reduce STRESS (which see) among sheep in paddocks, Stephen Williams recommends surrounding a system of paddocks by solid hedges and filled-in gates. 'The hedges are A-shaped and leafed to the ground and deflect noise upwards when they are alongside roads. In full leaf, they are high enough and solid enough to give perfect privacy for the sheep units they enclose. Various types of fences, hedges, and walls for subdividing the area into paddocks have been examined and, quite certainly, the open type wire fence is superior, even essential. The analysis of this matter reveals that the lambs like to keep their dams in view and are much more likely to forage in the forward paddock better and more widely if they can do this.'

PADS for horses' feet are made in several different shapes. They serve the purpose of minimising concussion; they prevent slipping, and protect injured or extremely sensitive frogs or soles; and to some extent they encourage the expansion of the frog in cases of contracted heels.

FROG-PADS are worn with a full-sized shoe, and consist of a leather sole, which fits between the shoe and the foot, carrying a thick rubber or composition pad over the frog and corresponding with it in outline. They are used to give protection to the sole and frog, and to encourage healthy growth of the frog.

BAR-PADS are somewhat similar to frog-pads, but they are worn with a half-shoe only, and reach across from the bar on one side of the foot to that opposite. The pad is usually made of rubber and gives a better grip on a slippery surface than when only a frog-pad is used.

PNEUMATIC PADS are made entirely of rubber and serve to protect a 'dropped sole ' from contact with stones, etc., on the ground. They have a depression on the foot surface into which the projecting portion of the sole descends, and are sometimes made with an air-chamber in the thickness of the rubber.

BRIDGE-PADS are made in the nature of a flexible steel bridge, running from one heel of the shoe across to the other, which carries one or two pads of rubber in the middle part. The ends of the steel bridge are riveted to the heels of the shoe and the pads rest across the frog on the foot. When in use the middle of the bridge breaks, so that there shall be no undue pressure upon the foot. When the weight of the horse comes on to the foot each half of the bridge-pad is firmly pressed against the ground, thereby constituting an anti-slipping device.

PAIN.—(For relief of pain, *see* ANALGESICS, ANÆSTHESIA.)

PAINT (*see* LEAD POISONING).

PALATE (*palatus*, the roof of the mouth) is the partition between the cavity of the mouth below, and that of the nose above. It consists of the *hard palate* and the *soft palate*. The hard palate is formed by the bony floor of the nasal cavity covered with dense mucous membrane, which is crossed by transverse ridges in all the domesticated animals. These ridges assist the tongue to carry the food back to the throat. The hard palate stretches back a little beyond the last molar teeth in animals, and ends by becoming continuous with the soft palate. This latter is formed by muscles covered with mucous membrane, and acts as a sort of curtain between the cavity of the mouth and that of the pharynx. In most animals it is short, and will allow food to be regurgitated back into the mouth, but this is not the case in the horse. In that animal it is long, and forms a division so arranged that food material can only pass from the mouth to the pharynx, and not in the reverse direction. It is owing to this anatomical peculiarity that the horse is not able to vomit through his mouth. Material brought up from the stomach must pass out by way of the nostrils. In race-horses, distressed breathing may arise as the result of inflammation or partial paralysis of the soft palate, which may be linked with paresis or paralysis of the vocal cords. Partial resection of the soft palate has been carried out as treatment for this latter condition. (*See Vet. Record* Feb. 2, 1963.) (*See also* GUTTURAL POUCH DIPHTHERIA.)

Prolonged Soft Palate is a recognised inherited abnormality of the short-nosed breeds of dogs, *e.g.* Boxers, Bulldogs, Pekingese, Pugs, Cocker Spaniel.

Symptoms.—Panting or, in extreme cases, a temporary loss of consciousness due to obstruction if the windpipe.

Severe injury to the hard palate is not uncommonly seen in cats which have fallen from a height.

PALATABILITY (*see under* DIET).

PALPEBRAL.—Relating to the eyelids.

PALPATION (*palpo*, I touch gently) means the method of examining the surface of the body, and the internal organs as to their size, position, shape, etc., by the method of feeling with the hand laid upon the skin gently manipulating the structures within reach.

P.A.M. — Pyridine-2-aldoxime methiodide. This has been recommended as an antidote to be given intravenously in parathion poisoning, in addition to treatment with atropine.

PAN- (πᾶς, all) is a prefix meaning all or completely.

PANCREAS (πάγκρεας), or the ' sweetbread ', is a gland which possesses digestive functions, situated in the abdomen, a little in front of the level of the kidneys and a little below them. It lies under the 16th and 17th thoracic vertebræ and to the right of the middle line of the body in the horse. When fresh it has a reddish cream colour, and resembles the salivary glands, being composed of a number of lobules loosely united together and not provided with a surrounding capsule. In the horse it possesses two ducts which carry its secretion to the first part of the small intestine, about 5 or 6 inches from the stomach.

Minute structure.—The gland resembles a salivary gland, being composed of large numbers of tubes of columnar cells bound together by loose connective tissue. These cells are arranged with one end abutting on a central lumen into which the secretion passes from the cells. Each group of tubes ends in a small duct, which unites with others to form, finally, one or other of the main ducts in those animals that possess two of these structures—horse and dog—and to form the pancreatic duct in those others that only possess a single duct—ox, pig, and sheep. These ducts open into the first part of the small intestine—*i.e.* the duodenum—with, or near to, the opening of the bile duct from the liver. The cells of an active gland show a clear zone remote from the lumen of the tube, and a granular zone near the lumen. This latter zone is filled with granules produced by the cells, which, with fluids, form the pancreatic juice. In addition to these main characters there are certain small clusters of cells, whose function is not completely understood, called 'cell islets'. They pour their secretion (known as 'insulin') into the blood-stream direct, and exercise control over the excretion of sugar in the urine, for when they are diseased, or when the pancreas is removed, diabetes results.

Function.—The most obvious function of the pancreas is the secretion of the pancreatic juice, which is poured into the small intestine to meet the food which has undergone partial digestion in the stomach. The juice contains alkaline salts and at least four ferments, viz. *trypsin*, which carries on the digestion of proteins already begun in the stomach; *amylopsin*, which converts starches into sugars; *steapsin*, which breaks up fats; and a substance that curdles milk. (*See* DIGESTION.) The less obvious function of the pancreas is that with which the cell islets are concerned; this has been referred to and is considered under HORMONES, ENDOCRINE GLANDS, and DIABETES, which see.

PANCREAS, DISEASES OF.—Among animals other than the dog, diseases of the pancreas are apparently uncommon, and when they are discovered it is (with the exception of diabetes) usually upon post mortem examination. When the cell-islets (*see* PANCREAS), however, which elaborate *insulin*, discovered in Canada by Dr. Banting, are diseased, or when their secretion is incompetent, diabetes results. (*See* DUCTLESS GLANDS, DIABETES.) Even where diseases of the pancreas, such as inflammation, suppuration, atrophy, tumour formation, etc., are diagnosed during life, treatment, unless it be surgical excision of the diseased part, is not possible.

Acute necrotic pancreatitis has been reported in obese dogs; the symptoms being increased tension of the abdominal wall, tenderness, or severe pain. Later a rise in blood sugar and shock may be evident. On post-mortem examination, the pancreas is found to be enlarged.

With chronic inflammation, thirst and polyuria may be accompanied by swelling of the abdomen and the passing of fœtid or fatty fæces. The pancreas shrinks. A ravenous appetite, large abdomen, fatty fæces, and an absence of body fat characterise atrophy of the pancreas.

PANHYSTERECTOMY (πᾶς, all; ὑστέρα, womb; ἐκτομή, excision).—An operation by which the uterus is completely removed.

PANLEUCOPENIA.—Feline Infectious Enteritis.

PANNUS (*see* EYE, DISEASES, p. 326).

PANOPHTHALMITIS (πᾶν, the whole; ὀφθαλμός, the eye) means inflammation affecting all the structures of the eye.

PANTOTHENIC ACID. — Associated with the vitamin B complex. (*See* VITAMINS.)

PANZOÖTIC (πᾶν, the whole; ζῷον, an animal) means a disease which affects all animals in an area.

PAPER.—Waste paper has been incorporated in ruminant diets with apparent success as a roughage.

In one trial, waste paper from an office was ground through a hammermill and incorporated in sheep rations at levels of 15, 30 and 45 per cent replacing equal amounts of chopped hay. At the 45 per cent level, paper was the only roughage in the diet and urea was added to balance the nitrogen at the various levels of paper addition.

Dry-matter consumption of 15 and 30 per cent paper rations was equal to the control, and the ration containing 45 per cent paper was eaten at about 95 per cent of the control consumption. (Nishimuta, J. F., & others (1969), *J. Anim. Sci.* **29** 642.)

PAPILLA (*papilla*, a nipple) means a small projection, and is applied to those tiny nipple-like buds which project into the outer covering skin from the deeper layers. It is also applied to other anatomical structures which have a similar shape, such as those of the tongue of the ox, the optic papilla of the retina, the renal papilla of the kidney, etc.

PAPILLOMA (*papilla*, nipple; *-oma*, termination meaning tumour) means a tumour composed of papillæ growing from the surface of the skin or mucous membrane. These may be malignant, but they are usually benign. (*See* TUMOURS.)

PAPULE (*papula*) means a pimple.

PARA- (*παρά*, beside) is a prefix meaning near, aside from, or beyond.

PARACENTESIS (*παρακέντμσις*) is a term applied to the tapping of the chest or abdomen for the removal of fluid. (*See* ASPIRATION.)

PARADONTAL DISEASE (*see* TEETH, DISEASES OF).

PARAFFIN (*parum*, little; *affinis*, akin) is the general term used to designate a series of saturated hydrocarbons, which were discovered by Reichenbach in 1830, and first produced by Young in 1850. The higher members of the series are solid at ordinary temperatures, some being hard and others soft. Lower in the scale comes petroleum, which is liquid at ordinary temperatures. Naphtha, petroleum spirit, and hydramyl, are members of the series lower still, which are very volatile bodies, and finally lowest comes methane or marsh-gas, which is a gaseous body.

These paraffins do not mix with water, nor do they form soaps with alkalis, and, unlike fats, they do not turn rancid with keeping. Bacteria will not grow on them, and they are accordingly non-infective for broken surfaces of the skin.

Uses.—Internally, only **medicinal** liquid paraffin is used; it is a gentle laxative, but has the disadvantage that it is liable to become tolerated by the system and lose its effect when given continually as a routine laxative. It was given in old dogs liable to impaction after eating bones. It should not be given regularly as it is said to absorb vitamin D and may cause rickets. Externally, the hard and soft paraffins are used in the preparation of various ointments and lubricants. They are not absorbed to the same extent as the animal fats, and are therefore not so suitable for the basis of a drug which requires to be absorbed so that its action may be made use of.

Methane is freely produced in digestive disorders of herbivorous animals, and constitutes the greater part of the gas which collects in the rumen of the ox affected with tympany of the rumen.

Kerosene has no place in animal treatment.

PARAGONIMIASIS.—Infestation with lung flukes of *Paragonimus* species in dogs, cats, foxes, mink. (*See* p. 648.)

PARAINFLUENZA 3 VIRUS.—Infection with this is widespread in sheep in the U.K. (*See also* INFLUENZA.)

PARAKERATOSIS.—The name applied to a scaly, elephant-like skin. The condition has been seen in pigs suffering from a zinc deficiency, following, *e.g.* a 'diet of maize, lucerne, limestone, and aureomycin'. It occurs in pigs fed dry meal *ad lib.*, and gradually clears up when a change to wet feeding is made. It often begins with a red pimply condition of the skin on the flanks, abdomen, etc. Thin, dry yellowish or greyish scales may be seen on the skin, which later becomes thickened. It responds to small doses of zinc sulphate.

PARALYSIS (*παραλύω*, I relax), in its widest sense may mean loss of nerve control over any of the bodily functions, loss of sensation, and loss of the special senses, but the term is usually restricted to mean loss of muscular action due to interference with the nervous sytem. When muscular power is merely weakened, without being lost completely, the word *paresis* is often used, as 'parturient paresis', which is another name for milk fever. Various terms are used to indicate paralysis distributed in different ways. Thus, *hemiplegia* is the term applied to paralysis affecting one side of the body only, along with the fore and hind limbs of that side; it is seen as the result of certain affections of the brain in dogs, very often following the more acute stages of chorea. *Diplegia* is used to mean a condition of more or less complete paralysis, in which both sides of the body are affected in the same manner. *Monoplegia* is the term applied to paralysis of a single limb, such as occurs in 'radial paralysis' in horses. *Paraplegia*, which is probably the commonest form of paralysis in animals, means that all the structures behind a certain level of the body are paralysed; this form occurs in broken back, typical azoturia, and certain affections of the spinal cord in or near the lumbar region. In paraplegia there is very often paralysis of the sphincter muscles of the bladder and rectum, so that urine and fæces are voided without any control from the higher nerve centres.

Paralysis should be regarded rather as a symptom than as a disease by itself. In the majority of cases it is inadvisable to keep an animal which has become affected with any extensive paralysis, for there is but a slight hope, and where recovery does occur it may take many months. During this time of waiting the animal must receive careful nursing, massage, electric treatment, etc., and even where these are conscientiously carried out recovery is problematical. Generally speaking, it is advisable, upon economic grounds, to slaughter paralysed animals the carcases of which may be used for human food, and extensively paralysed horses and dogs should be destroyed on humane grounds. (*See also under* RABIES.)

Varieties.—Paralysis is usually looked upon as being due to cerebral, spinal, or peripheral causes.

Cerebral paralysis.—These conditions resulting from brain troubles, such as apoplexy, encephalitis, tumour formation, fracture of the skull with depression of a portion of bone, etc., are accompanied by severe general or local paralysis, either

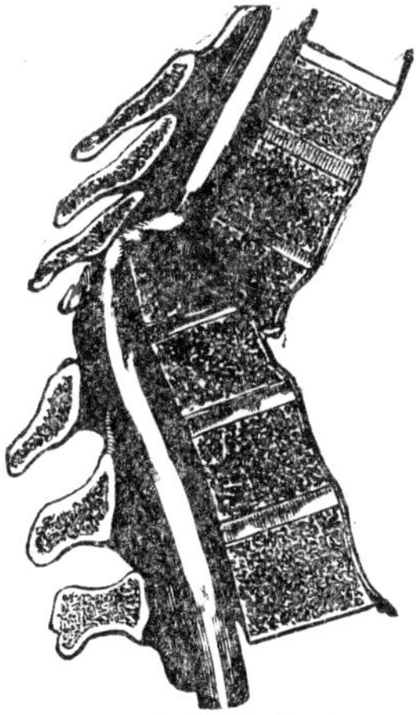

Fracture of the spinal column, with compression of the canal, which leads to paralysis of the parts behind the fracture. (Miller's *Surgery*.)

of the whole body (when death usually follows very rapidly), or of one side (hemiplegia). The animal lies upon its side, perhaps moving the uppermost limbs, but incapable of stirring those underneath. If assisted to its feet (smaller animals) it is unable to retain its balance, and falls violently to the ground. The paralysed members when examined are found to be flaccid, with the muscles totally relaxed, and passive movements are not resisted. Sensations of pain may be felt, however, and an indication that sensation is not destroyed is shown by raising the head, or struggling with the sound limbs when a pin-prick is made in a paralysed part. Unconsciousness or convulsions may accompany the paralysis, especially when extensive injury has been inflicted upon the brain from a blow, fall, etc.

In apoplexy the seizure is sudden, the animal falling to the ground when engaged in some sudden or severe exertion; in encephalitis there is usually some co-existing disease, such as influenza, strangles, distemper, etc., and the brain symptoms develop as a complication; in brain tumour formation the symptoms come on very gradually, and it may be weeks before any serious paralysis is noticed; with fracture and depression there is an immediate loss of power, just as when an animal is stunned.

Spinal paralysis or paraplegia is most often due to fracture of, or severe injury to, the vertebræ of the back, or to injuries involving the spinal cord. The weakest part of the column is at the junction between the last thoracic and the first lumbar vertebra, and it is in this part that fracture very frequently occurs. Horses that have struggled with their heads between their fore-legs when cast for operation, and small animals which have been run over by a heavy vehicle, usually suffer in this way. Concussion of the spinal cord, with perhaps hæmorrhage into the bony canal, which may result from falls, colliding with fixed objects, suddenly pulling up after galloping, severe blows, etc., may result in paralysis, but, if there is no great hæmorrhage or fissuring of the bone, recovery may occur some days or weeks afterwards. In this instance the paralysis is not complete. The absorption of toxic substances from the digestive tract, the presence of parasitic worms in young colts, azoturia, pressure upon the lumbar plexus from a pregnant uterus, exposure to a very hot sun or to an extremely low temperature, are all conditions which may result in partial or complete paraplegia; while lightning stroke, abscess formation in the cord, may also produce it. Animals usually possess the power of movement and have full sensations as far back as the level of the injury, but behind it there is neither muscular control nor feeling. An important feature of broken back is that very often the hind quarters of the body, as far forward as the level of the fracture, perspire profusely for some time after the injury occurs. A horse in this condition may make vigorous efforts to rise, and although the fore end of the body may be lifted, the hind-quarters lie inert, and the animal sinks down again. Breathing becomes distressed and the temperature usually rises. In complete paralysis death usually takes place in from 12 to 48 hours

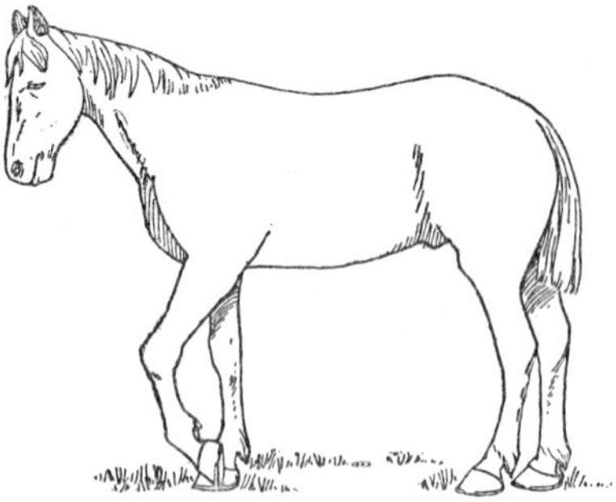

Diagram of a horse affected with paralysis of the radial nerve, commonly called 'dropped elbow' on account of the lowering of the elbow joint. The muscles which lie to the front of the fore-arm and those attached to the point of the elbow (which are all supplied by the radial nerve) are paralysed, giving the appearance shown in the figure.

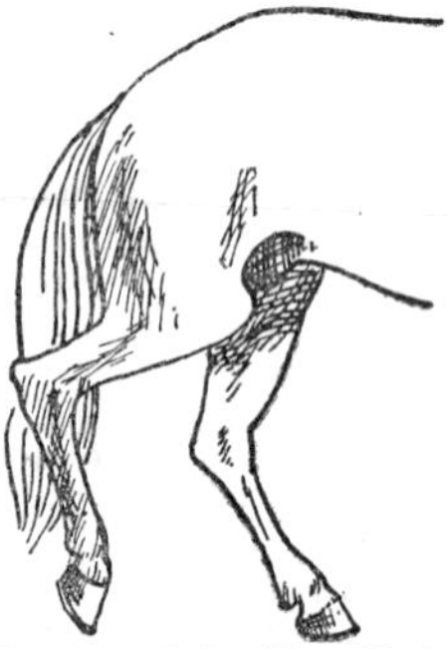

Crural paralysis. The stifle is impeded in flexibility and appears stiff. When weight is borne by the limb it results in a sinking of the stifle and difficulty in movement. It is caused by injury to the femoral nerve and is therefore frequently called 'femoral paralysis'.

after the injury. In partial paralysis the symptoms vary greatly, as would be expected considering the diversity of the symptoms. In the least serious type there may be little or nothing seen so long as the animal is standing or walking forward in a straight line, but upon making the animal turn suddenly or back a short distance, the hind-quarters droop or sink to the ground. In such cases full sensation is usually retained, and there may even be increased tenderness over the hind quarters. The treatment of incomplete cases demands the services of a skilled practitioner, for the nature of the drugs used, the curative measures adopted, and the variety of work advisable, vary with each case. (*See* INTERVERTEBRAL DISC, and, for horses, under COMENY'S.)

In *Peripheral paralysis* there is usually some injury to a nerve trunk, some affection of the nerve-endings in the muscle fibres, or perhaps a rheumatic condition of both muscle and nerve, which causes the condition. There are two very important forms of peripheral paralysis which affect the fore limbs of horses—'suprascapular' and 'radial paralysis'. The former of these is often called 'slipped shoulder', and the latter 'dropped elbow'. They are of sufficient importance to merit separate attention, and are described under SUPRASCAPULAR PARALYSIS and RADIAL PARALYSIS; to these headings reference should be made. 'Paralysis of the brachial plexus' results from collision with heavy bodies, from run-away accidents, from becoming cast and struggling violently, hæmorrhage into the axilla, or deep wounds in this region, such as are produced by stakes running into the front of the chest between the ribs and one of the fore limbs, etc. In each of these cases the important plexus of nerves of the fore-limb is injured. There is complete paralysis of all the muscles of the limb in most cases, but in some instances when one or more nerves have escaped, there may be only partial paralysis. 'Gluteal paralysis' is very uncommon. It consists of a marked wasting of the muscles of one hind quarter and a tendency to carry the limb out to one side. When the foot reaches the ground it does so with a peculiar tapping action. The causes of the condition are often unknown. In 'paralysis of the sciatic nerve' there is a loss of power in all the muscles of the thigh except those situated above and to the front of the stifle joint, *i.e.* the quadratus group. The limb hangs loosely and the animal jerks it forward when attempting to walk; although the stifle is advanced the hock and the fetlock remain flexed and the front of the foot comes to the ground. The animal may be able to bear weight, however, if the foot is placed in the normal position by the hand. When there is a severe injury to the side of the thigh from a fall, kick, or other similar cause, 'paralysis of the external popliteal nerve' (common peroneal) may occur; it results in an inability to extend the foot or flex the hock. When the horse is made to walk the limb is drawn out backwards into a position resembling that seen in dislocation of the stifle, but the fetlock is flexed instead of being fully extended. The limb is then carried a short distance forward and the foot comes to rest upon the ground on its anterior face instead of on the sole. By artificially posing the foot by hand, or by mechanical devices, some weight can be borne. In 'crural paralysis' (paralysis of the femoral nerve) the quadriceps muscles above the stifle, which normally extend that joint, are paralysed. When weight is put upon the limb the stifle sinks to the level of the hock or below it, all joints are flexed, and there is a peculiar drop of the hind quarter on the same side. So long as the opposite limb remains sound, however, the horse soon learns to make the necessary allowance for this inability to bear weight, and in time becomes able to walk better. Wasting of the affected muscles, however, is always severe, and the animal is unfit for work.

Treatment.—For general advice as to treatment the owner should consult a veterinary surgeon.

PARALDEHYDE.—A narcotic.

PARAMETER.—Normal levels of values, *e.g.* of calcium in the bloodstream of a particular species of animal.

PARAPHYMOSIS.—A constriction preventing the penis from being withdrawn into the prepuce. This is not uncommon in the dog, and is serious, for gangrene may occur unless relief is afforded. As a first-aid measure, swab the penis with ice-cold water. Surgical interference under anæsthesia may be necessary. The use of hyaluronidase in normal saline, by injection, has been recommended.

PARAPLEGIA (παραπληγία, paralysis crosswise) means paralysis of the posterior pair of limbs, and may be accompanied by paralysis of the muscles which control the passage of urine and fæces to the outside. (*See* PARALYSIS.)

It is seen following accidents involving injury to the spine—frequently in the dog knocked down by a car—and may also be associated with 'Disc' lesions. A rare cause is thrombosis of the femoral arteries. In the dog, this may occur suddenly—the animal playing one minute, and collapsing with a yelp the next. Absence of pulse in the femoral arteries assists a diagnosis. (*See also under* THROMBOSIS, COMENY'S.)

PARAQUAT.—This herbicide has caused fatal poisoning in man. Poisoning in the dog gives rise to lung œdema, congestion and consolidation.

PARASITES AND PARASITOLOGY

A parasite, according to the derivation of the word, from the Greek παράσιτος, means, freely translated, 'one who eats at another man's table'.

Parasitology, strictly defined, is that branch of biology which treats of both animal and plant parasites. The term is, however, usually applied to animal parasites. Vegetable parasites are treated separately and included in Bacteriology and Mycology.

The intimate association between animals may be divided into the following groups:

Commensalism is the association of species in which the one alone benefits but the other does not suffer.

Mutualism is the association of two species as a mutually beneficial partnership.

Symbiosis is any form of existence in which two different species of organisms live in close approximation; the term is often used in a restricted sense for an association which is of mutual benefit and at the same time obligatory.

Parasitism is the association of two organisms, one of which (the parasite) benefits by nourishing itself at the expense of the other (the host), but without normally destroying it. The following types of parasitic relations are recognised: 1 (*a*) ectoparasites, which live on the host; and (*b*) endoparasites, which live within the body of the host; 2 (*a*) accidental parasites, which are normally free-living animals but may live for a certain period in a host, *e.g.* rat-tailed larvæ; (*b*) facultative parasites, which are able to exist free or as parasites, *e.g.* blowfly larvæ; and (*c*) obligatory parasites, which are completely adapted to a parasitic type of life and must live in or on a host, *e.g.* most parasitic worms; 3 (*a*) temporary or transitory parasites, which pass a definite phase or phases in their life history as parasites and during which time the parasitism is obligatory and continuous, *e.g.* botflies, ticks; (*b*) permanent parasites, which always live for the greater part of their life as parasites, *e.g.* lice, tapeworms, coccidia, etc.; and (*c*) periodic, occasional, or intermittent parasites,

which only visit the host for short periods to obtain food, *e.g.* blood-sucking flies, fleas; 4 (*a*) erratic parasites, which occur in an organ that is not their normal habitat, *e.g. Fasciola hepatica* in the lungs; (*b*) incidental parasites, which, exceptionally, occur in an animal that is not their normal host; they are incidental only in this first host, *e.g. Dipylidium caninum* is incidental in man; and (*c*) specific parasites, which occur in a particular species of host or group of hosts, *e.g. D. caninum* is specific for dogs and cats. Specific parasites may be divided into (i) *stenoxenes*, which live in a species of host, or at most in a few closely related forms, *e.g. Tænia solium* in man, and (ii) *euryxenes*, which live in a wide group of hosts, *e.g. Trichinella spiralis* in about twenty different species of animals.

CLASSIFICATION.—In modern zoological practice all animals are given a generic and a specific name. This is called the 'binomial system'. The 'species' includes all forms of animals which resemble each other closely in every respect, and which interbreed and produce fertile offspring. Sometimes species are split into smaller groups called 'subspecies' or 'varieties'; but this practice is of doubtful value. Once a name is given to a species and is shown to be a valid one, it must be retained. This rule accounts for the present confusion in specific names in parasitology. Many of the species have been found to possess several specific names, and as the first valid name must be retained, many apparent changes have had to be made. Several species which resemble each other are grouped together in a 'genus', with one of the species selected as typical and called a 'genotype'. If this genus is valid, *i.e.* not preoccupied, it cannot be changed. It may be narrowed in its application, and some species transferred to new genera, but the genotype must remain with its original genus. Related genera are grouped together in larger groups as shown below, but in every case a type family and genus must be selected. The stem of this type genus must be used for the larger groups with its appropriate ending added.

Example.	Musca domestica.	
Species	*domestica*	
Genus	*Musca*	
(Tribe)	Musceæ	(*-eæ*)
(Subfamily) . .	Muscinæ	(*-inæ*)
Family	Muscidæ	(*-idæ*)
Superfamily . . .	Muscoidea	(*-oidea*)
(Section) . . .	Schizophora	
(Suborder) . .	Cyclorrhapha	
Order	Diptera	
Class	Insecta	
Phylum	Arthropoda	
Subkingdom . . .	Metazoa.	

Some of the above groups may be subdivided. Those shown in brackets are not always used. All zoological classification is merely an expression of opinion, and no two zoologists adopt identical systems. Specific and generic names are printed in *italics*; while the higher names are in Roman type. The name of an author who first names a species is written after the specific name. If his name appears in brackets it means that the species has since been removed to another genus, and the name of the person so removing it may follow that of the original author.

DISEASES DUE TO PARASITES.—The scientific name of a parasitic disease is formed by adding '*osis*' or '*iasis*' to the generic stem; *e.g. strongylosis* is the disease caused by the genus *Strongylus* in the horse and *Leishmaniasis* is the disease caused by the genus *Leishmania* in man and dogs. If more than one closely related genus is implicated the termination '*-id*' is sometimes added to the stem of the type genus of the group, before the usual termination; *e.g. strongylidosis* is the disease caused by the strongylid (or strongyle-like) worms in the horse.

Parasitic diseases are seldom caused by one or a few specimens, but as a rule depend on mass infestations. There are exceptions to this, however, as one *Ascaris* may obstruct the bile-duct with fatal results. Parasites, with few exceptions, do not spend all their lives in the animal body, but always require to spend a certain proportion of their life-cycle outside the host. They may cause damage to the host in the following ways:

(1) By abstraction of nourishment properly belonging to the host, *e.g.* many of the intestinal worms:

(2) By mechanical obstruction of passages or compression of organs, *e.g.* gapes (in chickens), hydatid, etc.;

(3) By feeding on the tissues of the host, *e.g.* blood-sucking worms or flies;

PARASITES AND PARASITOLOGY

(4) By production of toxins with varying effects, anæmia, cerebral symptoms, and so on. This subject is not well understood, but the toxins may belong to some of the following classes: excretory products of the parasites, digestive juices, or hæmolytic toxins. Probably most parasites are implicated, but the following are the best known: hookworms, bots and warbles, tapeworms, and ascarids;

(5) By actual traumatic damage, *e.g.* by piercing and destroying skin (ticks, mites, flies, etc.), by depositing eggs in the tissues (blood flukes, lung worms), by migrations of larvæ (*Ascaris* and *Trichinella*), by clinging to surfaces by means of sharp hooks (tapeworms), and in many other ways;

(6) By facilitating the entrance of bacteria; *e.g.* stomach worms in pigs allow the entrance of *Fusiformis necrophorus* (the necrosis bacillus);

(7) By transmitting diseases for which they act as intermediate hosts; *e.g.* ticks and babesiosis, etc.;

(8) By causing inflammatory or neoplastic reactions in the invaded tissues; *e.g.* pneumonia, gastritis, fluke adenomata in the liver, and so on. These are only some of the more obvious methods of injuring the host. Apart from the loss due to actual deaths, the depreciation in value of hides, meat, milk, and work is enormous, and, although less spectacular than a bacterial epizoötic, the loss is more constant, and in the aggregate is probably even greater than the loss due to bacterial diseases.

The drawings which follow of the various parasites are more or less diagrammatic, and are intended primarily as an aid to diagnosis. They show 'average' specimens, but considerable variations in size and outline exist in most parasites. All are magnified.

PROTOZOÖN PARASITES.—Protozoology is that part of biology which is concerned with the study of those animals consisting of only one cell. The animal kingdom is generally divided into two sub-kingdoms, Protozoa or non-cellular animals, and Metazoa or cellular animals:

The sub-kingdom Protozoa includes an enormous number of forms, all small and mostly free-living. Some, however, have taken to a form of life in which they are dependent on the efforts of other animals. Some live in dung—the so-called 'coprozoic forms'. Others have definitely taken up their existence in the animal body. In some cases they are actually of benefit to

PARASITES AND PARASITOLOGY

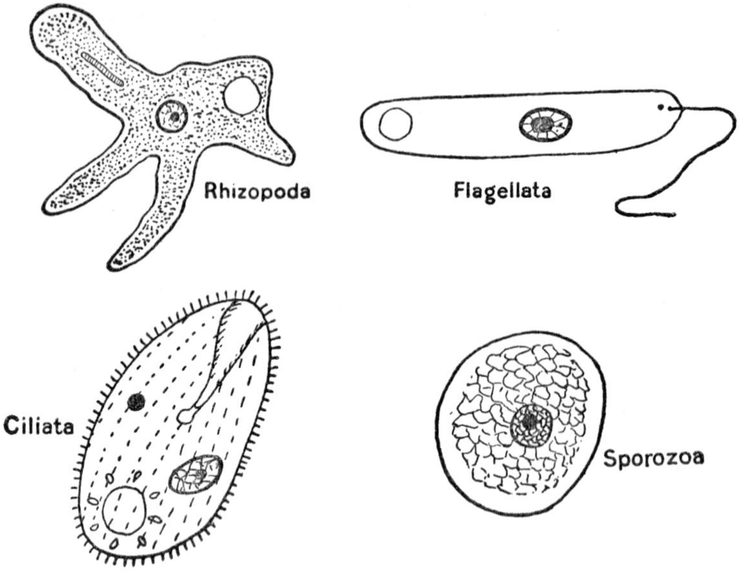

Types of Protozoa.

their host (symbiosis), in others they do no harm while doing no good (commensalism), but in others they are definitely harmful to the host animal (parasitism), and it is with this last group that we here mainly deal.

CLASSIFICATION.—Amongst others, there are four large groups or classes in the sub-kingdom Protozoa which contain species of veterinary interest or importance. Members of these classes may be easily distinguished by their mode of locomotion.

1. CLASS RHIZOPODA (=SARCODINA) includes the organisms which move and ingest food by means of temporary finger-like processes or pseudopodia. These forms are largely free-living, but the genus *Entamœba* is parasitic.

2. CLASS MASTIGOPHORA (=FLAGELLATA) includes the organisms which move by means of permanent whip-like processes called flagella. Many of the flagellates are free-living, but some are among the most important parasites of man and his animals. *Trypanosoma, Leishmania, Histomonas, Trichomonas,* and other less important genera belong to this group.

3. CLASS SPOROZOA includes those organisms in which there are no special organs of locomotion. They are exclusively parasitic in habit and at some stage in their development produce spores enclosing one or more sporozoites which carry the infection to new hosts. The group includes many important parasites

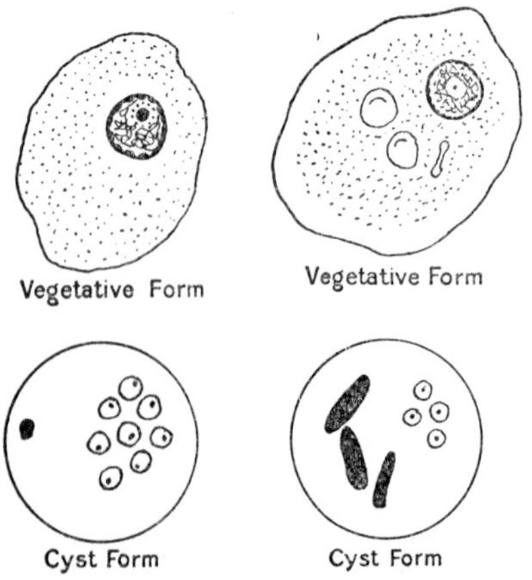

Entamœba coli. *Entamœba histolytica.*

such as *Babesia, Theileria, Anaplasma, Eimeria,* and so on.

4. CLASS CILIATA includes those organisms in which the organs of locomotion are cilia, or numerous small hair-like processes which move in rhythm. They possess these cilia in all stages of their development and comprise one of the most

highly evolved groups of the Protozoa. There is one important parasitic genus, *Balantidium*.

The parasitic genera will be treated in the above order.

ENTAMŒBA.—Two species of this genus may be met with in man and occasionally in dogs and cats: *E. coli* and *E. histolytica*. They have a close resemblance to the common amœba of the pond, but they are not found in their characteristic amœbic form outside the body. *E. coli* is a harmless commensal, while *E. histolytica* is the cause of human amœbic dysentery. The two parasites are figured (see above). *E. coli* shows feeble motility and never feeds on red blood-cells. Both forms are passed from the intestine in a cystic form, and the cyst of *E. coli* can be distinguished by its larger size and by the possession of eight nuclei in the ripe cyst, while *E. histolytica* has only four. In stained specimens the nucleus has the characteristic appearance shown in the figure.

It is interesting to note that while the cat can be easily infected by cysts of human origin, cysts are not formed in the cat. Accordingly, it is probable that these animals do not play any part in the transmission of the disease, and that infection always comes from man.

TRYPANOSOMA.—This is a genus of very minute flagellates usually found in

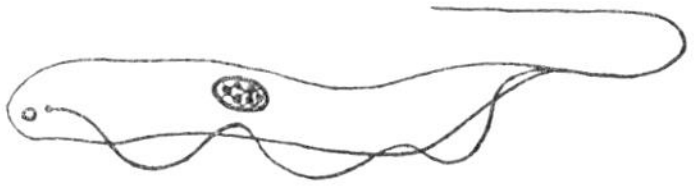

Diagram of Trypanosome

the blood of vertebrates. The body is of an elongated fusiform shape with a single flagellum and an undulating membrane. There are two nuclei—a large nucleus (macronucleus or trophonucleus) near the centre of the body, and a small kinetoplast (micronucleus) at the posterior end, remote from the flagellum. The flagellum is the continuation of the rim bordering the undulating membrane which arises near the posterior end. In some forms there is no free flagellum. Transmission is generally by the bite of an insect (except in the case of Dourine). The transmission may be mechanical, *i.e.* carried directly from an infected animal to an uninfected one by the bite of a blood-sucking fly, or cyclical, when the insect host is not infective for a definite time after ingestion of the parasite. In this case the parasite passes a definite part of its life-cycle in the fly. In many cases transmission may be both mechanical and cyclical. Thus, the tsetse fly may have two infective periods, one immediately after biting a sick animal and the second some time later (about 20 days) after the trypanosome has progressed to its infective stage along normal lines.

LIFE HISTORIES OF TRYPANOSOMES.—In the blood of the mammalian host the trypanosomes reproduce by splitting lengthwise (longitudinal fission). A quantity of blood is sucked up by the insect host, a species of *Glossina*, and in that host the flagellates undergo a definite developmental cycle. The location chosen by the parasite for its development varies with the species. Thus some will develop only in the salivary glands, others in the gut, and still others in the proboscis. The ingested trypanosomes take on the so-called '*crithidal*' form, *i.e.* the kinetoplast becomes anterior to the nucleus, and in this form multiplication by longitudinal fission takes place. After some time they assume the infective form, and are ready to be passed with the salivary fluids into the blood-stream of a suitable vertebrate host.

In the case of those forms which are mechanically transmitted no such cycle takes place. The ingested parasites remain in the proboscis for some little time, and if the fly bites another vertebrate within that time they are passed into the wound with the salivary juice of the insect. If no host is found within a fairly short period, the flagellates are destroyed by the fly's digestive fluids.

The diseases caused by trypanosomes are called *Trypanosomiases*, in addition to a number of local native names. The symptoms vary in individual cases; but there is always a more or less irregular fever, emaciation, weakness, and loss of condition, and enlargement of lymphatic glands. Frequently also there are skin lesions, while ocular and nervous symptoms are also common.

DISEASES CAUSED BY TRYPANOSOMES.—The more important of the trypanosome diseases in animals will now be briefly described.

'Baleri', 'Jinja', 'Nagana' (in part).

The causal agent of this disease is known as *T. brucei*.

(Synonyms: *T. pecaudi*, *T. rhodesiense*, and possibly *T. gambiense* and many others.) This species is polymorphic, *i.e.* long and short

PARASITES AND PARASITOLOGY

forms are found in the blood. It has a broad folded undulating membrane. The long forms have a long free flagellum and a pointed posterior end, while the short forms have a short or no flagellum and a rounded posterior end.

Transmission is by various species of *Glossina*, and in consequence the parasite

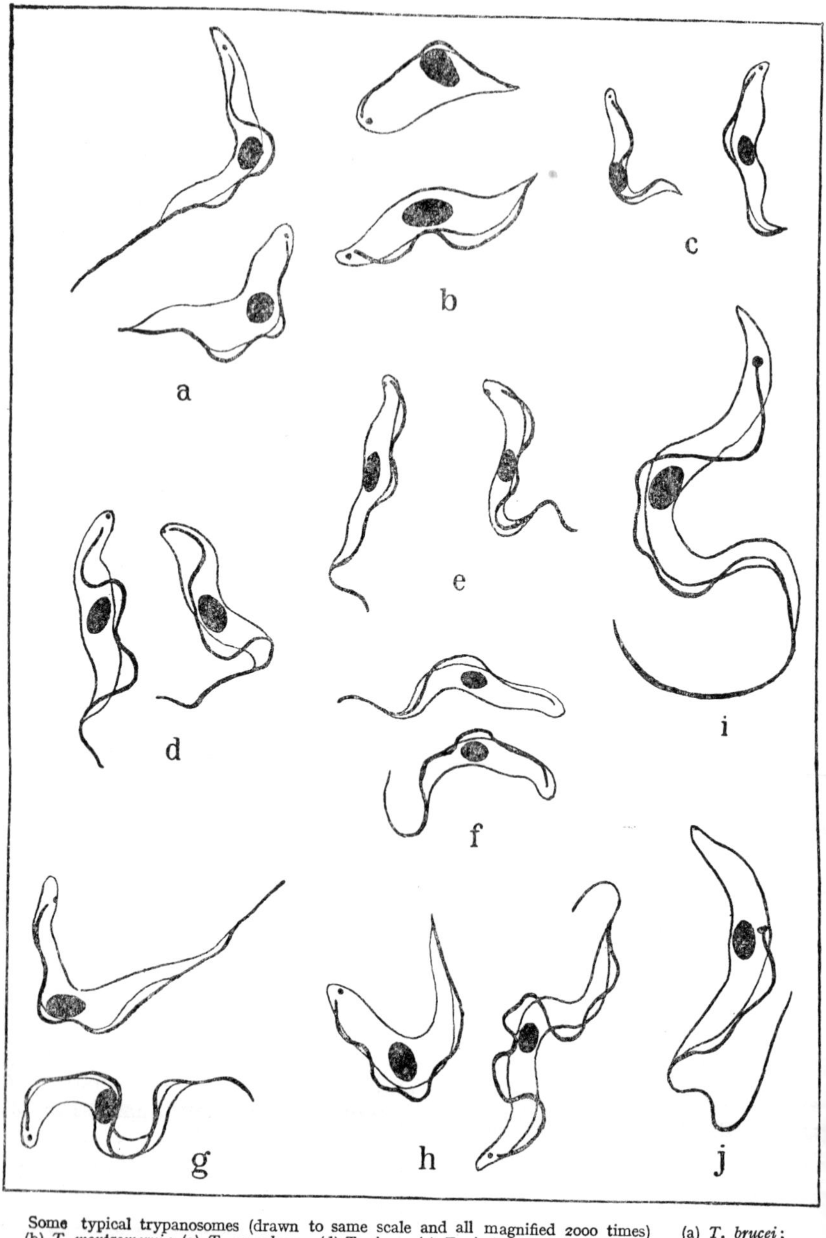

Some typical trypanosomes (drawn to same scale and all magnified 2000 times) (a) *T. brucei*; (b) *T. montgomeryi*; (c) *T. congolense*; (d) *T. vivax*; (e) *T. simiæ*; (f) *T. equinum*; (g) *T. equiperdum*; (h) *T. evansi*; (i) and (j) *T. theileri*.

PARASITES AND PARASITOLOGY

is limited to the African fly-belt. The animals affected are equines, sheep, goats, pigs, and dogs ; more rarely cattle.

Symptoms appear in horses in about three weeks after inoculation. There is a staring coat, progressive emaciation, œdematous swellings on the legs, and frequently a slight opacity of the cornea. The appetite remains good although the temperature is usually about 102°–104° F. The disease is usually fatal. In dogs the course is similar. In pigs the disease is stated to run a very acute course. In ruminants the disease is a chronic one with symptoms of anæmia. Cattle occasionally may act as reservoirs.

T. gambiense, the cause of 'sleeping sickness' in man, is identical with this form, being a strain which has become adapted to live in man.

'**Nagana**'. This is a native name applied somewhat loosely to any trypanosome disease of mammals in Zululand and refers to the state of depression and weakness characteristic of the disease. It is sometimes taken to apply to the disease caused by *T. brucei*, a disease primarily of equines, or to that caused by *T. congolense* which principally affects cattle, or to that caused by *T. vivax*, which also affects cattle. In scientific literature the name 'nagana' is valueless.

'**Nagana**' (in part), '**Paranagana**'. The causal agent is *T. congolense*, with numerous synonyms.

It is a smallish monomorphic species with a poorly developed undulating membrane and no free flagellum.

Transmission is by various species of *Glossina* and the parasite is restricted to the fly-belt, although it has once been reported from India. All domestic animals are affected, the disease being very acute in cattle and equines, but less so in the small ruminants. Local strains vary in virulence.

Symptoms occur in bovines in ten to forty days after infection. A progressive emaciation sets in, although the digestive functions remain more or less normal. The temperature rises at night to 106° F. and the temper becomes uncertain. Abortion is frequent. Unless treated, the animal dies.

T. montgomeryi only differs from the above by its greater width. It is found in the dog.

T. simiæ is related to *T. congolense* but is larger. It is pathogenic to pigs.

'**Souma**', '**Nagana**' (in part). The causal agent is *T. vivax*.

Like *T. congolense* this African form is monomorphic but is larger and has a free flagellum of varying length. It occurs most commonly in cattle, sheep, and goats, but also affects horses. The disease is similar to, but less virulent than, that caused by *T. congolense*; the average mortality is, nevertheless, high. Closely related to this species and probably identical with it is *T. viennei* (*T. guyannese*), which causes a fatal disease in cattle in Northern South America.

'**Surra**', '**Mbori**', '**El Debab**'.—The causal organism of this disease is *T. evansi* with numerous synonyms.

This is a monomorphic form which always possesses a flagellum and is of more uniform morphology than those of the African animal diseases. It does not undergo cyclical development in *Glossina* but is transmitted mechanically by various blood-sucking flies, such as Tabanids and stable flies. Experimentally, *Ornithodorus* ticks have transmitted infection. It is widely distributed in all the warmer parts of the world. It occurs mainly in wet weather.

It is found in all the domestic animals, but is most serious in equines and camels, when it is usually fatal. Cattle are more resistant. The average duration of the disease is about two months or less, while some cases have terminated in one or two weeks. Symptoms are generally visible in two to eight days.

Symptoms.—The symptoms at first are somewhat indefinite, with a slight fever and loss of appetite, and occasionally a localised urticarial eruption on the skin. This condition may disappear for a few days under suitable nursing, but in due course well-marked symptoms are found. The temperature is raised and the animal shows the typical signs of fever, usually accompanied by slight nasal catarrh and enlarged submaxillary glands. The animal rapidly loses flesh. In a few days the signs of fever disappear, and apart from the loss of flesh the animal seems quite well. This condition alternates with symptoms of fever accompanied by swellings in the pendulous regions, yellowish membranes, shallow abdominal respirations, but with an only slightly impaired appetite. Sooner or later the animal succumbs to one of the attacks, which gradually increase in severity. Towards the termination of the disease the animal shows a loss of power over the hind-quarters—possibly due to pressure of an exudate on the lumbar region of the spinal cord. In some cases the action of the heart becomes very accentuated just before the death of the animal and can be

 PARASITES AND PARASITOLOGY

heard several yards away. Death may be very sudden, or the animal may struggle violently in evident acute pain, and gradually die from exhaustion.

Treatment is not very satisfactory. Suramin is used in horses, and this or quinapyramine in camels.

T. hippicum is the causal agent of 'murrina' or 'derrengadera', a disease affecting horses and mules in the Panama Canal Zone. It is considered to be a variety of *T. evansi*, from which it is indistinguishable. Although transmissible by blood-sucking flies, particularly Tabanids, probably the most important means is by the vampire bat (*Desmodus rotundus*); a vicious blood-sucker which preys upon live-stock at night. Death of the horse usually occurs after several weeks or months, and the mortality is very high.

'Dourine', or 'Mal du Coit'.—The causal agent of this disease is *T. equiperdum.*

This species closely resembles *T. evansi* It is not usually found in the blood but in the local sores. This species is confined to equines, but unlike most of the species mentioned previously it occurs in temperate countries such as Europe and North America. It is absent from Britain, and has been stamped out in Canada. Transmission is by coitus.

Symptoms.—The symptoms fall into three stages. The first is characterised by œdema of the genitalia, often metastatic and sometimes with a discharge. Pain is shown in micturition. In about a month the second stage is seen, characterised by the appearance of 'plaques'. These look like discs of metal lodged beneath the skin in various parts of the body. They last for a very short time in any spot and are neither hot nor painful. A drop of blood from a plaque usually contains the parasite in small numbers. Anæmia, emaciation, and lassitude accompany the plaques. About the tenth month the tertiary stage, characterised by anæmia and paraplegia, is seen. Abscesses appear round the genital organs, and death soon occurs.

Diagnosis is difficult at first, and is only positive by demonstrating the trypanosome in the genital mucosa or plaque. Diagnosis is most conveniently carried out by means of a complement fixation test (similar to the Wassermann test for syphilis in man).

Treatment is not as a rule attempted, and infected animals are usually destroyed to prevent the spread of the disease.

'Mal de Caderas.'—The causal agent is *T. equinum.*

It is a long, slender monomorphic species with no kinetoplast but possesses a broad undulating membrane. It closely resembles *T. evansi.*

This species is only found in South America. Its mode of transmission is unknown. It is found mainly in equines, but ruminants and dogs may also be affected.

Symptoms consist of a gradual emaciation with a progressive anæmia and an irregular temperature. Conjunctivitis and keratitis are common, and a skin eruption is often seen on the shoulders, neck, and loins. The emaciation is progressive, with a characteristic weakness of the hind-quarters. Horses die in one to four months, but mules and donkeys are more resistant. Cattle only act as reservoirs, and show no symptoms.

Treatment: Suramin.

NON-PATHOGENIC TRYPANOSOMES.—*T. theileri* (Syn. *T. americanum*, etc.), This is a large form. The nucleus is oval and central, the kinetoplast is round and some distance from the posterior end, the undulating membrane is broad and folded, and there is a free flagellum. It is found in bovines in all parts of the world and is probably transmitted by several types of blood-sucking flies, Tabanids having definitely been incriminated.

T. transvaaliense, which is also found in cattle, has the kinetoplast midway between the nucleus and posterior end of the body. It is a variety of *T. theileri.*

T. ingens is a very large form found in cattle in Uganda.

T. melophagium is a parasite of sheep transmitted by the sheep ked. It has been found in Britain, and is doubtless of universal distribution.

LEISHMANIA.—This genus of parasites in smears from the spleen, bone-marrow, and so on, appears as a small round or oval body with a micro- and a macro-

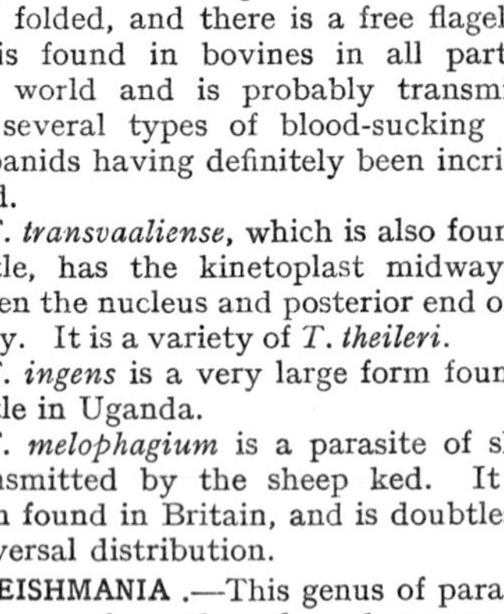

Leishmania as seen in spleen cells.

nucleus. In cultures, however, it develops a flagellum, and so is classed with the flagellates.

Canine Leishmaniasis, Canine Kala-Azar.—This is a disease of dogs and human beings in the Mediterranean region. The causal agent is *Leishmania donovani* and, while the method of transmission is not known with certainty, it is assumed that infection results from the bite of some insect in which cyclical development of the parasite has occurred. The probable vectors are species of the sand-fly (*Phlebotomus*).

Symptoms.—The disease may be acute or chronic. Acute symptoms are generally seen in young dogs. There is an intermittent fever (103°–104°), followed by loss of appetite, emaciation, motor disturbance of hind-limbs, and death in three to five months. Chronic symptoms may show some resemblance to dumb rabies, and may be found in the majority of dogs in an area. There is a progressive anæmia with muscular tremors, emaciation often with a sub-normal temperature. Death may occur in two years.

Treatment—Tartar emetic, given intravenously, has a markedly specific effect upon the parasite and has reduced the mortality of the disease.

Prevention is more important. All stray dogs should be destroyed, and the remainder severely restricted in their relationship with humans. Hygiene is most important.

'BLACKHEAD.'—This disease, also known as Infectious Enterohepatitis, occurs in turkeys, chickens, pheasants, grouse, and other birds. It is characterised by thickening of the walls of the cæca and by the formation of round, yellowish-green necrotic areas in the liver. This infectious disease is caused by a flagellate *Histomonas maleagridis*. (*See* BLACKHEAD.)

TRICHOMONIASIS.—The flagellates of the genus *Trichomonas* are usually pear-shaped, with 3 to 5 anterior flagella, an undulating membrane and, in some species, one free flagellum directed backwards. There is a definite cytostome, or cell mouth, and a hyaline rod-shaped supporting structure, the axostyle, which passes through the body to its posterior end and from which it usually protrudes. There is also a stiff basal fibre running along the line of attachment of the undulating membrane to the body. The nucleus is at the front end of the body. Reproduction is by binary fission. Species of this genus very commonly occur in the intestinal canal of many different kinds of animals and birds ; in many cases their disease-producing power is low.

Trichomonas fœtus is of importance as the cause of abortions, pyometra, and sometimes sterility in cattle in Europe, America, and elsewhere. The parasite is about 16μ long by 8μ wide, and is actively motile. It is transmitted as a true venereal infection in cattle, the cow becoming infected at coitus from an infected bull, or *vice versa*. After coitus with an infected bull, the cow may show

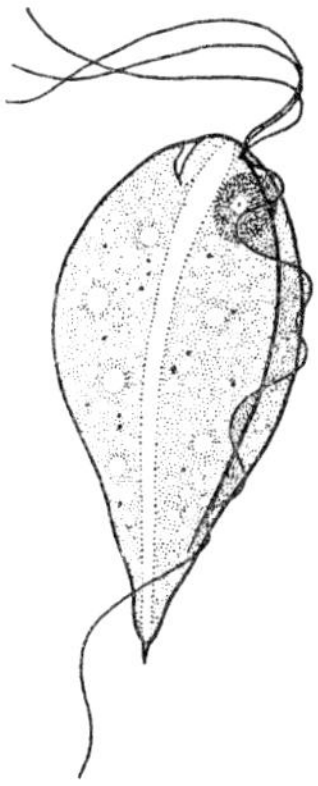

Trichomonas fœtus.

a transient vaginitis, which is often overlooked. If conception has not occurred, a chronic form of endometritis follows. If the cow is pregnant, the fœtus dies and is either aborted 1 to 4 months later or is retained in the uterus where it becomes macerated and a pyometra develops. There is apparently no specific remedy, and treatment consists in removing the uterine contents and douching with weak antiseptics. Spontaneous cure often occurs. Control of the disease includes the disposal of infected bulls, withholding all breeding operations on infected cows for at least three months, and the serving of non-infected cows and virgin heifers by a 'clean' bull. Freezing bull semen to —79° C., in the presence of 10 per cent glycerol, kills *Trichomonas fœtus* but allows the spermatozoa to survive. This method of deep-freeze commonly practised at A.I. centres, is one way of getting rid of the infection from semen.

Trichomonas suis.—This, it has been shown experimentally, can give rise to infertility and other symptoms in cattle similar to those caused by *T. fœtus*. The two organisms, which cannot be differentiated by the mucus agglutination test, may well be identical. The unwise disposal of pig manure on a dairy farm might lead to an outbreak of trichomoniasis.

SPOROZOA—This is a group of Protozoa which are all parasitic and produce spores at some stage of their life-cycle. It is divided into a number of orders, of which only two are important. These are the Hæmosporidia which are parasites of the red blood-cells, and the Coccidia which are parasites of epithelia.

HÆMOSPORIDIA.—This very important order includes the malarias of man and the piroplasms of the lower animals. The former, which are characterised by the production of a black pigment, are not treated here. The latter, which do not produce this pigment, are generally classified in four genera (in the domestic mammals) as follows :

Babesia (Syn. *Piroplasma*) ;
Nuttallia ;
Anaplasma ; and
Theileria.

It is probable that in the light of future research this classification will require revision. The genus *Nuttallia*, for example, should probably not be separated from *Babesia*, although the name is retained here to avoid confusion.

The diseases caused by these parasites are :

1. **Babesiosis (Piroplasmosis).** — Nearly all the domestic mammals suffer from infection with some species of *Babesia* ; sometimes more than one species may be present. The general symptoms are the appearance of fever in 8 to 10 days after infection, accompanied by hæmoglobinuria, icterus, and, unless treated, 25 to 100 per cent of the cases are fatal. Blood corpuscles may be reduced in number by two-thirds. Convalescence is slow and animals may remain 'salted' for three to eight years.

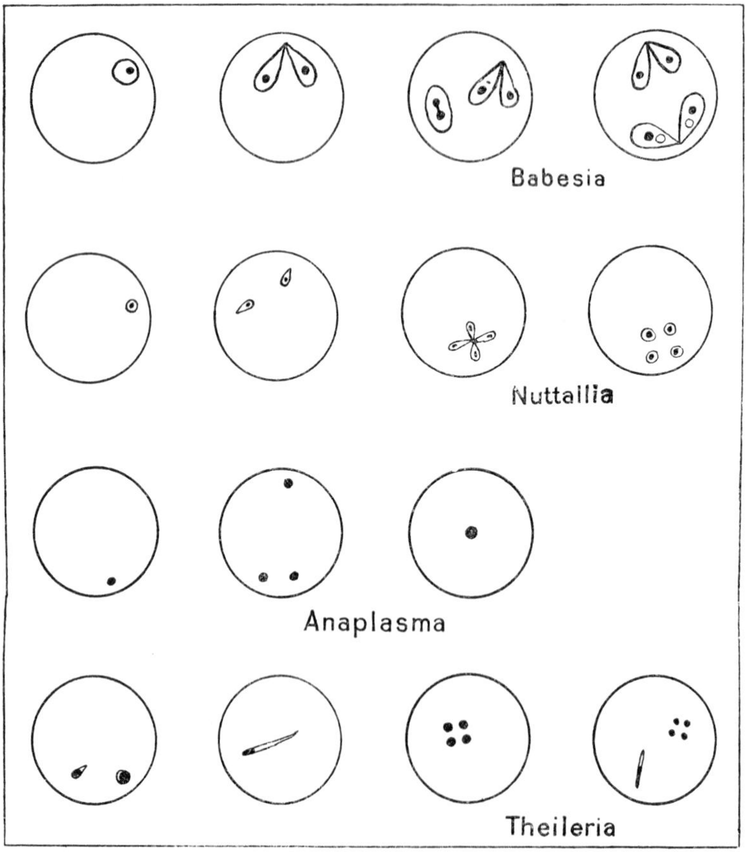

Types of Blood Sporozoa. The circles indicate the outlines of red blood-cells, in which these parasites are found.

PARASITES AND PARASITOLOGY

2. **Nuttalliosis.**—Only equines suffer from this disease. The symptoms are similar to babesiosis.

3. **Anaplasmosis.**—This disease is confined to cattle.

4. **Theileriosis.**—Infections with *Theileria* spp. are confined to cattle, sheep, and goats.

The above diseases are treated for convenience according to hosts.

BABESIA.—These are generally relatively large parasites within the red blood corpuscles and are pear-shaped, round, or oval. Multiplication is by division into two or by budding. Infected corpuscles frequently have two pyriform parasites joined at their pointed ends. Sexual multiplication takes place in the tick.

Transmission.—Development occurs in certain ticks which transmit the agent to their offspring. The various species are similar, but are specific to their various hosts. Thus the babesia of the dog will not infect the ox. The ticks should probably be regarded as the true or definite hosts, while the mammal is the intermediate host. The following species are important:

B. bovis	British and European red-water in cattle.
B. bigemina	Texas fever in cattle (not confined to America).
B. motasi	in sheep.
B. ovis	in sheep.
B. canis	Malignant jaundice in dogs.
B. gibsoni	in dogs.
B. vitalii	in dogs.
B. caballi	Biliary fever in horses.

NUTTALLIA.—These are smallish parasites, oval, sometimes pear-shaped, reproducing themselves in the form of a cross. Joined *pairs* are never seen, most cells containing only one parasite; a few contain cross forms.

N. equi occurs in the horse.

ANAPLASMA.—This is a very small parasite in the shape of a small granule of chromatin with no protoplasm. Evolution is unknown. It is found mainly in cattle. The species are:

A. marginale.
A. centrale.
A. ovis (possibly *A. marginale*).

THEILERIA.—These small, intracorpuscular parasites vary in shape, some being spherical, others ovoid, pear-shaped, or elongated rod-like. Division by binary fission within the blood corpuscle may occur, but has not been observed with certainty. It is believed that multiple forms represent multiple invasions rather than multiplication within the corpuscle. Multiplication occurs in the lymphatic glands and spleen where Koch's Blue Bodies, which are believed to be schizonts or asexual forms, occur. These divide and eventually produce forms which are ingested by the tick when it bites the mammalian host. Sexual multiplication occurs within the tick which transmits the parasite when it bites a new host.

There are several species in cattle and in sheep, including:

T. parva	East Coast fever in Tropical Africa.
T. mutans	Theileriosis in other lands.
T. hirci	Theileriosis in sheep.

BABESIOSIS IN CATTLE. — At the present day two or three types of babesiosis in cattle are recognised. They are due to:

(*a*) *B. bovis*, causing British Red-Water.
(*b*) *B. bigemina*, causing Texas Fever.
(*c*) *B. mutans*, which some regard as a species of *Theileria*.

British Red-Water, Bovine Hæmoglobinuria.—The causal agent is *Babesia bovis* (*B. divergens*). This is a small but typical babesia, and is sometimes placed in a subgenus, *Microbabesia* or *Babesiella*. When in pairs the elements diverge from each other, forming a fairly large angle, unlike *bigemina*, where the angle is small. This parasite is found in Europe, including Britain, North and South Africa, South America, and the East Indies.

Symptoms.—In some cases there is only a slight fever and hæmoglobinuria. Rumination may be affected. In more acute cases there is emaciation, icterus, diarrhœa followed by constipation, and anæmia, with a reduction in the blood-count to two millions. Death may result in three to four days. Only about 5 per cent of cases are fatal, and calves are more or less immune. The disease may recur during pregnancy with serious results.

Treatment.—Proprietory quinol-urea preparations (*e.g.* Acapron) have been found successful in a large number of cases. Good results are also obtained with tonics, stimulants, and nursing. There is no cross immunity with *B. bigemina*, *i.e.* animals immunised against Texas fever may contract British Red water.

PARASITES AND PARASITOLOGY

Transmission is by the following ticks :

Ixodes ricinus and *I. persulcatus*.

In this disease, as in all the tick-borne diseases, eradication of the ticks which convey the disease will result in the entire disappearance of the disease. Eradication of ticks is discussed under 'Ticks'.

Texas Fever.—The causal agent is *Babesia bigemina*.

This is the largest of the bovine forms. It is a typical babesia.

This parasite is found in Africa, America, Asia, Queensland, and Europe.

Symptoms.—The disease is recognised in an acute and a chronic form. The disease is essentially a pre-acute anæmia due to the breaking down of the red blood-cells. The liberated hæmoglobin is excreted by the kidneys and stains the urine (red-water). The temperature rapidly rises to 107° to 108° F. The parasites are now found in the blood, singly or in pairs. The temperature remains high, appetite and rumination cease, constipation is followed by diarrhœa, and rapid emaciation sets in. Hæmoglobinuria is usually seen about the second or third day of the disease. The parasites increase in number as the blood-cells fall from seven to two or three millions per cubic mm. Cerebral symptoms may be evident. The animal dies within three to ten days. On post-mortem examination the blood is bright red and abnormally fluid, while the tissues are paler. The spleen is enlarged from 2 to 4 times its normal size and is reddish-brown ('anthrax spleen'). The liver is swollen and pale and the gall-bladder is distended with thick, viscid, dark-coloured bile. The muscles are normal. The chronic form is similar but milder, and occurs in late autumn. Recovery is frequent, but convalescence is long (although it is stated to be very short in Argentine cattle).

Treatment is now fairly effectively undertaken by the intravenous injection of 100 to 200 c.c. of 1 per cent Trypan blue in the early stages of the disease.

Transmission is by :

Boophilus (*Margaropus*) *annulatus* (N. America).
B. microplus (S. America).
B. australis (many countries).
B. argentinus (S. America).
B. calcaratus (Asia).
B. decoloratus (S. Africa).
Rhipicephalus appendiculatus (S. Africa).
R. evertsi (S. Africa).
R. bursa (N. Africa).
Hæmaphysalis punctata (Europe).

Theileriosis.—Four species of this genus are usually recognised, but it is by no means certain that all are valid.

1. *T. mutans*, an almost non-pathogenic species producing premunition and persisting throughout life, and easily transmittable by inoculation. This occurs in cattle in Britain.

2. *T. annulata* is very similar to and may be identical with *T. mutans*; it is sometimes pathogenic. (Transmission is by *Hyalomma* spp.)

3. *T. dispar* always produces acute infection, causes 20 to 50 per cent mortality, and is transmissible by inoculation. Recovered animals are premunised; about 90 per cent of the parasites are round or oval. (Transmission is by *Hyalomma* spp.)

4. *T. parva* also always produces acute infection and causes 90 to 100 per cent mortality. It is very difficult to transmit the organism by inoculation, and recovered animals are immune. About 80 per cent of the parasites are rod-shaped. (Transmission is by *Rhipicephalus* spp.)

These four form a gradual series which cannot be distinguished morphologically. Koch's 'blue bodies' are rare in the first, and common in the last.

It is probable that the first and the last are true species, and the other two mere varieties.

East Coast Fever.—In tropical and East Africa this disease is caused by *T. parva*.

Symptoms.—The main symptoms are those of a toxæmia. There is fever, but no red-water, icterus, or anæmia. The blood-cells are not destroyed. The parasite multiplies in the lymphatic tissue, and from there invades the blood in such large numbers that almost every red-cell contains one or more parasites. Death is rapid (90 to 100 per cent of cases).

There is an incubation period of 6 to 20 days, and the disease lasts 6 to 20 days.

Animals can only be infected by lymphatic gland juice or by ticks. The parasite does not remain in recovered or immunised animals.

Chronic forms of the disease occur, with enlarged glands, especially in calves from immune cows.

Gall-Sickness (*pro parte*). Coast Fever of Europe and Asia. This disease is caused by *T. mutans*.

Symptoms.—There is a slight irregular fever of varying duration. Anæmia and

PARASITES AND PARASITOLOGY

loss of condition are noticed. The disease tends to be a chronic one, and in South Africa death is very rare. In North Africa and other places it may sometimes be fatal (5 to 10 per cent). The incubation period is 20 to 50 days. The parasite may be seen in the blood long after all symptoms have disappeared.

Anaplasmosis, Gall-Sickness (*pro parte*). The causal agent is *Anaplasma marginale* (*A. argentinum*). These are small, highly staining granules situated near the edge of the red blood-cells.

This parasite is found in Africa, Asia, Australia, S. Europe, S. America, and the southern States of N. America.

Symptoms. — The disease resembles Texas fever and frequently anaplasmosis coexists with babesiosis, but pure infections may also occur. It is characterised by acute anæmia, fever, jaundice, and degeneration of the internal organs; hæmoglobinuria does not occur as the rate of red blood-cell destruction is not fast enough to produce free hæmoglobin in the circulating blood. Young animals appear to be resistant, and cases in calves under one year old are rare. In older animals the disease may be acute or chronic, and in the former case they may die within 2 to 3 days after the appearance of the first symptoms. The disease starts with a high temperature of 105° to 107° F. and after a day or two anæmia and icterus appear, the temperature falling to normal or subnormal as death approaches. The mucous membranes are pale and yellowish; urination is frequent, but the urine is not blood-tinged as in Texas fever. The animal is usually constipated and diarrhœa is uncommon. In the more chronic cases the animals live longer, are weak, progressively emaciate, and show icterus and anæmia. The blood-cell count may fall from a normal of about 7 million to less than 1 million per c.mm. Mortality varies between 5 to 50 per cent, and losses are greatest in hot weather and in older animals. Experimentally, the incubation period varies from 20 to 40 days. Imported stock are the most susceptible to anaplasmosis. On post-mortem examination the blood is thin and watery, the tissues of the organs anæmic, the spleen enlarged with soft, dark pulp, the liver shows marked icterus, and the gall-bladder distended with dark green, mucoid bile.

A second species, *A. centrale*, in which the parasite is found in the centre of the corpuscle, causes a similar but milder and seldom fatal disease.

Transmission artificially may be by inoculation of blood from affected animals or those in a state of premunition. Natural transmission is by ticks, and various species of the following genera act as vectors: *Boophilus*, *Rhipicephalus*, *Hyalomma*, *Ixodes*, *Dermacentor*, and *Hæmaphysalis*. Infection is passed through the egg to the next generation of ticks. In addition, several species of Tabanid flies have been shown to be mechanical carriers provided the transfer of infective material from an infected to a healthy beast is immediate and within not more than five minutes. Certain mosquitoes have also been incriminated, but the Stable fly and the Horn fly apparently seldom, if ever, act as transmitters. The disease can also be transmitted through the use of common surgical instruments which have not been thoroughly sterilised after being used on an infected animal. Animals which recover from anaplasmosis are in a state of premunition, and remain carriers for long periods, probably for life.

In the South African States the less serious *A. centrale* has been found to give protection against the serious *A. marginale*, and both there and in other countries successful results follow its use as an immunising agent. In other areas where Texas fever and anaplasmosis frequently occur together, cattle are often immunised by blood of a bovine infected with *A. centrale*, which produces a mild infection, and with a mild form of *Babesia bigemina*. The inoculated cattle usually suffer from Texas fever first, as it has the shorter incubation period, and anaplasmosis later, and they then possess an increased tolerance for both diseases.

HORSES.—Equine Biliary Fever.—This disease is caused by two distinct parasites: *Babesia caballi* and *Nuttallia equi*. The former species resembles *Babesia bigemina* in size and morphology, and causes a disease similar to Texas fever but which is milder and more amenable to treatment than that caused by *Nuttallia equi*. *N. equi* is a smaller species than *B. caballi* and causes a disease which is highly virulent for adult horses and other species of the horse family, but is mild in young animals. Recovered animals are in a state of premunition, and inoculation of colts as a means of protection later in life is commonly practised.

Distribution.—The disease is found in Russia and various parts of Europe, India,

Africa, South America, and South Africa. In the two latter places *N. equi* seems to be present alone.

Symptoms.—At the beginning of the disease there is a sharp rise in temperature to about 107° F. During this period the parasites are multiplying in the blood. In a few days the temperature falls and anæmia sets in. In the horse this is usually masked by an intense icterus, though not in the donkey and mule. Hæmoglobinuria, and constipation followed by diarrhœa, are frequent symptoms, and are succeeded by rapid emaciation. The animal may die during the initial fever (2 to 5 days) or from anæmia and emaciation about the eleventh day or later. Complications are frequent.

Treatment.—Complete rest, an injection of Pirevan or Piroparv or of a broad-spectrum antibiotic.

Transmission. — In Southern Europe *B. caballi* is transmitted by *Dermacentor reticulatus* and *D silvarum*; in South Africa *N. equi* is transmitted by *Rhipicephalus evertsi* and *R. bursa*. Other species and genera of ticks probably act as vectors of *N. equi* in other countries.

SHEEP. — Ovine babesiosis, Carceag. — At least three species are implicated; there is a relatively large form, *Babesia motasi*, which is comparable to *B. bigemina* of cattle, and which produces a disease, often severe, with high temperatures, much blood-cell destruction, icterus, and hæmoglobinuria. This is the 'carceag' of Eastern and Southern Europe. The second parasite, of intermediate size and corresponding to *B. bovis* of cattle, is *Babesia ovis*. It produces a much milder disease with fever, jaundice, and anæmia, but recoveries generally occur. The small species is *Theileria ovis*, which appears to be similar to *T. mutans* of cattle, and is relatively harmless to its host. Animals recovered from *T. ovis* infection apparently develop a permanent and sterile immunity. The disease occurs in Europe, Africa, Asia, and North America.

Symptoms.—In acute cases the temperature may rise to 107° F., rumination ceases, there is paralysis of the hindquarters, the urine is brown, and death occurs in about a week. In benign cases there may only be a slight fever for a few days with anæmia.

Transmission.—*B. motasi*, *B. ovis*, and *T. ovis* are all transmitted by *Rhipicephalus bursa*.

A theileriosis, caused by *T. hirci*, has been described from sheep in Africa and Europe. It causes an emaciation and small hæmorrhages in the conjunctiva.

An anaplasmosis has also been noted in Africa and South America.

DOG. — Canine babesiosis, Malignant Jaundice.

Causal agent: *Babesia canis*. This is a typical babesia. It is found in Africa, Europe, India, and America.

Symptoms. — In five to fifteen days after inoculation there is a rise in temperature to 107° F. with emaciation, anæmia, and icterus. Hæmoglobinuria is not constant. Cerebral symptoms may be seen. The disease may be chronic, but the disease is frequently fatal particularly in imported dogs.

Treatment (*see* BERENIL).

B. canis is transmitted by:

- *Hæmaphysalis leachi* (S. Africa).
- *Dermacentor reticulatus* and *D. venustus* (Europe).
- *Rhipicephalus sanguineus* (many countries).

Another form of canine babesiosis, due to *Babesia gibsoni*, is found in India. The parasite is smaller than *B. canis* and also differs from it in the absence of the characteristic pairs of pear-shaped forms. The disease it causes has an insidious start, is chronic with severe anæmia and emaciation, but without hæmoglobinuria. *Rhipicephalus sanguineus* and *Hæmaphysalis bispinosa* are the tick vectors. Trypan blue appears to be of little value in treatment.

Nambyuvu, Peste do Sangue, Rangeliosis, Canine Yellow Fever.—The causal agent of this disease, which occurs in Brazil, is *Babesia vitalii* (sometimes also called *Rangelia vitalii*). It is possible that this parasite may really be the same as *B. canis*. The organisms are polymorphic, and often occur free in the blood at the end of the disease. They occur intracellularly in the endothelial cells of the kidney and less so in the lungs.

Symptoms.—The disease is found mainly in hunting dogs. It may run a mild course, but is usually acute or subacute. There is irregular fever and emaciation, anæmia, and icterus. At the close of the disease the icterus is general, with external hæmorrhages from the natural orifices and skin. The parasites are most frequent during the fever.

Treatment.—The use of Trypan blue is recommended.

Transmission is believed to be conveyed by *Amblyomma cayennense* and *A. striatum*.

COCCIDIA.—A number of species belonging to this order infect the domestic animals. They all belong to one of two genera.

(*a*) *Isospora*—in which the mature oöcyst contains *two* sporocysts, each with four sporozoites.

(*b*) *Eimeria*—in which the mature oöcyst contains *four* sporocysts, each with two sporozoites.

GENERAL LIFE CYCLE.—The oöcyst is passed to the exterior in the host's fæces. It consists of the zygote, which results from the union of the male and female elements, enclosed within a protective membrane or cyst wall. On the ground and in the presence of moisture, oxygen, and a suitable temperature development proceeds. The zygote splits into two or four sporoblasts (depending upon the genus), each of which becomes enclosed in a capsule to form oval sporocysts. The contents of each sporocyst divide into four (or two) sporozoites. Once this process of sporulation is completed the oöcyst is 'ripe' and capable of infecting a host, unsporulated oöcysts are not infective. When ripe oöcysts are swallowed by a suitable host, the action of the digestive juices on the cyst walls allows the motile sporozoites to escape and each penetrates an epithelial cell. Here each parasite increases in size and finally becomes a large rounded schizont. This divides into a number of small elongated merozoites which, escaping from the epithelial cell into the gut, attack new cells, and the process is repeated. The massive feeding stage in the cell before it starts dividing is called a trophozoite, and is usually a young schizont. Under certain conditions, however, some trophozoites develop into large female forms or macrogametocytes which, when mature, become macrogametes. Meanwhile certain other trophozoites develop into male cells or microgametocytes, which divide into a number of small microgametes. One of these unites with each macrogamete, and the resulting cell is called the zygote. The fertilised macrogamete, or zygote, then secretes a thick capsule around itself, forming an oöcyst which is discharged into the lumen of the organ (intestine or bile-duct) and thus escapes from the host in the fæces.

Coccidiosis in Cattle, Red Dysentery.

Causal agent : *Eimeria zürnii.*

This is believed to be the most important species affecting cattle. Developmental forms occur wholly in the large intestine and cæcum where considerable denudation of epithelium occurs, resulting in extensive hæmorrhage. The oöcysts are nearly spherical, and sporulation, under favourable conditions, takes place in from 48 to 72 hours. It is found in Europe, Africa, and North America. It is prevalent during the warm season, and attacks especially animals of two months to two years.

Symptoms are first seen in one to eight weeks after infection. There is a persistent diarrhœa which becomes hæmorrhagic. After about a week emaciation is evident, the temperature rises, and there are digestive disturbances. Milk is diminished or stopped. Passage of fæces is attended by straining or even eversion of the rectum. Death may occur within a fortnight or even earlier. Convalescence is slow. The lesions are mainly in the large intestine. Mortality may vary up to 50 per cent of the affected animals, but generally is not very high, at least in older cattle. Infection is usually introduced into a herd, or maintained in it, by carrier animals, and close-herding is the chief factor causing coccidiosis in cattle to become epidemic.

Treatment consists of isolation of all sick animals and careful nursing, with the use of demulcents and intestinal sedatives. Treatment by sulphamezathine or sulphaquinoxaline in daily doses for 3 days is generally satisfactory if begun early.

Coccidiosis in Sheep and Goats.

Causal agents : At least seven species of *Eimeria* occur in these animals, and mixed infections with two or more species is the rule rather than the exception. The various species are widely distributed and as a rule the clinical disease is seen in lambs and kids, seldom in the old animals which, however, may harbour coccidia. The relative pathogenicity of the different species is not precisely known, but it is probable that one species, *E. arloingi*, is concerned with most of the clinical disease.

Symptoms are those of a pernicious anæmia accompanied by diarrhœa and emaciation. There is no fever. The course of the disease may be very quick or may last several weeks. The lesions are mainly in the small intestine. The disease is a very serious one, but is not always recognised.

Treatment is on the same lines as for cattle.

Coccidiosis in the Dog and Cat.

The following species are known from the dog and cat :

Isospora felis.
I. rivolta.
I. bigemina.
Eimeria canis and *E. felina.*

Most of these parasites have been isolated from healthy animals. The majority of coccidial infections of dogs and cats are light, and there is little evidence of serious damage to the hosts. In some cases, however, there is diarrhœa and occasionally fatal dysentery.

Coccidiosis in the Rabbit.

Causal agents: At least five species of *Eimeria* affect the rabbit and, of these, two are common and destructive. *E. stiedæ* occurs in the liver, the others in the intestine, and all are specific for the rabbit and hare.

Symptoms.—Two forms of the disease may occur, and each may be acute or chronic.

(1) *Hepatic* form is caused by *E. stiedæ*. Sharply circumscribed white nodules found both within and superficially upon the liver of infected rabbits are characteristic of infections with this species. The naturally occurring disease is usually of the chronic type, and susceptibility is highest at 3 to 4 weeks of age and then declines, resistance being strong after 4 months of age. Affected animals frequently develop a pot-bellied appearance because of liver enlargement; there is dullness with icterus, and diarrhœa usually develops. In heavy infections rabbits may die within 3 to 4 weeks, while in more chronic infections death may be delayed for 6 weeks or more, or recovery may occur. Affected rabbits become very emaciated.

(2) *Intestinal* form is caused principally by *E. perforans*. The disease often appears in young rabbits as an infection of the peracute type. Diarrhœa is usually the first symptom to appear, and may be severe, lasting until the death of the animal, which occurs within 6 to 15 days. If diarrhœa ceases, polyuria usually develops; the animal becomes pot-bellied, loses appetite and weight, shows weakness of the hind-limbs and a soiled coat, and passes blood-stained fæces and in general presents a miserable appearance. Deaths from this species are usually high in numbers. *E. magna* also develops in the small intestine, and may, sometimes, be pathogenic.

Both the hepatic and intestinal forms of the disease may occur at the same time, and animals which recover may act as carriers.

Diagnosis.—In all coccidial infections the microscopic demonstration of oöcysts in the fæces is necessary. Freshly passed oöcysts are not sporulated, but if allowed to stand aside for a few days and not kept too wet, the fæces will usually yield sporulated oöcysts. The oöcysts of the different species vary slightly in shape and size and in other respects, but they are all more or less oval with a double contoured wall which often shows a thinner and flattened portion at one end where the micropyle is situated. A post-mortem examination shows white cheesy nodules, varying in size from a pin's head to a pea, in the liver, while the intestinal wall is usually thickened and inflamed, and white nodules may be found in it.

Treatment.—Sulphamezathine or sulphaquinoziline are worthy of trial and offer most hope of success. Good nursing is important.

Prevention is mainly a matter of cleanliness of food, water, and quarters. All newcomers and all young rabbits should be isolated.

Coccidiosis in the Fowl.

Causal agent: At least seven species of *Eimeria* have been found to occur in domestic fowls. Of these *E. tenella* and *E. necatrix* are highly pathogenic and destructive parasites; *E. maxima* and *E. hagani* possess virulence of a medium grade, and are usually associated with chronic infections, whereas *E. acervulina*, *E. mitis*, and *E. præcox* are nearly harmless. All, except *E. hagani*, are widespread, and several species often occur simultaneously in a single bird, and this condition usually occurs in older birds. Although coccidial infections are self-limiting, that is, birds surviving the original acute attack will completely recover and eliminate all traces of infection provided there is no reinfection, chronic coccidiosis frequently occurs and is due to repeated reinfections with the same or other species.

Symptoms.—*Eimeria tenella* (*E. avium*) appears to be responsible for most deaths from coccidiosis. It is limited to the cæca and sometimes the large intestine. Owing to extensive tissue destruction in those regions, gross hæmorrhage results and bloody diarrhœa is conspicuous as a symptom. In milder infections, affected chicks appear listless, mope, have ruffled feathers, and show a pale appearance about the head. Cæcal coccidiosis is most common in chicks of 5 to 7 weeks of age, but may also affect chicks as young as 1 week and older, growing birds. Outbreaks vary in severity, and up to 50 per cent of chicks in a group may die.

Eimeria necatrix produces, clinically, a prolonged, chronic, wasting type of

PARASITES AND PARASITOLOGY

disease, and occurs in birds several months of age and may cause serious damage amongst maturing birds. Two types of the disease are recognised, one of which is acute and may result fatally in 5 to 7 days. The other and more typical form is prolonged, and results in emaciation of the bird. Symptoms appear after the fourth day, and comprise inactivity, roughening of the feathers, loss of flesh, generally weakness, lameness, and drooping of the wings. Death may occur 5 days after infection, but it commonly takes place on the sixth and seventh days. Birds surviving the seventh day usually recover, but remain emaciated and worthless. The parasite attacks the small intestine mostly, but it is not uncommon to find the cæca also infected. Post-mortem examination shows the small intestine to be studded, often throughout its length, with whitish spots visible through the muscular and serous coats, and the intestinal contents are blood-stained mucus or dark-red blood clot.

Eimeria maxima attacks the middle portion of the small intestine which shows great thickening of the wall. There is no profuse hæmorrhage, and only exceptionally do severe spontaneous cases appear.

Treatment is now upon a much better basis than formerly. The administration of various 'sulpha' drugs will either kill the coccidia (coccidiocides) or arrest their development (coccidiostats). Of these sulphamezathine and sulphaquinoxaline are of value; as is also Nitrofurazone. These drugs are given in food or water. Their use requires care since they are capable of giving rise to symptoms of poisoning if given in wrong doses. Expert advice on methods and dosage should always be obtained and followed carefully. By these means an outbreak can now usually be readily controlled and heavy loss avoided.

Coccidiosis in Other Birds.

Turkeys are sometimes affected with species of *Eimeria*, but the diseases produced by them are of little practical importance. The chicken coccidia will not infect turkeys and those of the turkey will not infect chickens.

Coccidiosis in ducks occurs, but is of little economic importance.

In geese three species of *Eimeria* occur in the intestine. Rather severe outbreaks have been ascribed to *E. anseris*. A fourth, important species is *E. truncata*, which causes a severe form of renal coccidiosis. The disease affects goslings from three weeks to three months of age, and in heavy infections goslings may die within two or three days after symptoms are first seen. The mortality is often very severe, and may be 100 per cent.

CILIATA.—A large number of ciliates are found in the alimentary tract of different animals, but none appears to have any pathological effects.

Balantidium coli is a ciliate which often occurs in the pig's intestines, where apparently it produces no damage. Occasionally, however, in pigs that are debilitated for other reasons it causes a low-grade dysentery. It is pear-shaped, about 80μ long by 60μ broad, and possesses a large sausage-shaped nucleus and two contractile vacuoles. Reproduction is by transverse division and it is excreted as round or oval resistant cystic forms. It is of considerable importance as the cause of a severe dysentery in man. It is stated that infection can only occur by swallowing cysts, and that, in man, cysts are never found, so that infection can only take place directly from the pig. The organism is very refractory to treatment.

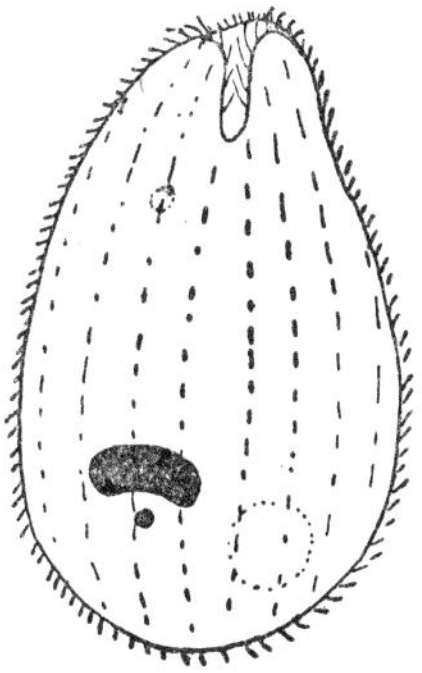

Balantidium coli.

SARCOCYSTIS.—These are organisms believed to be Protozoa, but possibly fungi. They occur in the striated muscle fibres of all the domesticated animals and in a number of birds. They are especially common in horses, cattle, sheep, pigs, and ducks. Many species have been described, often after the host in which they were found. There are very little grounds for their differentiation and, as they are not host specific, it is possible that they all represent a single species, *Sarcocystis miescheriana*. This form occurs in the pig, and is the name in general use and has date priority over all the other names.

In all hosts the organisms are very much alike in appearance, consisting of elongated, whitish, fusiform bodies known as 'Miescher's tubes'. All sizes may be seen from those just visible to the naked eye to others sometimes as large as a hazel nut. Within this body are a number of chambers filled with bean-shaped microscopic spores, called 'Rainey's corpuscles'. Little is known about the life-cycle or transmission of the organism which does not seem seriously to injure the host, even in heavy infections. Infection is very widespread, and sometimes in sheep and pigs there are so many cysts in the muscles as to lead to condemnation of the carcase. Cysts are especially common in the muscles of the œsophagus in sheep and in the heart muscle of cattle. The smaller cysts in the muscles may be mistaken for the encapsuled roundworm *Trichinella spiralis*.

GLOBIDIUM. — Closely related to *Sarcocystis* in appearance is a group of parasites which are found in the mucous membrane of the alimentary tract of herbivorous animals. *Globidium gilruthi* is common in sheep in Britain and other parts of the world, particularly in the wall of the abomasum. It appears as spherical bodies consisting of a thick wall which encloses enormous numbers of sickle-shaped microscopic spores not unlike those of *Sarcocystis*. The cysts may be seen by the naked eye as minute opalescent nodules beneath the mucosa and often surrounded by slight hæmorrhage. Nothing is known about the life-cycle or mode of infection, and in most cases the numbers of parasites are so small as to cause little damage; occasionally heavy infections occur. A species occurs in the intestine of the horse and another has been found in the skin and connective tissue of muscles of cattle.

SPIROCHÆTA.—These are organisms which are sometimes grouped with the Bacteria and sometimes with the Protozoa. Because of their close resemblance to organisms that are undoubtedly Bacteria they are generally regarded as such. They include some very serious parasites of man, but are not of the same importance in veterinary medicine.

Fowl Spirochætosis.—This is due to *Treponema anserinum*. The organism is also known as *Spirochæta anserina*, *S. gallinarum*, or *Borrelia gallinarum*. It is the cause of an important disease of fowls, geese, and occasionally ducks in tropical and subtropical countries including Africa, South America, Australia, and certain parts of Asia and of Europe. It is a loosely spiralled organism varying from ·008 to ·02 mm. in length, and is actively motile. It occurs in the blood of birds, especially the domestic fowl, and causes great losses amongst chickens. It is transmitted from one bird to another by ticks, generally *Argas persicus* and *A. miniatus*, occasionally by other species of *Argas*. The fowl mite, *Dermanyssus gallinæ*, has also been suspected as being a vector. Infection in the tick is hereditary, passing through the tick egg to the next generation. The disease may be acute or chronic. In the latter, birds become weak, emaciated, and anæmic, death following in 2 to 3 weeks. In the acute disease, which lasts 4 to 6 days, there are symptoms of acute septicæmia, fever, depression, profuse diarrhœa, emaciation, and anæmia. The mortality rate is very high. Recovery from the disease leaves the bird refractory to further infection for a considerable period of time. Control of the disease is by eradication of the tick vectors.

Other spirochætes are:

Treponema theileri which occurs in cattle, horses, sheep, and goats in Africa. It is found in the blood, particularly during the febrile stage of infection, and causes slight anæmia of a mild type. The disease produced is benign and seldom fatal, and symptoms resemble those of anaplasmosis, but are less severe. Transmission is by the ticks *Boophilus decoloratus*, *B. annulatus*, *B. australis*, and *Rhipicephalus evertsi*, and is hereditary through the tick egg.

Treponema suis or *T. suilla* occurs in pigs in Africa. It appears to be a tissue parasite associated with inflammatory and necrotic processes in various parts of the body and to gain entrance to the host through wounds.

Treponema cuniculi in rabbits causes a well-recognised, naturally occurring disease, often referred to as 'rabbit syphilis', in Britain, on the Continent, and in America. The organism, which does not affect humans, resembles that causing syphilis in humans, and has proved disconcerting to research workers investigating the human species in experimental rabbits. In the rabbit infection takes place during coitus, the disease being manifested by the appearance of nodules and superficial ulcers covered with thin, moist, scaly crusts and œdematous swellings of the surrounding tissues mainly in the region of the genitalia and also sometimes in the region of the nose.

Leptospira icterohæmorrhagiæ, the causative organism of Weil's disease in man and of enzoötic jaundice in dogs, measures about 7–14 μ long by 0·15 μ broad, and shows both rotary and undulating movements when examined under dark-ground illumination. It occurs in wild rats and field-mice. (*See* LEPTOSPIROSIS.)

Leptospira canicola is the cause of nephritis and uræmia in dogs, and of canicola fever in man. (*See* LEPTOSPIROSIS.)

HELMINTHOLOGY — Helminthology is that branch of Parasitology which deals with the parasitic 'worms'. This is an artificial group of animals which, for our purpose, we may divide into the following groups :

Phylum PLATYHELMINTHES—
- *A*. Trematoda, unsegmented flatworms, or flukes.
- *B*. Cestoda, segmented flatworms, or tapeworms.

Phylum NEMATHELMINTHES—
- *C*. Nematoda, unsegmented round worms.
- *D*. Goodiacea, horse-hair worms.
- *E*. Acanthocephala, thorny-headed worms.

Phylum ANNELIDA—
- *F*. Hirudinea, leeches.

There are various smaller unimportant groups of parasitic worms but only the Trematoda, Cestoda, and Nematoda contain many important forms.

A. TREMATODA.—Most, though not all, trematodes are flattish worms with either one or two suckers. They are primarily divided into two orders :

ORDER MONOGENEA : including chiefly ectoparasitic forms, occurring on fishes and other aquatic animals, and with a direct life-cycle.

ORDER DIGENEA : including the vast majority of flukes. They are endoparasitic forms having an indirect life-cycle complicated by metamorphosis and by the alternation of a sexual with one or more parthenogenetic generations. This group is divided into two suborders :

(*a*) Gasterostomata in which the mouth is in the middle of the ventral surface.

(*b*) Prostomata in which the mouth is at or near the anterior end of the body.

The flukes to be considered here all belong to the Prostomata and may, for convenience, be divided into three groups :

(1) Distomes, with one anterior and one more or less median ventral sucker.

(2) Amphistomes, with one anterior and one posterior sucker.

(3) Schistosomes, in which the sexes are separate, a condition not found in other flukes.

A typical fluke is flat and leaf-like with a terminal anterior mouth surrounded by the oral sucker. The ventral sucker, a more or less cup-shaped, superficial, adhesive disc with no aperture in it, occurs towards the middle of the body or at or near the hind end. There is no body cavity and the internal organs lie in a spongy tissue. The mouth leads back into the pharynx, a muscular sucking bulb, thence to the œsophagus and into a non-muscular bifurcated intestine. There is no anus. The excretory system consists of a network of vessels which open into an excretory vesicle, or bladder, discharging to the exterior by means of an excretory pore at the posterior end of the body. There is no blood system. With the exception of the Schistosomes, the trematodes are all hermaphrodite, *i.e.* each animal has both male and female organs. The male organs consist usually of two testes with ducts which join to form a common vas deferens which opens at the genital pore with a cirrus—the homologue of the penis in the higher animals. The female organs consist of an ovary, invariably single, an oviduct leading to a uterus, a shell-gland and two groups of yolk-glands.

The life-history of a typical fluke is as follows : The egg is usually passed to the exterior in the fæces of the host and under suitable conditions, chiefly of moisture and warmth, a small ciliated larva, called a 'miracidium', hatches from it. This larva, which is unable to feed and will die within some hours unless it finds a suitable host, gains access to the liver or some other special organ by actively penetrating the skin of an appropriate snail—

PARASITES AND PARASITOLOGY

usually a specific snail for any one parasite. In the snail's tissue it develops into a sac-like sporocyst which, by a process of budding from the internal lining of cells, gives rise to a number of elongated 'rediæ'. Each redia is a simple, cylindrical sac-like organism which gives rise, by budding of cells, either to another generation of 'daughter rediæ' or to 'cercariæ'. The cercaria, which resembles a miniature tadpole in general form, leaves the snail and, after leading a free existence in water or on wet vegetation for a short time, comes to rest on grass or other objects, loses its tail and becomes encysted within a protective covering and remains in this state until it is swallowed by the final host, in which it becomes a sexually mature fluke.

This life-history varies slightly with different flukes, but may be taken as typical. Variations will be noted under each species described.

A large number of flukes are known from the domestic animals; but only such forms as are of economic importance or are of frequent occurrence will be described.

FASCIOLA HEPATICA.—This is the common 'liver fluke' of sheep. (Other hosts are cattle, goats, pigs, rabbits, hares, horses, dogs, man, beavers, elephants, and kangaroos.) It is shaped more or less like a leaf, about 1 in. long, but considerable variations exist, and elongated forms are found. The anterior sucker is carried on a more or less distinct conical projection. The gut and the genital organs are all highly ramified, and yolk-glands are present on both sides of the body. It has been recorded from most herbivorous animals and from man; but it is in cattle and sheep that it is of most importance. It is generally found in the bile-ducts of the liver, but may be found in other organs.

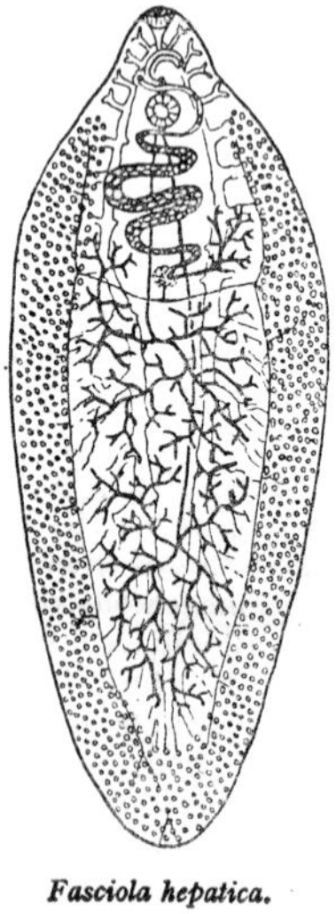

Fasciola hepatica.

The life-history is typical, the intermediate host being various species of *Limnæa*. Cercaria may be swallowed with drinking water or encysted on grass.

'Fluke Disease.'—This is a pernicious anæmia. The earliest symptom (in summer or autumn) is an apparent improvement in condition due to the stimulation of the liver as the flukes enter; but this is soon followed by a progressive emaciation. The animal feeds and ruminates less, swellings become visible in the pendulous parts, and diarrhœa is common. The skin and mucous membranes are paler, and the animal becomes weaker. Death may occur at any stage, but animals which survive till the spring usually recover—but never regain their original condition. The ducts in the liver are thickened and show as conspicuous white channels ('pipe-stem liver') in the softened liver substance, and may become calcified. The bile is usually thickened with dark flocculi. If a large number of cercaria are swallowed at about the same time, death is very rapid and the normal symptoms are generally absent. Very small flukes are found in the black liver, while a blood-stained fluid, oozing from the wounds made by the worms, is contained in the abdominal cavity. This severe form is usually found during a wet summer which has been preceded by a mild winter—conditions which favour the development of the intermediate host. The surest form of diagnosis is to kill a suspected sheep and examine its liver. Fluke eggs may be found in the dropping

Treatment is best given in late autumn when the adults have reached the liver. Before this they are not susceptible to drugs. Carbon tetrachloride is used for sheep only; also hexachlorothane. Carbon tetrachloride in 1 c.c. doses given to all sheep in a flock at monthly intervals from September to January, is necessary to control the disease in serious infestations. Where there is less trouble, two doses, in September and in November, usually suffice. Hexachloroethane has been used for cattle. (For more recent drugs, *see* LIVER FLUKES.) As enormous losses are caused by this disease, pre-

PARASITES AND PARASITOLOGY

vention is of the utmost importance. Sheep may with safety be put on to fields from which the intermediate host is absent, as infection can only take place through the snail. Copper sulphate (28 lb./acre with 4 parts sand) may be used to dress the land and so kill the Limnæas. Drainage is all-important, as the snail lives on marshy land.

Copper sulphate (1 part in a million of water) may be used to kill snails in water. It does not affect the snail eggs, and must be repeated in three months. In this dilution it is harmless to plants and mammals, but it may kill off fish. Muddy gateways, the areas around drinking troughs, and hoof-prints are also favoured by the snail.

FASCIOLOIDES.—This genus contains only one species. *F. magna*, the large American liver fluke. In general anatomy, this species resembles the common liver fluke, but differs from it in its larger size (up to 4 in.) and thicker form. It has no trace of an anterior cone, and the yolk-glands are practically confined to one side of the body; in consequence the fluke has a dark slaty ventral side and a light fleshy dorsal side. These points enable one to distinguish it easily from the other flukes.

The life-history is very similar to that of the parasite *F. hepatica*. It is found in North America, and is more common, though less serious, in cattle than sheep.

The symptoms are similar to those caused by the common fluke, but are rather more serious. Its larger size and its tendency to form cysts in the liver substance (not in the bile-ducts) make it a more formidable parasite. The appetite persists up to the time of death. The flukes appear to die *in situ*, rather than pass out in spring, as does *F. hepatica*. The cysts may become abscesses, and may be found in the spleen and lungs.

FASCIOLOPSIS.—This genus, which is found in the intestine and sometimes the stomach of the pig, dog, and man, resembles a large fasciola. It is a somewhat fleshy form with practically no anterior cone, but the gut shows no tendency to form secondary branches, and yolk-glands occur on both sides of the body. Probably only one species, *F. buski*, exists. It occurs in Asia.

The life-history is typical, the intermediate host being snails of the genus *Planorbis*. Infection is by eating water weeds containing cercaria.

The symptoms in the pig are not well

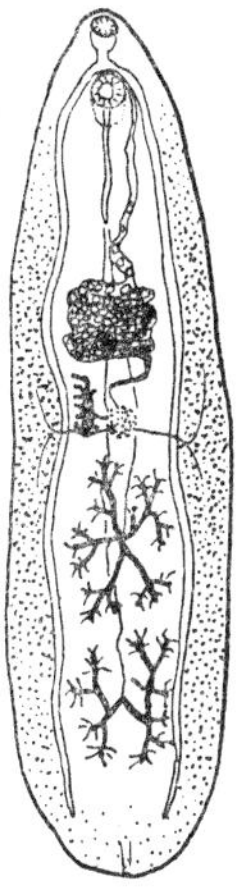

Fasciolopsis.

known. In man there are symptoms of anæmia and chronic diarrhœa, ascites and emaciation.

DICROCŒLIUM.—This genus is small and semi-transparent, the common species, *D. lanceatum*, being about ⅓ in. long. Its small size, its non-ramifying gut, and its compact genital organs situated anterior to the uterus are sufficient to distinguish this form from all related liver flukes. It occurs in all herbivores and in man, and is present in Scotland, Europe, and elsewhere. It is much less serious a pest than *F. hepatica*. It is carried by various land snails. In America, at least, a second intermediate host—the ant—is required; the ants being eaten by the grazing animal. Infestation of a heifer

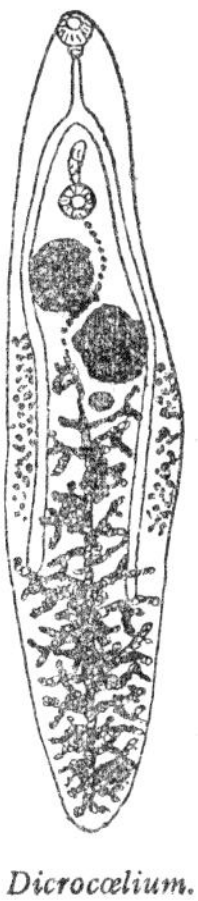

Dicrocœlium.

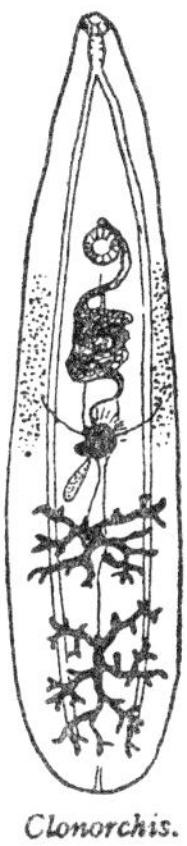

Clonorchis.

PARASITES AND PARASITOLOGY

with *D. dendriticum* was reported in Ireland in 1960.

CLONORCHIS.—*Clonorchis sinensis* is a common fluke of carnivores, pigs, and man in Asia. It is a small form somewhat resembling *D. lanceatum*, but can be easily distinguished from it by the possession of a pair of ramified testes in the posterior part of the body. The ovary is not ramified.

The first part of its life-history is on general lines, the molluscan intermediary being a species of *Bythinia*. The sporocysts give rise directly to cercaria which escape and encyst on various freshwater fish (*e.g. Carassius auratus*). Infection to mammals is by eating infected fish which are either uncooked or imperfectly cooked.

Closely related flukes are found in the liver of dogs in North Europe and North America. The symptoms are those usually associated with liver-fluke disease.

PARAGONIMUS.—Several species of lung fluke belonging to this genus are now recognised. These flukes are plump oval forms. The ventral sucker is situated just in front of the middle of the body. The flukes infect the carnivores, pig and man. Generally two flukes are found together in a cyst in the lungs. The presence of the flukes cause bronchitis, peri-bronchitis, and consolidation of portions of the lung. Lesions resembling tuberculosis may be developed, nodules also being formed round eggs. The flukes are found in America and Asia. Eggs are coughed up, swallowed, and passed out

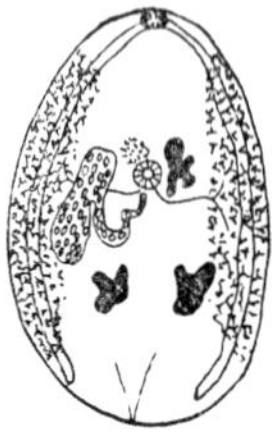

Paragonimus.

with the droppings. The cercaræ develop in operculated snails, and afterwards escape and encyst on freshwater crabs or cray-fish. These are eaten, and the adult flukes develop in the body. Treatment is unsuccessful. Diagnosis is by identification of the egg in the sputum or droppings.

SCHISTOSOMA.—The flukes of this genus live in the blood-stream of man and various mammals. They are peculiar in that the sexes are separate, and although occasionally found apart, are usually found with the female lying in a groove formed by the incurved edges of the male. The flukes live in the blood-vessels of

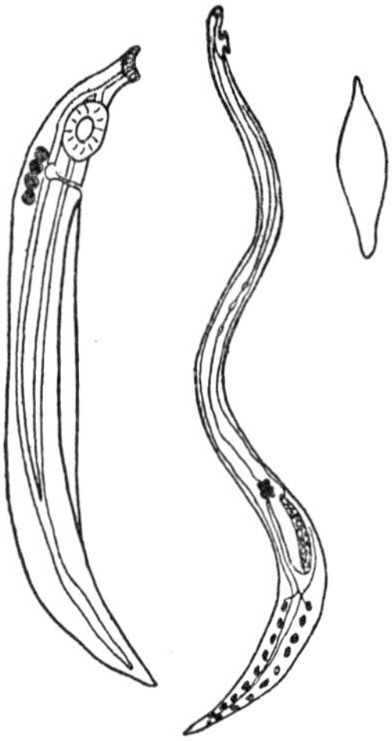

Schistosoma, ♂, ♀, and egg.

their hosts, in the portal vessels, mesenteric veins, or in the cystic or renal veins. The site seems to be constant for any one species. The ova, which in most cases have terminal spines, find their way to the exterior by burrowing through the wall of the vein and reaching the bladder or rectum. Although the pathology is only very imperfectly known in the case of the domestic mammals, there can be no doubt that the presence of the worms must cause considerable injury. Several species have been reported from the mammals in India, Africa, and Europe. One species, possibly two, of those found in domestic animals occur also in man.

The life-cycle differs from the typical case, in that the free cercaria may pierce the skin of its host instead of being swallowed. The cercaria also have bifid tails, and swim tail forwards.

AMPHISTOMA.—The amphistomes are fleshy flukes with the suckers at opposite ends of the body. They are found in ruminants, horses, and pigs. Those forms found in ruminants mostly occur in the rumen and are somewhat conical in shape. They are generally called '*Amphistoma conicum*', although several genera exist. These fall into two groups, one with and one without a ventral pouch.

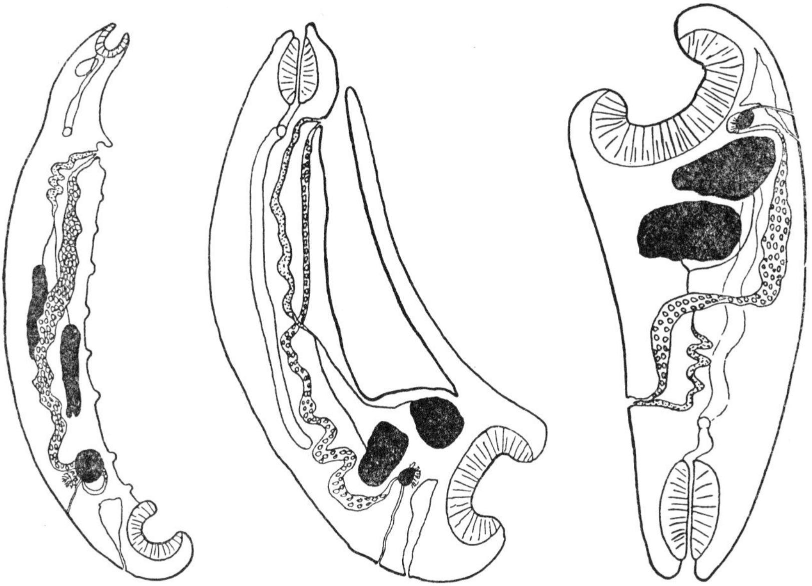

Sections through the three families of Paramphistomidæ. (Left to Right: Gastrodiscid Gastrothylid ; Paramphistome.)

They sometimes occur in very large numbers, and although they often appear to do little harm, the immature flukes may damage the duodenal mucosa of calves and cause rapid wasting. A peculiar species is found in the intestine of cattle in which the body is divided into two regions. It is not known whether this form is pathogenic or not.

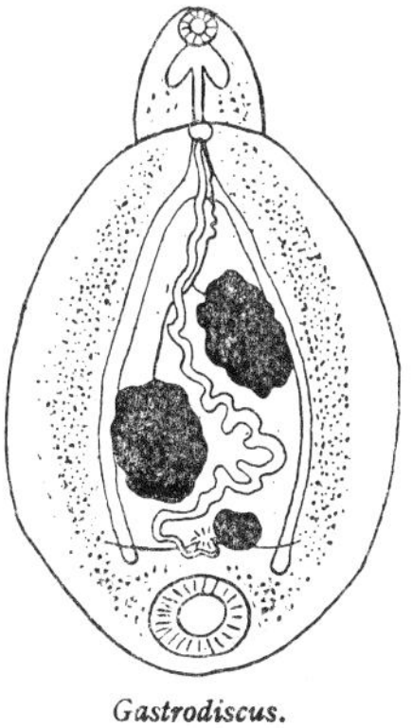

Gastrodiscus.

In the horse occurs a flat round fluke, *Gastrodiscus*, with the anterior sucker set on a conical projection. This fluke also occurs in considerable numbers with a consequent anæmia. The symptoms are, however, not very distinct.

In the pig occurs a similar but smaller

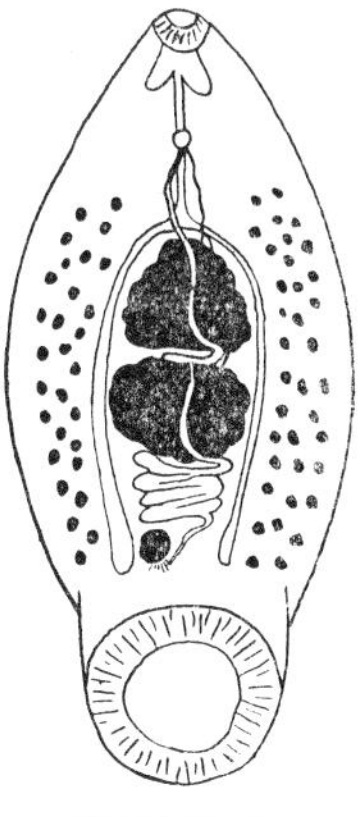

Homalogaster.

worm (*Gastrodiscoides*). It does little or no damage to the pig, but is of interest as being transmissible to man.

Little is known of the pathology of this group of worms, and they are included here because their comparatively large

PARASITES AND PARASITOLOGY

size makes them objects of interest on post-mortem.

B. CESTODA.—The Cestodes found in the domestic animals are long segmented forms without a digestive tract. Each consists of a head or ' scolex ', with four suckers or two sucking grooves, and in some cases also a number of hooks on a small terminal prominence or ' rostellum '. Behind this scolex, which is attached to the wall of the host's intestine, is a neck, which quickly gives place to a number of segments. These are continually renewed from the neck, and the older segments fall off and pass out with the droppings. The segments in each worm may be divided into three groups—immature, mature, and gravid. The immature segments are those nearest to the scolex, which contain only genital rudiments. The second are those which contain the mature genital organs, especially the male organs ; while the last group contain those farthest away from the head which have been fertilised and are more or less filled with eggs.

The mature segments contain male and female organs, consisting of the same essential elements as in the trematodes, while in the gravid segments these have more or less atrophied, and the uterus alone is important.

The excretory system consists of a system of longitudinal tubes, connected by transverse tubes at the posterior of each segment.

DIPHYLLOBOTHRIUM — *D. latum* is the broad tapeworm of man, the dog, and the cat. It is rare in Britain, but has a wide distribution. Several species are found, but this is the commonest. The genus can be recognised by the characteristic rosette shape of the uterus in gravid segments. The life-history is interesting. The ciliated larva liberated from the egg is swallowed by a crustacean, *Cyclops strenuus* or *Diaptonius* spp., in which it becomes an elongated form with a terminal sphere containing three pairs of hooklets, called a ' procercoid larva '. The crustaceans are swallowed by a fish, when the larva, migrating to the muscles, becomes an elongated infective larva called a ' plerocercoid '. The fish is eaten by a suitable host, and the adults develop. In man, the tapeworm may attain a length of 60 feet.

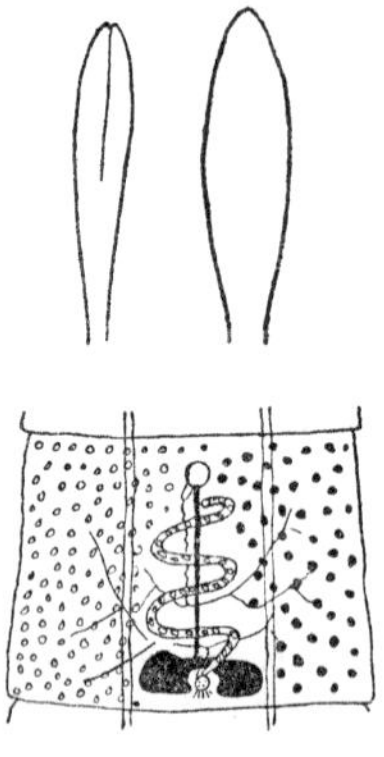

Diphyllobothrium. Head and segment.

The disease has received little attention in the domestic carnivores ; but it is probably similar to that in man, where it may cause a grave form of anæmia (bothriocephalus anæmia) associated with gastric and nervous symptoms. Treatment is on similar lines to other tapeworms.

D. mansoni is also widely distributed and has a similar life-history, but the infective stage is found in many hosts, including man, pig, and carnivores. It is common in frogs in Japan. The adult worm is found in carnivores.

TÆNIA.—This is the common genus of worms found in dogs and cats. The life-histories of the members of this genus are all on similar lines. When the highly resistant eggs are swallowed by a suitable intermediate host, there hatches from each a small ciliated larva, the onchosphere, after the shell has been dissolved by gastric juices. This larva penetrates the gut wall and forms a cystic stage. There are two types of bladder-worm formed, and the genus is sometimes split into two on this account. The genus tænia (*sensu stricto*) forms a cysticercus, a bladder-worm with only one head and which will develop into only one tapeworm. The genus multiceps, on the other hand, forms a bladder-worm containing many heads called a cœnurus, which will develop into several adult worms. The adults of both genera are very similar. The genus echinococcus forms the familiar hydatid or echinococcus, which contains numerous brood capsules, each containing many heads. That explains why an infection with adult echinococci is always a heavy one.

The bladder-worm, on being swallowed by its definitive host, develops into the adult form (or forms). The tapeworms cannot develop without an intermediate host. The following species of tænia are

PARASITES AND PARASITOLOGY

found in the dog. *T. pisiformis* (*T. serrata*) is one of the commonest. As in all tænias the hooks are of two sizes, and in this species the large hooks are very large (·22 to ·29 mm.). Its cystic stage, *Cysticercus pisiformis*, is found in the liver, mesenteries, or abdominal cavities of rabbits and hares.

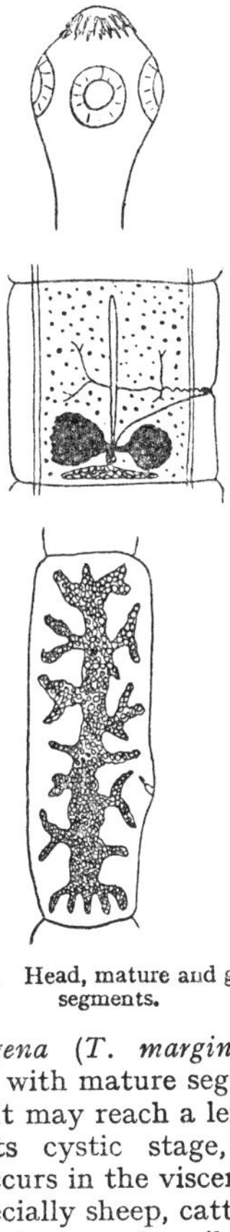

Tænia. Head, mature and gravid segments.

T. hydatigena (*T. marginata*) is the largest form, with mature segments wider than long. It may reach a length of over 16 feet. Its cystic stage, *Cysticercus tenuicollis*, occurs in the viscera of various animals, especially sheep, cattle, and pigs. It is a fairly large and easily seen form. There is always *some* risk of a fatal hæmorrhage from the liver in these animals.

T. ovis is frequently mistaken for the last form, from which it can be distinguished only by microscopical examination. Its cysticercus, *C. ovis*, is found in the muscles and organs of sheep and goats. It is a small form, easily overlooked.

T. multiceps (*Multiceps multiceps; T. cœnurus*) and the next species always occur in some numbers. It is a more delicate form than the others, semi-translucent, with smallish large hooks (·15 to ·17 mm.). The intermediate stage is a cœnurus, found in the nervous system of sheep and other ruminants and man.

T. serialis (*Multiceps serialis*) is a more robust form, its cœnurus being found in rabbits and hares. Only one species is common in the cat. *T. Tæniæformis* (*T. crassicollis*) has a very thick neck with very large hooks. The cystic stage, *Cysticercus fasciolaris*, is found in the liver of rats and mice.

Symptoms in Dogs.—Symptoms are frequently absent. By sheer numbers, tænias may cause impaction or even invagination of the intestine. Typically they cause an intestinal disturbance, capricious appetite, a general uneasiness, and even epileptiform fits (due to a toxin produced by the worms). The coat is staring, and the dog generally draws his hind quarters along the ground. Symptoms are very variable, but diagnosis is easy by examination of the fæces for eggs, assisted, if necessary, by a laxative.

Treatment is very important, not so much from the point of view of the dog; but because some of the species in their intermediate stages are dangerous to food animals. Farm dogs should never be allowed to harbour tapeworms. Regular examination and, if necessary, medicinal measures are necessary. If the dog has tapeworms, repeated doses of medicine are indicated until no more worms come away. All material passed should be burned.

There are several drugs used for the treatment of these pests. The best are perhaps arecoline hydrobromide, or acetarsol, which cause the expulsion of the worms in a very short time.

Dogs which hunt and those having access to slaughterhouse or knackery offal, whereby meat is eaten raw, are more liable to become infected with tapeworms and should receive regular treatment.

Symptoms in the Cat.—When present in numbers the cat loses its appetite, and becomes constipated, sometimes after a transient diarrhœa. The abdomen is retracted, and the animal becomes prostrate and may die in convulsions.

Gastritis or enteritis may be present.

Treatment is as in the dog.

Prevention is difficult, as the catching of mice is the function of most cats, and to prevent the catching of mice is the *only* preventive.

ECHINOCOCCUS.—*Echinococcus granulosus* (*Tænia echinococcus*) consists of only

PARASITES AND PARASITOLOGY

three or four segments, and measures under an inch long. Its larval stage is the hydatid found in all the domestic mammals, but most commonly in sheep, cattle, and pigs. As this develops in man, and is a very serious parasite, all infected dogs should be destroyed and no attempt made at treatment. All contaminated material should be burned.

DIPYLIDIUM.—A single species of this genus occurs in dogs and cats, called *D. caninum*. The worm may be easily recognised by the double genital pores in each segment and the cucumber-seed appearance of the gravid segments. The intermediate stage is a cryptocystis, an almost solid larval stage without the vesicle of the cysticercus, which is found in the biting-louse and the flea of the dog.

This species is more pathogenic than the tænias, as the head, with its several rows of hooks, is driven into the mucosa of the gut, and works through it, drawing the remainder of the body after it. This destroys the mucous membrane and causes a chronic catarrh. The gravid segments escaping from the anus cause pruritis, and are capable of movement in the fæces.

Treatment is as for the others, but the removal of this worm is more obstinate.

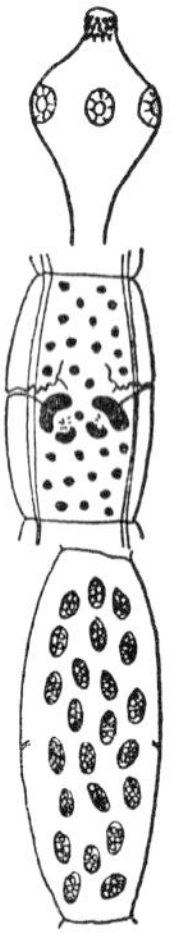

Dipylidium. Head, mature and gravid segments.

Prevention is by the destruction of ecto-parasites.

Bladder-worms.—The bladder-worms are the intermediate stages of certain tænoid tapeworms of man and the carnivores. They are found mainly in the herbivores, pig, and man.

Three types are found :

(*a*) *Cysticercus.*
(*b*) *Cœnurus.*
(*c*) *Echinococcus.*

Each type has the same basic construction, *i.e.* a bladder filled with fluid and one or more inverted tapeworm heads in vesicles in the bladder. In the case of the cysticercus the vesicle is comparatively small and contains only one head. The cœnurus is larger and contains several heads ; while the echinococcus contains a number of brood-capsules or vesicles each containing several heads. The cyst is surrounded by a thick striated membrane, and in addition a protective cyst is formed by the host round the bladder.

Cysticercus. — The cysticercus is the intermediate stage of the genus tænia of carnivores and man. The following are important.

C. bovis is the cause of measles in the ox. It is the intermediate stage of *T. saginata*, the unarmed tapeworm of man. As this species has no hooks on the scolex in the adult stage, so the larval stage has no hooks either. The cyst is small, not larger than a pea, and is found as a rule in the striped muscle. It occurs in order of frequency in the muscles of mastication ; heart, neck muscles ; intercostal and diaphragmatic muscles. It is more common in young than old animals. After some time the cysts calcify and degenerate, being no longer capable of infecting man. The cysts are rapidly killed in frozen beef. The condition in the ox is only realised on slaughter. The tapeworm may be 50 feet long

C. cellulosæ is the intermediate stage of *T. solium* of man, and is the cause of measles in the pig. The adult tapeworm is now very rare. The cysts are more delicate and translucent than *C. bovis*, and are somewhat larger. The head, moreover, has a double row of small hooks. The cysts are found in any organ ; but the following are the commonest locations ; tongue ; muscles of neck and shoulder : intercostal, abdominal, psoas and thigh muscles. The cysts ultimately undergo caseous degeneration and calcify. They live rather longer than *C. bovis*, and are not so easily killed in pork. Symptoms are absent in pigs. Man may also harbour the cysts.

C. ovis is the cause of measles in sheep, and is the intermediate stage of *T. ovis* of

PARASITES AND PARASITOLOGY

the dog. It resembles the last in appearance and size, and is often mistaken for it. It is non-infective for man.

C. tenuicollis, the intermediate stage of *T. hydatigena* of the dog, occurs in sheep, and occasionally other ruminants and the pig. It is a large form, resembling a sac about 1 inch in diameter, filled with a clear fluid in which projects a white object—the head and neck. Generally no symptoms are observed, but a severe infection may kill the sheep in the early stages by hæmorrhage of the liver.

Cœnurus.—The cœnurus is the intermediate stage of the genus *Multiceps* of dogs. It is a largish bladder containing a number of vesicles each with a single head. The most important form is—

C. cerebralis, the intermediate stage of *T. (multiceps) multiceps*. It is found in the central nervous system of sheep and other herbivores, and has been found in man. It may attain the size of a hen's egg, and is usually located in the brain. The bladder is semi-translucent, with numerous white spots showing through its walls—each being a larval head. There may be several hundred heads in a single cyst, and several cysts in the same animal.

Symptoms depend on the location of the cyst. Dullness, inappetence, fever, loss of sight, and emaciation are among the earlier symptoms. These occur in 10 to 20 days after infection, and if the sheep does not die, they subside. In 4 to 6 months a second series of symptoms appear. Loss of sight returns; the head is held in a peculiar position; and the animal moves in circles, always to the same side, or staggers or stumbles about, depending on the location of the cyst. The feet are lifted high, and the movements are impulsive. These symptoms are intermittent, but in some weeks give place to complete paralysis and death. If the parasite is located in the spinal cord, it is usually in the lumbar region with symptoms of paraplegia, debility, and progressive emaciation. Bladder and rectum are affected, and death takes place in 4 to 12 weeks.

Treatment consists in the surgical removal of the cyst. As a rule early slaughter is to be recommended.

The disease is known by various names, such as 'gid' or 'staggers'.

Echinococcus.—The echinococcus is the largest of the bladder-worms, and results from the smallest of the tænias, *E. granulosus* of the dog and cat. It consists of a more or less spherical cyst containing numerous vesicles, called brood capsules, each with several heads. Daughter cysts are also formed—often external to the mother cyst. The evolution of the vesicles is shown above. Hundreds of larval tapeworms may develop from a single egg. A second type of cyst is found in man in which the vesicles are never larger than a pea and are filled with a gelatinous

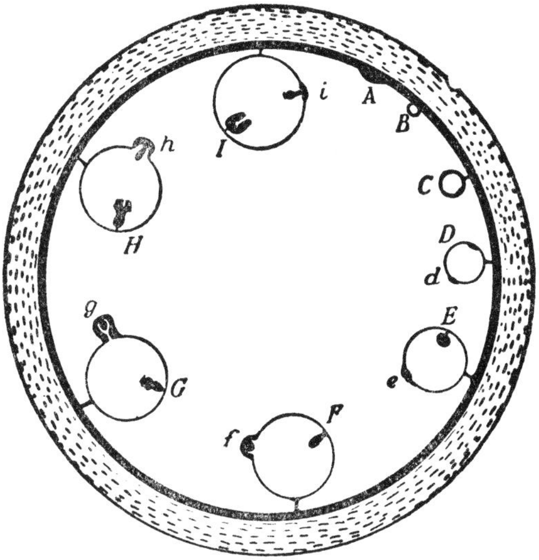

Diagram to show the evolution of the hydatid cyst and its brood capsules. The capital letter (*A* to *I*) show the usual development, while the small letters (*d* to *i*) show an alternative method.

PARASITES AND PARASITOLOGY

material. The vesicles have a honeycomb arrangement and are mostly sterile. Much confusion exists as to the different forms. The development of the hydatid is slow, but it may reach the size of a child's head.

Symptoms are very vague or even absent; and as the hydatid may be located in any organ, even these vague symptoms vary. It is common in the liver, with sometimes daughter cysts in the lungs. It is rarely fatal in the lower animals, but is a very serious disease in man. It is found in practically any of the domestic animals.

Prevention.—All the bladder-worms treated here develop from eggs passed by man or carnivores. Neither man nor the carnivores can be infected if denied access to infected meat or offal. Strict meat inspection can eliminate the parasites. It has been shown that wild carnivores, such as foxes, can play important parts in the spread of hydatid, and control may be rather more difficult. Farm dogs should be systematically examined for tapeworms and treated, the dog being confined until the worms are evacuated. The worms should of course be burned to avoid infecting stock.

Tapeworms in Horses.—Three species occur in horses, all belonging to the genus ANOPLOCEPHALA. *A. perfoliata* and *A. mammillana* are not uncommon in Britain, while *A. magna* is also sometimes encountered.

A. perfoliata, a stoutish worm with large head and no hooks, is reputed to cause large ulcers in the large intestine, although symptoms other than general unthriftiness have not been noticed. The fæces are coated with a blood-stained mucus, and the disease may be more serious than is generally supposed.

The intermediate host is a mite of the Oribated variety.

Tapeworms in Ruminants.—All the tapeworms of ruminants have four suckers and no hooks. In Moniezia and Helicometra the intermediate host is a free-living mite.

MONIEZIA.—This is the only genus found in Britain; but it is world-wide in its distribution. The segments of these worms are much broader than long; and the genital system, including the uterus, is double, with bilateral genital pores. The worms may attain a length of several yards, with a minute head little larger than a pin-head. Over 1000 worms have been recorded from a single host. Numerous species have been recorded, many of which are not valid. Two are common, *M. expansa* and *M. benedeni* (*planissima*). As a rule lambs of a few months only are infected. There is a mild anæmia with a staring coat. Although the appetite is good, the animals lose condition

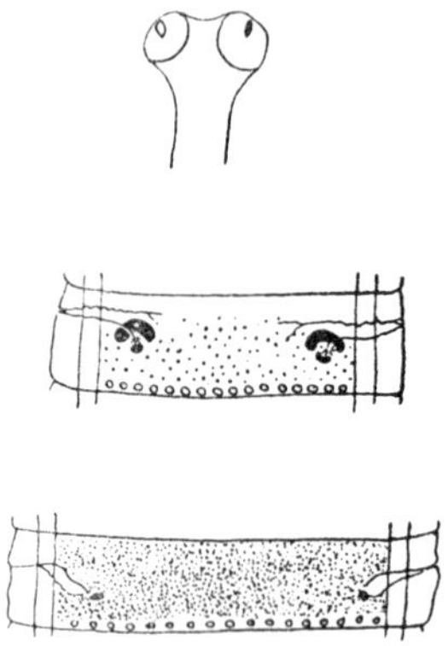

Moniezia expansa. Head, mature and gravid segments. In *M. benedeni* the circles are replaced by a straight line.

rapidly and growth is suspended more or less. Colic is frequent, and the bowels are irregular. Finally, a continuous diarrhœa supervenes and the animals die from exhaustion. If the animals recover, there has been a serious loss of growth which is often not recovered.

There is no well-established treatment for these worms. Best results are obtained with copper sulphate and sodium arsenite as used for hookworm. Copper sulphate alone and koussin have been tried with good results.

HELICTOMETRA.—This genus can be distinguished from *Moniezia* by the presence of a single uterus in each segment.

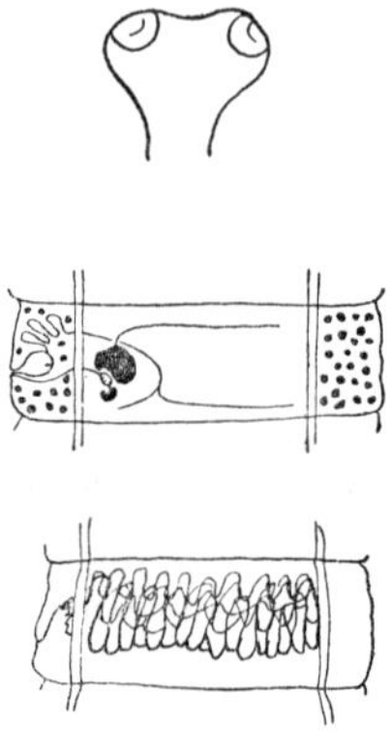

Helictometra. Head, mature and gravid segments.

PARASITES AND PARASITOLOGY

H. giardi is found in Europe, Australia, and Africa. It has no posterior fringe, and the testes are lateral. Genital organs are generally single. Is from 1 to 2 metres long.

A closely related form, *Thysanosoma actinioides*, is found in North America. This parasite can be easily recognised by the presence of fringes on the posterior border of each segment. It is about 30 cm. long, and is found in the liver. The symptoms caused are unthriftiness, diarrhœa, and emaciation. The wool is poor and the skin hide-bound. The sheep show general symptoms of malnutrition.

No successful cure is known.

Tapeworms in Poultry.—A number of tapeworms have been found in poultry, of which the commonest are *Davainea proglottina*, which has a larval stage in slugs and snails and is widely distributed, several species of *Raillietina*, with the larvæ in house-flies, dung beetles and ants; these are also common in many countries, *Amœbotœnia*, with larvæ in earthworms, and *Hymenolepis* of various species, some of which may be very numerous in individual birds.

Symptoms vary greatly; the worms are only likely to cause serious loss when present in very large numbers, and often they are only identified at post-mortem examination.

Treatment.—Male fern, arecanut compounds, and kamala are used with varying success, the latter in doses of 1 gram for a year-old fowl being useful.

C. NEMATODA.—The nematodes or round worms of the domestic animals all have separate sexes. The digestive tract consists of a mouth, œsophagus, a chyle intestine, and a rectum.

In most cases the female genital system is double, *i.e.* consists of two tubular ovaries, uteri, etc., opening to the exterior at a common vagina. In a few cases only one ovary is found.

In the male a single testes is found, which opens ln common with the rectum at a cloaca. Additional sexual organs in the male occur, such as one or two spicules, and an accessory piece. In certain groups are found adhesive organs for retaining the male in position during copulation.

The excretory system opens to the exterior at an excretory pore situated on the mid-ventrai line in the anterior region of the body.

Most nematodes lay eggs, but some produce living larvæ. The life-history may be direct or indirect, *i.e.* an intermediate host may be necessary. Those forms to be considered here fall into four super families.

(1) **Ascaridoidea,** forms with three lips.

(2) **Filaroidea,** slender forms with a simple mouth or two lips.

This super family of Nematodes may for the present purposes be divided into two families:

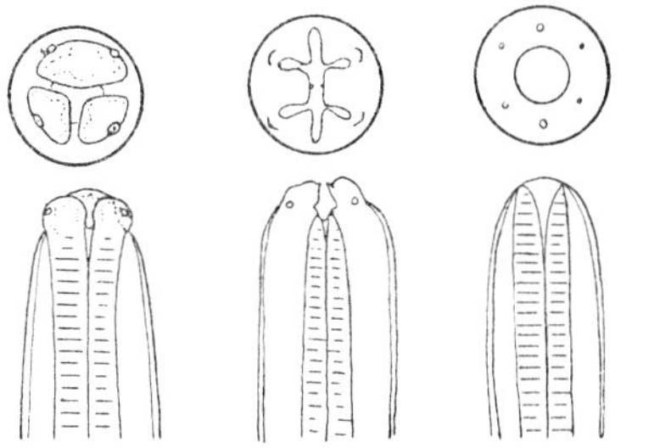

End-on and side view of head of ascarid.

Two groups of longish thin worms, *Spiruridæ* and *Filaridæ*. End-on and side views of head.

FILARIDÆ, which have round or hexagonal mouth openings without lips. All the forms to be found in the domestic animals live outside the digestive tract.

SPIRURIDÆ, which have generally bivalved mouth openings with more or less distinct lips. These forms live in the œsophagus or stomach. All the members of this group require an intermediate host.

(3) **Strongyloidea.**—This super family contains all those forms which have a caudal bursa in the male. This is an umbrella-like structure supported by a

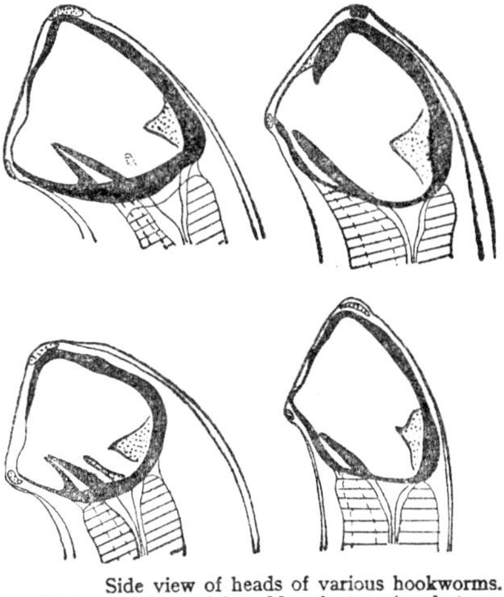

Side view of heads of various hookworms. Top row (left to right), *Monodontus*, *Ancylostoma*. Bottom row, *Necator*, *Dochmoides*.

PARASITES AND PARASITOLOGY

definite system of rays and used for clasping the female. All are smallish forms, but the great majority are more or less pathogenic to their hosts.

So far as is known, the life-cycle is always direct. The members of this group may be classified in the following families :

STRONGYLIDÆ.—This family includes those forms which have a terminal or subterminal chitinised buccal capsule. This is a highly organised structure, rigid, and often containing teeth. Closely related to this family are the œsophagostomes, which have a characteristic cuticular swelling near the head end.

ANCYLOSTOMIDÆ.—This family differs from the last in the possession of a dorsally opening buccal capsule. The Ancylostomidæ of the domestic mammals include the following genera :

Ancylostoma.—In this genus the dorsally turned head has the mouth opening protected by two or three teeth, while the other genera have cutting plates.

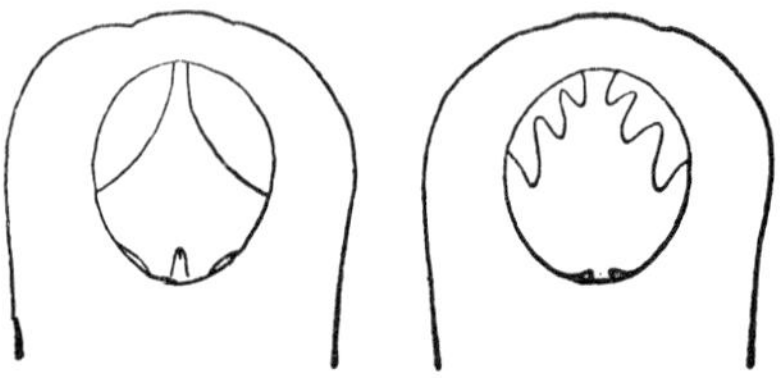

Diagram of mouth opening of the two groups of Hookworm. (Left) *Monodontus*, (right) *Ancylostoma.*

Dochmoides (Uncinaria).—This genus has one representative in carnivores. It has cutting plates, but no dorsal tooth.

Monodontus.—This genus and the following have cutting plates and dorsal teeth. This form has an asymmetrical bursa in the male.

Necator differs from the latter by having a symmetrical bursa.

In the pig is found a genus of hookworms which have no cutting organs to the mouth opening, called *Globocephalus.*

TRICHOSTRONGYLIDÆ are small slender forms living in the intestine and having no buccal capsule. *T. axei* may be found in the abomasum of ruminants and also in the stomach of horse, pig, and man. *T. tenuis* attacks poultry and game birds.

METASTRONGYLIDÆ resemble the last family, but live in the lungs, etc., and have atypical bursæ.

COOPERIA.—There are four species in this genus. They are usually reddish in colour, they suck blood, and their life-history resembles that of *Hæmonchus contortus.*

There are several other forms which do not fall into any of these families, and will be considered at the end of the part.

The pathology of all these forms is practically unknown. There is little doubt that the majority are not only blood suckers, but also producers of powerful toxins. In fact the anæmia which accompanies the disease is probably due as much to the latter cause as to the loss of blood.

(4) **Trichinelloidea.**—This is a small group containing whip-worms and the well-known *Trichinella* of pork. They are distinguished by the fact that the œsophagus consists of a tubular opening in a chain of cells, instead of being built up of a mass of cells as in the other forms.

HORSE. — I. Stomach — HABRONEMA.—Three species of this genus inhabit the stomach of the equidæ, in various parts of the world—one at least occurring in Great Britain. They all measure 1 to 2 cm. long, and are thin forms. The mouth has four lips, and there are lateral alæ to the body. The male has large caudæ alæ, two unequal spicules, and an accessory piece. The vulva is in the anterior part of the body.

In all the life-story is similar. The egg passes out with the droppings, and is swallowed by the larva of a fly. The egg hatches, and the worm larva reaches maturity in the body cavity or Malphigian ducts of the fly. It ultimately reaches the proboscis. When this organ comes into contact with any moist warm surface, the larvæ break their way through and become free on the surface. If this, for example, is the mouth of a horse, they are swallowed and develop into adults in the stomach. If it is an open sore, they cause the condition called ' summer sores ' (*see* p. 652). Infection of the stomach can also take place by the accidental ingestion of the fly in the fodder. The common intermediate host of *H. megastoma* and of *H. muscæ* is *Musca domestica,* the common house-fly ; while that of *H. microstoma* is *Stomoxys calcitrans,* the stable-fly.

H. megastoma is generally found in ' tumours ' on the stomach wall, while the others are found free on the mucous membrane.

' Gastric Habronemosis ' is the condition caused by the adults of *H. megastoma,* living in inflammatory tumours on the right sac of the stomacy. The tumour may be as large as a pigeon's egg, and in it is found, embedded in a caseous substance, the worms. The caseous substance is not necrotic tissue, but real pus.

Symptoms are not well defined, but the presence of a number of these nodules must seriously impair the gastric functions. The other two species do not cause the formation of nodules, but as they may be found embedded in the mucous membrane, they may cause a chronic inflammation of the stomach.

Treatment is not yet known, although carbon bisulphide has been recommended.

Prevention consists in destruction of flies and proper control of manure.

II. Small Intestine.—*Parascaris equorum.* (*A. megalocephala*).—This is the common large round worm of the horse. It is about as thick as a pencil, and may reach a length of over 20 inches, although normally about a foot long. The female is straight, while the smaller male has the posterior end curved. The head end has three prominent lips.

This parasite is universally distributed. It is usually found in the small intestine, and, unless present in large numbers, seems to cause little disturbance.

The life cycle is similar to that of the pig ascarid.

The symptoms produced are rather indefinite : colic, depraved appetite, irregularity of the movements of the bowels, and general unthriftiness. When numerous and when bunched up together as not uncommonly happens, they may cause mechanical interference with normal bowel movements, and have been known to cause intussusception and rupture. The larvæ which migrate to the lungs after hatching in the stomach, are capable of causing a catarrhal bronchitis or broncho-pneumonia, and probably cause some damage to the liver also, during their migration through this organ.

The eggs of this worm are capable of long periods of survival in favourable places, and the embryonated egg has been observed still living after 12 months in hay contaminated with horse dung. Diagnosis is by demonstration of the parasite or its egg in the droppings.

Treatment consists in the administration of such anthelmintics as sodium fluoride or carbon bisulphide, which are poisonous, and must only be given under veterinary advice.

Prevention.—Infection is caused by the horse eating fodder, etc., infected with eggs. Accordingly fæces should be removed at once, as should also soiled bedding, etc., to prevent the animal eating it and so reinfecting himself. Cleanliness and good feeding are important.

III. Cæcum and Colon — STRONGYLIDÆ.—The strongyle worms in the horse all fall into this family, and a large number of forms are known. The following are the important forms :

Strongylus.—This genus is characterised by the possession of a globular buccal capsule, the edge of which is fringed with a number of delicate leaf-like processes. The capsules may have teeth attached to its wall. Three species are known in the horse. They may be recognised by the shape of the buccal capsule. The largest is about 2 inches long; while the smallest is about ¾ inch long or less.

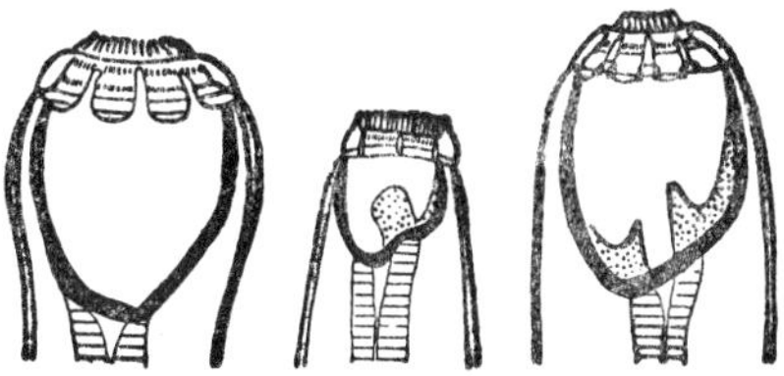

Strongylus (head). (Left to right) *S. edentatus*, *S. vulgaris*, *S. equinus.*

Triodontophorus.—This genus contains a number of species. They all have a globular buccal capsule with three teeth at junction of the œsophagus and buccal capsule.

Trichonema (*Cylicostomum*).—This genus has a cylindrical buccal capsule fringed with leaf-like processes. It contains a very large number of forms, most of which are of little importance as adults, but some of which are important in the larval stage. The pathology and symptoms caused by individual species is not well known.

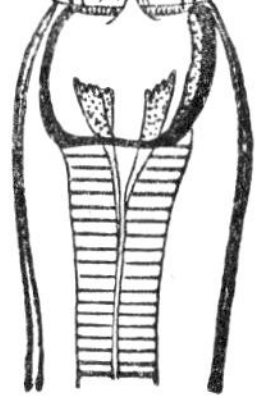

Triodontophorus (head-end).

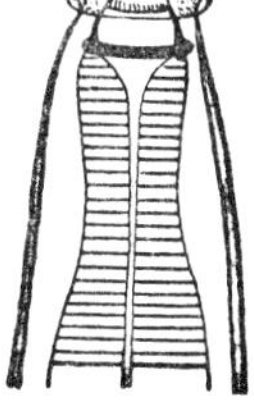

Trichonema insigne, a very common species (head-end).

STRONGYLIDOSIS.—As the strongyles in the horse seldom occur in a pure infection, the disease caused by their presence is usually called strongylidosis or sclerosto-

PARASITES AND PARASITOLOGY

miasis. However, some of the various subdivisions are known.

(*a*) Disease caused by presence of adults in the intestine and of immature forms of *Strongylus* and *Trichonema* encysted in the intestinal wall. Young animals of from 6 months to 2 years are most affected. The adults of the genus *Triodontophorus*, in the large colon, seem to be particularly virulent. The symptoms caused by these various conditions have not been differentiated, however. They consist of a progressive anæmia, with a resulting œdema and loss of condition. Diarrhœa is common. Colts become emaciated, with an irregular appetite. The temperature is irregular, but fever is usually absent. If the infection is heavy, death from exhaustion and anæmia results. On post-mortem examination numerous worms and worm cysts are found in the large intestine.

(*b*) Due to larvæ of *Strongylus edentatus*. The immature larvæ live sub-peritoneally, and under certain unknown conditions produce enzoötics in colts. The disease may be chronic, with progressive emaciation and anæmia, occasionally diarrhœa, but no fever or quickened pulse. Or it may be acute with a rapid feeble pulse, a temperature of over 106° F., and the colicky symptoms of peritonitis. The horses look towards their right flanks, and show a characteristic right torsion of the hind quarters as the off hind leg passes under the body. The symptoms increase, with ultimate death in a few days or weeks. There is no known treatment.

(*c*) Verminous aneurisms are frequently caused by *Strongylus vulgaris* in the cranial mesenteric artery. The young worms cause a local arteritis, atheroma, degeneration, and dilation of the vessel, together with a thrombus and aneurism. This causes a very violent and persistent colic which does not respond to the usual remedies. This condition may be suspected in all cases of habitual colic. Young foals of about 6 weeks of age may be affected when there has been a massive invasion of the tissues by many thousands of larvæ, but up to about 18 months or 2 years of age colic of verminous origin may occur. A not uncommon symptom is for the animal to roll over on to its back and remains for some moments with its legs up in the air or against a wall. Small emboli detach themselves from the large thrombus and obstruct the smaller vessels. This causes local areas of anæmia in the intestine and elsewhere, with consequent 'embolic' colic. Emboli or small fragments of thrombus may also cause intermittent lameness and even paraplegia.

The treatment of diseases due to the larval forms is impossible. Adult worms may be removed by the administration of phenothiazine in doses of from 10 to 30 grams, followed by daily dosage of 2 grams for the next 21 days. This method of using an initial large dose and a subsequent small daily follow-up dose is very effective in killing the adult worms and in rendering the eggs of any worms that may escape incapable of hatching.

OXYURIS EQUI.—This is the only species of *Oxyuris* found in the domestic mammals. It occurs in the horse. It is a stoutish worm about 2 inches long, much of the length being taken up by a long slender tail. The male is very small and seldom seen. It is whitish in colour. It is found in the large intestine and in all countries.

It does little harm to the horse by itself; but the female comes to the end of the rectum to deposit its eggs, which are ejected as a yellowish or greenish mass surrounding the anus. This may cause immense irritation to the animal, and so be the cause of considerable trouble. The animal, disturbed by the pruritis, is uneasy and sometimes more difficult to handle. He rubs his hind quarters on rough surfaces, and so soon renders them bare of hair and very unsightly.

Treatment is most effectively carried out by the use of salt or quassia enemata injected into the rectum once or twice daily.

PROBSTMAYRIA VIVIPARA.—This is a minute oxyurid worm frequently found in the large intestine of the horse. It occurs in Britain and the United States. It appears to be harmless.

IV. Lungs.—*Dictyocaulus arnfieldi* is the only worm found in the lungs of the horse. The male is about 3 cm. long, while the female is 5 cm. It has been found in many countries, including Britain. It is the cause of a verminous bronchitis which may be recognised by a cough and, if the worms are numerous, by loss of appetite and emaciation. Fatal cases have been seen in donkeys, a source of infection.

Treatment consists in good nursing with nourishing foods. The use of turpentine in linseed oil about twice weekly is recommended by some. Half an ounce in half a pint given by stomach tube is enough for an average horse of about 1000 lb. weight.

V. Connective tissue — ONCHOCERCA.— This genus occurs mainly in herbivores.

PARASITES AND PARASITOLOGY

They have a thick cuticle, with spiral thickenings on it in the female. They are very long, and usually coiled on themselves. The female has an obtuse tail, while the male has two unequal spicules and a variable number of caudal papillæ. The life-cycle is unknown, but they are probably carried by biting flies. *O. reticulata* is found in the horse, especially in tendons. It is common near the suspensory ligament, but is also reported in the withers. They may cause no symptoms, or may induce hypertrophy of the tendon or may cause 'fistulous withers'. *O. cervicalis* occurs in the ligamentum nuchæ of equines, and is often associated with poll-evil.

VI. Skin. — *Parafilaria multi-papillosa* (*Filaria hæmorrhagica*) is a smallish filaria, about 2 inches long, found subcutaneously in the horse and mule. It is whitish with a transversely striated cuticle which, in the head region, gives place to circular prominences. The two sexes are usually found side by side in the connective tissue.

The parasite is essentially an Eastern one, but is now found in many parts of the world.

It causes small hæmorrhages at various points under the skin. They rarely suppurate, and quickly disappear to reappear at another spot in a few days. They are absent during winter, but return in spring. They appear to do little damage to the host, other than occasionally interfering with the harnessing of the animal.

Treatment is not very satisfactory, as the life-history is unknown. Cleanliness is desirable, as also is the avoidance of pressure of harness on the affected parts. Recovery is usually spontaneous—often after several years—while deaths are uncommon.

'Summer Sores.'—This condition, which is common in all the warmer parts of the world, is caused by the larval stage of the worm *Habronema megastomum*, which lives normally in the stomach of the horse.

The sores are up to 1 inch in diameter, and may be present in any part of the body. They provoke an intense itching, which causes the horse to bite himself until extensive raw surfaces are produced. The sore is filled with a thin watery pus containing firm granulations which may be caseated. The larval worms are found in the centre of the mass.

The larvæ pass part of their life-history in the house-fly, and, on the proboscis of the fly touching any warm moist surface, they escape. This is normally the lips of the horse, and the larvæ proceed to finish their development after being swallowed. If the fly has been feeding on any wound, however, they escape into it. In other cases they seem to have reached the wound from contact with the dung on which the horse has been lying. At all events an existing wound is necessary, and if steps are taken to prevent any wounds being contaminated, this condition cannot exist.

Prevention.—Summer sores are evidence of neglect. All wounds should be kept clean. Iodoform and collodion are useful both as preventive and cure. Treatment by novarsenobenzol in an ointment applied to the sores is useful. Prevention also includes removal of the adult worms from the stomach, fly control, clean bedding, and destruction of larvæ in the manure. The disease is a serious source of loss, although not directly fatal.

RUMINANTS. — I. Œsophagus and Stomach — GONGYLONEMA. — This genus can be recognised by the presence of oval or rounded tubercles on the anterior part of the body. The tail of the male is spiral.

Two species occur in ruminants and one in pigs. They are found just below the epithelium in the thoracic third of the œsophagus. The intermediate hosts are various species of dung-beetles. The worms have no effect on their hosts, but render the œsophagus unfit for food.

HÆMONCHUS CONTORTUS.—This is the stomach worm or wire-worm of sheep and other ruminants. It is from ½ inch to 1½ inch long, and is about as thick as a pin.

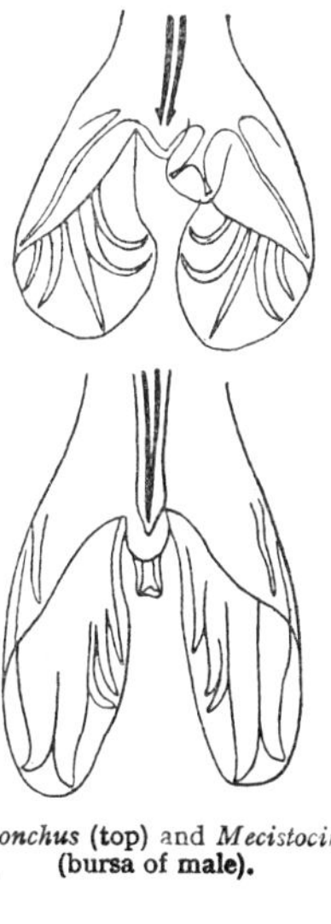

Hæmonchus (top) and *Mecistocirrus* (bursa of male).

PARASITES AND PARASITOLOGY

The female is larger than the male and is pointed at both ends. The uteri form a conspicuous spiral inside the worm and so give it its specific name. The genital opening is protected by a conspicuous flap. The male has a two-lobed bursa with a small asymmetrical dorsal lobule and two short spicules.

Closely related to this worm is another, *Mecistocirrus digitatus*, which so far has only been found in Asia. It differs from the stomach worm in having no genital flap in the female, and no asymmetrical lobule in the male. The male has long spicules. Its pathology is apparently similar to that of the stomach worm, and as it closely resembles that species in naked-eye appearance it has probably been mistaken for it in the part. Further investigation may show that it is more widely distributed than is thought. Hæmonchus is almost universal in its distribution, and is responsible for great loss in warm climates. It attacks all kinds of ruminants, and its usual habitat is in the abomasum, and occasionally the duodenum.

Life-history.—The life-history may be divided into two parts—free-living and parasitic. The egg passed in the fæces hatches, and the resulting larva very shortly moults and, escaping from its cast skin, continues to grow. In a few hours or days this larva also moults, but remains inside its cast skin, stops growing and feeding, and waits on a suitable occasion to enter a sheep or other animal. The previous stages, if swallowed, would die. This stage is accordingly called the infective stage. It can resist drying and adverse conditions, and may live for about a year. When swallowed, the larva casts the skin in which it had remained and, after further growth and moulting, becomes sexually mature. The sexes pair, and the female proceeds to lay eggs. The important stage from the point of view of prevention is the infective stage, and a knowledge of its biology is necessary in order to organise a campaign against it. It shows a tendency to migrate, and, under suitable conditions, it climbs grass blades and is thus more easily swallowed. Dryness and bright light send the larvæ back to the roots of the grass again. Accordingly infection takes place mainly at night and during dull wet weather.

Symptoms are at first indefinite. Animals are less active than usual and do not thrive so well, although the appetite remains normal. Anæmia, with its accompanying symptoms of paleness of the membranes and watery swellings under the jaw (' bottle-jaw '), becomes obvious. The fæces become dark and fluid, with evidence of pain in passing them. Death is rapid, especially in lambs, and may even occur before any symptoms have set in. In cattle similar symptoms are shown, but are generally much less severe and may even be absent.

Diagnosis.—The presence of the worm is most easily diagnosed by finding it in the fourth stomach of a dead or killed sheep. The stomach, after removal from the body, is carefully opened, and the reddish worms are easily seen with the naked eye as actively moving threads.

Prevention.—It has been found that larvæ, after being swallowed by a sheep, require a month to become mature and lay eggs. Therefore, if sheep are dosed monthly with drugs which kill the worms in the stomach, no fresh eggs reach the pasture. Those already there may live for about a year, so that if monthly dosing is continued for a year, the pasture will be freed. This plan has proved successful in South Africa, where the drugs originally used were copper sulphate and arsenic. At present, phenothiazine is widely used with great success, *Hæmonchus* being especially susceptible to its action.

OSTERTAGIA worms, which are of considerable economic importance, are peculiar in that while most infective larvæ living in the abomasum moult twice to become adults, some—especially perhaps those ingested by the calf during late summer and autumn—moult only once and remain as fourth-stage larvæ in a dormant state. They appear to be insensitive to anthelmintics. Later they develop into adults causing a winter outbreak of gastro-enteritis. Calves should therefore be dosed in September and moved to " clean " pasture.

II. Small Intestine — ASCARIS VITULORUM.—This large round worm of cattle is generally of little importance, but it may be a frequent and fatal parasite of calves in certain localities. The worm is about 6 inches to 12 inches long. It is probable that the symptoms in calves are due to a toxin secreted by the animal.

Infection is caused by means similar to *P. equorum*, but in some cases the evidence points to pre-natal infection from the mother. Our knowledge of the life-history of this parasite lends support to this theory.

NEMATODIRUS. — This is a common trichostrongyle genus found in large numbers in the small intestine of sheep. It is a very slender form under an inch long. In recent years nematodirus infestation has caused severe losses. Hexachlorethane has been used in conjunction with phenothiazine, as the latter alone has not proved effective, but greater success has been claimed for 'Frantin', a preparation of Bephenium embonate. Thiabendazole is effective; likewise Tetramisole.

The infestation is a 'lamb-to-lamb' one, and can be avoided—where practicable—by confining lambs to pasture which carried no lambs in the previous two seasons. Nematodirus species found in Britain are *N. filicollis*, *N. helvetianus*, *N. spathiges*, and *N. battus* (a parasite also of calves).

COOPERIA species are important.

Numerous other species of trichostrongyle worms are also found in the intestine, but their effects are still obscure.

'Hookworm in Ruminants.'—The species in ruminants are *Monodontus trigonocephalum* and *M. phlebotomum*. The former is found mainly in sheep, the latter in cattle. Both occur in Britain, and are almost universal in their distribution. The sheep form is very common in British sheep, but usually in small numbers. The clinical symptoms are not well known, but there is no doubt that in large numbers they may cause considerable damage. They are tissue feeders.

Symptoms to be looked for are anæmia, dropsy, and malnutrition — symptoms almost identical with those caused by stomach worm. They are, however, very difficult to remove; and if treatment for *Hæmonchus* is not attended with success their presence should be suspected. Petroleum benzine or carbon tetrachloride have proved successful drugs, and phenothiazine is very useful against all but the ascarids. For these sodium fluoride or carbon bisulphide are more specific.

III. Large Intestine—CHABERTIA OVINA is a parasite of the large intestine of

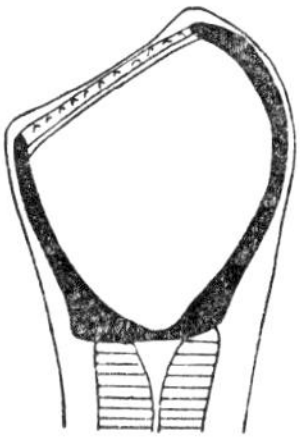

Chabertia (head).

ruminants. It has a large buccal capsule without cutting-plates or teeth, which opens ventrally.

It is a tissue feeder; but it is not definitely known whether it is pathogenic or not. It is a cosmopolitan species.

ŒSOPHAGOSTOMUM.—This is a genus of strongyle worms related to the horse forms, and found in ruminants and pigs. They are about an inch or so long, with a number of leaf-like processes surrounding the short cylindrical buccal capsule, with the cuticle of the head more or less inflated. Some species of these worms appear to be harmless; but *O. columbianum* in the sheep and *O. radiatum* in cattle are the cause of nodular disease of

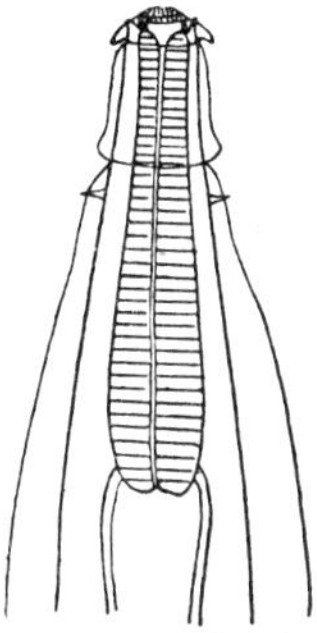

Œsophagostomum (head-end).

the intestine ('pimply gut'). If present in small numbers, the only result is to render the intestine unfit for sausage skins. If in large numbers, the symptoms are similar to those caused by the other intestinal strongyles, *e.g.* anæmia, emaciation, diarrhœa, and dropsy. The disease in this case often has a fatal termination. Prophylaxis is on general lines, and the bare-lot method has been used with considerable success. Lambs are kept on bare lots where there is no temptation to feed, and the ewes are admitted to nurse them when required. Other feed is supplied from raised troughs protected from fæcal contamination. Phenothiazine is effective. (*See also* 'THIN SOW SYNDROME'.)

TRICHOCEPHALUS.—This genus of whipworms occurs in the cæcum of various animals, and is of some importance. The worms have very slender necks with stoutish bodies. The necks are threaded through the mucous membrane of their host. The male has a spiral tail, while that of the female is bluntly pointed.

They may cause a low-grade inflammation at the point of insertion of the head and may admit bacteria.

IV. Lungs.—'Husk', 'Hoose', in Cattle.—Three species are known from this host, but only one is important, *Dictyocaulus viviparus*. The male is about 4 cm. long and the female is about 7 cm. Eggs hatch in the lung, and the larvæ, climbing up the trachea are swallowed, and pass to the exterior with the fæces. After moulting twice, they reach the resistant infective stage, and can live thus on pasture through the winter. When swallowed, they continue their development.

The symptoms and treatment are described under HUSK.

'Hoose' in Sheep and Goats.—Several species occur:

Dictyocaulus filaria is the largest and most common species. The male is about 5 cm. long and the female 8 cm. The infective stage is reached in about 10 days. Apparently lambs can be infected prenatally. This worm is cosmopolitan in its distribution. Its life-history is direct.

The symptoms are those of a verminous bronchitis, sometimes complicated by bacterial infection, but otherwise similar to those in bovines.

Protostrongylus (*Synthetocaulus*) *rufescens* is a red and much smaller form. The male is about 2 cm. and the female 3 cm. long. It is found mainly in Europe. These worms live in the bronchioles and in the pulmonary parenchyma, and cause a verminous lobular pneumonia. The eggs cause a diffuse nodular pneumonia. Cough is less prominent than in the above form, but breathing is difficult. Death is common in heavy infections. In both these cases, treatment is not successful as a rule.

The commonest parasite of the lungs of sheep in Britain and America is *Muellerius capillaris*, a form which is smaller than the other two, and which is the cause of the pseudo-tubercular verminous pneumonia so commonly seen in abattoirs. It is, however, much less serious than the other two, and is seldom the cause of death. Both the latter species are carried by land snails and slugs.

In 1954 a fourth species, *Cystocaulus ocreatus*, was recognised; and since then *Neostrongylus linearis*, a fine thread-like worm similar to *M. capillaris*.

V. Connective Tissues — ONCHOCERCA.—Several species occur in cattle in various parts of the world. They are the cause of 'worm nodules' or 'worm nests' so common in the ox in Australia. The nodules are oval, about the size of a pea to a walnut, with a firm surface. They are easily excisable from the surrounding connective tissue. In the fibrous capsule is found one or more of the long thread-like worms.

The nodules are found mainly in the brisket, but also occur in the flank and fore-quarters. They appear to cause little harm to their host, but as the capsule is a product of inflammation, beef containing worm nodules is condemned, and in Australia they have caused considerable loss in the export trade.

ELÆOPHORA.—This peculiar genus of worms is related to the last, but differs from it in the thickness of the cuticle, which is very deeply striated. The spicules have a terminal swelling. One species, *E. poili*, is known from the buffalo and cattle in Asia. They occupy encystments in the aorta, from which the tail end of female projects, while the male is completely covered.

They may cause parasitic aneurisms.

SETARIA.—Various species of this genus occur in the abdominal cavity of the domestic and wild herbivores. They measure about 2 inches to 6 inches long, and are very slender. Their embryos are found in the blood, and are probably conveyed to other animals by means of biting-flies (*Stomoxys*, etc.). The mouth is surrounded by a notched cuticular ring. The posterior end of both sexes is spiralled, closely in the male, loosely in the female.

Their pathogenicity, if any, is unknown.

DRACUNCULUS.—Only one species of this worm is found in the domestic animals, *D. medinensis*, the 'guinea worm'. It is found in India, Africa, and South America. The female is of considerable length, but is generally recovered from the host in small pieces. It is milky white in colour, smooth and without markings. Nearly the whole of the animal is occupied by the uterus, packed with coiled-up embryos. The worm occupies a subcuticular site, as a rule in the extremities, with the head-end projecting to the exterior. The larvæ are released by a prolapse of the uterus through the cuticle of the worm. They escape into the water, are swallowed by a cyclops in which they develop. The cyclops is in due course swallowed in the drinking water by a suitable host—practically any of the domestic animals will do—and larvæ are released by the digestive juices and proceed to their adult habitats. The worm may give rise to local abscesses, but as a rule is of little importance.

Treatment consists in the surgical removal of the worm.

VI. Eye. — THELAZIA. — Various species of this genus are found in the lacrimal gland and its ducts of the horse, cattle, and dog. They may be occasionally found in the conjunctiva or even the eyeball. They are small slender forms, never more than an inch long. There are no lips present, but there is distinct mouth cavity. The male has a curved tail without alæ and with numerous papillæ. The female vulva is near the base of the œsophagus. The worms are responsible for a certain amount of inflammation of the conjunctiva in cattle in tropical countries. The use of a weak antiseptic or of iodoform ointment is as a rule effective. If the worms are actually in the eye, surgical removal may be necessary, but the condition usually cures itself.

PIG. — I. Stomach — ARDUENNA AND PHYSOCEPHALUS.—These are two closely related genera frequently found together in the stomach of the pig. They may be found exceptionally in other hosts, such as donkeys, etc.

Arduenna strongylina is a small bright-red worm, the male being about 1 cm. long, while the female is double this length.

The caudal end of the male is curved in a single turn and supports two lateral alæ. The turn is absent in the female. It is found in Europe and America. A second and larger species occurs in China.

Physocephalus sexalatus is less common. It is more slender, and the tail of the male forms a distinct spiral instead of a single turn. Both genera have complicated mouth cavities with spiral thickenings in them.

The intermediate hosts are various dung-beetles. The worms are deeply fastened in the submucosa. The tissue is ulcerated and necrotic—probably due to secondary infections with *B. necrophorus*. The parasites are blood-suckers, and although little is known about their pathology, they are undoubtedly dangerous.

Symptoms.—The animal refuses food, drinks excessively, is very restless, and in general shows all the symptoms of a severe gastritis, with occasionally a fatal termination. Occasionally outbreaks become epizoötics of a rather serious nature.

Hyostrongylus rubidus is a small red trichostrongyle worm occurring in the stomach of pigs. It is by no means uncommon in Britain, and occurs also in America. When present in large numbers it appears to cause symptoms similar to the above. Its life cycle is direct. (*See also* ' THIN SOW SYNDROME '.)

II. Small Intestine — ASCARIS LUMBRICOIDES.—This worm is a very common parasite of pigs in all countries. It is similar to, but smaller than, the ascarid of the horse, having an average length of 6 to 12 inches. It is probably the most dangerous of all the parasites of the pig.

Life-history.—The adult female produces up to 80 millions of minute eggs, which pass to the ground with the droppings. These eggs have a remarkable vitality, and have been kept alive for as long as five years. The egg, in a few weeks after passing to the ground, develops an embryo, but this does not hatch until the egg is swallowed. When this happens, the larva, which is about $\frac{1}{100}$ inch long, bores through the intestine, reaches the blood-stream, and is carried through the liver and heart to the lungs. Here it remains for some days, but it finally climbs up the trachea and is swallowed. The larva which leaves the lung has grown to about $\frac{1}{10}$ inch in length. In the intestine it continues its development, taking about two and a half months to do so.

Symptoms.—In passing through the lungs a certain amount of bleeding is caused, and if the larvæ are numerous, pneumonia results. During this period the animal shows the symptoms known as ' thumps '. If it survives the lung symptoms, it often fails to grow properly and remains small and stunted—a piner. Carefully controlled experiments showed that ascarid-infested pigs, housed and fed under identical conditions with ascarid-free pigs of the same size, grew to less than half the weight of these animals. Ascarids are accordingly a very serious source of loss to breeders. The greatest damage is caused to young pigs, and if these can be protected during the first four to six months of their lives, losses can be considerably reduced. Clean farrowing-pens should be used, and it is inadvisable to allow access to the outdoor pens usually connected to these. Sows should be cleaned—the udder having special attention—and admitted to the pens a few days before farrowing. In one to two weeks after farrowing, the sow and the young pigs (in separate sides of a double crate) should be removed to a pasture which has not been previously used for pigs. No other pigs should be allowed access to this field, and the sows and their litters should not be allowed to leave it until the young pigs are about four months old (about 100 lb. weight). If the litters are of widely different ages it may be advisable to partition the field. Temporary shelters may be erected if necessary. It cannot be too strongly stated that permanent pig-yards are highly dangerous for young stock. Apart from the special treatment for the young pigs, cleanliness and the free use of disinfectants in the yards are to be recommended. Although less dangerous to adults than to young stock, ascarids are capable of causing considerable unthriftiness, restlessness, and emaciation.

Treatment for ' thumps ' is almost useless; but prevention on the above lines will reduce the need for treatment. The use of anthelmintics in dry powder form, given in dry mash, water being withheld for 3 or 4 hours afterwards, is now very common and generally quite successful. Since the sows are often the source of the worms in the younger pigs, a good plan is to dose the sows about half-way through pregnancy with the sodium fluoride and take strict precautions to disinfect the pens so as to kill eggs already passed to the outside. Thiabendazole is effective.

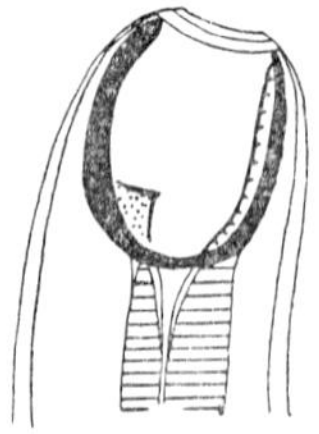

Globocephalus (head).

'Hookworms.'—Several species of hookworms occur in pigs: *Necator suillus*, a species closely related to the New World hookworm of man, and several species of the genus *Globocephalus* (Fig. 204). The latter genus can be identified by its smaller size—about ½ inch, and by the absence of cutting-plates at the mouth opening. The diseases caused by these parasites in pigs are not well known. The symptoms are those of anæmia and emaciation.

D. ACANTHOCEPHALA. — These are round worms without any alimentary canal. The anterior end is provided with a protractile appendage armed with hooks. Various species are known, but only one is of importance.

Macrocantorhynchus hirudinaceus is found in the small intestine of pigs. It is a whitish worm, the male being 5 to 10 cm. long, while the female is 20 to 35 cm. long. The neck is thin and the posterior region stout. The intermediate stages are found in *Melolontha vulgaris* (Europe) and *Lachnosterna arcuata* (America), two species of coleoptera. Infection is by eating an infected insect.

The parasite may cause a catarrhal enteritis or even actual perforation with peritonitis.

Trichuris suis, the pig whipworm, causes mainly subclinical disease in

PARASITES AND PARASITOLOGY

temperate climates, but in the tropics it may cause dysentery, anæmia, and even death. In the Americas up to 85 per cent of pigs may be infested; in some areas of the U.K., 75 per cent.

Experimentally, man has been infested with these worms which are indistinguishable from the human parasitic whipworm *Trichuris trichuira*, which infests millions of people.

Treatment in the pig can be undertaken with 'Shell Atgard' resin pellets containing dichlorvos.

III. Lungs.—In pigs two species are common, both belonging to the genus *Metastrongylus*. They are about the same size, 2 cm. in the male and 4 cm. in the female. Both species are common in Europe and America, and may occur in the same pig. They cause a verminous bronchitis and sometimes pneumonia. Young animals are more susceptible and may die from it. Both species are carried by manure-loving earthworms.

Treatment consists mainly in nursing and feeding. (*See also under* HUSK, treatment and prevention.)

IV. Muscles — TRICHINELLA SPIRALIS.— This is a small worm found in the intestine. The mouth is unarmed. The female produces living larvæ (0·1 to 0·16 mm. long) which migrate through the mucosa, reach the blood-stream, and are carried to various muscles. Here they pass into a cystic stage (the cyst being formed by the host), in which they remain until they are swallowed by some flesh-eating host or until they calcify and degenerate. In the intestine of the new host they reach sexual maturity and produce a new lot of larvæ, which in turn migrate to the muscles.

The normal hosts are carnivores (dogs and cats). Rodents may be infected, and rats can be a source of infection to pigs. Man may be infected from the pig. (*See under* TRICHINOSIS.)

Symptoms.—Depression, loss of appetite, persistent diarrhœa accompanied by colic. If the infection is serious the patient may die in several weeks from an entero-peritonitis. If not, the larvæ encapsulate, and may cause a transient stiffness with difficulty in swallowing.

Treatment is useless. Destruction is indicated.

Prevention is most important, and may be secured by rendering the sties rat-proof. A thorough system of meat inspection is essential in all infested countries.

PARASITES AND PARASITOLOGY

V. **Kidney.**—*Stephanurus dentatus* is a thickish worm of fair size, the male being nearly 3 cm. long and the female a little larger. It is found as a rule in the kidney fat of pigs, but also occurs in the liver and other locations in these animals and in ruminants. It is found in America and Australia, and is responsible for considerable damage. Its life-cycle is

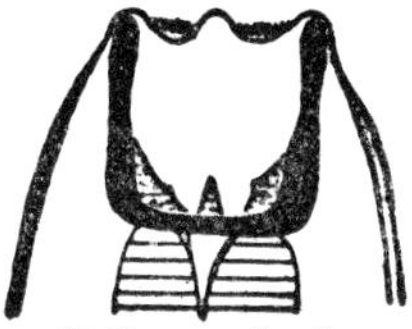

Stephanurus (head).

similar to that of the hookworms. Thiabendazole has proved effective in controlling this parasite.

DOG AND CAT.—I. Stomach.—SPIROCERCA.—*Spirocerca sanguinolenta* is found in tumours in the œsophagus and, less frequently, the stomach of the dog, in all hot countries and in Southern Europe.

It is a reddish worm. The male is 3 to 5 cm. long, with two unequal spicules in the spiral tail. The female is about twice this size. The intermediate hosts are various beetles and cockroaches. Seldom are more than six tumours present in one host, but they may reach the size of a pigeon's egg.

The disease is often undiagnosed during life, but in countries where it is common, the presence of the worm may be suspected from a frequent cough followed by repeated vomiting. They may result in death from exhaustion.

Treatment is useless.

Ollulanus tricuspis is a minute bursate nematode found on the gastric mucosa of cats in Europe. It is under 1 mm. long, and can only be seen on microscopical examination of scrapings from the stomach. It is the cause of a parasitic gastritis.

II. Small Intestine — Ascarids in Dogs and Cats.—Several species of ascarids occur in dogs and cats. They are largish worms, which when full grown are several inches long. The life-cycle is similar to that of *Ascaris lumbricoides* of the pig. They may be found in very young animals—in fact, pups are often infected prenatally. Over 2000 worms have been recovered from a single dog. They appear to be most dangerous about the third month of a pup's life.

Symptoms.—They cause emaciation, irregular appetite, colic, vomiting, and very frequently epileptiform fits. Owing to their peculiar life-history a larger infection may cause a serious pneumonia. They may penetrate the intestinal wall, and so cause a fatal peritonitis. They should be regarded as very serious and dangerous parasites, and some at least can be transmitted to children. (*See* TOXOCARA.)

Pathology.—Ascarids cause a hæmorrhagic enteritis, more or less severe. They in addition secrete a special toxin which is not yet fully understood.

Treatment.—Santonin is fairly effective. It is best given in several small doses after a 12-hours' fast. Oil of chenopodium may be used (1 c.c. for an average dog of about 20 lb.), and has given excellent results. It should be given just before or just after a dose of castor oil (1 ounce). Pure carbon tetrachloride has recently been introduced as a very effective drug. It has a larger margin of safety than chenopodium. All these drugs are dangerous, unless given under proper supervision. Dogs should not be dosed for worms while they have distemper.

In cats the symptoms are similar, but nervous symptoms are less common. Treatment is more uncertain in these animals.

'Hookworms in Dogs.'—Two species of hookworm are found in dogs: *Ancylostoma caninum* and *Dochmoides* (*Uncinaria*) *stenocephala*. The latter only is found in Britain. These are smallish worms, about ¾ inch long, found in the small intestine. The posterior end of the female is pointed, while that of the male has a bursa.

Life-history.—Eggs are passed to the exterior in the droppings and hatch in the soil or water. After several moults, the resulting larva becomes infective. This larva is able to gain access to the host either in the food or by penetrating the unbroken skin. It enters the bloodstream and is carried to the lungs. It then passes up the trachea and is swallowed. It completes its development in the small intestine, where it becomes mature.

Symptoms.—These parasites are specially common in hunting-dogs. The symptoms are those of emaciation, anæmia, and debility. There are generally digestive disturbances, with irregularity of the bowels. The animals look thoroughly poorly, with a staring coat, dull eyes, foul breath, and a general depression. Diagnosis may be confirmed by the dis-

PARASITES AND PARASITOLOGY

covery of the microscopic eggs in the droppings. (*See also under* HOOKWORMS.)

Prevention is of the utmost importance. The larvæ may reach the intestine either through the mouth or by burrowing through the skin. The kennels must be kept dry and clean, and sanitation must be strict. Isolation of all infected cases and quarantining of contacts. Diagnosis may be easily effected by demonstration of the ova in the fæces. Fortunately an excellent remedy has been found in carbon tetrachloride—a drug, however, which is unsafe in inexperienced hands.

In cats the species seem to be *A. tubæforme* and *A. braziliense*; but these have not been fully studied.

III. The whipworm *Trichuris vulpis* lives in the cæcum, occurs in the U.K., and gives rise to diarrhœa/dysentery, loss of condition and a harsh, staring coat.

IV. **Heart** — DIROFILARIA.—This genus is characterised by the large and conspicuous papillæ in the male tail. There are two species occurring in dogs and cats. *D. immitis* occurs in the heart of the dog and occasionally the cat. The female may reach a length of 30 cm., but the male is little more than half this size. It is found in Asia and, of recent years, in Britain. The embryos are hatched in the body of the female, and the young larvæ, passed into the blood-stream, are sucked up by a mosquito in which they develop. After a certain period they escape from the fly, when it attacks another dog, and entering the blood are carried to the heart, where they complete their development.

The worms interfere to a greater or less extent with the circulation. No symptoms may be shown; or the dog may suddenly die. Other symptoms include respiratory troubles, ascites, and so on. Various complications may be due to emboli, such as cough, dyspnœa, etc. Diagnosis is by demonstration of the microfilaria in the blood. **Treatment** is of no avail.

D. repens is an allied species found in the subcutaneous connective tissue of the dog. It also is transmitted by a mosquito, but appears to be more or less harmless.

V. **Kidney**—(*Dioctophyme renale*) *Eustrongylus renalis*.—The kidney worm of dogs and wild carnivores is a very large worm, reaching 1 metre in length, with a thickness of 1 cm. It is a blood-red colour. The male has a single spicule with a bursal collar surrounding it. The female has an obtuse tail, a single ovary, and the vulva near the mouth. It is generally placed in a super-family by itself. It is found in Europe and U.S.A. It occurs in the pelvis of the kidney, and gradually destroys the kidney substance, to leave only the wall as a cyst filled with a purulent fluid. The other kidney usually shows a compensatory hypertrophy. It is occasionally found in the bladder. Infestation follows the eating of raw fish.

Symptoms are indistinct, and if present, point to a unilateral nephritis. The worm's eggs are barrel-shaped and may be seen in the urine, under the microscope.

Treatment, even if diagnosed, is futile.

VI. BLADDER.—In the U.K. the bladder worm *Capillaria plica* is rare, and seldom gives rise to obvious symptoms. A severe infestation can lead to inflammation of the bladder and a mucoid discharge from vagina or prepuce.

VII. TRACHEA.—*Oslerus* (*Filaroides*) *osleri* occurs in the U.K. and gives rise to a sporadic but persistent cough, especially on exercise or if the dog is excited. Retching may be caused. Severe infestation can give rise to emaciation despite a fair appetite, laboured breathing, sleeping standing, and death in young dogs.

Another tracheal worm *Capillaria aerophilia* seldom gives rise to obvious symptoms.

VIII. **Lungs.**—A minute worm lives in the lungs of cats in Britain and elsewhere in Europe and America. It may cause a fatal form of parasitic pneumonia. The parasite (*Aelurostrongylus abstrusus*) is transmitted to cats by mice. In Africa, *Bronchostrongylus subcrenatus* is found.

POULTRY. — I. Intestine. — *Heterakis gallinæ* is a small worm, measuring up to ½ inch long, found in the cæca of poultry. In the small intestine of fowls occurs a larger worm, 1½ to 4 inches long, called *Ascaridia galli*. These worms cause symptoms of dullness, diarrhœa, anæmia, emaciation, and death from a subacute enteritis.

Treatment consists in the administration of carbon tetrachloride, phenothiazine, or 1 to 2 grains of calomel in bread to infected birds. The life-history is direct.

II. Lungs. — *Syngamus trachea*, the gape-worms of chickens, is somewhat related to the last species. The male and female are usually found in copula (Fig. 207), giving the worms a 'Y' appearance. They occur in the trachea of various birds, especially chickens. The female may be 2 cm. long, but is usually smaller. The eggs are coughed up and swallowed. On

PARASITES AND PARASITOLOGY

reaching the exterior they become infective in about 7 days. The eggs containing the infective larva or the larva itself is swallowed, and the young worm, reaching the trachea through the liver and lungs, rapidly develops. Eggs may be deposited within a fortnight after infection.

Symptoms are noticed only in young birds, and are those of choking, with a characteristic yawn and a shaking of the head. Death frequently results from asphyxia or exhaustion.

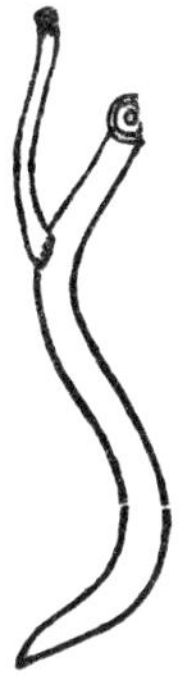

Syngamus. ♂ and ♀.

Treatment.—Thiabendazole, given in the feed, is an effective method of treatment.

Prevention consists in isolation, disinfection, and destruction of carcases. (*See also under* GAPES.)

E. HIRUDINEA. — he leeches are closely related to the earthworms. Like them they are segmented. Their extremities are provided with strong muscular suckers, the anterior one surrounding the mouth, which contains three or more saw-like teeth used to pierce the skin of the host. Certain salivary glands are present which secrete a substance used to prevent coagulation of the blood.

The important leeches are as follows :

Hirudo medicinalis is the well-known medicinal leech, a large form of various colours, measuring up to 12 cm. long. This species lives on the blood of any vertebrate.

H. troctina is also used medicinally.

Limnatis nilotica is found in North Africa and Southern Europe. It reaches a length of 10 cm. The ventral surface is dark ; but on the dorsal surface are six longitudinal stripes on a brownish-green background. It cannot penetrate skin, but on being taken in with water by men and animals, it attaches itself to the buccal mucous membrane. They produce constant small hæmorrhages, which sometimes cause a serious anæmia.

Treatment consists in the removal of the leech by surgical means or by the use of cocaine.

Hæmadipsa zeylanica occurs in Asia and lives on land. It is a clear brown colour with a yellow lateral stripe on each side and a greenish dorsal stripe. It has five pairs of eyes and three teeth. It lives in damp weather on the lower vegetation. They are small forms, about an inch long, but are very serious pests. The bite is painless but, as they occur in such enormous numbers, very deadly. They attack all vertebrates, and many different species of mammals have been killed by them through sheer loss of blood. Some parts of Asia have been cleared of mammals by this leech.

The following species have a proboscis instead of jaws :

Hæmenteria officinalis is the medicinal leech of South America.

Placobdella catenigera, occurring in the Mediterranean region, also attacks man and the domestic animals.

Parasitic worm control.—The ideal of ' worm-free ' animals is not likely to be achieved under modern conditions where the tendency is to more and more intensive production, concentration of grazing, and restriction of acreages for pasturage. Recognition of the general principle that the adult animal is the carrier and the young growing animal is the most susceptible to injury and disease from parasitic worms, enables general measures to be planned. Young animals of any species should *never follow* adults on a pasture ; they should always precede them or be kept separate as soon as weaned.

Dosing the animal may do good by eradicating adult worms, but it does not control the larval migrating forms, nor does it prevent the dosed animal from becoming re-infested in future.

Pasture treatment to kill worm-forms outside the body (eggs and larvæ which have hatched) is not yet practicable, but the ploughing up of old pastures, cropping them with a straw or root crop for 1 or 2 years and then sowing back to grass does eradicate the great majority of the eggs and larvæ, and disturbs or destroys many of the intermediate hosts (mites, slugs, snails, beetles, and other denizens of the soil surface).

Many modern drugs are much more effective and certain in their toxic actions on worms but all require to be used with care and it is strongly urged that veterinary advice should be sought. Further, no one drug is equally effective against all species of worms, and some drugs are useless against certain worm species. An endeavour should therefore always be made to determine which actual species of worms are present in a flock, stud, or herd, before therapeutic measures are launched. This can be carried out fairly accurately by having samples of fæces submitted to worm egg count and subsequent culture for species diagnosis.

After dosing is completed a second series of counts is desirable to check upon the efficiency of the dosing.

ENTOMOLOGY. — Entomology in the modern sense may be taken to mean the study of the PHYLUM ARTHROPODA, that division of the animal kingdom which includes the segmented animals, with jointed appendages and firm exo-skeletons.

The phylum is divided into five classes :

1. PROTOTRACHEATA, which includes only one very archaic genus, *Peripatus*.
2. MYRIAPODA, the centipedes and millipedes.
3. CRUSTACEA, which includes the crabs, shrimps, and so on. One genus, *Cyclops*, is of importance to the veterinarian.
4. INSECTA, a very large class, distinguished by the possession of six legs in the adult stage.
5. ARACHNIDA, members of which in the adult stage have eight legs. This class includes the spiders, ticks, and mange-mites.

INSECTA—GENERAL ANATOMY OF INSECTS.—The insects may be readily distinguished from all other arthropods by the division of the body into three distinct regions—head, thorax, and abdomen ; by the presence of three pairs of legs rising from the thorax, and of one pair of antennæ on the head.

The Head contains the sensory and feeding organs. The sensory organs consist of one pair of compound eyes, sometimes one or more simple eyes (ocelli), and the jointed antennæ. The mouth organs consist of :

(1) A median upper lip (*labrum*), which in blood-sucking forms is prolonged into a long style (*epipharynx*) ;

(2) A pair of upper jaws (*mandibles*) ;

(3) A pair of lower jaws (*maxillæ*), to which are attached a pair of *maxillary palps* ;

(4) A median lower lip (*labium* or *proboscis*), which is really a second pair of maxillæ fused together, and to which may be attached a pair of *labial palps*. The terminal portion of the labium often shows its double nature by being split into two small processes (*labella*) which are sometimes regarded as modified palps.

(5) A process from the mouth on which the salivary glands open. In the true flies this projects to form the single *hypopharynx*.

The Thorax consists of three segments, pro-, meso-, and meta-thorax, to each of which is attached a pair of legs. Typically, two pairs of wings are attached to the two latter segments, but in the Diptera or true flies the second pair of wings has been altered to form dumb-bell-shaped balancing organs called halteres. In some insects (fleas and lice) the wings are absent. The wings of insects are supported by ' veins ', the disposition of which is of importance in classification. Hairs and scales of various kinds may also be present.

The Abdomen is the segmented hind part of the body containing the digestive organs, and is usually without appendages other than hairs. The hind segments in the female are often modified to form an egg-laying organ or ovipositor.

Insects breathe by means of tracheæ, tubes supported by a spiral chitinous framework, which ramify through the body and open to the exterior through spiracles. The digestive system consists of a pharynx, œsophagus, stomach, intestine, and rectum. Reservoirs are present frequently, running from the œsophagus, and salivary glands open into the hypopharynx. Malphigian tubules, having an excretory function, are found at the posterior end of the intestine.

Reproduction.—The sexes are separate, and the female either lays eggs or the young are born as living larvæ. From the egg hatches a larva, which after several moults become more or less quiescent. This stage may be enclosed in a thin pellicle (mosquito) and be fairly active, when it is known as a pupa ; or, it may be, secrete a hard dark skin (butterfly) known as a chrysalis ; or spin a cocoon (flea) ; or remain in its hardened last larva skin (house-fly), called a puparium. In a few cases (lice) the young are like adults ; the larval stage is not evident. From this stage the mature insect (imago) emerges fully grown, and no further growth takes place. All growth in insects takes place in the larval stages.

ORDER DIPTERA—SIMULIUM.—The flies

of this genus are small thick-set hump-back flies—hence their name of buffalo-gnats. They are often black or reddish-brown in colour. The antennæ consist of ten or eleven segments without hair-whorls. The female mouth parts are short and stout, and are formed for cutting and stabbing. The females at certain times appear in swarms and attack cattle, horses, and other animals with fatal results.

The eggs are laid in water. The larvæ, which are aquatic and creep about like leeches, can only live in running well-aerated water. In still water they are asphyxiated. The larva when mature spins a silky cocoon which is attached to water weeds. In this the pupa lies loosely, breathing by means of extruded gill-tufts. The larval stage lasts for 3 to 4 weeks and the pupal stage for 1 to 3 weeks ; but the larvæ can live over winter and do not pupate until the following spring or summer. The fly is very active in Central

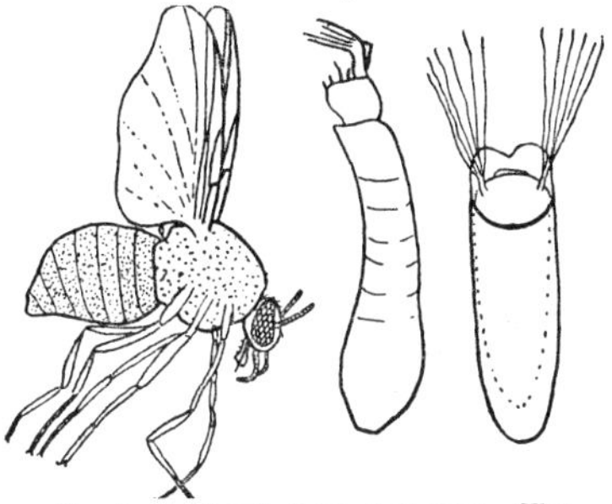

Simulium. Adult, larva, and pupa. The adult fly is magnified × about 10.

Europe, where cattle may die in 2 hours after attack. They show laboured breathing, stumbling gait, rapid pulse, and swellings in pendulous places. In less severe cases loss of appetite, abortion, depression, and temporary or permanent blindness may result.

In marshy areas, constant biting by these flies on the thin skin of the udder and between the thighs, may result in the production of crops of warts, particularly in young heifers feeding on marshlands or fields near streams.

It is unknown whether the fly produces a poison, or whether the symptoms are caused by an organism, or due to continual loss of blood.

Prevention.—As the fly lives in running water, applications of a heavy oil, which sinks, to streams in which the fly is breeding, is indicated. Weedy streams may be cleared, and draining may be useful. Tar repellents may be used for cattle, but require continual renewal. The use of DDT and gammexane products applied as sprays to the skin has given some protection against the fly, but the ideal chemical repellent has not yet been discovered.

Mosquito.—The mosquito, the carrier of malaria and yellow fever to man, is of comparatively little importance in veterinary entomology. It is, however, the carrier of worms of the genus *Dirofilaria* to dogs in Asia and elsewhere

THE TABANIDÆ.—The family of the gadflies is a large and important one, as the females are inveterate blood-suckers. They can be distinguished by the short antennæ of only three segments, the complicated venation of the wings, and the large prominent head, semi-circular in front and straight or even concave behind. The eyes are large, and during life finely coloured. The *female* mouth parts are formed for cutting and stabbing.

The eggs are laid in masses on leaves and plants near water. The larvæ are more or less aquatic, but towards maturity they live in damp earth or decaying vegetation. The larva is cylindrical, pointed at both ends, and with most of the segments carrying pseudo-pods or false feet. The pupa resembles that of a moth. In temperate climates development takes nearly a year. The males feed on plant juices, but the females are blood-suckers, and in addition carriers of various diseases, as for example, trypanosomiasis, swamp fever in horses, and filariasis in man.

The bite is painful, and causes much irritation to horses and cattle, causing runaways, decrease in milk yield, and so on. No remedies are really satisfactory, although nets have been used with some success on horses.

It has been noted that tabanids lower themselves to the surface of the water to drink. If the pools most commonly frequented by these flies are covered with a thick layer of paraffin oil, the flies are killed. If this plan is adopted early in the season the numbers can be kept under control.

Although about 1600 species are known, the majority are exotic, and only four or five genera are of importance.

TABANUS.—This genus has species in all parts of the world, and is familiarly known as the gadfly. The tooth on the antenna is characteristic. It can mechanically transmit surra and other blood

PARASITES AND PARASITOLOGY

diseases such as anthrax. Another species transmits swamp fever in horses.

Tabanus bovinus is the common British species; common American species are

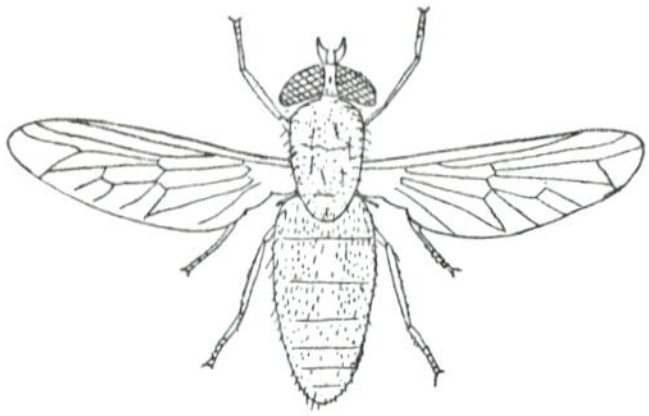

Tabanus. × 2.

T. atratus (the black horse-fly), *T. costalis* (the green head horse-fly), both of which cause much torture to horses and cattle. *T. striatus* (Philippines) has been proved capable of mechanically transmitting surra, but it only remains infective for 20 minutes after biting an infected animal.

HÆMATOPOTA.—This is also a world-wide genus. The species have smoky wings, and include the British clegg or horse-fly which, in addition to being a

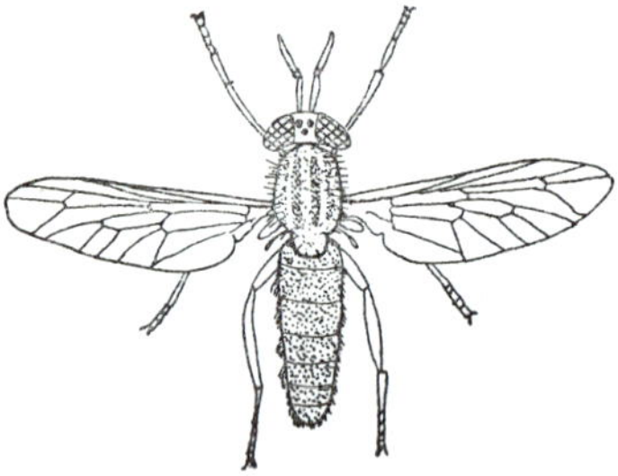

Hæmatopota. × 3.

veritable pest to horses, inflicts a very painful bite to man.

CHRYSOPS is distinguished by its long slender antennæ, and its green or golden eyes spotted with purple. It is found all over the world, including Britain. This genus is the carrier of the parasite of Calabar swelling in man. It also can inflict a very painful bite.

Flies.—The non-biting two-winged flies have an even greater significance to man and his animals than the biting flies. In the adult stages some are among the most important of disease carriers. *Musca domestica*, for example—the common typhoid- or house-fly—is one of man's deadliest enemies. As a carrier of typhoid fever, infantile diarrhœa, and similar diseases it is well known. It can also carry animal parasites, such as hookworm eggs and the larvæ of the stomach worm of the horse. The allied muscid flies are not less culpable. Every farmer knows the damage done to stock by maggots, the

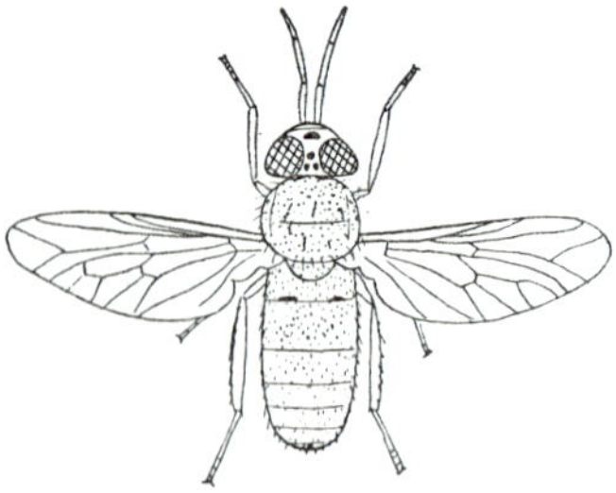

Chrysops. × 2.

larval stages of these flies. The allied family of œstrids also, containing the bot, warble, and nostril flies, causes damage amounting to millions of pounds annually.

To rid the agriculturist of these pests concerted action is necessary. A farmer

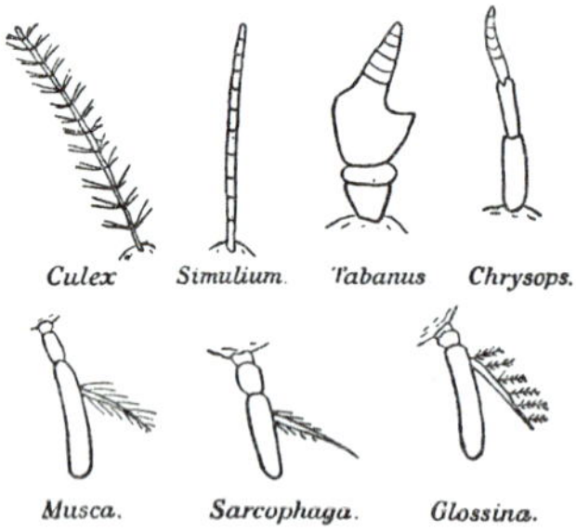

Antennæ of various flies. The small hair seen in the lower row is the 'arista'.

can rid his stock of worms and keep it free; but he cannot eliminate the fly without the co-operation of his neighbours. However, he can reduce the numbers by careful attention to manure disposal, general hygiene, and periodical examination of his stock.

MUSCIDÆ.—The flies belonging to this family are smallish to medium-sized flies. The type of this family is *Musca domestica*. All the members of this and related families have a small hair attached to the trisegmented antenna, called an arista. In this family this is feathered on one or both sides to the tip. In the allied family of flesh-flies it is only partly feathered.

PARASITES AND PARASITOLOGY

MUSCA DOMESTICA.—The great majority of flies found in houses belong to this species. It is a medium-sized fly with four black stripes on its back, and a sharp elbow in the fourth wing vein. The

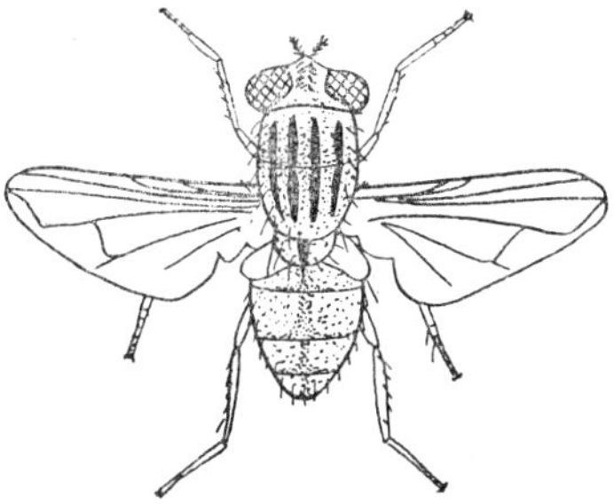

Musca. × 4.

eggs are laid, about 120 in a batch, preferably in horse manure, but occasionally in human or other excreta. They hatch in 24 hours, and the issuing larva (or maggot) feeds and moults and finally becomes full grown in 4 to 5 days. It leaves the manure at this stage, and crawls to a dry spot where it pupates. The puparia are more or less barrel-shaped and dark brown in colour. In 4 or 5 days

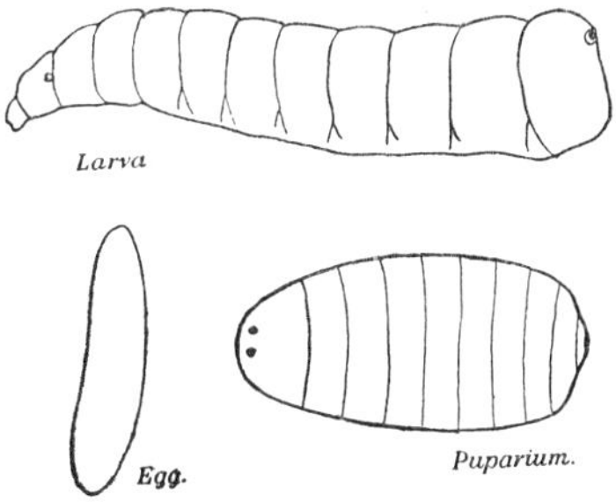

Diagram to illustrate the life-history of *Musca domestica.*

in summer the adult fly emerges. The shortest time on record between the laying of the egg and the appearance of the adult is 8 days; but 10 to 12 days is more normal. In 3 to 4 days the female is ready to lay eggs. The fly lives over the winter in the pupal stage, although in kitchens and warm places adults may be seen at every season of the year. The greatest length of life of a fly is 3 months.

The house-fly can transmit disease by swallowing bacterial spores, and either bringing them up in their vomit or passing them out in their fæces; or by carrying them about on its hairs and legs. Two species of stomach worm are carried by this fly, in which they pass part of their life-cycle. Among other organisms known to be carried by this fly are anthrax, tuberculosis, and many species of worm eggs.

Control.—Control by means of fly-papers, poisons, and traps are merely palliative, and preventive measures must be adopted. As the favourite breeding-place is horse manure, measures must be taken to render breeding in this medium ineffective. An excellent method is that of Hutchison. Manure is piled on a wooden framework on posts about 1 foot high. These posts stand in a concrete basin with 4-inch walls which is kept full of water. The manure is so placed as to cover the platform right to the edges. The fly is attracted to this place and lays its eggs on the manure. The larvæ grow, and on migrating to pupate fall into the water and are drowned. This method is stated to kill 99 per cent of the larvæ. A sump and pump to collect dead maggots and to keep the manure moist are desirable. A platform 10 feet by 20 feet on which manure is piled 5 feet high will hold the manure of twenty horses for 25 days. It has been found that manure 10 days old is unsuitable for the fly to breed in. After the first cost this trap costs nothing, requires little attention other than a weekly flushing, is very effective, and has no deteriorating effect on the manure. Of course a perfect sanitary system would entirely eliminate the fly, and to a certain extent the absence of *Musca* is a criterion of cleanliness. The use of fly-tight manure bins, the addition of chemicals to manure, and so on, are all good, but are useless unless carried out thoroughly. It is little use removing only part of the breeding-places and leaving others. In all cases thorough cleanliness of stables is essential, and concrete floors have much to recommend them.

Myiasis—Of very great importance to the veterinary surgeon and the agriculturist are those non-biting muscid flies which have taken on a parasitic existence in their larval stages.

Myiasis means the presence of dipterous larvæ (or other stages) in organs and tissues of the living animal and the disorders and destruction of tissue caused thereby. (*See* 'STRIKE'.)

The myiasis-producing flies are now usually divided into three groups—specific, semi-specific, and accidental.

Specific: This group consists of flies which *must* breed in living tissue. It includes:

Chrysomyia bezziana,
Cordylobia anthropophaga,
Wohlfahrtia magnifica,
Booponus intonsus, and all the *Œstridæ*.

Semi-specific: This group consists of flies which, normally breeding in carcases, *may* live in the living animal. It includes the blow-flies, the sheep-maggot flies, and some of the flesh-flies.

Accidental: This group includes all flies the larvæ of which, accidentally swallowed with the food, *may* live in the intestine.

The more important of the above flies are considered below.

The '**blow-flies**' — *Calliphorinæ* — are largish muscids of a metallic or yellow colour.

The '**common blow-fly**' or '*blue-bottle*' —*Calliphora* sp.—has reddish palps, black legs, and a bristly thorax. Their general colour is dark blue with lighter patches on the abdomen. The colour, however, is not lustrous. The ova are usually deposited in decaying animal matter, but occasionally in living tissue.

The '**green-bottle fly**' — *Lucilia sericata* —is the British sheep-maggot fly. It is also found in Australia and America.

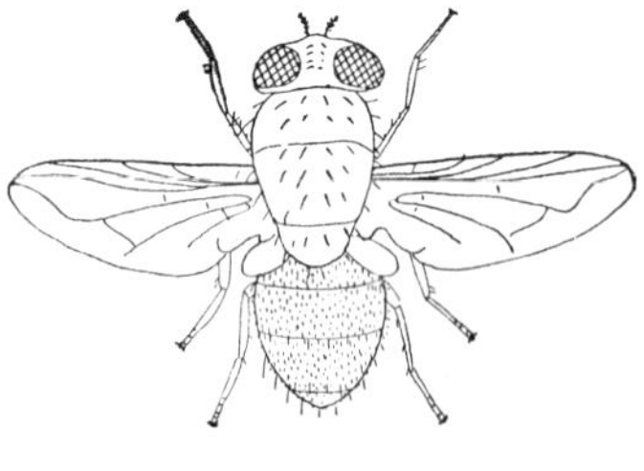

Lucilia. × 2½. This fly is larger than the house-fly and smaller than the blow-fly.

Lucilia cæsar, a common species in Europe, does not 'blow' sheep in this country, but does so in countries such as Russia, where other species are absent. Other species of *Lucilia* in India and Australia occasionally are also implicated.

These are of a bright metallic or bluish-green colour, with many strong bristles on the thorax arranged in two parallel rows. There are no stripes on the thorax or abdomen. The cheeks are not hairy as in *Calliphora*.

This genus blows wool, but occasionally infects wounds.

PARASITES AND PARASITOLOGY

Chrysomyia bezziana, found in India, Africa, and the Philippines, is a metallic greenish-blue blow-fly, closely related to *Lucilia*, but with dark transverse abdominal bands and with fewer and less-developed thoracic bristles. The metallic sheen is more brassy than in *Lucilia*. This fly breeds only in living tissue—in discharges from natural orifices, or in sores and cuts. Up to 500 eggs may be laid at one time. They hatch in about 30 hours, and the larvæ rapidly reach maturity, crawl out and pupate on the ground. Several other species of this genus are semi-specific myiasis flies, normally breeding in decaying matter. These include *C. albiceps*, a notorious sheep-maggot fly in Australia.

The '**screw-worm fly**' — *Callitroga americana*—in America, can be distinguished from the old-world species by the three well-marked blue dorsal stripes on the thorax and dark hairs on the abdomen. It is of a dark bluish-green colour, with a well-marked yellowish-red face. (*See also* FLY CONTROL.)

This species will lay eggs in decaying animal or vegetable matter, but will also oviposit in any diseased tissue, in wounds in the vulvæ of freshly calved cows, the umbilical cord of calves, and so on. The ova hatch in 24 hours, and the maggot matures in 4 to 6 days. The pupal stage on the ground lasts 3 to 10 days. The maggot resembles a blue-bottle maggot, but the deeply cut constrictions between segments and the prominent rings of spines give it its popular name.

As soon as the egg hatches, the larva starts burrowing into the flesh. It can penetrate the sound tissue of living animals, and may even lay bare the bones. Places likely to be attacked may be treated with 1 per cent to 3 per cent carbolic, while 5 per cent carbolic or creolin may be injected into the infected wounds.

Cordylobia anthropophaga is a specific myiasis fly in Africa, attacking many hosts. It is a dirty brownish-yellow blow-fly with blackish markings. There are few hairs on the cheeks, and the abdominal segments in the female are about the same length—a distinguishing point from the closely related Congo floor-maggot of man. The eggs are laid in dust and rubbish on which the host, usually a dog, is accustomed to lie. The small larva may live apart from the host for 10 days, but it must eventually burrow into the epidermis or die. It moults in this position, and forms a tumour below the skin with an opening to the exterior through which it breathes. The tumour does not suppurate unless the larva dies. The larva

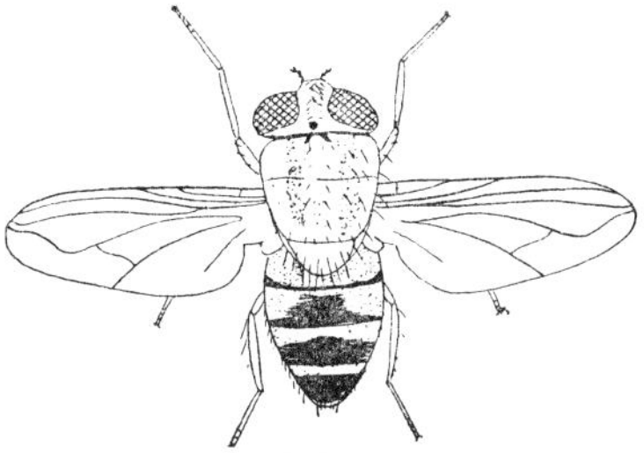

Cordylobia. × 2½.

emerges in about 7 or 8 days, and 2 or 3 days later it pupates. The adults emerge in about 20 days. This fly does not burrow into the deeper tissues. The scrotum is the most common site of the maggot, and it may become gangrenous. Other lesions depend on the site of the larva, *e.g.* blindness, etc.

Booponus intonsus is a light yellow specific myiasis fly found in the Philippines, which is somewhat allied to *Cordylobia*. It differs from that species, however, in having the arista not plumose, and in having many hairs on the face. It infects bovines and goats.

The eggs are laid on the hairs on the lower parts of the legs; and the larvæ make their way to the coronet and bury themselves in the flesh. The larvæ resemble the screw-worm, but differ from it in having the body irregularly covered with spines instead of a few irregular rows at the anterior part of each segment. It has conspicuous anterior spiracles; these are indistinct in the screw-worm. The larval period seems to last 2 or 3 weeks, when it leaves the host and pupates in the ground. The pupal life is 10 days.

The larvæ cause a considerable lameness with numerous superficial wounds and distortion of the horn.

The '**black blow-fly**'—*Phormia regina*—is common in Europe and America, but it is only in the southern United States that it blows wool, especially in winter. The adult is a greenish-black colour with no stripes on the back. It is less hairy than the blue-bottle. The eggs are laid on wool or old wounds, broken horns, and so on, as well as decaying carcases. The

larvæ hatch in 1 to 4 days. The larval stage lasts 3 to 4 days and the pupal stage 7 to 10. The fly reaches maturity in about a week.

The '**flesh-flies**' — *Sarcophidæ* — are closely related to the *Muscidæ*, but may be easily separated from that family by the fact that the distal part of the arista is bare. The body is more elongated than the blow-flies, and they are usually grey in colour, with a mottled abdomen and a striped thorax. They generally bring forth living larvæ instead of laying eggs. Two genera are important.

Sarcophaga spp.—These are large grey flies with red eyes and square chequered markings on the abdomen. The third segment of the antenna is long. All the species normally breed in decaying animal matter, but may be found in old festering wounds. They are found throughout the world.

Wohlfahrtia magnifica resembles the preceding genus, but has well-defined round spots on the abdomen. The third segment of the antenna is short and the arista is without bristles. It is widely distributed in Russia, Asia Minor, and Egypt. The larvæ never attack carcases, but are *always* found in wounds and natural cavities of living animals. The fly deposits living larvæ on sores and discharges.

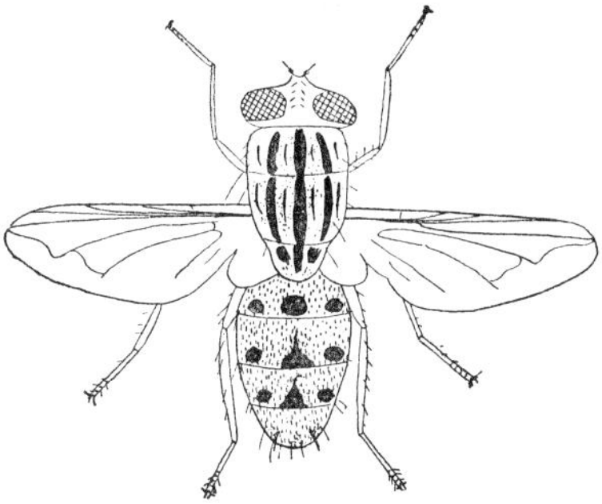

Wohlfahrtia. × 3.

In Australia the most important sheep-maggot flies are *Calliphora augur*, a large orange-coloured fly; *Calliphora stygia*, the common sheep-maggot fly, often called the 'golden-haired blow-fly'; and *Chrysomyia albiceps* var. *putoni*, the larva of which is known as the 'hairy maggot'.

INJURIES DUE TO MAGGOTS. — The injuries due to maggots may be roughly divided into two classes—larvæ attacking wounds and discharges, and larvæ attacking the wool of sheep. The first class of injuries are found on any animal, including man. The flies usually, but not always, select old sores. Some, such as *Chrysomyia americana*, the 'screw-worm', will penetrate into the sound tissue, and prefer fresh wounds or carcases. The infected wound usually has a watery discharge. The best line of treatment is to use chloroform to kill and pine tar to repel.

Prevention is most important and is obvious. (*See also under* MYIASIS.)

Cordylobia penetrates the unbroken skin and requires to be excised. Other genera prefer old foul wounds. The second class of injuries are found in sheep, and may easily develop into the first type. The wool maggots are a very serious pest. The eggs are laid in soiled wool and the larvæ feed close to the skin, which becomes inflamed, and the wool drops off. There is a strong odour, and more flies are attracted. The larvæ ultimately may enter the flesh and the sheep die.

Prevention.—Lambs should be docked to prevent soiling. Sheep should be shorn either before or shortly after lambing. Prevention of diarrhœa and careful supervision are very desirable.

Treatment.—Clip wool from infected parts, beginning outside the infected area and working inwards to prevent distributing the maggots. Apply concentrated dip or chloroform to the spots. Spraying the tail with weak dip gives a fair protection.

All the species treated above are carrion feeders and breeders. They and all their relations, whether already myiasis flies or not, should always be suspect; and numbers can be much reduced by destruction of carcases or by the use of poisoned bait.

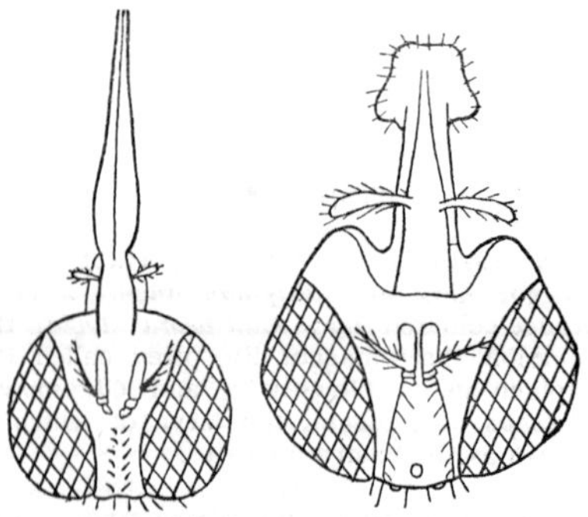

Front view of heads of *Musca* and *Stomoxys.*

PARASITES AND PARASITOLOGY

The Blood-sucking Muscid Flies.—These flies, which resemble the house-fly in general appearance, are responsible for an enormous amount of damage to farm animals. When one considers that they include such flies as the tsetse fly, the stable-fly, and the horn-fly, this is easily understood.

STOMOXYS.—This genus is mainly confined to Africa and Asia, but one species, *S. calcitrans*, the stable-fly, is world-wide in its distribution.

This fly resembles the house-fly, but can be distinguished from it by the possession of a distinct and obvious piercing

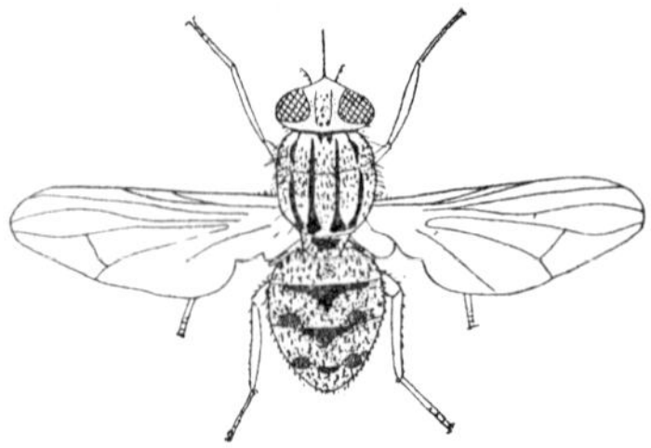

Stomoxys. × 3.

proboscis, by the arrangement of the wing veins, and by the absence of hairs from the dorsal side of the arista.

Stomoxys breeds in stable manure and in other places where moisture and organic material is found. The eggs hatch in 2 to 3 days, and the larva, which is similar to but smaller than *Musca*, becomes full-grown in 2 to 3 weeks. The pupal stage lasts 9 to 13 days. Development is more rapid in the tropics, where the time between egg and adult may be reduced to 12 days.

This fly is a serious pest to horses and other animals. It will also bite man. Apart from the extreme irritation of its bite, it can transmit anthrax, surra, and other diseases. It has recently been shown to be the intermediate host of *Habronema microstomum*, a worm parasite of horses.

HÆMATOBIA.—*H. stimulans* is a common blood-sucking parasite of cattle, and occasionally horses and man, in Europe. It resembles *Stomoxys*, but has spatulate palps as long as the proboscis, and has hairs on both sides of the arista. It breeds in fresh cattle dung. The larva becomes full-grown in 6 to 9 days, while the pupal stage lasts 5 to 8 days.

LYPEROSIA.—*L. irritans* is very closely related to *Hæmatobia*, but can be distinguished from it by the absence of bristles from the under side of the arista. It is found in Europe and America, and is spreading. It is a very serious pest to cattle, clustering round the base of the horns, a habit which gives the fly its popular name of horn-fly. The irritation caused by their bites is estimated to cause a drop in milk yield amounting in some

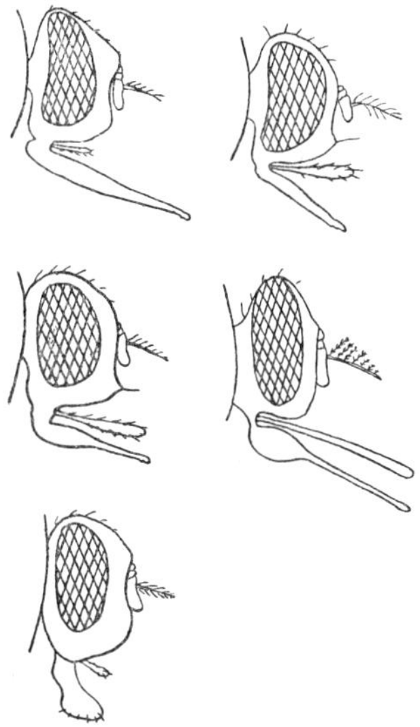

Heads (from side) of various flies resembling the house-fly. (Left to right), *Stomoxys*; *Hæmatobia*; *Lyperosia*; *Glossina*; *Musca*. Magnified.

cases to 50 per cent. The flies breed in fresh cow dung. Flies emerge in about 15 days after the egg is deposited. The maggots must have moisture, and can be destroyed by any means which will dry the manure quickly. The horn-fly seldom goes far from its host, and may be destroyed by attaching splash-boards to ordinary dippers. The fly leaves the cattle at the moment of entering the bath, but the dip, caught and flung back by the splash-board, drenches and destroys the flies. The hotter and more excited the cattle the closer the flies stick and the greater number killed. Any oily dip is suitable.

GLOSSINA.—The flies of this genus, the tsetse flies, are, with one exception (found in Arabia), confined to Africa. They are the notorious carriers of trypanosomiasis in man and animals. *Glossina* resembles a large stable-fly; but has a feathered arista, long slender palps, a slender shaft to the proboscis, and a peculiar wing

PARASITES AND PARASITOLOGY

venation. The life-history is unusual. The female produces one living larva at a time and deposits it when full-grown. It immediately pupates. One female produces only about a dozen larvæ in her life.

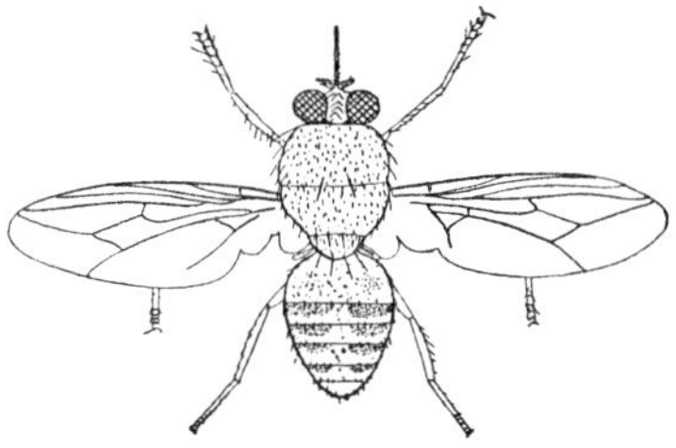

Glossina. × 2½.

Over a dozen species of glossina are known. The most important and the parasites carried are:

G. palpalis.—*T. gambiense*, *T. brucei*, *T. congolense*, *T. uniforme*.

G. morsitans.—*T. brucei*, *T. uniforme*, *T. capræ*, *T. simiæ*.

G. brevipalpis.—*T. congolense*, *T. brucei*, *T. capræ*.

G. longipalpis.—*T. vivax*, *T. congolense*.

G. pallidipes.—*T. brucei*.

G. tachinoides.—*T. vivax*, *T. congolense*.

The Bot and Warble Flies.—*Œstridæ*.—The bot family consists of hairy, heavy flies with rudimentary mouth parts. The female attaches the egg, or, in the case of the nostril flies, places the larva on a suitable host, and the remainder of the larval life is parasitic. When mature the larvæ leave the host and pupate on the ground.

These flies may be placed in three groups according to the habitat of the larva:

(1) In the alimentary canal—
Gastrophilus, the horse bot.
Cobboldia, the elephant bot.

(2) In the head sinuses—
Œstrus, the sheep nostril fly;
Rhinœstrus, the horse nostril fly;
Cephalomyia, the camel nostril fly; and others.

(3) In the subcutaneous tissue—
Hypoderma, the warble-fly;
Dermatobia, the macaw worm fly; and others.

These flies are of enormous economic importance, and the damage done by them must amount to millions of pounds annually.

GASTROPHILUS.—The flies of this genus are large and hairy, with large com-

PARASITES AND PARASITOLOGY

pound eyes and three ocelli. The females have an elongated ovipositor which is bent under the body when at rest. Four species are of importance.

G. intestinalis (*G. equi*), the common horse bot, has cloudy wings; it deposits its eggs on any part of the horse, but especially on the distal ends of the hairs. The eggs require moisture and friction (supplied by licking) before they will hatch.

G. nasalis (*G. veterinus*) is smaller, more hairy, and has a rusty coloured thorax. It oviposits usually at the proximal ends of hairs under the jaw. It lays one egg and flies to a distance, returning later to lay another. Its eggs sometimes hatch without assistance.

G. hæmorrhoidalis has a bright orange-red tip to the abdomen. It deposits its

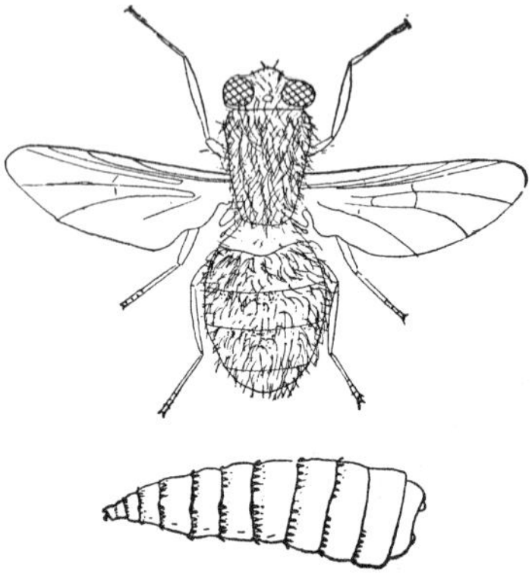

Gastrophilus. (Adult fly × 2½, and 'Bot' × 2.)

eggs only at the base of the small hairs on the lips of the horse. The eggs may hatch without moisture or friction.

G. pecorum resembles *G. intestinalis*. In colour it is yellowish brown to nearly black with brownish clouded wings. Its habits are similar to that species.

The distribution of the first three is universal, but the last seems to be restricted to Europe and South Africa.

The life-history of the species of this genus is not fully understood yet. Some of the newly hatched larvæ *may* pierce the skin or buccal mucous membrane. In any case the larvæ are found in various parts of the alimentary tract. Each species has its own special preference. *G. intestinalis* is usually found in the stomach, occasionally the duodenum; *G. nasalis* prefers the duodenum, but has been found in the pharynx and stomach; *G. hæmorrhoidalis* is found in the stomach, duodenum, rectum, and even in the anus; while *G. pecorum* usually occurs in the pharynx or stomach, but may be recovered from any part.

Bots when present in large numbers in the stomach or intestine, or even in small numbers about the pharynx and anus, may cause a considerable suffering to their host by mere mechanical obstruction. The adult fly worries the horse considerably, especially the species *G. nasalis* and *G. hæmorrhoidalis*, and may cause loss of condition.

Treatment. — Undoubtedly the best means of removing the bots is by means of carbon disulphide, administered in autumn and early winter by stomach tube and followed by warm saline. Some control can be achieved by regular removal of the 'nits' from the lower limbs of grazing horses during summer. Scraping off and burning, sponging with paraffin oil twice weekly, or singeing with a singeing lamp at the same intervals are all useful, more especially in foals and yearlings.

ŒSTRUS.—*Œstrus ovis*, the sheep nostril fly, is somewhat larger than the house-fly and is greyish yellow to brown in colour. It is found practically all over the world. It is still doubtful, however, whether it occasionally lays eggs, or whether it always produces living larvæ. The female hovers over and 'strikes' at the nostrils, and the young larvæ crawl up the nose, and may lodge in one of the sinuses of the skull. It remains there until fully grown, when it is sneezed out and pupates in the ground.

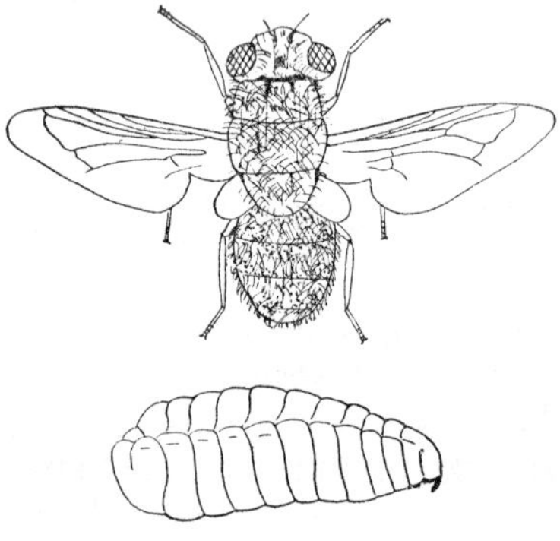

Œstrus. (Fly × 2; maggot × 1.)

The presence of the larvæ give rise to a condition known as 'staggers', 'false gid', 'grub in the head', and so on.

PARASITES AND PARASITOLOGY

There is a nasal discharge while the larva is working its way up. This ceases when the larvæ become stationary, but recommences when they descend. This is usually the only symptom; but the sheep may fall, the jaws and neck become rigid, eyes prominent, and the animal may die. This is uncommon, however. The larvæ may be removed surgically. Prevention is best carried out by means of an application of tar to the nostrils. This may be applied by means of a salt lick, access to which may only be obtained by smallish holes (2 inches) smeared with tar. Ploughing a single furrow across a sheep pasture, allows the sheep to protect their nostrils from the flies 'strike', and gives some measure of protection. Bayer 37342 was (1961) reported as effective against *Œstrus ovis*; a single drench being effective against all larval stages, without signs of poisoning.

RHINŒSTRUS. — *Rhinœstrus purpureus* (*R. nasalis*), the horse nostril fly, is common in Central Europe and North Africa. It is a smallish fly with the body covered with small tubercles, and is closely related to *Œstrus*. The female deposits a number of living larvæ at one time in the eyes or the nose of the horse (and occasionally man). The larvæ may be found about the cranial cavities or even in the pharynx or larynx. Russian Gadfly is a synonym.

HYPODERMA.—Two species of warble-flies, *Hypoderma bovis* and *H. lineatum*, are found in cattle (and occasionally in the horse). Both are very extensively found in Europe and America, and between them cause losses of many millions of pounds.

Hypoderma bovis is a largish fly with yellow hair just behind the head. The under part of the abdomen is nearly black, while the tail end is orange yellow. The legs have few hairs.

Hypoderma lineatum is rather smaller with a reddish-orange tail and rough hairy legs.

H. bovis lays its eggs in the sunshine, generally when the animals are running. One egg is laid on the base of each hair at a time and attached by means of a groove. The fly has a most terrifying effect on cattle, and causes them to gallop madly in all directions. *H. lineatum* irritates animals less than does *H. bovis*. The ova are generally deposited while the animal is lying in the shade. A number of eggs—up to fourteen—are laid on the same hair, and are often in full view.

In both cases larvæ emerge in several days and pierce the skin. They travel up through the connective tissue in some unknown manner and finally reach the back. Under the skin the larvæ form a small swelling (about the middle of winter), which moves about at first, but gradually becomes still and enlarges. A small opening appears in the centre through which the larva breathes. In spring the larva

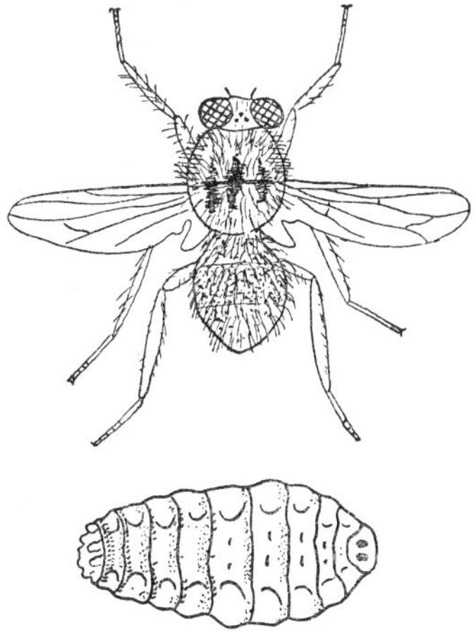

Hypoderma. (Fly × 2; and 'Warble' × 1½.)

falls to the ground and pupates. Several weeks later the adult fly emerges.

The presence of the larvæ may decrease the milk yield by 10 per cent to 20 per cent, cause a considerable depreciation in flesh near the points where the larvæ are, and enormously reduce the value of the hide. The adult fly also causes loss through the mad chasing about of cattle.

Treatment.—The grubs should be removed from the warble and destroyed. The larva should not be crushed in the warble as it contains a toxin which may cause the death of the animal if released in the body. By compulsory removal of all warble larvæ, the fly could be eliminated from the country. A special instrument for sucking out the larva is used in Denmark. A derris and soap dressing applied to the back has been found to be effective. In Britain, it is compulsory to dress the backs of cattle affected with warbles twice during early spring before they are mature. The dressing consists of 1½ ounces of derris resins (or ½ ounce of rotenone), 4 ounces of soap or soap powder, to each gallon of water. It is applied with a rough cloth or a brush. (*See also under* WARBLES.)

PARASITES AND PARASITOLOGY

DERMATOBIA.—*Dermatobia hominis*, the macaw worm-fly, is a parasite of cattle and other domesticated animals (and occasionally man) in tropical America. It is a medium-sized fly, grey or steel-blue in colour, with pale brown wings. The female lays its eggs on the body of some blood-sucking arthropod, usually a mosquito. This carrier attacks an animal 5 or 6 days later, and the larvæ, rapidly escaping from their shells, pierce the skin of the host, and form a local tumour near where they were deposited. In a month or so they emerge and pupate.

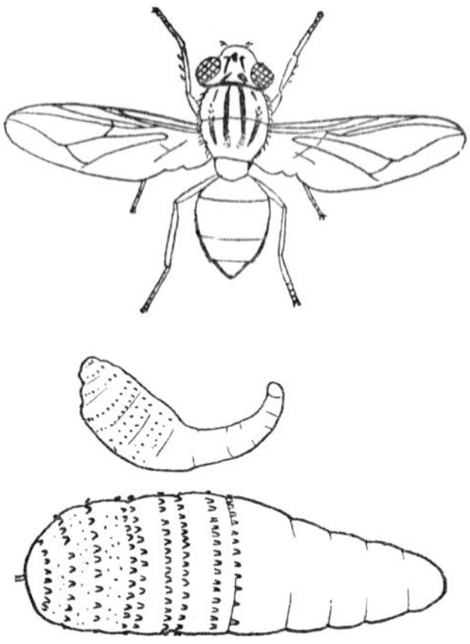

Dermatobia. (Fly and maggots × 1½.)

PUPIPARA.—This family, which includes the sheep ked and the New Forest fly, was so called because live larvæ are produced which pupate at once. The adults in this case are blood-sucking parasites with a hard integument with a broad neckless head and very stout legs ending in grasping claws. Wings are present or absent. The family is very completely adapted for a parasitic life. Two genera are important.

Hippobosca equina, the New Forest fly or horse ked, has wings which, however, are seldom used, the fly preferring to run swiftly between the hairs of the host. It is a typical member of the group.

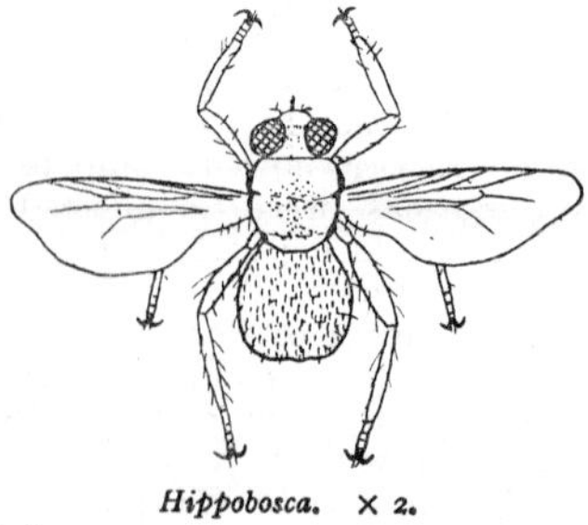

Hippobosca. × 2.

Melophagus ovinus, the sheep ked, is wingless, and lives on the wool and skin of the sheep. It is much larger than any of the lice, being a quarter of an inch long. It can easily be distinguished from the ticks by its tripartite body. It is a dark brown colour with a sharp biting proboscis. The nearly mature larvæ are laid on the wool and they at once pupate. The pupa may remain in the wool or fall to the ground. The young hatch in 19 to 24 days, and the females start to deposit larvæ in 12 to 23 days after emergence, and lay a larva every 9 days. The fly can live for about 12 days away from the sheep ; while the pupa can live for 6 weeks on the ground. The whole life-cycle may be completed on the sheep within 1 month.

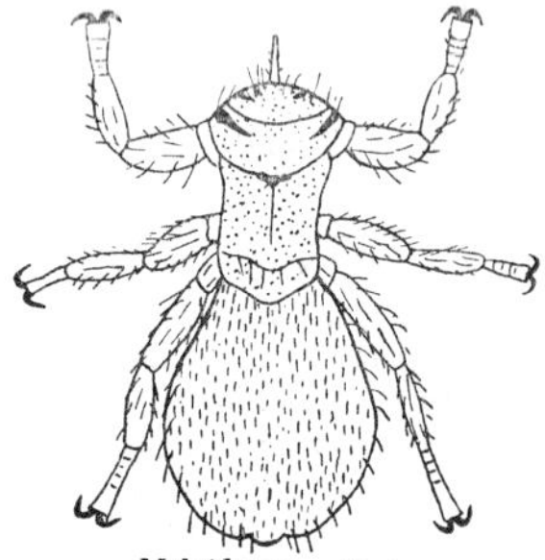

Melophagus. × 4.

Symptoms.—The ked is a blood-sucking parasite, and causes great irritation and loss of vitality if present in numbers. It causes loss by soiling the wool with its excreta and by the raggedness of the fleece resulting from the sheep biting and scratching at the pest. The fly is the carrier of a trypanosome which is, however, probably harmless.

Treatment.—Effective treatment is double dipping at an interval of 24 to 28 days, with an arsenic dip, but a single dip in a DDT or gammexane dipping solution, which leaves a residue effective for at least a month serves to kill adults and the newly emerged young keds from pupa cases. Consistent use of DDT dips has resulted in eradicating keds from many flocks.

Prevention.—As the pupa may live on the ground for 6 weeks, ground which has harboured ked-infested sheep should be kept free of sheep for at least that time· Contacts should be dipped, and fresh sheep should not be mixed with infected

PARASITES AND PARASITOLOGY

animals. Disinfection of woodwork, etc., with crude carbolic should be carried out. The ked may attack men while shearing and inflict a very painful bite.

ORDER SIPHONAPTERA. — This order, the fleas, is by some considered as an appendage to the Diptera ; but is now more generally recognised as a separate order.

The fleas are laterally compressed, wingless insects which are purely parasitic, and have mouth parts adapted for piercing and sucking. Both sexes are blood-suckers. Eyes may be absent, but when present are simple. The antennæ rest in pits behind and above the eyes. The female has a rounder abdomen than the male.

The eggs are laid on the floor or bedding. In a few days (2–12 in summer, but longer in winter) active footless larvæ are born. When full grown, the larva spins a cocoon inside of which the pupa lies, ultimately emerging as a typical adult.

Fleas are not of the same importance to the veterinary surgeon as to the medical man, to whom it is known as the carrier of plague.

Pulex irritans is the human flea, but is frequently found on dogs and cats, and occasionally pigs and horses.

Ctenocephalis canis is the dog and cat flea, but is often found on man.

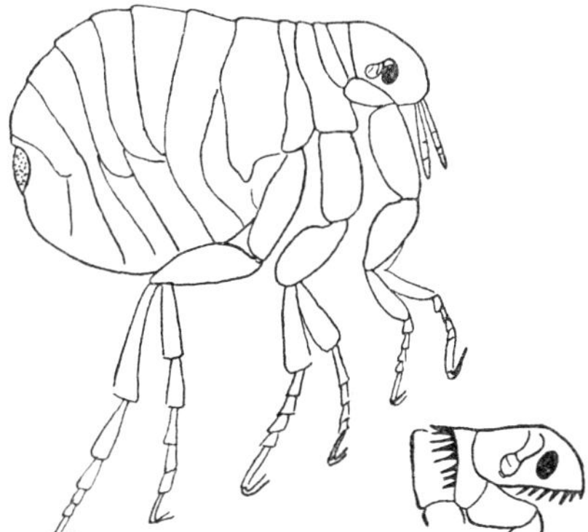

Pulex irritans. × 20.
Inset, head of dog flea.

It can be distinguished from the previous species by the two rows of dark bristles on its head. It can transmit *Dipylidium caninum*, and possibly *Leishmania*, to its host, in addition to being a considerable source of annoyance to dogs and cats.

Echidnophaga gallinacea, the 'sticktight' or chicken flea, is usually found attached in dense masses to the head of a fowl or the ear of a dog or cat. Man, horses, and cattle are occasionally infected. It is a common parasite throughout the Tropics and is frequently the cause of death in poultry. The female flea, after fertilisation, inserts its mouth parts into the cuticle of the host, and remains there. Ulcers may form ; and in any case the flea is difficult to move—a sterile needle with careful antiseptic dressing is indicated.

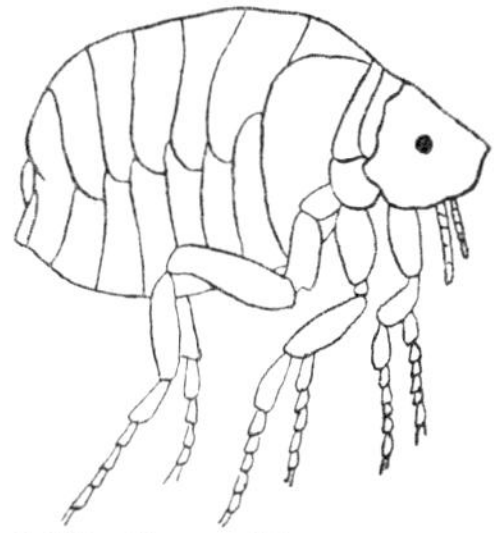

Echidnophaga gallinaceæ. × 30.

Tunga penetrans, the true jigger flea, differs only in slight details from the last species. The female, however, penetrates the skin, and lying in an inflammatory pocket with an opening to the exterior, becomes as large as a pea. It is found in Africa and America in man and all the domestic mammals, especially the pig.

The presence of the flea may, in addition to being very painful, give rise to ulceration and even gangrene.

The eggs are laid in the ulcers ; and the larvæ crawl out and pupate on the ground.

Destruction of Fleas.—Fleas can be destroyed on mammals by applications of gammexane or derris powder or shampoo, or DDT. The latter should *not* be used on cats. In all cases the bedding must be destroyed or disinfected and the surrounding floor boards and cracks cleaned thoroughly or the animal will shortly be reinfested. This is even more important than ridding the host of fleas. The 'sticktight' is best treated with a mixture of paraffin and lard (1 : 3) applied with care, or balsam of Peru, or sulphur ointment. Here again it is important to disinfect the premises. A similar treatment is necessary for the jigger flea.

LICE.—Two distinct families of lice are found on the domestic animals : the sucking lice and the biting lice. All the fowl lice belong to the latter family. The lice are wingless insects which undergo a direct development. The egg is laid on the body, glued to a hair or feather, and the young louse is, except for size, identical with the adult. There is no pupal stage, although several moults take place. The sucking lice belong to the order

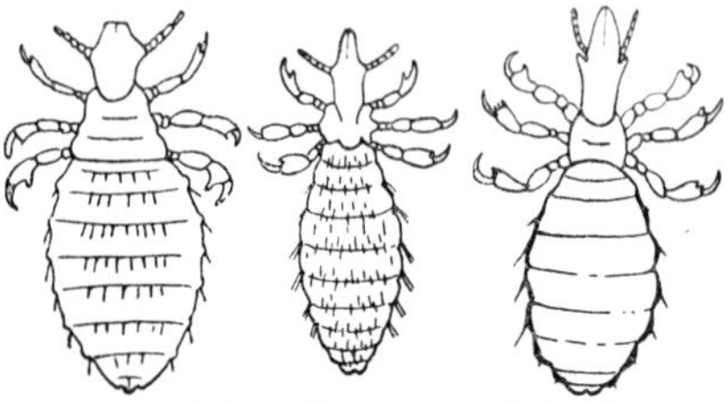

Sucking Lice. × 10. (Left, *Hæmatopinus* ; centre, *Linognathus* ; right, *Solenopotus*.)

SIPHUNCULATA. They are wingless insects, with compressed heads and strong claws. The mouth parts are constructed for sucking and are more or less pointed. Three slender stylets are enclosed in the proboscis. Three genera are found in the domestic mammals, none of them being able to live on man.

The biting lice belongs to the order MALLOPHAGA. The mouth parts are very different from those of the sucking lice.

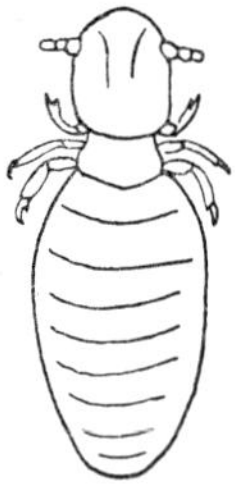

Biting Louse. × 15. (*Trichodectes*.)

They cannot suck blood, and the mouth parts consist of a pair of mandibles on the ventral side of the blunt head. In this order, as in the last, all the mammalian hosts, except the horse, has its own species. The horse has two species. Only one genus is found among the domestic animals, although a second genus occurs in the guinea-pig. The other genera are all bird forms.

Horse.—Only one species of sucking louse is found on the horse, called *Hæmatopinus asini*. Two species of closely related biting lice are also found : *Trichodectes equi* and *T. pilosus*. In *T. equi* the head is slightly longer than broad and the antennæ are set well back. In *T. pilosus* the head is broader than long and the antennæ are well forward, almost on a line with the anterior border. Sucking lice are more generally found at the base of the mane and tail, while the biting species are commonly on the lower parts of the body. They cause poorness of condition, itching, and loss of hair.

Treatment consists of cleanliness and applications of BHC powders. Two applications are necessary at an interval of about 10 days. Buildings, clothes, brushes, and grooming kit must be cleaned.

Cattle.—Three species of sucking lice occur on domestic cattle. These are *Hæmatopinus eurysternus*, *Solenoptes capillatus*, and *Linognathus vituli*. In addition, one species of biting louse occurs, *Trichodectes scalaris*. The sucking lice are found mainly on the head and shoulders, the biting lice on any part of the body. They cause itchiness and scratching which may produce thickening of the skin, and cause mange to be suspected.

Treatment.—Any dip, repeated at 10-day intervals, will kill the lice. Single dressings of BHC-containing dips or powders if thoroughly applied are also satisfactory. If only a few cattle are affected, the local application of a dip by spraying is recommended.

Sheep.—Two species of sucking lice occur on sheep : *Hæmatopinus ovillus* (on the body) and *Linognathus pedalis* (on the foot) ; and one species of biting louse, *Trichodectes ovis*. All are rather uncommon as a rule ; when they do occur the biting louse does the most damage to the wool by biting it. In addition, all cause irritation and itching. Lice must not be mistaken for the sheep ked, which is a very much larger insect.

T. ovis is common in Australia and New Zealand, where it causes considerable damage.

Treatment is best carried out by means of a dip, repeated in 10 to 14 days.

Goat.—The species of sucking louse *Linognathus stenopsis*, and one species of biting louse, *Trichodectes climax*, attack the goat.

Pig.—Only one louse is found on the pig, *Hæmatopinus suis*, a very large species which causes intense pruritus, which seriously interferes with fattening. Young pigs have been known to die from the loss of blood and the extensive irritation. The lice are usually found near the ears, inside the elbows and on the breast. Next to swine fever this is the pig's worst enemy.

Treatment.—Gammexane or derris or DDT preparations. The treatment should be repeated in 7 to 10 days. The use of 'rubbing posts', on which have been

PARASITES AND PARASITOLOGY

wound sacking soaked in crude oil, was a useful aid in controlling the pest.

Dog and Cat.—Two species of lice occur on the dog: a sucking louse *Linognathus piliferus*, and a biting louse *Trichodectes canis*. The latter is an intermediate host of *Dipylidium caninum*.

Trichodectes subrostratus, which although a biting louse, has rather a pointed head.

Treatment.—Dogs may be treated by the application of a gammexane or derris preparation (*see* FLEAS). Immersion for 10 minutes in a bath of weak derris solution will usually kill both adults and eggs.

All lice measures should be repeated three times at intervals of 8 to 10 days.

Poultry.—All the lice affecting birds are biting lice, six species of which are found in chickens. These belong to two families.

PHILOPTERIDÆ. — Antennæ with five segments, no palps, sluggish forms.

Goniocotes hologaster, 1 mm. long with a square head and angular temples.

Gonicotes abdominalis, 3 mm. long, with a semicircular head. Both these species are common.

Lipeurus variabilis, 2 mm. long, a long, slender, whitish species, with a large rounded head.

Lipeurus heterographis, with a head narrowed in front and a stouter body than the last species. It is not a very common form.

LIOTHEIDÆ.—Antennæ with four segments, palps present, active forms.

Menopon pallidum, 1½ to 2 mm. long and yellow in colour. This is the common hen louse.

Menopon biseratum is somewhat larger but less common. It is found on the head and anus of chickens.

Symptoms.—These lice feed on débris, but cause irritation by moving about. This makes the host restless, and causes weakness and debility.

Control.—Add sulphur and tobacco to the dust bath. Naphthalene or pyrethrum applied direct to the bird are useful. All must be used as very fine powder.

Treatment.—The best treatment is to sprinkle the birds individually with sodium fluoride powder, which may be mixed with flour or fine road dust to dilute it if desired.

ARACHNIDA.—This class differs from the class INSECTA in many important respects. For example, in the adult stage, eight legs are present; the body also is typically divided into two portions, a cephalothorax, corresponding to the head and thorax of the insects, which carries all the appendages, and an abdomen.

The paired appendages are:

(1) The *cheliceræ*, in front of the mouth;

(2) The *pedipalps*, on either side of the mouth; and

(3) to (6) The legs.

The eyes are always simple (if present), and the mouth is a slit. The class is a large one, and contains such diverse animals as all forms of spiders, mites, and ticks. The most important order from the point of view of the parasitologist is the acarina.

ORDER ACARINA. — This order contains the mites and ticks. The cephalothorax and abdomen are fused together. The anterior end of the body forms with the cheliceræ, a beak or *rostrum*. In addition to the cheliceræ there usually is found a rasp-like tongue or *hypostome* formed from a prolongation of the rostrum.

The female lays eggs which hatch and produce larvæ resembling the adults but having only three pairs of legs. The larvæ moult and become *nymphs* with four pairs of legs but sexually immature. After a third moult the adult is formed.

The **Ticks** (super-family IXODOIDEA).—All the species of this family are parasitic and are among the worst enemies of the

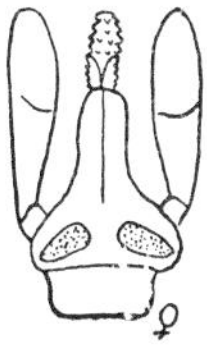

Head of female *Ixodes*.

domestic animals. The body is more or less oval. At the front end is a movable beak (*capitulum*) consisting of a strong flattened ring-like basal piece (*basis capituli*) surmounted by pedipalps, cheliceræ, and other mouth parts. The pedipalps act as a sheath to the more delicate mouth parts. Each chelicera consists of a long shaft with two strong hooks anteriorly, and is covered dorsally by a prolongation of the basis capituli. Ventral to the cheliceræ is the hypostome, a rasp-like prolongation of the basis capituli. It aids the cheliceræ in boring through the skin of its host. The skin of the tick may be hard or soft with localised thickened spots. Both hard and soft parts are formed from a substance known as 'chitin', as is the skin of all members of the arthropoda.

The four pairs of legs are attached to the ventral surface. Each consists of a swollen basal piece or 'coxa' and six segments, the last of which ('tarsus') ends in two claws.

The genital opening is situated near the middle line on the ventral side not far from the capitulum. On the same line, but posteriorly, is the anus. The spiracles open on conspicuous 'stigmata' behind and dorsal to the coxa of the third or fourth pair of legs. The male is smaller than the female, and often differs in other respects.

FAMILY IXODIDÆ. HARD TICKS.— In this family the dorsum of the body is more or less protected by a hard shield of chitin, and in some species the male has ventral plates also. The capitulum is anterior and easily visible from above. The pedipalps are rigid, and divided into four segments, only three of which are visible.

The female has a small scutum which only partly covers the body, whereas the

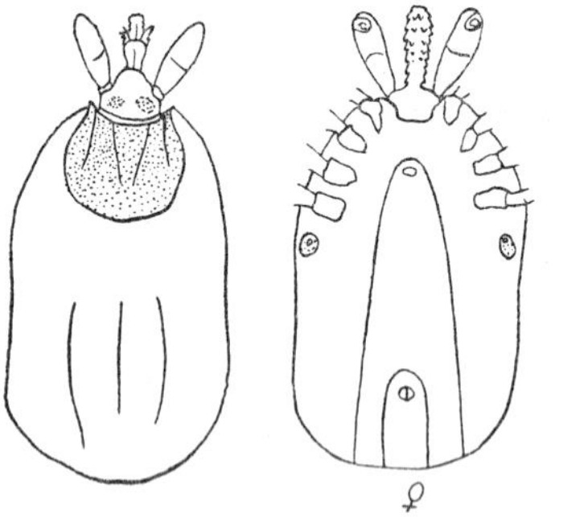

xodes. (Dorsal and ventral views of a small female. × 8.) In this and subsequent drawings of ticks only the fore parts of the legs are shown in diagrams of the ventral surface.

smaller male has the whole dorsum completely covered. The larvæ and nymphs of both sexes resemble the female.

The principal species attacking the domestic animals are dealt with below.

IXODES.—The ticks of this genus all have a conspicuous and groove arching in front of the anus. The rostrum is fairly long. Eyes and festoons are absent. The ventral surface of the male is more or less completely covered with non-salient plates, and the dorsal surface is inornate.

There are over fifty species in this genus, including the following:

(*a*) *Ixodes ricinus* attacks all the domesticated animals and is found in most

PARASITES AND PARASITOLOGY

parts of the world. This species may be recognised by the limbs of the anal groove diverging posteriorly. It is known locally as the 'castor-bean tick', the 'European sheep tick', and so on. It transmits louping-ill of sheep and red-water in cattle and possibly dogs. It is a 'three-host' tick, *i.e.* it leaves its host before

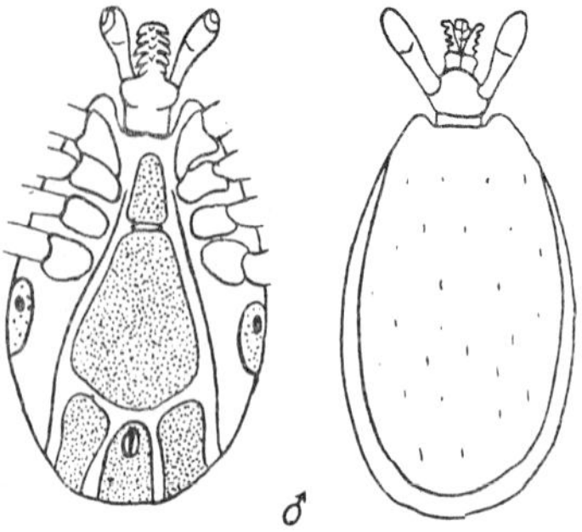

Ixodes. (Ventral and dorsal views of male. × 12.)

each moult, and then seeks a new host. In this way three animals are attacked by the same tick: one as a larva, one as a nymph, and one as an adult. The animals attacked need not be of the same species. This tick transmits 'tick-borne fever' in sheep, louping-ill, and causes 'tick paralysis' in sheep and cattle. It can also transmit *Babesia bovis* the cause of 'red-water'.

(*b*) *Ixodes hexagonus* attacks especially the dog, but is found on other hosts, especially sheep. It occurs in Europe, North Africa, and America; and is common on hunting dogs in France. It has two spines on the first coxa, whereas the first species has only one. In addition to being a transmitter of bovine babesiosis, it is thought to cause a fatal jaundice in dogs and to be a carrier of canine babesiosis.

(*c*) *Ixodes canisuga* is the common species found on the dog in Britain. It occurs also in Western Europe and North America. It has no spines on the first coxa. Like the last species only females are found on the host. It is known popularly as the British dog tick.

(*d*) *Ixodes pilosus* attacks all the domestic mammals in South Africa. It is a reddish-brown tick, with the body larger behind than in front. It is known locally as 'the russet tick', and is a causal agent of 'tick paralysis'.

(*e*) *Ixodes rubicundus*, another South African tick, which is found only on sheep, also cause 'tick paralysis'. It is uncommon, but may be distinguished from the last by the parallel sides to the anal groove.

(*f*) *Ixodes holocyclus*, in Australia and India, is found on ruminants, dogs, and pigs. The anal groove in this species converges posteriorly, and meets in the female. It is the cause of Australian 'tick paralysis', symptoms of which may appear within an hour of attachment.

HÆMAPHYSALIS.—This genus may be recognised by the salient external angle of the second segment of the short conical pedipalps. There are no eyes and no ventral plates present. The dorsum is inornate, although festoons are present on the posterior margins.

The following species are important:

(*a*) *Hæmaphysalis punctata* (*H. cinnabarina* var. *punctata*) is a common tick in Europe, North America, and North Africa on all the domestic animals. In

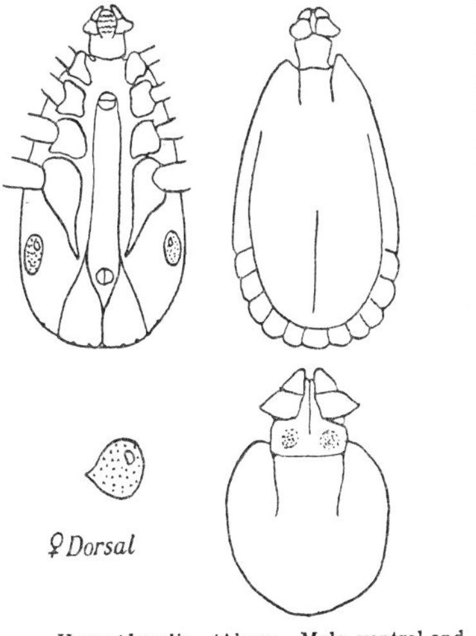

Hæmaphysalis. (Above—Male, ventral and dorsal surfaces. Below—Spiracle and shield of female.)

this species the outer angle of the pedipalps is blunt, although distinctly salient. The life-history is identical with that of *H. leachii*. It transmits *Babesia bovis* in Britain.

(*b*) *H. leachii* is a 3-host African species which has been found in Western Asia and Australia. It attacks carnivores, but is sometimes found on ruminants. In this species the pedipalps are broadly triangular. The external angle is very acute, and has a dorsal and a ventral tooth on its posterior border. In East Africa it is called the yellow dog tick.

PARASITES AND PARASITOLOGY

It is also known as the South African dog tick. The eggs hatch in about a month, and in a week the larvæ attach themselves to a host for 2 to 7 days and then drop off to moult a month later. The nymphs seek a second host, remain attached for 2 to 7 days, and, dropping off, moult in 10 to 15 days. The adults remain on the host for a few days, and the females oviposit in 3 to 7 days, after leaving the host. Winter is passed in the egg stage.

This tick transmits canine babesiosis and Q fever. The female sucks infected blood. The infection passes to the egg, *through* the larva and nymph to the adult, which alone is infective.

DERMACENTOR.—In this genus the body is elongate, and the rostrum short with coarse pedipalps. Eyes and festoons are present. The fourth coxa is very large and the first is bifid. There are no adanal plates although the anal groove is marked. The dorsum is usually ornate.

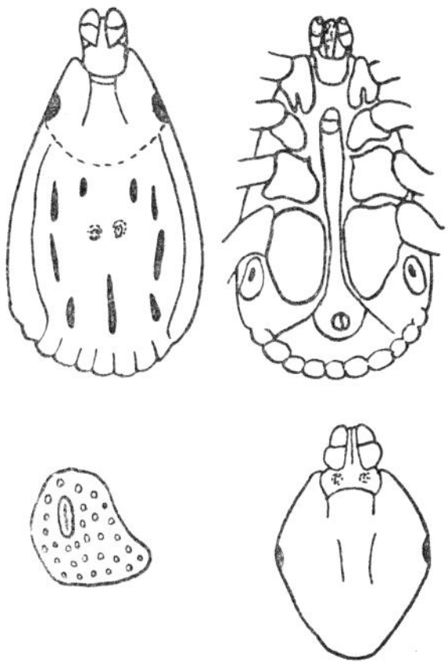

Dermacentor. (Above—Male, dorsal and ventral surfaces. × 5. Below—Spiracle and shield of female.)

The following species are important:

(*a*) *D. reticulatus* is common in Europe, but also occurs in North Asia. It attacks ruminants, and also the dog and the horse. It is occasionally found in Western England. It transmits equine and canine babesiosis.

(*b*) *D. variabilis* (*D. electus*) is found on dogs in North America. It also occurs on cattle and horses. It closely resembles *D. reticulatus*, but in that species a silvery white coloration is found laterally and posteriorly on the scutum, while in this

PARASITES AND PARASITOLOGY

species the coloration is yellow-white, and extends anteriorly, separated by a central brownish area. It is known as the American dog tick.

The eggs hatch in about a month, and the larvæ, attaching themselves to a host, engorge for 7 to 12 days and drop to the ground. After moulting the nymphs seek a second host, feed for 5 to 10 days, drop off and moult. The adults on a third animal feed for about a week, leave the host, and oviposit in 3 to 5 days.

(*c*) *D. occidentalis* occurs in Western North America on various domestic mammals. It is considered by some authorities to be *D. reticulatus* or *D. venestus*. It is called the Pacific Coast tick

(*d*) *D. venestus* is found in the Rocky Mountain District of North America. Adults are found on various mammals, including man. It is the transmitter of 'Rocky Mountain spotted fever' in man, and of canine babesiosis. It is the cause of American 'tick paralysis'. It is a three-host tick which usually takes two years for complete development, the winters being passed as nymphs or fasting adults.

RHIPICEPHALUS.—This genus can be distinguished by the oval body, hexagonal

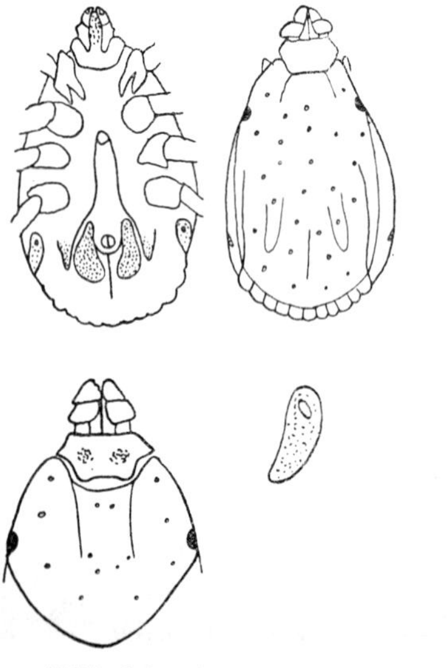

Rhipicephalus. (Above—Male, ventral and dorsal surfaces. Below—Shield of female and spiracle.)

basis capituli, short pedipalps and bifid first coxa. Eyes are present, as also are distinct festoons. There is an anal groove with two pairs of anal plates. The dorsum is usually inornate.

The following species are important:

(*a*) *R. sanguineus* is found in all parts of the world on dogs and ruminants. It is brown in colour. The scutum in the male leaves the edge of the back uncovered, and is irregularly pitted. It is known as the 'European brown tick' and also as the 'European dog tick'—a name shared with *Ixodes hexagonus*.

The eggs hatch in 17 to 19 days. The larvæ engorge in 4 days and moult 5 to 8 days later. The nymphs remain attached to a second host for 4 days and moult in 11 to 12 days. The adults feed on a third host for 7 to 21 days. Unfed larvæ will live for 9 months, nymphs for a third of this time, and adults for double the time. This tick transmits canine babesiosis in India and canine rangeliosis in Brazil. The following stages are infective: nymphs from infected adults, adults from infected nymphs, or adults from infected adults. It is stated to be the intermediate host of *Filaria grassi* of the dog.

(*b*) *R. appendiculatus* is found in Africa, where it attacks cattle, sheep, goats. It resembles the last species, but the first coxa is produced anteriorly and is visible dorsally, while a distinct tail-like process is present. The punctuations are small. It is called the 'brown tick', and is a 3-host tick.

Eggs hatch in 1 to 3 months, depending on the weather. The larvæ engorge for 3 to 7 days and, dropping off, moult in 16 to 21 days. The nymphs engorge on a second host for 3 to 7 days, drop off, and moult in 10 to 18 days. The larvæ can live for 11 months, the nymphs for 7, and the adults for 26 months without food.

This species transmits: East Coast Fever, Corridor disease, mild gall sickness, red-water, Nairobi sheep disease, louping-ill.

(*c*) *R. bursa* is found in North Africa and South Europe on all animals. It resembles the first species, but is much more frequently and closely pitted. It is a two-host tick, the larva moulting on the first host. The life-cycle has a minimum of 110 days. It transmits ovine babesiosis in Europe.

(*d*) *R. capensis* is found in South Africa on cattle, horses, and dogs. In it the scutum completely covers the male dorsum, and the pitting is very close. It is called the 'Cape brown tick'. The life-cycle is similar to the second species. It can transmit *Theileria parva*.

(*e*) *R. simus* is found in Africa on dogs and herbivores. The pores on the scutum are arranged in longitudinal lines, and are very large and uniform. The scutum is dark in colour. It is called the 'dark pitted tick'. Its life-cycle is similar to the second species. It can transmit:

(i) *Theileria parva.*
(ii) *Anaplasma marginale:* larvæ from infected adults.
(iii) *Theileria mutans.*
(iv) *Rhodesian fever.*

(*f*) *R. evertsi* in Africa may be found on all the domestic mammals except pigs. It has orange-red legs with round convex distinct eyes. The scutum is black and densely pitted. The under side of the males is red. The females are brown or reddish brown. It is called the red tick or the red-legged tick. The eggs hatch in about a month. The larvæ attach themselves to the ears and flank of a host, and after feeding and without dropping off moult. In 10 to 15 days they drop off and moult into adults on the ground in a little over 3 weeks. The adults are usually attached near the anus or scrotum. The larvæ can live for 7 months and the adults for a year without food. This 2-host species transmits:

(i) *Nuttallia equi:* adults from infected larvæ.
(ii) *Theileria parva:* adults from infected larvæ.
(iii) *Theileria mutans.*
(iv) Bovine babesiosis: adults from infected larvæ or larvæ from infected adults.
(v) Spirochætosis in herbivores: adults from infected larvæ.

BOOPHILUS.—This genus differs from the last in the practical absence of an anal groove and very indistinct festoons. The rostrum is very short. The first coxa is bifid, and two anal plates are present in the male.

(*a*) *B. decoloratus* is found on cattle and other animals in Africa. It is a 1-host tick, called the 'blue tick'. The eggs hatch in 3 to 6 weeks. The larva remains on the host until adult. The adults drop off in 22 to 38 days. Unfed larvæ can live for 6 months.

This tick, which may be a variety of *B. annulatus*, transmits:

(i) *Babesia bigemina;*
(ii) *Anaplasma marginale;* and
(iii) *Spirochæta theileri.*

(*b*) *B. australis* is found in Australia, India, Africa, and Tropical America. It is called the 'Australian blue tick'. It also is probably a variety.

(*c*) *B. annulatus* is the Texas fever tick, and is found in southern North America.

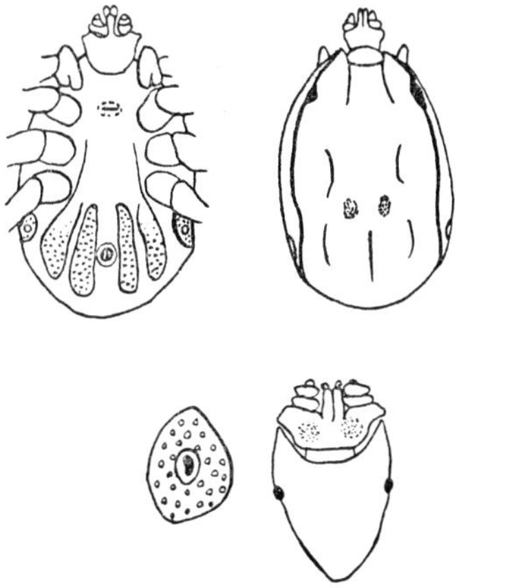

Boophilus. (Above—Male, ventral and dorsal surfaces. Below—Spiracle and shield of female.)

The eggs hatch in 20 days in summer to 200 days in winter. The tick remains on the host for 3 to 9 weeks. Eggs are laid in 3 to 5 days after dropping off. There may be three generations in a year. Larvæ will live for a maximum period of 8 months away from their host. It transmits *B. bigemina.*

HYALOMMA.—This genus has an oval body with longish pedipalps and distinct

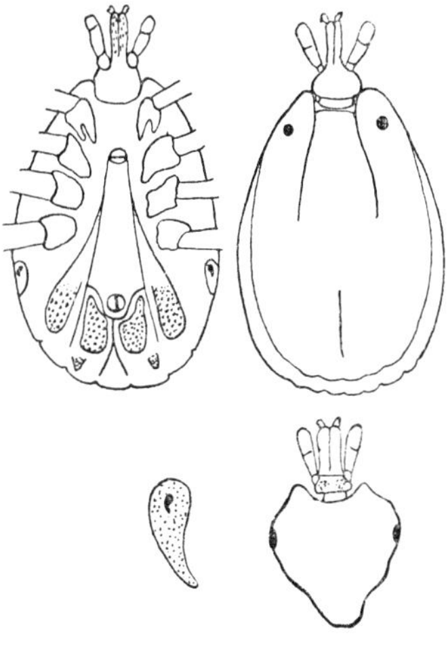

Hyalomma. (Above—Male, ventral and dorsal surfaces. Below—Spiracle and shield of female.)

PARASITES AND PARASITOLOGY

eyes. Festoons may be present. One or two pairs of anal plates are present in the male and two post-anal protrusions.

H. ægyptium is found on all the domestic animals in Africa, Southern Europe, and Asia. It has a brown scutum, a deeply cleft first coxa, and anal plates much longer than broad. Only adults are found on the domestic animals, the younger stages being found on small mammals. It is called the 'striped-leg tick', or the 'bont-leg tick'.

The eggs hatch in a month. The larvæ may moult on or off the same host in 4 to 15 days. Nymphs leave the host in 3 to 6 weeks after reaching it as larvæ. Females remain on for a week. Larvæ live for a year, nymphs 2 months, and adults 2 years without food.

This tick produces ulcerating sores in cattle, and is frequently the cause of lameness in sheep and goats owing to its attachment between the claws. It is believed to transmit both species of *Theileria*, and equine and bovine babesiosis.

H. truncatum, the African bont-legged tick, is usually a 2-host, occasionally a 3-host parasite. Cattle and goats are the main hosts. It transmits Sweating Sickness and Q fever.

AMBLYOMMA.—In this genus the body is broadly oval and the scutum of the adult

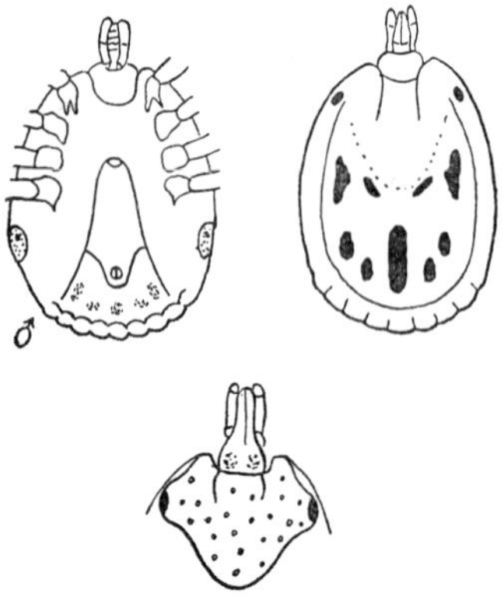

Amblyomma. (Above—Male, ventral and dorsal surfaces. × 7. Below—Shield of female.)

is generally ornate. The pedipalps are long and eyes are present. Festoons are generally present. Anal plates are absent, but small ventral plaques may be present.

(*a*) *A. hebræum* is an African tick attacking all the domestic mammals. It has a conspicuously marked scutum, yellowish with a red and blue tinge, and brown or black markings. The eyes are flat and flush with the body. It is called the 'bont tick'.

Eggs hatch in 7 to 10 weeks. The larvæ engorge for 4 to 20 days, drop off, and moult in 10 days to 4 months. The nymphs attack a second host, feed for 4 to 20 days, drop off, and moult in 2 to 4 weeks. The females engorge for 6 to 25 days, and remain on the ground for a month before ovipositing. Larvæ may live for a year, nymphs for 9 months, and adults for 2 years without feeding. This species causes ulcerating sores at the points of attachment, and is a frequent cause of sore teats. It conveys heart-water to ruminants.

(*b*) *A. variegatum* is an African species attacking herbivores. It has distinct convex eyes. The scutum is reddish yellow bordered with green with black markings. It is called the 'variegated tick'. Its life-history is as above. It also transmits heart-water.

A. lepidum, an African 3-host bont tick, apparently transmits no diseases but gives rise to unpleasant sores.

A. gemma, an African 3-host bont tick which infests cattle, camels, and other domestic animals. It can transmit both heartwater and Nairobi sheep disease.

(*c*) *A. cayannense* in South and Central America attacks all the domestic mammals. The eyes are flat and flush with the body. There are nine elongated white spots on the male scutum. It is a most vicious biter, and transmits equine nuttalliosis.

(*d*) *A. americanum* is similar to the last species, but the scutum is punctate and has a silvery white spot, giving it its popular name of the 'lone star tick'.

An American species of Amblyomma transmits *Anaplasma argentinum*.

Control of ticks (*see under* TICKS).

FAMILY ARGASIDÆ. SOFT TICKS.—This family is distinguished from the hard ticks by the absence of a scutum and by the fact that the males and females are almost indistinguishable. Looked at from above the capitulum is invisible in the adult, whereas in the *Ixodidæ* the head is always visible.

Only two genera exist in this family, *Argas* and *Ornithodorus*. *Argas* is distinguished by the possession of a well-defined striated edge; while *Ornithodorus* has a body with a blind edge in no way differentiated. The adults do not permanently attach themselves to one host, like the hard ticks, but resemble the bed-bug in habits. The female also generally lays more than one batch of eggs.

PARASITES AND PARASITOLOGY

Some ticks in this family are carriers of spirochætal diseases to man and birds.

ARGAS.—(*a*) *Argas periscus* (*A. miniatus*) is the well-known 'Fowl tick', or 'blue bug', or 'tampan'. It is practically cosmopolitan in its distribution.

It is essentially a bird tick; but will bite man and other mammals (horses and cattle) on occasion. It particularly attacks chickens. A large number on a fowl will suck so much blood that the bird will die from anæmia. Smaller numbers cause a milder anæmia, general poverty of condition, and a considerable reduction in egg-production. Young birds become stunted, and are more liable to contract disease. In addition it is the carrier of fowl spirochætosis, and fowl piroplasmosis.

The tick normally feeds at night, spending the day in crevices, and accordingly is seldom seen. This habit is similar to the bed-bugs, which also attack chickens. It is easily distinguished from this pest by the presence of eight legs—the bed-bug

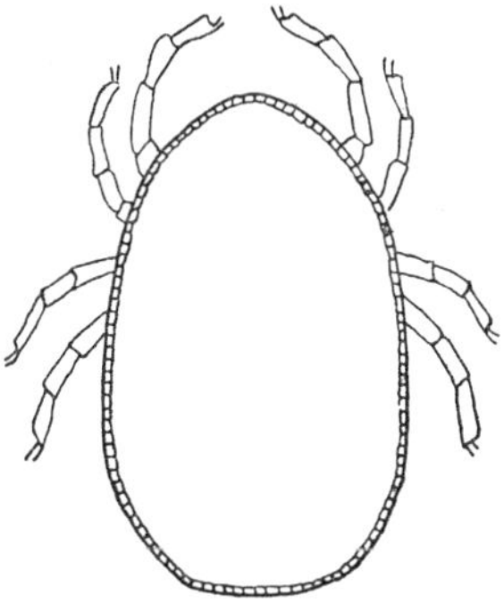

Argas. × 4.

being an insect, and in consequence having only six legs. The larval tick (seed tick) remains several days on the host, and is more frequently seen. The adults can live for two years without food.

(*b*) *Argas reflexus*, a closely related species, is found mainly on pigeons, but also attacks poultry and man. It is found in Europe, Africa, and America.

Control can be achieved with a BHC preparation.

ORNITHODORUS.—A number of species of this genus attack the domestic animals.

(*a*) *O. megninii* is the spinose ear tick of America and South Africa. The larvæ creep into the ear of some mammalian host, and in a few days moult. The nymphs, which are covered with minute spines, may live for 1 to 7 months in the ear, increasing in size from ⅛ inch to ⅝ inch. They finally drop to the ground, moult, mate, lay their eggs, and die. The adult is not parasitic. The eggs hatch in about 10 days. As many as eighty ticks have been found in one ear. The irritation is considerable and heavy losses may result.

As the ticks attack wild rodents, as well as all the domestic mammals, eradication is practically impossible. A mixture of 2 parts pine-tar and 1 part cotton-seed oil should be applied with a syringe to the external ear monthly in infective areas,

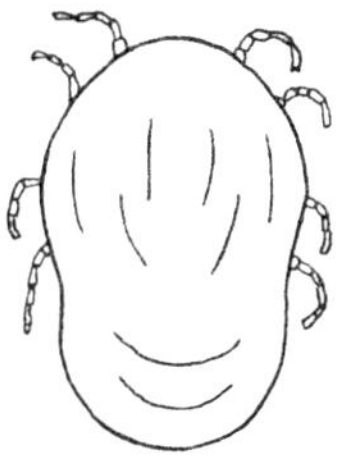

Ornithodorus. × 3.

where the irritation is pronounced. Cattle require half an ounce of this mixture for each ear; and more should not be given, as it will overflow and may cause blistering Hard wax in the ear should be broken up before application.

(*b*) *O. coriaceus* (*pajarœllo*) is a venomous species (found in Southern North America) which possesses a very painful bite.

FAMILY SARCOPTIDÆ.—This is a notorious family of small mites, belonging

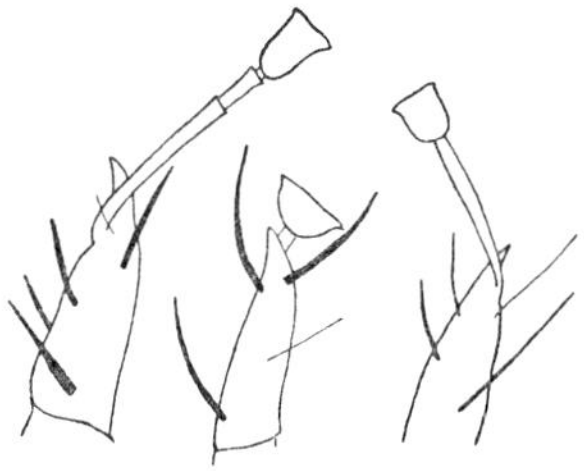

Legs of mange mites. (Psoropt, Chorıopt. Sarcopt.)

to the same class as the ticks. They are responsible for an enormous amount of damage to mammals and birds. The most important of the five sub-families is the Sarcoptinæ, containing the common *mange*

PARASITES AND PARASITOLOGY

mites. These are small ovoid mites, with no division of the body into cephalothorax and abdomen. Anteriorly there is a rostrum with a pair of cheliceriæ and short three-segmented pedipalps. The body possesses bristles, spines, and hairs at various parts. There are eight legs in the adult, two pairs anteriorly and two pairs posteriorly, the terminal segments of which end in suckers or hairs. These suckers have a diagnostic value.

The following genera are important. All are minute, and under favourable circumstances just visible to the naked eye.

SARCOPTES, with one species, *S. scabiei*, and numerous varieties. In this genus the male has suckers on all legs except the third pair, while the female has suckers only on the first two pairs. The other legs end in a very long bristle. These mites live in the skin of mammals.

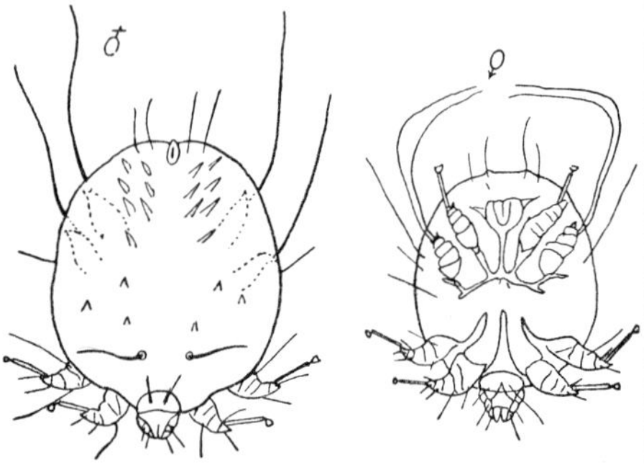

Sarcoptes. × 70.

NOTŒDRES is a closely allied genus found on carnivores. In it the anus is well on the dorsal surface, while in sarcoptes it is terminal. In both genera

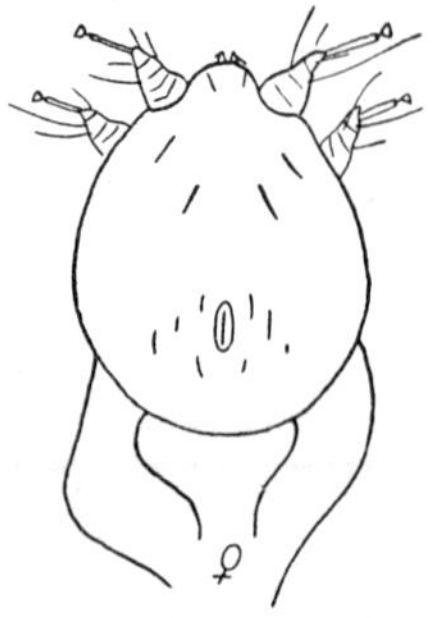

Notœdres. × 70.

the suckers are small and carried on long unjointed stalks.

CNEMIDOCOPTES, found in birds, has no suckers at all in the female, while the male has suckers on all feet. They otherwise resemble the first genus.

PSOROPTES.—In this genus the suckers are borne on segmented stalks. In the male, suckers are present on the first, second, and third legs, while in the female they are found on the first, second, and fourth legs. The male has anal suckers, which, in copulation, are attached to corresponding tubercles on the female. This genus lives on the skin. Two species are known.

CHORIOPTES (Symbiotes).—In this and the next genus, the largest suckers are carried on short unjointed stalks. Anal suckers are present in the male. Suckers are present on all the legs in the male, and on the first, second, and fourth pair in the female. One species is known, *C. equi*, with numerous varieties.

OTODECTES differs from the last genus in the absence of suckers on the last pair of legs in the female, while the posterior lobes in the male are less salient. It is found in the external ear, and one species exists.

Of the genera on mammals, numerous varieties of each species exist, but there appears to be no anatomical differences between them, and they are probably physiological differences rather than varieties.

The life-history in all the species is on similar lines. The egg hatches, either in the body of the female or after having been passed by her, and in 2 to 4 days gives rise to a six-legged larva. In 2 or 3 days the larva becomes a nymph, with eight legs, which, 3 or 4 days later, reaches the adult stage. Fertilisation takes place, and in 2 to 4 days the female starts egg-laying, the whole life-history from egg to adult taking from 7 to 11 days, and a new batch of eggs being laid every 10 to 14 days.

For convenience the parasites are treated according to hosts.

General Principles in Mange Treatment.—The patient should be at once isolated, and all 'in-contacts' examined carefully and at short intervals for any sign of the disease. All grooming kit, harness, etc., should be disinfected. Quarters must be cleaned out thoroughly and rendered free from eggs and nymphs. Bedding should be burned. Extensive mange is a symptom of neglect; and steps should be taken to prevent such neglect occurring (*e.g.* flocks should be brought in for periodic examina-

PARASITES AND PARASITOLOGY

tion, grooms and keepers cautioned, and so on). (*See also* DIPPING.)

Mange in the Horse.—In this host four varieties of mange occur.

Sarcoptic mange. — In this type the parasites burrow into the epidermis and make treatment difficult. The disease commences by the hair dropping out in patches with the formation of papules and an intense continuous itching. The hair becomes thin and broken, and abrasions are present. The skin is hard and folded. Emaciation is progressive, and finally death occurs from exhaustion. The disease especially attacks the thin-skinned areas, and under the harness, where the skin is thickened and the lesions are diffuse, but seldom hairless. It reaches its height in spring, and is at an ebb in late summer and autumn. Diagnosis is by demonstration of the parasite. It is the most serious form, and in Britain is a notifiable disease.

Treatment.—Gamma BHC at concentrations ranging from 0.01 per cent to 0.03 per cent is undoubtedly one of the most efficient mite killers. The organo-phosphorus compounds, diazinon and fenchlorphos are also effective. For the best results they should be applied by dipping or as saturating sprays, and for the sarcoptic manges particularly, two or more treatments may be necessary at intervals of 10 to 14 days.

Psoroptic mange.—Two varieties of this genus occur on the horse, one in the ear

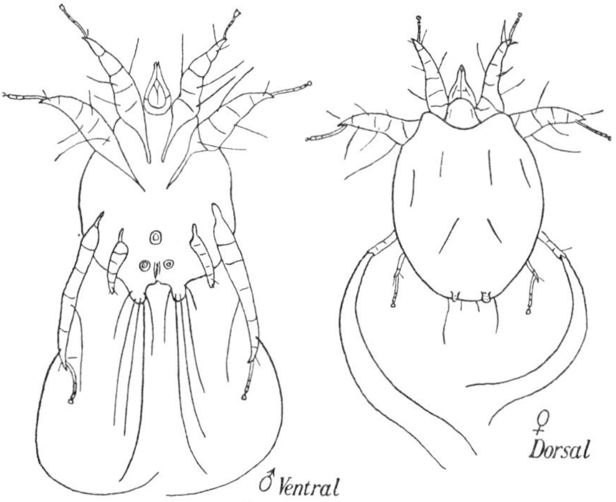

Psoroptes. × 70.

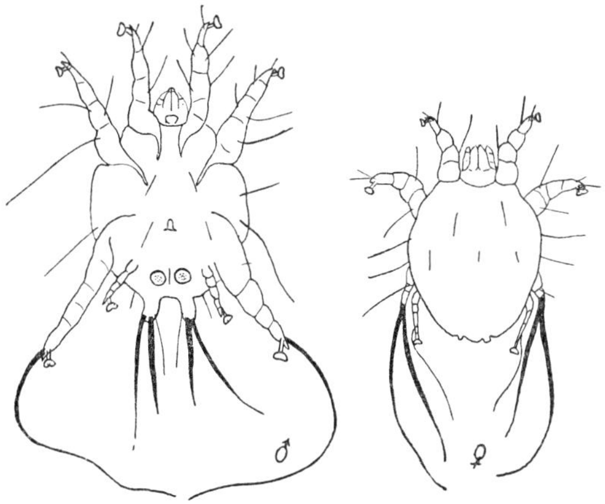

Chorioptes. × 70.

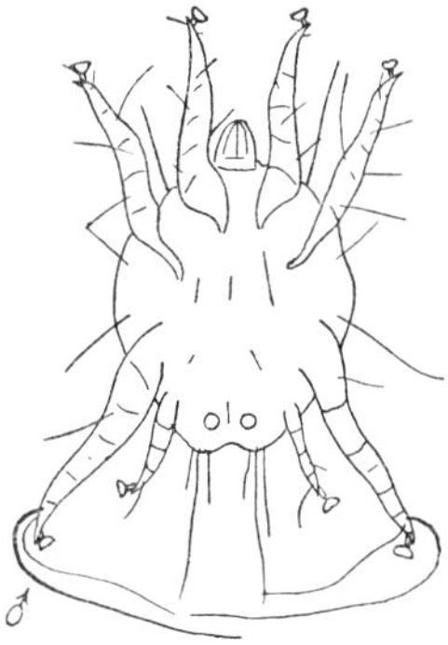

Otodectes. × 70.

and one on the skin. The lesions on the skin are localised at first, and usually start near the dorsal line where the hair is long. The patches are generally barer than in sarcoptic mange. The parasites bite the epidermis, but do not penetrate the skin. The serum which exudes forms a scab in which the parasites live. The disease is notifiable in Britain. Treatment is on similar lines to the last species. It is important to remember the presence of parasites in the ear, and to treat this part of the body also.

Chorioptic or symbiotic mange is usually confined to the legs or root of the tail. It is not notifiable. It causes great itching, stamping, and rubbing of one leg against the other. Papules, scabs, and even ulcers may be found. Treatment is similar to the last.

Mange in Cattle. — Sarcoptic mange is common in Britain and America and is the cause of 'dairyman's itch'. It is usually found on the head and neck, but may occur on any part of the body. Bulls are particularly liable to this form of mange.

Chorioptic mange is usually confined to the base of the tail, but may spread. It is unimportant.

Psoroptic mange, commences at the same spots on the neck and may extend to cover the whole body. It may cause intense itching but is usually not important.

Mange in Sheep. — Sarcoptic mange is usually confined to the head, and is seldom found on the woolly parts of the body. It tends to become more generalised in the goat. It is not important.

CHORIOTIC MANGE, caused by *Chorioptes bovis*, can be serious, especially in housed sheep overseas, and it is not uncommon in the U.K. Of 130 sheep received from South Wales at Weybridge 33 per cent were found infested. Lesions occur on the pasterns and interdigital spaces.

Psoroptic mange or 'sheep scab', occurs on all parts of the body covered with wool and in the ears. The life-cycle is typical, and can be completed in 13 to 16 days. The progress of the disease is in consequence very rapid. It is one of the worst of sheep diseases, and is notifiable in Britain. The mite feeds on the serum which oozes from the wounds made in the skin by its tiny mouth parts. The small punctures become inflamed and form a scab. The mite produces an irritating poison which causes the sheep to scratch and rub itself. This itching is usually the first symptom of the disease, and should be investigated *at once*. The skin becomes thickened and even ulcerated, the wool becomes detached and the sheep becomes emaciated. The itching causes the animal to rub itself against fences, and detaches the scab. This further spreads the disease, and permits secondary infections of the wound by bacteria.

Treatment is usually by means of double dipping at an interval of about 8 to 12 days, but which depends on local circumstances. In Britain a dip sanctioned by the Ministry of Agriculture must be used. If a commercial dip is used, it should be purchased *only* from a well-known firm and used exactly as directed. BHC dip is highly effective. Sheep should if possible be clipped before dipping (*see* DIPPING). In bad cases it is sometimes necessary to dip three times. The ears should also be treated.

Prevention.—In Britain dipping with, *e.g.* a BHC dip was enforced under the Sheep Scab Order, 1938, but has been abandoned by almost all local authorities since eradication of the disease.

Chorioptic mange, which generally attacks the feet, may cause intense itching, but is uncommon.

The "itch-mite" of sheep, *Psorergates ovis*, which occurs in Australasia, Africa, and North and South America, has not, so far, been found in Britain. This mite causes thickening of the skin and scurf formation. The growth of the wool fibre is affected and the fleece is further damaged by rubbing.

Mange in Pigs.—Sarcoptic mange starts on the head and gradually spreads all over the body, especially attacking the thinner skin. There is intense itching, the hair falls out, and the skin becomes covered with scab or with wart-like projections. It is found in America.

Treatment.—BHC preparations.

Mange in Dog and Cat.—Sarcoptic mange in the dog generally starts on the muzzle and spreads backwards. The symptoms are similar to the horse. The animal should be clipped and bathed with green soap. It may then be treated with a preparation of BHC or benzyl benzoate emulsion. If the infection is generalised treat one-half of the body one day, and the other half after 2 or 3 days. Turpentine, creosote, carbolic, tar, and lavender preparations should never be used on dogs.

PARASITES AND PARASITOLOGY

Notœdric mange in cats is similar to he last form in dogs. It is intensely rritating. It affects face, ears; occasion-.lly legs and external genitalia.

Benzyl benzoate and gamma BHC may rove toxic to cats and so one of the ulphur preparations or piperonyl but-xide is recommended.

Otodectic or auricular mange in Dogs nd Cats.—The parasite is the most fre-uent cause of irritation in the ears. It auses scratching and flapping of the ear. pileptiform fits and hæmatomata are requent accompaniments.

The eggs and larvæ are very resistant, nd survive under treatments which kill he adults. A 1 per cent solution of ammexane in liquid paraffin (medicinal) as been used with success. This softens he crusts, kills the parasites, and pene-rates far into the auditory meatus, to the valls of which it adheres. A few drops of he solution should be placed in the ear wice daily, the ear being then cleaned vith swabs of cotton-wool.

Mange in the Fowl. — **'Depluming cabies'** in fowls is caused by *Cnemido-optes lævis*, which lives at the base of the eathers, and so irritates the fowl that it ulls them out. The stumps left may be een to be surrounded with crusts.

Unlike mammalian scabies the disease s most active in summer. The affected pots and surrounding areas should be reated with sulphur ointment (1 : 4 of ard), or, if preferred, balsam of Peru in lcohol (1 : 3). This should be applied wice at 7 to 10 day intervals.

'Scaly leg' is caused by *Cnemidocoptes utans*. The feet and legs become enlarged nd crusted. The birds may become very me and even lose a toe. Destruction of fected birds combined with rigorous dis-fection is the most desirable method of radication. If this procedure is not con-enient, the scab should be removed with ap and water, the leg dried, and one of he preparations mentioned above used. his should be repeated in 3 or 4 days. ipping the legs in a mixture of equal arts of paraffin and linseed oil, repeating he treatment in a week, has been used ith success.

DEMODEX.—This is a genus of elongated ites which live in the follicles of the skin. number of species are recognised.

Demodex folliculorum is considered lentical with *D. canis*. It can infest an, cattle, and sheep, as well as dogs.

Demodex canis, the 'cause' of 'Follicu-r' or 'Black Mange' in dogs, is the most important species. The disease is apparently caused by a *Staphylococcus* introduced by the mite. The disease may assume a pustular or a squamous form. In the latter the skin is usually pigmented and the hair falls out in patches. It is generally chronic. In the pustular form the skin becomes reddened, hair falls out in tufts, pustules appear, a toxæmia sets in, and the animal becomes emaciated and dies. There is little pruritis, but the dog has a characteristic smell.

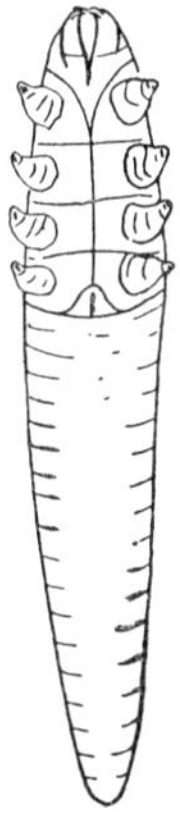

Demodex canis. × 150.

The disease often appears in the dog when 8–12 months old, usually first on the head, around the eyes and nose, and on or near the feet.

Treatment is usually unsatisfactory. The parasite lives in a very protected position and is difficult to reach. The best course may be euthanasia. If treatment is undertaken, the coat should be clipped short, and the skin washed with a sulphur soap such as Tetmosol. Various dressings have been tried, *e.g.* BHC, benzyl benzoate, fenchlorvos, and caparsolate sodium. It is best not to treat the whole area at once.

DERMANYSSUS GALLINÆ is the chicken mite of Europe and North America. It is whitish to red in colour. The complete life-cycle takes about 7 to 10 days.

The mite lives exclusively on blood. It is nocturnal in its habits, living in crevices during the day. It can live thus for 4 months or even longer without food. It is only found on birds when feeding. It causes a severe anæmia in poultry.

Eradication of the mite must be thorough. All wooden structures must be disinfected—crude petroleum is excellent, and if too thick may be thinned with paraffin oil. A painter's blow lamp is very useful for cracks. An insecticide, Sevin, is of use.

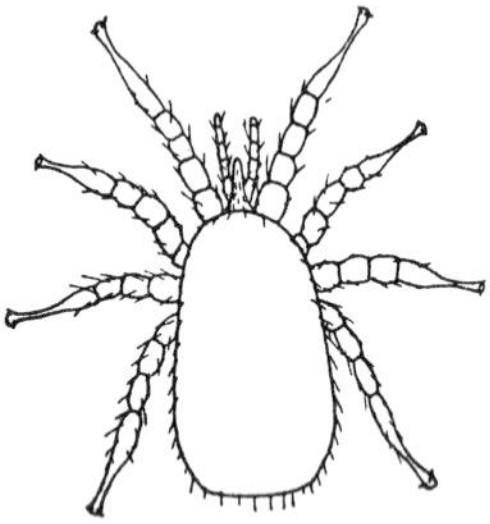

Dermanyssus gallinæ. × 35.

Although primarily a parasite of fowls, this mite will attack horses and other mammals, causing much irritation, with the eruption of papules and the formation of scabs. The mite, as it feeds only at night, may be overlooked as the cause of the disease. The proximity of fowls suffering from the mite may give a clue.

Also common in Britain, the northern fowl mite, *Ornithonyssus sylviarum*, causes scab formation, soiling of the feathers and thickening of the skin around the vent.

LIPONYSSUS BURSA, the tropical 'fowl mite', replaces the last species in th warmer parts of the world. Unlike it however, this species is found on th fowls and in the nest. It may feed durin the day. It also lays eggs and moult on its host. The symptoms are similar Dusting the bird and nest with sulphur i recommended.

Harvest mites.—The so-called 'harves mite' or 'chigger' is the larva of a specie of *Trombidium*. It is microscopic in size blood-red in colour, and in shape resemble a tick. The mite burrows under the ski of man and various animals, especially th dog and cat, and engorging with bloo appears as a red spot in the centre of a inflamed area. In 2 or 3 days the spo becomes a blister and ultimately a sca which falls off. The spot is extremel itchy.

Strong ammonia applied to the spot i the best cure, and dusting with powdere sulphur the best preventive.

Forage mites are occasionally parasite of the horse which live normally in th forage. They may cause considerab damage to the skin, but are usually easil killed.

CHEYLETIELLA.—Two members of th genus are of some veterinary importan in Britain, viz., *C. parasitivorax* an *C. yasguri*. These mites infest dogs, cat foxes, rabbits, hares. In the dog they a most frequently found on the nape of th neck, and down the back. Redness of th skin and intense itching may be caused-

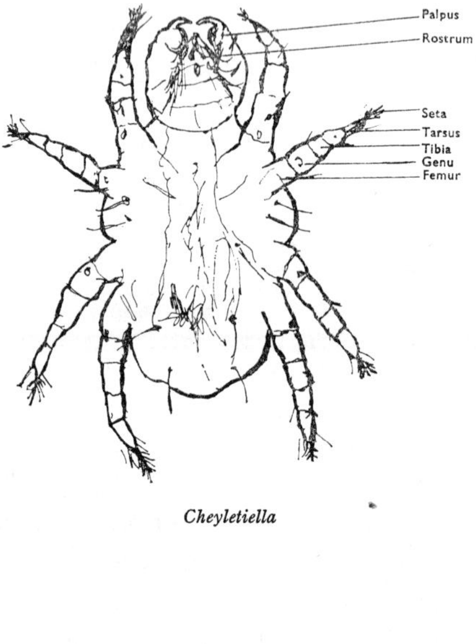

Cheyletiella

the latter symptom occurring in man also. Three dressings, at five-day intervals, with BHC, derris or pyrethrum, are recommended.

LINGUATULA SERRATA.—This parasite has a flat body shaped somewhat like a liver-fluke, but segmented. It is without appendages, but the head is provided with two pairs of hooks. In spite of its appearance and its popular name of 'Tongue Worm' it is not a worm but a very degenerate relation of the ticks and mites. It is found in the nasal passages of the dog and allied animals in various parts of the world. It is, however, apt to be overlooked in spite of its length of about an inch. The symptoms in the dog are ill-defined and its presence is seldom suspected. It sometimes causes fits and attacks resembling those of rabies, and is probably more common than reports indicate. The eggs are passed out with the fæces and are swallowed by some mammal—sheep or cattle are most commonly infected, but any animal may do. The eggs hatch in the stomach and the embryos encyst in some organ—liver, lungs, kidneys, and so on. The larvæ develop in these cysts, and then migrate through the body tissues until they reach one of the body cavities. They may perforate the intestinal wall and cause the death of the host from peritonitis. The subsequent parts of the life-history are unknown. The larval stage is very frequently overlooked in the intermediate host; but it may prove to be a very serious parasite, causing the death of the animal. It may infest man.

PARASITIC BRONCHITIS of cattle and sheep. (*See* HUSK.)

PARASITIC GASTRO-ENTERITIS OF CATTLE.—This is an insidious and economically important disease, and the cause of death in many calves and yearlings. It is now known that the output of worm eggs in the fæces does not bear any constant relation to the number of worms present. It rises to an early peak and then declines, and is not a reliable guide to the degree of infestation.

Cause.—Infestation with various species of round-worms, none of them much above one inch in length. (*See under* PARASITES.)

Symptoms.—A gradual loss of condition; a harsh, staring coat; sometimes, but not always, scouring; pale mucous membranes; progressive weakness and emaciation. In adult cattle, which acquire a high degree of resistance (only broken down when under-feeding, chilling, pregnancy, or massive contamination of pasture occurs), no symptoms may normally be shown, but nevertheless the animal's efficiency is lowered.

Treatment.—Dosing should not be delayed until the stock are weak.

Prevention.—Calves should be dosed once with an efficient anthelmintic in mid-July and moved to pasture which has not been grazed that season by other cattle. Doze again in the autumn.

PARASITIC GASTRO-ENTERITIS OF SHEEP.—It is likely that outbreaks in early lambs in March and April are the result of over-wintered larvæ. In one experiment, worm-free lambs were turned on to a pasture—'rested' during the winter—in the spring and became infested with 12 species of gastro-intestinal worms.

Treatment and prevention.—Routine use of, *e.g.*, Tetramisole.

PARASYMPATHETIC is another name for the autonomic part of the nervous system.

PARATHION is chemically diethyl-*para*-nitrophenyl-thiophosphate and is used for agricultural purposes to destroy aphis and red spider. In man and domestic animals it is a cumulative poison which readily enters the system through inhalation, by the mouth or by absorption through the skin. Animals should not be allowed to graze under trees sprayed with parathion for at least three weeks. In man symptoms of poisoning include headache, vomiting, and a feeling of tightness in the chest. Later there is sweating, salivation, muscular twitching, distressed breathing and coma. (*See* P.A.M. *and* ORGANO-PHOSPHORUS POISONING.)

In animals copious salivation and lachrymation, twitching, and increased intestinal movement are shown. Cattle are apparently tolerant of parathion, being able to break it down chemically.

The danger of spray drift, and the risk to dogs and cats wandering in sprayed areas, are obvious.

PARATHYROID GLANDS (*see under* THYROID).

PARATUBERCULOSIS.—A synonym for JOHNE'S DISEASE.

PARATYPHOID is a recognised disease in the foal (*see* FOALS), and in the pig (*see below*), and calf. Paratyphoid of cattle is associated with *Salmonella dublin* infection. (*See* SALMONELLOSIS.)

PARATYPHOID OF PIGS is not necessarily associated with *Salmonella* infection, as was once thought. Indeed, the causes are obscure. Cold and damp surroundings predispose to paratyphoid; anæmia may do likewise. Research suggests that infestation with *Œsophagostenum* worms may stimulate *Salmonella* organisms into activity.

Symptoms.—These vary very considerably according to the type of paratyphoid —and largely according to the age of the pig. (1) Pigs of from 6 to 12 weeks occasionally have circular dark red scabs on their flanks, etc., and usually die suddenly after several weeks. (2) Pigs from 2 to 4 months of age often show loss of appetite, dullness, diarrhœa, a 'dirty-looking' skin, and emaciation. (3) In pigs aged 4 to 6 months paratyphoid takes the form of pneumonia.

Diagnosis.—Paratyphoid must be differentiated from swine fever, but sometimes both diseases occur together.

Treatment.—Sulphathiazole and sulphaguanidine are of service in large doses. Nitrofurazone has been used in Sweden, given twice daily mixed in the food, with reported success.

Prevention can to some extent be effected by good hygiene and good feeding. A vaccine is available for use at 6 to 8 weeks of age.

(*See also* NECROTIC ENTERITIS *and* SALMONELLOSIS.)

PAREGORIC, or compound tincture of camphor, is a preparation of opium formerly much used for coughs in dogs. It contains, in addition to opium, aniseed, benzoic acid, and camphor. 'Scotch Paregoric' is a similar preparation of almost double the strength. Neither is safe for puppies.

PARENCHYMA (παρέγχυμα) is a term meaning originally all the soft tissues of the internal organs except σαρξ—the 'muscular flesh'. It is now reserved for the noble elements of an organ, *i.e.* the secreting cells, in the case of a glandular organ.

PARENCHYMATOUS is a term applied to diseases or structures connected with the parenchyma of an organ, as opposed to the interstitial principles. Thus there is *Parenchymatous mastitis,* in which the actual secreting cells of the udder are themselves inflamed, and *Interstitial mastitis,* where the fibrous and supporting tissues are inflamed.

PARENTERAL—(administration of a substance) other than via the digestive system, *e.g.* by injection.

PARESIS (πάρεσις, slackening) means a state of slight or temporary paralysis, also called 'fleeting paralysis'. (*See* PARALYSIS, GUTTURAL POUCH DIPHTHERIA.)

PARIETAL (*paries,* a wall) is the term applied to anything pertaining to the wall of a cavity; *e.g.* parietal pleura, the part of the pleural membrane which lines the wall of the chest.

PARONYCHIA (παρά, beside; ὄνυξ, the nail) is the term applied to inflammation near to the nail. It is sometimes applied to the condition which is more commonly known as 'Interdigital Abscess', which affects dogs. (*See also* RINGWORM.)

PAROTID GLAND (παρωτις) is one of the salivary glands. It is situated just below and behind the ear on either side, in the space between the angle of the jaw and the muscles of the neck. From its base commences a duct, the parotid duct, or *Stenson's duct,* which in the horse runs within the border of the mandible for a distance, and then turns round its rim to the side of the face in company with the external maxillary artery and vein, and ends by opening into the mouth opposite the anterior part of the third upper cheek tooth. In the ox the arrangement is similar, but the duct opens farther back; while in other animals it runs straight across the face instead of along the lower jaw bone.

The salivary glands are composed of collections of secreting acini held together loosely by a certain amount of fibrous tissue, but they do not possess a distinct capsule. (*See* SALIVARY GLANDS.)

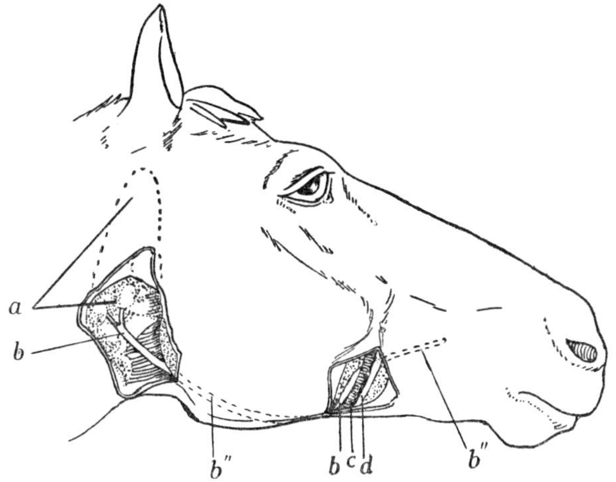

Diagram of the position of the parotid gland and of the course of *Stenson's duct* in the horse. *a*, The parotid gland, which in the upper part is indicated by a dotted line, and in its lower part is exposed to show the origin of the duct; *b*, Stenson's duct exposed where it turns round the lower jaw bone; *b″*, *b″*, its course before and after this; *c*, facial vein; *d*, facial artery.

PAROTID GLAND, DISEASES OF.—Apart from injuries, wounds, etc., the diseases of the parotids are few. Tumour formation may occur, especially in grey horses, when melanomata or melanotic fibromata form in and below the glands. When small and circumscribed they are best removed, but the operation requires great care to avoid injury to the large vessels and nerves that lie near the parotid.

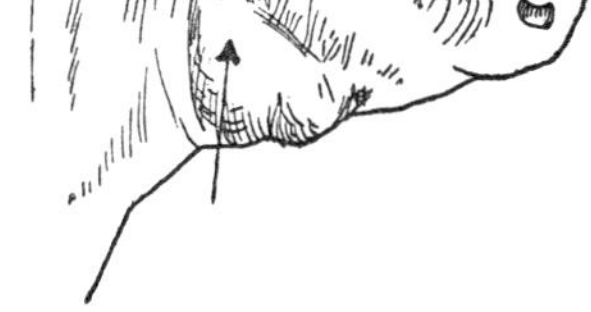

Diagram of inflammation of the parotid gland in the ox. The arrow points to the swelling, but the gland itself extends upwards to the level of the ear. The submaxillary gland is also swollen in this case.

Salivary calculi sometimes form in Stenson's duct from deposition of lime salts derived from the saliva. (*See* CONCRETIONS.) Abscesses below the gland are not uncommon in strangles, when they may cause pneumonia by bursting into the pharynx or larynx. Diffuse inflammation and swelling occur; there is severe pain on pressure over the gland; swallowing is difficult or becomes impossible; and in 1 to 2 weeks the abscess bursts either to the outside or inwards into the pharynx. From the pharynx pus may be insufflated into the lungs.

Parotitis means inflammation of the parotid gland. It is a common complication of influenza and strangles in the horse, and it may occur in the dog, when it is sometimes called 'mumps'. (*See under* MUMPS.) Generally speaking, parotitis in animals is a simple non-infectious inflammation of the gland, due to local irritation, infection, or injury from pulling on a tight dog-collar or neck-rope, is but seldom accompanied by general disturbances, and usually subsides after local fomentation and the application of stimulating liniments (such as soap liniment), and hardly ever leaves any complication.

PAROVARIUM is the name of rudimentary structures situated near the ovary, which are the remnants of the Wolffian bodies. The name Paroöphoron is also used. These structures are often the seat of cysts in the young adult. (*See* OVARY.)

PARRISH'S FOOD is the name of a compound syrup of the phosphates of iron, lime, potassium, and sodium. It is often given to young animals that are weakly or that are 'outgrowing their strength'.

PARTHENOGENESIS.—Birth from a virgin. This is a common method of reproduction among animals which have no backbones. It implies the division of an ovum, and its development into an embryo, 'by itself'; that is to say, without a male cell, or sperm, being in any way involved. Its occurrence has been reported in connection with the eggs of cat, ferret, and turkey. Living rabbits have been born to virgin does. It is now believed that, exceedingly rarely, parthenogenesis leading to the birth of young may occur under natural conditions; both in the rabbit and in other mammals.

PARTRIDGES (*see* GAME BIRDS, MORTALITY).

PARTURIENT LAMINITIS is laminitis occurring in connection with, or shortly after, parturition. When the uterus of the mare becomes inflamed, or when the fœtal membranes are retained after foaling, the feet frequently suffer. (*See* UTERUS, DISEASES OF; *also* LAMINITIS.)

PARTURITION (*parturio*, I bring forth) is the expulsion of the fœtus (and its membranes) from the uterus through the maternal passages by natural forces, and in such a state of development that, in domesticated animals at least, though not in the Marsupials, it is capable of independent life. The process is called 'foaling' in the mare, 'calving' in the cow, 'lambing' in the ewe, 'kidding' in the goat, 'farrowing' in the sow, and 'whelping' in the bitch. It is more likely to proceed successfully without than with human interference in the great majority of cases. It is not to be understood that human assistance should never be offered; there are many occasions when the judicious application of traction to a limb, or to the head and neck, will greatly assist the delivery of the foal or calf and relieve the dam of a considerable amount of suffering. To understand intelligently the indications for assistance, and to be able to give it to the best advantage, it is necessary to understand something of the process from the physiological and mechanical points of view.

Causes.—The living processes which are immediately the cause of the act are not perfectly understood. The increase in size of the fœtus, along with certain occult developments in the ovary, appear to combine in the production of a fatty degeneration of the placental cells (*see* PLACENTA *and* PREGNANCY), with the result that the interchange between fœtus and dam is less perfect and extensive. Some slight amount of irritation is probably set up in the uterus, and it is reflexly stimulated to contract and expel what becomes virtually a foreign body, *i.e.* the young adult animal.

The Forces of Expulsion.—The powers by which expulsion is achieved are exerted by the plain muscle of the wall of the uterus in the first place, and, secondly, by contraction of the walls of the abdomen which raises the intro-abdominal pressure. The total effect of this is called a *Labour pain.* At first the labour pains are weak, short, and infrequent. They gradually increase in strength, duration, and frequency, until, at the height of the act, they cause considerable distress to the dam. From this time onwards they diminish as gradually, and soon after the fœtal membranes have been expelled they cease altogether. In the early stages, all the force of the contractions is directed against the cervix of the uterus, and the pressure on the noncompressible amniotic fluid forces the membranes into the canal. This gradually dilates until a bladder-like piece of chorion (the outermost of the membranes) forces its way into and through the cervix. For a time the result of the following contractions is simply to dilate this opening still wider, until finally it becomes as wide as possible, and the uterus, cervix, and vagina form one continuous passage. About this time the chorionic bladder-like swelling appears between the lips of the vulva: this is popularly called the 'water-bag', and should on no account be interfered with. The head and fore-limbs soon become forced into the pelvis and external genital passage until the fore-limbs reach the level of the vulva. The water-bags soon burst (there are really two), and the contained fluid is discharged. There is often a pause in the series of labour pains at this stage—a provision of Nature whereby the dam gets an opportunity of resting and regaining her strength preparatory to the powerful and violent pains that are imminent. From this time onwards till the young is born the pains attain their maximum, both as to the force and duration of the contractions. They are all exerted upon the passive fœtus in an endeavour to drive it out from the abdominal cavity. The accessory contractions of the abdominal walls and the diaphragm come into play to a considerable extent. but the muscle in the uterine wall remains the chief expellant.

The head and fore limbs are gradually passed through the external genital canal to the outside where they become visible. The withers and shoulders of the young are now passing through the bony pelvis of the dam, and they correspond to the big end of a wedge whose smaller end is the fore legs and head. This wedge-like shape of the young completes the dilatation of the genital canal and makes delivery possible. It is often the case that some difficulty is experienced at this time, caused by the three bony points of the young (*i.e.* two shoulders and the withers) engaging the bony pelvis of the dam. This can generally be eased by pulling firmly but gently, first upon one and then upon the other fore limb, in a direction somewhat towards the dam's tail but out behind her. When each has cleared the brim of the pelvis they should both be grasped and pulled in a slightly downward direction toward the hocks, so that the withers of the young may clear the roof of the pelvis of the dam.

With a final supreme labour pain, which entails a maximum expenditure of the dam's energy, the chest and the abdomen, followed by the smaller hind quarters, are forced out, rather more rapidly than hitherto, and the young animal is born.

It is usually the case that the dam lies exhausted for some minutes after the birth of the young animal and the labour pains cease. She should be encouraged to lie thus and rest, as this is another of Nature's recuperative measures, and the attentions of the attendant should be given to the young animal. (*See later.*)

Stages in Parturition.—Although the act is really a continuous one it is customary to divide it into four stages: (1) The Preliminary Stage; (2) The Dilatation Stage; (3) The Expulsion of the Fœtus Stage; (4) The Expulsion of the Membranes Stage.

(1) The Preliminary Stage may occupy some hours or even days. The udder swells, becomes hard and tender, and a clear waxy fluid material oozes from the teats or may be expelled by pressure of the hand. The external genitals become swollen, enlarged, and flabby, and their lining is reddened. A clear, straw-coloured stringy mucus is secreted, which soils the tail and hind quarters. The abdomen drops and becomes pendulous. The quarters droop and the muscles and ligaments of the pelvis slacken. (This is popularly called the 'softening of the bones'.) The animal walks lazily and separates itself from its fellows if at pasture. It becomes uneasy; the mare whisks her tail, stamps, and moves about in an agitated manner; the cow bellows and becomes excited; the ewe bleats; the sow grunts; the bitch whines; and the cat emits a low cry. In all cases the animal, when at liberty, seeks a remote or an inaccessible place in which to bring forth its young, and some, such as the sow, bitch, and cat, prepare a bed or nest.

(2) Dilatation of the Cervix Stage merges with the preceding.—The uneasiness increases, and mild labour pains commence. The animal is sometimes somewhat distressed and may show signs of pain in its abdomen. It may lie and rise again several times, and in some cases a mare will show symptoms of colic, *i.e.* kicking at the belly, turning and gazing at her flanks, or wandering round in an aimless fashion. Meanwhile the labour pains have been getting more and more powerful and the intervals between them shorter, until the animal's attention is diverted from all else and is concentrated upon the matter in hand. The expression of the face becomes anxious and strained, the pulse is quickened, and the breathing distressed and rapid. When a pain has passed the animal calms down and remains so till the next takes place. After a variable time—from about ½ to 3 hours—the 'water-bag' appears at the vulva. It If tense and hard during a pain, but becomes slack and flaccid in the intervals. it is found to be empty at first, but the fore feet of the young animal can be felt in it later. At this time the cervix is fully dilated, and the third stage follows without any appreciable break in the sequence of events.

(3) Expulsion of the Fœtus Stage.—In this stage the severity of the pains is greatest, and the auxiliary muscles of the abdomen assist in the contractions. The animal may remain standing, may lie down in the recumbent position, or may alternately lie and stand. The back is arched, the chest expanded, and the muscles of the abdomen become board-hard with each labour pain. The animal may groan, or squeal or even scream with each effort. Frequently the rectum forcibly discharges its contents and the urinary bladder does

likewise. At each contraction the 'water-bag' protrudes farther and farther from the vulva until it finally ruptures in its most dependant part. There is a rush of fluid from the uterus to the outside and the animal has a period of ease. As already mentioned, Nature often calls a halt at or about this time. The fore feet, and the muzzle lying behind and over them, appear at the vulva, forming a kind of cone which dilates the softer tissues of the genital canal. In the larger animals the feet come first, but in the carnivora, where the head is very large, the head precedes the fore feet, which are tucked against the young animal's chest and sides. When the head has cleared the vulva there is usually another pause, which allows the tissues to become accustomed to the great distension, and prepares them for the still greater distension and strain that is soon to follow. The thorax and shoulders are now in the pelvis of the dam, and are driven slowly through it by the most powerful and painful of the contractions that occur during the process. As this part of the fœtus reaches the outlet of the pelvis there is generally a more energetic and painful effort than all the others—which pushes the fœtal trunk to the outside. This culminating effort may be so acutely painful and severe as to cause the bitch or cat to cry out. The expulsion of the remainder of the body is easy, partly because of its smaller size, and partly because the weight of that part of the fœtus which is already outside is considerable, and exerts a drag upon the rest still in the passage. (This is especially the case in those animals which give birth in the standing position.) In the mare the umbilical cord may rupture as the foal drops to the ground, or as the mare rises, but in some cases, where it is tougher than usual, it remains intact and pulls upon the membranes, so that they are born practically at the same time as the foal. In such cases the mare will usually gnaw through the cord with her teeth and so liberate the foal. It sometimes happens that a foal is born completely enveloped in its membranes; in such instances unless assistance is at hand to free the foal it will be rapidly suffocated. In the cow such things do not occur. The umbilical cord is much shorter and invariably ruptures before the hind limbs of the calf have passed to the outside, and owing to the cotyledonary attachment of the placenta the membranes are seldom born along with the calf. In the smaller animals, especially in the sow, bitch, and cat, the young are frequently born in their membranes, and these are licked away and cleared from the young by the dam, the umbilical cord being broken or bitten through in the process.

(4) EXPULSION OF THE MEMBRANES STAGE, or the 'delivery of the afterbirth', may occur with, immediately following, or not for some considerable time after, the production of the young in an animal.

Immediately after the young animal is born the uterus contracts and becomes smaller—a process known as 'Involution'—so that its capacity is decreased. The attachment between the membranes and the mucosa of the uterus is accordingly loosened and the placenta is ultimately separated from the uterus. These contractions also serve to force the membranes to the outside through the wide open cervix.

With the mare, owing to the diffuse and not very intimate adherence between the uterine mucous membrane and the placental membrane, the separation and the discharge of the envelopes are soon accomplished. In fact, if these are retained for more than a very few hours (4 or 6 or so), serious results are probable, but retention of the membranes is rare in the healthy mare.

In the cow, where the attachment is limited to the surfaces of the cotyledons and is very close, and where the shrinkage in the uterine wall (*i.e.* involution) does not tend greatly to upset the intimacy of the adhesion, the calf is never born in its membranes, and retention of these is more common. As a consequence, however, the cow is enabled to hold her membranes for quite a long time—in some cases until they actually decompose—without necessarily serious results. They are generally discharged within a few hours of the birth of the calf, but the time varies very much.

Animals which produce more than one young at a time generally discharge the membranes of each at the same time as or soon after it is born, with the exception of the last of the litter, whose membranes are occasionally retained in the extremity of one horn of the uterus.

In animals that are really uniparous (*i.e.* produce only one fœtus at a birth) but which have been modified by breeding so that they often produce two or more young, such as the sheep and goat, the membranes of the first twin come away with the second, and those of the second are expelled after it has been born.

With the possible exception of the ewe, the farm animals are all very liable to devour their fœtal membranes as soon as they are expelled, unless they are prevented from so doing. This may or may not cause some general disturbance, and has been known to produce choking in the cow. It is at least not advisable to allow them to do so, since the ingestion of a large amount of protein material, such as fœtal membrane, is likely to upset the digestive system, particularly of the herbivorous animals.

Early discharge of the membranes is very desirable, because so long as they remain in position they are likely sources of infection to the uterus, and they prevent that organ from returning to its normal. After they have been evacuated the involution of the uterus becomes more and more complete, until in a few days it has shrunk to less than half its former size. It never decreases so much as to return to its original virgin size, but it decreases enough to prevent easy access from the outside.

Duties of an attendant at Parturition.— As before mentioned, the majority of domesticated animals require little or no assistance in the actual feat of parturition, provided they are in a reasonably healthy and vigorous state. At the same time it is advisable that some one shall be at hand to give any help that may be necessary should some emergency arise, and as a rule the more artificially the animals are kept, and the further removed from the natural state, the more likely is it that the process will be difficult.

It is usual for an attendant to sit up with a valuable dam for a week or ten days before her time is up, firstly, lest she should produce her young previous to the scheduled date, and secondly, so that she may become accustomed to the presence of a human being with her at night-time before she actually gives birth. It is essential that this person shall not yield to the temptation of taking a few minutes' sleep, for frequently has a valuable mare foaled while the attendant slept, and many a valuable foal has been lost through failure to render some slight assistance. The mare should have been housed in the 'foaling-box' for a month or so previously, so that she shall feel quite at home (*see* PREGNANCY). and the ventilation, warmth, bedding, cleanliness, etc., should be as near an approach to the ideal as circumstances will allow. If possible, the cow should calve in a separate loose-box. Ewes frequently lamb out in the open and do quite well, but if the weather be cold or stormy, or if the ground is very wet, it is better to provide a 'lambing-pen', especially with Lowland breeds which have not the same hardiness as the mountain varieties. Sows should on all occasions have a sty or pen to themselves, for if other pigs are present the little pigs will most probably be eaten as soon as they are born. With bitches and cats the same principles apply, but the circumstances under which they are kept vary so much that it is difficult to lay down rules that may be applicable to all cases. With the pure-bred highly pedigreed toy creature, the preparations for whelping are often only slightly less than they are in the case of the birth of a human child, while the mongrel outcast is allowed to produce its puppies in any out-of-the-way corner of a shed or even in the open air, and between these two extremes there are all possible gradations.

For the larger animals the attendant will do well to provide himself with a proprietary antiseptic lubricant designed for vaginal use, and with Dettol for cleaning his hand and arm, when it may be necessary to insert the hand or arm into the vaginal canal.

When the act has commenced the attendant may require to soothe and quieten the dam if she becomes very excited, but beyond this the prospective mother should be left alone for some time. If all is going well the 'water-bag' will soon appear and later burst. No hard-and-fast rule can be laid down, but if the forelegs and nose of the fœtus do not appear in from 10 to 20 minutes in the mare, and in double that period in the cow, a simple examination should be made by the attendant to ensure himself that the presentation is a normal one. To do this he should strip, carefully wash his hands and arms in Dettol and thoroughly lubricate them with the special lubricant. He should gently insert his hand into the posterior genital passage and explore whatever presents itself to his hand. The two fore feet should be distinguishable in that part of the passage that lies lowermost when the dam is standing. Above them and slightly behind, the nose and mouth should be felt. These structures are often covered with fœtal membrane, but in a normal case can be located without difficulty. In such cases as this nothing

PARTURITION

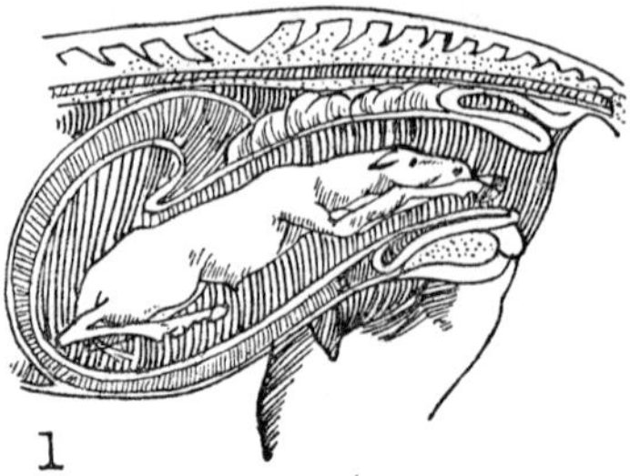

1

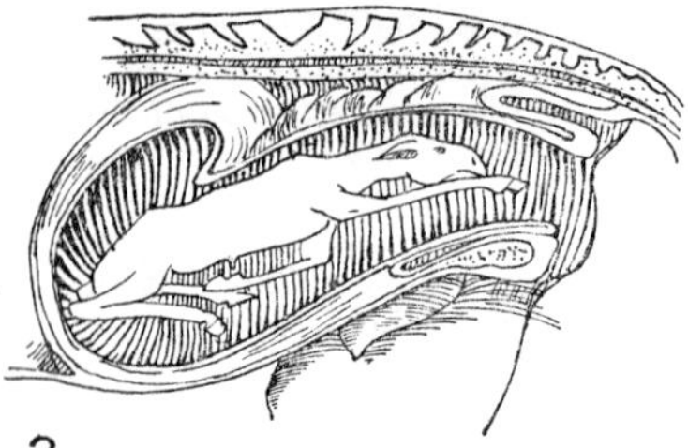

2

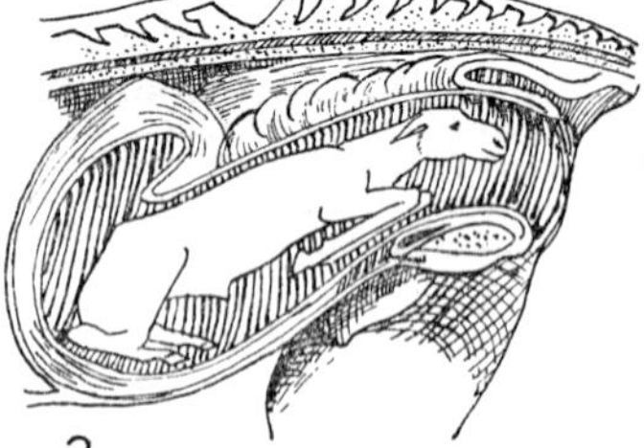

3

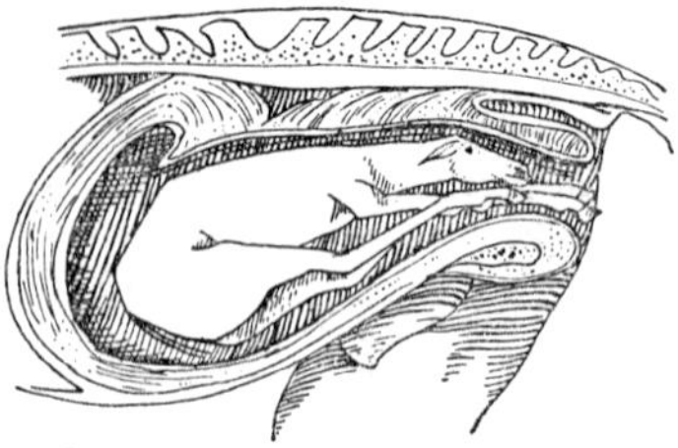

4

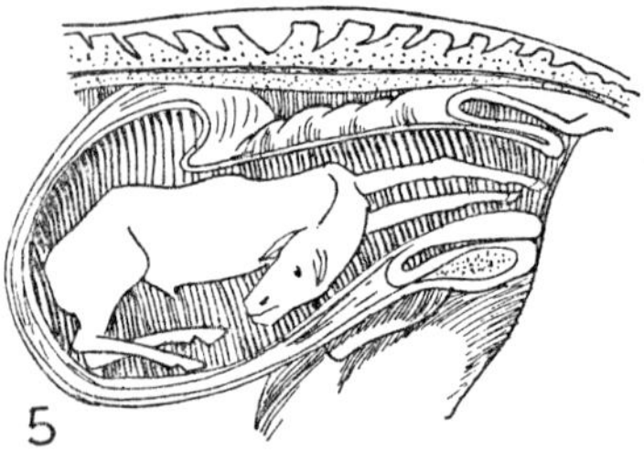

5

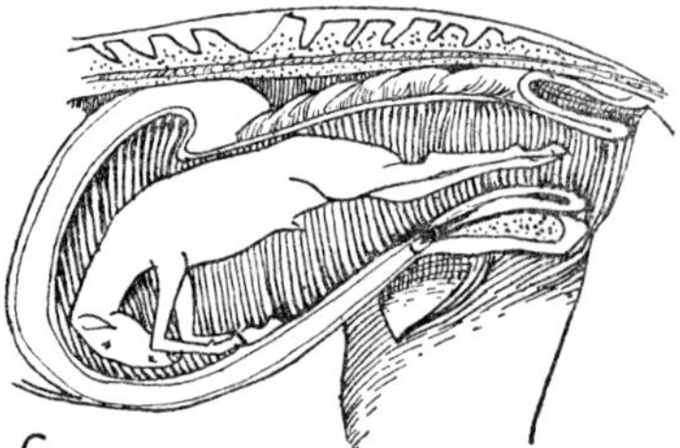

6

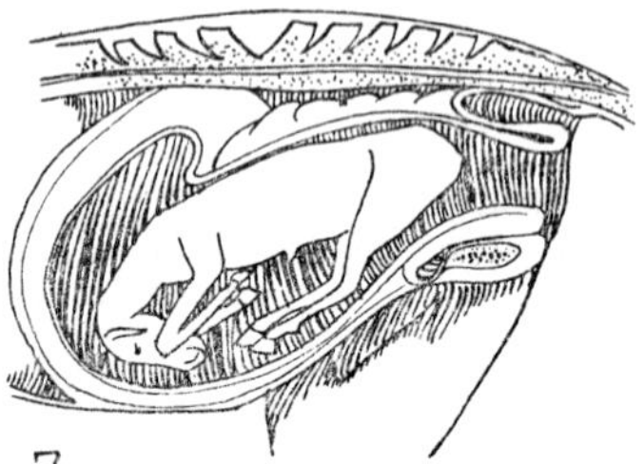

7

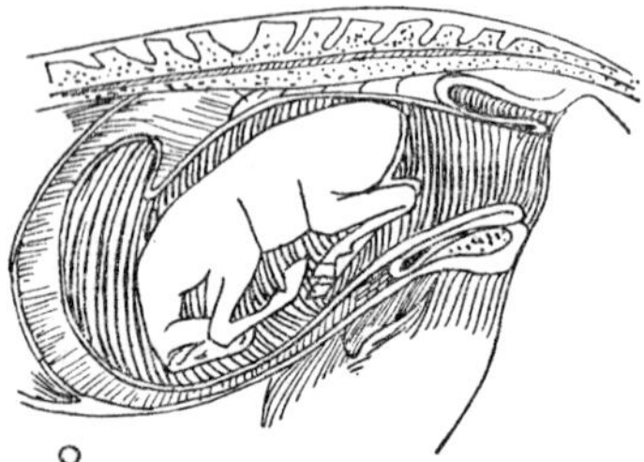

8

further need be done in the meantime; the dam will probably produce her young quite normally, and any attempts at assistance will only irritate and perhaps exhaust her.

It may happen, however, that one or both of the fore legs may be missing, or that the nose cannot be found. On introducing the arm still farther these parts can sometimes be discovered, and, by gentle pulling or readjustment, can be brought into the normal position. Before the process of parturition has advanced very far abnormal positions of the fœtus can be comparatively easily corrected, and serious trouble from subsequent jamming may be avoided. If all efforts at correction prove futile, no time should be lost in seeking skilled assistance, for the longer the dam is allowed to exert useless labour

 PARTURITION

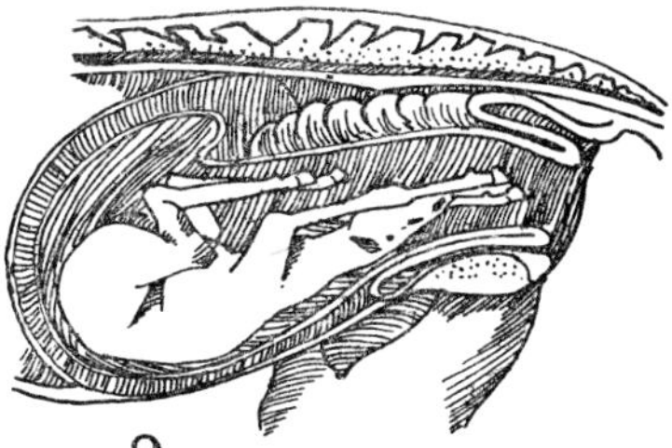

9

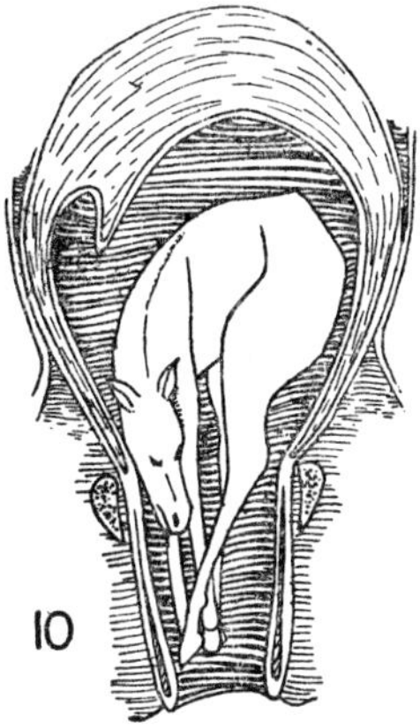

10

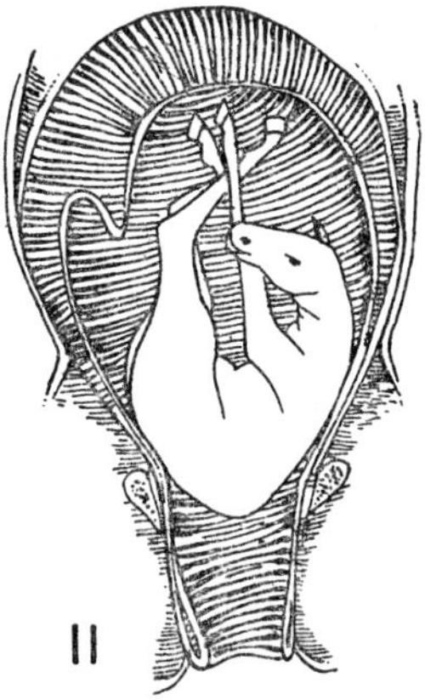

11

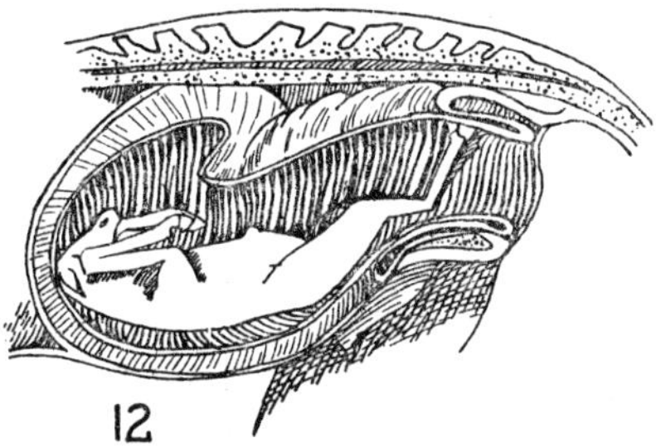

12

Different varieties of presentations of the foal. In other animals, except pig, dog, and cat (*see text*) similar presentations may be encountered.

1. Normal anterior presentation—nose and both fore feet in passage.
2. Anterior presentation with one fore limb retained completely. This should be brought forward by hand, or by passing rope round flexure of knee.
3. Anterior presentation with both fore limbs retained at the knees. Corrected as in No. 2.
4. 'Dog-sitting' presentation—nose and all four limbs presenting. The two fore limbs should be corded and the hind limbs repelled or pushed back.
5. Anterior presentation with head and neck retained. Delivery may often be effected by strong traction on fore limbs in foal, the head being pressed into the soft abdomen. In calf, owing to the short neck. this is not usually possible. Where possible, fore limbs should be corded, pushed back, and the head brought round by the hand or by hooks and cords.
6. Posterior presentation. Successful delivery often possible if the birth is speeded up by strong traction to avoid suffocation (*see text*).
7. 'Breech presentation.' Delivery difficult, foal nearly always dead. Cords in front of the foal's stifles and round buttocks may be applied if mare is large and foal small, but usually necessitates amputation of one or both hind limbs.
8. 'Thigh and croup presentation.' Cord round hocks may be successful in converting this into an ordinary posterior presentation. Quarters must be strongly repelled after hocks are corded.
9. 'Upside-down' anterior presentation. Occasionally delivery may be effected without adjustment, but assistance is always necessary. Removal of one or both fore limbs, with or without head and neck, often essential.
10. Ventral transverse presentation. This and No. 11 are the two worst positions in which foal can lie. Each case must be treated differently. Fore or hind limbs may be pushed back or brought forward according as they lie back in the passage or advanced. Removal of the foal in portions, a limb at a time, is often necessary.
11. Dorsal transverse presentation. Foal usually requires to be bisected and each half removed separately.
12. 'Upside down posterior presentation.' Delivery may be possible as soon as limbs have been adjusted, or amputation or version may be carried out.

pains with the fœtus in a position impossible of delivery, the more she will exhaust herself, the longer and the more difficult will be the act of parturition, and the less chance of survival will remain to the young animal.

Upon comparatively rare occasions none of the foremost positions of the body can be felt, but the two hind feet or legs (distinguishable by the difference between knees and hocks), and perhaps the tail of the young animal, are discovered. This is a posterior presentation, and as the head is the last part of the fœtus that will be born, respiration cannot begin until birth is complete, and the risk of suffocation is great. Accordingly, it is necessary to attempt to hurry the whole process by exercising a moderate amount of traction upon the hind legs. This is done by gripping them firmly by the hands above the fetlocks, or by applying a cord round that joint, and pulling in a gentle but firm manner without any jerks. The rope should be soft and clean, and should have been soaked in a mild antiseptic solution previously. The same advice as is given in a case of difficulty in the anterior presentation is offered in the posterior also; *i.e.* when matters seem to have proceeded beyond the powers of the attendant, or when the presentation is not normal, no time should be lost in seeking skilled assistance.

Attention to offspring.—As soon as the young animal is born and free from the maternal passages, it is absolutely essential to ascertain that the fœtal membranes are not obstructing its mouth or nostrils. It generally gives one or two spasmodic gasps or struggles, and then begins to breathe. Each respiration is shallow and weak at first, but in a very few minutes the breathing settles down to the normal.

Suspended animation. — Occasionally, foals and calves are born in a state of suspended animation, and vigorous measures are necessary to stimulate respiration. Artificial respiration, hanging the young creature up by the hind legs (so that mucus or saliva may escape from the respiratory passages), slapping it, and rubbing the surface of the body with wisps of straw or rough towels, should be carried out before life is despaired of.

The umbilical cord is, according to recent work carried out by the Equine Research Station, Animal Health Trust, best not interfered with.

'As a consequence of early severance of the cord the newborn foal is commonly deprived of 1000 to 1500 ml. of placental fœtal blood, whereas under "natural" conditions the amount concerned is probably well under 200 ml.

'It is suggested that apart from the possibility that specific illnesses might sometimes be precipitated by this blood loss, the general interests of the animal are better served when they are allowed to regain the blood, as they almost always do under natural conditions.

'Since the umbilical cord has a point at which it will rupture normally after a period during which mother and foal rest, and since hæmorrhage from either end of the severed cord is then extremely rare, it is suggested that the cord requires no human attention after a normal birth.

'Largely because it is not possible to state a time at which the transference of blood from the placenta is complete we would prefer that severance of the cord be left entirely to natural processes. We do not believe that the umbilical cord requires any human attention whatsoever provided it is allowed to break at the correct place and time (generally by the movement of the mare). Under normal circumstances there is no risk at all of hæmorrhage from the vessels in the navel stump, their retraction occurs in a way which is virtually impossible after cutting and provides an effective seal against both bleeding and (almost certainly) infection. It is difficult to imagine a worse procedure than leaving a substantial 'meaty' mass of umbilical cord at the navel as happens so commonly after cutting the cord with scissors. This provides an ideal medium for the passage of micro-organisms whose entrance to the abdominal portions of the umbilical vein and arteries are not hindered in any way by the 'sterile' piece of tape so frequently used to 'tie off' the stump. Almost as undesirable a procedure is the application of strong antiseptics (notably iodine) destructive as they are to tissues with which they come in contact.'

Drying the young.—If a young mare, for instance, does not at once commence to dry and cleanse her foal, a little salt rubbed over its coat may induce her to do so. Should the mother refuse to perform this office, the offspring must be dried with a towel, cloth, wisp of hay, etc., so far as is possible.

Suckling.—The first suck is of great importance. Within about half an hour the young of the domesticated animals are usually able to stand on their feet—although they are shaky at first—and as soon as they master this feat they make endeavours to reach the teat. The first milk contains a mild natural purgative, and it is essential that the newly born should obtain some of this as soon as possible. Colostrum promotes a secretion from the intestinal glands and stimulates peristalsis, so that the débris and black, gummy, fæcal material (called 'meconium') that has been lying in the bowels of the foal is evacuated and the way prepared for the digestion of food. When a dam dies before the foal obtains any of her first secreted milk, it is necessary to supply a substitute for the colostrum, such as castor oil and milk, or melted butter and milk.

Attention to the dam.—Where parturition has been easy and normal the dam rapidly recovers from her trying experience, and may be up on to her feet within a few minutes of the discharge of the fœtus. It is usually better to allow her to remain lying as long as she wishes while attentions are being paid to her offspring. It is good practice to offer a drink of chilled or warm barley-water or thin oatmeal gruel containing a tablespoonful of common table-salt, as soon after the act as convenient. Her system has undergone a considerable shock, and has lost quantities of fluid which should be replaced. The larger animals may require a rug if the weather is at all cold, and in all cases they should be given a thorough grooming and wisping after the drink. In from 6 to 3 hours or thereabout a pailful of bran mash and a little hay should be given.

When the dam is very exhausted by her labour it is necessary to administer stimulants. In addition, she should be warmly rugged and given plenty of bedding. If the birth of the young was difficult, and when the passages have been exposed to considerable strain by ropes and traction, it is advisable to apply woollen blankets rung out of very hot water by a wringer, to the whole of the external genital organs. These hot packs should be held in position for about 10 minutes, and replaced by others when they lose their heat. If all swelling is to be avoided it is essential to carry on the application of these packs for three or four hours at a time. Afterwards the parts must be covered with a warm and dry blanket, sewn in position on to the rug or a surcingle, to prevent any chilling. The loose-box must be warm yet well ventilated, and the mare should be encouraged to lie and rest as much as possible.

Subsequent management.—No oats or concentrated food-stuff should be given to the dam for the first two days after parturition ; her rations should consist of chilled water, bran mashes, and hay or green food given three times daily. After that time a gradually increasing amount of crushed oats and cut hay or chaff may be added to the mash daily, until at the end of a week or ten days she is back on to her usual diet. Gentle exercise is as necessary for the foal or calf as it is for their dams, and if the weather be suitable the dam and her progeny should be allowed out on to a sheltered meadow for an hour or so twice daily, after the first 3 or 4 days following the birth of the young. This period is gradually increased until in 2 weeks' time the pair may be left out from 9.0 A.M. till 5.0 in the evening, or even may be allowed to sleep out all night if the weather permits. In this connection it should be remembered that cold dry nights are much less harmful than those that are wet or foggy. Young animals of all species withstand dry cold very much better than wet cold, and it is inadvisable to allow foals or calves less than a month old to sleep out on a wet or marshy meadow. A useful method is to erect a covered-in shed in a corner of the meadow, containing a feeding-trough and well littered with straw, into which both dam and her offspring may retire whenever they wish. The amount of hand feeding which the dam receives must be judged according to circumstances. If the grass is rich and well forward, one feed of oats and hay may be sufficient after the first three or four weeks, but it is always better to err on the safe side and keep the dam in good general condition, for much of the subsequent quality of the offspring depends upon the start in life that it receives through its mother's milk, and if she herself is in poor condition her milk will be inferior.

If it be not too severe, the mare may be submitted to chain work for half a day at a time when the foal is from 2 to 3 months old. When the mare is at work the foal should be shut in a loose-box with a mate if possible, and given freshly cut green clover or lucerne. It is very important to avoid allowing a hungry foal to suck its mother when she is in a heated or sweating condition, for serious attacks of indigestion and diarrhœa are frequent results of such an indiscretion. If the mare returns to the stable hot and sweating—as she will when the weather is warm and before her condition is hardened—she should be given a feed of oats and a little hay and allowed to stand in a loose-box or stall for an hour until she has cooled down, before the foal is let out with her.

The general principles given above for the larger domestic animals are applicable to the smaller ones.

P.A.S. is the abbreviation for para-aminosalicylic acid, a drug which has been used in the treatment of tuberculosis in animals in zoological gardens.

PASSAGE (pronounced as in French) is a bacteriological term meaning the passing of a strain of organisms through a series of animals to decrease or increase virulence. For example, passage of cattle plague virus through goats is done to reduce its virulence for cattle, and is a technique used in the production of cattle plague vaccine.

PASTEURELLA is the name adopted by French scientists and others for organisms of the hæmorrhagic septicæmia group. The name was given to this class since the great French scientist Pasteur was the first to discover the organism responsible. He worked with the disease of fowl cholera, and for a time these organisms were known as the 'fowl cholera group'. They are now more frequently designated 'the pasteurella group', and the diseases they produce are called 'pasteurelloses', which include human plague. (A list of the group follows.) *Pasteurella septica* often infects cat-bites.

PASTEURELLOSIS OF CATTLE.—

Occurrence.—It is found in several parts of Europe, in Africa, India, and North America.

Susceptibility.—Cattle are the most susceptible animals, but buffaloes may also be affected. Wild deer, hogs, and even horses, donkeys, and goats may contract it, and in Egypt large numbers of donkeys as well as of cattle and buffaloes are lost annually. Rabbits, dogs, pigeons, and to a lesser degree guinea-pigs, are susceptible to inoculation.

Cause.—Infection with *Pasteurella multocida.* Isolated outbreaks occur from time to time in the same localities, and it is often of a seasonal character, but large tracts of country are not affected at once. The organisms live in the soil, specially when rich in organic matter. Drinking stagnant water, especially from pools which are low, is thought to be a cause. Any condition which renders the animal weak or unthrifty encourages infection. Abrasions to the mouths of such animals, which may be due to the hard maize-stalks, may accelerate infection.

Incubative stage.—After artificial inoculation the period of incubation is as short as from 6 to 24 hours—and by natural means it rarely exceeds two days.

Symptoms.—Suddenly occurring fever, which may reach 106° F. to 108° F., is one of the first signs. This is accompanied by symptoms of great nervous prostration, loss of appetite, cessation of rumination, congestion of the eyes, drooping of the ears, and rapid respiration. The heart and pulse rates are much accelerated; muscular tremors may be noticed, and the extremities of the body feel cold to the touch. The milk yield of cows rapidly falls off or ceases altogether. There are three distinct types of symptoms produced. (*a*) *The Cutaneous Form.*—In this, large œdematous swellings occur between the jaws, on the tongue, down the neck to the dewlap, even spreading as far as between the fore-legs. Breathing is very rapid and stertorous (noisy), the mucous membranes of the eyes take on a purple colour, and death may occur rapidly from asphyxia, but in any case is rarely delayed longer than from 12 to 48 hours. (*b*) *The Thoracic Form.*—This type is not so common in the ox, but is more often seen in wild deer. The lungs become the seat of acute congestion or of pleuro-pneumonia. The animal stands with back arched, is unwilling or unable to move, has a painful cough, and the breathing is very rapid and difficult. Constipation may be present at first, changing later into a blood-stained diarrhœa. Death usually occurs in from three days onwards. (*c*) *The Intestinal Form.*—In this form, in addition to the general symptoms there is acute gastroenteritis, giving rise to the passage of dirty fæces, brown in colour and mixed with mucus at first, but later with blots of blood, which may give rise to great straining (tenesmus). Œdematous swellings may complicate the symptoms, and death usually relieves the sufferer in a few days.

Course and fatality.—The disease runs a short course of from one to at the most eight days, but the majority of affected cattle die in from 3 to 4 days. Recovery is rare, from 85 to 95 per cent of affected animals dying.

Diagnosis.—Depending on the type of the disease, it may be confused with—

1. *Anthrax.* 2. *Cattle plague.* 3. *Contagious bovine pleuro-pneumonia.* 4. *Stiff sickness.* 5. *Black-quarter.*

Treatment.—Anti-serum, 100 c.c. to 250 c.c. daily, is reported to be effective, though obviously expensive. Sulpha drugs and penicillin are also indicated, but success is uncertain.

Preventive inoculation.—Cattle, or even

horses, can be hyper-immunised to the disease by repeated and increasing injections of pure cultures of the causal organism, but the use of vaccine is attended with risk.

PASTEURELLOSIS OF SHEEP.—**Susceptibility.**—Young sheep are the most frequently affected, especially after weaning, or in close association with some condition which lowers vitality.

Cause.—The *Pasteurella multocida* causes true hæmorrhagic septicæmia (described below).

Young sheep are liable to die from the acute septicæmic form, while older ones manifest a slower type of the disease, in which the pneumonic lesions predominate. Infection is thought to take place by means of the digestive tract through the ingestion of contaminated food or water. Dung, urine, and other discharges from infected sheep are virulent, and spread the condition through a flock. Sheep which have died from this disease are especially dangerous, and may infect the ground and keep up centres of infection if the carcases are imperfectly disposed of.

Incubative period.—This is short, as is the case for all diseases belonging to this category, rarely exceeding 1 to 3 days.

Symptoms.—The acute cases are ushered in by high temperature, great dullness and nervous depression, difficult respirations, muscular tremors, and sometimes by colicky pains. These are followed by rapid collapse and death in from 1 to 3 days.

In the less acute cases, similar but slightly milder symptoms occur. These are accompanied by a discharge from the eyes and nose, loss of appetite and absence of rumination, with signs of pneumonia or pleurisy and severe intestinal catarrh, either separately or conjointly. The tongue may swell up and the mucous membranes of the mouth show dark hæmorrhagic spots. Death usually occurs from weakness and cachexia in from a few days to 3 weeks. A few cases make an apparent recovery but are liable to a recrudescence of the pulmonary symptoms, leading to death from general debility. In the so-called chronic cases there is affection of the lungs accompanied by a chronic cough and often swelling of the joints, occurring along with a suppurative inflammation of the coronary band and sensitive laminæ of the feet. This form is the more common one in older sheep.

Course and fatality.—The duration is short in the case of young sheep, but runs into several weeks when old ones are affected, and the fatality is usually very high.

Diagnosis.—The acute form may be confused with anthrax, from which it must be distinguished by bacteriological means. Braxy has also been mistaken for this condition, but occurs chiefly in older sheep in the autumn and winter months, and the gastro-intestinal lesions are said to be more marked.

Immunisation.—Use has been made of a vaccine. A serum has also been prepared. (*See also* PNEUMONIA IN SHEEP for a description of Pasteurellosis caused by *P. hæmolytica* in Britain.)

PASTEURELLOSIS OF CATS.—Infection of cats with *Pasteurella pseudotuberculosis* (usually through eating infected birds and rodents) has been reported both in the U.K. and overseas.

Symptoms.—As a rule the cat becomes suddenly ill, with loss of appetite, vomiting, and diarrhœa; sometimes, however, the disease is at first mild, until the diarrhœa begins. Constipation may alternate with this. There is intense thirst, and emaciation is rapid.

Precautions.—The cat can be a source of infection to human beings.

Diagnosis.—This is not always easy during life. At *post-mortem* examination it has to be differentiated from tuberculosis.

PASTEURISATION OF MILK.—**High Temperature Pasteurisation** consists in heating the milk for 10 or 20 minutes at a temperature of 167° F. (75° Centigrade). This is sufficient to render harmless the germs of enteric and scarlet fever and diphtheria, and also bacteria which give rise to summer diarrhœa in children. It also affords a considerable measure of protection against tuberculosis.

Low Temperature Pasteurisation consists in maintaining the milk for at least half an hour at a temperature between 145° F. and 150° F. (63° to 65° Centigrade). This has the effect of considerably reducing the number of bacteria contained in the milk and very greatly delaying souring and similar changes. This procedure is sufficient for the sale of milk as ' pasteurised milk ' in England.

See also **Ultra High Temperature Treatment.**

PASTURE, CONTAMINATION OF.—This may occur in the vicinity of smelting works, (*see under* FACTORY CHIMNEYS), or as the result of droplets of chemical sprays being carried by the wind to adjoining fields. (For a list of chemical sprays, *see under* WEEDKILLERS *and* INSECTICIDES.) Contamination may also occur as the result of atomic fall-out. (*See* RADIO-ACTIVE FALL-OUT.) Bacterial contamination is exemplified by the presence of anthrax spores. (*See under* ANTHRAX.) Resting pasture for three weeks provides a measure of control of foot-rot; the organism responsible being unable to survive for more than a fortnight. For contamination by worm larvæ, *see* HUSK *and* PARASITIC GASTRO-ENTERITIS, and end of section below. For contamination by organic irrigation *see under* SLURRY. *See also* STRESS.

The average cow defecates about 12 times daily and each pat weighs about 2.5 kg.; in a 180 day grazing season, she will put about five tons of fæces (containing about 1,500 lb. dry matter) on to the pasture.

PASTURE MANAGEMENT is of the greatest importance in relation to diseases such as Bloat, Hypomagnesæmia, Parasitic Gastro-Enteritis of cattle, and Husk. (*See under these headings; also under* DEEP-ROOTING PLANTS, TOPPING, *and* WILTING. Controlled grazing is effected by means of an electric fence. (*See* Plate 4 *and* STRIP-GRAZING.) Rational grazing was the term applied by André Voisin to his system of intensively managed and highly productive grass from paddocks, and described in his book *Grass Productivity* (Crosby Lockwood & Son Ltd.). (*See under* PADDOCKS.)

It is important that heavy applications of nitrogenous and potash fertilisers to grassland should be made at the right time, or animals grazing there will be exposed to a greatly increased risk of hypomagnesæmia. (*See also* BASIC SLAG poisoning.) (*See also* HOOF-PRINTS).

The sudden (and harmful) change of diet which may occur when stock are turned out in the spring, or brought off pasture into yards for the winter, are discussed below.

In spring, it is a mistake to turn calves straight out on to grass. This means a sudden change from protein-poor food to the rich protein of the early bite, and the resulting effect upon the rumen will set them back. It is wise to get them out before there is much grass for a few hours each day; let them have hay and shelter at night to protect them from sudden changes of weather. Hypomagnesæmia, too, is far less likely under these circumstances.

Before yarding cattle in the autumn, it is wise to make a gradual change from sugar-poor autumn pasture to things like roots, and to accustom them to concentrates. Otherwise digestive upsets are very likely to occur.

It should be borne in mind that *Trichostrongylus axei* is a parasite common to cattle, sheep, goats, and horses, and grazing one species of animal after another in a field could give rise to a very heavy contamination with this one parasite. For a comment on 'clean pasture', *see under* PARASITIC GASTRO-ENTERITIS OF SHEEP.

Pasture grasses and herbs recommended by the Animal Health Trust, after preliminary trials, for **horses** are classified as under:—

Desirable species

Perennial Ryegrasses, Sceempter, Melle, Petra, Midas, S.23 and S.321, Timothy S.50 and S.48. Cocksfoot S.143, Crested Dogstail. Wild White Clover. Dandelion. Ribgrass. Chicory. Yarrow. Burnet. Sainfoin.

Probably useful (turf species which are also palatable)

Tall Fescue Alta. Canadian Creeping Red Fescue. Smooth Stalked Meadow Grass. Rough Stalked Meadow Grass.

Best excluded

Perennial Ryegrass S.24. Creeping Red Fescue. Brown Top. Meadow Foxtail. Red Clover.

PATELLA (*patella*, a small pan) is the name of the bone that lies at the front of the 'stifle joint', which is also called the 'knee-cap'. It lies in the tendon of the large extensor muscles of the joint, just above and in front of the true femoro-tibial joint. It is roughly pyramidal in the horse, with the apex of the pyramid pointing downwards. It is dislocation of the patella that constitutes the condition known as 'slipped stifle'. (*See* BONES.)

Dislocation of the knee-cap (Patella luxation) may occur as an inherited abnormality in certain breeds of dogs, *e.g.* Boston Terriers, Boxers, Bulldogs, Cairn Terriers, Chihuahuas, Wire Fox Terriers, Griffons, Pekingese, Maltese, Papillons, Pomeranians, Poodles, Labradors, Scotch Terriers, King Charles Spaniels.

PATHETIC NERVE is the fourth nerve arising from the brain and controlling the superior oblique muscle of the eye.

PATHOGENIC (πάθος, suffering; γεννάω' I produce) means disease-producing, and is a term applied to bacteria which have the power of producing disease.

PATHOGNOMONIC (πάθος, suffering; γιγνώσκω, I recognise) is a term applied to those signs or symptoms of a particular disease which are characteristic of that disease, and on whose presence or absence the diagnosis depends.

PATHOLOGICAL SPECIMENS, POSTING OF.—Specimens must be sent by letter post only, and marked 'Pathological Specimen'. They should be enclosed in a waterproof receptacle, *e.g.* a sealed polythene bag, and this should be surrounded with plenty of cotton-wool or sawdust, or other absorbent material in a strong box. For further information, *see* the Post Office Guide.

PATHOLOGY (πάθος, suffering; λόγος, a discourse) is the science which deals with the causes of and the changes produced in the body by disease.

PEAS, MUTTER (*see* LATHYRISM).

'PEAT SCOURS' is a name given in Australasia and Canada to molybdenum poisoning in grazing cattle. (*See* MOLYBDENUM.)

PECK ORDER.—This is the equivalent in poultry of the order of precedence described under BUNT ORDER.

PEDICULOSIS is the name given to massive infestation with lice. (*See* PARASITES.)

PELLAGRA (*see* BLACK TONGUE).

PELLETS (*see* CUBES).

PELVIS (*pelvis*, a basin) is the posterior girdle of bones by which the two hind limbs are attached to the rest of the skeleton. It is composed of two ilia, two pubes, and two ischia, united together by fusion into a basin-shaped whole (*see* BONES). Strictly speaking, it includes the sacrum and the coccygeal vertebræ. The two 'haunch bones' are the external angles of the ilia; the 'croup' is composed of the internal angles of these bones along with the spines of the sacrum; and the 'points of the buttocks' are the tuberosities of the two ischia. The pelvis is spoken of as having an 'inlet', formed by the brim of the pubes, and an 'outlet' posteriorly. In the living animal the outlet is occupied by the soft tissues forming the perineal region, except for the anus in the male and the anus and vulva in the female. The deep notch between the sacrum and the haunch bone is closed by the sacro-sciatic ligaments, upon which lie the gluteal muscles which give the quarters their shape. The pelvis varies in the two sexes: in the female it is broader from side to side, and deeper from above downwards, than in the male; this difference being chiefly necessary to allow of the act of parturition.

The contents of the pelvis are the rectum and urinary bladder in both sexes (except in the dog, where the urinary bladder is abdominal in position). In the male there is in addition the prostate gland and the seminal vesicles around the neck of the bladder and the beginning of the urethra; while the female pelvis contains the vagina, uterus, their appendages, and perhaps the ovaries.

In addition to these individual differences, there are variations according to the species of animal, and even according to the particular breed.

PELVIS, DISEASES OF (*see* ABDOMEN, DISEASES OF; and also see under the heading of the various pelvic organs).

PEMPHIGUS (πέμφιξ, a bladder) is a skin eruption which is characterised by the presence of large blebs on the surface of the body where the skin is thin.

PENICILLIN.—The first of the antibiotics, discovered by Sir Alexander Fleming in 1929. Benzyl penicillin is the sodium or potassium salt of the antimicrobial acids produced when the moulds *Penicillium notatum* or *Chrysogenum* (or related species) are grown under suitable conditions.

Purified penicillin salts occur as a white crystalline powder, readily soluble in water. Their therapeutic potency is expressed in International Units.

Following injection into the animal body, penicillin is rapidly absorbed and diffused in the blood-stream throughout the body, being excreted by the kidneys.

It is non-poisonous even in large doses and is effective against:

Staphylococci, causing local pyogenic inflammation as primary or secondary infections.

Hæmolytic streptococci, usually causing localised infections either primary or secondary.

Streptococcus equi, causing strangles in horses.

Streptococcus agalactiæ, *Streptococcus dysgalactiæ** *Streptococcus uberis*,* causing mastitis in cattle.

B. anthracis, causing anthrax.

Clostridium chauvœi, causing blackleg in cattle.

Corynebacterium renale, causing pyelonephritis in cattle.

Erysipelothrix rhusiopathiæ, causing swine erysipelas.

Actinomyces bovis, causing actonoymycosis.

Leptospira canicola, causing leptospirosis in dogs.

* to a slight extent.

Penicillin is of great value in the treatment of wounds for which it may, if necessary, be combined with one of the sulphonamides; and for the prevention of sepsis in surgery—both in cases where infection already exists and where there is risk of post-operative sepsis developing.

It is of great importance that penicillin should be used in full doses; otherwise there is a risk of strains of bacteria resistant to penicillin being developed. The *minimum* dosage for systemic administration is 2000 units per 5 lbs. body-weight or, in the large animals 50,000 units per 1 cwt.

'The long-established benzyl penicillin has the following shortcomings: (1) It is unstable in acids, and therefore cannot be given orally. This consideration, however, is of little importance in the veterinary field. (2) Organisms which produce penicillinase, and these are not uncommon, are resistant to benzyl penicillin. (3) It is active against only a narrow range of organisms. The new penicillins have been developed in order to overcome these drawbacks. Firstly, Phenethicillin potassium was developed as a penicillin stable in acids and which is an improvement on the older acid stable penicillin Phenoxymethylpenicillin, because after oral administration it gives twice as high a level in the blood. It is slightly resistant to penicillinase and is used in the veterinary field mainly in the treatment of mastitis involving susceptible strains of streptococci and staphylococci. Secondly, Methicillin; the main feature of methicillin is that it is resistant to penicillinase; it can, however, be given only parenterally. Methicillin should never be used in the treatment of infections caused by organisms susceptible to benzyl penicillin, since it is much less potent and may give rise to strains of organisms which show a penicillin resistance which is not due to the production of penicillinase. Moreover, methicillin actually stimulates the production of penicillinase. Thirdly, Cloxacillin; this penicillin is resistant to penicillinase, is stable in acids, but induces the production of penicillinase. Fourthly, Ampicillin; this is a most important introduction, because it is a penicillin active against both Gram-positive and Gram-negative organisms. It is useful particularly in the treatment of tetracycline-resistant coliforms, strains of *Proteus* and *Pseudomonas*, *Salmonellæ*, *Shigellæ*, and *Pasteurellæ*. It is not resistant to penicillinase, and is acid stable.

'Benethamine penicillin is a long-acting preparation, given by intramuscular injection as an insoluble suspension from which benzyl penicillin is slowly released. Benzathine penicillin has the same properties as benethamine penicillin, but is acid stable and can therefore be given by mouth to dogs and cats.

'While these long-acting preparations of penicillin eliminate the necessity for frequent administration, they do, however, present the risk of inducing resistant strains because they must by their nature provide a low level of penicillin in the tissues for a long period after their administration has terminated. This feature should be borne in mind when using them.' (Dr. F. Alexander, 1966.)

PENICILLIN IN MILK (*see* PENICILLIN, SENSITIVITY TO).

PENICILLINASE.—A penicillin-destroying ferment produced by certain bacteria, *e.g. E. coli*.

PENICILLIN, SENSITIVITY TO.—People handling penicillin suffer a risk of sensitisation, shown by skin lesions. In a limited survey, 4.3 per cent nurses working under local health authorities had become sensitised to one or more antibiotic. Some have had to abandon their profession. The same risk obviously applies to veterinarians. There is danger in the use of milk containing penicillin (*e.g.* milk from quarters of the udder treated for mastitis), especially in people sensitised to penicillin. Extremely severe skin lesions, and accompanying illness, have been caused in this way among farmers and others. A similar risk applies in the case of other antibiotics. (*See also under* MILK.)

PENIS (*penis*) is the male organ of copulation, down which passes the male urethra, which conducts the urine and the seminal fluids to the outside. It is formed of erectile tissue which contains many spaces which become filled with blood during the act of erection.

PENTOBARBITAL SODIUM.—A narcotic and anæsthetic. (*See* NEMBUTAL.)

PENTOTHAL SODIUM. — A short-acting barbiturate similar to NEMBUTAL.

PEPSIN (*pepsinum*) is a ferment found in the gastric juice which digests proteins by converting them into albumose and finally into peptones.

PEPTID is a term applied to a compound formed by the union of two or more amino-acids.

PEPTONISED FOODS are prepared with an extract made from the stomach or pancreas of the pig, so that digestion shall be more easily accomplished than otherwise. The extract, which contains the ferment *pepsin*, or, when made from the pancreas, the quadruplicate ferment called *pancreatin*, may be added to the food before feeding, or it may be given separately. Peptonised foods are sometimes used for dogs which have been affected with severe gastric complaints, and which accordingly may not be so well able to digest the protein principles of the food. The process converts the insoluble proteins into peptones, which is the first stage of true stomach digestion. (*See also* HYDROLISED PROTEIN.)

Peptonised foods should never be continued for any length of time, because by so doing digestion in the future may be compromised, since the digestive powers are liable to become inefficient from disuse.

PERCUSSION (*percutio*, I strike) is a method of making an examination of the deeper parts of the body by means of striking the area overlying such organs, either with the fingers of one hand or with an instrument known as a 'plessor', in such a way as to give out a note. According to the degree of dullness or resonance of the note, an opinion can be formed as to the state of consolidation of air-containing organs, the presence of abnormal cavities, the dimensions of solid or air-containing organs when these lie adjacent to each other, the presence of fluid in various parts, etc. Percussion is practised along with auscultation of the parts, and by considering the net results a fairly accurate estimation of the conditions can be given. (*See* AUSCULTATION.)

PERFORATION is one of the serious dangers attached to the presence of ulcerating conditions in the stomach and bowels. When a perforation from one of these hollow organs takes place into the peritoneal cavity, multitudes of bacteria, much ingesta, mucus, and other putrescible materials escape and set up peritonitis. (*See* PERITONITIS.) The immediate signs are a collapse of the patient, with, later, collections of gas or fluids in the abdominal cavity. It is not uncommon to observe vomiting in the horse when the stomach ruptures and the contents escape into the abdominal cavity; this is one of the very rare times when the horse is seen to vomit, and it is important accordingly.

PERFORMANCE TESTING.—A method of comparing strains or breeds of, *e.g.* beef cattle, by studying liveweight gains over a stated period with given rations.

PERICARDITIS.—Inflammation of the pericardium. Pericarditis has occurred for some years in piglets at grass in the Cambridge School of Veterinary Medicine's herd. The piglet, often in good condition and not anæmic, usually dies suddenly at about 2 to 3 weeks of age. Generally, only one or two pigs out of the litter succumb.

Traumatic pericarditis is common in cattle as a result of swallowing pieces of wire, nails, etc. (*See* HEART DISEASES.)

PERICARDIUM (περικάρδιος, near the heart) is the smooth lubricating membrane which surrounds the heart. (*See* HEART.)

PERIHEPATITIS (περί, around; *hepar*, the liver) means inflammation in the capsule of the liver and the peritoneum associated with it.

PERIMETRITIS (περί, around; μήτρα, the womb) means a localised inflammation of the peritoneum around the womb.

PERINEPHRITIS (περί, around; νεφρός, the kidney) means inflammation surrounding the kidney, and involving the loose connective tissue in the region. It often leads to the formation of an abscess.

PERINEUM (περίνεος) is the region lying between the anus and the genital organs in the male, and lying between the anus and the mammary region in the female of the horse, ox, sheep, goat, and pig. In bitches and cats the female genital organs lie lower than in other animals, and in them the perineum lies between the anus and the vulva.

Rupture of the perineum sometimes occurs in the cow at calving, when the fœtus over-distends the vulva. Suturing, under local anæsthesia, is usually required.

PERIODIC OPHTHALMIA.—Specific ophthalmia, or 'moon blindness', is a peculiar condition of the eyes of horses, due to inflammation of the uveal tract (especially of the iris and ciliary body) which is characterised by a remarkable tendency to recur time and time again.

Causes.—The cause is believed to be a virus. The disease is not at all common in Great Britain, but it is well known in America, and during the 1914 war was frequently met with in horses both on the Continent and in Great Britain. It is probable that collecting together large numbers of horses and keeping them under unhygienic conditions, such as was the custom in the old stage-coaching days, favour the occurrence of the disease. Damp surroundings, wet weather, and keeping horses in dark, ill-ventilated stables, appear to favour the disease, and in certain low-lying parts of Holland, Flanders, and America it is more common than in highly situated dry areas. Poor feeding and hard work have also been blamed, particularly in the case of young horses from 4 to 6 years old, which have been recently brought into towns for working purposes.

Symptoms.—In the first stage a horse which was apparently quite normal 12 hours previously is found one morning with the eyelids on one side half-closed; tears run from the eye down the face, and any effort to examine the eye is resented. Bright light is avoided, and the eyeball appears sunken in its socket. There is usually a certain amount of inflammation of the conjunctiva, and the deeper parts of the eye are also seen to be inflamed. The temperature may be a little above normal, but it is not usually greatly elevated. After this, other changes appear. The iris gradually loses its lustre, and appears of a dull yellow colour; the fluid in the anterior chamber of the eye (aqueous humour) becomes thick and turbid-looking; and the cornea becomes blurred. This period of inflammation may last up to 10 days, after which it gradually disappears and the eye returns to practically its normal appearance. Usually in three weeks from the first symptoms the eye shows but little wrong, except upon minute detailed examination. Then there is a period of normality which may endure for from 3 weeks to 3 months. Once again a second attack, perhaps in the same eye, perhaps in the other, occurs. The symptoms are essentially the same as in the first attack, but it takes longer for the eye to clear again. Each succeeding attack leaves the eye worse than before, until after several attacks the lens begins to show whitish streaks running through it, and the eyesight becomes impaired. Total blindness follows, the eye having an appearance suggestive of a cataract, and the skin of the eyebrow, above the upper eyelashes, becoming wrinkled in concentric lines.

Treatment.—Affected animals should be housed in a roomy shaded loose-box, or may be provided with an eyeshade when out in bright sunlight. The horse should be kept on light laxative food. In the acute inflammatory stage, warm salt-water fomentations are useful to allay the pain, and to stimulate resolution. Professional advice should be sought.

PERIOPLE (*see* FOOT OF THE HORSE, p. 350).

PERIOSTEUM (περιόστεος, round the bones) is the membrane surrounding a bone. The growth of a bone in its thickness is due to the action of the cells of this membrane forming fibrous tissue in which lime salts are deposited. (*See* BONE.)

PERIOSTITIS (περιόστεος, round the bones) means inflammation on the surface of a bone affecting the periosteum. (*See* BONE, DISEASES OF.)

PERIPHERY (περιφέρεια, the outer part) means the outer parts of the body as distinct from the central parts. Peripheral neuritis is an inflammation affecting the nerves in the outer parts of the body, the central nervous system being healthy.

PERISTALSIS is the name applied to the characteristic movement that takes place in the tubular organs of the body, such as the intestines, œsophagus, and the ureters. The movement is somewhat similar to the motion of a worm during progression, when viewed from the outside. It consists of firstly a slight dilatation of the calibre, associated with a small amount of shortening in length, then a vigorous contraction follows, the contraction taking place in a longitudinal as well as a transverse direction. The result is that the food material which is contained at any particular part is squeezed, mixed, and propelled forwards. In some parts of the bowel a reverse action takes place, by which the food is forced back towards the mouth. This is called ' reverse peristalsis ' and is seen particularly in the small intestines. (*See* INTESTINES.)

PERITONEUM (περιτόναιος, a stretched membrane) is the membrane lining the abdominal cavity, and forming a covering for the organs contained in it. That part lining the walls of the cavity is called the ' parietal ' peritoneum, and that part covering the viscera is known as the ' visceral ' peritoneum. The peritoneal membrane forms a closed sac, since both the visceral and parietal portions are continuous with each other along the roof of the cavity. One may understand its relationship to each of the organs by conceiving them to have been forced into this sac from above, in much the same way as the closed fist can be forced into a partially blown-up football bladder. Each organ is wrapped in a covering of peritoneum—its visceral layer—but the outer layer remains intact. In this way there results a fold of the membrane connecting the visceral with the parietal part, which is known as a ' ligament ', ' fold ', or ' mesentery '. (*See* MESENTERY, OMENTUM.) The folds of peritoneum passing from the roof of the abdomen and suspending various organs, and from one organ to another, are thus very complicated and difficult to describe without visualisation.

It has been stated that the peritoneum is a closed sac, but in the female there are two exceptions to this statement—the two Fallopian tubes or oviducts. Each of these has a small opening, leading into the uterus eventually, by which ova from the ovary can be passed into the uterus for expulsion or fertilisation. (*See* REPRODUCTION.) There is, however, no great opening by which fluids may be drained away, and there is always a small amount of lubricating fluid present in the sac as a consequence. The absence of any drainage makes inflammation of the peritoneum a very serious condition, for septic fluids, which might otherwise escape, remain to irritate and cause a spreading of the inflammatory condition to surrounding clean areas.

In structure the peritoneum consists of a dense, though very thin and elastic, fibrous membrane covered, on its inner side, with a smooth glistening layer of plate-like epithelial cells. Here and there between the cells are minute openings (stomata), each of which communicates with a lymphatic vessel, so that the fluid in the cavity is constantly being drained away into the general lymphatic circulation.

PERITONITIS means inflammation of the peritoneum or membrane lining the abdominal and pelvic cavities and covering their contained viscera. It may occur in an acute or a chronic form, and may be either localised to one part or generally diffused.

ACUTE PERITONITIS — **Causes.** — The direct immediate cause of acute peritonitis is always the invasion of the membrane by micro-organisms. It is very rarely primary, but usually occurs through a wound in the abdominal wall, in the stomach or intestines, uterus, bladder, etc., or through the spreading of inflammatory conditions from one or other of these parts, or from some other area of the body. It may follow castration, when the infection gains entrance by the inguinal canal ; it may occur from metritis, when the germs either pass through the wall of the inflamed uterus itself, or pass up the oviducts and escape by the openings of these tubes ; it may arise during a colic, when there is strangulation or twist of some part of the bowel ; it may occur through punctured wounds of the stomach, etc., such as are occasioned by foreign bodies in cattle, dogs, and cats ; inflammation, with or without rupture of the gall or urinary bladders, may lead to peritonitis, although in some cases rupture of these organs may occur without any accompanying inflammation. Stabbed wounds of the abdomen, penetrating injuries, such as are caused by a broken shaft, a prong of a fork, bullet-wounds, horn-gores from cattle, and the wounds caused by the tusks of boars, are other causes. Peritonitis may occur during the course of anthrax, acute tuberculosis, etc., when the organisms responsible for these conditions invade the peritoneal cavity and set up inflammation.

Symptoms.—There is usually the history of some pre-existing disease or injury, in which the abdomen has become implicated. The animal suffers great pain and is very much distressed, even before there are any definite symptoms which point to the abdomen as the seat of the trouble. In a short while, however, it becomes restless, looks round at the sides of the abdomen, paddles with the hind feet or paws with the fore, stands with the fore limbs apart, and moves as little as possible. Horses and cattle usually remain standing, but the smaller animals lie almost continually. The temperature is raised from 3 to 6° F., and the pulse is quick, small, and wiry. Fæces and arise are usually retained and lead to further complication, and vomiting in dogs is common. Pressure over the sides of the abdomen is painful, and the animal usually 'boards' the muscles of the abdomen, and may groan or grunt. As the disease progresses fluid may be thrown out into the cavity in great quantities, leading to dropsy or ascites. (*See* DROPSY.)

Treatment.—Operative treatment and drainage in the larger animals is seldom practicable, but it may be undertaken in dogs and cats. The cavity is opened and irrigated with penicillin solution, and penicillin and/or sulpha drugs may be given by injection. Hot fomentations to the abdomen relieve the acute pain. Nevertheless, in spite of what is done for an animal suffering from acute peritonitis, a fatal termination is by far the most common result.

CHRONIC PERITONITIS.—**Causes.**—Slowly forming abscesses in the liver of the ox, tuberculous lesions in the peritoneal cavity, foreign bodies in the reticulum of the ox, etc.

Symptoms. — There may be slight attacks of pain at times, but very often it is only after death that the condition is discovered. Ascites, or 'dropsy' of the abdomen, and a gradual loss of condition may be seen.

Treatment.—Surgical incision of the adhesions where they are present, is indicated. (*See* RUMENOTOMY.)

ASCITES or DROPSY (*see* DROPSY).

PERMANGANATE OF POTASH is a crystalline substance of brilliant purple hue. Permanganate of sodium is red in colour, and is the chief ingredient of Condy's disinfecting fluid, having an action similar to that of the potassium salt. Potassium permanganate dissolved in water is of a brilliant purple colour, and has a powerful oxidising action, in exerting which it disintegrates alkaloidal poisons and kills low forms of life, such as bacteria. It is itself decomposed as a result of exerting its oxidising powers, so that it gradually loses strength. *Green Condy's Fluid* contains sodium manganate which has a similar action.

Uses.—Permanganate of potassium is a cheap antiseptic which is used for dressing clean wounds in strengths of from 1 : 1000 to 1 : 200, dissolved in water. A solution which has a crimson tint (*i.e.* about 1 : 500 strength) makes a useful oxidising lotion for washing ulcers. In weaker solution still (about 1 : 1000), it is used as a uterine douche for all animals when septic conditions have arisen through retention of the afterbirth.

The permanganates are antidotes to poisoning by opium, strychnine, colchicum, oxalic acid, and snake venom. A pale pink solution of potassium permanganate is also a delicate test for the purity of drinking water; a drop or two allowed to fall into a glass of water should tinge the latter pink, but if the pink colour disappears, it indicates the presence of organic impurities.

PERNICIOUS ANÆMIA, or SWAMP FEVER, also called equine pernicious anæmia, is another name for the anæmia that affects horses in certain parts of America. (*See under* EQUINE.)

PERONEAL (περόνη, the fibula) is the name applied to the muscles, nerves, etc., that lie on the outer or fibular side of the hind limb.

PEROSIS (*see under* 'SLIPPED TENDON').

PEROXIDE OF HYDROGEN (*see* HYDROGEN PEROXIDE).

PERSPIRATION, or SWEAT, is an excretion from the skin, produced by microscopic sweat-glands. These glands are only present scattered over the surface of the whole body in the horse among the domesticated animals. There are certain parts of the skin which sweat more readily than others, *e.g.* the bases of the ears, under the forearm, and around the dock, and generally speaking, fore parts of the trunk sweat more quickly than do the hinder parts. Mules and donkeys do not sweat readily, and when they do it is generally confined to the bases of the ears. Oxen sweat at their muzzles very freely at all times, and only very rarely over the rest of the body. It is said that sheep perspire in hot weather when carrying a heavy fleece, and dogs and cats perspire through the pads of their feet only.

The process of perspiration continues always, but during ordinary conditions the moisture evaporates from the mouths of the sweat glands almost as fast as it is formed; this is known as 'insensible perspiration', and according to Colin amounts to about 14 pounds of water per day of 24 hours in the average horse. When the secretion is rapid and copious or the surrounding atmospheric conditions are not favourable to evaporation the animal visibly perspires and is said to 'sweat', and the process is called 'sensible perspiration'.

In horses there is a certain amount of complementary interaction between the kidneys and the sweat glands. For example, when the horse is sweating freely less urine is excreted by the kidneys, and *vice versa*. In this way it is known that the sweat consists to a very great extent of the waste products of the body, and by analysis it is found to consist of: water, 94·4 per cent; organic matter, 0·5 per cent; mineral matter, 5·1 per cent, so that its importance as an eliminating agent is great.

The excretion of organic matters is of some importance, because in a horse which perspires freely the loss of albumin per day is so much that condition is actually lost through excessive sweating in horses in soft condition. The only remedy for this is to prevent sweating by clipping. (*See* ANHIDROSIS.)

PERTHE'S DISEASE.—This name is given to a deformed condition of the head of the femur met with in children aged 3 to 8 years old. It simulates tuberculosis of the joint. The name is also applied to a similar condition recognised (by means of X-ray examination only) in the dog. The animal is noticed to be lame. The condition may clear up spontaneously within six months, but during that time drugs to relieve pain are indicated.

PERVIOUS URACHUS is a condition which sometimes occurs in foals generally of a weakly nature, and is due to failure on the part of the umbilicus to close at or before birth. In the condition, which is also popularly called 'leaky navel', there is a continual dribbling of urine and serum from the navel.

Before birth the urinary bladder is in direct communication with the fluid in the allantoic sac, and the fœtal urine which is formed escapes into this sac, thus preventing over-distension of the bladder. Immediately before the young animal is born, this communication is narrowed down to only a very small passage, and at birth it is either already closed, or it has practically ceased to function as a means of escape for the urine. With the tying of the umbilical cord, or with the shrinkage that follows exposure of this structure to the air, the urachus, which hitherto has connected the bladder with the outside of the foal's body, becomes quite impervious in the normal animal, and the urine now escapes by the urethra or natural passage to the outside. In pervious urachus this closure does not take place, and there is a continual dribble from the region of the umbilicus. The fluid tends to blister the skin of the surrounding area, and causes considerable discomfort, besides being very unsightly. Surgical treatment is necessary.

PESSARIES (πεσσός) are compounds of drugs made up with a basis of coco butter and some antiseptic element, which are used for introduction into the natural cavities of the body so that they may dissolve and liberate their active substances slowly. They are mainly used for the uterus and for the teat-canals of the mammary gland. In some instances pessaries are made with dry powders of the active antiseptics filled into gelatine capsules. (*See* SYNCRO-MATE.)

PET ANIMALS ACT, 1951.—A law relating to the licensing of pet shops and the conditions under which animals are kept there and offered for sale.

PETECHIÆ (Ital. *petechiæ*, flea-bites) are small spots on the surface of an organ or the skin, generally red or purple in colour and resembling flea-bites. They may be minute areas of inflammation, or they may be small hæmorrhages into the tissues on the surface of the area.

PETHIDINE.—An analgesic (pain reliever) used for dogs and cats.

PETRI DISH.—A shallow circular glass dish with lid in which bacteria are grown on a solid medium.

pH.—A symbol used to express acidity or alkalinity; pH7 being neutral, a higher figure being alkaline and a lower figure being acid.

PHAGE (*see* BACTERIOPHAGE).

PHAGOCYTOSIS (φαγεῖν, to eat; κύτος, a corpuscle) is the name applied to the process by which the attacks of bacteria upon the living body are repelled and the bacteria destroyed through the activity of the white blood corpuscles. (*See* ABSCESS, INFLAMMATION.)

PHALANX (φάλαγξ) is the name given to each of the main bones below the metacarpal and metatarsal regions. There are three in each limb in the horse, six per limb in the ox, twelve in the pig, and fourteen in the dog. In general each of the digits possesses three phalanges, but the first digit in each foot of the dog has only two as in the thumb and great toe of man. The horse has now only one functional digit left in each of its limbs.

'PHALARIS STAGGERS.'—A condition seen in Australia and New Zealand among cattle and sheep grazing on pasture dominated by *Phalaris tuberosa.* Cattle may show stiffness of the hocks and dragging of the hind legs. Similar symptoms are shown in sheep, with the addition of excitability, muscular tremors, and head nodding in the early stages. Dr. D. J. Richards has stated: 'It is thought that phalaris contains a specific nervous system poison which is normally destroyed in the digestive passage of the animal but, where there is a deficiency in cobalt, the destruction of the poison is impeded and the symptoms occur. Provision of oral cobalt seems to stimulate the growth of organisms in the digestive system which in turn destroy the toxin.

PHANTOM PREGNANCY (*see* PSEUDO-PREGNANCY, *also* 'CLOUDBURST').

PHARMACOPÆIA (φαρμακοποιέω, I prepare medicines) is an official publication dealing with the recognised drugs and giving their doses, preparations, sources, and tests. Most countries have a pharmacopœia of their own, that of Great Britain being known as the *Pharmacopœia Britannica,* or often called the 'B.P.' In the United States the official publication is the *United States Pharmacopœia,* often called the 'U.S.A.P.'

PHARMACOGNOSY.—The science of crude drugs.

PHARMACOLOGY.—The science of drugs, and especially of their actions in the body.

PHARYNGITIS means inflammation of the pharynx. This condition, although frequently referred to as a disease by itself, is in reality only a symptom. It is very frequently present in common colds in all animals, and is met with in strangles, influenza, distemper, etc. (*See* CHILLS AND COLDS; also above headings.)

PHARYNX (φάρυγξ) is another name for the throat, although the word 'throat' is often applied to the region about the corner of the jaws. The pharynx is an irregularly funnel-shaped passage situated at the back of the mouth, common both to the respiratory and digestive passages. It acts as the cross-roads between these systems. Into its upper part open the two 'posterior nares', by which air enters and leaves the nasal passages during respiration. Below is the opening from the mouth, known as the 'fauces'; while lower still is the entrance to the larynx—the 'glottis'. Situated most posteriorly is the beginning of the œsophagus, and on either side are the openings of the Eustachian tubes, communicating with the middle ear. (*See* EAR.)

The walls of the pharynx are composed of muscles which are the active agents of swallowing, along with a sheet of fibrous tissue known as the pharyngeal aponeurosis. On the inside they are lined with mucous membrane which is continuous with that of the several cavities which open into it. In young animals there are collections of lymphatic tissue in the pharynx, to which the name 'pharyngeal tonsil' is sometimes applied.

PHEASANTS (*see* GAME BIRDS, MORTALITY).

PHENACETIN is a coal-tar product. (*See* ANTIPYRINE.)

PHENAZONUM (*see* ANTIPYRINE).

PHENOBARBITONE (*see* LUMINAL).

PHENOL is another name for carbolic acid. (*See* CARBOLIC ACID.)

PHENOL-PHTHALEIN is a substance much used as an indicator in the testing of urine, gastric juice, etc., being colourless in an acid and a brilliant red in an alkaline medium. It is also sometimes given to dogs as a mild purgative. Phenol-sulphone-phthalein has been used as a test for the excretory powers of the kidneys; a known amount is injected into a muscle and the urine is tested by comparison of its colour with that of known standards during the next few hours. Phenoltetrachlor-phthalein is a coal-tar derivative used to estimate the functional power of the liver.

PHENOTHIAZINE.—A pale greenish-grey powder which darkens on exposure to light and is practically insoluble in water. In the body it is oxidised to colourless compounds which are excreted in the urine, and on exposure to air are converted to a red dye.

Phenothiazine has proved a valuable anthelmintic, being particularly effective against *Strongylid* worms in the horse, and against *Hæmonchus contortus* in sheep, cattle, and goats. It has been used in outbreaks of parasitic gastroenteritis in sheep and cattle, and is of great value as a routine preventive of heavy infestations in these animals. It is of no use against *Nematodirus*, however. In the pig it is effective against *Œsophagostomum* in the colon, and in poultry against *Heterakis* in the cæcum. It is not used in the dog and cat.

Phenothiazine may be administered in tablet form given with the aid of a 'balling gun', or special forceps, to sheep and goats; or as a drench. In the form of a powder it is conveniently given in dry food or mash to horses, cattle, and poultry. Fasting, and the giving of a purgative afterwards, are unnecessary.

Toxicity.—Young animals are more susceptible than older ones; sheep are more resistant than horses. Lambs under one month old, in-lamb ewes, or young foals should not be dosed with phenothiazine. In the horse cases of idiosyncracy have been reported, and overdosage has led to hæmolytic anæmia. (The reddish colour of the urine should not be confused with hæmaturia.) In cattle, symptoms of poisoning have been reported as dullness, weakness of the hindquarters, prostration, and coma. In calves exposed to bright sunlight following the administration of phenothiazine, a form of light-sensitisation and keratitis may occur, even in the United Kingdom. (*See also* THIABENDAZOLE, METHYRIDINE.)

PHENOTYPE.—In heredity this refers to all the individuals showing the same characters. The term can also mean the individual resulting from the reaction between genotype and environment.

PHENYTOIN SODIUM.—An anti-convulsant drug, more effective than the bromides and phenobarbitone.

PHEROMONE.—A chemical substance produced by one individual which affects the behaviour or physiology of another. The most obvious mammalian example is the odour which attracts the dog to the bitch ready for mating. In pregnant mice the odour of a strange male regularly causes fœtal resorption. Two compounds in the breath of a boar will stimulate a gilt or sow to display mating behaviour.

PHIMOSIS (φιμός, a muzzle), or PHYMOSIS, is the name given to a narrowing of the prepuce as the result of which protrusion of the penis is difficult or impossible. It is commonest among dogs, and relief is obtained by incising the narrowed aperture to make it larger.

PHLEBITIS (φλέψ, a vein) means inflammation of a vein. (*See* VEINS, DISEASES OF.)

PHLEBOTOMY (φλάψ, a vein; τέμνω, I cut) is the name for the operation of cutting a vein so that blood may be drawn. Formerly it used to be practised extensively not only among animals but in the human patient. In modern practice the vein is never cut but a hollow needle used when taking blood that is to be tested for the presence of disease; when immunised blood is being drawn from a hyper-immunised animal; and when it is imperative that the blood-pressure be reduced at once. The jugular vein is generally selected as being most accessible, and is raised by a cord passed round the neck to partially obstruct the circulation, a bandage or other pad being placed in the jugular furrow. In the dog the radial vein is used; in the pig an ear vein.

PHOLEDRINE SULPHATE.—A drug

which raises the blood-pressure, and is used in cases of heart failure after pneumonia or bronchitis and shock.

PHOSGENE.—This gas, first produced experimentally by John Davy in 1812 by the combination of carbon monoxide with chlorine in the presence of sunlight, has the formula $COCl_2$. Phosgene has a characteristic smell of musty hay, and is ten times more toxic than chlorine. The gas in the presence of water is converted into carbon dioxide and hydrochloric acid, and it is the latter which damages the lung tissues, giving rise to pulmonary œdema. Horses usually die between the 7th and 24th hour following exposure to the gas. Birds are highly susceptible. The gas may be liberated from chloroform, carbon tetrachloride, and paint strippers in the presence of heat. Stillbirths and heavy piglet losses followed the feeding in the U.S.A. of mouldy, weevily grain which had been fumigated with a mixture containing carbon tetrachloride.

PHOSPHATES are salts of phosphoric acid, and as this substance is contained in many articles of food, in bone, the nuclei of cells, as well as in the nervous system, quantities are continually excreted in the urine. The forms of phosphates that are excreted in the urine are phosphates of sodium and potassium which are soluble, phosphates of calcium and magnesium which become insoluble and are deposited when the urine is alkaline, and the double ammonium magnesium phosphate. Excess of phosphatic content in the urine leads, after a time, to the deposition of stones or calculi of a phosphatic nature in the kidneys, ureters, bladder, and urethra. Dogs and cats that are fed almost exclusively on fish of one kind or another frequently suffer from calculi in old age. (*See also under* PHOSPHORUS.)

PHOSPHORESCENCE of meat is a luminous condition due to the organism *Photobacterium phosphorescens*. The meat is apparently unchanged during the daytime, but in the dark it glows with a yellowish light. Fish, especially herring, show this condition normally, but sausages, pork, and occasionally beef may also exhibit the phenomenon. It is not associated with unwholesomeness.

PHOSPHORUS itself is not used in veterinary medicine.

Phosphorus is usually given in the form of one or other of the glycerophosphates, or hypophosphites of sodium, potassium, calcium, magnesium, or iron, which possess the tonic and nerve-stimulating actions of phosphorus without its dangers. (*See* PARRISH'S FOOD.) Preparations are used with calcium and dextrose in the treatment of 'Milk Fever'.

PHOSPHORUS DEFICIENCY.—This is seen in rickets, 'milk lameness', post-parturient hæmoglobinuria, and may complicate 'Milk Fever'. (*See under these headings and infertility.*)

PHOSPHORUS POISONING may occur in the dog and cat, either through puppies eating matches, or from animals gaining access to rat poison made with phosphorus.

Symptoms.—When an animal has been poisoned by phosphorus there is acute abdominal pain, vomiting, intense thirst, diarrhœa, and great dullness. The material vomited may be green in colour and is often luminous in the darkness. Collapse rapidly follows, and the animal dies in a few hours. Or, where less has been taken, death may not occur for two or three days. In chronic instances, where small amounts are taken over a considerable period of time, there is fatty degeneration of the liver and kidneys, abdominal disturbance with increasing loss of condition, jaundice, and extreme weakness.

Treatment.—An emetic should be given at once, so soon as the symptoms appear, such as sulphate of copper (bluestone) in doses of 5 grains to a collie or Airedale, and less in proportion to smaller animals. This induces vomiting, gets rid of the majority of the phosphorus, and renders inert what remains. In 15 minutes another dose of one grain dissolved in water as before should be given, and this should be repeated every quarter of an hour till four doses have been given. In all cases, *white of egg, milk, oils, and fatty substances* must be avoided, for these dissolve the phosphorus and render it able to be absorbed with greater rapidity. (*See also* **ORGANO-PHOSPHORUS POISONING**, which arises from contamination with certain farm chemicals.)

PHOTOPHOBIA (φῶς, light; φόβος fear) means a condition in which an animal, suffering from inflammation in the eye objects to a strong light falling upon the eyes.

PHOTOSENSITISATION (*see* LIGHT SENSITISATION).

PHRENIC NERVE (φρήν, the diaphragm) is the nerve which is concerned in supplying the diaphragm. It arises from the 5th, 6th, and 7th cervical spinal nerves, passes through the thoracic cavity, and ramifies in the muscular part of the diaphragm.

PHTHIRIASIS (φθείρ, a louse) means the condition of matted hair, scurf, dirt, and enlarged glands that results from a heavy infestation with parasitic lice. (*See* PARASITES.)

PHTHISIS, or PHTHYSIS (φθίσις) means wasting, and is generally applied to tuberculosis affecting the lungs. (*See* TUBERCULOSIS, PNEUMONIA.)

PHYCOMYCOSIS.—A rarely reported fungal disease of the intestines and/or lungs occurring in both domestic and laboratory animals. A monkey died from systemic phycomyosis in the U.K. (*Vet. Record* Nov. 6, 1965) after symptoms—loss of appetite, depression, and laboured breathing—observed over a 4-year period. For a case in a dog, see *Vet. Record*, June 21, 1969.

PHYLLŒRYTHRIN. — A substance formed in the rumen from chlorophyll by bacterial digestion. Some is absorbed and excreted in the bile, but when the liver is damaged in any way the phyllœrythrin may reach the peripheral circulation and give rise to Light Sensitisation.

PHYSOSTIGMINE, ESERINE, or CALABAR BEAN EXTRACT, is a preparation derived from the ripe seeds of *Physostigma venenosum*, a tree from West Africa. It is used for cattle and horses, but is unsuitable for administration to dogs.

Action.—When given hypodermically physostigmine exerts a rapid stimulating action on the muscular walls of the stomach and intestines, as well as on the secreting glands of these organs, resulting in the evacuation of fæces and an increased amount of fluid in the bowel contents. If the drug be given in large quantities paralysis of the nervous system takes place, although consciousness is maintained. The pulse-rate is slowed and the blood-pressure rises. Respiration is hastened at first and then slowed; the secretions from all the glands of the body are increased; the pupil is contracted, and intra-ocular pressure is lessened.

Uses.—The chief use of physostigmine is in the treatment of certain forms of colic in the horse, and in impaction of the rumen of the ox. It is most useful when a rapid evacuation of the contents of the bowels is desired, such as in stoppage affecting the large colon or cæcum. Externally, it is employed in cases of inflammation of the iris when adhesions are feared. It is then alternated with atropine which has the opposite effect, and is generally instilled into the pocket of the lower eyelid and massaged over the surface of the affected eye.

PHYTIN.—A substance present in oatmeal, maize meal (and in other cereals) antagonistic to calcification of bone, and thus a rickets-producing factor.

PIA MATER (*pius*, tender; *mater*, a nourishing structure, literally mother) is the membrane that closely invests the brain and spinal cord in which run the arteries and veins concerned in the nourishment of these structures. (*See* BRAIN, SPINAL CORD.)

PICA.— 'Depraved' appetite. (For causes, *see under* APPETITE.)

PICROTOXIN.—Used in veterinary medicine principally as an antidote to barbiturate poisoning.

PIÉTRAIN.—This Belgian breed of pig dates from about 1920, but the Breed Society was formed in the 1950s. There is uncertainty as to the origins of the Piêtrain, but it is thought that it stems from old native stock crossed with English breeds such as the Berkshire, Tamworth, and Wessex, and with the French breed Bayeux.

There is still some lack of uniformity within the breed, but a constant feature is the extreme development of the hams—perhaps the result of a mutation such as is believed to have occurred in a strain of Devon cattle. The Piêtrain is white with large black spots. It is a pork pig which gives high killing-out and lean-meat percentages, but it is slow growing and has, in comparison with Large Whites and Landrace, a somewhat high food conversion ratio.

The boars attain a weight of between 550 and 650 lb.; sows 600 lb. The sows are usually quiet and docile. Litter-size is smaller than that expected in the U.K.

PIG, THE, as seen by research workers: The fastest-growing of the domestic animals, prone to heart troubles and disease of the arteries, greatly affected in body by mental stress.

PIG, EXTERNAL PARASITES OF THE.—Half the bacon pigs examined at an abattoir were found to have external parasites—mange mites, lice, or forage mites; and a recent survey made at the Department of Veterinary Medicine, University of Edinburgh, suggests that 20 per cent of pedigree pigs and piggeries in Britain are infested with sarcoptic mange mites.

The itchiness and scurfiness of many infested pigs are attributed to the results of dry feeding or of a zinc deficiency, but pig breeders would be wise not to be in too much of a hurry to make this assumption.

A proper investigation by a veterinary surgeon would not merely pay for itself, but could effect a big saving; for mange can have an important effect upon food conversion ratios. Moreover, mange can actually kill piglets—and lead to stunting of others which do not succumb.

The use of a 0·1 per cent gamma BHC spray has been recommended by research workers. (The BHC sheep dip for scab protection is not strong enough, they found, for controlling mange in pigs.) In order to be effective, the spray must be directed at, and into, the ears, as these are a favourite haunt of the mites.

It is recommended that, once buildings have been cleared of the infestation, each new intake of pigs should be sprayed.

PIG HEALTH SCHEME.—This came into force in 1968, and was confined to the êlite and accredited herds of the Meat and Livestock Commission's Accreditation Scheme, and to candidate herds. The owners of these herds will be offered free veterinary advice on disease control and eradication, and a free quarterly visit of inspection by a ministry veterinary officer or his own veterinary surgeon. By means of these 'routine herd inspections, the examination of disease incidence, the use of readily available *post-mortem* data and by ensuring that expert advice is acted upon, the health scheme should make it possible to reduce significantly losses through disease'—Dr. D. R. Melrose.

Pig Health Control Association is a private enterprise mainly concerned with spreading knowledge of enzootic pneumonia in pigs, and with setting standards for herds claiming freedom from diseases. (*See also under* HEALTH SCHEMES.)

PIG-MEAL, SURPLUS.—Pig breeders who rear cattle and sheep should be wary of feeding surplus pig-meal to those animals unless it is definitely known that the meal does *not* contain a copper supplement. Sheep are very easily poisoned by repeated dosage of a copper supplement well tolerated by pigs, and the death of a heifer was reported after 5 months of supplementary feeding on pig-meal. Conversely, poultry meal medicated with nitrophenide against coccidiosis, should never be fed pigs. It has caused paralysis.

PIG POX (*see under* VARIOLA).

PIGEON-EYED.—(For this term, as applied to the horse, *see under* CONFORMATION DEFECTS.)

PIGEON POX VIRUS is probably a modified form of the fowl pox virus. It has a low pathogenicity for the fowl, and has been used to immunise the latter against fowl pox and roup.

PIGEONS in cities may constitute a hazard to public health, since many are infected with ornithosis. Some harbour *salmonellas*, and *Cryptococcus neoformans* has been isolated from pigeon droppings (but never from pigeons). Grain soaked in the narcotic chloralose has been successfully tried as bait; loss of consciousness beginning ten minutes or so after eating the bait.

Dieldrin is highly poisonous to pigeons. (*See also under* GAME BIRDS.)

In Scotland a herpes virus has been isolated from racing pigeons, and gave rise to conjunctivitis, rhinitis, and malaise.

In a U.K. outbreak among racing pigeons of Newcastle disease, the symptoms were :—depression, lateral deviation of head and neck, slight paresis of legs and wings with incoordination of movement. No symptoms of digestive or respiratory system involvement, such as is usual with

Newcastle disease (Fowl Pest) in poultry, were observed. (*See also* CLAY PIGEONS.)

PIGLET ANÆMIA.—A common cause of pre-weaning losses among housed pigs.

Cause.—The disease is associated with a deficiency of iron, and is aggravated by cold and damp. (A deficiency of copper and cobalt may sometimes also occur, it has been suggested.)

Symptoms.—Dullness, a pale whitish skin, scouring, and sometimes exaggerated heart-beats.

Treatment.—Turn sow and litter out to grass. Give an iron and copper preparation sold for the purpose.

Prevention.—If outdoor rearing is not desired, give a suitable iron preparation (with cobalt and copper, preferably) at 7 days of age. (A solution made by dissolving 2 oz. of commercial iron pyrophosphate in 1 pint of water is effective; a quarter of a teaspoonful being given daily for 4 or 5 days.) Place a fresh turf in the farrowing house. Acute iron poisoning, often leading to death within 24 hours, sometimes follows the injection or oral dosing of normally used iron preparations. To prevent this it is advisable to wait until the piglets are a week old when this danger is less; it is also wise to ensure that gilts' rations contain adequate vitamin E.

Supplements of calcium carbonate fed to fattening pigs from weaning onwards can cause iron deficiency, shown by reduction in blood hæmoglobin concentrations and rates of live weight gain. This effect is especially marked in litters with low weaning weights, probably because their reserves of iron are generally lower. Iron injections or dosing at weaning will overcome these harmful effects.

A secondary anæmia, due to blood-sucking lice, must be borne in mind.

PIGLET MORTALITY. — Causes include: Aujesky's Disease, 'Baby Pig' Disease, Piglet Anæmia, Hæmolytic Disease, Leptospiral Jaundice, Œdema of the Bowel, Paratyphoid, Streptococcal Meningitis, Swine Erysipelas, Swine Fever, Trembling, Enzoötic Pneumonia, Glasser's Disease, Talfan Disease, Atrophic Rhinitis, and transmissible gastro-enteritis (T.G.E.); also overlying by the sow. (*See also under* ILEUM, for another form of enteritis, *and* DYSENTERY; GASTRIC ULCERS *and* MUCORMYCOSIS; LISTERIOSIS; PERICARDITIS; DERMATOSIS; SPLAYLEG.) A list of diseases which affects pigs usually after weaning is given on p. 726.

PIGS.

HISTORY.—Domesticated pigs are believed to be the descendants of the native European Wild Boar (*Sus scrofa*) with probably an admixture of the blood of the closely related Asiatic species (*Sus vitatus*).

The earliest known remains of domesticated pigs belong to the very early Neolithic period, and are those of a small slenderly built animal (*Sus scrofa palustris*), which differed widely in all its characteristics from the Wild Boar. The remains in question are found in association with those of the so-called Celtic Shorthorn Ox (*Bos longifrons*) and of the Peat Sheep (*Ovis aries palustris*), which were also very small and ill-developed types. The generally accepted view is that probably all three of these early domesticated forms were brought to Europe, in an already domesticated form, from Asia. Hence the *Sus scrofa palustris* may most probably have been derived from the Asiatic *Sus vittatus*.

In later Neolithic times this early form of pig was displaced by another and much larger type whose remains indicate very close relationship with the native wild species; hence it is believed that Neolithic man either started afresh by domesticating the Wild Boar, or that he crossed the early form with wild specimens until it lost its original characteristics. In any case it is certain that the pigs of this country, during early historic times and up till the 17th century, were practically pure descendants of the European wild pig. They were characterised by long and rather narrow bodies and long snouts, and the coat consisted of strong bristles of a rusty colour.

During the 18th and early 19th centuries there were introduced into Britain considerable numbers of pigs belonging to a markedly different type, which originated at a very early date in China and South-Western Asia. This type, variously known as the Siamese or Chinese, and given the specific designation of *Sus indicus*, was of smaller size than the native stock; short-legged and round-bodied, with a short dished snout and a coat of soft hair. Its most marked economic characteristics were its early maturity and tendency towards rapid fattening. At the same time it was both less hardy and less prolific than the native type. The Chinese type was not long preserved in a pure state in Britain, but was widely employed for crossing with the native sorts, and it seems certain that all of our modern breeds have been influenced to a greater or less extent by the infusion of this Eastern blood. The influence is most clearly to be seen in the smaller and earlier maturing breeds such as the Middle White and the Berkshire, while it is least apparent in breeds such as the Tamworth and Wessex.

BRITISH BREEDS OF PIGS.

Eleven main breeds are now recognised in Britain. These are as follows :

White breeds :

The Large White.
The Middle White.
The Long White Lop-eared.
The Welsh.
The British Landrace.

Black and Black-and-White Breeds :

The Large Black.
The British Saddleback.
The Gloucester Old Spots.
The Berkshire.

Red Breed :

The Tamworth.

FOREIGN BREEDS. Pigs imported into the U.K. for commercial use and breeding trials, crossing purposes, etc., include: Duroc, Hampshire, Lacombe, Piétrain, Poland China.

It is only within the last 75 years or so that any particular care has been devoted to pig-breeding in Britain. Before 1884, when the National Pig Breeders' Association was formed, there were no herd books, and pure breeds, in the modern sense, can hardly be said to have existed. Even in the case of the Berkshire, which is frequently mentioned by old writers as far back as the 18th century, it is clear that the old type was rather variable in its characteristics, and was in the main quite unlike the breed that now goes under this name.

In spite of the fact that a few breeds, such as the Small White Yorkshire and the Small Black Breed, have become extinct within the last half-century, the number of recognised breeds in Britain has steadily increased during the same period. Thus, the Large Black Breed Society dates only from 1899 ; the Gloucester Old Spots Society from 1914 ; the Wessex Saddleback Pig Society from 1918 ; and the Long White Lop-eared Pig Society from 1922.

It has been frequently questioned in recent years whether the tendency to multiply breeds has not proceeded too far, and indeed it is difficult to see that more than half a dozen breeds are really necessary in order to meet all the requirements of the farmer as well as those of the consumer.

From the economic point of view breeds of pigs are ordinarily classified as bacon, dual purpose, and pork breeds. The classification is necessarily rather a loose one.

The modern trend is rather towards evolving hybrids, and certainly towards greater use of cross-breeding. For the production of pork or bacon, there is no point in using pedigree pigs, uncrossed.

In Britain there is, to quote Mr. J. White, Chief Livestock Officer, PIDA, ' A place in the industry for breeders who will specialise in producing high quality first-cross females for sale to commercial breeders. Not every breeder will be able to get into the Elite and Accredited Herds Scheme and a number of those outside the scheme may wish to pursue an interesting breeding programme. Those specialists would get pure bred females from one Elite or Accredited herd and a pure bred male of a different breed from another. They would cross the two to produce really good first-cross gilts which they would sell to commercial breeders. The commercial breeders would then use good tested boars or close relatives of such boars on the cross-bred females, and they could then expect the best of both worlds. They would cash in on the testing and selection that has been done for feed efficiency and carcase quality and, at the same time, they would have all the benefits of increased proficiency, improved mothering ability, and better growth rate that stem from hybrid vigour.

' It is a great mistake to think that any cross-bred pig will give better results than any pure bred, or that by crossing pigs one gets a bonus in all the economic characters. Strangely, hybrid vigour results in improvement in those characters which are very weakly inherited, and not at all in the characters that are highly inherited. So far as food conversion ratio and carcase quality are concerned, a cross-bred pig will give about the average of the two parents. For this reason it is very important to know that the pure bred animals used in producing the first-cross are of the highest possible quality. It is in such things as numbers born and

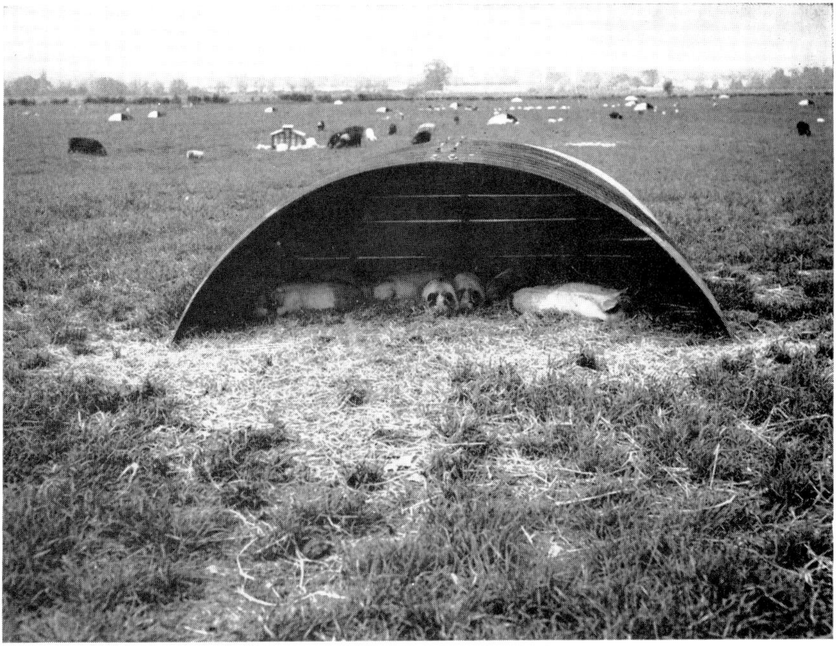

Economical housing on range: corrugated iron, wooden back.

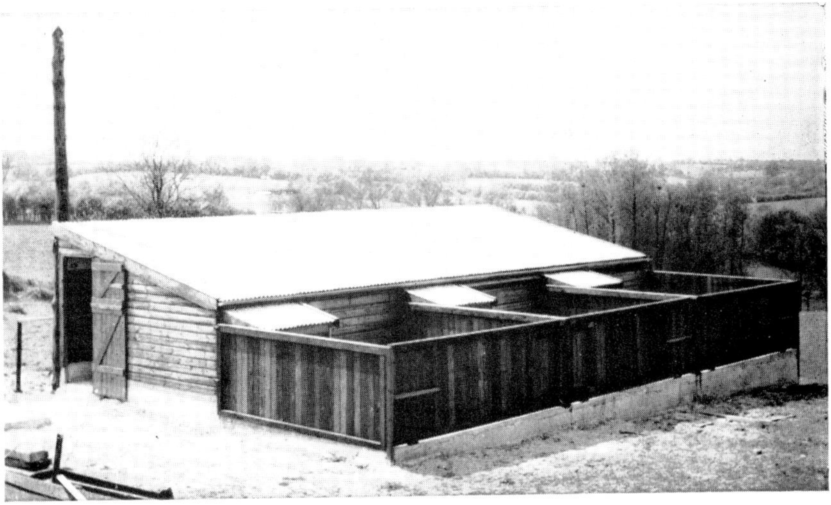

A Harper Adams-type pig parlour

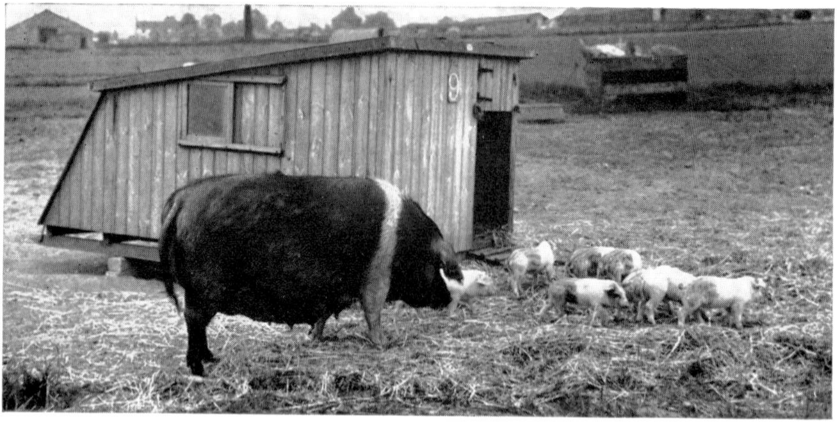

A farrowing house for outdoor use all the year round.

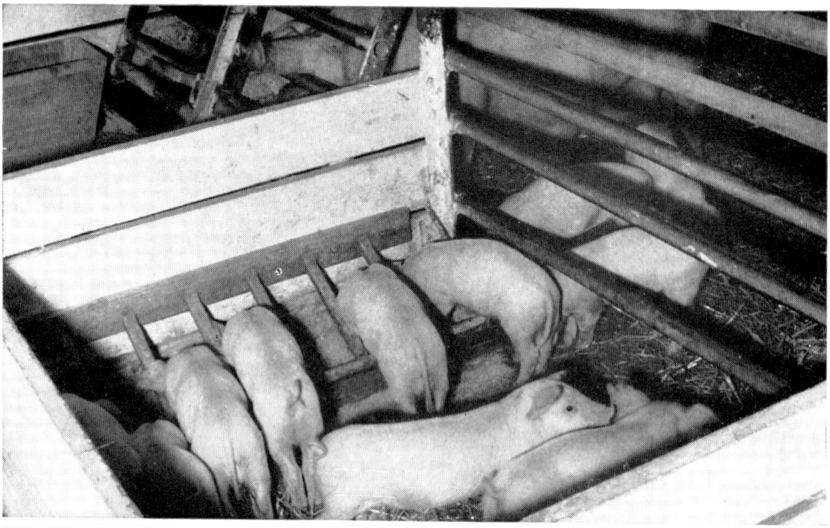

A creep to which the sow has no access. The piglets are Danish Landrace.

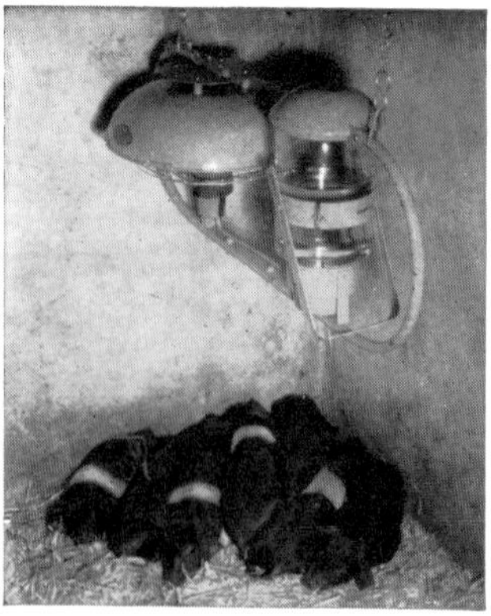

Infra-red electric lamps are commonly used in creeps. Here is an oil-burning alternative.

reared that one can expect improvement from cross-breeding.'

Leading hybrids include the Camborough female, and the Cotswold.

The Large White or Large Yorkshire breed was developed in the vicinity of Leeds about the middle of last century, and pedigree records trace back to the year 1884. The Large White is one of the largest of our breeds, being materially exceeded in weight only by the Lincolnshire Curly Coated. The breed is typically a bacon one, with great length of body, light shoulder, and smooth, neat, yet full, ham. It stands rather high on the leg and is somewhat narrow in build. The head is moderately long, the face slightly dished, but the snout not turned up; the ears, which are of medium size, incline forward but do not hang down over the face. The coat is moderately abundant and consists of rather fine straight hair. The Large White is common and very widely distributed throughout the northern half of Great Britain. It is largely bred in countries which cater for the British bacon trade, and has been exported to most pig-breeding countries in larger or smaller numbers. The Large White is a prolific breed, averaging frequently over eight weaned pigs per litter. It is also hardy and active but not remarkably docile. The breed produces excellent crosses with the Middle White, Berkshire, etc.

The Middle White was originally derived from a cross between the Large Yorkshire and the now extinct Small White or Small Yorkshire Breed. It has now been bred pure for over half a century and breeds quite true to type. This breed is among the smallest of British breeds, being slightly smaller than the Berkshire. The head is short and wide, the face dished and the snout turned up. The ears are rather short, erect, and fringed with long hair. The body is rather short, very wide of back and deep, on short legs. The shoulders are sometimes rather prominent and the jowl somewhat heavy. The ham is thick and well fleshed. The coat is longer and denser than in the Large White. The Middle White is very early maturing, and can be fattened and marketed at almost any age. The sows are reasonably prolific, and are good nurses. The breed, either pure or crossed with the Berkshire, is admirably adapted for producing young porkers, and crossed with the Large White or Large Black makes excellent small bacon.

The Welsh breed is somewhat similar to the last, but tends, on the average, rather more towards the bacon conformation, *i.e.* is longer and rather less plump in build.

The Large Black was officially established by the formation of a breed society in 1899. The old foundation stock, which had been kept tolerably pure for several decades prior to that time, was found partly in Devon and Cornwall and partly in Suffolk and Essex. The Large Black is slightly inferior in size, or at least in length of body, to the Large White. It is characterised by a deep side, light smooth shoulder, and long thick ham. The face is of medium length—shorter than in the Large White, but distinctly longer than in the Berkshire. The ears are long and lax, with the points hanging close together and level with the tip of the nose. The colour is a uniform jet black. The breed is both hardy and prolific, and is remarkably docile. The sows as a rule are excellent nurses. The breed is very well adapted for the outdoor system, grazing freely and taking moderate exercise. Under the indoor system it is said to give more trouble than others in the matter of leg-weakness. The breed crosses well with the Large White (for large bacon), or with the Middle White (for pork). The breed was originally confined to the southern parts of England, but is now very widely distributed over Great Britain. It also enjoys a considerable export trade.

The Essex and the **Wessex Saddleback** are two breeds which rather rapidly came to the front since the inauguration of their respective breed societies in 1918. They are believed to be of similar origin, it being claimed that both are nearly pure representatives of the original Old English Pig, with little or no admixture of Chinese blood. In conformation and in colour pattern they show only minor differences, and their separate existence was to the outsider rather difficult to justify. Amalgamation was for long discussed, and materialised in 1968. The **British Saddleback** is the new name.

The Gloucester Old Spots is native to the region embracing North Somerset, Gloucester, and part of Wiltshire. It is of large size, reaching weights comparable to those of the Large Yorkshire. The head is of medium length, rather similar to that of the Large Black. The ears are lax but slightly shorter than those of the Large Black, with the tips hanging rather wider apart. The colour is spotted—

clearly defined spots of black on white ground or *vice versa*, with the skin and hair colour corresponding. The coat is rather abundant, both long and thick, but straight and silky and with no strong bristles in the region of the mane. The Gloucester has been long bred and maintained under outdoor conditions, and is admirably adapted for outdoor feeding where grass forms a large proportion of the food. It isboth prolific and hardy, and can be fed for market at almost any age.

The Berkshire is one of the oldest established breeds, the breed society dating back to 1884. The face is short and the forehead markedly ' dished ', but the snout is not turned up. The ears are erect and rather short. The body is of medium length, very wide and deep, and carried on short legs. The loin is very thick and the ham heavily fleshed. The bone is fine. The colour is black, with white feet, a white tip to the tail, and a small but varying amount of white on the face. The coat is of medium length and density and of fine texture. The Berkshire is pre-eminent, like the Aberdeen-Angus among cattle and the South Down among sheep, for its combination of early maturity and quality of carcase, its record in open carcase competitions being in fact more remarkable than those of the breeds mentioned. Berkshire sows are not as prolific, on the average, as those of other breeds, and the young pigs in the early stages are rather slow growers. Berkshire boars are very largely used for crossing purposes, the Middle White sow being a favourite cross where young pork is the object in view.

The Tamworth is possibly the purest modern representative of the native English pig. It is found most numerously in the Midlands, particularly in the district about Birmingham. The breed is registered in the Herd Book of the National Pig Breeders' Association, and pedigrees trace back in most cases to 1884 or earlier. The colour of the Tamworth is reddish or chestnut, typically ' golden red hair on a flesh-coloured skin '. The snout is very long and straight. The ears are fairly large, rigid, and incline forward. The body is long, with fair depth of side and moderate width, on rather long legs. In other words, the conformation is tha described for the bacon type. The Tamworth is fairly prolific and hardy. It is late maturing, but the proportion of lean in the carcase is very high, and the quality of its bacon is high.

The Landrace.—Landrace pigs were first introduced into Great Britain from Sweden in 1949, and are descended from the indigenous white pig of Scandinavia and Eastern Europe. Improved by judicious selection based on progeny-testing, these hardy pigs were developed for bacon production ; the body being long and having other desirable qualities. At the time of writing, Denmark has never permitted export of her Landrace.

PIG BREEDING AND MANAGEMENT.—Skill and care in the selection of breeding-stock are essential to success in pig breeding, and there are certain qualities and characteristics to which close attention should be directed whatever the breed of pigs and whatever the economic object in question.

Of these one of the chief is the temperament of the animal. Breeding animals should be moderately active, so that they may have the natural inclination to take sufficient exercise to keep themselves in health yet without being restless. They should also be docile ; nervous and excitable sows often occasion great losses among their young at farrowing time. Milking qualities are also of first importance, and are too often neglected by the pedigree breeder with his eye on showyard success. There is a vast difference in the commercial value of litters at weaning time, according to the quantity of milk yielded by the sow. In this connection the number of teats should also receive attention. The number varies quite commonly from eight to fourteen, and since each piglet in a litter takes possession of a particular teat, the number of teats represents the maximum number of pigs that can be properly nourished by a sow. In the more prolific breeds the number in a breeding sow should ordinarily be not less than twelve, and even with the less prolific breeds, ten-teated animals should not be retained in the herd. Prolificness itself is a quality that should be bred for ; if the average litter in a herd can be maintained at eight or nine, a good profit from breeding may be anticipated, whereas with five or six no measure of success in other directions will make the breeding of pigs for commerical purposes a success. This is another quality which tends to be neglected in pedigree herds, where showyard results are too often taken as the criterion of success. Constitutional vigour and ability to make rapid growth are other points of obvious importance. (*See* GENETICS—HERITABILITY OF CERTAIN TRAITS.)

Gilts or Yelts, as young females are

called, are ordinarily put to the boar for the first time at the age of eight to twelve months, so that the first litter is dropped when the animal is from twelve to sixteen months of age. Where maintenance charges are low and where non-intensive systems are in use the older age is perhaps preferable, as the gilt is then better grown and may be expected to produce and rear a better litter. Boars may be used for breeding at from seven to nine months according to size and development. Œstrus occurs, in females that are in good thriving condition, at all seasons of the year, except when the animal is pregnant or nursing. The period of gestation is about sixteen weeks; the time allowed for nursing varies from seven to twelve weeks, and œstrus generally recurs within ten days, and very commonly on the third or fourth day, after the litter is weaned. The whole breeding cycle is thus completed in from twenty-four to twenty-eight weeks, and it is often possible to arrange for sows to produce two litters a year regularly throughout their breeding life. The normal breeding life is five or six years, but exceptionally good breeders are sometimes kept much longer, and twelve years or more is not unknown.

As regards the general system of management, pigs may be kept under the out-door system or the indoor system or a combination of the two. Under the out-door plan, sows with their litters, and groups of from four to a dozen young stock, are given fenced paddocks, commonly of about half an acre in extent. Cheap wooden huts with some 80 square feet of floor space are provided as shelter and the pigs run out and in at will. The advantages of this system are that the pigs get ample fresh air and exercise, keep healthy and grow well; if the paddocks are capable of carrying grass, coppice wood, etc., the pigs have always a certain supply of green food at hand, and are thus able to look after their own requirements as far as vitamins and ash ingredients are concerned. Moreover, the necessary equipment is much cheaper than where substantial permanent buildings are included.

Plate 11 shows Mr. Richard Roadnight's system of economical housing on free range. Apart from some instances of cannibalism, the system provides healthy pigs but it is one which requires ample land.

On the other hand, while pregnant sows and the older sort of stores, etc., do admirably out of doors in most districts, quite young piglets often thrive badly, in the bleaker areas, during the winter months. To afford more protection the fold-unit system may be adopted. In this, each hut, measuring about 8 feet by 8 feet is provided with a stout wooden floor and has an open fold about twice the above length and of the same width attached to it. The whole is movable and can be moved to fresh ground at the necessary intervals. A number of fold-units of this type are usually arranged in a line and move across the field, utilising the crop in a regular manner.

Fattening pigs, if correctly fed indoors, make substantially greater live weight increases than those fed outside. The indoor system, by reason of the smaller space involved, is less expensive in labour, but has the drawback that the pig is absolutely dependent on the ration with which he is supplied; any deficiencies in the mineral or vitamin supply or other errors in rationing lead to serious losses. Pregnant sows thrive best when they have a free range and ample exercise.

HOUSING.—This varies from the simplest to elaborate controlled-environment buildings. Special types of house are often used for farrowing, for rearing up to the time of weaning, and then for fattening; but this multiplicity may involve four or five moves during the pig's life (*see under* STRESS), with a severe check in growth rate and often the triggering off of disease. Accordingly, Dr. D. W. B. Sainsbury has strongly advocated the use of farrowing-to-finish pens.

However, relatively few fatteners breed their own pigs. Bought-in pigs are best kept away from other stock on the farm for 3 or 4 weeks. Dr. Sainsbury has commented: 'My impression is that pigs do much better at this period if they are kept as far away from their dung as possible, and this is one reason why slatted floors and floor feeding rarely work at this stage.

'A popular way of achieving good accommodation at this time is to provide a simple covered straw yard allowing about 10 sq. ft. per pig of total area preferably with part of the area "kennelled" to give a warm sleeping area. If the latter is raised and dark it will usually be kept clean, and the dung placed in the lighter and lower strawed area. Suitable sized groups are of 25–30 weaners and a lean-to yard will be as cheap a method of housing as any, particularly with *ad lib.* feeding from large hoppers.

'An alternative procedure is required by the farmer who cannot use straw or other bedding and there are a number of designs of kennel-type pens with covered or uncovered yards where the muck can be readily cleared away, sometimes with tractor or squeegee, sometimes with a hose to wash it down a drain. An essential of this system is to have pigs in small and separated groups perhaps no more than 20 to a pen.

'After the conditioning period, the usual practice is to finish the pigs under more intensive conditions. This often involves keeping pigs in litter-less pens and there is little doubt that this is the type of environment that can be conducive to tail biting and cannibalism.'

Ventilation.—*at pig level*—becomes all the more important in such circumstances. 'Railed or Weldmesh pen fronts or sides are often preferred as they allow a much better circulation of air in a low-roofed building in particular. Their advantages do not stop there. Many farmers find that it is difficult to get the younger pig dunging in the passage rather than the pen. A sure help is a gate of Weldmesh or of bars, as a new group will appear to follow the habits of its older companions on the other side of the gate.'

Some of the advantages of farrowing in huts are obtained with a modified Solari pen. Dr. Sainsbury comments: 'A major complaint about this design is that it makes access to the creep difficult. A way round this is to build a covered uninsulated passage way behind the pens to allow access above the creep for easy handling of the piglets. This, however, does materially add to the cost and brings it back towards the totally enclosed building.'

(*See also* ROUNDHOUSE, Plates 11 and 12, HOUSING OF LIVESTOCK, INTENSIVE LIVESTOCK, PRODUCTION, SALT POISONING, SLURRY.)

It should be added that it is wise to have separate sections or units which can be cleaned and disinfected between batches.

The pregnant sow may run with others, receiving only a light ration, until within a few weeks of farrowing. The food during this period may be moderately bulky, and it often suffices, if the sow be running on good pasture, to supply about 2 lb. per day of any of the ordinary concentrates such as maize or barley meal or sharps. Where good pasture or other green food is not available care must be taken that protein and minerals are ample. To this end fish meal, meat-and-bone meal, or ground limestone and steamed bone flour, are often included in the diet. When perhaps two or three weeks from farrowing the sow should be removed to the farrowing pen, so that she may have ample time to settle down. Proprietary sow and weaner meals may be fed.

As soon as the signs of approaching parturition are observed (*e.g.* the gathering of litter to make a nest) all long litter should be removed and oat or wheat chaff or chaffed straw substituted. The animal should be disturbed as little as possible, and ordinarily only her regular attendant should approach her. If she becomes nervous or excited there is a risk of her killing her piglets, which should therefore be removed to a well-littered box and kept apart from the sow until she has settled down. The incisor teeth of the young pigs may require to be nipped off in order to avoid irritation of the teats of the sow.

As regards the number of piglets in a litter, the number born varies from one or two to over twenty, and very commonly from six or seven to twelve or fourteen. The number retained should ordinarily not exceed ten in the case of a first litter and twelve or at most fourteen (according to the number of teats) in the case of subsequent litters. Transference of piglets at birth to other newly farrowed sows may often be made successfully, but in case such are not available surplus piglets should be reared artificially (*see* WEANING), or killed, those sacrificed being, of course, the weakest. With indoor-reared piglets, it is highly necessary to give each member of the litter a preventive of iron deficiency anæmia, which is otherwise liable to occur. (*See* PIGLET ANÆMIA.)

The age for weaning piglets is usually eight weeks. Where for any reason the sow is not wanted for breeding again immediately, the period of suckling may be extended by an additional week or two. In countries with a severe winter climate, where only spring litters are satisfactory and where consequently only one litter per annum is bred, the last course is that normally followed. (For early weaning, *see under* WEANING.)

About seven days after weaning the sow will generally come on heat, and should normally be served at this time. Exceptions may be made in the case of animals in very reduced condition or where immediate breeding would bring the resulting litter at a bad season of the year. November should generally be avoided, as pigs born in that month are ready for weaning in mid-winter, and are often unsatisfactory.

Piglets should have a comfortable and draught-proof sleeping place, and should at all times be provided with a dry bed.

FEEDING.—A great variety of food-stuffs are used for pig feeding, but a majority of those commonly employed are far from forming balanced rations. For example, barley, maize, and potatoes are deficient in protein; wheat offals are seriously deficient in lime, and most of the cereals are lacking in vitamin A. Many unsatisfactory results are directly attributable to badly balanced rations. (*See* CONCENTRATES.)

The growing pig needs at least ten amino-acids in order to form body proteins, but if any of these is missing then the process does not take place satisfactorily and protein is excreted. Moreover, a balanced protein, containing all essential amino-acids, will be partly wasted if the energy content of the ration as a whole is inadequate. For this reason, in the young pig's ration it is essential to have some animal protein, of which white fish meal is the best.

In the creep feed (*see* CREEP-FEEDING), at least 15 per cent should be present, reducing to 10 per cent or not below 7 per cent during the growing period. For the fattening pig, when protein deposition is low, a good quality vegetable protein will suffice. Breeding stock with a high protein requirement should be provided with about 10 per cent as animal protein.

If white fish meal is included, it will provide much of the necessary minerals; but if other proteins are used a reliable pig mineral mixture should be added. The ration should provide about 0·65 per cent calcium, 0·45 per cent phosphorus, 0·5 per cent common salt, and trace elements, including zinc, are necessary. It is advisable to provide vitamins A and D also—and this applies not only to pigs indoors, receiving little or no greenstuff or sunshine; but also to sows at pasture, where the grass often provides insufficient vitamin A. The vitamins best added as a special preparation according to the manufacturer's recommendations. (*See* RATIONS, ANTIBIOTIC SUPPLEMENTS, COPPER SUPPLEMENTS, SOW'S MILK.)

The digestive system of the pig is not well adapted for dealing with fibrous and bulky foods, and a large proportion of the ration must consist of materials with a low fibre content.

Hard grains should be ground. Household refuse, damaged potatoes, heated grain, etc., should be steamed. The cooking of sound food-stuffs is not to be recommended, as their digestibility is lowered thereby and no compensating advantage is gained. Potatoes, however, require to be steamed if any considerable quantity is being fed.

Ordinary meals may be given either dry or soaked, and in the former case are often supplied by means of self-feeders. These permit the pig to feed at will without fear of wastage, and give satisfactory results for fattening animals if they be of some age and if they have opportunities for sufficient exercise.

Floor feeding, Dr. D. W. B. Sainsbury has commented, has a connection with vices. If pens are dirty and the food goes on top of this muck a scouring, uncomfortable pig can be the result—and it does not seem to take long for the other pigs to set about the weakened individual. Also if ventilation is bad, the dust from meal fed on the floor can appear to induce coughing and fractiousness—in pig and even in pigmen—which is an intolerable state of affairs.

A virtually automatic system of liquid feeding *via* pipelines is not uncommon in large, modern piggeries. Dry meal may be delivered from hoppers in pre-arranged quantities and at set intervals by means of a time-switch.

Experiments have shown that dry-fed pigs took 10 days longer to reach bacon-weight and 0.2 lb. more food for each 1 lb. live weight gain, as compared with wet feeding.

Good results have been obtained by feeding moist barley from a Harvestore tower silo.

A method practised at Harper Adams College is for weaners to be brought into the fattening house at 8 weeks old, and there they have meal from self-feeders. At 100 lb. live weight, the *ad lib.* feeding ceases, and the pigs are trough-fed twice daily. Water is run into the trough (from a conveniently placed tap) and the meal is placed on top, being mixed with the water by the pigs themselves. They are given as much as they will clean up in 20 minutes, subject to a limit of 7 lb. per head per day. (*See* RATIONS.)

The feeding for the last two or three

weeks before slaughter must be arranged with a view to avoiding any deleterious effect on the quality of the carcase. Certain foods such as maize, linseed, etc., produce a soft, oily, and sometimes yellow-tinted fat; fish meal is liable to impart a characteristic fishy taint, and excessive quantities of whey, wet distillery by-products, etc., tend to make the flesh soft and watery.

The percentage of dressed carcase to live weight (the head being included and the carcase unskinned) reaches about 70 in the case of four- or five-month-old animals, about 75 per cent for average baconers (7 months or 200 lb. live weight) and over 80 in the case of larger and fatter animals. (*See also under* FARROWING RATES, ARTIFICIAL INSEMINATION, ROUNDHOUSE, HOUSING OF ANIMALS, BEDDING, FLOOR FEEDING.)

PIGS, DISEASES OF (*see under the following headings:* AGALACTIA; ANÆMIA; ANTHRAX; AUJESKY'S DISEASE; BRINE POISONING; CLOSTRIDIAL ENTERITIS; ENCEPHALOMYELITIS OF PIGS; EPERYTHROZOÖN; GASTRIC ULCERS; HÆMOLYTIC DISEASE; HEAT STROKE; LEPTOSPIROSIS; LISTERIOSIS; MANGE; MASTITIS; MENINGOECEPHALITIS; MILK FEVER; MULBERRY HEART; NECROTIC ENTERITIS; ŒDEMA OF THE BOWEL; PARATYPHOID; PERICARDITIS; POST-PARTURIENT FEVER; PYELONEPHRITIS; RHEUMATISM; RHINITIS, ATROPHIC; SALMONELLOSIS; SWINE DYSENTERY; SWINE ERYSIPELAS; SWINE FEVER; SWINE INFLUENZA; TAIL SORES; TALFAN DISEASE; TESCHEN DISEASE; TOXOPLASMOSIS; TRANSMISSIBLE GASTRO-ENTERITIS; TRICHINOSIS; TUBERCULOSIS; ENZOÖTIC PNEUMONIA. For causes of death among unweaned pigs, see list of diseases, etc., given under PIGLET MORTALITY.) (*See also* FOOT-ROT, GLASSER'S, 'GREASY PIG' DISEASE, STREPTOCOCCAL MENINGITIS, ŒSOPHAGOSTOMIASIS; VOMITING AND WASTING SYNDROME; 'BABY PIG DISEASE'.)

PIGS, NAMES GIVEN ACCORDING TO AGE, SEX, etc.—The naming of pigs at various times in their life, and according to their age, sex, etc., varies in different areas; the following gives the most usual names:

Bussen, Bust, or *Broken Pig* — ruptured.

Sucking, Suckling, or *Sucker Pig*—an unweaned pigling.

Cad Pig or *Ratling*—the smallest in a litter and generally the last born. It is also called a 'Rit', 'Crit', 'Dilling', 'Timothy', 'Rutland', or 'Ritling'.

Gummer, Gunner, or *Runner*—weaned pig.

Store Pig—a pig between the time of weaning and being fattened.

Hog—a male pig after being castrated.

Stag, Steg, or *Seg*—a male castrated late in life.

Gilt or *Yelt*—a female intended for breeding purposes, and up to the time that she has her first litter.

Open Gilt—a female before the operation of removal of the ovaries has been performed.

Closed Gilt—a female after ovariotomy has been performed.

Boar, Bran, or *Hogg*—an uncastrated male.

Sow—a breeding female after the first litter.

PIGS, SEDATION OF.—Sedation is useful to prevent fighting after the mixing of litters or re-grouping of pigs; to 'cure' fighting after it has broken out; to make the aggressive sow accept her litter; to facilitate castration, nose-ringing, detusking, etc. Among drugs used for this purpose is Azaperone, an ingredient of 'Stresnil' and 'Suicalm', claimed to be virtually non-toxic, and short-acting.

PIGS, TRANSPORT OF.—The use of containers for the transport of pigs can reduce the risk of infection being carried on to a purchaser's farm. One crate can hold a complete little group, and keep the pigs from coming into contact with the sides and floor of the lorry—which are often not properly cleaned and which can seldom or never be sterilised.

PILES, or HÆMORRHOIDS, consist of an inflamed and varicose condition of the veins of the anus and rectum. It is not common in animals, and usually only occurs in old fat dogs. It is never such a serious and painful condition as in the human subject, and is frequently amenable to treatment by gall and opium ointment.

PILLS form a convenient method by which medicines may be administered to dogs, cats, and horses, although in the latter animals they are generally called 'balls'. The pill is made up with a suitable basis (or excipient), and the active ingredient is incorporated by thorough kneading or working. Many of the pills for canine work are subsequently coated with chocolate or sugar so that they leave a pleasant taste in the mouth. Most pills are machine-made and dispensed by chemists according to prescription.

Administration.—Pills are given by placing the fingers of the left hand around the dog's upper jaw, opening the mouth with the small fingers of the right hand, and depositing the pill, held between the thumb and forefinger, or between the first and second fingers of the right hand, at the back of the mouth as far back as will ensure that it cannot be brought forward again into the mouth. Dogs can be dosed with pills by cutting a chocolate in two nearly equal parts, removing the contents from the centre, substituting the pill, re-forming the chocolate, and giving it to the dog. Another method, not quite so satisfactory, is to smear the pill with butter, hold the dog's jaws forcibly apart, and drop the pill into the back of the mouth, after which the jaws are shut and held together until a swallowing movement takes place. Pills may also be given by putting them in the centre of a piece of meat, and tossing it to the dog, so that he swallows it without chewing.

To be of use, pills must readily dissolve in the digestive canal. (*See* BALLS, TABLET, etc.)

PILOCARPUS and PILOCARPINE (*see* JABORANDI).

PIMPERNEL POISONING.—The Scarlet Pimpernel (*Anagallis arvensis*) has been credited with causing serious illness and even death to animals eating it, but it is not often that this pretty little plant is taken in sufficient quantity to be dangerous. It is very commonly found in the bottom of cereal crops, and grows with vigour in wheat and oat stubbles. Sheep 'shacking' stubble-fields, or other animals put on to them to eat the green growth, may be affected where there is an abundance of Pimpernel and a scarcity of other green food. On the Pacific coast of America the plant is known as the 'poison weed', but it is probable that its composition varies on different kinds of soils. It contains at least one glucoside (probably two) known as *Cyclamin*, and there are quantities of a saponin-like substance present also. It has depressant effects upon the nervous system.

PINEAL BODY is a small peculiar structure situated in a deep recess of the midbrain. Its function is not known, but it occupies a position similar to the third eye in certain of the lower vertebrata, as for example the lizard, *Hatteria*.

'PINING' (or 'PINE') was a term formerly used to describe any progressive loss of condition in sheep, but nowadays —together with 'vinquish'—it is usually reserved for cobalt deficiency. This occurs in many parts of the world, is known as Bush Sickness in New Zealand, and has been reported in areas of Scotland, Northumberland, Devon, and North Wales, where tracts of land are cobalt deficient.

Symptoms.—Progressive debility, anæmia, emaciation, stunted growth, lustreless fleece, sunken eyes from which there is often a discharge. Mortality may reach 20 per cent. Symptoms are not always as definite and clear-cut as this description suggests, however, and in many instances a 'failure to thrive' is all that is observed or suspected.

Diagnosis.—This is usually based on the history of the flock, and may be confirmed with the aid of the soil chemist and by improvement following cobalt administration. A differential diagnosis between 'pining' and worm infestation must be made, though both may co-exist.

Prevention and Treatment may be effected by the provision of cobalt licks or top-dressing the soil with cobalt sulphate (2 lb. per acre).

'PINK-EYE' is the colloquial name for infectious keratitis of cattle caused by *Moraxella* (*Hæmophilus*) *bovis*; and also for Equine Viral Arteritis.

'PINK TOOTH'.—The colloquial name for congenital PORPHYRIA in South Africa.

PIPERAZINE compounds are used in the treatment of roundworm infestations in domestic animals, including pigs, poultry, and horses. They are of low toxicity and can be given in wet or dry food.

PIROPLASM (*see* p. 636).

PITANGUEIRAS.—A breed of cattle: $\frac{5}{8}$ Red Poll and $\frac{3}{8}$ Guzera (itself originally a Red Poll Brahman) developed in Brazil with Red Poll semen from the U.K.

PITCH POISONING.—This has occurred

with fatal results in pigs after eating clay pigeons, and after contact with tarred walls and floors of pig pens. The symptoms are: inappetence, depression, weakness, jaundice, anæmia.

PITUITARY BODY, or GLAND, or the HYPOPHYSIS, is a small oval body about an inch in diameter, attached to the base of the brain and situated in a depression in the upper surface of the sphenoid bone called the *Sella turcica.* It is a ductless gland, which elaborates hormones, adding these to blood circulating through it. The hormones produced by its anterior lobe regulate growth, control the thyroid gland, the suprarenal cortex, the organs of reproduction, and probably the parathyroids, and induce lactation.

Hormones from the posterior lobe affect blood-pressure, the contractility of plain muscle, and the function of the kidney. (*See also* DUCTLESS GLANDS, HORMONES, PARTURITION.)

PITUITRIN.—An injection prepared from the posterior lobe of the pituitary gland, and containing two distinct fractions; one affecting the blood-vessels and the other the uterine muscle. These fractions are named the 'pressor' and 'oxytocic' principles, respectively. Pituitrin is used in cases of uterine atony, uterine hæmorrhage, pyometra, intestinal atony, and in cases of shock and collapse following severe injury or operation.

In the horse, pituitrin may produce inhibition of the smooth muscle of the gut, and fatal constriction of the coronary vessels. In human medicine, the whole extract is no longer used because of the fear of 'pituitrin shock'; the oxytocic fraction only being employed. (*See* HORMONES, ENDOCRINE GLANDS.)

PITYRIASIS (πίτυρον, bran) is the name of a bran-like eruption that appears on the surface of the skin. *Pityriasis rosea* was recorded in 72 out of 120 litters sired by a certain Landrace boar. Lesions resembled ringworm, were red, and lasted 10 weeks.

'PIZZLE ROT'.—A disease mainly of Merino sheep in Australia. (*See under* BALANITIS.)

PLACENTA (*placenta*, a cake) is the technical name for the afterbirth. Strictly speaking, placenta means the medium by means of which the mother nourishes the fœtus. It is composed of three parts: chorion, amnion, and allantois. (*See* AFTERBIRTH, PARTURITION, REPRODUCTION.)

PLAGUE, AVIAN (*see* AVIAN PLAGUE).

PLAGUE, or BUBONIC PLAGUE, is the name of an infectious disease of man and rats and mice, caused by *Pasteurella pestis.* It has not been recorded as affecting the domesticated animals in temperate climates, at least.

The main characters of plague are fever, swelling of the lymphatic glands, a rapid course, and a very high mortality. At the time of the 'Great Plague' ('Black Death') in 1664–65, 70,000 people died in London out of a population of 460,000. A small outbreak occurred in Glasgow in 1900, but was quickly suppressed.

The intermediate link between the infected rat and man is the rat flea. (*See also* CATTLE PLAGUE *and* PASTEURELLOSIS.)

PLANTAR.—At the back of the hind-limb.

PLANTAR CUSHION is the dense fibro-fatty rubber-like structure which lies immediately above the frog in the foot of the horse, and is one of its most important anti-concussion or shock-absorbing mechanisms. (*See* FOOT OF HORSE.)

PLASMA is the name applied to the fluid portion of the blood.

PLASMA SUBSTITUTES (*see* DEXTRAN, GELATIN).

PLASMODIUM GALLINACEUM. — *Plasmodium gallinaceum* causes 'bird malaria' in poultry imported into Ceylon, India, etc., with death following quickly upon symptoms of fever, congestion of the comb. Local birds have immunity.

P. duræ causes death in turkey poults similarly in Kenya.

PLASTIC 'BONES'.—A fractured scaphoid in the right hind leg of a racing greyhound has been successfully replaced by a plastic replica of a scaphoid bone. For a further use of plastics, *see under* HOOF REPAIR.

PLATE CULTURE.—The growing of bacteria in a medium contained in a Petri dish which gives a large surface.

PLATING is the cultivation of bacteria on flat plates containing nutrient material. The term is also applied in surgery to the method of securing union of fractured bones by screwing to the sides of the fragments narrow metal plates which hold them firmly together whilst union is taking place. (*See* Plate 6.)

PLEURA, or Pleural Membrane (πλευρά, a rib) is the name of the membrane which covers the external surfaces of the lungs and lines the inside of the chest walls. The membrane is continuous on either side of the body ; that is, each lung is furnished with its own pleural membrane, one layer of which covers the lung and the other is reflected off to line the inside of the chest wall. Where the two pleuræ meet each other in the middle line of the thoracic cavity they form a fenestrated membrane which is generally called the mediastinum and which, in the horse, is important, because fluids or air in the pleural cavity on one side can pass through it to the other side of the chest. (*See* Lungs.)

PLEURISY, or **PLEURITIS,** means inflammation of the pleuræ, or serous membranes investing the lungs and lining the interior of the thoracic cavity.

The pathological changes which the pleura undergoes are :

(1) Inflammatory congestion and infiltration of the pleural membrane, which may spread to the tissues of the lung on the one hand, and to those of the chest wall on the other.

(2) Exudation of fibrin on the pleural surfaces. This exudation is of variable consistence, sometimes composed of thin and easily separated pellicles, or of extensive thick masses or strata, or again, showing itself in the form of a tough fairly thick membrane. It is usually of a greyish-yellow colour, and, microscopically, consists mainly of coagulated fibrin along with epithelial cells, and both red and white blood corpuscles. Its presence causes roughening of the two pleural surfaces, which, slightly separated in health, may now be united by bands of fibrin extending between them. These bands may break up or may become organised by the development of new blood-vessels and by the formation of fibrous tissue, and, adhering permanently, may obliterate the pleural cavity throughout a greater or less space, and interfere with the free play of the lungs during respiration.

(3) Effusion of fluid into the pleural cavity is the last stage. This fluid may vary in its characters. Most commonly it is clear or only slightly turbid, of yellowish-grey, yellowish-green, or yellowish-red colour (sometimes straw-coloured), sero-fibrinous, and contains flocculi of solid fibrin. In some cases, generally those where complications have occurred, or in which the general resistance of the animal is low, the fluid may be deeply coloured, bile-stained, purulent, or rarely it contains bubbles of gas from decomposition. The amount varies. In the horse there may be as much as 10 gallons ; in dogs and cats there may be as much as from 1 to 3 pints. When a large amount is present it may fill the pleural sac to distension, and, pressing upon the lungs (which float above it), may embarrass the functions of respiration and heart action. In some cases the heart may be dislodged from its normal position and become pushed to the opposite side of the chest (especially in dogs) ; while in occasional instances even the liver is forced backwards. In favourable cases the fluid is absorbed more or less completely and the pleural surfaces united by adhesions ; or all traces of the pleurisy having disappeared, the membrane returns to its normal condition.

It should be observed that in very many cases of pleurisy there is but little effusion, the inflammation being associated with the exudation of fibrin. To this form the term *dry pleurisy* is very often applied. Pleurisy may affect only a very small localised area of the pleural membrane of one side (especially in the horse), or parts of both sides may become attacked, or, in the most serious types, practically the whole of the pleural surfaces of both lungs may be involved.

Causes.—Practically all cases of pleurisy among animals are due to the activity of organisms which have gained access to the pleural membranes, either through the chest wall from wounds, or from internally. They may arrive by the blood-stream, they may come from inflammation situated in some adjacent organ or tissue, they may enter from inflammation in the abdomen (*e.g.* during peritonitis), or they may invade the pleura from the lungs. Occasionally, pleurisy in the ox is due to the penetration of a foreign body from the second stomach. A number of cases in cattle, dogs, and cats particularly, are due to the activity of the tubercle bacillus, which causes a dry pleurisy in cattle, but is associated with considerable effusion in the smaller carnivores. In the horse, pleurisy very often accompanies or complicates an attack of strangles, pneumonia, and equine influenza.

Symptoms.—Two forms of pleurisy can be recognised as the result of the symptoms shown by an animal: the acute and the chronic.

Acute pleurisy generally commences suddenly with a sharp attack of pain, during which the animal becomes distressed, dull, and remains almost stationary. Some sweating is often noticed in the horse, and shivering fits (rigors) are seen in all animals. The temperature rises, and may stand at almost any point between 103° F. and 107° F. The pulse at first is hard and wiry, but soon becomes full and soft. The manner of breathing changes. The chest walls become fixed, and the flanks and abdominal muscles labour and heave. The rate of respiration is often many times faster than usual, and there appears to be an inability to expand the lungs fully. The diaphragm moves excessively and carries the abdominal contents backwards and forwards, so that the abdomen appears to be engaged in respiration instead of the chest. This phenomenon is almost characteristic of pleurisy, and is known as *abdominal respiration*. The excessive movements of the abdominal muscles cause the line of the rib cartilages to stand out prominently, and the appearance of this *pleuritic ridge* is another almost characteristic feature of the disease. As would be expected, it is more easily recognised in a comparatively lean horse than in other animals, and may not be discernible in a fat bullock or hairy dog. The animal exhibits pain when its chest walls are pressed upon, and horses and cattle may grunt when compelled to turn sharply. The early painful stage of the acute type may last for from 12 to 48 hours, after which fluid is thrown out and the pain subsides. Before this, however, a short, sharp, 'hacking' cough generally makes its appearance, particularly in the horse. As the fluid collects, the cough becomes less troublesome, but the difficulty in breathing increases. When pleurisy remains confined to one side of the chest cavity, the larger animals, if they lie at all, will generally lie on the sound side during the early stage. As fluid is thrown out, however, they prefer to stand, or when they lie, it is upon the affected side, so that the sound lung can move more freely. These tendencies are not so readily observed in dogs and cats. Upon examination of the side of the chest by percussion and auscultation the veterinarian can usually determine to what level the fluid has risen, but there are cases in which it is not possible to do this. As a general rule, pleurisy is very serious when the level of the fluid effusion is above a line drawn one-third the way up from sternum to spine. The greater majority of cases with as much as or more fluid than this end fatally, but it by no means follows that the majority of acute cases where the fluid is below this level will recover. Pleurisy is always a serious disease; it may cause death in two days, or not until three or four weeks have passed. Recovery may, in other instances, begin after several days.

Chronic pleurisy may be either of the 'dry' type, in which there is but little effusion, or it may be accompanied by effusion. Both varieties may follow an acute attack, or they may arise slowly and without the acutely fevered stage seen in the latter. (*See* TUBERCULOSIS.)

In the dry form the symptoms are vague, and only very careful examination of the chest can reveal the presence of the disease. There is, generally, a certain amount of loss of condition, an irregular appetite, and loss of strength, so that horses and dogs become easily tired upon slight exertion. Periodic attacks of difficulty in breathing, with or without a cough, may be seen, and, between attacks, the respirations are found to be faster than usual. Horses often 'grunt', when threatened with a stick; and cattle may sigh or groan when rising or lying. In the majority of cases adhesions form between the visceral and parietal layers of the membrane; considerable amounts of fibrous tissue are laid down, and the bands so formed embarrass the free movements of the lungs, so that when the animal is called upon to move quickly breathing becomes more hurried than normally; race-horses and hunters become 'short in their wind', and both they and racing dogs (whippets and greyhounds, for example) lose distance, and never again come quite up to their previous form.

Treatment.—Pleurisy is one of those diseases which does not readily lend itself to 'first-aid treatment'.

Expert advice should be sought upon all occasions, for cases of pleurisy benefit by early tapping of the chest to remove the fluid. It is important to establish the presence or absence of tuberculosis. (*See also under* PNEUMONIA *and* NURSING OF SICK ANIMALS.)

PLEURODYNIA (πλευρά, rib ; ὀδύνη' pain) means a painful condition of the chest wall. It is a symptom of pleurisy ; it may be due to fractures of the ribs ; it is sometimes seen in tumours affecting the chest wall, and it is commonly manifested by pressing the fingers into the spaces between the ribs in intercostal rheumatism.

PLEURO-PNEUMONIA means a combination of pleurisy with a pneumonia. Acute pneumonia is often accompanied by some amount of pleurisy, which is largely responsible for the painfulness which accompanies pneumonia. (*See* CONTAGIOUS BOVINE PLEURO-PNEUMONIA.)

PLEURO-PNEUMONIA, CONTAGIOUS BOVINE (*see* CONTAGIOUS BOVINE PLEURO-PNEUMONIA).

PLEXUS (*plexus*, braid) is the name applied to a network of nerves or vessels, *e.g.* the brachial and sacral plexuses of nerves and the choroid plexus of veins within the brain.

PLICA (*plica*, fold) is the term applied to various folded structures in the body.

PLUMBISM (*plumbum*, lead) is another name for chronic lead poisoning. (*See* LEAD POISONING.)

P.M.S.—Pregnant Mare's Serum.

PNEUMOGASTRIC (πνεύμων, lung ; γαστήρ, stomach) or **VAGUS** (*vagus*, wandering) **NERVE**, is the tenth cranial nerve. This nerve is remarkable for its great length, and for the attachments which it forms with other nerves and with the sympathetic trunks. It arises from the side of the medulla, passes out of the skull, runs down to the jugular furrow of the neck, where, along with the sympathetic, it accompanies the carotid artery to the entrance to the chest. From this point the right and left vagi differ from each other in their course. They both pass through the chest cavity, giving branches to the pharynx (which run up the neck again), to the heart, bronchi, œsophagus, etc. Each nerve then splits into two parts and the two upper branches fuse with each other to form the dorsal trunk, the lower branches behaving similarly to form the ventral trunk. These two branches now pass through the diaphragm, with the œsophagus, into the abdominal cavity, and end by giving branches to the stomach, duodenum, liver, and various ganglia near by.

PNEUMONIA (πνεύμων, lung), or inflammation of the lung substance. There are several different forms, but since to describe them all would be to invite confusion and involve repetition, they will be described under three headings : viz. *Acute lobar* (or *croupous*) *pneumonia* ; *Catarrhal, lobular*, or *broncho-pneumonia ;* and *Chronic, fibrous, interstitial pneumonia*, or *pulmonary cirrhosis*. In addition to this classification pneumonia is sometimes spoken of as *parasitic*, when it is caused by minute worms in the lungs of cattle, sheep, and pigs (*see* HUSK) ; *septic*, when the already inflamed areas in the lungs are invaded by septic organisms, setting up gangrene of the lungs ; *purulent*, when quantities of pus are produced in the lungs ; or *mycotic*, as in aspergillosis in fowls (*see* ASPERGILLOSIS). (*See also* ENZOOTIC PNEUMONIA OF PIGS, *and* CALF PNEUMONIA.)

ACUTE LOBAR PNEUMONIA.—This is the disease commonly known as 'Inflammation of the lungs'. It derives its name from its pathological characteristics, which are usually well-marked. The changes which take place in the lungs are three. (1) *Congestion*, or engorgement, in which the blood-vessels become greatly distended ; the lung is voluminous and heavier than normal, and of a dark red colour, and the air-capacity of the lung is reduced. The air cells, however, still contain air, and a piece of lung will float in water. The congestive stage is seldom seen, since it only lasts 12 to 36 hours, and is hardly ever fatal. (2) *Red hepatisation*, so-called from its resemblance to liver tissue. In this stage there is poured out from the gorged pulmonary blood-vessels into the air sacs a quantity of blood-plasma, red and white blood-cells, and other material, which obliterate the lung cells, and render intake of air impossible in the areas affected. The smallest bronchioles are often also filled. The exudate rapidly coagulates into a solid jelly-like mass, which completely excludes air and presses upon the blood-vessels. When cut, the surface has an appearance somewhat like red granite ; it is firm, but brittle ; and when a piece is placed in water it sinks at once. It is to the character of the exudation, consisting largely of coagulated fibrin, that the name 'croupous' is due. This stage lasts usually about two days and then the third stage follows. (3) *Grey hepatisation*. In this stage the lung still retains its liver-like appearance, except that its colour is grey—somewhat like grey granite. The consistence is less firm than in the second stage, but portions of lung still sink in water. The appearance is due to the invasion of the coagulated exudate by white blood corpuscles. The stage of grey hepatisation usually lasts for an indefinite length of time, and gradually merges into what may be called the stage of *resolution*. The coagulated exudate becomes gradually liquefied and absorbed, so that in time the lung cells get rid of their contents and resume their normal functions. In those cases which terminate unsatisfactorily, however, instead of absorption, the liquefied material suppurates, and abscess or gangrene results.

Lobar pneumonia may diffusely affect one or both lungs, or it may be confined to localised areas in the lower parts of the apices. The more extensive the affected areas are, the more serious is the condition.

Causes.—Acute lobar pneumonia is probably always due to an invasion of the lung by virulent organisms, or by normally present organisms at times when the vital resistance of the body, and of the lungs in particular, is low.

Symptoms.—At first, little beyond a very high temperature, accelerated respiration, and a rapid pulse, can be discovered wrong with the animal, and sometimes horses may show such slight symptoms that they are sent out to work as usual. (Such cases generally end fatally.) In from 12 to 24 hours the breathing becomes more laboured, food is refused, the horse appears dull, and the pulse is found to be quick, full, and bounding. Shivering fits, often of great severity, attack the animal, and the coat stares. Later, the surface of the body regains its normal temperature and the shivering ceases. About the second day of the attack the breathing changes to a series of short, quick pants. The neck is outstretched, the nostrils are dilated, and the sides of the chest can be seen 'lifting'. Coughing is not marked unless the animal is made to perform some strenuous work, or is greatly excited; it is never so distressful as in cases of bronchitis. As a rule, a nasal discharge appears; at first it is thin and watery, and later it becomes thick, mucoid, or whitish and purulent. If the discharge assumes a putrid offensive odour it is usually taken as an indication that gangrene has set in.

During the course of an attack of acute pneumonia a horse prefers to remain standing, since in the recumbent position great pressure is put upon the lung space, and respiration becomes most difficult. Cattle lie more, usually upon the affected side; they grunt and grind their teeth. Dogs and swine remain lying almost continually, unless pleurisy accompanies the pneumonia, when they often sit upon their hind-quarters, but keep their fore-end upright. Only when exhaustion is great will any animal stretch itself out upon its side, and when one does so it should be considered as an unfavourable symptom.

There is not so definite a crisis as is seen in lobar pneumonia in human beings, but, in favourable cases, on about the fifth to the eighth day a marked change for the better can often be discerned, and the animal slowly returns to normal. Signs which are to be considered very grave are as follows: a foul-smelling reddish discharge from the nose; an absolute lack of appetite or thirst; a *sudden* fall in the temperature to normal or below it; an apparent improvement occurring suddenly; rapidly progressive weakness accompanied by staggering movements and a very low carriage of the head; slate-coloured conjunctiva; and prostration.

Treatment.—If there is any disease in which everything must be sacrificed in favour of a full and free supply of *fresh air*, it is pneumonia. Immediately the warning signs of the disease are noticed the animal must be removed from its surroundings and housed in some place where there is an unobstructed supply of fresh air, and, if possible, sunlight. The farm animals should be put into a large airy (even cold) loose-box, provided with plenty of bedding, and left with a supply of clean cold water. If the weather is cold a warm rug should be applied and fastened loosely over the chest. Bandages and a long hood may be added in the case of horses, and a second rug may be necessary in the case of those animals which are accustomed to wearing one rug normally. Owing to the danger of a case being of a contagious nature it should be isolated, and, if possible, one attendant should be detailed to look after it. Food is of great importance. (*See* NURSING OF SICK ANIMALS.) So far as medicinal treatment is concerned, penicillin may prove of great value. Expectorants may be necessary in some cases; heart stimulants are needed in others. Applications of mustard or other counter-irritants favour recovery in some cases, but only unnecessarily distress highly nervous animals. Febrifuges are of assistance at times, but may do harm if used to excess. The one golden rule in the medicinal treatment of pneumonia in all animals is '*Do not drench*'. Any medicines should be given hypodermically, or should be mixed with a little spice and added to the food, or in the form of balls or pills.

LOBULAR, or BRONCHO-PNEUMONIA. (*See also under* BRONCHITIS.)—This differs from the last in several important points. The inflammation is more diffusely scattered throughout the lungs, attacking a few small lobules here and there instead of being localised to one or more large lobes, as occurs in croupous pneumonia. At first the affected patches are dense, with a bluish-red appearance tending to become grey or yellow. When seen under the microscope, the air vesicles and the finer terminal bronchioles are found to be crowded with a multitude of cells, the result of the inflammatory process, but there is no fibrinous exudate, such as is seen in the lobar form. In favourable cases recovery results from absorption of the products, but, on the other hand, they may undergo degenerative changes, abscesses may form, chronic interstitial pneumonia may develop, or the affected areas may become almost solid with a caseous material. In human beings, tuberculosis (phthisis) may result from already present centres of infection, and the same change may be met with in the ox, pig, and dog. (Tuberculosis of the lungs is very rare in the horse.) Broncho-pneumonia very often succeeds an attack of bronchitis. It frequently attacks animals in which some specific disease has already become established : thus it may complicate attacks of strangles, glanders, influenza, etc., in horses ; tuberculosis in cattle ; swine fever or tuberculosis in pigs ; distemper in the dog, etc. It may be set up as the result of infection with either animal or vegetable parasites, such as in parasitic bronchitis in cattle, sheep, and pigs, aspergillosis in fowls. Actinobacillosis has been recorded as the cause in rare instances in cattle, and the migration of the immature stages of the ascarid worm of the dog or pig has also produced it.

In addition, the inhalation of irritant gases, the insufflation of medicinal irritants, food, etc., and direct injury to the lung substance by penetrating bodies, such as broken shaft splinters, bullets, the prongs of forks, or other sharp-pointed bodies, may cause it.

Predisposing causes, such as cold, chills, general debility, standing for long periods in slings, or lying for long periods on the ground, etc., are also liable to act by lowering the vital resistance of the lung tissues and allowing the ever-present organisms to attack them.

Symptoms. — The temperature rises to from 103° F. to 105° F. or may be higher in severe attacks. The breathing becomes gradually more and more distressed, and is often accompanied by a short moist cough and a whitish thick catarrhal discharge from the nostrils, which is present from the start. The pulse is fast and strong, and the general impression is that the animal is seriously ill, but not so acutely affected as in cases of the lobar type. Appetite is suppressed ; milk-production is lessened or may cease ; rumination is suspended in cattle and sheep ; the head is extended, and breathing may be through the mouth in some animals. In the dog the lips are often blown out and sucked in alternately with each respiration. The cough is usually frequent and troublesome, and in the later stages it may occur in paroxysms of such severity that they rapidly exhaust the animal. During the resolution stage the cough may bring a copious nasal discharge to begin with, and finally a 'cast' may be expelled. These 'casts' are agglutinated collections of the catarrhal material, which have moulded themselves to the inside of a bronchial tube, and during the process of shrinking and liquefaction have loosened and, being disturbed from their positions by the cough, are forced into the trachea, through the throat, and finally to the outside by the nostrils. They are much commoner in cases which have followed bronchitis than in others. Occasionally they may be bifurcated, but as a rule they are in the form of short cylinders.

The course of lobular pneumonia may last for an indefinite period ; sometimes it proves fatal in three or four days, or it may last for several weeks, passing into a stage of chronic interstitial pneumonia, or ending in recovery. The majority of ordinary cases generally recover from the acute symptoms in the course of two weeks. Relapses may occur, however, and an animal which has been progressing favourably for some days may suddenly become much worse, and even die, if the care in its nursing and general management is relaxed for a little.

Treatment.—As for Lobar Pneumonia. (*See* NURSING OF SICK ANIMALS.)

CHRONIC, FIBROUS, INTERSTITIAL PNEUMONIA, or PULMONARY CIRRHOSIS, is a slow inflammatory change affecting chiefly one portion of the lung tissue, viz. its fibrous framework. The changes produced in the lung by this type of pneumonia are marked chiefly by the growth of nucleated fibrous tissue around the walls of the bronchi and blood-vessels, which spreads to such an extent as to invade and obliterate the air-cells. The lung, which is at first enlarged, becomes shrunken, dense in texture, and solid, any unaffected portions becoming emphysematous (*i.e.* blown out to a larger size than normal). The bronchi are dilated, the pleural membranes are thickened, and the lung substance is often pigmented. In later stages the lung tissue breaks down and cavities are formed. Perhaps the commonest cause of fibroid pneumonia in animals, however, is invasion of the lung tissues by parasitic worm larvæ, or by echinococcus cysts.

Symptoms.—Breathlessness, inability to perform prolonged or strenuous work or exercise, a short troublesome cough, which is often mistaken for asthma, general weakness and debility along with loss of condition, and a staring coat. There is seldom any rise of temperature, or any marked respiratory acceleration so long as the animal remains at rest. Animals may die from mere exhaustion during the course of chronic pneumonia.

Treatment.—Owing to the gross amount of tissue alteration which is characteristic of this form of pneumonia, it is impossible to treat the condition with any success.

PNEUMONIA IN CALVES (*see* CALF PNEUMONIA).

PNEUMONIA IN SHEEP.—In Britain a disease which has spread much in recent years is pneumonia caused by *Pasteurella hæmolytica*. This organism commonly lives in normal sheep, and causes disease only when the animal's resistance is weakened by bad weather, transport from one farm to another, movement from a poor to a richer pasture, or perhaps by a virus. In some outbreaks, where the disease takes an acute form, a sheep which seemed healthy enough in the evening may be found dead in the morning. Usually, however, the shepherd sees depressed-looking animals with drooping ears, breathing rather quickly and having a discharge from eyes and nostrils, and a cough. Death often occurs within a day or two. The last sheep to be involved in the outbreak tend to linger for several weeks, looking very tucked-up in the meantime, with a cough and fast breathing. A vaccine is available. (*See also* MÆDI, JAAGSIEKTE.)

PNEUMO-PERITONEUM. — Distension of the abdominal cavity with gas following rupture of the uterus has been reported in cattle.

PNEUMOTHORAX (*πνεῦμα*, air; *θώραξ*, the chest) means a collection of air in the pleural cavity which has gained entrance through a hole or wound in the chest wall. (*See* LUNGS, DISEASES AND INJURIES OF.)

Pneumothorax is not uncommon in the dog which has fallen out of a window, or been run over or hit by a car. Distressed breathing and cyanosis are, following an accident, suggestive of pneumothorax.

Mild cases may be accompanied by mild symptoms, and spontaneous recovery may occur. Severe cases may die. Treatment includes aspiration of the air. (*See also* COLLAPSE OF LUNG on p. 519.) (For further information, see *Veterinary Record*, Nov. 28, 1959, p. 859.)

'POACHING'.—Especially on heavy land, with high stocking rates, wet weather can bring serious poaching problems. (*See* DAIRY HERD MANAGEMENT.) At gateways deep mud, in winter often at near freezing temperatures, can lead to foul-in-the-foot and mastitis.

PODOPHYLLIN is a resin derived from the root of *Podophyllum peltatum*, a plant of the United States and Canada. It is a mildly acting purge in small doses. In large doses it is a drastic purgative.

POIKILOCYTE (*ποικίλος*, manifold; *κύτος*, cell) is the name applied to a malformed red blood corpuscle found in the blood in various types of anæmia.

POINTS OF THE HORSE.—Through long usage certain names, generally expressive rather than elegant, have been applied to certain parts of the surface of the body of the horse, and are used almost exclusively in popular phraseology. A list of them will be found below. The names of most of the regions are self-explanatory and will be passed over without comment; where names are commonly employed which have been handed down from earlier days, and which apparently have no connection with the parts they indicate, a brief explanation will be given.

From the muzzle to the tail the points are as follows :

Muzzle : the region of the upper lip.
Nostrils.
Bridge of nose.
Face.
Forehead.
Forelock : the tuft of hair which hangs forward from between the ears.
Poll or *Nape of neck :* the region lying between the ears and a little behind them.
Crest : the upper part of the neck from which grows the mane.
Withers : the highest part of the back immediately behind where the neck joins it. The withers are formed by the longest of the spinous processes of the thoracic vertebræ.
Back : from behind the withers to the head of the last rib.
Loins : the region of the lumbar vertebræ. The loin of the ox was ' knighted ' during Charles the First's reign as ' Sir Loin ', since it was the finest quality beef in the carcase ; hence ' sirloin ', which is the flesh in the region of the lumbar vertebræ.
Croup : the region of the sacrum.
Point of croup : the highest point of the croup, formed by the internal angles of the ilia.
Dock, or *root of tail.*

When viewed from behind the following points are seen :

Buttocks : the masses of muscle lying one on either side of the anus and extending downwards to the level of the stifle.
Point of buttock : the prominence formed by the ischial tuber. This is also called the ' angle of the buttock '.
Gaskin, or *Second thigh :* the swell of muscle on the side of each limb, between stifle and hock.
Achilles' tendon, or ' Hamstring ', the large tendon which is attached to the ' point of the hock '.
Point of hock : the uppermost extremity of the hock, formed by the tuber calcis (calcaneus).
Hock : the complex joint formed between the tibia, bones of the hock, and the metatarsal bones.
Back tendons of the hind limb : the flexors, deep and superficial.
Hind cannons : the metatarsal bones between hock and fetlock.
Fetlock : the joint between the lower end of the large metatarsal bone and the first phalanx with its sesamoids. Originally this name was used for the lock of hair behind the joint, *i.e. feet-lock,* now corrupted to ' fetlock '.
Ergot : the horny callosity situated at the back of the fetlock joint.
Long pastern : the first phalanx.
Pastern joint : between the first and second phalanges.
Bulbs of the heels.
Coronet.
Hoof, frog, etc.

When viewed in profile, the following points are seen :

Side of face.
Parotid region : behind the edge of the lower jaw, just where the head joins the neck.
Jugular furrow : the groove above the windpipe, reaching down the under part of the neck.
Neck.
Shoulder : the region of the shoulder-blade (scapula).
Point of shoulder : the prominence formed by the upper extremity of the humerus.
Arm : the region of massive muscles lying over the humerus.
Elbow : between humerus and radius and ulna.
Point of elbow : formed by the olecranon of the ulna.
Forearm.
Knee.
Fore cannon : the metacarpal bones.
Ribs and side of chest.
Abdomen.
Flank.
Point of hip, or *of haunch :* prominence formed by the external angle of the ileum.
Thigh : the region on the side of the hind quarter bounded by the croup above, the buttocks behind, the flank in front, and the gaskin below.
Stifle joint : the joint between the femur, patella, and tibia.
Gaskin, hock, cannon, etc., as already described.

When viewed from a front aspect, the following points are seen :

Muzzle.
Lower lip.
Root of neck.
Point of sternum : the anteriormost part of the sternum.
Chest.
Axilla : on the inside of the elbow.
Chestnuts : in front, above the knee on the inside of the limb, and behind on the inside about a hand's-breadth below the point of the hock.

POISONING.—This usually results from the poison being swallowed. In a few instances poison may be taken in through a wound of the skin, or even through the unbroken skin, *e.g.* when dipping sheep, and occasionally malicious cases of poisoning by hypodermic injection have been recorded, but these are not common. Malicious poisoning is most frequently carried out against dogs and cats, although horses and ruminants also sometimes suffer, but the nefarious practice of poisoning an opponent's animal is, in the civilised countries, fortunately very rare. The use of poison to control vermin —rabbits, foxes, rats, mice, etc.—is commoner, and when the poisoned bait is accessible to domesticated animals, cases of poisoning in them may result. It should be remembered that the exposure of such poison above ground constitutes a punishable offence.

The constituents of common and commercial rat-poisons are mentioned under RAT POISONS (which see).

Many cases of poisoning result from the careless use of sheep-dips, paints, weed-killers, insecticides, which, either in powder, paste, or solution, are left about in places to which animals have access. Cattle are notoriously inquisitive, and will lick at anything they find, sometimes with fatal consequences.

It is perhaps not widely enough realised that cattle seem to like the taste of lead paint—one heifer helped herself to a whole pint of it—and that very small quantities spattered on the ground can kill several beasts. Even the contents of old, discarded paint tins can be lethal. In one instance, children found such tins and scraped out the residue on to pasture, killing five yearlings. In another instance, cattle licked out old paint tins on a rubbish dump in a pit to which they found their way. A recently-painted fence is also a danger; and it is worth while getting a farm-worker to clear up behind any plumber using red-lead.

Thirsty cattle will drink almost anything. Diesel oil and a copper-containing spray liquid have each caused death in these circumstances. Salt poisoning is certainly no myth, and pigs should never be kept short of drinking water.

Some insecticides, such as TEPP and Parathion, are totally unsuitable for use on livestock. Fatal poisoning of a herd of cattle sprayed with TEPP has been reported from Texas. A farmer in Ireland used aldrin as an orf-dressing, and killed 105 out of 107 lambs. Fatal poisoning of cattle has also occurred through the application to their backs of a carbolic-acid-arsenic preparation against flies. Near chemical works, grass, etc., may become impregnated with such substances as copper, lead, or other metals and lead to chronic poisoning of any animals grazing near by. The same thing applies in orchards after spraying of fruit-trees. Pasture may be contaminated by spray-drift or dusting operations, particularly from the air, and the chemicals used may cause poisoning. This applies also to other treated green crops which animals may eat. DDT and BHC and other insecticides (used in home and garden) of the CHLORINATED HYDROCARBON group may poison birds, cats, and dogs. (*See also* ORGANO-PHOSPHORUS POISONING *and* FARM CHEMICALS.)

The use of pitch (the poisonous ingredient of clay-pigeons) or coal tar on the walls and floors of piggeries is a cause of poisoning. Some wood preservatives cause Hyperkeratosis.

Unfortunately, a comparatively common cause of poisoning results from indiscretion on the part of owners or attendants in the use of patent or other animal medicines.

Fodder Poisoning.—Excess of fodder beet may cause scouring in both pigs and cattle, and the after-effects may be serious. In sows just farrowed the milk supply may almost disappear. Beet tops have caused the deaths of cattle when given unwilted, and even when wilted they should be strictly rationed. Kale and rape must likewise be used sparingly and not constitute an animal's sole diet; hay in particular being necessary in addition. Deaths have occurred in horses and cattle restricted to rye-grass pasture. Sheep have been fatally poisoned by feeding them surplus pig-meal containing a copper supplement; a heifer likewise. Pigs have been poisoned by giving them medicated meal intended for poultry and containing nitrophenide against coccidiosis. Which all goes to show that medicated feeds are by no means always interchangeable be ween different species of livestock. (*See* GROUNDNUT MEAL.)

The use of surplus seed corn for pig-feeding has led to fatal poisoning—the mercury dressing having been overlooked! (*See also* DIELDRIN *for poisoning from seed dressings.*)

Hay contaminated with foxgloves or ragwort is a source of fatal poisoning. Silage contaminated with ragwort has similarly caused death. Silage contaminated with Hexœstrol has caused abortion. (*See under* HORMONES IN MEAT PRODUCTION.)

Poisonous plants growing in pastures, in swampy or marshy places, in the bottoms of hedges, on waste land and in shrubberies and gardens, are other very fruitful sources of poisoning. In the early spring, when grass is scarce, and when herbivorous animals are let out for the first time after wintering indoors, the tender succulent growths attract them, often with serious consequences. Similar results may be seen during a very dry summer when grass is parched.

Clippings from shrubs, especially from yew, rhododendron, aconite, boxwood, lupins, laurel, laburnum, etc., should never be thrown 'over the hedge', because in some of these the toxic substances are most active when the clippings have begun to wither, and animals are very prone to eat them in this condition. It is a safe rule to regard all garden trimmings as unsafe for animals, with the exception of vegetables, such as cabbages, turnips, etc.

POISONS.—

Varieties.—Strictly speaking, bacteria and their toxins, the products of decomposing or damaged food-stuffs, the harmful substances produced by insects, worms, and other parasites, and certain animal products like snake venom (known as *zootoxins*), should be included here, but these are dealt with elsewhere (*see* BACTERIOLOGY; BITES; etc.). Leaving these out of account, we may classify poisons either according to their source or to their mode of action. (*See also under* RAT POISONS.)

Classified according to source they are: *animal*, like cantharides; *vegetable*, like yew, deadly nightshade, or hemlock; *mineral*, such as arsenic or corrosive sublimate; and *aerial*, like chlorine gas, carbonic acid gas, etc. But this classification includes in each group substances with the most diverse actions, and a more practical arrangement is made by grouping them according to their mode of action, as follows:

(1) *Irritants*, which generally have an irritant action upon the stomach or bowels;

(2) *Narcotics*, which affect the brain and spinal cord, inducing stupor or narcosis;

(3) *Narcotico-irritants*, which produce, first of all, an irritant effect upon the stomach or upon the nervous system, and later act as narcotics.

(1) **Irritants** include the class of corrosives, very often considered separately, since their action is more concentrated than irritants. They may be so active as to cause corrosion, ulceration, and even perforation of the organs with which they come into contact. The chief *corrosives* are the strong mineral acids, sulphuric, nitric, and hydrochloric; the caustic alkalies, caustic soda and potash; their carbonates in strong solution, and ammonia; and certain strong salts or concentrated solutions of these, such as perchloride of mercury (corrosive sublimate), pernitrate of mercury, etc.; and carbolic acid in strong solution. Among the *irritants* are included the vegetable acids, some acid salts, such as tartar emetic; white arsenic (arsenious acid), yellow arsenic (orpiment), acetate of lead (sugar of lead), subacetate of copper (verdigris), sulphate of copper (blue vitriol), arsenite of copper (Scheele's green or Paris green), chloride of antimony (butter of antimony), chloride of zinc (Burnett's disinfectant), nitrate of silver (lunar caustic), bichromate of potassium, sulphate of iron (green vitriol or copperas); also the leaves, roots, berries, or resins of many plants, when taken in considerable amounts such as colocynth, savin, gamboge, aloes, croton oil, elaterium, nux vomica, etc.

(2) **Narcotics** are mostly drawn from the vegetable kingdom. Few poisons have a purely narcotic action, most producing also signs of irritation, such as vomiting, delirium, excitement, or convulsions. The simple narcotics include opium and its preparations (for the dog only; excitement and delirium are noted in cases of poisoning by opium compounds in the other domesticated animals), prussic acid (hydrocyanic acid), cyanide of potassium, alcohol, ether, chloral, chloroform. Most poisonous gases also belong to this class, the chief among them being carbonic acid, carbon monoxide, sulphuretted hydrogen, phosphuretted hydrogen, phosgene, ammonium sulphide, and other sewer gases. The amount of these which is present in the atmosphere is normally very small, but in the neighbourhood of chemical works, sewers, etc., the amount may be sufficient to cause illness to small animals continually breathing them, and even to result in death.

(3) **Narcotico-irritants** form a very large group in which the individual substances cause very varied symptoms of irritation, such as excitement, delirium, convulsions, vomiting, nausea, or indigestion. The group includes fluoroacetate, carbolic acid (weaker solutions), oxalic acid, binoxalate of potash (salts of sorrel), nux vomica and strychnine, meadow saffron (*Colchicum autumnale*), white hellebore (*Veratrum album*), green hellebore (*Veratrum viride*), foxglove (*Digitalis purpurea*), monk's-hood (*Aconitum napellus*), henbane (*Hyos-*

cyamus niger), deadly nightshade (*Atropa belladonna*), black or garden nightshade (*Solanum nigrum*), woody nightshade or bittersweet (*Solanum dulcamara*), potato tops and seeds (*Solanum tuberosum*), tobacco (*Nicotiana tabacum*), Indian tobacco (*Lobelia inflata*), thorn apple (*Datura stramonium*), spotted hemlock (*Conium maculatum*), water hemlock or cowbane (*Cicuta virosa*), water dropwort (*Œnanthe crocata*), five-leaved water hemlock (*Phelandrium aquaticum*), fool's parsley (*Æthusa cynapium*), yew leaves and berries, especially when slightly withered (*Taxus bacata*), laburnum pods, bark and leaves (*Cytisus laburnum*), etc., and very many species of poisonous fungi, toadstools, etc.

Symptoms.—The symptoms of each of the more common poisonous agents are given under their respective headings, but the general train of symptoms of each group of poisons will be briefly mentioned here.

Irritant poisons produce acute abdominal pain, vomiting (when possible), purging, rapidly developing general collapse, and often unconsciousness, perhaps preceded by convulsions. The mouth in many cases shows signs of the presence of the irritant, being inflamed and sensitive when examined. There may even be areas of corroded mucous membrane visible on the tongue, cheeks, or gums.

Narcotics produce excitement at first, unsteady movements, interference with sight; and later, stupor and unconsciousness appear; coma, with or without spasmodic or convulsive movements, supervenes, and death occurs in many cases almost insensibly.

Narcotico-irritants produce symptoms of irritation in the first place, and later, delirium, convulsions, and coma.

As a general rule poisoning should be suspected when an animal becomes suddenly ill, soon after feeding, when put out to pasture for the first time in the season; after dipping, or when a change of food has recently taken place. Newly purchased samples of food-stuffs, when bought from a firm without a reputation, may be followed by an outbreak of illness, and such results point to the inclusion in the food-stuff of some harmful substance. It is false economy to purchase cheap food-stuffs of uncertain composition.

It should be remembered that no matter how strong circumstantial evidence seems to be, it is always essential that a post-mortem examination be made, and that if necessary samples of the stomach contents, portions of the liver and perhaps other organs, should be submitted to a qualitative and quantitative chemical examination by an analyst, before a suspected case of poisoning can be considered to be definitely proved. The necessity for this procedure is obvious when legal proceedings are contemplated.

Treatment.—With regard to the treatment of poisoned animals the owner is advised to place himself in the hands of a qualified person as soon as may be, and be guided by his advice. There is difficulty in answering the question, 'What is to be done when an animal (or animals) appears to have been poisoned?' Under the heading ANTIDOTES will be found a list of the commoner poisons and their chemical or physiological antidotes, but the difficulty is to ascertain which poison has been responsible for the symptoms. In such cases it is always wise to adopt general principles of treatment which are applicable to practically all forms of poisoning. These are as follows:

(1) *Prevent more poison being taken*, by having all animals under the dangerous conditions removed from contact with the suspected poisonous substance. House the affected in a safe place, away from others, and give only food and water of known purity.

(2) *Prevent absorption, or render inert any poison on skin or in stomach.* Skin applications, dips, etc., should be washed off at once by warm soapy water. The stomach should be cleared by giving an emetic to the pig, dog, or cat; and by using a stomach-tube, or stomach-pump, for horses and cattle, to introduce large quantities of a demulcent fluid, such as thin oatmeal gruel, barley water, or even warm water alone. These fluids dilute the poison and tend to soothe the irritated or inflamed areas, and where the nature of the poison is known they serve as vehicles in which the appropriate antidotes may be administered.

Emetics which may be safely used are —pig, a dessert-spoonful of mustard in a cupful of water; dog, a strong salt solution (ordinary household salt); cat, hypodermic injection of apomorphine, or the salt solution.

To hinder absorption in the horse, ox, or sheep, $\frac{1}{2}$ an ounce for the larger and $\frac{1}{4}$ of an ounce for the smaller animals of tannic acid, or double these amounts of powdered oak bark, oak galls, strong black tea or coffee which has been *boiled*, or catechu thoroughly stirred up in thin gruel, may be given. These substances, all of which contain tannic acid or tannates, are especially useful against vegetable poisons. In cattle, where a very rapidly acting poison, such as yew, has been taken, the immediate operation of opening the rumen and removing the ingested poison by hand, becomes urgent. When much gas formation occurs the rumen may have to be punctured by trocar and cannula.

(3) *Neutralise the effects of the poison taken.* To counteract the effects of irritants, use demulcents (oatmeal or starch gruel, barley water, linseed tea, olive oil, castor oil, milk, milk and eggs, or liquid paraffin). Yellow phosphorus is an exception to this rule; oily substances favour its absorption and must be avoided; copper sulphate should be given instead. Against narcotics, stimulants are needed; *e.g.* strong coffee or black tea, given by the mouth as a first-aid measure. When convulsions appear, it is often necessary to administer an anæsthetic or anti-convulsant drug.

(4) *Promote excretion.* An oily purgative (except where phosphorus is suspected) will very often clear away unabsorbed material from the bowels and prevent further absorption. Copious enemata of warm (or even hot) soapy water hasten the movements of the bowels and assist evacuation. The administration of common salt in the food or water induces thirst and assists in the elimination of absorbed poisons by the kidneys. Certain drugs, such as iodide of potassium, assist in the expulsion of lead and mercury compounds from the body. And judiciously regulated exercise, when the animal is strong enough, does much to quicken the circulation and assist in elimination.

Perhaps the best advice that can be given to owners whose stock of medicine is not great, or whose confidence is not strong, is to take all precautionary measures, keep the animals as quiet as possible, and send an urgent message to their local practitioner, and be guided by his advice. (*See also under* ANTIDOTES, and under the respective headings of the various poisonous plants.)

POISON WEED (*see* PIMPERNEL).

POLAND CHINA.—A breed of pig from Ohio, U.S.A. Colouring is black with six white points (feet, tip of nose and tail). Rapid growth and good meat production are characteristics of the breed.

POLIOENCEPHALOMALACIA.—A disease of cattle, sheep, and pigs, characterised by dropsy of the brain. It may affect up to 25 per cent of the stock, and up to 90 per cent may die in feedlots in N. America. It appears similar to the effects of salt poisoning in pigs.

Muzzle twitching, opisthotonos, blindness, and inability to stand are symptoms observed in affected calves in Britain. (*See also* CEREBROCORTICAL NECROSIS which closely resembles the above.)

POLIOMYELITIS OF PIGS.—This disease is distinct from that of human beings and is possibly identical with TALFAN DISEASE.

POLL (*see* p. 735).

' POLL EVIL ' is an old, colloquial name sometimes incorrectly applied to any swelling in the poll region, but which should be reserved for a sinus following infection of some of the deeper tissues and giving rise to pus-formation. It may result from an injury which displaces a chip of bone from the atlas. Apart from this, and its situation, ' Poll Evil ' resembles Fistulous Withers.

Causes.—Self-inflicted injuries such as striking the poll against the top of a doorway, or falling backwards with the poll striking the ground; blows, such as from a whip-handle; bridle pressure.

Fusiformis necrophorus has been associated with some cases and may have gained entrance through damaged skin. It has been suggested that some cases may arise through infection without injury. *Brucella abortus* and the worm *Onchocerca reticulata* have each been found, and the former is now believed to account for some cases of Fistulous Withers.

Symptoms.—A painful swelling on one or both sides with, after a time, the appearance of one or more orifices exuding pus. The animal resents the part being touched and, if the *ligamentum nuchæ* is involved, avoids downward movement of the head.

First-aid measures include the use of an antiphlogistine poultice and the placing of food at a level which the animal can reach without pain.

Treatment may necessitate the removal of any dead tissue and the surgical enlargement of any openings to allow free drainage. Antibiotics may be used to overcome the infection.

POLLED.—Inherited hornlessness of an animal belonging to a normally horned breed, e.g. Hereford cattle. (*See* SCUR.)

POLYCYTHÆMIA (πολύς, many ; κύτος, cell ; αἷμα, blood) is the name given to a marked excess in the number of red blood corpuscles.

POLYDIPSIA (πολύς, much ; δίψα, thirst) is excessive thirst.

POLYMORPH (πολύς, many ; μορφή. form) is a name applied to certain white cells of the blood which have a nucleus of varied shape. (*See* BLOOD.)

POLYNEURITIS (πολύς, many ; νεῦρον, nerve) means an inflammation of nerves or their sheaths occurring in different parts of the body at the same time. (*See* NEURITIS.)

POLYPUS (πολύπους, many-footed) is a general term applied to tumours which are attached by a stalk to the surfaces from which they spring. The term only applies to the shape of the growth and has nothing to do with its structure or to its nature. Most polypi are benign, but some may become malignant. They are generally of fibrous tissue in the centre covered with the type of epithelium that is found on the surface from which they spring. In animals, the common situations where they are found are in the cavities of the nostrils of horses and cattle, and sometimes of dogs ; in the vaginæ of the females of all animals, where they sometimes interfere with successful coition ; in the interior of the bladder, uterus, bowels, and stomach. As a rule they are easily removed when situated in accessible regions, but those in the internal organs are at times inoperable, or at the best require a major operation for their removal.

POLYURIA (πολύς, much ; οὖρον, urine) is a condition that commonly affects the horse when fed on mouldy, or otherwise unwholesome, hay or fodder, in which a much greater amount of urine is passed than is usual. It is a simple condition which rapidly clears up when the causal material is stopped.

Polyuria is also a symptom of diabetes, and it occurs in certain forms of inflammation of the kidneys, especially in the early stages of pyelonephritis affecting cows after calving, when infection has travelled into the bladder, up the ureters, and so into the kidney. (*See* KIDNEY, DISEASES OF ; URINE.)

POLYVALENT VACCINE.—One prepared from cultures of several strains of the same bacterial or viral species or from different species. A single vaccine can now protect against eight diseases.

PONDS (*see* LEECHES, ALGÆ POISONING, COCCIDIOSIS, JOHNE'S DISEASE).

PONIES ACT, 1969.—This regulates the export of ponies (*i.e.* horses not over 14½ hands in height other than foals travelling with their dams where these are over 14½ hands), which must be of certain minimum values, *e.g.* £40 for a Shetland or £100 for a pony over 12 hands. A 10-hour rest period and a veterinary examination before ship/air travel are required. (*See also under* HORSES, BREEDS OF.)

PONS, or PONS VAROLII, is the so-called 'bridge of the brain'. It is situated at the base of the brain in front of the medulla, and behind the cerebral peduncles, and appears as a bulbous swelling not unlike a small curved artichoke. It is mainly composed of strands of fibres which link up different parts of the brain.

POPLITEAL (*poples*, the ham) is the name applied to the region that lies behind the stifle joint, and to the vessels, lymph glands, nerves, etc., lying in this region. It is protected laterally by the biceps femoris, posteriorly by the semitendinosus and the gastrocnemius, and internally by the gracilis and semitendinosus tendon ; consequently it is seldom that its vessels or nerves are injured.

POPPY POISONING in Great Britain is not at all common, partly because the opium poppy does not grow wild in any profusion in pastures, and partly because the common red poppy (*Papaver Rhoeas*) does not contain opium. It grows very commonly in crops of oats, barley, and beans in some parts of the country, but the plant has died down to a mere brown stalk by the time harvest begins, and, even when oat straw containing large amounts of poppy stalks is cut into chaff for feeding, it does not seem to cause any harm when eaten. Fatal cases of poisoning have rarely occurred, but the green flowering plant, when eaten in quantity by cattle, may cause excitement, indigestion, stupor with a low temperature, slowed respiration, and death from asphyxia.

Treatment.—A brisk oily purge should be given, and measures taken to ward off the stupor, as given under OPIUM).

PORKER.—In Britain, porkers weigh 100-190 lb. (liveweight). 'Heavy Hog' weight is 260 lb.

PORPHYRIA (*see* BONE, DISEASES OF, *and* HEXACHLORO-BENZENE).

PORTAL VEIN (*porta*, an entrance) is the large vein which carries to the liver the blood that has been circulating in many of the abdominal organs. It is unique among the large veins of the body in that on entering the liver it breaks up into a capillary network, instead of passing its blood into one of the larger veins to be carried back to the heart. It is formed by the confluence of the anterior and posterior mesenteric with the splenic vein in the horse, and by the union of the gastric and mesenteric radicles in the ox, and, from a point behind the pancreas and below the vena cava, it runs forwards, downwards, and a little to the right, to reach the *porta* of the liver. Here it divides and subdivides in the manner usual with an artery. (*See* LIVER for further course, and DIGESTION.)

The blood that is carried to the liver by the portal vein is that which has been circulating in the stomach, nearly the whole of the intestines, the pancreas, and the spleen.

POSOLOGICAL.—Relating to dosage.

POST- is a prefix signifying after or behind.

POSTHITIS (*see* BALANITIS).

POST-MORTEM EXAMINATION (*see under* AUTOPSY).

POST-PARTUM.—Following parturition.

POST-PARTURIENT FEVER of sows occurs, as a rule, 2 or 3 days after a normal farrowing. The animal goes off her food, is slightly feverish, and apt to resent suckling by her piglets. The udder is hard; the hardness beginning at the rear and extending forward. A watery or white discharge from the vagina is not invariably present. The uterus may not be involved at all. Treatment by antibiotics and pituitrin is successful if begun early. (*See also* UTERUS, DISEASES OF.)

POST-PARTURIENT HÆMOGLOBINURIA.—This disease is seen in high-yielding dairy cows soon after calving.

Symptoms.—These are sudden in onset and include red-coloured urine, loss of appetite, and weakness. Fæces are firm. Breathing may be laboured. Death may occur within a few days.

Cause.—This is associated with a phosphorus-deficient diet.

Treatment.—Blood transfusion, a suitable phosphate preparation intravenously, or bone-meal by mouth.

(*See also under* KALE.)

POTASH, or POTASSA, is the popular name for carbonate of potassium. Hydrated oxide of potassium is generally known as caustic potash, and its solution (usually 5 per cent) is called liquor potassæ. Potash is prepared by burning wood, washing the ashes with water, and evaporating the solution to dryness. The remainder contains 60 to 80 per cent of carbonate of potassium, which is used to obtain many of the other salts of potassium.

Potash fertilisers are best not applied to pasture land in the spring shortly before grazing, owing to the increased risk of HYPOMAGNESÆMIA (which see).

POTASSIUM is a metal which, on account of its great affinity for other substances, is not found in a pure state in Nature. Its salts are used to a very great extent both in human and animal medicine, but as their action depends in general not upon the metallic radicle, but upon the particular acid with which each is combined, their uses vary greatly and are described elsewhere. Thus for the action and uses of potassium bromide *see* BROMIDES, for those of potassium iodide *see* IODIDES, for those of potassium permanganate *see* PERMANGANATE OF POTASH, for those of the bicarbonate *see* BICARBONATE OF SODA, for those of the citrate and tartrate of potassium *see under* CITRIC ACID, and for those of the nitrate of potassium *see* NITRATE OF POTASH.

All salts of potassium are supposed to

have a depressing action on the nervous system and on the heart, but in ordinary doses this effect is so slight as to be of no practical importance. The corresponding sodium salts can be used if preferred. **For intravenous injections, however, potassium salts must not be used as they are liable to be rapidly fatal ; sodium salts must be used instead.**

The solid tissues of plants and animals (protoplasm) contain a considerable amount of potassium salts, but the fluids of the body, blood, saliva, bile, etc., contain salts of sodium, calcium, etc. When potassium salts are taken in excess, they are rapidly excreted from the body, and thus by stimulating the functions of the kidneys and bowels they increase the amount of urine passed and act as gentle purgatives. The solubility of potassium salts is greater than that of sodium salts, and it is therefore supposed that since the amount of potassium in the herbivorous animal's body is generally considered to be greater than the amount of sodium salts, and as uric acid can be kept dissolved more easily when combined with potassium than when united to sodium, this explains why herbivorous animals are not at all commonly affected with gout (due to deposition of uric acid crystals in joints and other parts of the body).

Potassium sulphate has purgative actions similar to but weaker than those of Epsom salts, and is sometimes used in conjunction with them ; potassium chlorate has a soothing action on inflamed mucous membranes, and is used to add to electuaries for sore throat in the horse ; potassium acetate is a diuretic and febrifuge, used in fevered conditions to promote action of the kidneys and to reduce excessive acidity of the blood.

POTATO HAULM.—The use of arsenites for destroying the haulm was a dangerous practice. Cattle have died as a result of straying into a field recently sprayed with arsenites, and the same danger applies to other stock, including dogs which may be poisoned after licking their coats. In Britain it was agreed that after the 1960 harvest, the use and manufacture of arsenite potato-haulm destroyers should cease.

POTATO POISONING.—The common potato—*Solanum tuberosum*—is a member of a Natural Order to which belong a number of very poisonous plants. The potato tubers themselves are not usually considered dangerous for live-stock, so long as they are wholesome, but the haulms and sprouted, diseased, old, or 'greened' tubers may give rise to poisoning both in man and the lower animals. The haulms are most dangerous just after flowering. Both the haulms and the tops contain varying quantities of *solanin*, an alkaloid, which is also found in the poisonous plant Bittersweet—*Solanum dulcamara*. The tubers when perfectly sound are practically harmless unless taken in excessively large quantities, but even they contain a definite amount of solanin in the skin and eyes. When boiled, the alkaloid is dissolved out in the water, and does no harm.

Old, rotten, frosted or sprouted potatoes are another serious source of poisoning, and many cases are recorded where cattle, horses, and pigs have suffered from eating them. In most cases the potatoes need to be fed for some little time before symptoms of poisoning result, but in other cases —especially where large amounts have been taken — poisoning may appear rapidly.

Symptoms.—In horses, after feeding on unsound tubers, staggering movements, loss of appetite, excessive thirst but inability to drink, constipation followed by foul-smelling diarrhœa, stertorous breathing, and a rapid feeble pulse, have been noticed. Death occurred quietly in some cases ; in others there was distress. Cattle show an inability to rise, cessation of lactation, salivation, and vomiting in some instances, dryness of the muzzle, but no tympanitis, moaning, or grunting. In calves, there is recorded prostration, drowsiness, and signs of narcotic poisoning. Pigs have shown loss of appetite, dullness, exhaustion, absence of perceptible pulse, watery diarrhœa, low temperature, and coma.

Cases on the continent of Europe have exhibited peculiar skin lesions. They occurred after the green haulms had been eaten by cattle, and consisted of eczematous ulcerated areas occurring on the scrotum of the male and the udder of the female. In addition, there were ulcers in the mouths of some animals, and blisters about the hind limbs which suggested foot-and-mouth disease, except that considerable quantities of pus were produced.

The most constant symptoms appear to be loss of appetite, prostration or interference with movement, a weak pulse, a low or subnormal temperature, and depression almost as marked as sleep.

Loss of condition is noticeable when small amounts have been taken for some considerable time.

Treatment.—A drench containing equal parts of strong black coffee or tea and linseed gruel should be given at once, and followed by an oily or saline purgative. Where possible copious enemata of warm soapy water should be given. Injections of strychnine are advised by some.

POTENTIATION.—The increased toxicity arising from the combined action of two chemical compounds. For example, if one destroys the liver enzyme which renders the other safe. One hundredth of the lethal dose of each compound may then prove fatal. (*See* MALATHION.)

POULTICES AND FOMENTATIONS.—Poultices are soft, moist, warm applications used for the surface of the body, when it is desired to effect emollient, relaxing, and softening effects. Fomentations are applications of warm or hot fluids, usually containing some antiseptic and soothing agents. Both applications act to a great extent in the same way; they soften the parts with which they come into contact, soothe irritated nerve-endings, relax spasmodically contracted muscle fibres, and, after being applied for some time, they cause dilatation of the vessels of the part they cover, and increase the circulation through it. These applications are therefore useful in all stages of inflammation to soothe the pain and promote resolution, or in the late stages, when pus is forming, to hasten the formation of an abscess. (*See* ABSCESS.)

Varieties.—These include a mixture of kaolin and glycerin, made into a paste, incorporated with an antiseptic, and applied hot upon a piece of gauze or cotton-wool to the part. A proprietary preparation of this nature is on the market, made up in conveniently sized tins, containing directions for its use, which can be considered fully reliable and satisfactory to use by an owner instead of a poultice. It goes by the name of 'Antiphlogistine'.

Hot fomentations are usually made by cooling boiling water down to a temperature that can be easily borne by the bare elbow, wringing a piece of flannel or blanket out of the water, and applying it to the part. As the animal becomes used to the heat, more and more hot water is added, until it becomes uncomfortably hot. At first the wrung-out cloth is used, but later the inflamed part may be swabbed by the wet cloth, which is held in contact with the skin for a minute or two.

POULTRY, DISEASES OF (*see under* ASPERGILLOSIS, AVIAN DIPHTHERIA, AVIAN ENCEPHALOMYELITIS, AVIAN LISTERIOSIS, AVIAN PLAGUE, AVIAN TUBERCULOSIS, BUMBLE-FOOT, CAGE LAYER FATIGUE, COCCIDIOSIS, CRAZY CHICK DISEASE, *E. Coli*, EGG-BOUND, FAVUS, FOWL CHOLERA, FOWL PARALYSIS, FOWL TYPHOID, GAPES, 'HÆMORRHAGIC DISEASE', MONILIASIS, NEWCASTLE DISEASE (Fowl Pest), OMPHALITIS, PARASITES, PULLET DISEASE, PULLORUM DISEASE, ROUP, SALMONELLOSIS, SLIPPED TENDON, SYNOVITIS, 'TOXIC FAT DISEASE', C.R.D., GUMBORO, BRONCHITIS, NEPHROSIS, LIVER/KIDNEY SYNDROME, MAREK'S DISEASE.)

POULTRY HEALTH SCHEME.—In the U.K. this came into operation on Jan. 1, 1966, and the objective is to maintain healthy sources of poultry stock to the benefit of both egg- and meat-producing flocks. Poultry breeders and hatchery owners in Great Britain with a prescribed minimum flock size or incubator capacity, and who meet certain standards required under the Scheme, are eligible for membership. The main benefits to members are the free *post-mortem* service for their flocks and the opportunity to obtain free veterinary advice. Copies of the Scheme can be obtained from the Ministry of Agriculture, Hook Rise, Tolworth, Surbiton, Surrey.

POULTRY AND POULTRY KEEPING.—These have, so far as large-scale production is concerned, undergone great changes in recent years. Many of the older breeds and strains of poultry have given way to more efficient hybrids. Increasingly there is a move towards intensive production of layers or broilers in controlled-environment houses. Formulation of poultry foods for optimum production has advanced, too, and well-balanced proprietary compounds are extensively used.

Hybrids.—The following have done well in Britain: Double-A1, Babcock 300, CH20, Honegger, Shaver 288, Sykes 3, SW20, Thornber 606, Sterling White Link.

Large-scale production.—Information will be found under CONTROLLED ENVIRONMENT, HOUSING OF ANIMALS, BROILERS, INTENSIVE LIVESTOCK PRO-

POULTRY AND POULTRY KEEPING

DUCTION, BATTERY SYSTEM, NIGHT LIGHTING, CANNIBALISM, DEEP LITTER, EGG YIELD, etc.

Hen Yards are nowadays preferred to large pens for birds kept intensively, and are often adapted from old bullock yards. Protection from cold winds and rain is necessary. The high cost of straw is sometimes a disadvantage; gravel, shingle or sand from a beach, or clinker, may be used. The system is labour-saving and does not involve great capital expenditure.

Housing.—Competitive broiler and egg production has now led to highly expensive (though economic) and elaborate buildings. The main features are described under CONTROLLED ENVIRONMENT HOUSING and HOUSING OF LIVE-STOCK. A comfortable weatherproof house is of the greatest importance. It may be of wood, stone, or brick. The material, shape, and design are of little consequence provided certain conditions are fulfilled.

What follows relates to housing where high capital expenditure is not possible or desirable.

Size.—A minimum of 3 sq. ft., and if possible 4 sq. ft., per bird should be allowed.

Height.—A very high house is apt to be cold and draughty, while a very low one is difficult to ventilate and troublesome to clean. From 6 ft. 6 ins. to 7 ft. at the highest point to 4 ft. 6 ins. or 5 ft. at the lowest should be allowed.

Ventilation.—There must be good top ventilation. The amount to be given depends a good deal upon the situation and exposure. Houses of the open-fronted type may prove to be too draughty for exposed wind-swept districts. For such places a pitched roof is rather to be preferred to a lean-to. Dampness in a house may be due to faulty ventilation.

Light.—The maximum amount of light and sunshine should be aimed at. Fowls will not shelter during the day in a dark house. Additional windows should be placed a few inches above the level of the floor, if possible at the east and west sides. This means that the floor will always be light, and the birds will always be encouraged to scratch for grain buried in the litter. (*See also* NIGHT-LIGHTING.)

Litter.—The floor should be covered to a depth of a foot or more with clean dry litter, such as straw. (*See* DEEP LITTER.)

Perches.—These should measure 2 ins. by 2 ins. and have the edges on the upper surface smoothed off. They should be all on one level about 2 ft. 6 ins. from the floor, and made to drop into sockets. About 6 or 8 ins. below the perches should be placed a removable dropping board. This keeps the floor clean and prevents upward draughts. They must be cleaned regularly, and lightly sprinkled with sand or peat moss litter.

Nests are best placed on the same sides as the windows, so that the light does not shine directly into them.

Houses should be regularly cleaned and sprayed with disinfectant from time to time, or they may be lime-washed.

Runs.—Fresh clean ground is very necessary. If birds remain too long in one place the ground becomes foul, and the egg-yield and the birds' health soon suffer. Where space permits (as on farms) the birds may be kept on free range in portable houses. When the ground round the house becomes dirty the house may be removed to another place. In this way the fowls always have clean land. Where the birds are to be penned, not more than 100 to the acre should be allowed if the runs are to be permanently occupied. A more economical method is to allow two runs to each house. As soon as one run begins to show signs of wear the birds are shifted into the other one. The vacated run (if in grass) may be limed and allowed to rest for a few months, or it may be dug up and cropped. The value of clean grass runs containing abundance of clover cannot be estimated, and every care should be taken to keep the grass in good condition and to encourage the growth of the clover. Where this alternate method is adopted it is safe to keep at the rate of 250 birds to the acre. Small earth runs are difficult to keep clean. The top layer of soil may be removed from time to time and fresh earth or sand put in its place. Sea sand is an excellent material for covering the surface of small runs.

Hatching and Rearing.—The time to begin hatching depends on the breed, the strain, and the poultry-keeper's requirements. Quick maturing breeds, such as Leghorn, Ancona, and good laying strains of White Wyandottes, Rhode Island Reds, and Light Sussex, will, if properly fed and managed, lay at 5 or 5½ months, so that if pullets are wanted to lay in October, chickens should be hatched in March or April. It is generally considered that birds hatched early in the year have more natural vitality and mature more rapidly than those hatched later. Against this must be the fact that in very cold weather and in exposed districts the percentage of

POULTRY AND POULTRY KEEPING

fertility may be low in the first two months of the year, and there may be heavy mortality in the rearing of the chickens unless adequate protection can be given. June or even July chicks may be brought on to lay if they are well fed. As soon as the days begin to get short, these late-hatched chicks should be fed by lamplight, otherwise they are not getting sufficien food to make their full growth. Where only a few chickens are to be raised, or where very special eggs are to be set, the hen is to be preferred to the incubator. It is sometimes difficult to get broody hens early in the season, and in such cases **Silkies** make excellent sitters and mothers. They are small eaters, their eggs are of fair size, they lay a small batch, and then go broody almost irrespective of the season. A silkie hen can cover from 6 to 8 ordinary eggs.

Brooders.—Bottled gas is much used nowadays for heating brooders, and has advantages over paraffin burners. Infra-red heating, especially the dull-emitter kind, is popular where reliable electricity supplies are available, and enables the chicks to be readily observed. (*See also* HAY-BOX BROODERS which enable the chicks to be kept for a shorter time in the rearing house.)

Rearing Houses.—These should be well ventilated but free from floor draughts, well lit by windows, and spacious enough. Allow half a square foot per chick up to a month old.

Drinking Water (*see under* CHICKS) must be constantly available.

Trough Space.—Six lineal feet of trough space per 100 chicks should be provided until the birds are 3 weeks old ; ten feet per 100 chicks at from 3 to 6 weeks old ; twelve feet at from 6 to 12 weeks old ; sixteen feet at from 12 to 16 weeks old, and twenty feet thereafter.

Bought-in Stock.—If buyers insist on 'Accredited' stock, they can be almost certain of avoiding trouble from Pullorum disease (Bacillary Whit Diarrhœa) and from Fowl Typhoid.

When chicks are bought as day-olds, mortality should not exceed 3 per cent by the third week. Losses exceeding 5 per cent indicate the need for an investigation ; and several dead chicks should be sent to a laboratory for a *post-mortem* examination.

Chick Feeding.—There is no longer support for the old idea that chicks must not be fed for the first 48 hours. It is better to feed day-olds on arrival (otherwise they pick at their bedding) and to allow them ample cold water. Feeding appliances must be of a good design and not placed in a dark spot where chicks may fail to find them.

Proprietary crumbs, or mash or meal, may be fed. Limestone grit and oyster shell should *not* be given with these. (*See under* GRIT.) Day-olds do not need this unless they are to be fed on grain or to be put on grass when very young. Grain should not be fed *ad lib.*, but rather as a twice-daily scratch feed, until chicks are about a month old.

The following materials have been used in poultry feeding :

Sussex ground oats.
Barley meal.
Maize meal, maize germ meal.
Wheat and millers' offals.
Rice bran.
Linseed cake meal.
Coconut cake meal.
Palm Kernel cake meal.
Sunflower cake meal.
White fish meal, Herring meal.
Meat meal.
Dried skimmed milk.
Dried buttermilk.
Dried whey.
Dried grass or lucerne meals.
Dried yeast.
Molasses.
Synthetic vitamins A, B_1, B_2, D_3, and E.
Concentrates of carotene.
Anti-oxidants.

Dirt, dampness, and overcrowding are the chickens' worst enemies. Coops and brooders should be moved constantly, so that the chickens have fresh clean ground to run on. After the birds have been removed from the rearing ground, the land should be dressed with burnt lime at the rate of 40 cwt. to the acre. The cockerels should be separated from the pullets as soon as it is possible to differentiate them. The pullets need plenty of space both in their houses and in their runs. It is best to get them into their winter quarters by August or September and not move them again, as changes of all kinds are apt to check laying. As a preventative of soft-shelled eggs, 2 per cent steamed bone flour or bone meal may be added to the mash. Pullets should begin to lay in October or November if hatched in good time. Trap-nesting should be adopted wherever it is possible, as it is important to find out the winter records of the pullets. A good winter record (for 4 months) is from 30 to 40 eggs, but birds of good strain, properly managed and fed, will produce up to 70 or 80 eggs. A good flock average for the year is 180, but there are, of course, instances of birds producing up to 300 eggs in their first year.

Feeding.—Where fowls have access to good grass runs, and especially where these contain a fair proportion of clover, they can themselves correct any faults in a badly balanced ration, but birds on earth runs, or kept purely on the intensive system, are entirely at the mercy of the poultry-keepers, and their diet must be carefully considered. An excess or deficiency of any one substance in the ration may cause derangement of the digestive system of the bird, and so may affect egg-production. Birds, especially those kept in confinement, often suffer from a deficiency of some sort. **Modern carefully formulated proprietary foods have been developed to obviate all known deficiencies in housed birds.**

The amount which a fowl will eat must depend on the breed, the condition of the bird, whether she is laying or not, and the conditions under which she is kept. The bird's appetite is the best guide, but a rough rule is to allow about 2 oz. of grain and 2 to 2½ oz. of mash per bird per day. For a grain food a mixture of two parts oats and one part cracked maize may be recommended. The grain should be lightly buried in the litter, so that the birds have to work for it. The mash may be fed either wet once a day, or dry in hoppers, so that the fowls can help themselves.

(*See under* **RATIONS.**)

POULTRY WASTE, DRIED.—This has been fed to beef cattle as part of their diet, especially in the U.S.A. The product is very variable in its content—droppings being the main ingredient; but litter, feathers, broken eggs may also be present. From a veterinary point of view there may be dangers—high levels of copper or arsenic, for example, used in broiler diets; also high calcium carbonate levels. Crude protein content may vary from 15 to 35 per cent, crude fibre 12 to 35 per cent.

POWDERS form the simplest method by which medicines are prescribed. They are prepared by reducing the dry substances to a fine powder in a mortar with a pestle, and portioning the mixture into appropriate amounts, according to the dose, etc., and wrapping the separate doses in white paper. Substances which are very powerful and have a small dose are generally diluted with some inert substance such as powdered sugar, linseed, etc.

Administration.—Powders are most easily given in the food whenever the animal will take them. Failing this the larger animals will sometimes not refuse a powder if it be given in a little damp bran, especially if some fenugreek powder is added. Some horses will take powders when they are given in the drinking water or in a bran mash. Cattle can generally be persuaded to take them in a meal drink, especially if some milk is added. Linseed or hay tea is useful to disguise the taste. It is sometimes possible to induce the dog to take a powder by making it into a pill with butter or lard, or by spreading it on to a piece of bread and butter and offering it to the dog.

POX (*see* VARIOLA).

P.P.D.—'Purified Protein Derivative'. (*See under* TUBERCULIN.)

P.P.L.O.—Pleuro-pneumonia-like organisms; *i.e.* similar to those which cause contagious bovine pleuro-pneumonia. (*See* MYCOPLASMA.)

A blood agglutination test is available in the U.K. for those wishing to establish P.P.L.O.-free flocks of chickens and turkeys.

P.P.R.—'Peste des petits ruminants' is a disease of goats and sheep, but not cattle, resembling Cattle Plague and occurring in West Africa.

PRECARDIAL or PRECORDIAL REGION is the region of the chest cavity that lies in front of the heart.

PREDNISOLONE.—A drug which raises blood-sugar levels and has been used in the treatment of agalactia in sows. (*See* CORTICOSTEROIDS.)

PREDNISONE.—This has been recommended for use in serious cases of pneumonia in dogs associated with a virus infection. (*See* CORTICOSTEROIDS.)

PREGNANCY DIAGNOSIS TESTS.—During pregnancy the urine in the human female and in the mare and cow undergoes a change. In the human female a substance elaborated from the anterior pituitary gland is excreted in the urine.

This, because of its property of stimulating the ovary, is known as the *gonadotropic* hormone. After suitable preparation, if a sample of urine is injected into immature female rats or mice, certain well-defined changes (the formation of hæmorrhagic follicles in place of normal Graafian follicles) occur in their ovaries if gonadotropic hormone is present. It is upon this principle that the human pregnancy diagnosis test—the Zondek-Ascheim test—is based. The reaction may in some few cases be given as early as 12–14 days after conception has occurred, but most cases cannot be determined until at least three weeks to one month have elapsed. The accuracy is very high.

In the mare and cow no large amount of gonadotropic hormone is excreted in the urine, but another substance—the female sex hormone, œstrin, or œstrone—is present during pregnancy. This can also be identified by the use of test animals—mice or rats. After injection of small amounts of urine, the œstrin, if present, produces a characteristic change in the epithelial cells of the vagina which can be smeared and stained.

In the mare, reactions may be obtained as early as the 42nd day after service, but more often the amount of œstrin present remains low until about the 60–65th day, when the concentration rises rapidly. In the cow, the quantity of œstrin in the urine during pregnancy varies very considerably. Generally, by the 90th day at least, the amount is sufficient to yield the reaction, but in some cases individual cows fail to give a reaction even at 175 days after service.

In Norway, a very accurate test for the early diagnosis of pregnancy in the sow has been evolved, based upon the quantity of œstrin in the urine. The test takes an hour and is expensive.

The Capon Test.—The Brown Leghorn capon has also been used to test the presence of œstrin in a sample. The breast feathers of the capon are normally black. After injection of œstrin, a salmon-coloured bar appears across the width of the growing feather. This reaction by suitable microscopic preparation can be obtained within 48 hours in a strongly positive case. (*See also under* MUCUS for another test.)

Ultrasonics are being used for pregnancy diagnosis in ewes—and also in sows. The method, adapted from the echo-sounder of marine application, has not the dangers for the fœtus of X-rays and is claimed to be over 90 per cent accurate.

Vaginal biopsy is a technique now being applied to large pig herds on a commercial scale.

Pregnancy in the bitch cannot be diagnosed in the early stages. From 24 to 32 days is the best time for abdominal palpation; after 35 days pregnancy may be difficult to recognise by this means; though occasionally posterior fœtuses can be felt at 45 to 55 days—when the fœtal skeleton can be palpated. Auscultation of fœtal hearts in the final week of pregnancy will differentiate pregnancy from pyometra and show that the fœtuses are alive. Pregnancy has to be differentiated also from pseudo-pregnancy, ascites, adiposity, and diabetes mellitus.

PREGNANCY EXAMINATION of cattle is carried out by means of rectal palpation, but requires expert knowledge not only of anatomy but of physiology and pathology. It is not always a simple matter and an accurate diagnosis not always achieved. The dangers of attempts by herdsmen and other untrained people to carry out such an examination include: rupture of the heart of the embryo calf; perforation of the rectum; and abortion due to mal-handling of the ovaries.

PREGNANCY and GESTATION.—The uterus, the ovaries, and the whole of the tissues of the mother are influenced directly or indirectly during pregnancy, but the gross changes exhibited, with certain exceptions, subside quickly after the birth of the young. The minor alterations which persist throughout life, such as increased size of the mammary glands, enlargement of the uterus, and of the whole of the genital canal, are not generally obvious except after repeated breeding, and in from 4 to 6 weeks the dam has returned to the normal to all intents and purposes, always excepting the flow of milk in the mammary glands. In most uniparous animals—producing one young at a time—the horn of the uterus which becomes pregnant greatly enlarges and becomes straightened out so as to be practically continuous with the body of the uterus, and the non-pregnant horn appears as a small appendage projecting from its side; in the multiparous animals, however, both horns usually carry a share of the number of the young, and both are consequently nearly alike in size. The pregnant horn (or horns) develop an intricate and very complete vascular system

PREGNANCY AND GESTATION

The uterine arteries increase to a great size, and together they form a very perfect plexus in and around the wall of the uterus, thereby ensuring an even and regulated blood-flow for the needs of the young. As the organ gradually increases in size to accommodate its contents, the broad ligament, which supports it from the roof of the abdomen, increases in length and strength to allow the uterus to move farther and farther forward and downward in each animal, so that eventually it may occupy the greater part of the abdominal cavity. At the same time there is a very great increase in the muscular coat of the uterus. Not only do the individual muscle fibres greatly hypertrophy, but it appears that there is an increase in their numbers as well. The walls of the organ become firmer, stronger, and thicker, and better able to accommodate the extra weight of the young. The lining mucous membrane also shows well-marked changes. In those animals which have a diffuse placenta, *e.g.* mare and sow, the mucous membrane over the inside of the uterus is thickened, very vascular, and in it are found the crypts which receive the villi of the chorion (outermost fœtal membrane). In the ruminants the characteristic cotyledons enlarge and multiply. These are mushroom-like elevations projecting into the lumen of the uterus, with crypts scattered over their convex crowns (cow), or over their concave crowns (ewe and goat). In the dog and cat, the zones where intimate connection between dam and fœtal membrane occurs show a corresponding hypertrophy and increased vascularity.

Duration of Pregnancy.—This varies greatly in different species and to some extent in different individuals. Certain differences can be ascribed to definite causes, but in many cases no satisfactory explanation can be given why one animal of a breed carries its young for a longer or shorter period than another of the same size, age, and appearance. Male fœti are carried longer than females. A mare served by a thoroughbred stallion will carry its foal longer than when served by a poorly bred sire. The same applies to service by the stallion ass. Debility, weakness, or illness in the dam shortens the duration of pregnancy. (*See the* TABLE *on next page.*)

Signs of Pregnancy.—When well advanced the typical signs of pregnancy are well enough known to the majority of livestock owners, and require no mention here, but in the earlier stages they are not always so clear, and for the first few weeks in the larger animal it is often difficult to diagnose pregnancy by clinical signs.

The chief changes and differences to be looked for are as follows:

Cessation of œstrum.—In the majority of cases, but not in all animals, the female exhibits no desire for the male after conception occurs. There are many instances, however, when service is allowed until late on in pregnancy, and there may be all the usual signs of œstrum evident on each occasion. In such cases abortion of the fœtus may occur, or no harm may result. When the *bull* refuses to serve a cow which is apparently in season it may be taken as a strong sign that she is pregnant.

Alteration in temperament.—Vicious, troublesome, or easily excited mares generally become very much more tractable and quiet after conception, whereas if they are served and do not conceive they are frequently more intractable than previously. The same signs are sometimes seen in the cow.

Fattening tendency.—In the sheep and the cow particularly, condition markedly improves during the first few weeks of pregnancy—a fact which is often used for the advantage of the feeder—but during the latter stages when the abdomen has increased in size the opposite effect is seen in all animals.

Easily induced fatigue.—In the later stages, pregnant animals almost always show a decreased capacity for exercise or work. They become easily fatigued, mares perspire sooner, and a general sluggishness becomes apparent. Pigs and dogs show an increased desire to rest as much as possible.

Enlargement of the abdomen, which occurs in every direction, is a most important sign of pregnancy; it occurs at about the same rate as the rate of development of the young, which is greatest towards the end of the period. It descends or 'drops', the flanks become hollow, the spine appears more prominent, and its line tends to become flat or even concave in the thoracic and lumbar region, the muscles of the quarters appear to fall in, making the haunches and the root of the tail appear more prominent, and the pelvis tilts into a more vertical position.

Enlargement of the mammary glands commences very soon in pregnancy in those animals which are bearing young for

PREGNANCY AND GESTATION

the first time. The glands become larger, firmer, and more prominent; teats appear, wrinkles are lost, and about the end of the period a little thin yellowish viscid fluid may be easily pressed from them. In breeding animals the mammary glands actually decrease in size during the first period of pregnancy, and it is only towards the end that they increase. Cows in milk and mares with their foals gradually ' dry off ', giving less and less milk until by about the end of the 7th month in cows, and the 8th or 9th in mares, the milk secretion has become very little, and the animal may be dry altogether.

Increase in weight is, of course, a *sine qua non* of normal pregnancy, but practically it is not a great deal of use since it necessitates periodic weighings, and the result may be falsified by coincident gains or losses in the general condition of the dam which are due to other causes.

' *Quickening* ' is the term applied to the signs of life exhibited by the fœtus in the uterus. In the mare these movements are seen in the left flank; in the cow in the right flank. They may be induced by giving a drink of cold water, especially in the morning, or after work or exercise; they may be seen if the dam is made to trot for a short distance and then is allowed to remain still for a few moments; turning a mare sharply round in a small circle to the right side, or a cow to the left, and observing the opposite flanks in each case, may induce them; or they may be observed immediately after the dam rises from the ground. In the smaller animals they are not usually seen because of the relatively smaller size of the fœti, but by pressing the hand on the right side of the abdomen of the ewe about the level of the stifle and a little in front of it, they may sometimes be felt.

Manipulation of the abdomen in the smaller animals—especially in the bitch and cat—yields reliable evidence of pregnancy. (*See* PREGNANCY DIAGNOSIS.)

Rectal or vaginal examination is also a most important means of diagnosing pregnancy, but is only applicable to the larger animals. By these methods the existence of pregnancy can often be established from the 3rd month onwards. Owing to the risk of inducing abortion the owner is not advised to attempt vaginal examination, which is essentially an expert procedure.

Auscultation, which consists in listening on the wall of the abdomen for the beating sounds of the fœtal heart, is a method of determining the presence or absence of pregnancy which has sometimes been applied to animals, but without the success that is claimed for it in human beings. The sounds of the intestines in the horse and those of the stomachs in cattle, mask

PERIODS OF GESTATION

Animal.	Average Period.		Shortest Period.	Longest Period
	Months. (Calendar.)	Days.	Young Born Alive.	Young Born Alive.
Mare	11	340	307	419
Ass	12¼	374	365	385
Cow	9	283	200	439
Ewe and Goat	5	144 to 150	135	160
(Merinos	..	150.)		
Sow	4 months or 3 months 3 weeks and 3 days	116 to 120	110	130
Bitch	2 months	58–63	55	70
Cat	8 weeks	55	—	—
Elephant	2 years (nearly)		—	—
Zebra	13 months or over		—	—
Camel	45 weeks		—	—
Rabbit	32 days		—	—
Guinea-pig	63 days		—	—

the faint rhythmic pulsations of the fœtal heart. (*See also under* PREGNANCY DIAGNOSIS.)

Care of the dam during pregnancy.—In all species of animals exercise (or work) is essential if the vigour of the dam is to be retained, and if her circulatory, digestive, muscular, and nervous systems are to be maintained in a fit state for the strains they will have to withstand at parturition. Food is of great importance. It should be perfectly wholesome, as plain as possible, given liberally so that the fœtus may be well-nourished. All irritant or stimulating spices, unduly laxative or purgative substances, and unusual foods should be avoided. No sudden changes in the ration should be made. Cooked foods should not be given to the larger animals, and in each animal it is better to give an extra feed each day rather than unduly to increase the quantities given at each feed. This avoids excessive distension of stomach and intestines which may lead to nausea and indigestion. A plentiful supply of cold clean water is a necessity for the pregnant dam (with the exception of sheep, which generally get all the water they require from the herbage and possibly by absorption of rain from the skin). Water is essential to supply the fluid required for the 'water-bag' (fœtal fluids) which is derived from the maternal blood, and it is needed for the increased activity in the mammary gland, especially towards the end of pregnancy.

PERIODS OF DEVELOPMENT DURING PREGNANCY.

Stage of Pregnancy.		Mare.	Cow.	Ewe and Goat.	Sow.	Bitch.
I.	Duration of Period Length of fœtus .	14 days Ovum $\frac{1}{12}$ in.	14 days Ovum $\frac{1}{12}$ in.	14 days Ovum $\frac{1}{15}$ in. to $\frac{1}{20}$ in.	14 days Ovum $\frac{1}{15}$ in. to $\frac{1}{20}$ in.	10 days Ovum $\frac{1}{15}$ in. to $\frac{1}{20}$ in.
	Stages in development . .	Fertilised ovum has reached uterus from oviduct.				
II.	Duration . . Length of fœtus .	3 to 4 weeks ½ in.	3 to 4 weeks ⅛ in.	3 to 4 weeks ⅛ in.	3 to 4 weeks ½ in.	10 days to 3 weeks ⅛ in.
	Stages . . .	Traces of fœtus appear; head, body and limbs are discernible by end of this period.				
III.	Duration . . Length of fœtus .	5 to 8 weeks 2⅛ in.	5 to 8 weeks 1¾ in.	5 to 7 weeks 1¼ in.	4 to 6 weeks 1¾ in.	3 to 4 weeks 1 in.
	Stages . . .	First indications of hoofs and claws visible as little pale elevations at ends of digits.				
IV.	Duration . . Length of fœtus .	9 to 13 weeks 6 in.	9 to 12 weeks 5½ in.	7 to 9 weeks 3½ in.	6 to 8 weeks 3 in.	5th week 2½ in.
	Stages . . .	Stomach well defined in foal, pig, and puppy; differentiation of four stomachs in ruminants at end of this period.				
V.	Duration . . Length of fœtus .	14 to 22 weeks 13 in.	13 to 20 weeks 12 in.	10 to 13 weeks 6 in.	8 to 10 weeks 5 in.	6th week 3½ in.
	Stages . . .	Large tactile hairs appear on lips, upper eyelids, and above eye. Teats visible in female fœtuses.				
VI.	Duration . . Length of fœtus .	23 to 24 weeks 2 ft. 3 in.	21 to 32 weeks 2 ft.	13 to 18 weeks 1 ft. 2 in.	11 to 15 weeks 7 in.	7 to 8 weeks 5 in.
	Stages . . .	Eyelashes well developed. A few hairs appear on tail, head and extremities of limbs.				
VII.	Duration . . Length . .	35 to 48 weeks 3½ ft.	33 to 40 weeks 3 ft.	19 to 21 weeks 1½ ft.	15 to 17 weeks 9 to 10 in.	9th week (8th in cat) 6 to 8 in. (kitten 5 in.)
	Stages . . .	Fœtus attains full size. Body becomes gradually covered with hair, hoofs and claws complete, but soft.				

A certain amount of special attention should be given to pregnant dams of each species of animals, and below some indications of these special precautions are given. *The mare* should if possible be treated absolutely as usual until the time that her abdomen begins to increase in size. Up till this time she can do the usual farm

PREGNANCY AND GESTATION

work without any danger. She may still be kept at work, harrowing, drilling, rolling (not in the shafts), etc., until about the middle of the 10th month, when turned out to grass. The field should be as level as possible, and shelter should be provided from extremes of weather. By the time she has reached the middle of the 11th month she is at grass every afternoon, but can be gently worked during each forenoon. Where two or more mares are in-foal at the same time it is very advisable to work them in pairs, for then not only do they go at a more even pace, but they become accustomed to each other, and when turned out together later on with their foals they are less likely to disagree. With saddle horses, harness work is preferable to riding, as much as possible; if such mares must be ridden they should not be galloped, jumped, ridden over rough ground or up or down steep slopes, spurs should be discarded, and upon no occasion should the mare be subjected to a severe use of the whip. During the last month an extra feed per day should be given, and if clover, or better lucerne, hay is available it should be given in preference to other kinds of hay. Lucerne, being rich in lime and magnesium salts, provides a plentiful supply of these for the mare's milk, as well as for the developing foal. During this last month it is well to allow the mare to sleep in the foaling-box, so that she may become accustomed to it, and settle better. The box should previously be thoroughly cleaned out, its walls scrubbed with boiling water containing Jeyes' fluid (or other suitable disinfectant), and when dry, it should be lime-washed to a height of 6 feet from the ground. This precaution is especially necessary where joint-ill exists upon a farm premises. In the south of Great Britain, or when or where the climate is mild, mares may, with great advantage, be allowed to foal out of doors in a clean pasture. Grooming should on no account be neglected, but harsh wisping or curry-combing should be prohibited. Cruel treatment on the part of groom or stable-boy should be sternly suppressed. With young mares foaling for the first time it is very advisable that they should be hand-rubbed about the flanks, belly, and udder, so that they may lose the natural ticklishness in these parts, and allow the foal to approach them without danger. Powerful purgatives should be avoided, but the food given should be gently laxative; for this purpose the addition of pulped roots, carrots, bran, or treacle to the food is good. (For further information see under PARTURITION.)

The cow is usually allowed to calve in a loose-box. There is no doubt that were cows heavy in calf given more exercise there would be far less trouble at calving. At about the end of the 7th month of pregnancy milking cows should be dried off, so that the substances which are destined for the nourishment of the calf in the uterus shall not be diverted to the udder. All rough treatment, chasing by dogs, crowding through narrow doorways, exposure to severe weather, or the unwanted attentions by the bull, should be guarded against from the 7th month onwards. Drastic purgatives and narcotics must be avoided, on account of the danger of inducing abortion.

Ewes may either be kept out on the hill, or brought down to lower land, and housed in a lambing-pen during the last week or so of pregnancy, but otherwise little special attention is necessary. Chasing by dogs, crowding through gateways, and all other forms of rough treatment are to be avoided. Care is needed when catching. Heavy in-lamb ewes should not be turned up to have their feet dressed.

Sows greatly benefit from having access to an old pasture or paddock, where they will not be disturbed by other animals, and where they may take as much exercise as they desire. But at night they should have a clean, warm, dry bed to sleep on. Pregnant sows are best fed individually or in twos; otherwise some sows get more than their fair share, while others suffer from under-feeding. Wet, cold floors and cold, draughty premises predispose to mastitis and agalactia.

Bitches must be given regular exercise, and as they are often not inclined to take exercise of their own accord it may be necessary to compel them to do so. Food should be of good quality, not too rich in fatty substances, and not too dry. An occasional small amount of minced raw or cooked liver serves to keep the bowels active, and also supplies a stimulus to the mammary glands. At night the pregnant bitch should have a warm dry box containing an old pillow or cushion and a towel where she may make a bed when the desire to do so comes upon her. Failing these, she should be given a thick wheat-straw bed in a stable or outhouse. (*See also* SUPERFŒTATION, BREEDING OF ANIMALS, PARTURITION, etc.)

PREGNANCY, FALSE (*see* PSEUDO-PREGNANCY *and* 'CLOUDBURST' (in goats)).

PREGNANCY, TERMINATION OF.—With a pregnant bitch or sow, for example, there are three possible outcomes: (1) she may have her litter; (2) she may abort; (3) resorption of the fœtuses may take place. (*See* RESORPTION.)

PREGNANCY TOXÆMIA IN EWES.—An acute metabolic disorder occurring during the last few weeks of pregnancy; or, perhaps it would be more correct to say, a number of disorders—one of which may be acetonæmia.

Causes.—In the more typical outbreaks, several factors are usually reported. The ewes are generally in good bodily condition, are carrying twins or triplets *in utero*, or have a particularly large single lamb. They are on good rich grazing, seldom getting much exercise. Bad weather, *e.g.* a fall of snow, has often occurred previous to the outbreak. It has been claimed that the disease can be produced experimentally by a short period of starvation during advanced pregnancy, and that ewes which become fat during the first three months of pregnancy are especially susceptible.

Symptoms.—The condition is typically an intoxication leading to coma and death. The first symptoms are incoordination of movement, the animal lagging behind others when driven, stepping high, and often staggering and falling. In another hour or two the ewe lies down and can only be induced to rise with difficulty. She stands swaying and will fall or lie down again almost immediately. In general appearance she is dull, hangs her head, her eyes appear to be staring—owing to widely dilated pupils—and breathing is laboured or stertorous. Fluid may be copiously discharged from the nostrils. Acetonæmia may be present, giving rise to the characteristic odour from breath and urine. A comatose condition develops. Death occurs within 1 to 6 days.

Prevention.—Owners have been advised to take the ewes for a walk over ploughed fields, fallow ground, or even along a road for an hour or two each day. Good results have followed. In addition, it has been recommended, that after the pre-tupping flush, ewes should be kept in store condition for the first 3 months of pregnancy.

Treatment.—Ewes should be dosed at once with glycerine (2 tablespoonfuls) in water; or glucose (2 oz. in ½ pint of warm water) or, preferably, glucose solution may be given intravenously.

PREGNANT MARE'S SERUM (*see under* PREGNANCY DIAGNOSIS TESTS *and* HORMONES).

PREISZ-NOCARD BACILLUS (*Corynebacterium ovis*). (*See* CASEOUS LYMPHADENITIS, ULCERATIVE LYMPHANGITIS.)

PREMATURE BIRTH (*see* ABORTION and PARTURITION, *and the table on* p. 749).

PREMEDICATION (*see under* PRENARCOTISATION).

PRE-MILKING (*see under* PRE-PARTUM MILKING).

PREMUNITION, which is a term meaning, broadly speaking, 'forearmed', is used in relation to the type of resistance shown by cattle, and possibly other animals against severe illness caused by trypanosomes. Animals which are premunised are *infected* with trypanosomes but are not *affected* by trypanosomiasis.

There are two types recognised: (*a*) Natural premunition, which occurs inside or in close proximity to a fly-belt, and (*b*) Artificial premunition, which results from the administration of a sub-sterilising dose of a trypanocidal drug. Unfortunately, it seems very probable that, at least in the majority of cases, natural premunition only gives protection against one local strain of trypanosomes, and cattle which are thus premunised against a local strain may succumb when exposed to infection with a different strain of the same species; if, for instance, they are moved out of one fly-belt to another. The occurrence of intercurrent diseases of other varieties may also lead to a breakdown in premunition. Similarly, artificial premunition can only be relied upon to protect against a single strain. Hornby admirably sums up the position by saying that '*for animals to be able to survive in all fly-belts they must be resistant under all conditions to all strains of all species of trypanosomes*'. It is obviously exceedingly difficult to achieve such protection as this by artificial means. (*See also* TSETSE FLY.)

PRENARCOTISATION.—The use of a

narcotic prior to inducing general anæsthesia. (*See* CHLORPROMAZINE.)

PRE-PARTUM MILKING.—Milking a heifer or cow a few days before the birth of her calf. Where this is practised, the calf when born must be provided with colostrum from another cow.

PREPOTENCY.—The ability of one parent, in greater degree than the other, to transmit a characteristic (*e.g.* high milk yield) to the offspring.

PREPUCE.—The foreskin or skin covering the end of the penis.

PRESBYOPIA (πρέσβυς, an old man; ὤψ, the eye) is the general term used to indicate the changes that normally affect the eye in old age, quite apart from any disease. The most important of these changes is a diminution of the natural elasticity of the lens of the eye, resulting in an impaired power of focussing objects near at hand.

PRESCRIPTION (*praescriptio*, an order) means the written order given by a practitioner to a chemist or dispenser for the compounding of medicines necessary in the treatment of a case. The prescription is written in Latin, a usage which has been handed down from mediæval times.

In March 1969 the British pharmaceutical industry adopted the metric system, and manufacturers changed to the 5 ml. (millilitre) dose; the old-fashioned and inaccurate 'teaspoonful' and 'tablespoonful' doses disappearing from labels. For human use, new 5 ml. spoons are supplied by dispensing chemists.

PRESENTATION means the appearance in parturition of some particular part of the young animal's body at the cervix of the womb. This is normally an anterior presentation, with the fore limbs and the head appearing first, but in a certain number of cases the breech may present first. (*See* PARTURITION.)

PRESSOR is the term applied to anything that increases the activity of a function, for example, a pressor nerve or pressor drug. Producing a rise in blood-pressure is its most common meaning.

PREVENTIVE VETERINARY MEDICINE.—This is the keynote of modern veterinary practice, and is of increasing importance in these days of intensive livestock husbandry and of very large units. (*See* HEALTH SCHEMES FOR FARM ANIMALS.)

PRICKING BY NAILS (*see* INJURIES FROM SHOEING).

PRIVET POISONING is very rare, and only occurs when horses and cattle have free access to privet hedges, or break into gardens and shrubberies containing this common ornamental shrub. Privet—*Ligustrum vulgare*—contains a glucoside—*ligustrin*, which causes loss of power in the hind legs, dilated pupils, slightly injected mucous membranes, and death in 36 to 48 hours.

Treatment.—All animals should be removed from contact with the plant, and the affected ones housed in a comfortable loose-box. A drench containing tannic acid, or strong black coffee or tea, should be given while awaiting the arrival of a skilled practitioner who will advise treatment according to the symptoms shown.

PROBANG.—A rod of flexible material designed to aid removal of foreign bodies from the œsophagus. (*See* CHOKING.)

PROCAINE HYDROCHLORIDE is used in solution as a local anæsthetic, and for epidural anæsthesia (which see). It is also known under the names of Novocain and Kerocain. A synthetic product, it is, generally speaking, as effective as cocaine (except for anæsthetising the cornea, for which cocaine is preferable) but far less toxic and safer to use, besides not coming under the Dangerous Drug Act regulations. It is often combined with adrenalin, in order to lessen hæmorrhage during minor surgery.

Given by intravenous injection, procaine hydrochloride has been used in cases of pruritus in dogs. Occasionally, relief from scratching lasts only a few hours, but in other cases it is reported that relief lasts several days, often until the cause has ceased to act.

Toxicity.—Excessive amounts of procaine hydrochloride cause stimulation of the central nervous system. In the horse 5 mgm. per lb. bodyweight gave rise to nervousness (tossing of the head, twitching of the ears, stamping of the feet, snorting, or neighing), while muscular inco-ordination and convulsions follows larger doses. In the dog, 20 mgm. per lb. caused salivation and vomiting, with muscular tremors and inco-ordination.

Procaine penicillin.—The procaine salt

of penicillin is often used, the concentration of penicillin in the blood remaining for a longer period, and the injection being less painful.

PROCTITIS (πρωκτός, the anus) means inflammation or only irritation situated about the anus or rectum. It is a frequent symptom of the presence of parasitic worms in almost all animals.

PRODROMAL (πρόδρομος, running before) is a term applied to symptoms of a disease which are among the first seen but not necessarily characteristic.

PROGENY TESTING.—A method of assessing the value of, *e.g.*, a bull as a sire, by examining the milk yield, etc., figures for an unselected sample of his daughters. Dam-daughter comparisons may show whether a high-yielding cow can transmit her capability to her progeny, but these comparisons are valid only under identical systems of feeding and management.

PROGESTERONE.—A sex hormone obtained from the *corpus luteum*.

PROGESTIN.—A proprietary brand of progesterone.

PROGRESSIVE RETINAL ATROPHY.—In the U.K. there is a joint scheme operated by the British Veterinary Association and the Kennel Club to reduce the incidence of this disease in any breed of dog; and certificates are issued to dog-owners. (*See* EYE, DISEASES OF.)

PROGLOTTIS is a term applied to the joint of a tape-worm.

PROGNOSIS (πρόγνωσις) is the term applied to a forecast of the probable outcome and course of an attack of disease, particularly with regard to the prospect of early or late recovery. It is based upon the nature of the attack, the severity of the symptoms, and the condition of the animal.

PROJECTILE SYRINGE.—Fired from a crossbow, this instrument is useful for administering sedatives, etc., to wild animals.

'PROJECTILE VOMITING.'—This term is used when the vomitus is thrown 2 or 3 feet from the body—a symptom of pyloric stenosis in the dog.

PROLACTIN.—A hormone associated with lactation.

PROLAN A is a follicle-stimulating hormone obtained from the pituitary of the pig. PROLAN B is a luteinising hormone from pig and sheep pituitary glands.

PROLAPSE (*prolabor*, I sink down) means the slipping down of some organ or structure. The term is applied to the displacements of the rectum and female generative organs, which result in their appearance to the outside.

The best plan is to seek professional assistance at once. (*See* UTERUS, DISEASES OF; RECTUM, DISEASES OF.)

PROLAPSE OF OVIDUCT.—This condition is fairly frequently met with in fowls, particularly in birds which have been laying heavily. It is nearly always associated with some aberration from normal of the cloaca or oviduct, irritation resulting and causing the bird to strain. Occasionally it is seen after an endeavour to pass a large or malformed egg, yolk concretion, etc., and in cases known as 'egg bound'. It is also sometimes met with in cases of vent gleet. The prolapsed oviduct appears as a dark red swelling protruding from the vent. Other birds are attracted by the swelling and peck at it, frequently leading to evisceration and death. Treatment consists in removing the affected bird from the flock. The prolapse should be washed with warm water containing a mild antiseptic, and then gently pressed back into the abdominal cavity after first removing the egg or other foreign body, if the presence of such can be detected. It greatly aids return to have the bird held head downwards by an assistant. After returning the prolapse, cold water is sometimes injected to reduce the swelling and to quicken contraction of the oviduct wall. The bird should be kept quiet for a day or two, fed on a laxative diet, and then may be returned to the flock. Occasionally, the prolapse reappears, and treatment must be repeated.

PROLONGED SOFT PALATE.—An inherited abnormality of dogs. (*See under* PALATE.)

PROMAZINE HYDROCHLORIDE.—An effective sedative and prenarcotic, administered to the dog by intravenous or intramuscular injection. (*See under* CHLORPROMAZINE.)

'PROMINTIC'.—A drug used against worms in cattle and sheep. (*See* METHYRIDINE.)

PRONTOSIL.—A reddish crystalline powder; the forerunner of the sulpha drugs.

PROPHYLAXIS (προφύλαξ, an advanced guard) means any treatment that is adopted with a view to the warding-off of disease. Thus, inoculation.

PROPIONATE, SODIUM.—A bacteriostatic and fungicide which has been recommended in the treatment of obstinate infections of the conjunctiva and cornea.

PROPYLENE GLYCOL has been used in the treatment of acetonæmia in cattle.

PROSTATE GLAND is one of the accessory sexual glands that lies at the neck of the bladder in the male animal, and partly surrounds the urethra at that point. It is of importance because of the great increase in size to which it is prone, especially in dogs. When greatly enlarged not only does it interfere with the free passage of urine to the outside, but it may obstruct the passage of fæces. At times it causes a very troublesome incontinence of urine when abnormally large in size. In such cases the use of stilbœstrol is helpful; otherwise operation of castration is necessary. When the testicles are removed the activity of the gland ceases and it undergoes atrophy.

Apart from this gradually occurring hyperplasia of the gland in dogs over 5 years old, enlargement may be due to an acute infection, when evidence of pain (with arched back and a stiff-legged gait) may be added to the symptoms. Cancer of the prostate is rare in the dog; cysts sometimes occur.

PROTARGOL is a preparation of silver with an albuminous substance, possessing great astringent and antiseptic properties. It is used in inflammatory conditions of the eyes or of mucous membranes, in strengths varying from 1 part in 200 to 1 in 25 of distilled water.

PROTECTION OF ANIMALS (ANÆSTHETICS) ACT, 1954 (*see under the heading* ANÆSTHETICS). (*See also under* LAW.)

PROTEIN CONCENTRATES.—Products specifically designed for further mixing, at an inclusion rate of 5 per cent or more, with planned proportions of cereals and other feeding stuffs either on the farm or by a feedstuff compounder.

PROTEIN EQUIVALENT.—This provides the measure of the value of a feeding-stuff, taking into account the protein content plus the non-protein nitrogen content, capable of being converted into protein by the animal's digestive system. It is expressed as a percentage. For example, the protein equivalent of linseed cake is 25 per cent; *i.e.* 100 lb. of the cake is equivalent to 25 lb. of protein and potential protein. The protein equivalent of grass silage is about 2 per cent; that of kale, 1·3 per cent.

PROTEIN, HYDROLISED.—A mixture of amino-acids and simple polypeptides prepared by enzyme digestion of whole muscle. A valuable source of protein used in cases of shock, malnutrition, convalescence, fevers, chronic nephritis, etc. It may be given by mouth or injection.

PROTEIN SHOCK.—A reaction following the parenteral administration of a protein. (*See* ANAPHYLAXIS.)

PROTEIN THERAPY.—Treatment by means of injecting a foreign protein (*i.e.* one not occurring in the animal's own tissues).

PROTEINS are the flesh-forming principles present in greater or lesser amounts in most foods. They are also known as 'proteids', 'albuminoids', or 'nitrogenous principles', the latter name being used on account of the presence in them of nitrogen. Generally speaking, this class contains the foods of animal origin, though many vegetables, notably the leguminous kinds (peas, beans, tares, clovers) and various nuts, contain vegetable protein.

Nitrogenous food is necessary to replace the daily loss through wear and tear of muscle, and to build up body tissues in the growing animal. It therefore follows that animals which are called upon to do much heavy or fast work, and consequently to expend their tissues at a fast rate, require more protein in their rations than do those which live a less strenuous existence. The proportion of available protein to other nutritive substances in the ration, known as the 'protein ratio', is an important fact to be borne in mind when rations are being computed for animals. This and other aspects of proteins are considered under DIET, and sections are also included under PIGS, SHEEP, etc.

PROTHROMBIN.—A substance formed in the liver with the assistance of vitamin K, and essential for the clotting of blood.

PROTOPLASM (πρῶτος, first; πλάσμα, form) is a viscid, translucent, glue-like material containing fine granules, and composed mainly of proteins, which makes up the essential material of plant and animal cells, and has the properties of life.

PROTOZOA (πρῶτος, first; ζῶον, animal) is the name given to the animalcules, for the most part microscopic, which consist of one cell only, in distinction to all other members of the animal kingdom, which possess more than one cell and are therefore known as 'Metazoa'.

PROTOZOÖN PARASITES are extremely important in that they are parasitic upon the higher animals and man, in which they cause disease. Malaria, tsetse-fly disease, surra, nagana, mal du coit, mal de caderas, red-water fever, Texas fever, and other 'tick diseases', have as the causal organism one or another form of protozoa. (*See* 'Parasites', under above headings.)

PROUD FLESH is the popular name given to the unhealthy granulations which sometimes arise perhaps around an inflamed ulcer, when a wound is greatly infected and the discharge copious, or at the edges of a sinus. It can be checked by the application of a caustic astringent.

PROXIMAL is a term of comparison applied to structures which are nearer the centre of the body or the median line, as opposed to more 'distal' structures.

PRURITUS (*prurio*, I itch) is the name applied to the symptom of itching which is a prominent feature of most parasitic skin diseases, and of Aujesky's Disease and Scrapie.

PRUSSIC ACID, or HYDROCYANIC ACID, is a very deadly poison with a sweetish smell and a sweet but stinging taste.

As a poison it acts with great rapidity, especially when used as the Scheele's acid, which is double the strength of the ordinary prussic acid, and contains 4 per cent of hydrocyanic acid in solution in water. It was once greatly used for the destruction of dogs, and when properly employed is useful for this purpose though far from ideal. Human experiences suggest that, despite convulsions and cries, it is humane. It should only be used by responsible persons, and precautions should be taken that none of the acid is spilled, or comes into contact with the mouth, eyes, nose, or a wound in the skin. If such should happen the person should *at once* wash the part with hot water, and dry with a towel immediately afterwards, and should remain in the open air for a few minutes. This precaution is very necessary, for as little as 5 drops may cause an adult person to fall to the ground writhing in convulsions, if he should receive it in the mouth; and though fatal effects may not necessarily follow this small dose, it is very dangerous. (See next section for treatment.)

Prussic acid is found in nature in the leaves of the Cherry Laurel (*Prunus lauro cerasus*), in the kernels of many stone fruits, in almonds, etc., and under the action of warmth and moisture it may be produced in vegetable substances which contain a cyanogenetic glucoside, such as 'Java' beans (which are differently known as Rangoon beans, Burmah beans, Lima beans, Paıgya beans, etc.), *Phaseolus lunatus*, linseed cake (certain kinds), maize, etc.

PRUSSIC ACID POISONING is liable to occur when an overdose of prussic acid is given in error, when animals have eaten quantities of laurel leaves, or have taken, some time previously, considerable amounts of some substance containing a cyanogenetic glucoside (see previous section).

Symptoms.—Since the drug is very volatile and diffusible, its action is very rapid. When a fatal dose has been administered either by the mouth or otherwise, there is at first an increase in the number and volume of the respirations, occasionally accompanied by coughing. Then, a few moments later, the animal utters a cry (especially dogs and cats), and falls to the ground. The limbs and body generally become stretched out to their fullest extent, all the muscles being rigid, and the respirations cease during this phase. Gradually, the tense muscles slacken, and the whole body becomes limp. A few shallow or sighing respirations occur, and, after a few feeble beats, the heart ceases and the animal is dead. Upon occasion, when less acid has been taken, the heart may continue to beat for some minutes after apparent death, and during this time it is often possible to resuscitate the animal by artificial respiration. (*See* ARTIFICIAL RESPIRATION.)

With the larger animals, where poisoning has resulted from eating one or other of the substances mentioned, the symptoms of prussic acid are not so constant. There may be no symptoms until from half to one hour after eating the substance, and then there is a sudden onset of great excitement, salivation, slight diarrhœa, quickened pulse and breathing, and muscular spasms, passing into paralysis and causing prostration. Death or recovery follows very rapidly, owing to the nature of the poison, which, being volatile, is quickly absorbed, and also quickly eliminated by the kidneys and lungs.

Treatment consists in dragging the animal out into the open air as rapidly as possible, and commencing artificial respiration *at once*. For so long as the heart can be felt beating, it is advisable to persist in this measure, and to give inhalations of ammonia and oxygen, and to douche the head and neck with cold water. (*See* ANTIDOTES.)

PSAMMOMA (ψάμμος, sand) is the name given to a small hard tumour of the brain.

PSEUDO- (ψευδής, false) is a prefix put to the name of certain well-known diseases to indicate other conditions whose symptoms closely resemble those of one of the other diseases in question, although the real nature of the two maladies is quite distinct.

PSEUDO-CYESIS is another name for PSEUDO-PREGNANCY (which see).

PSEUDO-LEUKÆMIA.—This is not a single entity but rather a group of diseases—all of which bear a close resemblance to leukæmia although there is no increase of white cells in the blood.

The infective, malignant granulomata (Hodgkin's disease of man) has not been proved to occur in domestic animals.

Granulomata—when they occur as a generalised disease of the lymph-adenoid system—may resemble clinically true leukæmia. Tuberculosis may be a cause.

Lympho-sarcomatosis is not uncommon in animals.

The lymph glands, spleen, and liver are usually enlarged in pseudo-leukæmia, and there is anæmia.

PSEUDO-PREGNANCY is a condition commonly seen in the bitch, but probably occurring in all breeding female animals to a lesser degree. In it the physical signs of pregnancy are exhibited in the absence of fœtus or fœtuses. The abdomen increases in size, the uterus becomes swollen and turgid, its walls are thickened, and in extreme cases mammary development may occur, and milk may be secreted. The bitch may actually make a bed and prepare to litter.

In time, since no fœtuses are present, the organs and tissues return to their normal state without the occurrence of parturition ; heat returns, and successful breeding may occur subsequently. The cause of pseudo-pregnancy is believed to be due to excessive or irregular secretion of a hormone from the corpus luteum, which should normally only be produced in quantity after fertilisation has occurred. The condition can—where necessary—be treated by injection of the appropriate hormone. (*See* REPRODUCTION, BREEDING, 'CLOUDBURST' of goats, etc.)

PSEUDOMONAS PYOCYANEA.—This organism is a motile, gram-negative rod, 1·5 to 3 μ long. It flourishes in suppurating wounds, and has been found in cases of otitis in the dog. It has also been reported as causing outbreaks of disease in turkey poults and other birds.

Chronic mastitis, with diarrhœa and wasting resembling Johne's disease, has been caused in a cow by *P. æruginosa*.

PSEUDO-RABIES.—A name occasionally used for AUJESZKY'S DISEASE.

PSEUDO-TUBERCULOSIS is a name often applied to caseous lymphadenitis of sheep. (*See* CASEOUS LYMPHADENITIS.)

PSITTACOSIS is a disease of parrots and man which is due to what was formerly regarded as a virus. (*See* VIRUSES.) It can be readily transmitted to fowls, mice, and guinea-pigs.

Symptoms.—Affected parrots may not show any symptoms for some considerable time after contracting the infection, but when once the symptoms have appeared illness becomes marked, and death occurs in a very few days. The birds are listless and dull ; a hæmorrhagic diarrhœa is often seen, and a catarrhal condition of the nasal passages and eyes may be shown in the later stages of the disease. (*See also* ORNITHOSIS.)

In the U.S.A. psittocosis agents have been isolated from calves with arthritis. Death usually followed 2 to 10 days after the first signs of stiffness and enlargement of joints.

PSOAS (ψόα, the loin) is the name of two muscles, *Psoas major* and *Psoas minor*, which lie along the roof of the abdomen immediately beneath the last two or three thoracic and the whole of the lumbar vertebræ, and stretch into the pelvis. The psoas minor is inserted to the *psoas tubercle* of the ilium, and the psoas major runs to the inner or lesser trochanter of the femur in common with the *iliacus* muscle. The action of these muscles is to bend the pelvis on the rest of the trunk, or if those of one side of the body are acting alone, to bend the posterior part of the trunk towards that side. The act of crouching preparatory to kicking is accomplished by these muscles and others, and they are largely concerned in the movements of galloping. Disease or injury, such as a severe sprain, is shown by a difficulty in walking both forwards and backwards, by a crouching appearance of the back, and by extreme difficulty in rising from the ground.

PSORIASIS (ψώρα, scurf) is a chronic inflammatory skin disease with scurf formation. (*See* MALLENDERS.)

PTOMAINE POISONING (πτῶμα, a dead body) is the general name given to cases of poisoning following upon the eating of meat, fish, cheese, or other animal substance which has undergone some decomposition. Naturally, dogs and cats, among the domesticated animals, suffer most from this form of poisoning, and it is probable that it is very much more common than is generally supposed. The serious effects produced are usually due to the formation of animal alkaloids, known as *ptomaines*. Their chemical analysis proves them to be closely related and very similar to the poisonous alkaloids found in plants. Among animal alkaloids are *collodine*, contained in decaying mackerel; *muscarine*, derived from putrid fish; *mytilotoxine*, from decomposed mussels; *tyrotoxicon*, which is sometimes contained in old musty cheese. *Xanthine* and *creatinine*, which can be extracted at any time from urine, are bodies of a similar nature; and the dog's urine, according to some authorities, contains a poisonous base known as *cynosine*. During the chemical analysis of the organs of dogs suspected of having been poisoned by some more common poison, there are sometimes found substances which act in most respects (but not in all) like well-known vegetable alkaloids; thus, there have been described 'corpse-strychnine', 'corpse-conine', 'corpse-delphine', and a substance very similar to morphine. Others of a very poisonous nature, which may be found in ordinary decomposing animal flesh (especially in the early stages), are: *neurine*, *trimethylamine*, and *sepsine*. These are, however, not always stable, and may themselves become altered or split up into harmless bases.

Symptoms.—Slight attacks of vomiting and diarrhœa, accompanied by varying degrees of fever and drowsiness or torpor, from which a dog recovers in 24 hours, may in reality be mild cases of ptomaine poisoning. In more severe cases the alkaloids act as narcotico-irritants, causing severe attacks of vomiting shortly after a feed, a high temperature, great depression, prostration, and even death.

Treatment.—Castor oil should be given in order to remove from the body the offending material. In more severe cases an emetic is required, and the animal should be placed under the attention of a veterinary surgeon.

PTOSIS (πτῶσις, a fall) means a drooping of the upper eyelid due to paralysis of the third or oculomotor nerve, which actuates the muscle that raises the upper eyelid. It is commonly seen along with facial paralysis, which is due to paralysis of the facial nerve, and is commonest in the horse after accidents to the head. It may be so severe as to make vision difficult, and it only disappears gradually. Ptosis may be a symptom of GUTTURAL POUCH DIPHTHERIA.

PTYALIN (πτύαλον, saliva) is the name of the ferment contained in the saliva, by which starchy food-stuffs are changed into sugars, and so prepared for absorption.

PTYALISM.—Salivation.

PUBERTY is the period in the life of the animal when it attains sexual maturity and becomes capable of propagating its species.

Animal.	Average Age at which Puberty occurs.
Mare . .	15 to 18 months.
Cow . .	12 ,, 14 ,,
Ewe, Goat, Sow . .	8 ,, 12 ,,
Bitch, Cat . .	7 ,, 12 ,,

Note.—Males usually reach puberty slightly in advance of females, on an average from 2 or 3 months sooner.

PUBIS is the bone that forms the lower anterior part of the pelvis. The pubes of right and left sides meet each other at the 'symphysis of the pubes', which in old age is no longer a separable union, bony fusion having taken place.

PUBLIC HEALTH (*see* SANITATION, DISINFECTION, DISPOSAL OF CARCASES, MILK, FOOD INSPECTION; PENICILLIN, SENSITIVITY TO, and the list of diseases given under the heading ZOONOSES; etc.).

PUERPERAL APOPLEXY (*puerperus*, bringing forth children) is another name for milk fever. (*See* MILK FEVER.)

PUERPERAL FEVER (*puerperus*, bringing forth children) is a name sometimes applied to septic metritis following parturition. The name is taken from human medicine. (*See* UTERUS, DISEASES OF, *and* POST-PARTURIENT FEVER.)

PUERPERIUM (*puerperium*) is a name borrowed from human medicine, and used to indicate the two or three days or more immediately following parturition, when the dam's body tissues generally are recovering from the strain of the act of parturition, and when the milk flow is attaining to its normal condition. The chief changes that occur are: diminution in size and volume of the uterus; return of the abdomen to its usual size; increase in the general activity of the dam following upon a period of comparative sluggishness; decrease in the amount of colostrum in the milk, and an increase in the amount of milk secreted. The period is a somewhat critical one when parturition has been difficult or when abortion has occurred. (*See* UTERUS, DISEASES OF; PARTURITION; PREGNANCY.)

'PULLET DISEASE.'—A pyelonephritis; identical with 'visceral gout nephritis'.

Symptoms include loss of appetite, diarrhœa with watery or whitish evacuations and *sometimes* darkening of the comb. Birds appear drowsy. About 10 per cent die. The cause is unknown; perhaps a virus.

PULLORUM DISEASE OF CHICKS (BACILLARY WHITE DIARRHŒA).—Is an acute, infectious, and highly fatal disease of chicks, causing much loss during the first 2 weeks of life. Adult fowls, especially laying hens, act as 'carriers' and transmit infection through their eggs to the chick before hatching. They may also spread infection in their droppings.

Cause.—The disease is caused by *Salmonella pullorum*, which is found in the ovary and oviduct of carrier hens, which are birds which themselves contracted the disease when young, but which survived. The disease is a true 'egg-borne' disease, and since only one infected egg in a large number can, if it hatches successfully, infect many or most of the chicks in a batch, it can be realised that incubator hatching and artificial foster-mother and brooder rearing, where perhaps several hundreds may run together, is a very important factor in causing the disease to spread. With eggs hatched by hens the spread is of only small dimensions, since only a particular clutch can be infected from each infected egg.

Intensive methods of management instead of extensive or range methods also favour spread by concentrating the infection upon a limited area of soil or floor, or in the poultry houses, coops, brooders, etc.

In addition to direct infection from birds on the same farm, outbreaks have been traced to the use of 'clear' eggs from incubators used to add to chick food, and to the use of shells from eggs purchased for domestic use, which without being cooked are sometimes broken up and used as a mineral addition to chick mash.

Symptoms.—The symptoms are not very characteristic at first, but young chicks are noted to be uneasy, cheeping continuously in a weary manner, dull and generally unlike the normally alert, active young chick. Down is ruffled and the chicks are unsteady on their feet. Later, a yellowish or whitish diarrhœa occurs and the down feathering around the vent becomes gummed and sticky. However, in acute cases, no diarrhœa may be seen. Death occurs suddenly after only 12 hours' to 2 or 3 days' illness, but as the outbreak develops, each case becomes a little less severe, and chicks affected in the later stages may survive, as may older chicks infected from outside sources.

Birds which survive establish an immunity, and it is by a blood agglutination examination that these can be identified. Though they are themselves immune they carry the germs in their bodies and can serve as a menace to the healthy flock.

Infected chicks may infect the hens used to brood them, but adults generally recover to become 'carriers' as already described.

It should be noted that in spite of the name of this disease, diarrhœa is not a constant symptom in all outbreaks. Moreover, diarrhœa which is not distinguishable from that associated with this disease may occur from other causes, such as bad feeding or management. To reach an accurate diagnosis, laboratory examination of sick or dead chicks is necessary, though a history of many deaths among newly hatched chicks, some of which show diarrhœa, pneumonia, a mottled or congested liver, and other lesions, should always be regarded as very suspicious.

Treatment.—In most cases it is not satisfactory to attempt treatment when an outbreak is confirmed. Death rate is always heavy (80 per cent or more), and survivors become a constant danger to the rest of the flock. It is generally cheapest to destroy and burn all the chicks in the hatching, thoroughly disinfect incubators, coops, foster-mothers, etc., and all movable appliances which have been used for the chicks. Fumigation with formaldehyde gas (generated by pouring commercial formalin on to potassium permanganate crystals) is effective for fumigating incubators and incubator houses.

Prevention.—This can be achieved by testing all birds, eggs from which are to be used for hatching, by the 'B.W.D. Agglutination Test'. Any positive reactors are eliminated, preferably by being killed for food purposes, to avoid spread of infection if sold to other establishments.

The negatives are moved to fresh, clean ground and a second test a month later is desirable, and if further reactors are found, monthly tests are carried out until an all-clear pass is obtained.

When a flock has had all the positive birds eliminated, and when certain other regulations have been fulfilled, it may qualify for 'accreditation' under the scheme of the Ministry of Agriculture. Annual testing is necessary to prevent the recurrence of infection and the subsequent spread of the disease through the clean flock. Precautions must be taken to prevent reinfection from the purchase of new birds, eggs for setting, etc.

The agglutination test can either be done with the co-operation of a laboratory, when samples of each bird's blood must be collected and sent away for test, or the 'rapid' test can be carried out on the farm itself.

General.—There are some points of general importance regarding pullorum disease which should be kept in mind.

(i) Infection may be present on a farm without any signs of illness being seen among the 'carrier' birds, so that the appearance of the flock is of no guidance in establishing the presence of infection.

(ii) Eggs from 'carrier' hens do not always hatch into chicks which become clinically affected. The number of infected eggs varies from only 5 per cent to about 40 per cent of those laid by a carrier, and the healthy eggs will hatch into normal healthy chicks. If all the eggs set are, by accident, healthy ones, there will be no outbreak in the hatching. It is, however, only rarely that this will occur, though when the number of 'carriers' in a flock is few it may readily occur once or twice in a season.

(iii) One blood test cannot be relied upon to clear an infected flock, and the reintroduction of infection from other sources must be constantly guarded against.

The Ministry of Agriculture Laboratories are excellently equipped to deal with samples and to carry out the necessary post-mortem examinations.

PULMONARY DISEASES (*see* LUNGS, DISEASES OF).

PULPY KIDNEY DISEASE IN LAMBS attacks lambs between about 3 weeks and 18 weeks of age, particularly those which are thriving. The disease has recently been seen in lambs under a week old. It occurs in Britain, America, New Zealand, etc.

Cause.—A bacterial intoxication of intestinal origin. It seems probable that more than one strain of organism may be involved, but in this country *Clostridium Welchii*, Type D (*B. ovitoxicus*, Bennetts), in the bowel has been shown to be responsible. In all probability the high protein feeding acts as a predisposing cause, rendering conditions in the bowel particularly suitable for the production of toxin. Anti-serum will protect against infection.

Symptoms.—As a rule the affected lambs are found dead without having previously been noticed ailing. Usually the lambs in the best condition are the first to be affected. The loss may be very heavy, especially with the larger earlier maturing breeds. Post-mortem examination shows striking changes in the kidney, which are different from those encountered in almost any other condition. They are soft in consistency, mottled in colour, and the cortex is jelly-like or almost semi-fluid. The liver usually shows hæmorrhagic spots on its surface and is markedly congested. There may be diffusely scattered small hæmorrhages over the peritoneal surface of other organs. In adult sheep the disease is known as Enterotoxæmia (which see), and the 'pulpy kidney' lesions are absent.

Prevention.—It is recommended that immunity be maintained by autumn vaccination, with a second dose of vaccine in the spring, 'preferably about 10 days before lambing, unless the ewes are to be moved to a better pasture prior to lambing, when the second dose should be given before the move is made. These two doses should protect the ewe through the spring months and allow her to pass to the lamb *via* the colostrum sufficient antibodies to protect it for the first 8 to 12 weeks of life. That temporary immunity in the lamb should be converted to an active one by the use of vaccine . . .'

PULSE (*pulsus*, a blow). The forcing of blood from the heart into the elastic arteries of the systemic circulation brings about a pulsation in them. This may be better understood when it is remembered that the beating of the heart drives blood out from the left ventricle into an already full aorta, in which it is imprisoned by the closing of the aortic semilunar valves. To accommodate this extra blood the aorta dilates, and the blood already in it moves onwards throughout the course of the vessel, and through the larger branches to which it gives origin. The wave of dilatation also travels along the course taken by the blood, and is therefore distributed along all the larger arterial trunks. If the fingers be laid over any of these latter, which lie near the surface in the horse, a periodic thrill or 'pulse' can be felt, occurring about 35 to 45 times per minute. What is spoken of as *the pulse* is this periodic pulsation occurring in one or other of the arteries which lie near enough to the surface to be felt without great difficulty, but a pulse can be felt wherever an artery of a large or medium size lies near the surface. These pulsations get less and less as the wave passes into smaller and smaller branches, until finally in the minute capillaries they are lost. For this reason, and because the pressure is much lower, pulsations are not felt in the veins.

The pulse-rate varies according to the state of the animal's health, being faster in fevers, and slower and weaker in debilitating non-febrile diseases; according to the age of the animal (faster in the very young and very old); according to the climate, bodily condition, and under other circumstances. During and immediately after exercise it is greatly increased, but in health it subsides rapidly subsequently. During sleep and unconsciousness it is slower.

In the horse the pulse can be easily felt about half-way between the angle of the lower jaw and the lower incisor region, where the facial artery turns over the edge of the lower jaw-bone, and also on the inside of the fore-arm at the level of the elbow-joint, where the radial artery crosses immediately over the bone. In the ox it may be felt along the lower jaw, and also under the root of the tail. In the sheep it is taken on the inside of the thigh or at the cheek, in the pig inside the thigh if the animal is not too fat, and in the dog on the inside of the fore-arm or, better, on the inside of the thigh, where the femoral artery is superficial. It will not always be felt the first time in these situations, but if no pulse is discovered after a few moments, the fingers should be shifted a little distance farther upwards, forwards, or backwards, and after a few moments' search it will usually be found.

The normal pulse-rates of the domesticated animals at rest are as follows:

	Per minute.
Horse	36 to 42
Ox	45 ,, 50
Sheep } Pig }	70 ,, 80
Dog	90 ,, 100
Cat	100 ,, 120

and of certain other animals as follows :

	Per minute.
Elephant	25 to 28
Camel	28 ,, 32
Buffalo	40 ,, 45
Reindeer	60 ,, 65
Mouse	130 ,, 150

If the above table is studied it will be seen that, roughly speaking, the smaller the bulk of the animal the faster the pulse. The same principle applies to animals of one species but of different sizes or of different breeds ; *e.g.* the pulse of the Shire stallion is usually about 35 per minute, while that of the Shetland pony in 45 or more. These facts must be taken into account when counting the pulse of any given animal. (*See also under* HEART.)

PUPIL (*pupilla*) is the opening in the centre of the iris of the eye through which the rays of light pass to the retina. (*See* EYE.)

PUPPING (*see* WHELPING, PARTURITION).

PURGATION is now recognised to involve dangers which include potassium depletion.

PUPPIES, NEWBORN, INFECTION IN.—A virus has been found by American research workers to be responsible for a fatal disease of new-born pups. It has been successfully transmitted experimentally, when it caused death in 6 to 9 days.

Symptoms.—Mild diarrhœa, vomiting, acute abdominal pain. (*See* FADING.)

PURGATIVES (*purgo*, I cleanse) are drugs or other substances or measures which produce evacuation of the bowels.

Varieties and actions.—Purgatives are divided into several groups, according to the manner and degree of violence with which they act.

Laxatives are those which gently stimulate the bowels and render the evacuations more frequent and liquid, without producing any griping or colicky action. Small doses of linseed oil, Epsom salts, Glauber's salts, roots, green food, treacle, and bran mashes for the larger animals, and small doses of cascara, liquid paraffin, mixed saline salts (such as ' Kruschen '), in the smaller animals, are among the most common. Most vegetables or fruits (which possess a considerable amount of indigestible fibre) also act in the same way.

Simple purgatives or *aperients* are rather more powerful than the former class, producing more frequent and fluid evacuations, not always unaccompanied by pain or discomfort. Examples of this class are castor oil, syrup of buckthorn, cascara, or calomel for the pig, dog, and cat. (*See also* DIHYDROXYANTHRAQUINONE.)

Drastic purgatives cause a violent action of the bowels, usually accompanied by pain and straining. In large doses they produce an inflammation of the lining mucous membrane of the bowels, and therefore they should never be included in first-aid measures undertaken by animal owners themselves. Such obsolete purgatives include croton oil, gamboge, podophyllin, elaterium, eserine, arecoline, and barium chloride.

Saline purgatives are salts of the alkaline metals and alkaline earths. They include sulphates of potassium, or sodium (Glauber's salts), and of magnesium (Epsom salts) ; sodium potassium tartrate (Seidlitz powder, for dogs only) ; and occasionally citrate of magnesium. Of these, Epsom and Glauber's salts are by far the most common and useful. Saline purgatives are most useful in cattle and sheep ; in the horse they are chiefly used in small doses to induce an aperient rather than a purgative action, and in dogs with certain exceptions, or unless given in small doses, they are liable to produce vomiting. When given to cattle they should be dissolved in warm water, to which treacle has been added, and, afterwards, a tablespoonful of ground ginger stirred into the jug used for mixing will usually prevent the griping action which may otherwise follow.

Purgatives produce their effects in different ways ; some stimulate the action of the bowels (peristalsis) ; others irritate the mucous membrane and thereby induce the glands to pour out a greater amount of secretion ; some hinder absorption ; and others still produce a solution in the intestines of such concentration that fluid is encouraged to flow from the mucous membrane by osmosis. The majority of the substances mentioned act in more than one of these ways, although one action in each is preponderant. Further, certain purgatives act all along the intestinal canal, such as Epsom salts and castor oil, while others have no action until the large intestine is reached (such as cascara).

PURPURA HÆMORRHAGICA (*purpura*, purple), which is also known as Petechial fever, Anasarcous fever, and used to be called 'scarlatina of the horse', is an acute or subacute fevered condition, usually following some other disease, in which small purple hæmorrhages occur in the mucous membrane of the nasal passages, eyes, etc., in parts of the skin, and in certain of the internal organs, and in which bilaterally symmetrical, dropsical swellings of the lower parts of the body and the head are common. The disease is commonest in the horse and members of the horse tribe, but it has also been described in the ox, and a disease similar to it has been recorded in dogs. As

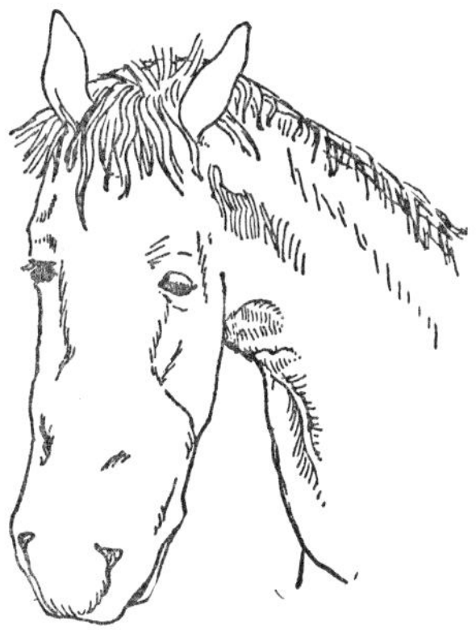

The appearance of a horse's head showing swelling of the upper jaw, nostrils, and upper lip, due to purpura. The eyelids are also swollen, causing the eyes to be kept half-closed, which changes the expression of the face. The swellings are usually bilaterally symmetrical, and affect the limbs and lower parts of the body as well.

already noted, it usually follows some other disease (such as strangles or influenza), and makes its appearance when the symptoms of the primary disease are subsiding and when the horse appears to be recovering satisfactorily.

Cause.—The cause of purpura is unknown. It is a disease which may be of an allergic nature—the reaction to streptococcal protein. It is not possible to reproduce the disease by injections of blood from an actual case. The disease is not contagious, although several horses in a stable may be affected at or about the same time.

Symptoms.—Appear suddenly; often overnight. They consist of purple-coloured spots (known as 'petechiæ' when small, 'vibices' when somewhat larger, and 'ecchymoses' when of considerable size) scattered over the mucous membranes of the nasal passages, eyes, inside the lips, and within the lips of the vulva of the mare. These vary from the size of a pin's head to almost as large as a two-shilling piece; they are not greatly raised above the surface of the surrounding membrane, and are not usually painful to the touch. A blood-stained discharge from the nose is usually found. At the same time, swellings, very often the same on each side of the body, are found on the limbs, the breast, the eyelids, and almost always about the muzzle and nostrils. These swellings may be diffuse from the first, or they may begin as isolated circumscribed flat prominences about the size of a duck's egg, which coalesce in the course of a day or more. The swellings are cold, painless to the touch, and when pressed with the point of the thumb a little pit remains afterwards for some moments.

The horse is dull, hangs the head, loses its appetite, moves stiffly and with difficulty, and if the swellings of the nostrils are large, shows rapid and laboured breathing. Swollen lips may prevent a horse from feeding or drinking, swollen eyelids may hinder or prevent vision, and a swollen sheath in the male may make the act of urination difficult or impossible. The temperature does not usually rise very high, but remains between 102° F. and 104° F.; the pulse is soft, feeble, generally rapid, and may be very irregular—an indication of the loss of tone and weakness of the heart. Complications, such as pneumonia, convulsions, paralysis of the hind-quarters, etc., are not uncommon.

The percentage of recoveries is not large in well-marked cases, and even where death does not occur, complete recovery takes a long time, and relapses are common. It is said that cases showing nervous complications *always* end fatally, and the same may be said of those with pneumonia.

Treatment.—The most careful nursing and feeding are essential in all cases of purpura. (*See* NURSING OF SICK ANIMALS.) Medicinal treatment should be under the direction of a veterinary surgeon. Good results often follow the intravenous injection of an antihistamine.

After apparent recovery the horse must have a long period of convalescence.

PUS (*pus*) or MATTER, is a thick, white, yellow, grey, greenish, reddish, or bluish fluid, which is found in abscesses and sinuses, and on the surfaces of ulcers and inflamed areas where the skin is broken. Its colour and consistence vary according to the variety of organism that is present in the part, and to the multitudes of pus corpuscles that form, with serum from the blood, the bulk of the discharge. The pus corpuscles are modified white blood corpuscles that have left the blood-stream by diapedesis (under the compelling action of the presence of an irritant in the tissues), together with the superficial cells from mucous membrane or granulation tissue that have died and been cast off under the influence of the inflammation of the part. (*See* ABSCESS, PHAGOCYTOSIS.)

PUSTULE (*pustula*) means a small collection of pus occurring in the skin, or immediately below it. (*See* ABSCESS.) 'Malignant pustule' is the name applied to the form that anthrax most commonly takes when it affects the human being.

PUTREFACTION (*putrefacio*, I make rotten) is the change that takes place in the bodies of plants and animals after death, and in the course of the process various offensive and poisonous gases and other substances are formed. (*See* PTOMAINE POISONING.)

The first sign of putrefaction is the appearance of a greenish tinge in the skin covering the lower part of the abdomen, visible on the second or third day after death during hot weather, or in three or four days in cold weather. In about a week the surface of the skin becomes brownish, and the hair or fur can be easily pulled out by the roots. In from two to three weeks the skin is a uniform brownish colour and is beginning to give way, breaking up easily when handled. (These changes are, of course, irrespective of the action of the maggots of the various blow-flies, rats, 'burial beetles', etc.; when these are at work the changes are more rapid and mutilation is excessive.) By the end of a year none of the organs are recognisable, and in from 4 to 7 years bodies buried in sand have lost all trace of soft tissues, only the bones remaining.

When bodies decompose in water, particularly in that drained from peaty soil, the skin becomes white and sodden and the changes occur more slowly. Sometimes, under these circumstances, instead of going through the usual changes, the body tissues undergo a process of saponification, and are converted into a mixture of soaps, fatty acids, and volatile substances, which is called *adipocere*. Once formed, this does not readily undergo further changes.

The hot dry air of deserts, or a strong draught of cold air, may prevent putrefaction, and cause a kind of mummification, through gradual drying, which preserves the body for a time. A striking effect is seen in the bodies of animals which have died from taking large doses of arsenic or antimony, even after having been buried for weeks, especially in a dry soil; the internal organs of such bodies have been found to show a fresh and brightly coloured appearance which would lead an observer to conclude that they had only recently died. This is due to the antiseptic action of these two metallic substances, deposited in large amount in the internal organs.

PYÆMIA (πῦον, pus; αἷμα, blood) means a form of blood-poisoning in which abscesses appear in various parts of the body, due to the entrance of pus into the blood-stream.

PYELITIS (πύελος, a vessel) means a condition of pus-formation in the kidney which produces pus in the urine. It is due to inflammation of the part called the *pelvis of the kidney*, which is connected with the ureter. The condition is commonest among cows after calving, when infection has reached the bladder, invaded the ureters, and has arrived at the pelvis of the kidney.

PYELONEPHRITIS.—This term is used when both the pelvis and much of the rest of the kidney are involved, as described under PYELITIS.

CONTAGIOUS BOVINE PYELONEPHRITIS is a specific infection of cattle caused by *Corynebacterium renale*, giving rise to inflammation and suppuration in kidneys, ureters and bladder. As a rule, only one cow in a herd is attacked—though others may be carriers. The passage of blood-stained urine and abdominal pain are symptoms. Penicillin is useful in treatment. Otherwise, death may occur (sometimes after several weeks).

In the pig, an infectious pyelonephritis is caused by *C. suis*.

PYLORIC STENOSIS.—This occurs as a rare congenital defect in the dog. Only liquid food can pass into the stomach. ' Projectile vomiting ' is a symptom. The defect can corrected by means of surgery. (*See* PYLORUS.)

PYLOROSPASM means spasm of the pyloric portion of the stomach. This interferes with the passage of food in a normal, gentle fashion into the intestine, and causes distress from half an hour to three hours after feeding. It is associated with severe disorders of digestion.

PYLORUS (πυλωρός, gate-keeper) is the name of the lower opening of the true stomach. Exit of food from the stomach is guarded by a strong ring of muscular tissue called the *sphincter of the pylorus*, which opens under nervous activity and allows escape of small amounts of partly digested food material into the small intestine. (*See* STOMACH ; DIGESTION ; INTESTINE ; etc.)

PYO- (πῦον, pus) is a prefix attached to the names of various diseases to indicate that, in the disease in question, the formation of pus-forming cavities or abscesses is a characteristic. For instance, in pyo-nephritis there is inflammation of the kidney with the formation of small pockets of pus in the outer parts.

PYOGENIC (πῦον, pus ; γεννάω, I produce) is a term applied to those bacteria which cause the formation of pus, and so lead to the production of abscesses.

PYOMETRA.—A collection of pus in the uterus : a condition not uncommon in maiden bitches, and occurring in all species. (*See* p. 973, *under* CHRONIC METRITIS.)

PYORRHŒA, which means a ' flowing of pus ' in the strictest sense, but is the term commonly applied to ' Pyorrhœa alveolaris ', which is septic inflammation of the gums, in which suppuration is produced and ultimately interference with the integrity of the teeth. It is a common condition in aged dogs and cats, but does not often affect the other domesticated animals. In the majority of cases it follows upon the collections of tartar. These incrustations harbour under their edges numerous organisms, which, when the mucous membranes of the gums become abraded, gain an easy access into the oral ends of the tooth sockets. Pus is produced as the result of the inflammation set up, and the breath of the animal acquires a somewhat characteristic foul odour of a most persistent nature. Pyorrhœa may also arise independent of the presence of incrustations of tartar, when it presents an appearance as though the gums were eroded around the roots of the affected teeth. In this form it is extremely difficult to relieve, short of extracting the teeth (which themselves may be quite healthy).

Treatment.—Rational systems of feeding, and the occasional provision of a hard bone, which cannot be splintered, to ' clean ' the teeth, should prevent the formation of tartar. The removal of tartar once a month by means of tooth-scalers and the subsequent use of an antiseptic mouth-wash, tends to keep pyorrhœa in check, but when once it has become established it is advisable to have the dog's mouth thoroughly examined by an expert practitioner, who will extract any teeth that may be necessary.

PYOSALPINX.—Distension of a Fallopian tube with pus.

PYRAMIDAL DISEASE is the name applied to an exostosis affecting the pyramidal process (extensor process) of the third phalanx of the horse's foot. It is usually found in association with low ringbone. (*See* RINGBONE.)

PYRETHRUM FLOWERS, when powdered, are used as an insecticide, but are less effective for use on animals than BHC or derris powder. They, and their active principles, are, however, of value in fly control, especially where a resistance to insecticides such as DDT has become established. Pyrethrum is useful where DDT and other chlorinated hydrocarbons are too poisonous for safe use.

PYREXIA (πυρέσσω, I am fevered) means fever. (*See* FEVER.)

PYRIDINE is an alkaloidal substance derived from coal-tar, tobacco, etc. It is added to methylated spirit in order to render this unpleasant to drink.

PYRIDOXINE.—Vitamin B_6.

PYROGALLIC ACID is a substance derived from gallic acid which is sometimes used in the treatment of parasitic skin diseases. It stains the surface of the skin, and hair growing on it, a deep brown colour.

PYRUVIC ACID.—An organic acid which is an intermediate product in carbohydrate and protein metabolism. Excessive quantities accumulate in the blood-stream in cases of vitamin B_1 deficiency.

PYURIA (*πῦον*, pus; *οὖρον*, urine) means pus in the urine produced by suppuration in some part of the urinary tract; perhaps kidney, perhaps ureter, bladder, or urethra. (*See* URINE.)

Q

Q FEVER.—A disease first recognised in Australia in 1935. It is caused by *Coxiella burneti*, which gives rise to illness resembling food-poisoning or influenza with headaches in man. Infection in domestic animals is frequently unaccompanied by symptoms, though pneumonia and abortion in sheep and goats have been attributed to it. In the United Kingdom a preliminary survey shows that 2581 farms in England, 553 in Wales, and 240 in Scotland are infected. It has been found possible to isolate the parasite from 3000-gallon milk tankers, but pasteurisation destroys the germ. In a village outbreak in Germany the source proved to be dogs returning from the fields with infected ticks. Handling, or coming into contact with, the fæces, urine, fœtal membranes of infected cattle, or sheep, are the means—in addition to drinking raw milk—whereby much of the illness from Q Fever in humans is caused. Q Fever is common in Italy.

In a recent survey, sera from cattle and sheep in the north-east of Scotland were tested for antibodies to *Coxiella burnetii*. Approximately 1 per cent of 4,880 cattle had antibodies to the organism. These potentially infected cattle were distributed throughout the area. Two flocks of sheep were tested; in one flock 30 per cent of sheep had antibodies, while the other was negative. The flock with the high prevalence of *C. burnetii* antibodies appeared to be associated with an outbreak of human Q fever on that farm.

QUADRICEPS (*quattuor*, four; *caput*, a head) means having four heads, and is the collective name applied to the powerful muscles situated above the stifle-joint. These are: medial and lateral *vasti*, and the *rectus femoris*; the fourth muscle (*vastus intermedius*) in the horse is so blended with the medial vastus that it has lost its autonomy.

QUARANTINE (Ital. *quaranta*, forty) means that principle employed for the prevention of the spread of infectious disease by which an animal or animals, along with boxes, rugs, kennels, and other appurtenances, which have come from infected countries or areas, are detained at the frontiers or ports of entrance, or at other official centres, before being allowed to mix with the stock of the country.

The regulations dealing with quarantine of animals are altered from time to time, and so information on the matter is best obtained direct from the Government department that deals with live-stock in a particular country. (*See* RABIES.)

QUATERNARY AMMONIUM COMPOUNDS are among the important newer antiseptics, and they have found widespread application in dairy hygiene. Cetrimide—or cetyl trimethyl ammonium bromide—is an example. It is used in 0.1 per cent solution for washing cows' udders, teats, and milkers' hands, being effective against *Streptococcus agalactiæ*. In higher concentrations it acts as a detergent. (*See also* HIBITANE.)

QUARTER HORSE (*see* AMERICAN QUARTER HORSE).

QUARTER ILL is another name for black-quarter. (*See* BLACK-QUARTER.)

QUASSIA is the wood of *Picræna excelsa*, a large West Indian tree, which is cut into chips and called 'quassia chips'. Its virtues depend on the presence of an active principle, *quassin*, which is excessively bitter and irritant. An infusion is sometimes used for injection into the rectum to expel oxyurid worms in the horse.

QUEENSLAND ITCH.—This is caused by sensitisation to bites of the sandfly—*Culicoides robertsi*. The lesions resemble those of mange, and are seen usually along the animal's back. Antihistamines are useful in treatment.

QUEY.—A heifer.

QUICKLIME is another name for calcium oxide. Quicklime is an irritant caustic capable of causing severe burns when applied to the wetted skin or to a moist mucous membrane surface. Its antidotes are weak watery solutions of the vegetable acids, such as vinegar, dilute acetic or oxalic acid, and demulcent oily dressings.

Quicklime has in the past been recommended for the disinfection of poultry runs where disease has been present, but its effectiveness is in some doubt.

QUIDDING, or ' CUDDING ', is the name given to that condition in horses, depending upon injuries to the mouth or diseases of the teeth, in which food is taken into the mouth, chewed repeatedly, and then expelled on to the floor of the stall or into the manger. It may result from the teeth being too sharp, irregular in height, uneven in alignment, or from permanent teeth pushing the temporaries out from the gums ; it may arise when the gums, cheeks, or tongue have been injured or are diseased ; or it may arise in paralysis of the throat, or some other condition which causes inability to swallow.

Symptoms.—In quidding, masses of thoroughly chewed food are found in the stable, and if the horse is watched when eating long hay, it will be seen to reject it after having first spent some time in chewing. The mouth should be examined, and the cause of the condition corrected by whatever measures are necessary. (*See* MOUTH, DISEASES OF ; TEETH, DISEASES OF.)

QUINIDINE is an alkaloid obtained from cinchona bark and closely related in chemical composition and in action to quinine. It is used in the form of quinidine sulphate.

QUININE is an alkaloid obtained from the bark of various species of cinchona trees. This bark is mainly derived from Peru and the neighbouring parts of South America. It contains four alkaloids, of which *quinine* is the most active and important, the others being *quinidine, cinchonine,* and *cinchonidine.*

Quinine is usually used in the form of one of its salts, *i.e.* sulphate, hydrochloride, or hydrobromate of quinine. These are slightly soluble in ordinary water, but very soluble in water containing a small amount of a dilute mineral acid.

Action.—Quinine lessens the activity of all low forms of life, especially of a protozoön nature. It is a specific against the parasite which causes malaria in human beings. It causes a lowering of temperature in fevers. It stimulates the muscular wall of the uterus.

Uses.—These have dwindled. Before the advent of the sulpha drugs and antibiotics it was much used in influenza, strangles, colds, inflammation of the uterus, distemper, and similar conditions. It is still sometimes used in the treatment of pyometra in the bitch. It is sometimes given as an intramuscular injection. Owing to its very bitter taste it is seldom that it will be taken in the food.

Toxicity.—' The dog is very susceptible to quinine and becomes blind at plasma concentrations readily tolerated by man.' (*Lancet,* Feb. 6, 1965.)

QUITTOR is the name given to a condition of the ungual or ' lateral ' cartilages of the horse's foot, in which the cartilage is the seat of some suppurative process, and in which there is an opening in the region of the coronet from which pus or sanious fluids are discharged.

Causes.—The condition is due to injury, in which the cartilage is either broken or bruised, or is infected with organisms. It commonly occurs in the fore feet, but it may also be seen in the hind feet. Horses that work in pairs and are careless in turning may tread upon their own or their neighbour's coronets, inflicting wounds with the calkins, frost studs, or sharp edges of their shoes, or perhaps breaking the uppermost edges of the cartilages. In other cases, quittor may arise from frostbite of the region of the coronets, burning with caustics or hot agents, or from pus burrowing upwards from a suppurating corn, sandcrack, under-run sole, picked-up nail, etc.

The cartilage is very delicate, having a poor blood-supply, and is not able to protect itself against attack by organisms as are other tissues that are better supplied with blood, so that even slight injuries in the region of the coronets should always receive careful attention and be treated with antiseptic applications until healed.

Symptoms.—In all cases there is a greater or lesser degree of lameness according to the severity of the lesion. Animals that have been injured near the coronets, instead of getting better and going sound in a reasonable time after the infliction of the injury, remain lame, and if there is an opening on to the surface, the area goes on discharging for weeks after the occurrence of the accident. In some cases the original wound heals up, but later the side of the coronet swells and becomes tender to pressure. In a few days the swelling will burst and liberate a certain amount of pus, but there is no tendency towards healing. There is usually only one opening to the surface, but occasionally there may be several.

The opening is devoid of hair round its margin, red and angry-looking, and a small amount of greyish thin pus with an objectionable odour is continually oozing from the orifice. When the condition has arisen from infection lower down, there are signs of the presence of this latter when the sole of the foot is examined.

In serious cases the pus burrows inwards and forwards as well as coming to the surface, and unless the condition is checked, the capsule of the coffin joint may become infected, when the horse will be unable to put its foot to the ground. In such cases as the latter, the temperature of the horse rises several degrees, food is refused, and there are all the usual signs of fever, but there are seldom general systemic symptoms with uncomplicated cases of quittor.

Treatment.—The advent of sulpha drugs and antibiotics have made treatment easier and speedier; otherwise it often takes months of treatment before a cure is effected. There are several methods of treatment suitable for different cases. When of recent occurrence, and the opening small and the discharge slight, good results often follow the injection of antiseptics with a special syringe, the nozzle of which passes down to the depths of the cavity. The liquid is syringed into the sinus several times daily, and great care is taken to ensure that any fresh infection is avoided, by the use of moist antiseptic packs. In resistant cases the only resort is the radical operation of surgical removal of the whole of the diseased cartilage. This is usually attended with good results, but it is liable to lead to some slight deformity of the foot afterwards. In all cases, the sooner operative or other methods are applied the less tedious will be the treatment, and the greater the hopes of recovery.

R

RABBITS act as hosts of the liver fluke of sheep, and of the cystic stages of some tapeworms, e.g. *Tænia pisiformis, T. serialis.* Rabbits have been used experimentally as incubators for sheep's eggs. (*See* TRANSPLANTATION OF MAMMALIAN OVA.)

Breeds of domesticated rabbits used for table purposes include: the New Zealand white, the Californian, and the Dutch rabbit.

RABBITS, DISEASES OF.—These include tuberculosis (usually caused by the bovine strain; pseudo-tuberculosis, caused by *Pasteurella pseudotuberculosis rodentium*; 'snuffles', corresponding to the human cold; Schmorl's disease or necrobacillosis; rabbit syphilis ('vent' disease); hæmorrhagic septicæmia; rabbit pox, salmonellosis, myxomatosis, toxoplasmosis, listeriosis. Impaction of the colon and appendicitis occur.

RABBIT FUR MITE.—This is believed to cause itching in dogs and man. (*See Cheyletiella parasitivorax.*)

RABIES (*rabies*, madness), HYDROPHOBIA, or 'MADNESS', is a specific inoculable contagious disease of virtually all mammals, including man; and occasionally it occurs in birds. It is characterised by nervous derangement, often by a change in temperament, with paralysis occurring in the final—and sometimes in the intermediate—stages.

Rabies occurs in all continents with the exception of Australasia and Antarctica. In parts of southern Europe, *e.g.* Greece, southern Italy, dogs remain the principal vectors; in a few countries in Europe cats attack more people than do dogs. In Asia and South America dogs are still the most important vectors, but in many countries wild animals provide a reservoir of infection, and infect dogs and cats and farm animals—which in turn may infect man, who is an incidental host of the disease. (*See* Table of vectors.)

Public health.—Rabies is virtually always fatal in the human being, and there is danger not only from being bitten by rabid animals, but also from contamination by their saliva of wounds, cut fingers, eyes, etc. Scratches may convey infection as well as bites.

People have died from rabies following attacks by rabid dogs, cats, foxes, wolves, badgers, skunks, racoons, mongooses, bats, rodents, etc.

In the U.K., as in most other countries, rabies is a Notifiable Disease, and must be reported to the Ministry of Agriculture or to the police. Bitten persons should seek medical advice immediately.

Rabies in Wild Animals—Principal Vectors in Various Regions

Europe	FOXES, ROE-DEER, BADGERS, MARTENS Bats (Yugoslavia, perhaps Germany)
Asia	WOLVES, JACKALS Bats Mongooses
N. America	FOXES SKUNKS, COYOTES Bats
Central America	Bats
S. America and Trinidad	VAMPIRE BATS

Cause.—A virus, present in saliva from affected animals. When it is injected into the tissues, either naturally (from a bite) or artificially, the virus passes along the nerves and reaches the central nervous system. The time elapsing between infection and onset of symptoms varies greatly with the location of the bite, its severity, and—no doubt—the quantity of virus in the saliva. In the most rapidly developing cases the symptoms may be shown as early as the ninth day after being bitten, and at the other extreme cases have appeared several months after the accident. It is owing to this fact that the 6 months' period of quarantine insisted upon in Great Britain is something of a compromise. The average incubation periods in dogs, sheep, and swine are from 15 to 60 days, in horses and cattle from 30 to 90 days. In young animals the period of incubation is shorter than in adults.

Symptoms.—(1) **Dog.**—There are two distinct forms of rabies in the dog—the *furious* and the *dumb*; but it is probable that these are in reality two stages only. It is customary to consider three stages in the development of typical symptoms. (1) *Melancholy:* The preliminary dull stage is often not noticed, or, if it is, only scant attention is paid to it. The habits of the dog change. It becomes morose and sulky, indifferent to authority, disregards its usual playthings or companions, shows a tendency to hide in dark corners, and may appear itchy or irritable as regards its skin. Noisy, boisterous animals become quiet and dull, while animals that are normally of a gentle, quiet disposition may become excitable. After 2 or 3 days of such behaviour the next stage is reached. (2) *Excitation:* The symptoms as described above become exaggerated, and there is a tendency towards violence. The dog pays no attention to either cajoling or threatening. It becomes easily excited and very uncertain in its behaviour. Food is either disregarded completely or eaten with haste. Sometimes there is difficulty in swallowing, but the intense horror and dread of water (hydrophobia), which characterises the disease in man, is not exhibited. After a time the appetite becomes deranged. The dog refuses its ordinary food, but eats straw, stones, wood, coal, carpets, pieces of sacking, etc., with great avidity. If the animal is shut up in a kennel, it persists continually in its efforts to escape. Should it be released, or should it escape, it almost invariably runs away from home. It may wander for long distances. In its travels it bites and snaps at objects which it encounters, real or imaginary, animate or inanimate, but it will seldom go out of its way to bite. The animal may take a sudden dislike to some part of its own anatomy; upon occasion it will seize a paw or a part of its hind quarters in its teeth and inflict serious injuries. The face has a vacant stare, the eyes are fixed and expressionless, and the pupils are dilated. This stage lasts from 2 to 4 days, unless the dog's strength gives out sooner, and the next stage appears. (3) *Paralysis:* The characteristics of the last stage in the train of symptoms of rabies are those of paralysis, especially of the lower jaw and the hind quarters. The dog begins to stagger in its gait, and finally falls. It may manage to regain its feet when stimulated, but soon falls again. The lower jaw drops, the tongue lolls out of the mouth, and there is great salivation. The muscles of the throat and larynx are soon involved in the progressive paralysis,

The *dumb* form of rabies consists of this paralytic stage; the stage of excitation having been omitted. The *dumb* form is the more common in the dog. Barking ceases—hence the name.

(2) **Cat.**—In this animal the *furious* form is more common than in the dog. The aggressive stage is most marked, the animals attacking other animals and man with great vigour, and attempting to injure their faces with teeth or claws. Sometimes the rabid cat will at first show extra affection. The course of the disease is usually shorter than in the dog.

(3) **Cattle.**—These animals are usually affected through having been bitten by a rabid dog. The stage of excitement is short and the dumb stage is most evident. Affected cattle behave in an unusual manner; they stamp or paw, bellow, salivate from the mouth, break loose, and may do much damage. Rumination and milk production cease, muscular quiverings are seen, sexual excitement is noticed, and there is a great loss of condition. Exhaustion soon follows and paralysis sets in. Death occurs in from 2 to 6 days or more after the commencement of the condition.

In the U.S.A., in 1953, the number of confirmed cases of rabies in cattle totalled 1012. In Central and South America, cattle are infected with a paralytic form of rabies by vampire bats.

(4) **Sheep, goats, and swine.**—The sheep and the goat are affected in a manner similar to cattle, but the stage of excitement is shorter or absent, and the dumb paralytic stage is more often noticed. Pigs become excitable, may squeal, show muscular spasms, before paralysis.

(5) **Horse.**—In the horse, which is not often bitten by a rabid dog, the stage of excitement is quite distinct, but there is less tendency for the animal to do damage, although the manger or other fixture in the stable may be seized with the teeth and bitten. Thirst is usually excessive, but there is difficulty in swallowing. Depression and paralysis of the hind quarters and of the throat set in, and death occurs in 3 or 4 days after the onset of the symptoms.

Diagnosis.—The routine examination for Negri bodies has now in many countries been superseded by the fluorescent antibody test, with confirmation by mouse inoculation if necessary.

Treatment.—Once the symptoms of

rabies have appeared in an animal, recovery is practically impossible (except in 'Oulou fato', which see). For public health reasons treatment of rabid animals is not allowed.

Prevention.—Various vaccines are used for immunisation as the table shows. Mass vaccination of dogs is carried out in many countries as a control measure; and in Central and South America cattle on ranches are vaccinated against vampire-bat transmitted rabies.

Vaccine	Strain of Virus	Tissue used for Preparation of Vaccine	For use in:
Live virus:			
LEP	Flury, 40–60 egg passage	Chicken embryo	Dog
K	Kelev, 60–70 egg passage	Chicken embryo	Dog and cattle
HEP	Flury, above 180th egg passage	Chicken embryo	Cattle, cat, and dog
Nervous tissue	Fixed	Central nervous system	Man, dog, cattle, and other animals
Inactivated:			
Duck	Fixed virus	Duck embryo	Man
Nervous tissue	Fixed virus	Central nervous system	Man, dog, cattle, and other animals

Vaccines prepared from tissue culture cells		
Live virus:		
ERA	Pig kidney	Cat, dog, cattle and other animals
HEP-Flury	Dog kidney	Cat, dog, and cattle
Inactivated:		
Fixed	Hamster kidney	Cat, dog, cattle, and other animals

It must be remembered, however, that no vaccines are 100 per cent effective, that certificates of vaccination can be forged, and that consequently it is still essential to control the import of animals, whether vaccinated or not, and to enforce quarantine measures in countries where the disease is not endemic.

Control of rabies in Britain.—From 1902 until 1918 no cases occurred in the British Isles, but in that year an infected dog was smuggled from the Continent, and the disease obtained a fresh hold for a period of a little more than 3 years. Britain had been free since then, but in 1969 a dog released from quarantine 10 days earlier showed symptoms of rabies and bit two people at Camberley, Surrey; and a second case occurred in 1970. Several cases have also occurred in recent years *inside* British quarantine kennels, and in 1965 there was a case in a recently imported leopard in quarantine at Edinburgh Zoo. In Britain, in 1969, the danger of allowing the importation of rabies-susceptible exotic animals, for sale as pets or for research, was officially recognised, and the quarantine regulations amended to include monkeys, mongooses, etc.

In 1969 an Order was made extending the quarantine period from 6 to 8 months; 1970 the quarantine period extended to 12 months. In March 1970 the import of dogs and cats, except from Ireland, the Channel Isles and the Isle of Man, was banned.

This could be regarded as an interim measure pending the recommendations of the Waterhouse Committee, and following several cases of rabies.

Following publication of the Committee's Report in 1971, six months' quarantine was re-imposed in place of the ban on imports. All dogs and cats must be vaccinated in quarantine—whether previously vaccinated or not. (This last measure was adopted partly in order to minimise the risk of rabies being spread within quarantine kennels.)

RACHITIS (ῥάχις, the spine) is another name for rickets. (*See* RICKETS.)

RADIAL PARALYSIS, or 'DROPPED ELBOW', is the name given to that condition in which, through injury to the radial nerve in the fore limb, certain of the muscles of the elbow and knee are incapable of action through being paralysed. The condition is commonest in horses and dogs, though it may be seen in any of the domesticated animals.

Causes.—Probably the majority of cases are due to a fracture of the 1st rib on the same side of the body, the broken ends of the rib lacerating the nerve-fibres as they pass the rib, or pressing against them. In other cases the origin of the paralysis seems to be situated in the end-plates of

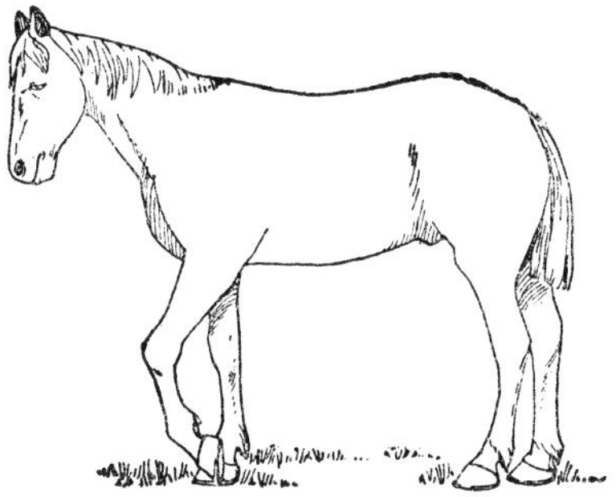

Radial paralysis, or 'dropped elbow', in the horse's near fore limb. The limb cannot be advanced, weight cannot be borne by it, the extensor muscles of the knee and elbow being paralysed.

the nerve-fibres where they are distributed to the muscles, and in some cases a neuritis involving the radial nerve, or a tumour pressing upon it at some part of its course, is responsible for producing the condition. Some authorities hold that radial paralysis can be, and often is, produced through the fore limb of the horse having slipped violently to the outside ('side-slip'), or having been extended either forwards or backwards to too great an extent, and having put an undue strain upon the comparatively inelastic nerve, which has resulted in a certain amount of tearing of its fibres. In this way can those cases of incomplete radial paralysis be explained.

Symptoms.—In a typical case the horse stands with the elbow dropped lower than normally, and with the knee, elbow, and fetlock joints flexed. Little or no pain is felt, unless there is a fractured rib, or some inflammatory condition which has caused the paralysis. The limb is held in the position assumed at the commencement of a stride, but the animal is incapable of advancing it far in front of the sound limb. No weight is borne upon the leg, the muscles are flaccid and soft, and if the horse is made to move forward it either does so by hopping off and on to the sound fore limb, or it may fall forwards. If the hand be forcibly pressed against the knee, so that the limb is restored to its natural upright position, the horse is able to bear weight upon it and may lift the other limb from the ground, but as soon as the pressure is released, the joints fall forward again. Sometimes the toe is rested upon the ground, but at other times the horse stands with the wall of the foot in contact with the ground. In cases that are not so severe, the flat of the foot may rest on the ground, and the limb can be advanced forwards to a considerable extent.

Treatment.—The majority of such cases as these will recover in a few weeks. In all cases sufficient time must be allowed for the nerve-fibres that have been injured to grow down and regain control of the muscles. Shoeing with a shoe which has a plate projecting forwards from the toe to an extent of about 4 to 6 inches, helps to keep the foot flat upon the ground and to straighten out the flexed joints. Exercise in a flat field, or in a large yard or barn, etc., also assists the condition, the horse soon learning to hop about in a fairly efficient manner. Patience on the part of the owner is essential.

'RADIATION SICKNESS'.—Dogs exposed to radiation following a nuclear explosion will vomit as a result of gastroenteritis, become dull and lose their appetite. This may return after a day or two, but leucopenia develops, and may be followed by hæmorrhage or septicæmia.

RADIO-ACTIVE FALL-OUT, following the explosion of hydrogen bombs, etc., or accidents at atomic plant, may be dangerous to farm livestock on account of the radio-active iodine and strontium released. After the accident at Windscale, radio-active iodine alone contaminated pasture in the area. (*See also below and under* HYDROGEN BOMB EXPLOSIONS.)

RADIO-ACTIVE IODINE.—Cattle grazing pasture contaminated by fall-out pick up ten times as much radio-active iodine as do people in the same locality, according to American reports. Much is excreted in the milk, and much concentrated in the thyroid glands.

Feeding-stuffs or pasture contaminated by fall-out containing radio-active iodine and strontium may give rise to illness in cattle. Digestive organs may be damaged, changes in the blood occur, and deaths follow within a month or so, after a period of dullness and scouring. (*See below.*)

RADIO-ACTIVE STRONTIUM.—Whereas the half-life of radio-active iodine is a matter of days, that of strontium is thirty years. Following the grazing of contaminated pasture or the eating of other contaminated feed, radio-active strontium is excreted in the milk, but much of it enters the bones and is liable to set up cancer many years afterwards. (*See above.*)

RADIO PILLS or telemetering capsules have been developed for research purposes. A radio transmitter, the size of an ordinary drug capsule, can give information concerning pressure, temperature or pH within an organ. Price (1961) about £10.

RADIUS is the inner of the two bones of the fore limb. In the horse and ox particularly, the radius forms the main bone of this part, the ulna being much smaller and not taking part in weight-bearing. (*See* BONE.)

RAGWORT POISONING causes losses among cattle and sheep in Great Britain, Canada, and New Zealand. It is the cause of the 'Pictou cattle disease' of Canada, and of 'Molteno cattle disease' in South Africa. The plant (*Senecio Jacobæa*, or sp.) is very often fed off by sheep when it becomes too plentiful in grass land. In the United Kingdom fatal poisoning has followed the giving of hay contaminated with ragwort; death occurring many weeks after the last mouthful. The death of 28 head of cattle was caused 2 to 4 months after feeding ragwort-contaminated silage.

Effect: Cirrhosis of the liver, inflammation of the 4th stomach, and other lesions. The symptoms are: 'Severe and strained purging; fæces yellowish to dark brown; cows cease to give milk; abdominal pain, groaning; animal may go mad and charge any one approaching, or lie with outstretched head, drooping ears, staring coat, and dull glaring eyes; death usual within 3 days from the commencement of purging'. Acute ragwort poisoning may also occur, causing death in 5 to 10 days. (*See* LIVER, DISEASES OF.)

Milk from a cow which has eaten ragwort may be dangerous to children, causing liver damage.

RAINFALL may infiuence outbreaks of HYPOMAGNESÆMIA, BLOAT.

RÂLES, or MOIST SOUNDS, are sounds heard by auscultation of the chest during various diseases. They are divided into two main classes: (1) *Crepitant* or *vesicular râles*, which are heard in the first stages of pneumonia, and are sharp, fine, crackling noises noticed during inspiration only. They are due to the glueing together of the walls of the air alveoli by the exuded semi-fluid material, and the sudden expansion of these when air enters the lung. (2) *Mucous râles* are produced in the bronchial tubes or in cavities in the lungs, and are due to the passage of air through mucus, serum, blood, etc., that may be contained in them. They are heard during expiration as well as during inspiration, and may be described as bubbling or gurgling sounds similar to that which water makes when it issues from a narrow-mouthed bottle.

RANCIDITY of cod-liver oil or other fish oils, etc., can be extremely dangerous. Rancid mash may bring about deficiencies of vitamins A, D, and E, with acute digestive disorders and death in chicks. Growing and adult birds may also suffer losses from this cause; with osteomalacia, and decreased egg production. (*See also under* VITAMIN E.)

RANGOON BEANS (*see* JAVA BEAN POISONING).

RANULA (*ranula*, a little frog) is the name given to a swelling which sometimes appears below the free portion of the dog's tongue. It is caused by a collection of saliva in one of the small ducts that carry saliva from the glands below the tongue, or farther back, into the mouth, and when of some size a ranula may cause considerable interference with feeding. It is treated by incision or excision, and is usually not serious.

RAPE POISONING occurs in animals which are not given hay or other food in addition to rape. Poisoning can be extremely serious, especially in sheep. Symptoms include dullness, red-coloured urine, and blindness.

A form of light sensitisation called 'Rape Scald' occurs in sheep on rape. Swelling of the head occurs, there is irritation leading to rubbing, the ears may suffer damage. Jaundice may occur.

RAPHE (ῥαφή, seam) means a ridge of furrow between the halves of an organ.

RAREFACTION OF BONE.—This means a decrease in the mineral content.

RAT-BITE FEVER.—This is a disease recognised in man and caused, following the bite of a rat (or, sometimes, dog, cat, mouse, weasel, or squirrel), by infection with either (1) *Spirillum minus*; or (2) *Actinomyces muris.* In the case of the latter, the incubation period may be 2 or 3 weeks. In addition to fever there may be an extensive rash.

RAT POISONS are of many kinds and careless use of them may give rise to poisoning in domestic animals. They include: phosphorus, zinc phosphide, strychnine, barium salts, red squill, antu, fluoroacetate (1008), thallium, warfarin, and so-called 'viruses' which may contain strains of *Salmonella enteritidis*. (*See also under* some of these headings and *under* POISONS.)

RATIONS FOR LIVESTOCK: Dairy Cattle.—

Winter rationing.—The home-grown foods available naturally vary from farm to farm. Farm-mixed rations often make good use of barley. Proprietary compound feeding-stuffs are well balanced and formulated to contain all necessary ingredients such as vitamins, trace elements, etc., and are nowadays extensively used. Proprietary barley balancers and straw balancers are also much used (*See also under* WINTER DIET.)

Calves.—*See* CALF-REARING.

Maintenance and 1-gallon rations for cows of Friesian breed or similar:

(*a*)	Hay	18
	Brewer's grains	10
	Dried sugar beet pulp	4
(*b*)	Hay	18
	Dried sugar beet pulp	4
	Silage	50

with parlour-fed concentrates, 3½ lb. per gallon, for both (*a*) and (*b*).

Maintenance plus 2:

Ryegrass/lucerne haylage	*ad lib.*
Brewer's grains plus minerals	15 lb.

with 4 lb. hammer-milled maize fed in parlour for every additional gallon.

A ration for dairy cows used at Boxworth Experimental Husbandry Farm for many years:

Rolled barley	12 cwt.
Sugar beet pulp	2½
Kibbled beans	4
Groundnut meal	1½
Minerals	½

This ration is fed at the rate of 4 lb. per gallon to Friesian cows.

Summer rationing.—Grass is the standard summer food for cattle. On a good, well-managed pasture—where over-stocking is avoided—young, leafy grass will supply enough protein for high yielders, but they will require additional carbohydrate. This may be supplied in the form of cereals, *e.g.* 4 lb. for each gallon of milk over about 4 produced per day. If the pasture is less good, cereals will be required for each gallon over 3.

Mr. Kenneth Russell recommended that in April, cows grazing young, leafy grass 4 to 6 inches high for 4 hours daily, should receive 7 lb. hay and cereals (plus a mineral mixture) at the rate of 4 lb. for each gallon over 3. In May, with unrestricted grazing of grass 8 or 10 inches long at the pre-flowering stage, the hay is discontinued; the cereal ration remaining as before. In June and July, with grass at the flowering stage, the cows receive balanced concentrates for yields over 2½ gallons (June), then over 2. In August, grazing aftermath (or green fodder during a drought), the cows receive concentrates for each gallon over 1. In September, with young aftermath or maiden seeds, there is a hay ration of 7 lb. (or 28 lb. kale) plus concentrates for yields over 2 gallons per day.

Rations for beef cattle (*see under* BEEF).

Rations for Pigs :

Creep Feed	*Per cent*
Barley meal	40
Flaked maize	30
White fish meal	15
Wheatings	15

Breeders and Growers *	*Per cent*
Barley meal	70
White fish meal	10
Wheatings	10
Ground maize	10

Fatteners *	*Per cent*
Barley meal	75
Soya bean meal	5
Wheatings	20

* Plus mineral and vitamin supplements.

Rations for Sheep (*see under* SHEEP, and FLUSHING OF EWES).

Rations for Poultry :

Chicks to 12 weeks	*Per cent*
Maize meal	23
Ground barley	10
,, oats	10
,, wheat	20
Wheat bran	13
Grass meal	5
White fish meal	10
Soya bean meal	5
Dried yeast	1½
Ground limestone	1
Salt mixture	½
(10 parts of common salt, 1 of manganese sulphate)	
Vitamin pre-mix	1

Layers'/Growers' Mash (Balancer for grain)	*Per cent*
Ground wheat	30
,, barley	25
Wheat middlings	8
,, bran	5
Grass meal	8
White fish meal	3
Meat and bone meal	3
Soya bean meal	10
Ground limestone	3
Steamed bone-flour	2½
Salt mixture	½
Vitamin pre-mix	2

Rations : Theoretical Basis for Calculation.—It is customary to regard the ration as being composed of two parts : (*a*) the 'maintenance' part, which provides the material for all vital activities and makes good the normal wear and tear of the body without causing increase or decrease in live weight ; (*b*) the 'production' part, which supplies the materials used for increase in body size, fat production, growth of the fœtus, and milk production.

It is usually said that for maintenance of a dairy cow weighing 1,000 lb., the ration should contain 6 lb. Starch Equivalent, and 0·6 lb. Protein Equivalent—a ratio of 10 to 1.

The production part of the ration (for milk of 3·5 to 4 per cent butterfat) should be, per gallon, 2·5 lb. Starch Equivalent, 0·5 lb. Protein Equivalent—a ratio of 5 to 1.

By referring to a table giving the estimated food values of average samples of various food-stuffs, it is then possible to calculate what the ration should, in theory, be.

Dry Matter Content of foods is important, and tables for this should also be consulted. An 8-month-old calf will require about 12 lb. of dry matter per day, supplying about 5 lb. of Starch Equivalent. A dairy cow weighing 10 cwt., will require the equivalent of about 29 lb. dry matter—more with dry foods. (*See also* DIET.)

RATS are important from a veterinary point of view as carriers of infection to cattle, pigs, dogs, etc. Examples of rat-borne diseases are : Aujeszky's Leptospirosis, Salmonellosis, Ringworm, Trichinosis, and Foot-and-mouth.

R.A.V.C.—The Royal Army Veterinary Corps, which has a long and honourable history. An Army Veterinary Service was established in 1796 ; this became the Army Veterinary Corps in 1906 ; the title of 'Royal' being bestowed in 1918.

A History of the R.A.V.C. 1796–1919 was compiled by Major-General Sir Frederick Smith, K.C.M.G., C.B., a former Director-General, Army Veterinary Services, and published by Baillière, Tindall & Cox. A second volume, by Brigadier J. Clabby, was published in 1963. (J. A. Allen & Co.)

R.C.V.S.—The Royal College of Veterinary Surgeons, 32 Belgrave Square, London. The governing body of the veterinary profession in the United Kingdom. (*See also* REGISTER.)

REACTION.—A response to a stimulus

of some kind. Allergic reaction is one based upon hypersensitivity to an antigen. The reaction in the tuberculin test—indicating that the animal's body has been sensitised by the presence of tubercle bacilli, and manifested by local inflammation—is another example.

RECESSIVES (*see* GENETICS).

RECTUM (*rectus*, straight) is the terminal part of the large intestine. It commences on a level with the anterior opening of the pelvis and extends to the anus, passing through the upper part of the pelvic cavity. In most of the domesticated animals it possesses a dilatation, known as the ' ampulla ', which serves to collect the fæces that are slowly passed into it from the colon, and holds them until time and circumstances are convenient for their evacuation to the outside. The anus, the actual opening to the outside. is held tightly shut by a strong ring of muscular tissue of an involuntary nature, called the ' sphincter of the anus ', until the accumulation of fæces in the ampulla is such that it begins to cause discomfort to the animal. The nerve endings in the ampulla send messages to the higher nerve centres in spinal cord or brain, and secondary impulses are sent by the nerves which control the sphincter down to the muscle fibres of which it is composed, resulting in the relaxation of the sphincter and the passage of fæces to the outside. In structure it is similar to that of the other parts of the intestine. (*See* INTESTINE.)

RECTUM, DISEASES OF.—With the exception of the dog the domestic animals are comparatively free from disease of this part of the alimentary system. In the larger animals the calibre of the rectum is large enough to ensure that any obstructing materials will negotiate the rectum when they reach it, but in the dog and cat it very frequently happens that pieces of bone, string, wool, and other foreign materials will become impacted a few inches within the rectum even though they have been passed through the rest of the alimentary canal without great difficulty. The affected animal attempts to pass fæces, but after considerable efforts fails to do so. If the impacted material contains spicules of bone or other hard material every effort at defecation causes the animal to cry out with the pain. It may run away in a frenzied manner, and strongly resents having its hind-quarters handled. In some cases the animal appears to be mad, and the owner may suspect that it is affected with rabies. In a few cases the animal's temperature rises, it becomes very dull and depressed, refuses food, shows great thirst, but can retain little or nothing upon its stomach. In rare cases the animal may vomit formed fæces, and its breath always has a very objectionable odour. As a rule the removal of the offending matter is effected by the administration of an enema of glycerine, oil, or soapy water, and the introduction of the lubricated finger. Hard masses are broken up and taken away in portions if too large to remove whole. A mild laxative should be given by the mouth after the impacted material has been cleared from the rectum, and the dog should receive a soft semi-fluid diet for some days afterwards.

INFLAMMATION of the rectum may follow impaction, or it may commence as the result of an injury. The animal frequently strains, and the owner may surmise that it is constipated, but exploration reveals the absence of fæces. It is treated by the introduction of gall and opium ointment, etc.

ABSCESSES, tumours, ulcers, and piles may also affect the rectum, but they are not common.

PROLAPSE of the rectum may occur in any animal, but is especially common in the smaller animals. A portion of the gut is protruded from the anus to an extent of a few inches. It appears as a tumorous swelling of a bright-red appearance, cold to the touch, and usually covered with mucus or fæcal material. There is usually some straining when the condition is of recent origin, but after a time the animal appears to become used to the protrusion of the piece of bowel, and only strains when it is handled or when attempts are made to return it. Anæsthesia may, of course, be necessary. Sometimes a piece of the small intestine is contained within the prolapse, and its return is difficult or impossible. As the condition is a serious one, expert advice should be sought, rather than that the owner should attempt to return it himself. Rupture of the mucous membrane, lacerations, and other injuries are always followed by inflammation of the rectum, even when it is successfully returned. It may be gently bathed with warm water containing common salt in solution (5 per cent) while awaiting assistance. An operation, in which the rectum is sutured to some part of the abdominal roof, is sometimes necessary to prevent its recurrence after replacement. Prolapsed rectum is not uncommon in the horse, as the result of severe straining, *e.g.* during colic, or parturition in mares, and the above remarks apply equally to the horse as the dog. Sometimes it may be easily returned by placing the neck of a quart bottle within the central depression that is always present, and pressing slowly and cautiously in a forward direction, the tail being held out of the way by an assistant.

In some instances amputation of the protruded portion becomes necessary, especially if it has been outside for some considerable time and has become gangrenous.

RECURRENT LARYNGEAL NERVE is a branch of the vagus nerve which leaves the latter at different points on the right and left sides of the body. On the right side it leaves the parent nerve opposite the 2nd rib, curves inwards round the subclavian or the costo-cervical artery, and runs up the neck on the lower surface of the trachea and below the carotid of the same side. In the case of the left, the branch leaves the vagus where that nerve crosses the arch of the aorta, winds inwards around the concavity of the aortic arch, and runs up the neck in a position similar to that of the right side. Both nerves supply the muscles of the larynx which are concerned in the production of voice and in maintaining the glottis open during ordinary and forced respiration. The left nerve is important, because it is held that, owing to the course round the aortic arch, it is liable to be tugged during vigorous pulsation of the latter, and paralysis of the muscles of the larynx on the left side may result. Whether this is so or not it is a fact that the majority of cases of ' roaring ' in the horse are affected on the left side only, and roaring is due to paralysis of the muscles that hold the vocal folds out of the line of the stream of air passing in and out of the trachea. (*See* ROARING.)

RED SQUILL.—Preparations of the dried ground bulbs of the sea onion, *Urginea maritima*, are used for poisoning rodents, baits being made up to contain 10 per cent Red Squill. Domestic animals refrain from eating such preparations owing to the smell and taste. Symptoms of poisoning include profuse vomiting in the pig but not in the cat, according to one report (*Vet. Rec.* 19/2/55), excitement, muscular inco-ordination, and convulsions. Poisoning in rodents by Red Squill may be agonising and very prolonged.

RED URINE.—Causes of red discoloration of the urine include: Red-water Fever, Leptospirosis, Post-parturient Hæmoglobinuria, Azoturia, infection with *Clostridium hæmolyticum*, the eating of frosted kale and rape, dosing with phenothiazine, Pyelonephritis, poisoning by turpentine, and the drinking of very large quantities of water.

RED WORMS.—The common name for Strongyles. (*See* STRONGYLIDOSIS, p. 658.) These can cause severe anæmia, unthriftiness, and debility. (*See under* FOALS, DISEASES OF; *also under* ANEURYSM.) Thiabendazole is a useful drug for the removal of red worms in horses. (*See also* METHYRIDINE.)

REDE, or ' RENNET STOMACH ', is the popular name given to the abomasum, or 4th stomach, of ruminants. It is possessed of true digestive glands which are absent from the 1st, 2nd, and 3rd stomachs.

' REDFOOT '.—A condition seen in new-born lambs, in which the sensitive laminæ of the feet become exposed owing to detachment of the overlying horn. The cause is unknown, no treatment effective, and the lambs soon die.

REDUCTION of a fracture or hernia means restoring the part to its normal relation.

REDUPLICATION is a term applied to a duplication of the normal heart sounds as heard by auscultation. There are heard a first and a second sound in a normal heart-beat, and in the above condition one or both of these may be doubled. It is probably due to the fact that the two sides of the heart are not acting together, and is found in certain diseases of the heart, such as obstruction of the valve between the auricle and ventricle on the left side of the organ (the mitral valve).

RED-WATER (British Isles), also called HÆMOGLOBINURIA, and BOVINE PIROPLASMOSIS, is a disease of cattle due to the presence in the blood of a protozöon parasite which attacks the red blood corpuscles, destroying their envelopes and liberating hæmoglobin, which is excreted by the kidneys and colours the urine reddish or blackish. It occurs mainly in the south and west of England, in the north and west of Scotland, and practically all over Ireland, but it is also seen at times in districts that are not included in these areas. It is common in low-lying, rough-pastured, and moorland districts, where ticks, which harbour and transmit the parasite, can find abundant shelter and suitable breeding places. Cattle are exclusively attacked from the age of about 3 months upwards, but young calves are practically immune. One attack gives a great degree of immunity, and cattle that have been bred upon infected farms, and from infected cattle, are more resistant than those brought from a clean district. It is more prevalent in the spring and autumn months, since the ticks are then at their maximum activity. (*See under* PARASITES, p. 682.)

Cause.—*Babesia* (*Piroplasma*) *bovis*. This is transmitted by the common tick, *Ixodes ricinus*, and occasionally by *Hæmophysalis punctata* which occurs in any numbers only in the south of England. A similar disease in America is due to *Babesia* (*Piroplasma*) *bigemina*. (For further details of the relations between ticks and parasites, and for the life-history of the parasites, etc., *see under* PARASITES, p. 637.)

Symptoms.—Two varieties of the disease are recognised: an acute and a mild form.

The *acute type* is sudden in its onset and frequently fatal. The animal becomes very dull and depressed, separates itself from the rest of the herd, moves slowly or not at all, grunts, groans, arches its back, salivates freely, grinds its teeth, and often staggers and falls. The coat becomes hard and staring, the skin is dry and often hide-bound, and there is almost always a profuse, watery, violent diarrhœa. The temperature rises to a great height (*e.g.* 105° to 107° F.), the pulse is fast and weak (often 100 per minute), and the respirations are laboured, blowing, and rapid (80 to 100 per minute). The visible mucous membranesare pale and wrinkled, and parts of the skin may be cold and others hot. After a day or two the animal's distress becomes less acute, and the most alarming symptoms subside. The signs of fever, however, are still evident, and the ox is still in a serious condition. The urine usually shows some degree of coloration, which varies from a clear reddish claret to a deep dark brown or black—almost like stout. It is generally frothy when passed, and the froth remains for long periods. Some cases rapidly recover and the urine clears up in a very short time, but in others its high colour persists for perhaps a week or ten days. Cows in milk give much less than usual, and what is secreted may be tinged a pink colour.

The duration of acute attacks varies, but it is seldom that the high temperature lasts for more than a week. Death may take place in from 3 to 5 days, or later on, when it is usually due to exhaustion.

In the *mild type* the urine is not usually highly coloured ; there is only slight dullness and loss of appetite. The animals are ill for a week or ten days, and the only marked sequel is anæmia.

There are *irregular forms* of red-water met with at times, in which the general symptoms are similar to those seen in the typical acute attack, but the urine does not become discoloured. Many of these cases end fatally.

There may be an attack of red-water following calving. In such cases the parasites are very difficult to demonstrate in the blood-stream, and the trouble is not always recognised as being red-water.

Treatment.—The affected animals should be quietly taken from the pastures and shut up in loose-boxes or cattle sheds, where they are protected from rigours of the weather. Plenty of water should be provided, for thirst is usually excessive.

Injections, either into the blood-stream by a vein, or under the skin, of Acapron or Piroparv give good results. A combination of iron, ammonia, and nux vomica is useful as a tonic and stimulant to blood formation during the later stages.

Otherwise, the animal should be kept comfortable, fed upon laxative, nourishing, easily digested foods, and not allowed out again until convalescent. All ticks upon their bodies should be removed, either by hand-picking or by daily spraying with a suitable parasiticide. Preventive measures: *See* TICKS, CONTROL OF

Calves can be immunised by inoculation with blood of recovered animals, being subsequently housed for 2 weeks. They become carriers.

RED-WATER (**U.S.A.**), also called Bacillary Hemoglobinuria, or icterohemoglobinuria, occurs in California, Colorado, Idaho, Louisiana, Montana, Nevada, Oregon, Texas, and Utah.

Cause.—*Clostridium haemolyticum.*

REFLEX ACTION is one of the simplest forms of activity of the nervous system. For the mechanism *see* NERVES.

Reflex acts are usually divided into three classes.

Superficial reflexes are well instanced in the sudden shivering movement that is seen when a fly or other insect settles upon the skin of a horse, particularly in the region of the back of the shoulder. The lightest impression is received by the sensory fibres of the part, and almost simultaneously the motor nerves actuate cutaneous or 'skin muscle', which contracts and causes a shiver to pass over the area.

Deep reflexes are seen at their greatest perfection in the wild, fighting animals. Impressions of the surroundings are received by means of special tactile apparatus, such as the whiskers of the cat tribe, and, without any actual brain control, the movements of the body are altered by messages sent from the area of the spinal cord which, fractions of a second before, received the warning impulse from the 'end organs'. The time taken for the passage of these impulses is quite beyond human imitation. The animal's life may depend upon the rapidity or otherwise of the dodging movement that is necessary to avoid the rush of a charging lion, for example. The time taken for the animal to become aware of the presence of its foe and to leap away at full speed is so short that in popular parlance it is said to 'vanish'—a word that only inadequately expresses the marvellous speed that can be exhibited by certain wild animals, which is due to reflex action.

Visceral reflexes are those connected with various organs, such as the narrowing of the pupil when the eye is exposed to a bright light.

Reflex action takes place without the necessary intervention of the brain which occurs in 'considered action'. The impulses are carried by the sensory nerves to a part of the spinal cord in the vicinity, are changed there from sensory impulses to motor impulses, and are then sent by the motor nerves to the muscles concerned in the action that is to be effected.

REFUSE AND SEWAGE DISPOSAL (*see* POISONING, SWILL, SEWAGE, MANURE HEAPS, *and* SANITATION).

REGIONAL ANÆSTHESIA.—This consists in the anæsthetisation of a region of the body by means of a local anæsthetic solution injected either into the connective tissue surrounding a sensory nerve trunk or into the spinal canal. (*See* EPIDURAL ANÆSTHESIA, ANALGESICS.) The most common example of perineural injection is Plantar Block in the horse.

REGISTER OF VETERINARY SURGEONS, THE, lists members of the profession who qualified in the United Kingdom. It may be consulted in some public libraries or is obtainable from the Royal College of Veterinary Surgeons, 32 Belgrave Square, London. (*See also under* VETERINARY SURGEONS ACT, 1948.)

REGURGITATION (*re*, back; *gurgus*, a whirlpool) is a term used in two distinct connections, first in connection with the heart, and secondly with the stomach. So far as the heart is concerned the term is used to indicate a condition in which as the result of valvular disease the blood is not completely driven out of the heart on contracting, and when it begins to dilate again, the valve, instead of preventing a re-entrance of that same blood by closing, allows a certain amount of the newly expelled blood to regain the heart cavity. The valves affected are said to be 'incompetent', and they generally show the presence of hard fibrous nodules along their free edges, which prevent accurate apposition, or else the natural elasticity is lost and they close incompletely.

In connection with the stomach the term regurgitation is used to denote that physiological process by which animals that ruminate are able to pass food from the stomach back into the mouth with ease and celerity. (*See* RUMINATION.) The word regurgitation is also applied to the process by which food reaches the throat or nasal cavity from the stomach in the horse tribe, where true vomiting does not occur.

RELAPSE (*re*, back; *lapsus*, slipping) means the return of a disease during the period of convalescence. Most relapses are due to errors in diet, exercise, or management on the part of the owner of an animal, or to undue exposure to extremes of climate. A relapse occasionally occurs when antibiotic or sulpha drug treatment of an infectious disease is stopped—the infection having been suppressed but the animal's powers of resistance not having been stimulated to establish a sufficient degree of immunity. Some forms of lameness are particularly liable to relapses, especially those associated with sprains of tendons or ligaments. This has given rise to the saying that 'horses with sprained tendons should not be worked until a week after they *appear* to be better'.

RENAL.—Relating to the kidney.

RENNET is a substance found in the stomach of the calf, which possesses the power of curdling milk. Its activity is due to the presence of a ferment called *rennin*, which coagulates the caseinogen of the milk, producing a new material called *casein*. (*See* MILK.)

REOVIRUS.—The name derives from the words 'respiratory enteric orphan virus'. Reoviruses have double-stranded ribonucleic acid (RNA), and will replicate and produce changes in cells of cattle, pigs, dogs, cats, rabbits, monkeys, and man. (*See also* CALF PNEUMONIA.)

REPAIR of tissue after injury is described under WOUNDS, and for the repair of special tissues *see under* BONE, MUSCLE, NERVE, etc. (*See also* HOOF REPAIR.)

REPRODUCTION (*re*, again; *productio*, I lead forth, or I produce). Among the higher animals reproduction is always the result of intimate association between male and female. (Parthenogenesis—birth from a virgin—is possible among some of the lower creatures, *e.g.* the liver fluke, worms, etc., and even the rabbit under experimental conditions, and may, *exceedingly rarely*, occur under natural conditions in mammals. (*See also under* PARTHENOGENESIS.))

Ovulation—This is the process of the extrusion of a mature ovum from the ovary. Each ovum is formed within a Graäfian follicle in the ovary, and as development proceeds the follicle gradually approaches the surface of the ovary, upon which it produces a slight bulge. The cavity of the follicle contains fluid, and at one part of the wall of the follicle there is a little heap of cells called the cumulus, which supports the ovum. In the process of time—either corresponding to the occurrence of œstrus, or else as the result of coition with the male (*e.g.* rabbit and ferret)—the Graäfian follicle bursts, and the ovum is expelled by the rush of the escaping fluid. (*See* OVARY.) The cavity of the Graäfian follicle becomes filled with special cells to form the *corpus luteum*, and the ovum begins its interesting career as an absolute entity. In normal circumstances the fimbriated and dilated funnel-shaped end of the Fallopian tube, or oviduct, is applied to the point at which a follicle will burst, so that upon escape of its ovum this latter may be caught and retained. The dilated end of the oviduct is usually known as the vestibule, and it is in this part that the male germ cell *usually* meets the ovum and fertilises it.

Coition.—The act of coition or copulation, which consists of the introduction of the male ejaculatory organ (penis), in a state of erection, into the posterior genital canal or vagina, is the normal method by which the male germ cells are introduced into the female genital tract. As has been mentioned under ŒSTRUS (which also see), service by the male is only allowed during the period of œstrus by the females of the majority of species of higher animals. At other times there is little or no desire exhibited by the male, and all attentions are resented by the female. Such an arrangement prevents undue promiscuity among animals, and acts as a check upon the breeding of animals at times and seasons which are unsuitable or inconvenient for the rearing of the young. Artificial methods of domestication have to some extent modified the frequency and duration of œstrus, so that the domestic animals, sheltered under the protection of man, breed more frequently than do the majority of wild animals of similar species.

During the act of coition both sexes experience a pleasurable sensation which, through reflex nerve action, results in a pouring out of mucoid secretion from the glands in the cervix and vagina of the female, and in the male causes a sudden secretion from all the accessory sexual glands and an evacuation of millions of spermatozoa from either the testes or the epididymi, where they are stored for use. There is now little doubt that the point of the penis is not actually introduced into the cervix of the uterus, but it is at least certain that if not actually introduced it is brought into very close contact with the posterior opening of the cervix. The uterus, under the nerve stimulus already mentioned, becomes erect, and upon its relaxation at the termination of the act, a certain amount of aspiratory action is exerted upon the male ejection, which is accordingly sucked through the cervix into the cavity of the uterus. Much of the semen remains in the vagina, and may even be expelled to the outside, but, such is the profusion of Nature, this does not greatly matter, for the majority of the spermatozoa are, in any case, superfluous. Only one sperm is required for the fertilisation of each ovum, and it is seldom that more than 12 ova are matured and fertilised at one t me; in fact, in the mare and cow it is rare that more than one ovum needs to be fertilised at each service.

During one ejaculation of an adult vigorous stallion about 80,000,000 sperms are released. As soon as the sperms are free in the uterus or vagina, they commence to travel towards wherever the ovum is situated. This they accomplish by a kind of wriggling movement of their tail parts, which drives them onwards always in one direction. They are attracted to the ovum by a powerful attraction to which the name 'chemotaxis' is applied.

Fertilisation.—Somewhere in the oviduct, generally in its vestibule but not necessarily so, the spermatozoa arrive in the region of the waiting ovum. It is the fate of one single spermatozoön only, to penetrate the wall of the ovum, and immediately that has happened the wall becomes impervious to the hosts of late-coming sperms, which ultimately perish.

The spermatozoön, having penetrated the ovum, loses its tail, which is no longer required, and lies within the protoplasm of the ovum. The essential parts are the head and middle piece, the former of which contains the all-important chromosomes in its nucleus, and the latter of which contains a body known as the 'centrosome', which is to direct and control further activity. The nucleus of the ovum and that of the head of the sperm now fuse, each contributing half the number of chromosomes that are to be found present in nearly all the cells of the future young animal. The fused body is known as the *segmentation nucleus*, and from it, when it begins to divide, all the body cells of the embryo are formed. The process of the formation of the young embryo is considered under EMBRYOLOGY, to which further reference should be made. (*See also* TESTIS, OVARY, ŒSTRUS, BREEDING OF ANIMALS, PREGNANCY, PARTURITION, PARTHENOGENESIS, etc., and PLATE 8.)

RESECTION (*resectio*, a pruning) is the name given to an operation in which a part of some organ is removed, as, for example, the resection of a piece of dead bone, or resection of a part of the intestine which is diseased; resection of a rib in thoracotomy; aural resection done to overcome chronic disease of a dog's ear.

RESERPINE.—A tranquiliser, which lowers the blood pressure and has been used for this purpose in turkeys. (*See* AORTIC RUPTURE.)

RESISTANT STRAINS.—This phrase is commonly used of bacteria which are not sensitive to antibiotics, or of insects which are not killed by, *e.g.* DDT.

RESISTANCE TRANSFERABILITY (*see under* ANTIBIOTIC RESISTANCE).

RESOLUTION (*resolvo*, I loosen) is a term applied to infective processes, to indicate a natural subsidence of inflammation without the formation of pus.

RESORPTION.—Re-absorption. Resorption of the fœtus occurs, *e.g.* in heifers receiving a high calcium and low phosphorus diet. It may occur in the sow with Aujesky's disease, and is by no means a rare occurrence in the bitch.

RESPIRATION (*respiratio*) is the process by which air passes into and out of the lungs with the object of allowing the blood contained in them to absorb oxygen after having given off its carbon dioxide and water vapour. It is probable that other complex poisonous substances are also given off from the blood and exhaled into the air; for instance, the peculiar sweetish odour of the breath of cattle fed upon turnips is probably due to one of such poisonous substances. The combustion, upon which all bodily activity depends, takes place throughout the whole of the body wherever the blood is carried. The oxygen necessary for this combustion is taken in through the lungs, loosely combined with the hæmoglobin of the red blood corpuscles, and carried throughout the body by the blood-stream. The carbonic acid gas (CO_2), produced by the union of carbon from the food with oxygen, and the water vapour (H_2O), produced similarly by union with hydrogen, are collected by the blood, carried to the lungs, and are there diffused out into the air cells, to be exhaled with the next expiration. For the composition of air, etc., *see* AIR, VENTILATION, etc.

Mechanism of respiration.—For the structure of the respiratory apparatus *see* AIR PASSAGES, LUNGS, etc.

The air passes rhythmically into and out of the air passages, mixing with the air already contained in the alveoli of the lungs, and afterwards being expelled. The drawing in of breath is known as 'inspiration', and the discharge as 'expiration'.

Inspiration is due to muscular effort which enlarges the chest in all three dimensions, so that the lungs have to expand in order to fill up the vacuum that would otherwise be left. The expansion of the lungs lowers the pressure of the air contained in them, and, to keep the balance even, air rushes in from the outside through the air passages. In most vertebrates, except birds, the lungs are not normally attached to the walls of the chest, but are rather suspended in them from their 'roots', so that there is no direct pull upon the lungs when the chest cavity increases in size. The increase in size of the chest from before backwards is mainly effected by a drawing back and a flattening of the dome of the diaphragm, whose muscular fibres contract with each inspiratory movement. The vertical diameter of the chest is increased during inspiration through the downward tilting of the sternum. This movement is best seen in the dog when it is out of breath; at other times, and in other animals, it is so slight that it escapes detection. The transverse dimension of the chest increases when any one of the ribs behind the first 2 or 3 are forcibly pulled forward by muscular action. Each rib only moves a small amount, but the mass effect of the series is very considerable. The muscles which bring about these changes in ordinary inspiration are the diaphragm, the intercostal muscles which are situated in two layers between each rib and its two neighbours, and possibly the levators of the ribs, and the serratus muscles. During forced inspiration, such as occurs during pneumonia or when an animal is out of breath, in addition to the above muscles the following are concerned: the latissimus dorsi, the scaleni, the muscles of the larynx, and those that dilate the nostrils.

Expiration is in ordinary circumstances merely an elastic recoil, the diaphragm moving forward and the ribs settling back into their original positions, partly through muscular action, and partly through the elasticity of their cartilages. It occupies a slightly longer period of time than does inspiration. In forced expiration the abdominal walls lift and compress the abdominal organs so that they force the diaphragm forwards and press upon the lungs, and at the same time the ribs are brought forcibly back into their original positions. The net result of these actions is to effect very considerable pressure upon the contents of the chest cavity, and if the larynx is partly closed, *e.g.* during a cough, or when voice is produced, the amount of energy required is considerable.

Nervous control.—Respiration is usually either an automatic or a reflex act, each expiration causing sensory impulses to be sent up to the higher nerve centres, and resulting in motor impulses being sent down to the muscles which carry out the process of inspiration. A very large number of nerves are involved in respiration, and these are to a great extent controlled and governed by a centre in the medulla, known as the 'respiratory centre'. This centre is capable of initiating and transmitting impulses which result in the movements of respiration, without any consciousness, or assistance from the conscious centres.

Although the respiratory centre is itself capable of carrying on respiration, it is in its turn liable to be controlled by the higher conscious centres. This is seen particularly well in human beings, where it is possible to 'hold the breath', or inhibit respiration for considerable periods, when diving under water, for example.

Rate of respiration.—The speed of the respirations varies with many internal and external factors. It is faster during rises of temperature, in fevers, after violent exercise, or even after mild exercise (though it soon returns to normal upon cessation); during powerful emotions, such as fear, anger, sexual excitement, etc.; during very cold or very hot weather; when the body condition is very fat, or when radiation is obstructed, through too thick a covering of wool, fur, etc., or too much clothing. It is also faster during extremes of temperature, especially in hot weather, and when the diet contains excessive amounts of fat, and in the later stages of pregnancy.

It is slower than normal during resting, either when merely lying or when sleeping; in cases of unconsciousness from shock, disease, or from the action of powerful anæsthetic or narcotic drugs; and it is also slower during certain diseased conditions in which the whole of the bodily activities are slowed down, *e.g.* in milk fever.

The normal rates in adult domesticated animals are as follows:

Horse . . .	8–12 per minute.
Ox . . .	12–16 ,, ,,
Sheep and goat .	12–20 ,, ,,
Pig . . .	10–16 ,, ,,
Dog . . .	15–30 ,, ,,

In each case the larger the particular animal the slower does it breathe, other things being equal; for instance, a Shetland pony respires about 12 times per minute, while a Shire stallion respires only 8 times; also, the young of any species breathe faster than do adults; and females breathe faster than males—especially during pregnancy.

Gaseous changes.—As already mentioned, the chief exchange between the blood and the atmospheric air is one in which CO_2 leaves the blood-stream and is exhaled, and oxygen is taken up from the air by the blood. In addition, considerable amounts of excess water vapour and other waste products (*e.g.* marsh gas in cattle) are eliminated by the lungs. The elimination of water vapour is particularly well seen on a frosty day when 'steam' can be noticed leaving the nostrils of a warm-blooded animal.

The composition of the atmospheric air varies according to local conditions—climate, altitude, proximity to manufacturing centres and to the sea-coast, etc., as well as depending upon the efficiency or otherwise of the ventilation in a building. An average composition is given as follows:

Oxygen . . .	20·93 per cent.
Nitrogen . . .	78·09 ,, ,,
Carbon dioxide .	·03 ,, ,,
Argon . . .	·94 ,, ,,
Neon, Krypton, Xenon, Helium, Hydrogen	Traces amounting to 0·01 per cent.

In addition, there are variable amounts of ammonia, nitric and sulphuric acids, ozone, water vapour, soot, dust, débris from manufacturing processes, tar, sulphur gases, etc., according to the locality, proximity to sea-coast, etc. (*See* SMOG.)

	Inspired air.	Expired air.
	Per cent.	Per cent.
Nitrogen . .	78·09	78·09
Oxygen . .	20·93	16·02
Carbon dioxide .	·03	4·38

When this air is taken into the lungs its composition is altered, so that upon leaving the lungs its CO_2 content is about 4 per cent greater and its oxygen content about 4 per cent less.

Quantity of air.—The lungs do not by any means completely empty themselves at each expiration and refill at each inspiration. An amount equivalent, in respiration, to about $\frac{1}{10}$ of the total air in the lungs passes out and is replaced by the same quantity of fresh air, which mixes with the stale air in the lung substance, with each complete respiratory cycle. This amount in the horse is about 7 pints (4 litres), and is known as the *tidal air*. In times of repose the amount of air that passes into and out from the lungs of a horse during an hour is from 80 to 90 cubic feet, but during vigorous exercise ten times this amount will be dealt with. During the same period an average horse will use up from the tidal air about 3½ cubic feet of oxygen, and will produce about 3 cubic feet of carbon dioxide. Ventilation may be expressed as the arrangements for the carrying away of the carbon dioxide and the supplying of fresh oxygen to take the place of what has been used, without the production of a draught. And since the horse will require to be supplied with at least 3½ cubic feet of oxygen every hour, and will need to have removed from the stable 3 cubic feet of CO_2, the inlets and outlets must be of such size as will allow the movement of a sufficiently large stream of air to meet these demands. (*See* VENTILATION.)

Irregular forms of respiration.—Apart from mere changes in rate and force, the respiration is modified in various ways under certain conditions. *Coughing* is a series of violent expirations, during each of which the larynx is at first closed until the pressure of air in the lungs and lower passages is considerably raised, and then suddenly opened, so that the contained air is released under pressure and rushes to the outside; its object is to expel some irritating object from the air passages. *Sneezing* is a single sudden expiration, which differs from coughing in that the sudden rush of air is directed by the soft palate up into the nose in order to expel some source of irritation from the nasal chambers. It is particularly well exhibited by the dog which has inhaled an irritant gas.

Yawning is a deep slow inspiration followed by a short expiration, the air being taken in by the open mouth as well as by the nose. *Hiccough*, which occurs in the horse (where it is usually called 'spasm of the diaphragm '), and in dogs, is due to a sudden spasmodic contraction of the diaphragm, along with a sudden closing of the larynx, producing a sound not unlike a very loud heart-beat. *Hyperpnœa* is a term applied to the slightly increased frequency and depth of respiration occurring during gentle exercise, or from some mild stimulus to the respiratory centre. *Dyspnœa* means that there is distinct distress in breathing, due to a more powerful stimulus to the respiratory centre, and is usually characterised by convulsive movements of the chest and diaphragm. It is frequently the forerunner of asphyxia. *Apnœa* is seen when there is a hyper-oxygenation of the tissues, and consequently no further immediate demand for oxygen. It consists of a complete cessation of the respiratory movements without the exhibition of any distress. It is artificially produced in human beings when a diver takes ten or twelve deep breaths before entering the water, where he must hold his breath. It is not commonly seen in the domestic animals, but the seal and other diving animals have developed the power of inducing apnœa to a very marked extent. (*See also under* ASTHMA, ROARING, VOICE, etc.)

RESTRAINT.—In order to examine an animal thoroughly for signs of injury or disease; in order to carry out inoculations, or even to administer a narcotic, some form of restraint is often necessary. There are those who look upon all means of restraint which may necessitate the infliction of a small amount of pain as unnecessary and cruel, but the enlightened owner should realise that the application of proper methods of restraint does not imply cruelty, and that the discomfort caused may obviate danger to human life or limb; in other words, while restraint may be an evil, it is at least necessary.

It must not be understood that the following methods may be used indiscriminately upon any and every animal; quite the contrary. A method that is sufficient to restrain one animal may prove aggravating to another; *e.g.* while the common twitch may serve for a heavy draught gelding, it is very likely to cause a thoroughbred stallion to be more restive than ever. A person who finds it necessary to employ some means of restraint should first of all consider the temperament, age, breed, and, if possible, the individual characteristics of the animal, as well as the purpose of the restraint, before deciding upon what methods will be employed. Firm gentleness, a kindly spoken word, and a hand-pat, with a little coaxing or urging, will very often allay an animal's fears, but there are those of a surly morose nature which will not respond to gentleness, and will only recognise mastery when they are cowed by a show of might; it is to such particularly that such methods as will be described here are applicable.

Horses.—The usual halter, head-stall, or bridle is generally sufficient to control broken horses that are to be handled or examined without the infliction of pain. In some cases it may be necessary to tie the animal to a ring in the wall or manger, or to the heel-posts, but it is better in such cases to take a couple of turns round the ring and have a man hold the end of the rope. It is at times useful to apply two halters, the second one being reversed with the shank on the off-side of the head, and to back the horse into a stall, and either tie him to each pillar, or have two men hold him. For measures which involve handling of the hind parts of the body, it is usually advisable to have one of the fore feet picked up and held (preferably that upon the same side of the body as the operator is to work). Sometimes it is necessary to strap up a fore foot either with a piece of rope or with a stirrup leather. The pastern is looped in each case, and the ends are passed over the fore-arm after the knee has been flexed. Such a procedure should not be carried out upon ground which may inflict injury to the fully flexed knee-joint if the horse

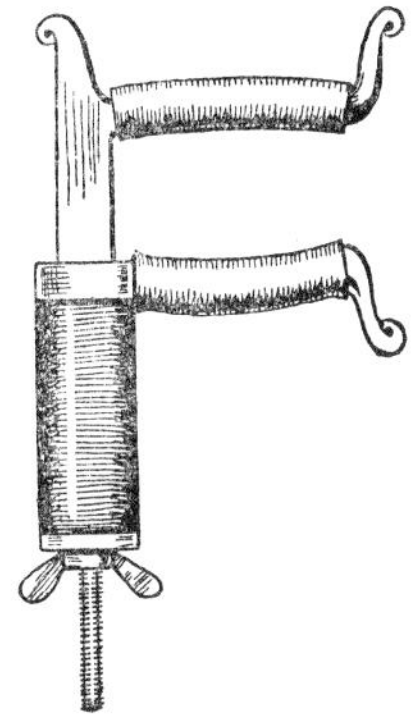

Varnell's movable mouth-gag for the horse. The two bars are covered with rubber to prevent injury to the gums when the gag is in use. The ' butterfly ' nut below the handle adjusts the space between the jaws.

should struggle and fall. When more severe measures are needful it is usual to have the horse secured by an ordinary *twitch*. This consists of a loop of soft rope threaded through a ½-inch hole near the end of a stout piece of wood. Holly or blackthorn makes the best twitch stick, although a pick-handle serves very well,

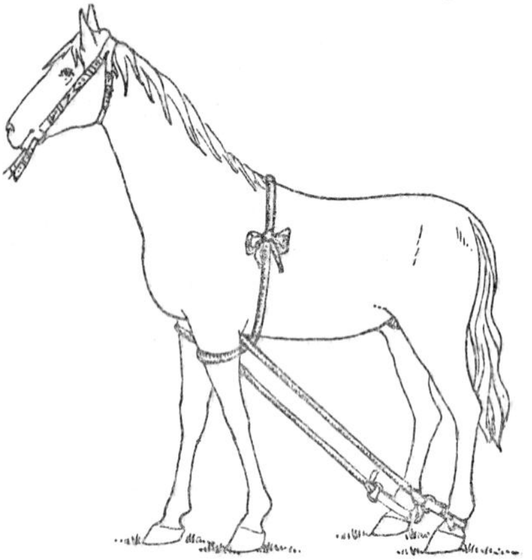

A method of arranging a rope to prevent a horse kicking with the hind feet, and to obviate danger to the stallion during the service of vicious mares.

and cotton rope, binder twine, or plaited horse-hair are best for the loop. The twitch is applied to the upper lip as a rule, where it acts by compressing the plexus of sensory nerves situated there and drawing the animal's attention to this part away from other parts of the body. A twitch should not be applied to an ear or to the lower lip. *Galvayne's twitch* consists of a slip-knot or running noose at the end of a length of rope, the noose being adjusted around the poll and above the upper incisor teeth but under the upper lip. It may be used when the upper lip is torn or when the horse will not allow the application of an ordinary *twitch*.

Blinders, *blinkers*, or *winkers* are useful at times when the horse ' sees too much ', *e.g.* when boxing nervous horses on the railway, or when excitable animals are being taken through traffic or are being led at shows among strange animals. Generally speaking, it is better to use such as do not completely blind the horse (*i.e.* blinkers), but which prevent vision to the sides and behind.

Side-sticks are merely rods which have holes or straps at each end ; one end is tied or strapped to a surcingle and the other to the head-collar. One or two may be used. They prevent a horse from getting his head round to bite at his feet, clothing, or the attendant, limiting lateral movement but allowing vertical movement. *Cradles* or *beads* is the name of a series of parallel rods strung on to two cords at intervals, and so arranged round the horse's neck that it is unable to flex the neck to any extent. The appliance is used for preventing a horse from biting at its limbs after blistering.

Cross reins are reins or ropes which cross at the withers, the ends being respectively fixed to the head-collar and the surcingle on either side. They prevent a horse from getting his head too far round to the sides, and are better tolerated than cradles. (*See also* TRANQUILLISERS, ANÆSTHETICS.)

Cattle.—The ox is an animal of much less intelligence than the horse, and can never be made to learn to the extent that a horse can. It is consequently much more often necessary to restrain it forcibly. For this purpose a cattle crush, either of a commercial pattern or one improvised by farm labour, is useful (*see* CRUSHES) for inoculations, etc. As a rule, if the head be firmly secured an ox will remain quiet. In the case of comparatively quiet cattle, milk cows, etc., it will generally suffice if an assistant takes the animal by the nose. The thumb and middle finger of one hand are inserted into the respective nostrils, and the nasal septum is pinched between them. The other hand may steady the horn, or may be placed under the jaw. The animal's head is now twisted round in towards its shoulder, the neck being forcibly bent, and the assistant's back kept pressed against

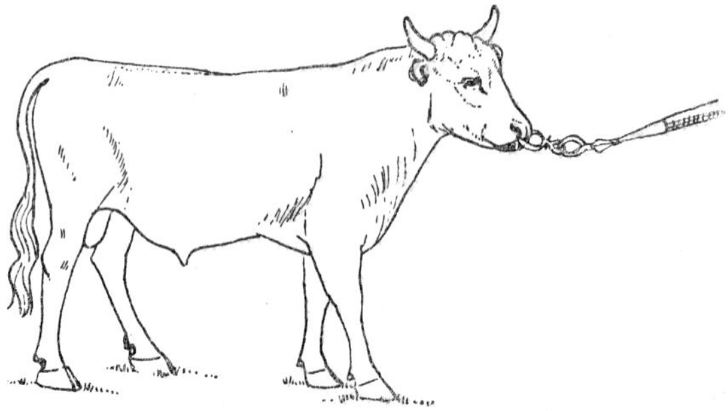

Method of controlling a young bull by means of bull-holders (' bull-dogs ') and a bull-pole or bull-leader. Where the bull has been rung and wears a ring the catch of the bull-pole is snapped into it.

the shoulder. In this position the majority of adult quiet cattle can be easily held. For bulls and those cattle that are more difficult to control it is usual to use a pair of *bull-holders*, '*bull-dogs*', '*bull-tongs*', or if the animal is already rung (with a copper or aluminium ring), to attach a rope or *bull-leader* to the ring in the nose. In some cases an ordinary cart rope may be thrown round the base of the horns, or

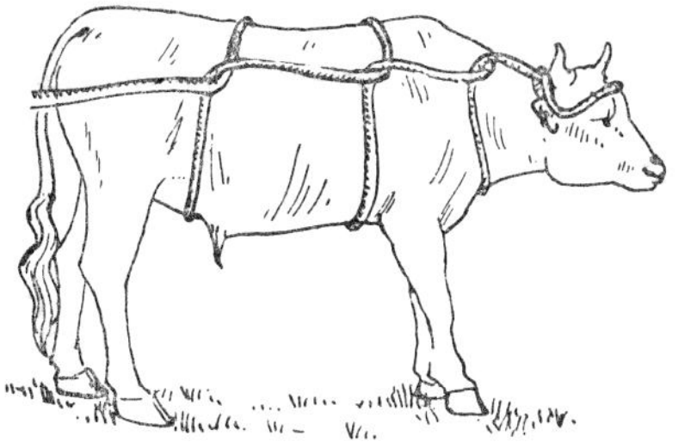

Method of arranging rope for casting ox. The loop is passed round the base of the horns first, and thereafter half-hitches are adjusted in the positions shown. One man steadies the head, and two men exert a steady pull on the end of the rope behind the animal. In a short while its legs fold under it and it sinks to the ground. where it is secured by tying the feet.

round the necks of polled cattle, the long end being passed round a post or rail and pulled tight as the animal is made to approach the fixture. For drenching purposes it is necessary to keep the head and neck in as straight a line as possible to obviate the risk of choking. With quiet cattle the person administering the drench passes his arm over the nose in front of the horns and places his fingers in the opposite side of the animal's mouth, using the other hand to manipulate the drenching horn or bottle. If an assistant is needed he should stand on the opposite side of the beast and take the horns in his hands so that he may tilt the head upwards and at the same time keep the head and neck straight out. A pair of bull-holders may be inserted into the nostrils, and have a rope attached to them which is passed over a beam and the head pulled up as much as may be necessary. Sometimes a rope may be looped round the base of the horns, crossed over the face, and passed through the mouth, and either held above the level of the animal's head, or thrown over a beam and held by an assistant. To prevent cows kicking while being milked there are various devices used for immobilising the hind legs. A rope may be tied to one leg above the hock and then passed round the other, and back to the first leg again, in a figure-of-eight manner. A stirrup leather may be first passed round one leg above the hock, and then two or more turns are taken round the other, and the buckle is finally fastened to the outside. A rope may be attached round the fetlock or above the hock on the milking side, and then fastened to a ring, etc., in the wall behind the cow. For lifting one hind leg, a pole, broom handle, etc., may be placed in front of that hock and behind and above the other. Two men take hold of the ends of the pole and pull the leg upwards and backwards, at the same time steadying the animal's balance by leaning against its thighs with their shoulders. For the fore feet it is usual to pass a rope round the cannon or above the heels and over the back to the opposite side, where it is held by an assistant.

Sheep.—For most purposes the sheep may be turned up into a position in which it sits upon its rump, by placing the left hand round under the neck from the near side, and the right hand over the back to seize the wool of the abdomen, lifting the animal's fore end off the ground and twisting its hind legs from under it. In this position its feet may be dressed, its fleece may be examined, etc. With in-lamb ewes it is not advisable to turn them owing to the possibility of doing them damage; they may be held against a wall or fence by an assistant while their feet, etc., are being dressed. Sheep stocks are sometimes used; they consist of two stakes or poles driven into the ground about 6 inches from each other, between which the sheep's head is pushed, and pieces of rope or cord are finally tied from one stake across, above and below the neck, to the other stake. Or a Y-shaped piece of wood may be used in a similar manner. It may occasionally be necessary to tie three legs of a powerful ram or ewe while the fourth is being dressed, the sheep lying on the ground meanwhile, but this is not commonly carried out except during shearing operations. Shearing tables are now used.

Pigs.—The adult pig is proverbially a difficult animal to handle and restrain, especially when the handling involves pain or discomfort, but small piglings are easily held by the hind legs with the hands, while the knees grip the dependent head. With large sows and boars it is wise to remember that they are apt to be vicious with strangers, and to use a shield of wood or a hurdle to prevent a rush by the angry animal. A short-handled broom does equally well. Either may be thrust in front of the charging animal, and each gives some protection. The best method of securing a large pig is to drive it into a corner of the sty and pen it there with a door, gate, or heavy hurdle carried by two men, and held so that the pig has no room to turn while a noose is dropped over its head and pulled tight round its jaws, and another is secured to a hind leg above the hock. The ends of these ropes are then passed round a post or a rail in the fence and pulled tight when the pig is released from its corner. Pigs possess considerable strength, and it usually takes three or more men to deal with a large savage animal. A shepherd's crook is sometimes useful for securing a hind leg, but must be used with care lest the limb is bruised by the steel head.

Dogs and Cats.—These animals are usually more easily restrained than some of the larger animals because of their intimate association with man, but there are certain animals that present much difficulty when angry or excited. A kind word and a caress will often be necessary to gain the animal's confidence before attempting to examine it, and, wherever possible, severe methods of restraint should be avoided except as a last resort. The animal which gazes up into a person's face with an expression of interest and frankness will generally allow itself to be handled without any trouble, but the sly-looking creature which watches every move of one's hands out of the corner of its eyes should be treated with respect. The human voice often exercises a wonderful amount of control over an excitable animal, and there are certain people who appear to possess the faculty of immediately gaining almost any dog's confidence and of being able to do anything with it.

However, it is always wise in any case of doubt to take no risks. The safest way of dealing with a dog is to muzzle it first. An ordinary leather or wire muzzle may be used, or a *tape muzzle* may be applied. This latter is simply a piece of tape or a bandage about 3 feet long whose middle is wound round the dog's nose, the ends being crossed under the jaw and tied round the neck or on to the collar. A clove hitch may be taken round the jaws and the ends fixed in the same way, or a loop may be made and a stick or pocket knife used to tighten the loop round the jaws in the manner of a tourniquet. It is sometimes also necessary to tie the two fore legs together to prevent the dog from removing the tape muzzle by using his fore feet to scrape it off. With bulldogs, and those with a short face and a pug nose, it is better to tie the tape round the jaws, finishing with the ends above the nose, tying them together there, and then passing the ends back to the collar.

Cats can be rolled in a sack or towel and the part required exposed by folding back the sack, or they may be pushed down the sleeve of an old coat as far as necessary. With cats it is important to prevent them from using their claws, which inflict injuries more often than do the teeth. (*See also under* TRANQUILLISERS, ANÆSTHETICS.)

RESUSCITATION, ARTIFICIAL (*re*, again ; *suscito*, I arouse). (*See* ARTIFICIAL RESPIRATION.)

RETCHING is an ineffectual attempt at vomiting, generally characterised by some amount of pain, and taking place when the stomach is in an irritable condition but empty. (*See* VOMITING.)

RETENTION OF AFTERBIRTH, or 'HANGING THE CLEANSING', is one of the untoward sequels of parturition, and is liable to occur in any of the domestic animals. The condition in the mare, and the appropriate treatment, is described under UTERUS, DISEASES OF, and the reader is referred to that section. Retention of the fœtal membranes is commonest in the cow, but this animal possesses great powers of resistance, and serious consequences are not so frequent as they are in other animals. Normally, the membranes should be expelled in from ½ to 4 or 5 hours after the birth of the calf, but owing to the intricate cotyledonary attachment in the ruminant, and especially in cattle, they are often retained for long periods. (*See* PARTURITION.) It frequently causes little or no obvious disturbance to the cow at the time, but subsequent service by the bull is not successful. It is commoner after difficult parturition, and in those cows whose general vitality is low, than in opposite circumstances.

Symptoms.—The symptoms of retention are very obvious in typical cases: one portion of the fœtal membranes hangs from the lips of the vulva attached to what remains inside the cavity of the uterus. The amount that has been passed to the outside may only appear as a few inches, or a large mass reaching to the cow's hocks may be seen. In some cases there are no parts of the membranes visible externally, but there is usually an odour of decomposition evident. Upon occasion, where a cow has calved in the open field, or in a loose-box with no supervision, no membranes may be found, but this does not necessarily mean that the membranes are retained, since in some cases cows will devour them unless restrained. During the first day after calving the membranes in an ordinary uncomplicated case are fresh, slimy, and pinkish in colour. There is no objectionable smell, and the cow is not distressed. After the second day the external portions undergo decomposition; the colour becomes greyish, and the membranes are often stained with dung; an offensive irritating often chocolate-coloured discharge makes its appearance and soils the hind quarters and tail of the cow. The cow, after this, begins to show a certain amount of uneasiness. She stands with her back arched, frequently switches her tail and paddles with the hind feet. Her milk production may fall off a little, and she may be dull and refuse her food. The abdomen becomes tucked up, and the skin hidebound. In some cases she groans and grunts when passing her fæces, which are dry and passed less frequently than normally. These symptoms in a cow which has calved but shows no external signs of retention of the afterbirth, should be taken as an indication that she has not cleansed. About the fourth or fifth day the cow either recovers, or else becomes attacked with a metritis. In cases that appear to recover the membranes undergo liquefying decomposition and are gradually eliminated from the uterus, and the resistance of the mucous membrane is sufficiently great to prevent any severe inflammation of the uterus. In such instances masses of semi-dissolved membrane, looking like pieces of wet cobweb, are passed out at intervals, and can be found behind the cow along with quantities of greyish foul-smelling discharge; the mucous membrane of the vagina is inflamed, and the cow resents having her hind quarters examined.

Treatment.—What is given under PARTURITION and under UTERUS, DISEASES OF, which concerns strict cleanliness both during and after calving, is of great importance in preventing retention of the afterbirth, or in avoiding infection where retention has already taken place. These sections should be referred to in this connection. When the membranes have been retained the common practice in many parts is to remove them immediately, but this is not always advisable. It is certainly not advisable that a mass of decomposing fleshy material should be allowed to hang from a cow's uterus for a longer time than is absolutely necessary, but too hasty attempts at removal are often followed by serious results and even the death of the cow. Individual cases require different methods of treatment, but as a general rule the membranes should not be removed until they can be displaced *without difficulty, and without distress to the cow.*

In modern practice stilbœstral injections have largely displaced manual removal, with its attendant risks. Manual removal consists of introducing the hand and arm which have been previously cleansed as far as possible by thorough washing in an antiseptic solution, and a subsequent rinsing in strong salt and water. Each cotyledon is grasped as it is reached, and the adherent membrane is peeled off from its surface with the fingers and thumb. At the same time steady traction should be exerted upon the protruded membranes from the outside. After removal it is customary to douche out the uterus with a suitable antiseptic solution, and to introduce one or more uterine pessaries (*see* section ' Metritis ', UTERUS, DISEASES OF).

In the sow and bitch the membranes that are liable to be retained are those belonging to the fœtus that is born last, which occupied the extremity of one or other of the horns of the uterus, but the condition is rare in each of these animals. Stilbœstrol injections may be indicated.

It is most advisable that owners of animals which have retained their afterbirth after parturition should seek skilled advice wherever possible.

RETENTION OF FÆCES (*see* OBSTRUCTION OF BOWELS).

RETENTION OF URINE (*see* URINE).

RETICULOCYTES.—Newly formed red-blood corpuscles in which a fine network can be demonstrated by special staining methods. They are typically found in anæmic conditions and indicate an effort of the blood-forming tissues to restore the red-blood corpuscle count to normal levels.

RETICULUM (*reticulum*, a little net) is the name of the 2nd stomach of ruminants.

It lies in front of and a little below the level of the mass of the 1st stomach towards the middle line of the body, and has a wide entrance from the 1st stomach, and a smaller one into the 3rd stomach. Its mucous membrane lining is thrown into large numbers of little pockets, or cells, some of which are hexagonal in outline, some square and some triangular, and most of which possess smaller secondary cells in their cavities. (*See also* FOREIGN BODIES IN RETICULUM, p. 885.)

RETINA (diminutive of *rete*, a net) is the innermost and light-sensitive coat of the posterior part of the globe of the eye. (*See* EYE.)

RETINA, ATROPHY OF. — Occurs especially in Night Blindness, a disease partly hereditary—in Red Setters, etc.

RETRO- (*retro-*, backward) is a prefix signifying behind or turned backward.

RETROPHARYNGEAL ABSCESS is the name given to an abscess occurring at the back of the throat in the region behind the pharynx. It is commonest in the horse, where it is due to the presence of the organisms that cause strangles in the lymphatic gland. Such abscesses generally make swallowing difficult or impossible until they burst, which they frequently do into the cavity of the pharynx, whence the pus is swallowed. (*See* STRANGLES.)

The retropharyngeal glands in the ox and pig may be affected with tubercular abscesses when the disease is located in the lungs or anterior parts of the body.

RHABDOVIRUS.—A group of bullet-shaped viruses which includes the rabies virus and that of vesicular stomatitis and Marburg disease.

RHEUMATIC FEVER is another name for acute rheumatism.

RHEUMATISM.—A general term indicating disease of muscles, tendons, joints, bones, or nerves, resulting in pain and disability.

Rheumatism is seen in dogs, pigs, and horses most commonly, but it affects all of the domesticated animals. Young animals are most often attacked by the acute type, especially young pigs and puppies, and adults by the muscular form and by chronic or articular rheumatism.

Causes.—It appears probable that it is associated with the absorption of toxins from the alimentary canal (mouth, stomach, or intestines), or from some other seat of bacterial activity, and that these toxins cause a localised inflammation in some area of the body which is exposed to overwork, chill, or some other devitalising circumstance. Amongst factors which at least exercise a predisposing effect upon the body are damp, cold surroundings, lack of sunlight, exposure to draughts.

Symptoms.—In the *acute type*, which is perhaps commonest among young pigs and puppies, the symptoms develop rapidly. There are the usual signs of fever ; the temperature is very high, and the pulse and respirations are increased in rate ; the animals are dull, and one or more of the joints of the limbs is held stiffly and is obviously painful.

In the *muscular type* the condition also appears rapidly. (*See under* MUSCULAR RHEUMATISM, p. 574.)

In typical *chronic rheumatism*, which is also called *articuiar rheumatism*, the chief changes are usually in the joints, which become swollen and stiff, due to a deposit of new bone round the edges of the joint surfaces. It has been suggested by some that ringbones and spavins in horses are merely localisations of articular rheumatism. It is at least certain that the appearance, history, and progress of rheumatic arthritis in man is extraordinarily like what is seen in ringbones in the horse. In some cases the heart becomes affected with vegetations upon its valves during chronic cases, this organ develops a murmur, and there is evidence of incompetency of its valves. In other instances the muscles may be affected in a manner somewhat resembling what is seen in the acute form, but the symptoms are less severe, and an almost characteristic peculiarity is that the lameness is ' fleeting ', *i.e.* it affects one limb one day and another the next, etc.

Treatment.—There is no absolute specific, although certain drugs have enjoyed a great reputation in the alleviation of this disease, especially salicylates. Phenyl-butazone has been used with reported success. (*See also* CORTISONE.)

RHINITIS (ῥίς, the nose) means inflammation of the nose. (*See* NOSE.)

RHINITIS, ATROPHIC.—This term cannot be precisely defined, but Done (1962) stated : ' Atrophic rhinitis (the macroscopic lesion) is the product of a severe persistent inflammatory reaction in the nasal mucosa of a growing, and therefore very young pig, and as such is non-specific with regard to ætiology.'

Although it has been suggested that this condition is hereditary or nutritional in origin these may be only predisposing or accessory factors. The generally accepted view is that in the first 2 or 3 months of life the rapidly growing nasal structures are extremely liable to attack by infectious agents but quite often recovery from these is complete. In herds with severe disease, however, the condition may progress to give rise to the marked displacement or atrophy of the turbinate bones and also to an associated pneumonia.

There may be several agents causing the primary inflammatory reaction. One histologically identifiable cause is inclusion-body rhinitis (I.B.R.).

A survey carried out in 1956–57 in the U.K. showed that the incidence of atrophic rhinitis varied from 2·8 per cent in 926 pigs over 6 months of age passing through a slaughterhouse to 40·3 per cent in 3754 pigs from herds known to have atrophic rhinitis; in another 5268 pigs not considered to have this disease 10 per cent of the snouts showed definite microscopic abnormalities.

RHINITIS, INCLUSION-BODY (I.B.R.).—A contagious disease of pigs encountered in America and Europe. It was first reported in Britain in 1954, but by 1962 had ceased to be regarded as serious. The cause is a virus.

Symptoms.—The acute form is to be found in piglets 2 or 3 weeks old, when there is no deformity of the snout to be seen and not always an overflow of tears. Sneezing is perhaps the most common symptom. The eyelids may be puffy, and sometimes the piglet has a copious discharge from its nose and breathes through its mouth. The disease can be so mild that symptoms pass unnoticed, or so severe that death occurs within a week. In some outbreaks the mortality is 10 per cent or more, and survivors suffer a growth check from the disease which continues in the sub-acute form.

Atrophy of the turbinate bones and distortion of the snout are frequent but not invariable sequels—depending perhaps upon the secondary invaders involved, the bone conformation of the pig, etc. Brown tear stains may be observed.

Treatment.—At present there is no effective treatment and a slaughter policy, though no longer enforced, is a wise precaution on the owner's part. The disease ceased to be notifiable in 1962 in the U.K.

Diagnosis.—This may be confirmed by microscopic examination of scrapings from the mucous membrane from the nose, stained by Giemx or methylene blue, during the first fortnight of the illness. After that, inclusion-body cells are not found.

It should be noted that deformity of the snout may occur in the absence of the virus of Inclusion-Body Rhinitis.

RHINOSPORIDIOSIS.—A chronic disease of the nasal mucous membrane, and associated with polyp-formation leading to difficulty in breathing, caused by a fungus *Rhinosporidia seberi*. The disease occurs in cattle and horses, in the U.S.A., S. America, Australia, and India.

RHINOTRACHEITIS, INFECTIOUS.—A disease of cattle recognised in the U.S.A. in 1954. It is also called Infectious Bovine Rhinotracheitis, or I.B.R. for short. It is caused by a virus which may damage various parts of the body, accordingly giving rise to varying groups of symptoms; but in the 1962 U.K. outbreak the main symptom was a profuse discharge from the eyelids with matting of the hair around them. A discharge from the nose was another symptom, observed particularly in white-faced animals. In the U.S.A., it appears to be very sudden in onset, with excessive salivation and a temperature rising to 108 degrees in some cases.

I.B.R. is sometimes associated with a fatal pneumonia, and sometimes with an infection of the female genital system. In other outbreaks it has amounted to nothing more than conjunctivitis. A mortality rate of 3 per cent has been quoted in the U.S.A., but this figure is likely to vary from outbreak to outbreak. The disease may closely resemble Mucosal Disease, with which at one time it was thought to be possibly identical, and also Malignant Catarrh.

An outbreak among store cattle in England has been reported (1962).

The disease has been recognised in Canada, New Zealand, and Germany.

At least one strain of the virus is neurotropic and has caused encephalitis in calves in Australia.

(*See also under* FELINE.)

RHODODENDRON POISONING is not common. There are about 20 varieties which have been recorded as causing poisoning in sheep, cattle, goats, and even man. The toxicity is not equal in all varieties, however, and it appears that when only small amounts have been taken there is little likelihood of serious consequences. The shrubs contain a glucoside called *Andromedotoxin*; symptoms resemble those of ACONITE POISONING.

RHONCHI, or DRY SOUNDS, sometimes also referred to as 'DRY RÂLES', are continuous sounds heard during breathing by auscultation of the chest, when there is some constriction of the bronchi. (*See also* RÂLES.)

RIBOFLAVIN.—A component of vitamin B_2. (*See* VITAMIN B_2.)

RIBONUCLEIC ACID.—A substance which appears to influence the nature of cell development. In some experiments it has been shown that RNA from malignant cells will cause normal cells *in vitro* to show characteristics of malignancy; and the converse is possible.

RIBS are the long bones which together form the cage of the thorax. Their numbers vary in the different animals, according to how many thoracic or dorsal vertebræ are present, as follows: horse, 18 pairs; ox, 13 pairs; pig, 14 or 15 pairs; dog, 13 pairs. In any of these animals an extra rib (often called a 'floating rib' because it possesses little or no cartilage to unite it to the costal arch) may be present on one or both sides of the body. The first 8 of these in the horse and ox, the first 7 in the pig, and the first 9 in the dog, have cartilages which are united to the sternum, and are called *sternal ribs*, while those farther back in the series in each case have cartilages which do not reach the sternum, but form an arch by overlapping each other, and are known as *asternal ribs*.

Each rib possesses a 'head', by which it is joined to the anterior part of the vertebra to which it corresponds in number, and to the posterior part of that immediately in front, and this is succeeded by a 'neck', and a short distance farther down the shaft is a 'tubercle', which articulates with the transverse process of the vertebra to which it corresponds. The rest of the rib is composed of a long curved flat shaft, whose curve varies according to the position of the rib in the chest, being greatest about the middle of the series, and also according to the animal to which it belongs; *e.g.* greater in the horse than in the ox. Immediately posterior to each rib runs the intercostal nerve and blood-vessels which are situated in a little groove along the borders of each rib. In life the ribs are attached to each other by the intercostal muscles to form the continuous wall of the chest. (*See* BONES.)

RICKETS, or RACHITIS, is a deficiency disease of young animals characterised by a tendency towards the formation of enlarged extremities of the long bones, and a bending of their shafts. Dogs, pigs, lambs, foals, and calves are all affected, the first two more frequently than the other species of domesticated animals. It has also been met with in intensively managed poultry establishments where chicks are deprived of sunlight.

Cause.—Rickets is an aphosphorosis essentially, which may be caused by a deficiency of either vitamin D or phosphorus, or in some cases both these.

Absence of sunlight is a contributory cause and animals kept in dark buildings, especially if inadequately fed, are prone to rickets. Avoid repeated dosing with liquid paraffin, or yeast in excess. A diet consisting largely of oatmeal or maize meal, such as is commonly the lot of sheepdogs, results in rickets. (*See* PHYTIN.)

Symptoms.—The typical changes consist of the development of bony swellings upon the ends of the long bones of the limbs, where they meet other bones to form joints, and the production of swellings at the point where a rib joins its rib cartilage, *i.e.* along each side of the chest about two-thirds the way down from the spine. If the hand is placed flat along the side of the animal and moved backward and forward a series of bony swellings, to which the name of a 'rosary' has been applied, can be easily distinguished in a typical case. In most cases, especially in puppies, there is also a tendency for the shafts of the long limb to bend in an outward direction under the influence of the weight of the body. In advanced cases there is also some digestive disturbances, the animal becoming affected with diarrhœa and indigestion, and a dropsical condition of the abdomen ('pot-bellied') usually develops.

Treatment.—This consists essentially in giving the animal cod-liver oil (for the sake of its vitamin D content), or—if expense is no objection—halibut-liver oil. The latter involves less bulky doses, and the content of vitamin D is often better standardised and to be relied upon. Administration of calcium phosphate in the absence of vitamin D will not be found effective. Sunlight and ultra-violet radiation are beneficial, but vitamin D in the food is the essential remedy. At the same time *avoid* the continuous administration of either yeast or liquid paraffin.

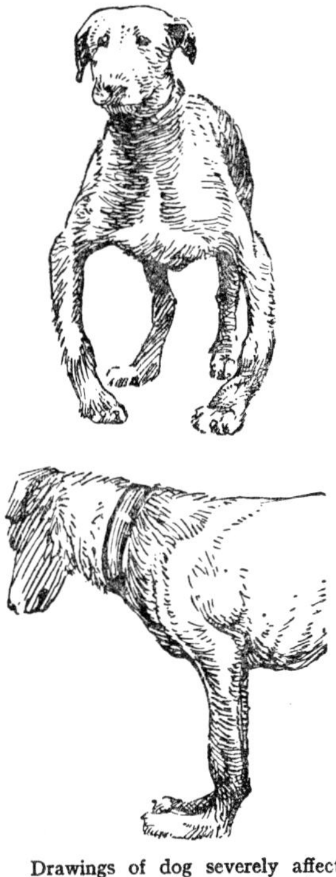

Drawings of dog severely affected with rickets. In the upper diagram the outward bending of bones of the fore limbs is well seen. The lower diagram shows the thickness of the carpal joint greater than normal, and the collapse of the digit, resulting in plantigrade instead of digitigrade gait.

For the larger animals, vitamin D itself is recommended.

Local treatment of the enlarged bones is not usually either necessary or advisable, but where there is very serious bending of the shafts of the long bones it may be necessary to support them by elastic or other bandages. (*See* PLATE 2.) (*See also* OSTEOMALACIA.)

RICKETTSIA.—The generic name for a group of minute micro-organisms which may be said to be intermediate between the smallest bacteria and the filterable viruses. 'They have certain characteristics in common with Gram-negative bacteria; but their failure to grow in ordinary culture media, and their multiplication intracellularly, show that their metabolic requirements are more akin to those of the filterable viruses.' (Topley and Wilson, 1964.) They flourish in the alimentary canal of ticks, lice, etc. One causes TICK FEVER.

RIDA.—A disease of sheep involving the nervous system.

RIDEAL-WALKER COEFFICIENT.—Expresses the comparative efficiency of antiseptics, as based on the R.W. Test, taking carbolic acid as unity. It does not take into account the influence of body fluids upon the efficiency or otherwise of the antiseptic.

RIDING ESTABLISHMENTS ACT, 1939.—This empowers local authorities to authorise a veterinary surgeon to inspect premises and horses, and to prosecute in the event of unfit horses being used.

RIFT VALLEY FEVER, or **ENZOÖTIC HEPATITIS,** is a disease of sheep, cattle, goats, camels, and man which occurs in Africa. It is caused by a virus. The vectors include mosquitoes.

Lambs are particularly susceptible, while a common feature of most outbreaks has been heavy abortions among pregnant ewes. In young lambs, between birth and 7 days old, the mortality may reach 80 per cent or more. The disease also attacks older sheep, but the death-rate in them is less.

Symptoms.—The affected lambs become dull and listless; they prefer to lie, and get steadily weaker during the day that they are first noticed ill, and as a rule are dead 24 hours later.

The disease is transmissible to mice, and in man causes fever.

RIG, RIDGLING, or CRYPTORCHID.—A male animal in which one or both testes do not descend into the scrotum from the abdomen at the usual time. A retained testis gives rise to a certain amount of unnatural irritability of the animal, probably due to an excessive secretion of the interstitial cells of the usually imperfect male gonad (*i.e.* testicle). Hormone treatment may be tried. (*See* HORMONES, HORMONE THERAPY.) Otherwise, when retention persists later than the second year in the horse it is always advisable to perform an operation, in which the scrotum is opened and a search made in the abdomen for the missing testicle. In the majority of cases it will be found at the upper end of the inguinal canal, but there are some cases in which it is found in other parts of the abdominal cavity. (*See also under* MONORCHID.)

RIGORS (*rigor*, stiffness).—Shivering fits. When prolonged, a fit of rigors is generally accompanied by an elevation of the temperature, and may be the warning sign of the approach of some disease or fever, such as influenza, mastitis, or lymphangitis. *Rigor mortis* is the name given to that stiffness which rapidly sets in after death, generally within 3 or 4 hours, and passes off at the end of a few days or sooner.

RIMA (*rima*) is a term, meaning a crack or fissure, applied to any narrow natural opening, *e.g.* rima glottidis, the space between the vocal cords.

RINDERPEST (*see* CATTLE PLAGUE).

RING-BONES.—A term used to mean any bony exostosis affecting the interphalangeal joints of the horse's foot, or indeed any bony enlargement in the same region. A precise definition of 'ring-bone' has never been enunciated in such a manner that it will satisfy all critics, but, since to a great extent all forms of bony growth in the foot are serious, this is not such an important matter. So-called 'ring-bone' is divided into at least three types: (1) *High ring-bone*, where the pastern joint (*i.e.* between the long and short pastern bones) is the seat of the disease; (2) *Low ring-bone*, where the deposit occurs round the coffin-joint, between the short pastern bone and the coffin-bone; and (3) *False ring-bone*, where the enlargement occurs upon the shaft of one of the bones and does not involve the edges of a joint surface. In addition, some authorities consider that a *traumatic form* of ring-bone may occur, which is less serious than any of the others. From the point of view of etymology it would appear that the term 'ring-bone' should be restricted to conditions in which a partial or complete *ring of bone* is formed round one or other of the joints, and that all other bony enlargements affecting the surface of the shaft of the bones, but not involving the edges of the joint surfaces, should be called *exostoses*. Difficulty arises, however, when examining a horse's foot, in determining exactly whether the joint surfaces are affected, or are likely to become affected, in any particular given case. The term 'false ring-bone' is also somewhat misleading, because it is not uncommon for a bony exostosis, which commences upon the shaft of the bone, to spread gradually upwards or downwards and ultimately involve one or other of the joints and become quite as serious as the so-called 'true ring-bone'.

Causes.—The causes of ring-bone have never yet been efficiently demonstrated, and a good deal of the evidence brought forward to support one or another theory is circumstantial. At present it is considered that most ring-bones are produced through concussion, acting along with some hereditary factor which implies an inherent lack of power of resistance in the bones themselves, or which produces some irregularity in the conformation of the limbs and throws extra strain upon the phalanges. It seems likely that heredity plays a part as a predisposing cause, for foals born from parents which are thus affected very often become subjects of ring-bone when they become adult, and the more generations of affected ancestry a foal has the earlier will the disease manifest itself. Some authorities hold that ring-bones are manifestations of rheumatism—*i.e.* rheumatoid arthritis—affecting the horse, and that in a horse with a rheumatic tendency the bony enlargements will certainly develop irrespective of concussion or any other exciting factor. A vitamin D deficiency has been suggested also as a possible cause.

Strains and blows upon the surfaces of the bones of the digit will produce exostoses from inflammation of the periosteum, but in such there is usually no tendency to fixation of the joint involved, and they are often called 'traumatic ring-bones', to distinguish them from other forms. In the same way bony enlargements may result from the healing of partial fracture of small portions of the phalanges, and it is probable that such are commoner than is generally supposed, more particularly in light-legged horses.

Symptoms.—The symptoms of most ring-bones are vague, and an owner often cannot remember exactly when the horse first showed symptoms, because in the

RING-BONES

early stages nothing more than a fleeting lameness was seen, and little or no attention was paid to it. 'The horse has been habitually stiff on commencing work in the mornings for some time past, and as the day wore on the lameness has disappeared.' These symptoms become more and more marked until eventually the horse will go lame all day if it is worked, or becomes too lame to take out of the stable. In some cases work exaggerates the lameness from the very first, especially upon hard paved roads, and it is always worst during work in later stages when bony enlargements have made their appearance. To begin with, the lameness is usually unaccompanied by any heat or pain in the limb, and no bony outgrowths can be felt, but after a time one or other of the joints becomes enlarged, and the cause of the lameness becomes obvious. It must be understood that it is only in the case of high ring-bones (around the pastern joint) that the exostosis can be felt; when the lower (coffin) joint is affected there is at first no outward visible or palpable sign; but after a time the hoof alters in shape, becoming distinctly bulged or 'buttressed' at the coronet. This latter effect is due to the fact that in low ring-bone the extensor or pyramidal process of the coffin-bone is usually involved, and the deposit of bone upon it pushes the coronet, and the wall which grows from it, in an outward direction ('pyramidal disease'). At times the alteration in the outline of the hoof is not by any means regular: it may be bulged at any point from one heel to the other, denoting that there is a deposit of bone wherever there is a bulge.

The main difference between 'true' and 'false' ring-bone is that in the former the ossifying process extends around one or other of the two joints of the digit, while in the latter the deposit occurs upon the shaft of the first or second phalanx. It is not always easy to distinguish between the two forms in the living animal, because of the difficulty of palpating past other hard tissues in the region, but where a discrete enlargement is felt above the pastern joint, and where there is no obstruction to passive flexion and extension of this joint when the horse's foot is picked up, it may be considered that the condition is one of 'false' ring-bone. This does not, however, preclude the possibility of a 'true' ring-bone forming afterwards, for the process of exostosis may extend so as to involve a joint sooner or later.

In 'true ring-bone' the joint that is affected almost always ends by becoming stiff (ankylosed), owing to fusion between its complementary bones and obliteration of the joint having occurred. In this state the horse may become fairly sound, because the pain occasioned by movement

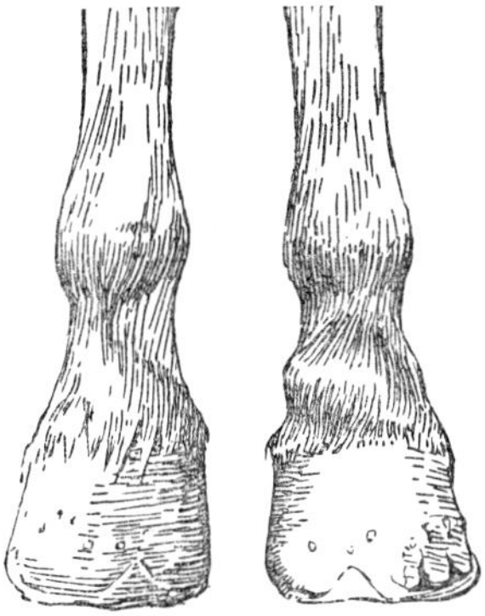

The appearance of ring-bone around the first interphalangeal joint (high ring-bone) of the near fore foot of the horse. The normal off fore limb is also shown for comparison.

at the joint has disappeared, but the gait will always be stiff and stilted. Light horses so affected are incapable of great speeds, and even the draught animal working at a slow pace becomes less agile and nimble on its feet.

Where a ring-bone results from a severe injury, such as a violent blow or a fracture, lameness is apparent at once. Instead of subsiding in the course of a week or 10 days with appropriate treatment, such a variety of lameness as is complicated by ring-bone formation persists. The horse recovers from the original injury to a certain extent, but it is not until the ossification process is complete that it will be able to go at all sound or be fit for work, and before this occurs the bony enlargement will become obvious.

In addition to instances such as these already given, there are some cases where ring-bones form, in which no symptoms of lameness or even stiffness are noticed.

With regard to the incidence of the disease, it is more common in the fore feet than behind, probably owing to the greater stresses to which the former are subjected; and it occurs oftener in the heavy breeds than in light horses. It is not commonly seen before four years of age, but it may develop at any time after that, and it is very often seen in horses that are 'aged'. Shetland and other ponies are remarkably free from the disease, even in old age, and the same remark applies to the Arab, but no breed is immune.

Treatment.—Once exostoses have formed it is quite impossible to remove them, and an absolute cure is never effected. In the early stages of 'true ring-bone' the horse should be rested from work, and should receive cold applications to the feet and lower limbs twice daily. If possible, it should be turned out to grass in a level field, or it may be turned out into a yard or reed. If it must remain indoors it does better in a loose-box well bedded with peat-moss or sawdust. The foot should be examined, and any overgrowth of horn at toes or heels reduced. As a rule a flat shoe, below which is placed a leather sole stuffed with Stockholm tar and tow, should be applied. After a week or a fortnight of such treatment the cold applications should be stopped.

More harm than good results when blistering is carried out indiscriminately. In the early stages blistering increases the blood-supply, favours the production of more exudate, and stimulates the bone-forming cells to produce a larger exostosis than would otherwise form. In all cases it is better to give Nature time and *not to blister.*

If the deposition is large and well defined, and if the lameness does not improve after such treatment, the only means of affording relief is to carry out the operation of double plantar neurectomy or median neurectomy. This does not materially alter the enlargement, but it cuts off the pain sensations passing up to the brain, and allows the horse to work for some months afterwards in favourable cases.

Where there is a discrete 'false ring-bone' the alleviation of pain, and the chances of at least partial recovery, are more probable than in 'true ring-bone', but the risk of the former merging into the latter must never be forgotten. Treatment is upon the same lines as that given for the 'true' forms; the rational reduction of the horn of the hoof so that a true balance is obtained between outside and inside, to avoid any undue strain, is of the greatest importance.

If a partial fracture is suspected, the horse should be put in slings in a stable for a time, and the affected foot should be bandaged in plaster of Paris, or with pitch bandages, to immobilise the separated portions of bone as much as possible. Finally, after the horse has recovered from lameness, it is necessary to allow at least 3 weeks' rest before it is again returned to its work.

RINGER'S SOLUTION consists of sodium chloride, 9 grams; calcium chloride 0·25 gm.; potassium chloride, 0·42 gm. per litre.

'RINGWOMB'.—This is the colloquial name for a condition which sometimes complicates lambing, and is due to failure of the cervix to dilate. Usually, the *os uteri* will admit one or two fingers, which can feel what seems like a firm ring.

The shepherd may recognise the condition on seeing a small portion of fœtal membrane protruding from the vulva. The ewe remains in good health (but does not lamb) until death and decomposition of the fœtus occur.

Manual dilation of the cervix is practised by some veterinary surgeons. Should this prove impossible, Cæsarean operation is the only alternative. (*See* UTERUS, *and* PARTURITION.)

RINGWORM and FAVUS, which are called by other names, such as HERPES, DERMATOMYCOSIS, TINEA, etc., are contagious skin diseases caused by the growth of moulds or fungi, which live either upon the surface of the skin or in the hairs of the areas affected. Ringworm may affect any of the domesticated animals, but it is probably commonest in young store cattle when they are enclosed in buildings during winter, and in pet cats and kittens. Dogs and horses are also frequently affected, but the disease is not often seen in the sheep and pig, and when it does occur it is usually due to one or other of the parasites which normally affect other animals. Favus affects the dog and cat, the mouse and rat, rabbits sometimes, and fowls occasionally. It is characterised by the formation of scales which have a depression in their centres, giving an appearance suggestive of a honeycomb (*favus*, honeycomb).

Ringworm and favus in the domesticated animals are caused by parasitic fungi which belong to the family GYMNOASCIDÆ.

Lesions generally.—Ringworm appears in the form of patches of dry, raised, crusty skin, from the surface of which the hairs have fallen and upon the surface of which there are scales or scabs. The patches are often more or less circular, but in bad cases large irregular areas may be produced, which result from the coalescence of adjacent areas. In cases of favus, in

RINGWORM AND FAVUS

the raised patches there are cup-shaped depressions which bear some similarity to a honeycomb, from which they get their name.

As a rule, the first manifestations of either ringworm or favus is that the skin becomes reddened and inflamed, and a little whitish, greyish, or yellowish serum exudes from its surface. This soon dries into a crust or scale which glues together the hairs over the part, and eventually falls off. Later, more crust is formed in the same manner, and with each successive crust formation the skin thickens and wrinkles.

Predisposing causes.—There are two important contributory causes of ringworm, which it must be remembered can be avoided: viz. (1) over-crowding of animals into unhygienic, badly ventilated, dark buildings; and (2) general debility, resulting from bad feeding. In addition, youth must be considered a predisposing cause, for more often are young than adult animals affected. Season also has some influence upon its spread, for it is seldom that it is troublesome during the summer, but it occurs freely during the dark days of winter and early spring. Carelessness in the use of grooming-tools—*e.g.* when the implements are used for any and all animals indiscriminately, and when the skin surface becomes scarified through friction from too severe use of the curry-comb or dandy brush—also tend to foster the spread of ringworm through a stud of horses. Changing of harness and clothing from one horse to another is a fruitful source of its spread. The presence of vermin (rats, mice, or rabbits), which are preyed upon or killed by dogs and cats, is responsible for these latter animals developing lesions in some cases.

Results of Laboratory Examination for Animal Ringworm 1955–66 (Inclusive)
Data in Terms of Number of Premises on which Infection was Detected

	Infected	*Epidermophyton floccosum*	*Microsporum canis*	*M. equinum*	*M. gypseum*	*Microsporum* spp.	*T. equinum*	*T. gallinae*	*T. mentagrophytes*	*T. persicolor*	*T. simii*	*T. verrucosum*	*Trichophyton* spp.	Unidentified
Horse	251		1	78	2	1	130		6			19	14	
Cattle	223											199	24	
Dog	44	1	18		1	1			16	1		1	4	1
Cat	31		24			1			6					
Pig	3								2			1		
Goat	3		1						1			1		
Sheep	3											2	1	
Chicken	3							3						
Total	561	1	44	78	3	3	130	3	31	1		223	43	1

(The above simplified table is reproduced with acknowledgements to the Central Veterinary Laboratory, Weybridge.)

Ringworm in the horse may be due either to parasites belonging to the class *Trochiphyton* or to *Microsporum*. In cases due to the former, the first affected areas are usually confined to the head, neck, withers, and sometimes to the root of the tail. The hair becomes matted in patches about the size of a five-shilling piece, and in the centre of each patch appears a bare area from which the hair has fallen off; this gradually extends until the whole area is denuded. The skin becomes raised and scurfy, and greyish-white crusts are formed; at times there may be grey or yellow scales adherent to begin with, but becoming detached later. As time progresses the area becomes normal again, but new patches develop around the original lesion, until in a few weeks large areas of the body are covered with the lesions. There is usually little or no itchiness, except when due to *Trichophyton mentagrophytes*, where little pustules are formed below the crusts, but in badly neglected cases which are kept under dirty conditions, and when the horses are not well fed, there may be a considerable amount of wasting of condition accompanied by itchiness.

When the horse is affected with ringworm due to *Microsporum* parasites practically any part of the body may be attacked.

Ringworm in cattle is of only one form and is due to *T. verrucosum*. It is very common among young animals in autumn, winter, and early spring, especially if they are kept indoors. The head and neck are most often affected, especially the eyelids, lips, ears, and above the jaws, but it may occur anywhere on the body. The lesion begins as a raised ring-like patch on which the hairs stand erect. In a day or so the hairs fall off, and the surface of the skin becomes covered with masses of scales heaped up into a greyish-white or greyish-yellow crust. The areas are usually very numerous and often become confluent, so that large areas become bare of hair and present roughened, crusty, hard, dry surfaces with a tendency towards pronounced wrinkling of the skin around and between them. Where calves are very extensively affected with ringworm there is always a good deal of loss of condition and itchiness.

When **sheep** are affected there is almost always a great deal of itchiness which may be mistaken for the itch caused by scab mites, ked, ticks, or other parasites. The fleece becomes matted, and falls out in circular patches over the shoulders, neck, and chest.

Ringworm in the dog may be one of four varieties: *Trichophyton, Microsporum, Oidmella*, or *Oospora*, the last named causing favus. The lesions produced by the first three of these are very similar in all respects to those seen in horses and cattle, but there is nearly always a certain amount of irritation which leads to scratching and sometimes to tearing of the skin. In favus caused by *Oospora canina* the lesion appears as a raised circular patch upon whose surface there is a pale yellow crust with little depressions (honeycomb) scattered through it. The skin in such cases is often very much thickened.

Ringworm in the cat is of three kinds: due to *Trichophyton, Microsporum*, and *Achorion*, the latter producing favus. When due to the first two of these the symptoms and lesions are similar to what is seen in other animals. (*See* Plate 14 *and* ONYCHOMYCOSIS.) Favus is usually contracted from mangling mice affected with mouse favus (*A. quinckeanum* or *A. arloingi*), although it may also be due to *A. Schœnleinii*—the favus of man. The lesions are chiefly confined to the fore-paws and the head and the neck, though they may spread to other parts of the body. Itchiness is usually absent. The areas affected vary in size from that of a pin's head up to a shilling or so, and are not always regular in outline. The skin is thickened and the edges are raised. When newly formed, the covering crust is yellow and soft to the touch, but when old it is grey and powdery. The characteristic cup-shaped depressions are seen in most cases, but when affecting the claws they may be absent.

Ringworm due to *Microsporum canis* Bodin is of considerable public health importance. It is often overlooked by owners; affected cats being a danger to children.

Favus in the fowl, due to *Trichophyton gallinæ*, affects the comb, wattles, and other parts of the fowl's head. It commences as small whitish or greyish round patches which vary from the size of a millet seed to half an inch in diameter. In some cases the scales are yellowish or even yellowish-brown in colour.

If the condition spreads down to feathered parts the feathers become dry, brittle, and break off at the surface of the skin, leaving large bare areas. There is always a most disagreeable odour from fowl favus, so much so that it is at times referred to as 'foul favus'.

Treatment of ringworm.—In the first place all affected animals should be isolated, and, if possible, looked after by separate attendants. The buildings occupied by them should be cleaned out, and the walls, mangers, and other fittings and infected objects should be disinfected.

Cats and dogs should, if possible, be excluded from a stable or byre where ringworm exists, for these animals are liable to become themselves infected and act as means of spreading the disease to other animals. Vermin should be exterminated. All young affected stock should be especially well fed so that their general vitality may remain high.

It should be remembered that practically all forms of ringworm of animal origin are liable to be contracted by human beings, and precautions for washing and disinfecting after handling affected animals should not be neglected. Where pets are diseased they should be removed from contact with children and young people who do not understand the danger of infection. It should be borne in mind that people may become infected through contact with dogs and cats, etc., which to the naked eye in ordinary light do not show lesions. (*See* WOOD'S LAMP.)

Oral administration of griseofulvin is the best and simplest method.

Cattle and horses can be given a supplemented feed. This makes possible group treatment, and avoids handling of infected animals; thus reducing the risk of infection being transferred to man.

Otherwise, treatment consists, in the first place, of removing the hair from around the lesions, collecting it and burning it; soaking the scabs in hot soda and water, or caustic potash in water (a 10 per cent solution in either case), removing them with a spoon or piece of wood, and burning them; and, finally, painting the raw surfaces with some reliable dressing of which there are many. A choice may be made from the following: gentian violet solution; undecylenate ointment; isoquinolinium chloride lotion, which has given rapid and good results in the treatment of ringworm in cattle. A dichlorophon spray is a convenient method of treatment, and can be used to assist scab removal instead of the soda solutions; re-spraying being then repeated.

Dressings should be carried out twice a week for a fortnight for cattle and horses, and by then the most of the fungus will be killed, but the cases should not be considered cured until there is a level crop of new hair over each of the areas. For the smaller animals it is better to use the dressings once every second day.

In all instances it is very important to remember that ringworm spreads from the centre outwards, and the edges and margins of the areas should be especially well dressed.

R.N.A. (*see* RIBONUCLEIC ACID).

ROAN (*see* GENETICS).

ROARING AND WHISTLING IN HORSES.—These two terms, which indicate an abnormality in the manner of breathing, are employed to describe a weakness of the larynx in which unusual sounds are produced. They are similar to each other in so far as their production is concerned, but they differ from each other with respect to the pitch of the note, which is higher in whistling than in roaring. In each case the noise is made when the animal takes in breath, and expiration is unaltered. The sound is produced by an interference with the stream of air passing through the larynx on its way to the lungs. As a rule it is caused by vibration of the slackened vocal folds on one or both sides of the larynx, occasioned by complete or partial paralysis of the muscles which move the arytenoid cartilages outwards, but it may also be produced artificially by a too tight throat-lash, or by a bearing-rein which causes too much arching of the neck. A large number of respiratory diseases may give rise to a temporary roaring due to inflammation and thickening of the mucous membranes lining the larynx. GUTTURAL POUCH DIPHTHERIA (which see) may have a permanent effect.

The horse that is affected with either of these conditions is generally able to perform easy work at slow paces without distress, but when made to pull very heavy loads, or when galloped for some distance, in each of which cases respiration is markedly exaggerated, the sounds indicated become more obvious and are more easily detected. During laboured respiration the opening into the larynx is normally made wider to allow a greater volume of air to pass in and out, and in the roarer or whistler this increase does not take place, or only takes place imperfectly. As the air is sucked in through the glottis it comes against the slackened vocal fold and causes it to vibrate and give out a high or low sound, according to the tensity of the muscles which move the arytenoid cartilage to which it is attached. (*See also* LARYNX.)

A horse that whistles may develop into a roarer, but it is most unusual for a roarer to change into a whistler.

The only reliable test for a horse's wind is to make it perform some kind of work which will very considerably disturb its respiration and make it breathe sixty or more times per minute. A period of idleness and heavy feeding previous to the test will very often exaggerate the noise produced and make it more obvious; on the contrary, regular exercise and judicious feeding will frequently cause the sound to become so modified that its detection is difficult.

While most cases follow such conditions as colds, strangles, influenza, pharyngitis or laryngitis, pneumonia, purpura hæmorrhagica, etc., roaring or whistling may also arise spontaneously in a very short time from unknown causes; it may be the result of heredity; or in rare cases it may be produced through the horse having been previously fed upon lathyrus peas. A variety of roaring is also met with during cases of 'grass disease', obstruction of the nasal passages, and in other conditions. If it appears in a horse over six years old it is usually less serious than in one below that age.

Whistling is generally less serious than roaring, since it frequently remains stationary; roaring, on the contrary, usually tends to become worse with the lapse of time. When severe, roaring usually gives rise to a loss of condition, since its presence precludes adequate oxygenation of the blood in the lungs, and even though horses are well fed and managed they often remain thin and starved-looking. The distress from laboured respiration reacts upon hearts and lungs, and the whole body functions are impaired.

Treatment.—Only surgical measures have any beneficial effect of a permanent nature upon roaring or whistling, and there are some cases in which, even after the usual operative treatment, no marked improvement occurs. The operation performed is one in which the vocal fold is encouraged to adhere to the wall of the larynx out of the path of the entering stream of air, by stripping the lining membrane from a little pouch which lies between the vocal cord and the laryngeal wall. In some cases the operation of tracheotomy is carried out instead: in this, a silver tube is inserted into the trachea at a lower level than the larynx, and the air is able to enter and leave through the tube instead of through the larynx. Tracheotomy is of most use in race-horses and hunters affected with roaring.

Both roaring and whistling are unsoundnesses.

ROCHELLE SALT, or TARTRATED SODA, is another name for the tartrate of sodium and potassium, a saline purge, which forms the chief constituent of Seidlitz powder.

ROCK SALT is the name of the salt incrustations that are obtained from salt-mines. Broken into lumps, the rock salt fulfils the need of all types of herbivorous animals. It is placed in the mangers and on pastures, either loose or in containers. It should be provided at all times. (*See also* SALT LICKS.)

ROCKY MOUNTAIN FEVER, which is also called Rocky Mountain Spotted Fever, is a disease of man due to a Rickettsia.

Rocky Mountain fever affects human beings usually between March and July, but the Rickettsia is actually present in many wild animals in which it is non-pathogenic. The onset of fever is sudden, and in 2 to 5 days a rash appears over the whole body, including the palms of the hands. The rash changes to a sort of mottling—petechiæ, scattered over the skin, which gives the condition its name of 'spotted fever'. Mortality may be up to 90 per cent (in Montana) of affected persons. There is an animal reservoir of the Rickettsia responsible, and wild ground rodents and wild goats have been mentioned. The infection is transmitted by ticks, especially *Dermacentor andersoni*—the Rocky Mountain Wood Tick.

RODENT ULCER (*rodo*, I gnaw) is the name given to a form of cancer. (*See* CARCINOMATA AND SARCOMATA.)

RODENTS.—Rats and mice are important from a veterinary point of view on account of the diseases which they may transmit to domestic animals. For examples, *see* AUJESKY'S DISEASE; SALMONELLOSIS; LEPTOSPIROSIS; RINGWORM, FOOT-AND-MOUTH DISEASE. (*See also under* RAT POISONS.)

RŒNTGEN RAYS (*see* X-RAYS).

ROMPUN (*see* XYLAZINE).

'ROPY MILK' (*see* MILK).

ROSE BENGAL PLATE TEST.—A simple and quick screening test used in the diagnosis of brucellosis in cattle. Sera giving positive results may then be tested by means of the Serum Agglutination Test and Complement Fixation Test.

ROTENONE.—The insecticidal principle of Derris root.

ROTHERA'S TEST.—A modified version of this test for ketones in milk or urine requires the following reagent: ammonium sulphate 100 grammes; anhy-

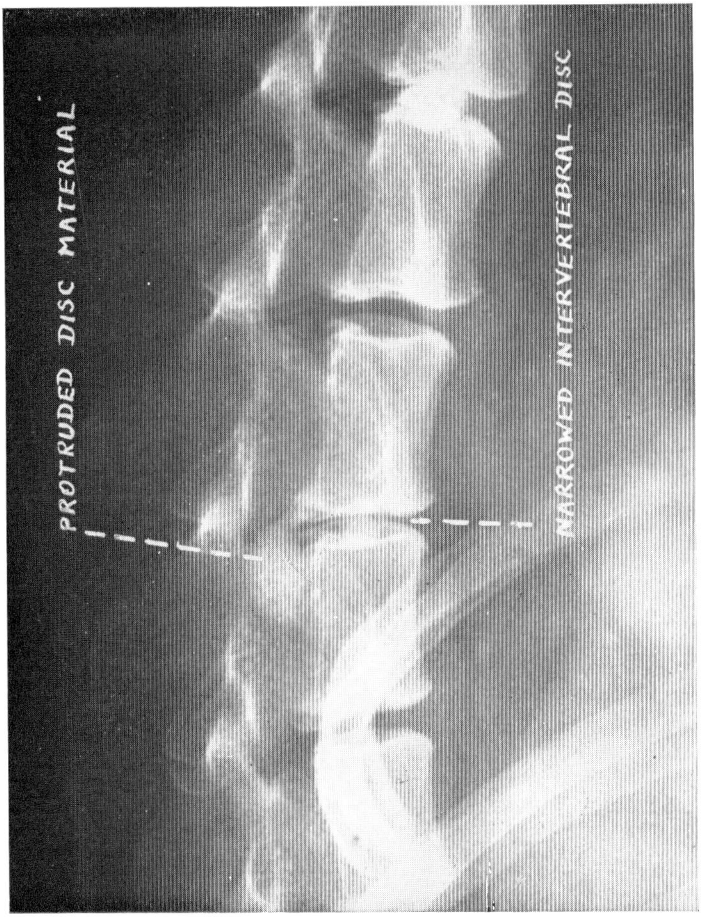

A ruptured intervertebral disc in the dog, shown by X-rays.

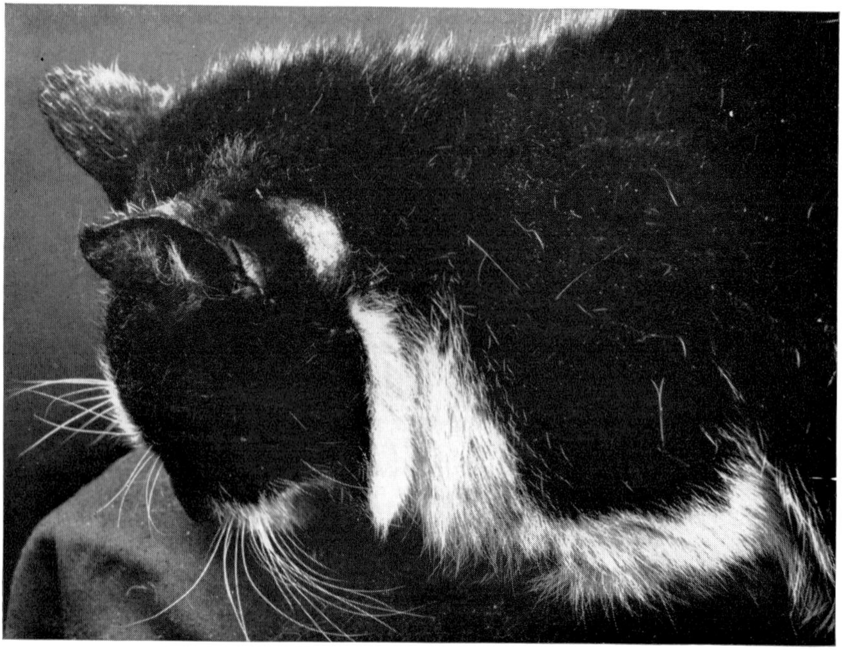

Ringworm in the cat: a whitish, scaly lesion can be seen to the right of the ear, above the white fur.
See RINGWORM.

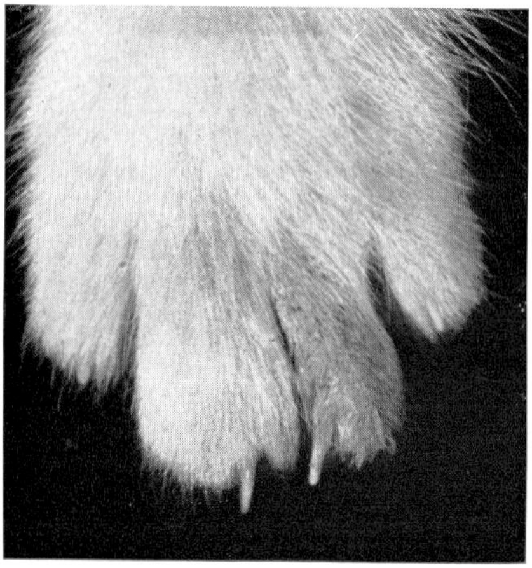

A bare, scaly patch on a kitten's toe due to ringworm—transmissible to Man.

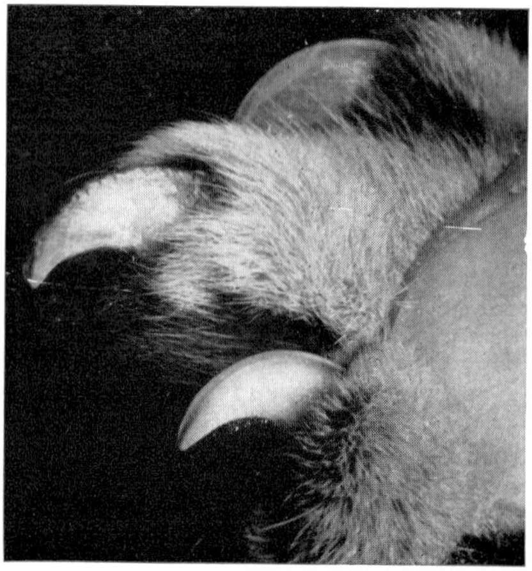

The roughened appearance of an infected claw. *Microsporum canis* Bodin was responsible in each case.

(*With acknowledgments to Dr. C. J. La Touche and the University of Leeds.*)

drous sodium carbonate, 50 grammes; sodium nitroprusside, 3 grammes.

If the bottom half inch of a test-tube is filled with this powder, and a little of the fluid to be tested run down the side of the tube, a red colour will develop after three or four minutes if ketones are present as with acetonæmia.

projection which will act as an anti-slipping device in winter. The calkin of each inner heel is sharpened to a chisel-like point whose direction is the same as that of the line of flight of the foot, *i.e.* longitudinally; and the calkins on the outer heels are laid transversely across the foot. In this way side-slipping is prevented.

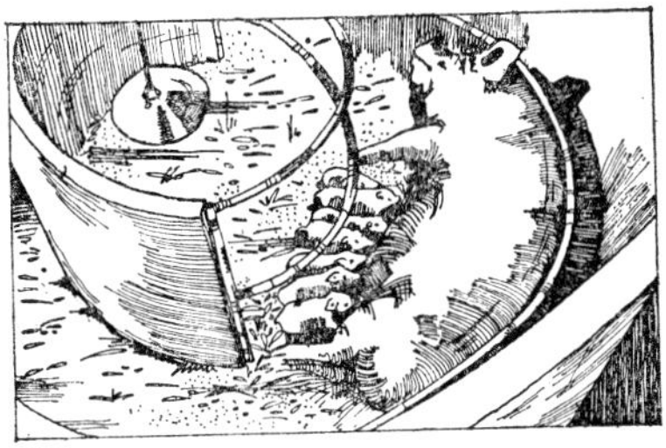

The New Zealand Pen: a drawing showing the position which the sow voluntarily assumes, and, below, a plan for the pen's construction.

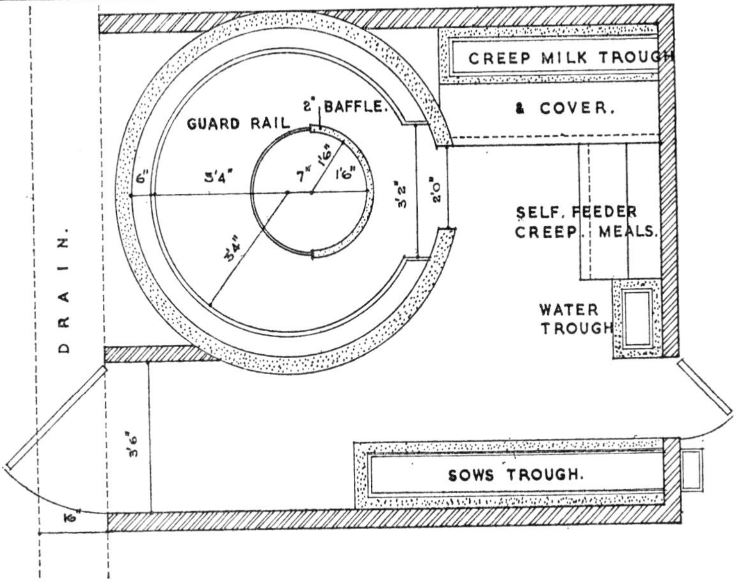

ROUGHAGE.—By this is meant food of a bulky and fibrous nature, such as hay and straw. These have a low water-content, and are in a sense the opposite of succulents, *e.g.* kale, silage. (*See also* 'FIBRE' *under* DIET.)

ROUGHING, strictly speaking, consists of removing the shoes from a horse's feet and turning down a short length of metal at each heel to form a calkin (provided such does not already exist), and sharpening the turned-down calkin to provide a

'Roughing' is also sometimes loosely used to indicate any anti-slipping device, such as the use of frost-studs or cogs, or frost-nails.

ROULEAUX is the term applied to the columns into which red-blood corpuscles collect as seen under the microscope. The appearance somewhat resembles a pile of stacked coins.

ROUND HEART DISEASE causes sudden death of poultry in apparently good condition. The cause is unknown.

A greatly enlarged heart is seen *post mortem*.

ROUNDHOUSE.—A type of circular farrowing pen devised in New Zealand. A variant of the original described in *Agriculture*, consists of a circle of hardboard, about 8 feet in diameter and 4 feet high, bolted to a light iron framework and fitted with an internal creep rail. A smaller circle, about 3 feet in diameter, made partly of hardboard and partly of tubular rails, is fitted eccentrically within the larger one, and the whole is fastened with bolts to the concrete floor of the piggery. The smaller circle which is warmed by an infra-red lamp, acts as a creep for the piglets, while the sow is kept in the space between the two circles. Because of the shape of this space, the sow invariably lies in the same position, with her udder towards the piglets' creep. This gives the piglets the maximum degree of safety. (See illustration above.)

ROUND WORMS.—These can be the cause of anæmia, wasting, gastro-enteritis, bronchitis and pneumonia, aneurism, convulsions, and blockage of the intestine. Some are of public health importance. (*See* TRICHINOSIS, TOXOCARA.) For hosts, life-histories, etc., *see* PARASITES.

ROUP (*see* C.R.D.).

ROUS SARCOMA of chickens. This is produced by a virus. (*See under* CARCINOMA AND SARCOMA.)

-RRHAPHY (ῥαφή, seam) is a suffix meaning an operation in which some opening or tear is closed by stitches.

RUBARTH'S DISEASE (*Hepatitis contagiosa canis*).—This is named after the Swedish scientist Rubarth who, in 1947, described for the first time a disease in dogs which he called, on account of its contagious nature and the damage caused to the liver, *Hepatitis contagiosa canis*. This is now commonly known as CANINE VIRUS HEPATITIS (which see). He regarded this disease, on the basis of the microscopical findings, as identical with Fox Encephalitis which had been known in America for some seventeen years previously.

RUBBER BANDS.—These sometimes get, or are put, on to the legs of cats (and possibly dogs), where they may remain unnoticed until the continual pressure has destroyed the skin beneath the band and caused damage to the underlying structures. Gangrene or loss of use of the limb results.

A successful prosecution has followed the application of rubber bands to cows' teats in the U.K.

Rubber rings have been used for the castration of lambs and calves, and for the docking of lambs. (*See* ELASTRATOR, etc.)

'RUBBER JAW'.—A condition seen in the dog in some cases of chronic nephritis. It may be associated with enlargement of the parathyroid glands. Softening of the bones of the skull, particularly the jaw, occurs, and in a severely affected part the bone can be cut with a scalpel. There is resorption of bone and its replacement by vascular fibrous tissue. 'Rubber jaw' is not, of course, seen in all cases of chronic nephritis, though some changes may be detected microscopically.

RUBBER PADS are made to fit below a horse's shoe to give protection to the foot, to minimise concussion, and to prevent slipping upon smooth surfaces. They are of two varieties: *frog-pads*, in which the pad only covers the frog of the foot; and *bar-pads*, in which the pad reaches across the heels from one bar to the other, and which are worn with a half-shoe only. In each instance the rubber pad is attached to a leather or rubber sole whose outer circumference lies between the lower part of the wall and the foot surface of the shoe, and through which pass the nails which hold the shoe in position.

RUBEFACIENTS (*ruber*, red; *facio*, I make) are a class of blistering agents that are mild in character. (*See* BLISTERS.)

RUMEN, 'PAUNCH', or 1st stomach, is the name applied to the 1st stomach of ruminants. It lies on the left side of the body, occupying the whole of the left side of the abdomen and even stretching across the median plane of the body to the right side. It is a capacious sac which is subdivided into an upper or *dorsal sac*, and a lower or *ventral sac*, each of which has a *blind sac*, at its posterior extremity. These divisions are defined by the presence of grooves on the outside of the organ and by pillars or ridges internally. The whole organ is lined by mucous membrane which possesses a papillated, stratified, squamous epithelium containing no digestive glands, but mucus-secreting glands are present in large numbers. Its entrance is through the œsophagus, and its exit is into the reticulum or 2nd stomach through the *rumeno-reticular orifice*.

Coarse, partially-chewed food is stored and churned in the rumen until such time as the animal finds circumstances convenient for rumination. When this occurs, little balls of food are regurgitated through the œsophagus into the mouth, and are subjected to a second more thorough mastication. Each bolus is chewed from 30 to 60 times and mixed with copious amounts of saliva, to be again swallowed and pass onwards into other parts of the compound stomach.

RUMEN FLUKES.—In North America the species commonly found is *Paramphistomum cervi*. The flukes do little or no damage to the rumen but may cause severe inflammation of the duodenum, causing scouring and unthriftiness ; occasionally death. In the U.S.A. this disease is not regarded as of much economic importance. (*See* PARASITES.)

RUMEN, ULCERATION OF.—In calves ulcers in the rumen may be associated with lesions of the liver caused by *Fusiformis necrophorus*. (*See also* STOMACH, DISEASES OF.)

RUMINAL DIGESTION.—In the rumen, bacteria break down the cellulose (which forms the structural materials of plants, and starch by means of enzymes, and convert them into fatty acids. The bacteria fall a prey to the protozoa which, besides digesting starch, thus perform the useful task of converting plant protein into animal protein. This becomes available to the cow when the protozoa are, in their turn, destroyed further down the digestive tract and themselves digested. (*See also under* FIBRE on p. 257 in the section on DIET, *and under* LACTIC ACID.)

RUMINATION, or 'CUDDING', is the process whereby food taken into the stomachs of ruminants is returned to the mouth, subjected to a second more thorough chewing, and is again swallowed. Rumination is supposed to be a modification found necessary by the ancestors of ruminants, which allowed them to eat herbage with great celerity in fertile feeding-grounds, only chewing it sufficiently to allow of convenient swallowing, thus enabling them to retreat from the fertile areas (which were the hunting-grounds of large and rapacious carnivores) to open plains or barren regions where the food could be subjected to a more thorough and leisurely mastication, and whence the animals could view the approach of marauders from afar and take measures to ensure their individual safety, or, if need be, the safety of the whole herd. Whether this is or is not true, it would appear that some such provision as rumination were necessary when the coarse nature of the food and its indigestibility are remembered. Practically all herbivorous animals possess some special modification in their alimentary systems which allows food eaten to be retained and subjected to a more prolonged and thorough digestion than is the case in other animals, and rumination is a means to this end in the ruminating herbivora.

The act occurs at intervals of from 6 to 8 hours, and occupies a longer or shorter time according to the nature of the food and the amount taken at the last meal. It usually commences about half an hour after feeding ceases, and probably continues until all the coarser constituents have been re-chewed, or at least until the animal is disturbed. This fact is of considerable importance practically ; cattle and sheep should be allowed at least 2 hours' rest after feeding before they are subjected to any severe exertion. Disregard of this is a fruitful contributory cause of stomach disorders in both cattle and sheep.

The act of regurgitation appears to be in reality a complex one, but it may be briefly summarised as follows :

(1) The tension of the œsophagus relaxes, partly by dilatation, and partly through an inspiratory movement of the diaphragm (the glottis being temporarily closed) which reduces pressure in the thorax.

(2) The rumen and the reticulum powerfully contract and squeeze upon their contents.

(3) The abdominal muscles contract and raise the intra-abdominal pressure.

The direct result is that ingested foodstuffs are forced from the area of high pressure (*i.e.* the rumen and reticulum) through the open œsophagus into an area of lower pressure (*i.e.* into the thoracic portion of the œsophagus). When a small quantity, sufficient to form a bolus or 'cud', has entered the œsophagus, the lips of the œsophageal groove and the muscles in the vicinity close the terminal part of the œsophagus, and there commences an antiperistaltic movement which conveys the ' cud ' upwards past the closed glottis, underneath the soft palate, and so into the mouth. Excess fluid is immediately squeezed from the mass and swallowed, and chewing movements commence at once. Each bolus is chewed from 30 to 60 times according to its consistency, size, and to the nature of its constituents; coarse straw or hay fodder requiring the longest time. The chewing occupies from ½ to 1¼ minutes, and then the bolus is rolled up by the dorsum of the tongue and again swallowed. In from 3 to 6 seconds another bolus has reached the mouth, and so the process is continued. The fate of each bolus of food after having been swallowed appears to be the subject of considerable controversy; some authorities hold that it passes onwards into the 3rd stomach; others that it may travel as far as the 4th stomach when of fine consistency; while most believe that the boli are in great part returned to the 1st or 2nd stomach, to be mixed with the remainder of the food and perhaps passed up for a third mastication later on. A great deal depends upon the nature of the food and upon the amount of fluid present in the rumen.

' RUN-BACK '.—This must be avoided by means of back fences. (*See under* STRIP-GRAZING.)

RUNCH (*see* CHARLOCK POISONING).

'RUNNERS'.—This is an old, popular term for hounds unable to gallop properly. ' Runners ' are usually recognised as such when they return to hunt kennels at about 7 months old after being walked; and they are then often culled from the pack. Technically, the condition is known as osteochondrosis of the spine. Symptoms include: poor muscular development in the spinal region, poor bodily condition, an unnatural gait, and often inability to jump a fence successfully negotiated by the rest of the pack. Some curvature and rigidity of the spine may also be observed. It seems that this is, in part at least, an inherited defect of foxhounds.

RUNT PIGS.—Many of these can be reared with the help of antibiotic supplements. (*See* ADDITIVES.)

RUPTURE (*rumpo*, I break) is a popular name for hernia. (*See* HERNIA.) The term is also applied to the tearing across of a muscle, tendon, ligament, artery, nerve, etc. Rupture of the aorta is a cause of death in male turkeys 5–22 weeks old.

RUSSIAN GAD-FLY.—*Rhinœstrus purpureus.* This attacks horses in Europe and N. Africa.

RUSSIAN SPRING-SUMMER VIRUS causes an encephalitis of man and goat, caused by a virus and transmitted by the tick *Ixodes ricinus* in Russia, Poland, and Czechoslovakia.

RYE-GRASS poisoning has caused the death of cattle and horses restricted to grazing rye-grass pasture. (*Lolium perenne.*) In New Zealand and Australia, a fungus present on the rye-grass may cause facial eczema. A staggering gait—and convulsions—may occur in cattle and sheep on rye-grass pasture giving rise to the colloquial name ' Rye-grass staggers '.

RYZAMIN-B.—A proprietary syrup made from rice-polishings, used in vitamin B. therapy.

S

SABULOUS.—Gritty, sandy.

SACKS may be a means of passing infection from one farm to another, for when empty they are put to many uses. Poisoning has occurred through contamination of feeding-stuffs by sacks previously used for sheep-dip. For these reasons, non-returnable paper sacks have advantages over jute sacks.

SACRUM (*sacer*, sacred) is the part of the spinal column lying between the lumbar region and the tail. It consists of 5 vertebræ in the horse and ox, 4 in the sheep and pig, and 3 in the dog and cat, fused together in each case. It is roughly triangular in shape in all animals, and forms the roof of the pelvic cavity, lying midway between the two 'points of the hip' or 'haunch bones'. It gives a firm foundation on the spinal column to which the pelvis and its appendages—the hind limbs—are attached.

SADDLE-GALLS are formed through uneven pressure upon the back by some part of the saddle. They may be found in the middle line, immediately over the upper ends of the spinous processes; they may occur on either side of the middle line where the fore arch of the saddle-tree presses; or they may be found just behind the elbow, when they are caused by badly fastened girths, and are often called 'girth-galls'.

The injuries consist of raw areas from which the hair has been rubbed or chafed off, and later, ulcerous sores form through constant pressure, irritation, and infection of these raw areas. Or, alternately, patches of the skin, varying in size from an inch in diameter to almost three inches, may become hard and leathery, pus being formed underneath. These are known as 'sitfasts', on account of the difficulty of freeing them from the underlying more or less healthy tissue.

Treatment.—Attention must first of all be paid to the saddles. They must be kept clean and free from adherent grease and hair by washing or brushing weekly. They should fit evenly all over the back, and the stuffing or padding should be adequate to protect the skin from pressure by the rigid framework of the saddle-tree. The hollow of the arch of the saddle should never press upon the middle line of the back, and the girth should never be fastened with the skin folded under it. Superficial injuries where only the hair and surface epithelium of the skin are rubbed off may require a day's rest. Ulcers and sitfasts necessitate rest from work for a longer period. Suppurating sores must be cleaned by clipping the hair from their margins, and frequently require cauterising to encourage healing from a new, healthy raw surface. Copper sulphate (bluestone) crystals do well for this purpose. Thereafter, the area is treated as an open wound, antiseptic dressings being applied daily. Iodoform dusting-powder does well as a dressing. Sitfasts must be completely removed before healing can take place. Where they are large it is necessary to inject a local anæsthetic and excise the piece of dead skin, thereafter treating the wound as an infected open wound.

As a preventive of sore backs, horses with naturally thin skins should have their backs swabbed with spirit, or a strong solution of salt and water, immediately after coming in from work, and, if sweating, it is sometimes advisable to leave the saddles on the backs, with the girths unfastened, for a few minutes, to cool off.

SAGITTAL (*sagitta*, arrow) is the term applied to a structure or section running transversely across the trunk or a limb.

ST. JOHN'S WORT.—This plant, *Hypericum perforatum*, which may be present in hay or lucerne, does not lose its poisonous character when dried. It causes LIGHT SENSITISATION (which see) in cattle, sheep, and pigs, especially in Australia.

SAL VOLATILE is another name for aromatic spirit of ammonia, a liquid possessing some stimulating powers for the intestinal canal, heart, and bronchial tubes. It is a common constituent of colic drenches, when it is used to dispel the gas which collects in parts of the alimentary canal, which it effects by stimulating the walls of the hollow organs to a vigorous contraction.

SALICYLIC ACID and the **SALICYLATES** are prepared either synthetically, or, when a pure compound is wanted, from oil of wintergreen or oil of sweet birch. Salicylic acid is an external antiseptic, the ointment, though expensive, sometimes being used for ringworm. Like quinine, salicylates inhibit the movements of protozoön organisms. Internally, the acid is absorbed as the salicylate of soda, and the action of the salicylates is mainly antifebrifuge, lowering temperature, and acting to some extent as internal antiseptics. They are chiefly used in the treatment of rheumatic conditions in both horses and dogs, distemper, strangles, and influenza. *Bismuth salicylate* is useful in diarrhœa in dogs proceeding from irritation or mild catarrh of the small intestines; *aspirin*, which is acetyl-salicylic acid, has almost replaced the other salicylates for the treatment of rheumatism in dogs, and is given in distemper and other specific fevers; *salol*, a compound of salicylic acid and carbolic acid, is an internal antiseptic which has no great irritant properties; and certain powerful drugs, which are mainly used as hypodermic injections, such as physostigmine, are combined as the salicylate.

Salicylate poisoning has occurred in young animals following overdosage.

It has been found in human medicine that repeated administration of salicylates may give rise to anæmia following slight internal hæmorrhages. In the cat, gr. 5 daily may prove fatal within 12 days. (*Vet. Record* Nov. 16, 1963.)

SALINE (*see under* NORMAL SALINE).

SALINE PURGATIVES (*see* PURGATIVES).

SALIVA (*saliva*) is the fluid which, normally, is always present in the mouth, and is secreted from the salivary glands, especially copiously, immediately before and during feeding. Saliva contains much mucus, a considerable amount of serous fluid, ptyalin—a ferment which acts on starches (changing starch into dextrin and maltose), a certain number of corpuscles similar to the white corpuscles of the blood, and in samples taken from the mouth there are always large numbers of the usual bacterial inhabitants of the mouth, which vary according to the particular animal from which the sample is taken. Notwithstanding the specific starch ferment contained in the saliva, which is said to be absent in animals such as the dog and ox, the chief action appears to be one of lubrication, rather than one of digestion of the starch in the food. This is particularly the case in dogs, which bolt their food before time has been allowed for enzyme action to take place, and in cattle swallowing their food for the first time; in them, however, it appears probable that during rumination the ptyalin (if present) acts upon the starch in a more efficient manner, although, even at the best, the action is never so thorough as in man, where the greater majority of the starch in the food is not enclosed in a cellulose envelope as is the raw starch in the food of animals.

The amount of saliva secreted during the 24 hours of a day on which an ox is fed on a dry ration, such as hay and oats, is enormous: according to Colin it may be as much as 12½ gallons. In the horse the same observer gives the daily amount as 9½ gallons. It will thus be seen that the salivary glands, from which the saliva is produced, are very active organs.

An excessive flow of saliva is seen when there is any non-specific painful condition affecting the mucous membrane of the mouth, throat, or pharynx; when the teeth are diseased; in certain digestive disturbances of the stomach; in foot and mouth disease, actinomycosis, and rabies; after chronic poisoning by mercury, iodide of potassium, or arsenic; and after the administration of certain drugs which stimulate the action of the salivary glands, such as arecoline, pilocarpine, etc.

SALIVARY GLANDS are the glands situated near, and opening into, the mouth, by which saliva is manufactured. They include the *parotid gland*, lying in the space below the ear and behind the border of the lower jaw; the *submaxillary gland*, lying just within the angle of the lower jaw. under the lower part of the parotid; and the *sublingual gland*, which lies at the side of the root of the tongue. Each of these glands is paired, so that actually there are six glands, not all of which function at the same time. Each gland is made up of branching tubules closely packed together, and supported by a framework of fibrous tissue. These tubes are lined by cells which secrete the saliva, and from their interior come ducts which, uniting with one another, ultimately form the large ducts which open into the mouth. In the horse the duct from the parotid (' Stenson's duct ') commences at the lower part of the gland, runs forward within the space between the halves of the lower jaw to the anterior edge of the masseter muscle, winds over the edge of the bone, on to the side of the face, and after an upward course of about 2 inches perforates the cheek, and opens into the mouth opposite the 3rd upper cheek tooth. The submaxillary duct (' Wharton's duct ') runs forward along the inner face of the sublingual gland to pierce the floor of the mouth opposite the lower canine tooth. From the sublingual about thirty small ducts emerge on the floor of the mouth below and at the sides of the tongue. In the other animals these ducts follow somewhat different courses.

Roughly speaking, it may be said that the secretion from the parotid is mainly, if not entirely, serous or watery in character, and has the function of mixing with and softening the food during chewing, while in man it contains ptyalin ; from the submaxillary and sublingual the secretion is mucinous or mixed, and has the function chiefly of a lubricant for rendering the food slippery for swallowing.

The salivary glands are not subject to any great variety of diseases, probably because of their protected position and comparatively simple structure. Like all other tissues they are sometimes affected with inflammation, generally arising from wounds or injuries from without, or from the development in the vicinity of a strangles abscess in the horse. This may affect either the parotid or the submaxillary. In dogs and in horses they are liable to be the seat of tumour formation.

In the horse, calculi may form in either the parotid or in the submaxillary duct. At first there is merely a slight deposition of the salivary salts, but as time goes on this becomes larger and larger, until later it may grow so large as to hinder the free flow of saliva into the mouth, and eventually it may cause complete obstruction. Surgical removal is, in such cases, imperative. Occasionally, both in horses and cattle, pieces of chaff, awns of barley, etc., may become wedged in the oral end of the parotid ducts, and if present for any length of time may set up inflammation and cause occlusion of the orifice. Saliva goes on being secreted until the whole duct becomes greatly dilated, and appears as a fluctuating swelling along the border of the jaw. In some such cases an artificial opening into the mouth will relieve the condition ; in others, it is necessary to inject substances which will cause the parotid to cease functioning. The parotid on the opposite side enlarges, and takes on the function of both. (*See also* PAROTID GLAND.)

SALLENDERS (*see* MALLENDERS).

SALMONELLOSIS.—Infection with organisms of the *Salmonella* group—is of importance from two distinct aspects : (1) food poisoning in man, and (2) disease in domestic animals.

In Cattle and Calves.—Salmonellosis and brucellosis have four points in common—both are important from the public health point of view, both can lead to abortion in cattle, to a carrier state likely to perpetuate infection on the farm, and to considerable financial loss to the farmer.

While the salmonella group of bacteria includes over 1,000 different serotypes, the two of most importance to the dairy farmer are *Salmonella dublin* and *Salmonella typhimurium*. Either can produce acute or subacute illness in adult cattle and in calves.

S. typhimurium infection is of greater public health importance, and is a notorious cause of outbreaks of food poisoning in man. In 1944, in the West Riding of Yorkshire, no less than 79 households, involving 162 people, suffered from food poisoning as a result of this organism being excreted by an apparently healthy cow ; and there have been many outbreaks since that time.

An outbreak of this same infection involved over 200 cows on a single farm, and led to the death or slaughter of 29 of them, with a cost (including loss of production) put at £15,000.

S. dublin infection may be associated with abortion, sometimes without any other symptoms being observed, but more often in the course of the illness. Another characteristic of this particular infection is that animals which recover may excrete the organism for years. Besides this carrier state, which may keep infection on the farm, there is also a latent carrier state in which the organism remains dormant within the animal until it is subjected to some stress or superimposed disease, and then excretion of the organism occurs and fellow members of the herd become infected.

Symptoms.—The two infections are usually very similar and can be distinguished only by laboratory means. In the acute form of the disease, the cow becomes dull, feverish, goes off her food, and the milk yield suddenly drops. Scouring is usually severe, and the animal may pass blood and even shreds of mucous membrane from the intestine. Death may occur within a week. If treatment is delayed, mortality may rise to 70 per cent or so; whereas early treatment can bring the death rate down to 10 per cent. In animals which recover, scouring may persist for a fortnight, and it may be several weeks before the cow is fit again.

The sub-acute form in adult cattle runs a milder course and, indeed, the infection may exist without any symptoms being shown. A latent infection may become an overt one following stress of any kind or when another disease becomes superimposed—sometimes masking the symptoms of salmonellosis itself. A liver fluke infestation may be a precipitating factor.

Salmonellosis may run through eight calves out of a batch of 10, and kill four of them. Some calves collapse and die without ever scouring; others become very emaciated as a result of persistent scouring. Pneumonia, arthritis, and jaundice may be among the complications; and occasionally the brain is involved, giving rise to nervous symptoms. The disease is now widespread across the country, and especially prevalent among calves in East Anglia.

S. typhimurium infection seldom persists from one season to another on any particular farm because there are fewer 'carrier' animals than there are with *S. dublin*; it is often brought on to the farm by calves brought in from markets and suffering from the effects of stress, rough travelling conditions, lack of food or a change of diet. The infection occurs in many species of animal including, as the name suggests, mice.

S. dublin infection arises mostly from other cattle. It can be spread from farm to farm via slurry and streams. Mr. L. E. Hughes, M.R.C.V.S., and colleagues in the Ministry's veterinary service have pointed out that infection may enter even a closed herd if it is grazing flooded pasture land.

It was shown in 1969 that *S. dublin* could survive in slurry for at least 12 weeks. In 1971 Mr. C. R. Findlay, of the Veterinary Investigation Centre, Newcastle upon Tyne, described some experimental work which gave a longer survival time. The material used was 'summer slurry' from a 150-cow dairy herd mostly at grass but making some use of a cubicle house, and with dairy and wash-down water included in the effluent. Three bins were filled with nine gallons of this liquid, which was seeded with *S. dublin*. One bin was then covered, one was left uncovered and exposed to rainfall, and the contents of the third were spread on to a grass plot nine square yards in extent.

S. dublin had been recovered regularly from both tanks for five months after inoculation; and while it could not be recovered from the grass two weeks after spreading, the organism was isolated from soil cores five months after spreading.

It is also known that salmonella organisms can survive for six months or so in dung and litter, and *S. dublin* can survive for up to 307 days, if not longer, on dung splashes on a wall, so that thorough cleaning and disinfection of buildings are necessary, and reliance must not be placed on a simple 'resting period' between batches of calves.

Results of a 1957 survey suggested that organic fertilisers may be a source of some of the unexplained outbreaks of salmonellosis. Of 123 samples, bought mainly in retail shops, 50 were positive for salmonella; bone-meal being the most heavily contaminated product.

Another source is animal feeds. The tallow used in some calf feeds is sometimes contaminated; and the same is true of other ingredients of animal origin.

There is not much which the farmer can do about feeds and fertilisers, but preventive measures which can be taken include keeping rats and mice off feed, avoiding pig and poultry effluent for organic irrigation, having piped drinking water for

SALMONELLOSIS IN 1969

	S. dublin	*S. typhimurium*
Wales	997	16
South-West	1,162	118
South-East	309	105
East	179	40
E. Midlands	234	25
W. Midlands	427	33
Yorkshire/Lancs.	328	31
North	444	86
Total	4,080	454
Ratio	9	1

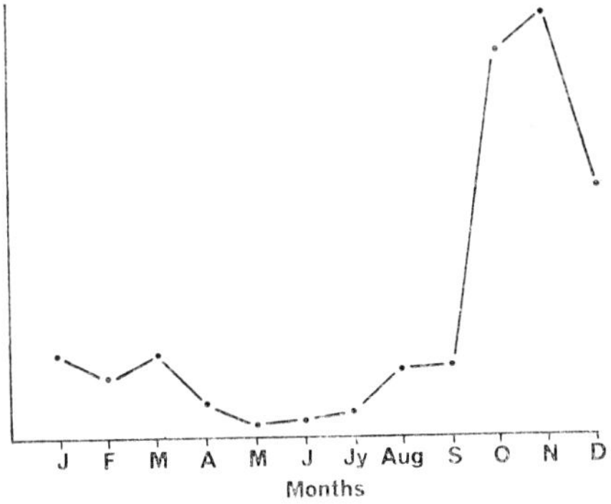

Seasonal incidence of salmonellosis (with acknowledgements to the *British Veterinary Journal*)

cattle, and not buying in through markets or dealers but rather from farms with a known health record. Disinfection has already been mentioned. The earlier housing of cattle in the autumn may help, and it is important not to neglect liver fluke infestation which can sometimes act as a 'trigger' to outbreaks of salmonellosis in which the infection was hitherto latent.

Treatment.—Drugs used include furazolidone, chloramphenicol, and ampicillin.

Prevention.—Apart from wise buying and energetic disinfection, a vaccine is useful, and can be safely used in calves one week old and upwards. Protection lasts for about 6 months. As a routine preventative, antibiotics and antibacterials are, in the view of Mr. Hughes and his colleagues, best avoided.

In pigs.—The term 'salmonellosis' is now usually reserved for a severe septitæmia. *Salmonella choleræ suis* causes this; symptoms including fever, huddling together, purple discoloration of ears, unsteady gait, *sometimes* scouring. The same organism may give rise to a chronic infection with scouring. The organism can infect man.

A live vaccine is available for prevention on farms where this infection is a recurrent problem. It is called 'Suscovax'.

Infection with *Salmonella dublin* sometimes occurs in pigs, and may give rise to dysentery.

More common is infection with *S. typhimurium.* This causes fever, scouring, vomiting, unsteady gait, usually in younger pigs than the first-named organism. Sulphamezathine has proved useful in treatment.

In horses.—*S. typhimurium* has caused serious outbreaks of food-poisoning in young horses.

In dogs.—Illness may be mild, with fever and malaise; or there may be severe gastro-enteritis and death. Many *Salmonella* organisms infect dogs. It is possible for a dog to become a symptomless carrier of *S. typhimurium* and to infect people. (*See Vet. Rec.* for Nov. 22, 1969.)

In cats.—Infection with *Salmonella enteritidis* and *S. typhimurium* may be set up following the catching of infected rats and mice. For this reason cats should not be allowed to lie on uncovered foodstuffs.

In poultry.—Over 50 members of the *Salmonella* group have now been isolated from poultry in this country, and several have caused outbreaks of disease in broiler plants. (*See* PULLORUM DISEASE, FOWL TYPHOID.)

Arthritis, due to a variant strain of *Salmonella pullorum*, gives rise to a mortality of 5 per cent or so, as a rule, but in one outbreak 200 deaths occurred in a 1,000-bird unit. Apart from lameness and swelling of the foot and hock joints, symptoms include poor feathering and under-development. Deaths can be expected between the ages of 10 days and 5 weeks.

It was found that survivors did not react to a blood test carried out with standard *S. pullorum* antigen, but reacted strongly to antigen prepared from the variant strain. This probably accounts for carrier birds having remained undetected in the past.

A survey conducted in 1957 suggests that organic fertilisers may be a source of some of the unexplained salmonellosis outbreaks in Man and farm livestock. Of 123 samples of fertilisers, bought mainly in retail shops, 50 were positive for salmonellæ; bone-meal being the most heavily contaminated.

Salmonellæ will remain alive for periods of up to 6 months or more in dung and litter. Therefore such material should be stacked so that heating occurs; no animals should have access to the heap.

SALMONELLOSIS OF DUCKS.—Several varieties of Salmonella, including *Salmonella ærtrycke*, *Salmonella enteriditis*, and *Salmonella anatum*, have been isolated from outbreaks of disease in ducks. Ducklings are more susceptible than adult birds, and mortality in them may be very high.

This condition is of great importance since the causative organisms belong to the 'Food poisoning' group. Fatal cases of food poisoning in man have been traced to the ingestion of duck eggs. (The organism may be recovered from the eggs laid by affected ducks.)

Should untoward losses occur amongst ducks, several bodies should be sent to a laboratory for post-mortem and bacteriological examination. In the event of a positive diagnosis, a sample of blood should be collected from each bird and subjected to the agglutination test, all birds reacting being destroyed and disinfection of the premises carried out.

SALOL (*see* SALICYLIC ACID).

SALPINGITIS (σάλπιγξ, trumpet) is inflammation in the Fallopian tubes or oviducts, sometimes the cause of sterility in cattle. (*See* STERILITY.)

SALPINGO- (σάλπιγξ, a tube) is a prefix indicating a connection with either the Fallopian or Eustachian tube.

SALT is the general name applied to chemical substances in which a metal is substituted for the hydrogen of an acid. 'Common salt' is sodium chloride; 'Epsom salts' is a popular name for magnesium sulphate; 'Glauber's salts' is the name given to sodium sulphate; 'salts of lemon' is applied both to potassium binoxalate and to oxalic acid, each of which is a poison; 'salts of sorrel' is another name for oxalic acid; 'rock salt' is native sodium chloride as obtained from salt-mines.

Sodium chloride, or common salt, is necessary for all animals for blood formation and digestion. It is also a useful appetiser, and is commonly incorporated in animal feeding-stuffs in carefully measured proportions.

A 10-cwt. cow needs $\frac{3}{4}$ oz. salt a day for maintenance and a further $\frac{1}{8}$ oz. for every gallon of milk produced. Therefore, a 700-gallon cow requires about 30 lb. of salt yearly.

SALT LICKS.—Salt is necessary for animals and on some pastures or under some systems of management they may not obtain sufficient. To obviate this danger, salt licks are commonly provided. In some salt licks traces of iodine are incorporated and sometimes also other 'trace elements' such as copper, manganese, cobalt, magnsieum. (*See also* ROCK SALT.)

SALT POISONING has been reported in both pigs and poultry. It is essential that pigs are not kept short of water, or given too salt food.

An outbreak, reported from Scotland, involved piglets aged six weeks brought indoors from field arks at weaning. A proprietary meal was fed dry. The water bowls in the house were not very accessible, and some of the piglets were not strong enough to depress the levers. Two days after being housed, 23 out of the 32 piglets were showing symptoms of salt poisoning, and some died.

Symptoms.—Often a number of pigs are found dead without symptoms having been observed, the remainder being weak and very thirsty. Vomiting and diarrhœa may occur. (For other symptoms, *see under* MENINGOENCEPHALITIS.)

In poultry, adult birds show excessive thirst and diarrhœa, with sometimes cyanosis of the wattles, somnolence, and sudden death. In young birds gasping and ascites may occur. (*See* BRINE *also.*)

SAND COLIC is a form of colic due to the collection in the cæcum and colon of quantities of sand. It may be caused through feeding horses with food contaminated with sand; horses grazing on the seashore or along tidal mud flats learn that the sand contains salt, and may lick up large quantities of it in their endeavour to get the salt. The symptoms set up are chiefly those of colic with impaction. (*See* COLIC.)

Cattle feeding on the seashore take in with their food quantities of sand, which in some cases may be so great as to hinder the movements of the rumen (where the sand always collects), and, by upsetting digestion, may cause unthriftiness and even emaciation. As much as a barrowful of sand has sometimes been removed from such animals, by operation through the flank.

SANDCRACK is a pathological condition affecting horses' feet, in which a deep fissure or crack forms at some part of the wall of the hoof, extending downwards from the coronet, and usually involving the whole of the thickness of the wall. It may extend from the coronet down to the shoe, or it may not be so extensive as this. In the hind feet sandcrack is commonest at the toe, and in the fore feet on the inside quarter, but it may appear at any part of the wall both before and behind.

Causes.—Anything which interferes with the proper nutrition of the horn at the coronet predisposes to sandcrack, the actual splitting of the horn occurring as the result of the strains put upon the foot. Treads on the inside of the coronet, occasioned by hurried turning when at work, are frequent causes in the fore feet, and continual pressure on the coronary matrix by the second phalanx, especially when the toes have been allowed to grow too long, appears to be the commonest cause in the hind feet. In addition, undue or repeated rasping of the wall by the blacksmith, which renders the horn brittle, a naturally dry condition of the feet, repeated wetting and drying of the horn, and leaving the toes or heels too long when shoeing, are other causes. A predisposition to sandcrack may be inherited.

Symptoms.—The presence of the crack is the most important symptom. It may be simple, in which case there is no discharge and the edges appear dry; or it may be complicated by inflammation and suppuration when pus is produced between the edges of the horn. In severe cases there may be considerable swelling at the coronet immediately above the sandcrack. Lameness may or may not be present. It may be due to the inflammation, or it may be caused by the pinching of the sensitive structures between the two edges of the crack. Lameness in a toe-sandcrack is characterised by a sudden jerk when the horse lifts the foot (not unlike stringhalt), a period of suspension, and then a careful placing of the foot on the ground, well forward and generally heels first. Where necrosis of the surface of the bone has set in, the horse may be unable to put the foot to the ground, but such cases are usually only the result of gross neglect.

Treatment. — Simple sandcracks, in which the whole thickness of the wall is not split, and where there is no pus formation, are usually easily dealt with by cutting a transverse groove deeply through the wall immediately above the crack at the coronet, and at the same time taking measures that will ensure the immobility of the crack. To effect the latter, there are several methods. A nail may be driven transversely through the crack and clenched at both ends, in exactly the same way as an ordinary horseshoe nail is clenched. A clip, made like a staple with very short prongs, may be fastened across the crack, in one or two places. A shoe with bar clips which fit inside the bars on either side (*i.e.* into the lateral clefts of the frog) may be applied; this is a means of preventing the normal expansion and contraction of the heels during progression, which is responsible for the movements of the edges of the crack. (*See* HOOF REPAIR.)

With complicated cracks, where inflammation is acute and lameness is present, it is necessary to reduce the inflammatory process by the use of hot antiseptic footbaths for a day or two previously. With all such cases it is advisable to place the animal under veterinary attention.

SANGUINEOUS (*sanguineus*) means containing blood.

SANITATION and DRAINAGE.—Advice can be obtained from books on farm buildings, or from Local Authorities, or the Ministry of Agriculture, as appropriate. (*See* SEWAGE, SLURRY.)

SANTA GERTRUDI.—This breed of cattle are ⅝ Shorthorn and ⅜ Brahman in origin.

SANTONIN is a yellow or white crystalline powder obtained from 'santonica', also known as 'worm seed', the dried flowers of *Artemisia maritima*, which is brought from the Levant. It was used as an expellant for round worms in all animals, but has little or no action on tape worms.

As in the case of most other remedies for worms it must be preceded by at least 24 hours' fast, for the presence of food in the bowels prevents the action of the santonin from being fully exerted upon the worms present. (*See* PARASITES.)

SAPO is the Latin name for soap.

SAPROPHYTE (σαπρός, putrid; φυτόν, plant) is the term applied to organisms which live usually upon decaying and dead animal or vegetable matter often in soil, and produce its decomposition.

SARCO- (σάρξ, flesh) is a prefix signifying flesh or fleshy.

SARCOCYSTS (*see* PARASITES, p. 643).

'SARCOID'.—A tumour which resembles histologically a sarcoma, but which is regressive in character, disappearing within a matter of months. It has the appearance of a reddish button, raised about an ⅛th of an inch above the surrounding skin. It affects the dog

SARCOMA (σάρκωμα, a fleshy growth). (*See* CARCINOMA *and* SARCOMA, *also* TUMOURS.)

SARCOPTES are members of a class of parasitic acari, which cause mange in animals and man. (*See* PARASITES, p. 688.)

SAUSAGE.—Discarded portions of sausage, or sausage-skin, can be a source of infection when fed, unboiled, to pigs, etc. Foot-and-mouth disease has been transmitted in this way. African Swine Fever and Swine Fever could similarly be spread by this means. (*See* SWILL.)

SAVAGING OF LITTERS by sows.—Various causes of this have been suggested, including: an inherited tendency; absence of any straw for nesting purposes; a painful udder; insufficient time to have become used to her farrowing quarters; and fright resulting from the use of a farrowing crate. (*See* PIGS, SEDATION OF.)

SAWDUST (*see under* BEDDING).

SCAB is the name given to the crust which forms on superficial injured areas. It is composed of fibrin which is exuded from the raw surface, together with blood corpuscles and epithelial cells entangled in its meshes. Healing takes place naturally under this protection, and the scab dries up and falls off when healing is complete. (For 'SHEEP SCAB', *see* p. 690).

SCABIES is the name given to the results of infection of the body with sarcoptic mange mites. (*See* PARASITES, p. 688.)

'SCAD.'—A colloquial name for a transitory lameness, in sheep, which may follow frost. (*See* 'SCALD.')

'SCALD'.—Inflammation between the digits of young sheep, causing acute lameness. Its onset is said to be associated with frosts and moisture. Recovery may occur spontaneously under dry conditions. The term is vague, however, and has been used to include the non-progressive form of foot-rot. It has to be differentiated from foot-and-mouth disease. (*See also* 'SCAD' *and* OVINE INTERDIGITAL DERMATITIS.)

SCALDS (*see* BURNS).

SCALY LEG is a condition of the legs of fowls in which large, hard, irregular scales are formed on the featherless parts, as the result of the action there of mange mites called *Sarcoptes mutans*, var. *gallinæ*. This parasite attacks hens, turkeys, and cage birds, but is very rare in aquatic birds. The foot is generally first affected, and then the condition spreads upwards, until, in a severe case, the whole of the unfeathered part of the leg is covered with irregular horny scales, and may be more than twice its normal thickness. There is considerable itchiness, more marked at night than during the day, and the bird persistently pecks at the scales, irritating them and making the condition worse.

(*See also* PARASITES, p. 691.)

SCAPHOID.—A small bone present in the carpus and tarsus. In the racing greyhound, fracture of the right hind scaphoid is a common accident. Treatment has included the removal of bone fragments and the successful insertion of a plastic 'scaphoid'.

SCAPULA, or SHOULDER BLADE, is the large, triangular, flat bone that lies on the outside of the front of the chest, to which are attached many of the muscles that unite the fore limb to the trunk. It is not directly connected with the side of the chest by any bony attachment, but is able to slide backwards and forwards over the surface of the ribs. On its outer surface it is crossed by a definite ridge running longitudinally at a small angle with the vertical when the animal is standing at rest in the normal position. This ridge can easily be felt in all but very fat individuals. At its lower end the scapula possesses a cup-shaped depression into which the head of the humerus fits to form the shoulder joint. At the opposite (*i.e.* the uppermost) side of the triangle the bone has a crescentic cartilage attached. On the inner aspect of this cartilage, and to the surface of the bone next the chest, is the attachment of the inverted fan-shaped ventral serratus muscle, whose other attachments are to the last four or five cervical vertebræ and to the first eight or nine ribs. This muscle, and its fellow of the opposite side, form the sling-like support by which the body is suspended between the two fore-limbs. Great freedom of movement and a well-sloped scapula form two of the necessities of speed, and are considered good points in race-horses and hunters. (*See also* BONES.)

SCAR.—The remains of a healed wound, ulcer, or breach of tissue. A scar consists essentially of fibrous tissue, covered by an imperfect layer of skin when on the surface of the body. The fibrous tissue is formed from connective tissue cells at the edges of the lesion, as well as from connective tissue corpuscles that wander into the granulating wound during its repair. It is at first soft, well supplied with minute blood-vessels, and easily bleeds when damaged, but later, it becomes hard and dense, loses its blood-vessels, and generally contracts, causing a puckering of the surrounding surface. The specialised structures, such as hairs, sweat, or other glands, etc., do not grow again, and consequently these are absent from a scar. This fact is one that is important from the point of view of the purchase of animals. For example, when a horse has fallen and 'broken his knees' and these have healed, and the horse is subsequently exposed for sale, intending purchasers should be very certain of the circumstances which occasioned his fall. The scar remains as an indelible mark; proof that he has at one time fallen, and logically, having fallen once, he may do so again; indeed, he may be so given to falling as to be unsafe to drive, and should be avoided accordingly. Needless to say, various devices are resorted to by the unscrupulous dealer so that the scar may be hidden or obliterated, such as the smearing of tar, burnt cork, or lamp-black over the area, etc., but these are so obvious to the watchful that only seldom do they mislead. The unchangeableness of the scar is made use of in the branding of both cattle and horses, and special marks of ownership are common. Horses that have been possessed by the government of a country for military or other purposes are generally marked on the shoulder or the hip, as witness the mark of the 'Broad arrow' on those used by the British Army.

Scars may be situated in such a position that they interfere with the functions of organs, and are liable to cause trouble when they contract. For example, the scar tissue that remains after injury to the uterus during difficult parturition may contract so much that subsequent service by the male is impossible until the scar has been surgically treated, or the scar that remains after injuries to the teats of milking cows may contract during the dry period so that when lactation recommences the milk will not flow until the obstruction has been removed. (*See* BONES, FRACTURES, NERVES, REPAIR OF, etc.)

SCARLET PIMPERNEL (*see* PIMPERNEL POISONING).

SCHEDULED DISEASES (*see under* NOTIFIABLE DISEASES).

SCHISTOSOMIASIS.—Infestation with flukes which live in the blood-vessels of ruminants, pigs, dogs, cats, and man, who can become a host through skin contact with water contaminated by the intermediate host snails. It occurs in Brazil, Caribbean islands, Surinam, and Venezuela. (*See* p. 648.)

SCHIZO- (σχίζω, I divide) is a prefix signifying splitting.

SCHMORL'S DISEASE (*see* NECROSIS, BACILLARY).

SCHRADAN.—An organo-phosphorus insecticide used in agriculture and a potential danger to farm livestock. (*See also* PARATHION.) Symptoms of poisoning may include vomiting, lachrymation, salivation, straining, twitching, distressed breathing, and coma.

SCIATICA (ἰσχίον, the hip) means pain connected with the sciatic nerve which runs down the thigh.

SCIRRHOUS CORD is a condition in which there is a chronic fibrous enlargement of the cut end of the spermatic cord in castrated horses. In most cases the castration wound does not completely heal, but a small sinus discharging a thick white pus persists. The discharge may cease later, but the swelling of the cord goes on increasing slowly in size, until eventually it may be nearly as large as a man's head. Before the swelling has increased far, however, *e.g.* when about the size of an apple, it is usual to find that one or more new sinuses have appeared, and the discharge from each of these is seen on the horse's hind feet and about the stall. In extreme cases the swelling extends upwards through the inguinal canal and into the abdomen, and a mass weighing as much as 100 lb. may sometimes be encountered on *post-mortem* examination. The treatment is entirely surgical.

SCIRRHUS (σκῖρος, a hard tumour) is a term applied to a growth or to other hard fibrous conditions of various organs.

SCLERA, or **SCLEROTIC COAT** (σκληρός, hard) is the outermost hard fibrous coat of the eye. (*See* EYE.)

SCLERITIS means inflammation of the sclerotic coat of the eye.

SCLERODERMA (σκληρός, hard; δέρμα, the skin) is a condition of the skin occurring in certain trypanosomiases (diseases due to tiny parasites called 'trypanosomes') in which large areas of the skin become hard and insensible. The areas are called 'plaques', and are commonest in dourine. (*See* PARASITES.)

SCLEROSIS (σκληρός, hard) means literally 'hardening', and is a term applied to conditions in which portions of organs become hard and useless as the result of inflammations which produce excessive amounts of fibrous tissue. The term is particularly used in connection with the nervous system. When it occurs in other organs or parts the term 'cirrhosis' or 'fibrosis' is used, but they each refer to the same pathological condition. (*See* CIRRHOSIS.)

SCLEROTIC COAT (*see* EYE).

'SCOTTIE CRAMP'.—A condition apparently confined to the Scottish Terrier, and occurring usually for the first time at 4 to 8 months of age. There is cramp following exercise. In mild cases the animal may be seen to be in difficulties when negotiating steps; in severe cases a hundred yards' brisk trot will cause the animal to double up and collapse, and in a few instances excitement without exertion will give rise to cramp. Mild attacks often become worse, reaching a maximum severity at 12 or 15 months of age. At 2 or 2½ years of age the dog may have outgrown 'Scottie Cramp'. The cause is unknown. Intravenous injections of calcium borogluconate, or parathyroid extract administration, have been recommended. The condition could be eliminated by breeders.

SCOURS, SCOURING.—Diarrhœa. Scouring is not, of course, a disease in itself, but merely a symptom which may indicate nothing more than the results of a chill or an 'error of diet'. In adult cattle the best first-aid measure is to feed only hay. If scouring persists beyond 48 hours in spite of this treatment, veterinary advice should be obtained so that a diagnosis may be made.

Calves may be affected with 'WHITE SCOURS' (which see) or *Salmonella dublin*, which gives rise to a blood-stained diarrhœa and often death.

Adult cattle may scour as the result of certain specific diseases, including JOHNE'S

Disease, Coccidiosis, Tuberculosis, Salmonellosis (*see under* these respective headings), parasitic gastro-enteritis (*see under* Parasites), and 'Black Scours'. Scouring leads to Dehydration (which see). (*See also* Soil-Contaminated Herbage with reference to sheep.)

'Black Scours' (*Winter Dysentery*) occurs in housed cattle during the winter and early spring. The infection may spread along a road to several farms.

Cause.—*Vibrio jejuni.*

Symptoms.—Watery, black diarrhœa affecting half or even the whole herd. Severe cases with the passage of blood are sometimes met with. The disease is responsible for a loss of condition and loss of milk, and it may kill calves. The period of incubation is 3 days to a week, and the scouring usually lasts for 3 days.

SCOURING IN PIGS.—The causes of this are numerous and include:

iron deficiency; high fat content of sow's milk at about third week; stress, caused by, *e.g.*, long journeys; cold, damp surroundings; change of diet; vitamin deficiencies; poisons; viruses, *e.g.*, TGE, swine fever; bacteria, *e.g.*, *E. coli* (some strains), *Vibrio coli*, *Salmonella choleræ suis*, *Salmonella dublin*, *Clostridium welchii*, *Erysipelothrix rhusiopathiæ* (the cause of erysipelas); protozoa, *e.g.*, *Balantidium coli*, *coccidia*; fungi; yeasts; worms.

E. coli is regarded as being associated with a high proportion of outbreaks of scouring, but as it can be obtained from the gut of virtually any healthy pig, its precise importance and role are still somewhat controversial. *E. coli* vaccines have been administered to sows before farrowing on farms where scouring is a problem.

Scouring piglets need plenty of drinking water, for there is always a danger of Dehydration. (*See also* Antibiotic Supplements, Sow's Milk.)

SCRAPIE is a disease of sheep mainly confined to the districts of the English and Scottish Borders, to Spain, France, and Germany. Sheep imported into Australia, New Zealand, Canada, and the U.S.A. have brought the disease with them. It has been well known by Border farmers for generations, but until comparatively lately had not received much attention from research workers; and even at the present time the nature of the disease is a matter of controversy.

All breeds of sheep appear to be susceptible, but it is difficult to be dogmatic about which are mostly affected, since much secrecy surrounds the incidence of the disease.

Rams, ewes, wethers, and very occasionally lambs are affected; the majority of cases occurring in sheep stock between the ages of 2 and 3 years. Accordingly, the young ewe stock on a farm furnishes most of the cases.

Two beliefs have been held with regard to its transmission: that copulation is responsible for its spread, or that prenatal infection must be held blameworthy. If the former view is correct, the incubation period is about three months, since ewes generally show the first symptoms about two months before lambing; and if the second view is accepted, the period of incubation must extend to 1½ years to 2 years. It has also been held that transmission may occur through contaminated pastures and possibly through the eating of each other's afterbirths by ewes at lambing time.

Experimentally, scrapie has been transmitted to goats, mice, rats, and hamsters.

Cause.—This is still undetermined. The disease is always more important in purebred flocks, and its incidence said to increase with in-breeding—factors suggesting that heredity plays a part. Indeed, it has been described as an inherited defect, related to a widespread disease of muscle. Previously, and since, there has been support on scientific grounds for the theory that an infective agent is responsible. Transmission experiments have been successfully repeated by independent research workers, and seemed to indicate a virus as the cause—except that the material used is still effective after heating to 100° C. and no known virus can survive such treatment. An explanation for this has been suggested, however—the virus being not in a pure state but within tissue fragments, of a resistant nature, which protect it.

A view put forward in 1968 was that 'the scrapie agent is present in an inhibited form in normal mice, and in a released form in scrapie-affected mice, and that an unmasking process would provide an alternative explanation to the self-replication that has been so difficult to explain because the scrapie agent does not apparently contain nucleic acid.' (Nature, **218**, 102).

A possibility is that the infective agent

is a protein which stimulates infected cells to produce more of itself.

Symptoms.—The late Sir Stewart Stockman stated: 'The symptoms of the disease can best be described in relation to the stages of the disease. The *first stage* usually lasts about three weeks, more or less. At this time the symptoms are intermittent, and the sheep must be shepherded in order to observe them. The affected animal frequently changes its position, separating itself from the others. It eats as usual, but will sometimes drink large amounts of water, if available. It often ruminates in the upright position, holding the head high. The pupil of the eye is dilated, and the look fixed. When moved, the scrapie sheep often turn this way and that, in an excited, stupid fashion; then they trot away in front, lifting the fore feet high. When put in a loose-box, jerky movements of the ears, eyelids, muscles of the lips, shoulders, and thighs are noticeable. The *above stage* is characterised by twitchings and excitability. Later, there is occasional straining, and passage of small quantities of fæces and urine, and the twitchings become more marked. If chased, the animal may suddenly fall down, lie for a few minutes, and then get up again and move away. This might be called the *second stage*, and lasts to about the sixth week of noticeable illness. Then itching begins along the back to the root of the tail, becomes more intense, and extends to the sides, shoulders, and limbs (*third stage*). Towards the end, sheep appear almost demented by the itching. The thirst is intense. The animals emaciate rapidly, get weak in the hind quarters, and become paralysed. Affected sheep may live for a fortnight or longer if fed. From start to finish the disease appears to last from three to four months.'

In a typical case in Great Britain, the most striking and easily seen symptom of scrapie is the torn, ruffled, and untidy appearance of the fleece, and when very severe, the bruised or scratched condition of the skin. In many cases, especially those occurring during the late spring, the fleece may be almost entirely rubbed off against fences, posts, trees, or may be greatly removed by the mouth. In addition, the condition of the sheep is noteworthy; whereas the remainder of the flock may be in fair bodily condition, the scrapie sheep are thin, gaunt, and apt to become weak on their legs, lagging behind when going uphill, and losing their foothold when descending.

Occasionally, when startled, as for instance, when being moved by dogs, or when a gun is fired near the unwary scrapie sheep, convulsive seizures are seen, usually lasting from 3 to 5 minutes, and leaving the animal temporarily dazed.

Prevention.—In the present state of our knowledge it would appear that the best advice that can be given is to breed *as much as possible from a clean stock*, and where conditions will allow, *to use rams for the main flock only when in their third year*. Logically, only ewes older than three years should be used for breeding, but to carry out this in most of the hill flocks would be to deplete the numbers of lambs to too great an extent.

SCREW-WORM FLIES.—These belong to the sub-family *Calliphorinæ*, which includes the greenbottles, bluebottles, and the flies which cause 'Strike' or Blowfly Myiasis in British sheep. The American screw-worm fly deposits its eggs only in fresh wounds, but another species lays its eggs only in wounds already invaded by larvæ of other flies. The tumbu fly of tropical Africa, *Cordylobia anthropophaga*, is noteworthy for larvæ which penetrate the skin. 'Congo floor maggots'—the larvæ of another African screw-worm fly—themselves suck blood (a rare if not unique example of insect larvæ sucking blood) and infest various animals besides man. (*See also* p. 674. *and* 'STRIKE'.)

SCROTAL.—Relating to the scrotum.

SCROTUM is the pouch of skin in which the testicles are lodged. It consists of a purse-like fold of skin that is generally hairless, within which each organ has an investment of muscle-fibres, several layers of fibrous tissue, and a serous membrane called the 'tunica vaginalis'.

SCUR.—A loose, horny growth, not attached to the skull, at the site normally occupied by a horn in a horned breed of cattle.

A bull calf with a scur, or with a bony protuberance beneath the skin at the horn site, is not a pure polled animal. Without these, a bull can be expected to breed true as regards the polled character; this can be checked by a progeny test of the bull mated to horned cows—the result should be polled heifer calves or bull calves with scurs or bony protuberances, but no calves with horns.

'SCURVY RICKETS' has been recorded in the dog. It did not respond to treatment with vitamins A and D and vitamin C (ascorbic acid) had little effect; but fresh orange juice had a remarkable effect.

SEASON (*see* ŒSTRUS).

SEAT-WORM is another name for the thread-worm or oxyuris. (*See* PARASITES, p. 658.)

SEAWEED.—A source of agar and a food grazed by sheep on the seashore and sometimes given to horses and cattle. A source of iodine and other trace elements and (in the case of brown seaweeds) of vitamins A, B_1, B_2, C, and D. Animals do not take readily to seaweed as a rule, nor are they able to digest it well at first, but after a few days it usually proves an acceptable supplement to the ration.

SEBACEOUS GLANDS (*sebum*, grease) are the minute glands that are found alongside each of the hairs, whose mouths open into the hair follicles a little below the point at which the hair emerges from the skin. These glands secrete an oily substance which serves to keep the hair from becoming too brittle, and gives it its glossy appearance. They are liable to become invaded during several of the parasitic diseases, especially the manges and follicular mange in particular, and in such cases the hair becomes harsh and dry and is easily broken or shed altogether.

SEBORRHŒA (*sebum*, grease; ῥέω, I flow) is the name given to a group of diseases of the skin in which the sebaceous or oil-forming glands are at fault. It is shown either by accumulations of dry scurf, or by the formation of an excessive oily deposit on an otherwise healthy skin.

SECRETIN is the name given to a hormone secreted by the mucous membrane near the commencement of the small intestine when food comes in contact with it, which, on being carried by the blood to the pancreas, stimulates the secretion of pancreatic juice.

SECRETION (*secerno*, I set apart) is the name given to the material that is formed by a gland as the result of its activity. For example, saliva is the secretion of the salivary glands, gastric juice that of the glands in the walls of the stomach, pancreatic juice that of the pancreas, bile that of the liver, etc. Some so-called 'secretions' are really 'excretions'; that is, they are composed of substances for which the body has no further use, for instance, the urine and the sweat. For further details see under the various headings of the organs, also URINE; DUCTLESS GLANDS; SALIVA; *and* SWEAT.

SEDATIVES (*sedo*, I calm) are drugs or other measures which soothe over-excitement of the nervous system, whether the effects of pain, delirium, muscular spasm, or fear, etc. Those that soothe pain are called 'anodynes', sedatives for delirium or fear are known as 'hypnotics', and sedatives, for spasm are called 'antispasmodics'. (*See also* TRANQUILLISERS.)

SEED CORN, dressed with a mercury dressing, has been fed to pigs with fatal results.

Dieldrin seed dressings lead to poisoning in wild birds and, indirectly, have killed dogs, cats, and foxes which have eaten poisoned birds. (*See also under* GAME BIRDS.)

SEEDY TOE.—A condition affecting the hoof of the horse, in which there is a separation of the wall from the laminar matrix below, and the formation in the space so produced of a dry, crumbly, friable variety of horn, which bears some resemblance to pumice-stone. It may occur at any part of the wall of the foot, but is commonest at the toe; it may extend from the ground surface upwards, for only a short distance, or right to the coronet. It may be narrow or wide, and only one or several parts may be affected at the same time.

Cause.—Pressure of some kind is usually considered to be responsible for producing seedy toe, a very common cause being a tightly hammered-back toe-clip, or a tightly driven nail. In some instances, however, the cause is obscure.

Symptoms.—In most cases the condition exists for some time before it is recognised, and is generally first noticed by the blacksmith when paring down the wall prior to fitting a new shoe. Lameness is only seen when the extent of the separation is large, or when foreign matter becomes forced up into the space, and causes pressure upon the sensitive matrix.

When struck with a hammer the affected

part of the foot gives out a hollow resonating note, and the margins of the separated area can usually be fairly well determined by this means. In many cases an ordinary horseshoe nail can be passed up into the diseased horn under the outer crust of the wall with little or no resistance, and may serve to indicate the extent of the affection.

Treatment.—Where only a small area is affected which does not extend far up the wall, the diseased horn may often be pared away from the lower surface by means of a narrow-bladed searcher, without interfering with the integrity of the outside of the wall, but in more extensive cases it becomes necessary to lay open the whole of the affected part by removing the outer crust of apparently healthy wall. All the soft friable horn should be cleared away and the cavity disinfected. The shoe should be provided with a bar across the heels, and immediately below the affected part the pressure should be relieved by paring away the lower edge of the wall. In many cases where the toe is affected benefit will accrue from removing completely a portion of the web of the shoe immediately below the seedy toe. (*See* Hoof Repair.)

SEITZ FILTER.—An asbestos composition disc used in bacteriological work.

SELENIUM.—Sodium selenate is used by horticulturists as an insecticide, and accordingly there is a possibility of toxic effects occurring in animals. Sterility results, and also loss of hair. These symptoms are also observed in parts of the U.S.A. and Eire where the soil contains an excess of selenium. In the acute form of poisoning, animals may be found wandering aimlessly or in circles. Paralysis precedes death.

Selenium is a trace element. It has a curative effect in Muscular Dystrophy and has been used in the treatment of skin disease. (*See also* Vitamin E, Lathyrism *and* Trace Elements.)

Retention of the afterbirth in a dairy herd in the north of England was associated with a selenium deficiency.

SELLA TURCICA is the name applied to the deep hollow on the upper surface of the sphenoid bone in which the pituitary gland rests.

SEMEN.—The fluid produced by the male reproductive and accessory organs. (*See under* Artificial Insemination.)

SEMINAL VESICLES. — (*See under* Testicle, Actino Bacillosis).

SENILITY (*senilis*, old). (*See* Age.)

SENKOBO.—Cutaneous Streptothricosis, caused by *Actinomyces congolensis*, occurring in tropical Africa in cattle, sheep, goats, and horses. The hair stands erect and matted on small threepenny-bit-sized patches along the back. Moist, raw areas are left, then crusts form, and eventually a 'crocodile-skin' effect is produced. The disease occurs in association with tick infestation, and can therefore be controlled by means of a BHC dip.

SENNA.—A standardised preparation of this household laxative has been recommended in treating or preventing constipation in pigs—especially in pregnant sows. A sub-laxative dose of 3 g. is recommended during the farrowing period.

SENSIBLE LOSS OF HEAT.—This is the heat which animals lose by convection, conduction, and radiation. It does not include heat lost by vaporising water from the skin and respiratory passages.

SENSITISATION is a term used in several ways. Sensitised vaccine is a vaccine in which the bacteria have been exposed to contact with the immune serum prepared against them, and then washed free from the latter before injection. Such a vaccine is supposed to produce immunity more quickly and to be less irritating than a plain vaccine. Sensitisation of an animal means the production of a certain degree of anaphylaxis by a particular protein, vaccine, hormone, etc. (*See also* Light Sensitisation; Allergy; Antihistamines; Antibiotics.)

SEPSIS (*see* Antiseptics).

SEPTICÆMIA (σηπτικός, putrid; αἷμα, blood).—A condition of the blood-stream when bacteria are circulating in it. It is a very serious condition, because the organisms and the products of their activity (toxins) become widely distributed throughout the tissues, and practically every organ is affected by them. In most cases, septicæmia terminates in death.

Causes.—Extensive wounds or inflamed areas, especially in bones, joints, or blood-vessels, may become secondarily infected with some strain of virulent organisms (of which there are many), and, finding conditions favourable, these germs rapidly multiply, until they reach the general circulation. Infection following difficult parturition, the wounds caused by picked-up nails in the feet of horses, infection of arge raw areas which have been scalded or burnt, phlebitis following the operation of bleeding etc., are liable to be complicated with septicæmia and end fatally. In some cases death does not occur so readily, but abscesses break out in various parts of the body, due to infection with less virulent organisms. This condition is more correctly termed ' pyæmia '. In addition to the above conditions, septicæmia is characteristic of specific diseases, such as anthrax, braxy, and swine erysipelas, while in each of the diseases which belong to the class of ' hæmorrhagic septicæmias ' infection of the blood-stream is a marked feature.

Symptoms.—In many cases, especially when the animal is in a weakened state, sudden death, preceded by a very high temperature, may be the only sign of the presence of septicæmia. Rigors (shivering fits) may occur ; the horse may break out into a sweat ; respiration and heart action may be greatly distressed ; and there may be small hæmorrhages about the size of a pin's head on to the visible mucous membranes. Popularly, the term ' blood poisoning ' is usually applied to all forms of non-specific septicæmia, and is a good indication of the actual condition, there being literally poison in the blood.

Treatment.—Antibiotics and/or the sulphonamides, and antisera (where appropriate) are given.

SEPTUM.—A thin wall dividing two cavities or masses of tissue.

SEQUELÆ (*sequor*, I follow).—Symptoms or effects which may follow disease or injury. Thus pneumonia may follow a simple influenza, roaring may follow strangles, and chorea may follow distemper.

SEQUESTRUM (*sequestro*, I separate).—A fragment of bone which, in the process of necrosis, has been cast off from the living bone and has died, but still remains in the tissues. A sequestrum generally results from a fracture in which the bone has been broken into more than two pieces. The piece of dead bone generally remains in contact with, or surrounded by, the living newly formed bone, but should pus or serous discharge form, it burrows into the surrounding soft tissue, finally reaching the outside and bursting through a sinus. This sinus generally continues to discharge pus until the sequestrum is removed. (*See* BONE, DISEASES OF.)

SEROUS MEMBRANES are smooth, glistening, transparent membranes that line certain of the large cavities of the body and cover the organs that are contained in them. The chief of the serous membranes are : (1) the peritoneum, lining the cavity of the abdomen ; (2) the pleuræ, one of which lines each side of the chest and surrounds the corresponding lung ; (3) the pericardium, in which the heart lies ; and (4) the tunica vaginalis, one on each side, enclosing a testicle.

The name of these membranes is derived from the fluid which moistens their surfaces and which is derived in its turn from the blood or the lymph. Every serous membrane consists of a ' visceral portion ' which closely envelops the organ concerned, and a ' parietal portion ' which lines the wall of the cavity. These two portions are continuous and, where the reflection from the wall on to a certain organ takes place, the supporting band is generally called a ' ligament ' or ' mesentery '. The parietal and visceral parts are constantly rubbing against each other, and perfect lubrication is ensured by the small quantity of fluid always present During inflammations of serous membranes the amount of fluid is often increased to an enormous extent, and may interfere with the freedom of movement of the organs contained in the cavity. Thus, in some forms of pleurisy in the horse, literally gallons of the fluid exudate may be found in the chest cavity, and the lung is compressed out of its normal shape. (*See* PERITONEUM.)

SERUM (*serum*) is the fluid which separates from blood, lymph, and certain other fluids of the body, when the process of clotthing takes place in them.

Serum is a clear, yellowish fluid, containing, in addition to water, about 8 to 9 per cent of proteins, mainly serum-albumin and serum-globulin, with smaller amounts of salts, fat, sugar, urea, uric acid, and other extractives, as well as very small amounts of protein-like substances which are of the greatest importance in the prevention of disease. (*See* IMMUNITY *and* SERUM THERAPY.)

Serum is also obtained from lymph upon coagulation, and from the fluids which are poured out in cases of pleurisy and dropsy of the abdomen, as well as in certain other diseased conditions of body cavities.

The serum that is used for administration in tetanus, swine fever, anthrax, and other diseases is produced by artificially immunising animals against these diseases. (*See* SERUM THERAPY.)

SERUM GONADOTROPHIN (*see* HORMONES).

SERUM SICKNESS.—In human medicine this term is applied to the fever, glandular enlargements, œdema, pain in the joints, which occur 8 to 12 days after the injection of a 'foreign' serum. Immediate reaction, denoting sensitisation by a previous injection of the same kind of serum, is regarded as anaphylactic shock.

SERUM THERAPY.—When bacteria gain entrance to the body they multiply—under circumstances favourable to them—but exert their harmful effects not, as a rule, by directly attacking the tissues, but through poisonous substances produced by their growth and activity. These substances are of a chemical nature, and are known as 'toxins', and different organisms produce different kinds of toxins. The presence of toxins in the body, in small amounts at least, stimulates the body cells to produce other substances, called 'antitoxins', which by a process allied to chemical neutralisation deprive the toxins of their hurtful actions. Small amounts of snake venom, and the alkaloidal principles of certain vegetable drugs, possess a like power of so stimulating the body tissues that they produce nearly similar antitoxic substances. That these toxins and antitoxins react together in a manner similar to chemical neutralisation can be proved by mixing them together in a vessel and injecting the result into a susceptible animal. This toxin-antitoxin, as it is called, is then harmless.

When an animal is repeatedly inoculated with gradually increasing amounts of a bacterial toxin (or in some cases with the devitalised organisms themselves), a time arrives when it will withstand infection by doses of virulent organisms which would ordinarily prove fatal to it, and will tolerate doses of the toxin many times larger than would ordinarily kill it. Such an animal has been artificially immunised against that particular disease. For instance, if a horse is given graduated doses of tetanus toxin in ever-increasing quantities, there comes a time when it can withstand a dose several hundred times larger than would kill an ordinary horse. Further than this, if that horse's blood be withdrawn from it, allowed to clot, and the serum which is expressed from it is collected, it is found that it will protect another horse, or a person, against tetanus, when it is injected in appropriate doses. In this way infection of wounds by the *Clostridium tetani* can be rendered harmless by forestalling the production of tetanus toxin in the body by the administration to the animal of doses of tetanus antitoxin from artificially immunised horses.

Different toxins act on different tissues. For example, the tetanus toxin acts specifically upon the cells of the nervous system, and it is probable that the nervous tissue cells produce the tetanus antitoxin, or anti-tetanic serum.

With regard to the products that break up bacteria—bacteriolysins—it is maintained by some authorities that they are formed within the bodies of the polymorphonuclear leucocytes (a variety of the white blood-cells), since the bacteria are generally enveloped by the protoplasm of these white cells before they are broken up. (*See* PHAGOCYTOSIS, ANTIBODIES, COMPLEMENT.)

The use of sera, either as curative measures or as preventives against disease, is briefly discussed under the headings of those diseases to which they are applicable. (*See* ANTHRAX; BLACK QUARTER; DISTEMPER; CATTLE PLAGUE; SWINE FEVER; SWINE ERYSIPELAS; TETANUS, etc.)

SERVICE PERIOD.—An 85-day service period would appear to be the optimum number of days between calving and successful service. If the trend of heat periods after calving is detected at about six weeks, checked again around nine weeks, the cowman can, with a fair degree of accuracy, be on the look-out for bulling at or about the 12th week (or 84–85 days).

Very early service *may* produce prolonged infertility.

SEVIN.—An insecticide used against the chicken mite.

SEWAGE.—Human excreta should not be used for manuring pasture, as the eggs of the tapeworm *Tænia saginata* can survive for weeks and give rise to cysticercosis in cattle. (The eggs are not destroyed or filtered off in *all* sewage plants.) (*See also* SLURRY, COPPER POISONING in sheep.)

SEX-DETERMINATION by treatment of semen. (*See under* ARTIFICIAL INSEMINATION.)

known, no Y-borne gene in any way influences the expression of a character the gene of which is resident in the X, has been exploited commercially in order to identify the sex of chickens at the time of hatching.

For example, if a gold cock (gold is a recessive plumage colour character found in the Rhode Island Red, Brown Leghorn, and various other breeds of poultry) is mated to silver hens (silver is the alternative dominant plumage colour character found in such breeds as the White Wyandotte and Light Sussex, but not in the White Leghorn) the colour of the

A gold cock (sX) (sX) × (SX)Y a silver hen—

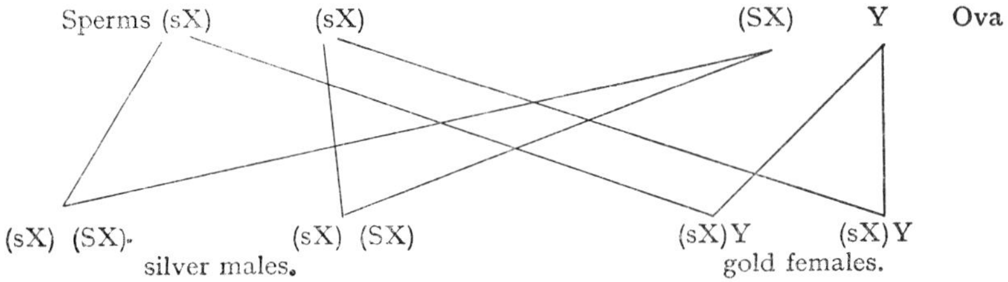

SEX-HORMONES (*see* HORMONES).

SEX-INVERSION.—Animals which at birth, and for a variable period afterwards, are of normal sexual structure and function, but which later in life acquire properties of the opposite sex, are said to undergo sex-inversion. This has been seen in Ayrshire cows permanently kept indoors.

SEXING OF CHICKS.—It was shown conclusively by Japanese workers that it is possible to distinguish male and female day-old pure-bred chicks by reference to sex-differences in the size of the cloacal papilla. Experts in this technique practise their art with amazing rapidity, and guarantee that the error shall not be more than 10 per cent. A new instrument, one end of which is inserted into the cloaca, enables the user to see through the cloaca wall and carry out sex differentiation after a much shorter period of training than with the above method.

SEX-LINKAGE.—The fact that in the case of birds, the female, having the sex-chromosome constitution XY, receives her single X-chromosome from her father, whereas the male, being XX, receives an X-chromosome from each of his parents, coupled with the fact that, so far as is

down in chicks, on hatching, falls into two classes, silvers and golds, and of these the silvers are the males and the golds are the females. Or, if a self-black cock is mated to barred hens (Plymouth Rocks, for example, but not Campines) then the chicks on hatching will be of two kinds, those with a white spot on the top of the head which are males, and will be barred when they grow up, and those without this occipital spot, which are females, and will not be barred when adult. In both cases the female offspring exhibit the plumage characters of their father, whilst the males are, in respect of plumage colour, like their mother.

The explanation of this peculiar criss-cross type of inheritance is that the genes for the characters known as gold and silver are carried by the X-chromosomes, and that in any X-chromosome only one gene for either gold or silver can be present. Because such genes are distributed to the egg and sperm cells in exactly the same way as the chromosomes which bear them, the characters to which they give rise are sex-linked.

If the letter 's' represents the hereditary factor or gene for *gold*, and 'S' that for the alternative dominant *silver*, and the brackets indicate that a particular gene is resident in a particular X, the principle may be expressed as follows:

The male chicks are male because they have received an X-chromosome from each parent, and are silver because, though they possess one gene for silver and one for gold, silver is dominant to gold. The females are female because they receive only one X-chromosome and are gold because, since their father was gold, the X-chromosome they receive carries the gene for gold.

The exploitation of the facts of sex-linkage in poultry breeding has so far, as will have been recognised, required the crossing of two breeds or of two varieties of one breed (*e.g.* Red Sussex cock and Light Sussex hens), but this disadvantage has been overcome by the creation by Professor Punnett of Cambridge of the Cambar breed, in which males can be distinguished from females by reference to the fact that of the sex-linkage genes, the male, having two X-chromosomes, can show a double dose, as it were, of a character, whilst the female, with but one X, can show only one.

Recently, out of a comprehensive study of herd books, the suggestion has emerged that sex-linked factors are involved in the inheritance of high milk yield, and experiments are proceeding which have been designed to examine its validity. If it should prove to be well founded, considerable changes in breeding practice may be expected, for, as will be understood, it would follow that a son would not possess the good or bad qualities of his father since (and in this matter the mammal differs from the bird, for it is the male that is XY and the female XX) the son received his single X-chromosome, and therefore the genes resident therein from his mother. (*See also* GENETICS AND HEREDITY.)

SHARPS, CALKS, COGS, or FROST-STUDS are small pointed studs which are inserted into holes prepared for them in horses' shoes to prevent slipping in frosty weather. There are two varieties: the first has a shank which is tapered slightly to fit into a corresponding recess in the shoe; the second has a round shank upon which a thread is cut to correspond with a similar thread in the recess of the shoe. It is said that the screwed frost-stud or sharp was invented by Thomas Carlyle. Those of the first variety are driven into the recess with a hammer, while those of the second type are screwed in with a spanner. In the screwed-shank types it is usually necessary that the threaded recess shall be kept patent by means of a 'blunt-sharp', or 'blank'. The pointed ends are made in various forms: chisel-shaped, pyramidal, rounded cones, or in the form of a capital letter O, N, H, or X, which allows the sharp to be used for some time without becoming blunted.

SHEARING.—In Britain, the usual time for shearing is May in the southern counties, early June on upland semi-arable farms, and during July in mountain flocks.

The newly shorn sheep is very sensitive to cold. This is particularly so with machine shearing 'which in the most professional of hands leaves a fleece of about 6 mm. depth compared with about 12 mm.' after hand shearing (Dr. K. L. Blaxter). In Australia, late winter and early spring shearing of ewes has led to a high mortality, so that the practice is being abandoned or the usual shears replaced by 'snow combs' which leave a longer fleece. 'In Britain, losses of weight or poor gains in lambs shorn during the summer can largely be attributed to an effect of cold.'

In the U.S.A. trials have been carried out with a drug, cyclophosphamide, (or cytoxan, to use another name for it) which causes the wool to loosen so that it can easily be plucked (in much less time than that required for shearing and without the skill needed for the latter). The sheep is left naked and unprotected against cold, and the possibility of undesirable side-effects or toxic residues has yet to be investigated.

'SHEATH ROT'.—A disease of sheep in Australia. (*See* BALANITIS.)

SHEEP: Names given according to age, sex, etc.—There are probably more names for any given class of sheep than is the case among any of the other domesticated animals, and it is almost impossible to give a list that will include all the various designations that are used, but the table following gives a list of commoner terms.

SHEEP, BREEDS OF

Introduction.—Sheep are maintained, generally speaking, with the object of producing both wool and mutton.

Hardiness, prolificness, milking capacity of the females, activity, are all important. What will constitute the most profitable type must be carefully considered in relation to local conditions. Broadly speaking, mutton constitutes the more valuable commodity in countries that have good local markets—*e.g.* Britain; whereas in regions that are far removed from markets —*e.g.* the central parts of Australia—wool becomes the main product. Again, on good arable land, where food is abundant throughout the year, the most highly improved and earliest maturing types can be kept; whereas on mountain grazing the main effort of the breeder must be concentrated on maintaining or improving the hardiness of the breed even at the sacrifice, it may be, of other desirable qualities.

BRITISH BREEDS OF SHEEP.—British breeds offer a wide choice of types, adapted to almost every conceivable set of conditions under which sheep are maintained in the country, from the highest mountain grazings in Scotland and Wales to the richest lowland pastures, like Romney Marsh or the dry arable farms of the Wolds.

At the 1965 Oxford Farming Conference, Mr. N. R. Woods of New Zealand House, London, gave a friendly but frank appraisal of the British sheep industry, and his criticisms could be summed up as 'too much tradition'. This applied to our 40 breeds of sheep, and the size of our flocks. He pointed out that a reduction (possibly by amalgamation) in the number of breeds would give immeasurably greater opportunities for breeding, culling, and selecting according to defined performance standards. In New Zealand they manage with two breeds and a cross—Merino, Romney,* and Merino-Romney—which between them thrive from sea-level to an altitude of 5000 feet, and in areas with a rainfall varying from 12 to 200 inches.

Mr. Woods found it surprising that our hill flocks number no more than 400 ewes; a size which, to-day, implies a labour cost of 30s. per ewe. In New Zealand the farmer himself will commonly look after a flock of up to 1000 or 1200 ewes, and will hand-feed them as a matter of course during the winter months. Mr. Woods referred to the reluctance of hill farmers here to feed their sheep even in the face of a more severe winter. In the name of 'hardiness —whatever that might be'—prolificacy, lamb performance, and wool were sacrificed.

* But see COOPWORTH, a breed formed in 1968.

With this we strongly agree. Work at the Hannah Dairy Research Institute has shown the wisdom of feeding starchy concentrates to obviate the hill ewe burning up her own tissues in order to keep warm and alive in very cold weather.

There was already, before this Conference, a move towards the development of new breeds of sheep in Britain. For example, Mr. Oscar Colburn had produced his COLBRED (which see), and Mr. J. Brian Cadzow had been working in Scotland. He started with the Finnish Landrace, a prolific breed, crossed with the Dorset Horn to give out of season lambing. The Ile-de-France is being used because of its fame as a mutton producer to bring in the live-weight gain factor, and the Westfalen is brought in for its great milking capacity. These last two breeds are used in long-term experiments. (*See* CADZOW IMPROVER RAM.)

The aim of the first development is to produce a ewe which will live long and average two lambings a year; giving four to five lambs a year or more.

Since that time Thornber-Colburn have put on the market hybrids such as the TC1 sold entirely on specification with no reference to breeds involved. This is likely to be the future trend.

In the U.S.A. the Morlam has achieved 6 lambs in 2 years.

The British breeds are commonly classified as Longwools, Downs, other Shortwools, and Mountain breeds.

The longwools have, with certain exceptions that will be noted later, the following characteristics in common: they are of large size, have white faces and legs, and are hornless. The fleece is heavy, consisting of long strong combing wool of good lustre. The length of the staple may be anything from 7 or 8 up to 18 or 20 inches, and the mean diameter of the fibre may be from 0·040 to 0·050 of a millimetre. The wool is of a clear white colour, and dark fibres are rare. In conformation the longwools are distinguished by great breadth of back, which is flat and thickly covered with meat; the leg of mutton is, however, less well developed than in, for instance, the Downs. The mutton is comparatively poor in quality, being coarse in grain, poor in flavour, and liable to contain excess of fat. The longwools are adapted to the more fertile types of farm, where pastures are productive and food plentiful. They are quiet in temperament and less active than the other types. The longwool breeds include the Leicester, Border

Leicester, Lincoln, Wensleydale, Kent or Romney Marsh, Devon Longwool, South Devon, and Roscommon.

The Downs, as a class, are smaller than the longwools, although the largest representatives are larger than the smallest of the longwool group. They have dark faces and legs, and are hornless. The fleece is densely set on the skin, and consists of fine short wool with a fine ' crimp ' and a soft handle. The length of staple is from 2 to 5 inches and the mean diameter typically about 0·025 to 0·030 of a millimetre. The colour of the wool is creamy, and black or brown fibres occur in some breeds rather frequently. The back is not so broad as in the longwools, but the hind quarter is well developed and the leg of mutton is large and thick. The mutton is of good texture and flavour and well mixed, without excess of fat. The Down breeds are suited to the lighter and drier types of soil at moderate elevations with a high proportion of arable. They include the Southdown, Suffolk, Hampshire, Dorset Down, and Shropshire. The Ox-

NAMES OF SHEEP GIVEN ACCORDING TO AGE, SEX, ETC.

Periods.	Male.		Female.	Remarks.
	Uncastrated.	Castrated.		
Birth to weaning	Tup lamb Ram lamb Pur lamb Heeder	Hogg lamb	Ewe lamb Gimmer lamb	A sheep until weaning is a lamb
Weaning to shearing	Hogg (also used for the female) Hogget (also used for the female) Haggerel or Hoggerel Tup teg Ram hogg Tup hogg	Wether hogg Wedder hogg He teg	Gimmer hogg Ewe hogg Sheeder ewe Ewe teg	Hogget wool is wool of the first shearing
First to second shearing	Shearing, or Shearling, or Shear hogg Diamond ram Dinmont ram tup One-shear tup	Shearing wether Shear hogg Wether hogg Wedder hogg Two-toothed wether	Shearing ewe Shearling gimmer Theave Double-toothed ewe Double-toothed gimmer Gimmer	' Ewe ', if in-lamb or with lamb ; if not a 'barren gimmer'; if not put to a ram is a ' yeld gimmer ' (Scotland)
Second to third shearing	Two-shear ram Two-shear tup	Four-toothed wether Two-shear wether	Two-shear ewe	A ewe which has ceased to give milk is a ' yeld ewe '; taken from the breeding flock she is a ' draft ewe ' or a ' draft gimmer'
Third to fourth shearing	Three-shear ram Three-shear tup	Six-toothed wether Three-shear wether	Three-shear ewe Winter ewe (Scotland)	
Afterwards	Aged tup or ram	Full-mouthed, full-marked or aged wether or wedder	Ewe	After fourth shearing ' aged ' or ' three-winter '

ford, although generally included amongst the Downs, differs from the others in important points, and is best regarded as an intermediate or middle-woolled breed.

The other shortwools include the Dorset Horn and the Western or Wiltshire Horn (whitefaced, horned), the Ryeland and Devon closewool (white-faced, hornless), and the Kerry Hill (speckled-faced, hornless) which are broadly similar, in fleece and conformation, to the Downs.

The mountain breeds are of small size; active and hardy; and are mostly somewhat slower in maturing than the other classes. They tend to be narrower of back, particularly at the shoulder, than Down or lowland breeds, but the mutton is usually of very fine quality. In respect of fleece and other characteristics the mountain breeds have little in common. The more important breeds are the Scotch blackface, Cheviot, Swaledale, Herdwick, Lonk, Welsh Mountain, Exmoor, and Dartmoor; there are various other types of breeds of greater or less local importance.

THE LONGWOOL BREEDS.—**The Leicester** was the oldest, or at least was the earliest to be improved, of the longwool breeds, and in its improved form was used to a greater or a less extent in forming or in improving most of the others. The credit for the formation of the New Leicester belongs to Robert Bakewell of Dishley, the first great British stock-breeder. Starting with the Old Leicester, a large, ungainly, slow-maturing sheep, whose sole good point was its long, fine, lustrous fleece, Bakewell, during the period between 1755 and 1775 applied his new system of selection combined with close inbreeding, and had by the latter date produced what was essentially a new breed, short-legged, squarely built, wide backed and symmetrical, with vastly improved early maturity and tendency to fatten. Doubtless Bakewell allowed his breed to deteriorate in respect of weight of fleece, and also in prolificness, but these faults have been eliminated by subsequent generations of breeders.

In most respects the Leicester may be regarded as typical of the group to which it belongs. It is a middle-sized longwool, smaller than the Lincoln or Cotswold, but larger than the Romney Marsh and comparable in size with the largest of the Downs, such as the Suffolk and Oxford. The head is wedge-shaped, the nose rather narrow and slightly Roman; the hair on the face and ears white, with a bluish tinge and occasional black specks, which are more marked on the ears. The nostrils black, the forehead covered with wool, the ears rather long and thin. The neck is short, thick at its junction with the shoulder, and carried almost horizontally. The fore-end is of great width, and the back broad, square, and thickly fleshed, but the hind quarter is sometimes lacking both in length and in symmetry. The fleece is of typical fine long combing wool, dense on the pelt, curly, and lustrous. Ram tegs commonly clip about 14 lb. of wool, and ewe flocks may average 9 or 10 lb.

The breed is fairly hardy and of good fecundity. It is very early maturing, but the mutton of pure-bred specimens, unless those killed as lambs, shows the same faults as that of the longwool breeds generally. The rams are impressive sires and are excellent for crossing with the smaller and leaner types of ewe; *e.g.* with Masham (Wensleydale—blackface mountain cross).

The breed is now to be found chiefly in the North and East Ridings of Yorkshire (especially the Wold district) and in Durham. Abroad it has found a good deal of favour in Tasmania, New Zealand, Australia, and to a somewhat less extent in Canada and the United States.

The Border Leicester was derived from the English Leicester, either solely by selection or, according to other authorities, by selection accompanied by a slight infusion of Cheviot blood. In any case it has been bred pure, as a distinct breed, for over a century, and has been recognised as distinct since 1869, when it was given separate classification by the Highland and Agricultural Society. It differs from the English Leicester in being somewhat longer of leg and lighter in build; in having the head bare of wool, and narrower behind the ears; the nose more aquiline in shape; the neck longer, and the carriage of head much higher and more stylish. The ears, too, are carried higher. The bone is somewhat lighter and the hind legs below the hock are free from wool. The fleece has the same general character, but separates into somewhat more distinct locks or 'pirls' of about finger size.

The Border Leicester is more active and probably somewhat more hardy and prolific than the English Leicester. The clip is probably rather lighter, under comparable conditions. On account of its thin head the Border Leicester is specially suitable for crossing with small mountain ewes, which are liable to give trouble in lambing when mated to other large breeds. The breed is maintained almost entirely for the purpose of producing rams for crossing with Cheviot or blackface mountain ewes. The mutton of the pure-bred sheep is of no more than average longwool quality, but that of the crosses with these leaner breeds is very satisfactory.

Border Leicesters are to be found in practically all lowland districts from Northumberland and Cumberland to Caithness and Orkney and are quite numerous in Northern Ireland, but the chief breeding centre is South-Eastern Scotland and Northumberland. The breed has gained a very considerable amount of popularity in New Zealand and Australia, and numbers have been exported to many other countries.

The Lincoln constitutes perhaps the most extreme form of the longwool type —the largest, the longest, and heaviest woolled, and, as breeders of other varieties have it, the coarsest of the group. It is an old breed, and for long the breeders refused to introduce any outside blood such as that of the New Leicester, which was earlier brought to perfection and which was used in the improvement of longwool sheep almost everywhere in England. Eventually, about the beginning of the 19th century, a certain amount of crossing did take place, the immediate effects of which were to improve the Old Lincoln in symmetry and early maturity, but materially to diminish the length of staple and the density of fleece. However, after several generations of selection, the old wool character was recovered and the benefit of the Leicester blood at the same time retained.

The Lincoln is the biggest of our British sheep ; indeed it is the biggest to be found anywhere. While perhaps no taller than the Cotswold or the South-Devon, it excels both in width and in depth of body. Massiveness of build rather than size is its most striking characteristic. Mature rams occasionally weigh over 400 lb., and the average of the wethers exhibited at Smithfield is about 300 lb. at 21½ months.

Face and ears are white, with occasional dark spots on the latter ; and the nostrils are black. The head is proportionate to the size of the body, wide between the eyes, and the profile nearly straight. There is a tuft of the long wool on the forehead. The shoulder-top, back, loin, and hind quarters are very wide and flat on top, and the whole conformation very square. The bone is rather large. The wool is of great length—up to 20 inches, very dense on the pelt, and divided into staples as broad as two fingers. It is stronger and coarser in character than Leicester wool, but finer than that of the Cotswold or South Devon. Rams frequently clip between 20 and 28 lb., and ewes often more than a stone, but 16 and 12 lb. respectively would represent good flock averages.

The Lincoln naturally requires fairly good pasture and abundant food. It is fairly prolific, but probably not quite so early maturing as the Leicester. The mutton of the pure-bred aged sheep is of poor quality. It is for crossing purposes that the Lincoln is most valuable, and especially for crossing with the merino the breed is prime favourite. Its popularity for the last purpose depends on its large size, great capacity for laying on fat, and its heavy fleece of uniform pure white wool. So useful has the Lincoln-merino cross been found that lately the cross-bred type has been fixed in a breed—the Corriedale. British breeders depend largely on the Australian and South American export trade, with the result that the prices for Lincolns show very violent fluctuations from year to year. The breed is found mainly in Lincolnshire and the adjoining parts of Yorkshire.

The South Devon, a local breed of considerable merit, is a large but somewhat loosely built sheep with strong bone and a heavy fleece ; the latter approaches that of the Lincoln in character but tends to be coarser, particularly at the breech. The breed is hardy, the lambs are very rapid growers, and the proportion of lean meat in the carcass is said to be very high. The habitat is South Devon and Cornwall.

The Devon longwool, which is native to Devon and Somerset, is considerably smaller than the last, attaining somewhat less than average longwool weight. It has, however, the same capacity for rapid early growth, so that lambs of the breed are nearly as heavy as those of the largest in the group. The fleece is heavy ; it is finer and generally denser than that of the South Devon.

The Devon closewool is the product of crosses between this breed and the Exmoor Horn.

The Wensleydale is a sheep of about average longwool size, somewhat narrower of back than most of the related breeds and rather long in the neck. The fleece is open, dividing into small separate locks of about pencil size, and is long and silky, with a beautiful lustre. The breed yields the finest quality of true lustre wool. The

Wensleydale is active and hardy, well adapted to live and thrive under semi-upland conditions, and produces probably the best mutton of all the longwools. In its native Yorkshire, and throughout the North of England and South-West of Scotland, the Wensleydale is largely employed for crossing with blackfaced mountain ewes, the cross-breds being known in Yorkshire as 'Mashams' (after the town of that name), and in Scotland as 'Yorkshire crosses'. For this purpose the breed comes into competition with the Border Leicester, producing a hardier but later-maturing lamb than the latter. The Wensleydale is also the favourite breed for crossing with Herdwick ewes. The steel-blue face and legs are a very striking peculiarity of the breed.

The Kent or Romney Marsh is the smallest and, in some ways, the least typical of the longwool group. It is long bodied and short legged, with rather frequently a 'tied-in' appearance behind the shoulder. The fleece is dense and uniform, finer in quality than that of the other longwools, but lacking both in length and in lustre. Through long adaptation to the peculiar conditions of Romney Marsh the breed has become singularly resistant to foot-rot and also to liver fluke. In its home district it is almost exclusively grass fed, receiving hay during winter, with sometimes a very few mangolds during the lambing season. Romneys show no natural tendency to flock, but scatter widely over their allotted pastures and graze singly. The breed has proved extraordinarily successful in New Zealand, and is by much the most numerously represented of our British breeds in that country. It crosses well with the merino.

The Romney Halfbred has been developed, by crossing Romney Marsh ewes with North Country Cheviot, for economic fat lamb production.

The Roscommon is the only breed of sheep native to Ireland. It is large, standing on rather long legs, produces mutton of good quality, but is rather slow maturing. The fleece has rather less length than that of the typical British longwool, but is dense and of good quality. Few remain.

THE DOWN BREEDS.—**The Southdown** occupies a position among the Down breeds analogous to that of the Leicester among the longwools; *i.e.* it was the earliest improved and contributed a good deal to the improvement of all the other breeds in its group. If we except some of the true mountain and moorland types, such as the Exmoor and the Welsh, the Southdown is the smallest British breed, reaching rather less than two-thirds of the weight of the Lincoln. The general conformation is compact and blocky with a wide firm back and an exceptionally thick leg-of-mutton. The head is short and wide, the ears small. The face and legs, which are partially woolled over, are of a uniform light greyish brown. The wool is exceedingly dense on the pelt, very short, and is the finest in quality that is produced in Britain. The clip is not heavy, but is greater than might be judged from the appearance of the fleece, reaching ordinarily about 4 or 4½ lb. in the case of breeding ewes. The Southdown is very early maturing and produces mutton of unsurpassed quality, the joints being thickly fleshed and the meat tender and of excellent flavour. The breed and its crosses have received a very large proportion of the awards in carcase competitions both at home and abroad. In Britain the Southdown is not widely dispersed, being common only in the south-eastern counties. It has been quite largely exported to other sheep countries.

The Suffolk, which was produced originally by crossing the improved Southdown with the now extinct Norfolk horned, is widely distributed throughout the lowland districts of Britain. It is one of the largest of the Downs, and nearly similar in weight to the Leicester. The head is cleanly cut, and, with the legs, is free from wool and of a pure lustrous black. The ears are carried rather low and are fairly long. The neck is of a fair length; the back is inclined to handle a little hard, lacking the layer of subcutaneous fat that is so quickly formed by the longwools, but the leg-of-mutton is exceptionally full and fleshy. The wool is of typical Down quality and of fair length and good density, but is liable to contain a high proportion of dark fibres. The lambs are sooty grey or nearly black when born. Although the carcase is somewhat less compact and fleshy than that of the Southdown, the mutton is of excellent texture and flavour. The Suffolk is very prolific, a fall of 160 or 170 lambs per hundred ewes being not uncommon. The ewes are good milkers. Rams of this breed are largely used for crossing with longwool, half-bred, and other ewes.

The Hampshire was derived originally from two old local types, the Berkshire Knot and the Wiltshire horned (the latter of which is still extant), crossed with the

Southdown. It is a large sheep, but little inferior in size to the Suffolk and Oxford. The face is deep brownish black, and is woolled down to the level of the eyes, or a little lower. The head is wide and rather heavy, the ears large and carried low. The general conformation is a little rough, the shoulder being on the heavy side, but the mutton is of good quality and full of lean meat. The fleece is short and not very dense, the clip being rather light in relation to the size of the sheep. Dark fibres are rather common. The Hampshire is hardy and thrives well on poor land, while, on the other hand, it stands forcing well, the lambs on heavy feeding making very rapid gains. The ewes are not notably prolific. Hampshires are very largely kept as commercial sheep in the South Midlands and South of England, particularly on the arable farms on the chalk formation. The breed has been quite widely exported, but has not become prime favourite in any of the larger sheep countries.

The Oxford Down is in the main a product of the crossing of the Cotswold with the Hampshires, and in most of its characters is intermediate between the two breeds. It is a large sheep, probably on the average heavier than the Suffolk, and thus exceeding all the other Downs. The face is greyish brown, with a topknot of longish wool. The conformation is square and blocky, with something of the flat back, strong rump, and lighter thigh that distinguish the longwools from the Downs. The fleece is of the middle-wool type, fairly dense and of fair quality, though coarser than that of the other Downs. The Oxford is prolific and fairly hardy, but requires the better sort of land with fairly abundant food. The mutton tends to become coarse and greasy in older sheep, and the breed is best suited to produce either fat lambs or tegs in the early winter. The Oxford is still most numerously represented in Oxfordshire and Gloucester, but the breed is largely kept in Scotland for the purpose of producing rams for crossing, the usual cross being with the half-bred (Cheviot × Border Leicester) ewe.

The Dorset Down may be fairly accurately described as a small and rather refined type of Hampshire. It is a middle-sized Down breed, slightly larger in frame and of nearly the same weight as the Shropshire. The colour of face is distinctly lighter than in the Hampshire, being a good rich brown. It is less numerous than the other Down breeds.

The Shropshire was produced by crossing the Southdown with old types native to Staffordshire and Shropshire, especially those of Morfe Common and of Cannock Chase. It is numerously represented in Canada and the United States, but has virtually disappeared from Britain and New Zealand.

THE OTHER SHORTWOOLLED BREEDS.—**The Dorset Horn** is a very old, white-faced and pink-nosed breed, native to Dorset, Somerset, and the Isle of Wight. Both sexes are horned. In size it is comparable with the Shropshire, though it is less compact and blocky than the latter breed. The conformation is not strikingly good, many of the sheep being rather loose in the shoulder and long and slack in the back, and yielding a somewhat rough carcase. The grain and flavour of the mutton are, however, excellent. The wool is nearly as fine as that of the Southdown, and being of a clear white colour (as opposed to the creamy tint of Down wool), and free from dark fibres, it commands a very high price. The fleece is not specially dense, and the clip is consequently rather light. A striking peculiarity of the breed is that the ewes will take the ram as early as May, so that it is possible to have lambs by October, which can be fed for the Christmas market. A proportion of the ewes will breed twice a year, but it is better to mate only once. The production of house lamb in this country has very greatly declined with the development of the New Zealand lamb trade, and the commercial importance of the Dorset's peculiar quality has therefore diminished. The ewes are prolific and excellent milkers, and the breed, being native to rather poor semi-upland country, is active and hardy.

The Western or Wiltshire Horn is a very ancient breed that has recently been increasing in numbers. It somewhat resembles the Dorset Horn, but carries practically no wool, the coat being of short hair like that of a goat, white in colour with dark spots. The conformation is rather rough, but the sheep are hardy and the young lambs grow with great rapidity. The majority of existing flocks, which are all small, are found in Northamptonshire. Wiltshire rams are rather largely used in North Wales and Anglesey for crossing with draft Welsh Mountain ewes.

The Ryeland is another old breed whose home country is the poor and rather wet district (Ryelands) in southern Herefordshire. The Ryeland has been described as resembling in appearance a white-faced Southdown. Actually, however, it is considerably larger framed and somewhat bigger boned, less blocky and compact, and has a somewhat longer head and larger ear. The quality of mutton is first class, though the sheep can easily be made too fat for the modern taste. The fleece is of very fine quality, and the breed has often won premier place in open wool classes in competition with the Dorset Horn and Southdown. The length of staple is greater than in the last-mentioned breed, and the clip is on the average considerably heavier. The Ryeland is, like the Romney Marsh, highly resistant to foot-rot and liver fluke. The breed is increasing in popularity, and a considerable number of flocks have been established in widely scattered areas in Britain, from Kent to Cumberland and Scotland.

The Kerry Hill (Wales) derives its name from the Kerry Hills of Montgomeryshire, but is now fairly widely distributed in the West Midlands. The face and legs are speckled black and white. The breed is middle-sized, nearly equal in weight to the Shropshire. The fleece shows good length and is comparable in quality to that of the Shropshire, though it is commonly less uniform over the body, and notably rather coarse on the breech. The ewes are very prolific and are excellent mothers. Rams are used for crossing with Welsh mountain ewes, and Kerry Hill draft ewes are frequently crossed with Shropshires, in order to produce early fat lambs.

MOUNTAIN BREEDS.—The blackfaced, horned, and strong - woolled mountain breeds, of which the Scotch Blackface, the Herdwick, Swaledale, and Lonk are the most important, appear to have had a common origin. The earliest known home of the type was the Pennine country in the North of England.

The Scotch Blackface now occupies most of the true moorlands and heather mountains throughout Scotland. The breed has been kept in the Southern upland area for many hundreds of years, and was introduced into the North and West Highlands during the 18th century, displacing the earlier soft-woolled and tan-faced Celtic type. The face and legs are either black or black and white (' brockit '). The size of the breed naturally varies greatly according to the quality of the soil and the elevation of the particular grazing. But under good conditions the Blackface is a sheep of medium size, larger than some of the Downs. The conformation is generally good, though, like most other true mountain breeds, it has narrow shoulders and rather a sharp wither. Early maturing qualities are remarkably highly developed, lambs being frequently sold fat off the hills during August. The quality of the mutton is exceedingly good, the breed being a frequent winner of championship honours in the Smithfield carcase competitions. The wool of the modern show type is long, strong, and rather hairy in character, though fairly free from kemp. Many commercial flocks have somewhat finer wool, but generally speaking the quality is so coarse that the wool can only be utilised for the manufacture of carpets and other coarse materials, and brings a low price. The fleece is of fair weight, clips from ewe flocks under mountain conditions varying from 3½ to 5 lb. per head. The breed is of course exceedingly hardy, thriving on the poorest of mountain grazings at elevations of up to 2000 and 3000 feet. Ordinarily the ewe hoggs or tegs are wintered in the low country (but on grass only), while the ewes remain on the hill-sides and receive no artificial food except a little hay in times when the ground is covered with hard frozen snow, so that natural food cannot be reached. Under mountain conditions the ewes are of course not very prolific 80 to 100 lambs per 100 ewes being a satisfactory crop. Draft ewes kept under lowland conditions twin freely, 140 or 150 per cent of lambs being not uncommon. On the higher and poorer grazings pure-bred Blackface lambs are generally bred, while on better land at lower elevations the ewes are commonly crossed with Border Leicester or occasionally with Wensleydale rams, the crosses making very useful commercial sheep for winter and spring feeding.

The Swaledale, which is the common variety of Blackface in Yorkshire and East Lancashire, is somewhat shorter woolled, especially in front, than the Scotch type. The face is black, with a pronounced ' mealy ' or grey ring round the nose, while the legs are mottled or grey. The head is not so strong as in the Scotch Blackface. The breed is well adapted to its own locality and is quite as hardy as the northern variety.

The Lonk, which is found farther south

in the adjacent parts of Yorkshire, Derbyshire, and Lancashire, is a softer-woolled variety, larger and somewhat higher on the leg and with a longer tail than the Scotch Blackface. The face and legs have on the average more white. The Lonk is distinctly less hardy than the Swaledale or Scotch Blackface, the ewes being commonly kept in enclosed fields during winter, and receiving hay.

The Cheviot, although originally confined to rather a narrow area on both sides of the Scottish Border, and although still bred in the greatest perfection in the Cheviot country, is now very widely distributed. It occupies the bulk of the grassy hill land throughout Scotland, and in particular is very numerous in Caithness and Sutherland. Great numbers of draft ewes are taken south annually, and the breed is quite frequently seen in the Midlands and Southern English counties. The Cheviot is of medium size, white-faced, and normally hornless, though horns occasionally appear on the rams. The head is rather short, thick, and strong at the bridge of the nose. The hair on the face is wiry and the nose dark. The ears are short and carried very high, giving the sheep a characteristically alert appearance. The wool commences abruptly behind the ears, standing out sharply as a kind of ruff. The body is of good length with often rather a light fore-quarter and sharp wither and sometimes a tendency to be slack in the back. The wool is of good quality, of middle length (about 4 inches), and fairly dense and uniform. It is normally used for manufacture into tweeds. Kemp is liable to occur, but is usually small in quantity. The quality of the mutton is excellent, the cross with either the Southdown or Suffolk being a favourite one for producing show carcases. The breed is very hardy, though less so than the blackface, and the ewes are good milkers and excellent mothers. There is considerable variety of types within the breed. North Country (Caithness and Sutherland) sheep are larger framed, somewhat more loosely built, and considerably finer woolled than the Border type. Many flocks of Cheviots are kept on hill grazings, receiving no hand feeding except a limited amount of hay in periods of storm. Other flocks are kept as ' park sheep '—*i.e.* on enclosed land—and these generally receive a limited ration of roots during the latter part of the winter. In park flocks the older ages of ewes are generally crossed with Border Leicester rams, and the same cross is employed on the better sort of hill grazings. The product is the well-known ' half-bred ', which forms the great bulk of the ewe stock on the arable sheep farms of the North of England and South of Scotland.

The Herdwick is found in the Fell District of North Lancashire, Cumberland, and Westmorland. This area includes some of the poorest and bleakest mountain pasture in Britain, and the Herdwick is, in keeping with the natural conditions of its home country, probably the hardiest of all English breeds. It is a small breed. The rams generally bear medium-sized horns, while the ewes are hornless. The face and legs of the lamb are of a deep bluish-grey colour, becoming gradually paler and sometimes white with age. The wool is more or less mixed with grey in many cases, is coarse and strong, and frequently contains kemp. The clip averages perhaps 3 lb. for ewe flocks under typical conditions. The mutton is of very fine quality, though the breed is somewhat slow maturing.

The Welsh Mountain, which is found throughout the mountainous districts of Wales, most numerously in the North, is the smallest of British breeds, reaching little more than two-thirds of the weight of the Southdown. The males only bear horns. The face is either white or of a light tan shade, the latter being commoner. The body is rather long and the fore-quarter light, with a somewhat sharp wither. The fleece is short and close, and contains a large proportion of very fine wool, but is generally rather lacking in uniformity, with a coarse breech, and often a proportion of kemp. Ewe flocks give an average clip of perhaps 2½ lb. The mutton ranks in quality with that of the Southdown and Scotch mountain breeds. The breed is hardy, but the ewes are often wintered on the lower ground, going back to the open mountains after lambing. The older ewes when taken to low country districts produce excellent fat lambs to Southdown, Shropshire, Kerry Hill, or other rams of the larger and earlier maturing breeds.

The Exmoor Horn or **Porlock** is another small breed, larger only than the Welsh Mountain. It is horned in both sexes, with white face and legs and a dark nose. The sheep are long bodied, often somewhat slack at the heart-girth, with a rather characteristic rounded conformation. The fleece is of good depth of staple and of good density and quality, somewhat similar to that of the Cheviot. The clip may average 4½ lb. for ewe flocks. The mutton is of fine quality.

The Dartmoor is a large moorland breed which has many of the characteristics of a longwool. The breed is ordinarily hornless in both sexes; the face is white with black spots, the latter more or less concentrated about the nose. The fleece has somewhat the same character as that of the Wensleydale, being very long, curly, lustrous, and rather open, and the weight of fleece is comparable to that of the longwools. Breeding ewes run on moorland pastures during summer, but are generally wintered on enclosed land, with roots and hay. (*See also* COLBRED.)

SHEEP BREEDING AND MANAGEMENT.—The increasing rise of hybrids, referred to under SHEEP, BREEDS OF (British) is one new trend. Another is the in-wintering of sheep—one aspect of the current move towards intensive livestock production.

Other developments.—Sheep management has undergone change due to other economic factors. For example, a full-time shepherd is now expected to look after 1,000 rather than only 400 ewes.

Then again, in the U.K. the market for mutton, except for processing, has disappeared, and virtually the sole requirement is lamb. Lightweight carcases of under 40 lb. are in demand. Fat is not wanted.

It may prove possible to reduce the present high costs of zero-grazing and then use this to prevent the high wastage (up to 40 per cent) of grass trampled underfoot.

Greater use may be made of the various forms of creep-grazing in order to obtain higher stocking rates.

A plan put forward by the Grassland Research Institute, Hurley, involves rearing lambs artificially from day-old, keeping ewes on high/marginal land leaving lusher lowlands for growing stock.

Research at the G.R.I.—Dr. C. R. W. Spedding has listed three ways by which productivity can be raised: (a) by growing more herbage (or other sheep foods) per acre; (b) by ensuring that more of what is grown is eaten by the sheep; and (c) by improving the efficiency with which the sheep convert their food into meat and wool. The last really means improving the sheep.

'With bred varieties of grasses and legumes, and liberal use of fertilisers, very high levels of herbage production can be achieved. Sheep performance—especially that of lambs—has been better on legumes than on grasses. Sainfoin and lucerne have proved most effective but, on balance, a ryegrass/white clover mixture will generally give the greatest total production with sheep.

'The main disease hazard is excessive worm-infestation, especially in lambs that receive less milk than they could readily use. Ensuring good milk output from the ewe is therefore important, but this may not be enough for twins and triplets. The problem remains greatest where high stocking rates and high lambing percentages are combined. Possible solutions include better use of modern, efficient anthelmintic drugs, the use of grazing management and supplementary feeding of the lambs. Weaned lambs do best when they have plenty of herbage, provided that its quality is also high, especially in terms of digestibility.

'Since food costs may amount to 60 per cent of the total costs of sheep production, the efficiency with which food is converted is bound to be important. In a lowland ewe flock, most of the food is consumed by the ewes—the lambs eat about 10 per cent of the total, if they are singles, and up to 25 per cent if they are twins. In other words, the proportion of the total food that goes towards meat production depends chiefly on the number of lambs per ewe.

'A ewe requires so much food for the year, whether she produces any lambs or not: for a little more food she can produce 30–40 lb. of lamb carcase, and for a little more again, nearly twice as much meat. Wool production is still important—and will remain so whilst sheep production is not very profitable and whilst the wool can be sold—but it is on meat production that the British sheep industry of the future will surely rest.

'The most important factor at present appears to be the number of lambs per ewe per year. What we want, it seems, is a small ewe (thus reducing the food bill—cheaper still if the food comes from cheap by-products), crossed with a large ram to produce a lot of lambs that will achieve heavy carcase weights.

'Experimentally, we have been producing large litters (up to 6) by hormone injections and breeding more than once a year (in some animals) by hormones and by light treatments. There is no reason to suppose, however, that all these things cannot be done by ewes bred for the purpose.

'It is *unlikely*, nevertheless, that eweg will be bred that are capable of rearins all the lambs they can produce, under the intensive stocking conditions needed to make the best use of the heavily fertilised pastures.

'For this reason, and to ensure that loss of young lambs is minimised, a great deal of work has been done to develop methods of artificial rearing for lambs. We are now at the stage where large-scale rearing, housed or in the field (weather permitting), either fully-automated or managed by simple methods, can be visualised in practice.

'By feeding cold milk substitute at a high level, it is possible to achieve faster growth rates in lambs than are normally achieved, even in singles, on the ewe. The problem is that the cost of the milk substitute is currently too high to do this unless the lambs are extremely cheap and other costs are minimal. It is therefore a technique to be applied to the lambs that the ewe cannot rear or fatten at the level of stocking, fencing and supplementary feeding dictated by the whole farming system and its economics. This might be all lambs in excess of two per ewe, or in excess of one in very intensive conditions.

'The next major problem is to devise cheaper diets or combinations of diets on which to rear and finish lambs.

'Ultimately, there will be several different ways of combining the new techniques into economically viable husbandry systems. Some will involve housing for all or part of the year, for ewes and/or lambs; some will depend largely on grazing.'

(*See also* SYNCHRONISATION OF ŒSTRUS).

In-wintering.—In Scotland the in-wintering of sheep denotes a revival rather than an innovation, for it was, of course, the usual practice on many hill farms until a change was made to transferring the sheep to a lowland farm for the worst of the winter. Now that such an arrangement has become too expensive or otherwise proved impracticable, the ewes are being housed again on hill farms. It is, however, on mixed farms in England that in-wintering is chiefly gaining popularity, and it is here a part of the general process of intensification affecting livestock production. A flockmaster of some 30 years' standing has commented: 'If more live lambs are reared because of closer supervision and the avoidance of bad weather hazards, then there is every justification for the use of permanent buildings for flocks which lamb in the December to April period.'

Professor Cooper has emphasised that the biggest single cost in fat lamb production is flock depreciation. With winter housing, it is possible to retain ewes to a greater age, as a result of their being spared the stress arising from exposure in severe weather, and of their having their food provided for them. He has also commented, with reference to the lowlands: 'The case for in-wintering only really arises with high-intensity stocking on land subject to poaching.'

Mr. L. J. Williams has commented: 'The floor space allowed per sheep will depend basically on the size and breed of the animals and whether or not they are entirely confined to the shed for 24 hours of the day. Some upland flock masters allow the mountain lambs to run out of the shed during the day time and only hold them in the shed during night time, while others will argue that this practice has nothing to commend it. Furthermore some lowland flockmasters in low rainfall areas manage quite well with only 50 per cent cover over the sheep holding area. As a general guide, however, and based on the assumption that there is complete coverage and that the sheep are completely confined, mountain lambs require only 6 to 7 sq. ft. and lowland ewes 10 sq. ft.

'Portable feeding racks or boxes have two main advantages: they can be easily removed to give an unobstructed floor area should this be necessary, and they can be used to divide the flock into sizeable units—generally about 70 upland sheep or 50 lowland.

'There are two types in general use. The first, which is more often used for upland sheep, consists of a hay rack with a small concentrate trough below. The rack should not be too flat otherwise hay seeds will get into the eyes of the sheep and cause serious trouble. The other feeder is of the box type where a metal grille or wooden ladder can be used to prevent the hay being wasted.

'These box troughs have the advantage in that they can be used by the shepherd to walk down to feed the flock—a real advantage where large heavy sheep are involved. As to trough lengths a space

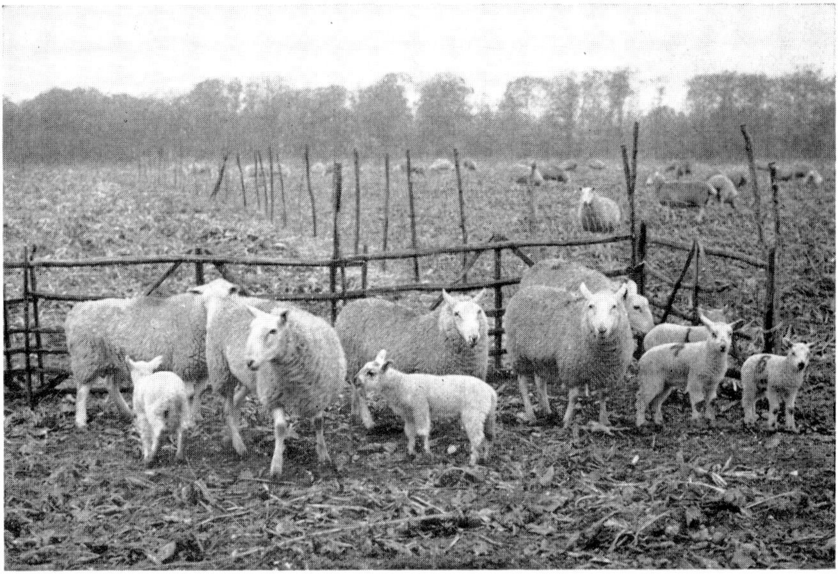

October lambs: a second crop in the year obtained by means of hormone injections.
(*An Esso photograph.*)

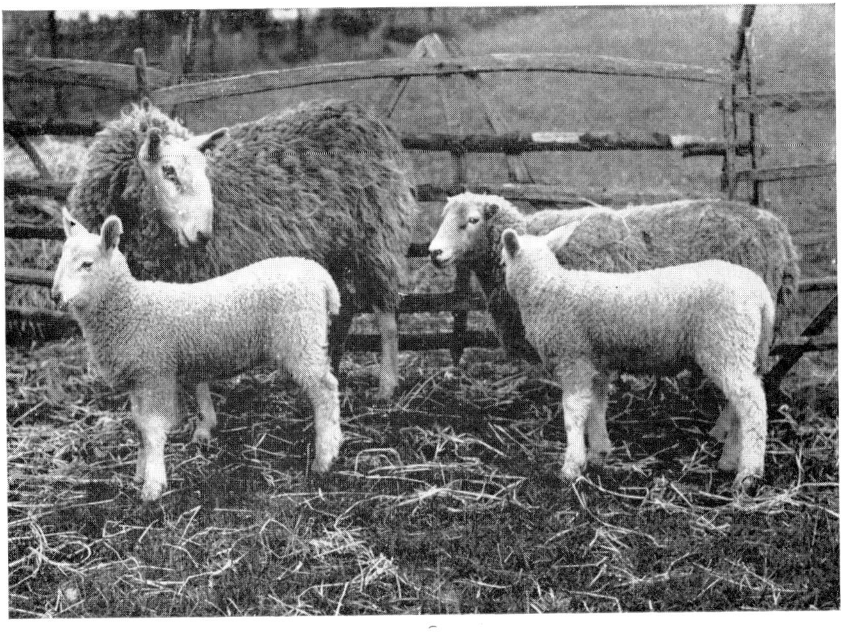

Twins from different mothers. One of two eggs was removed from the Border Leicester ewe and transplanted into the Welsh ewe.

See TRANSPLANTATION.

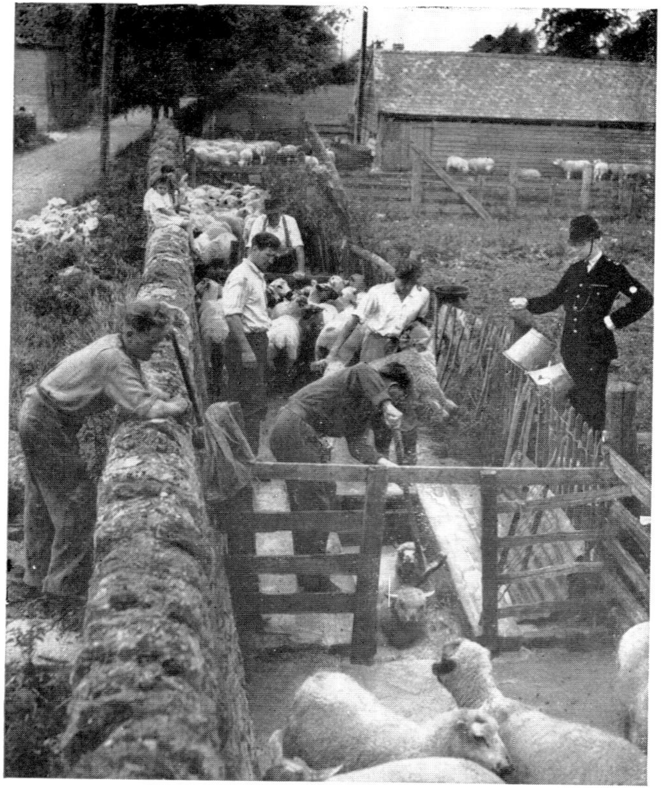

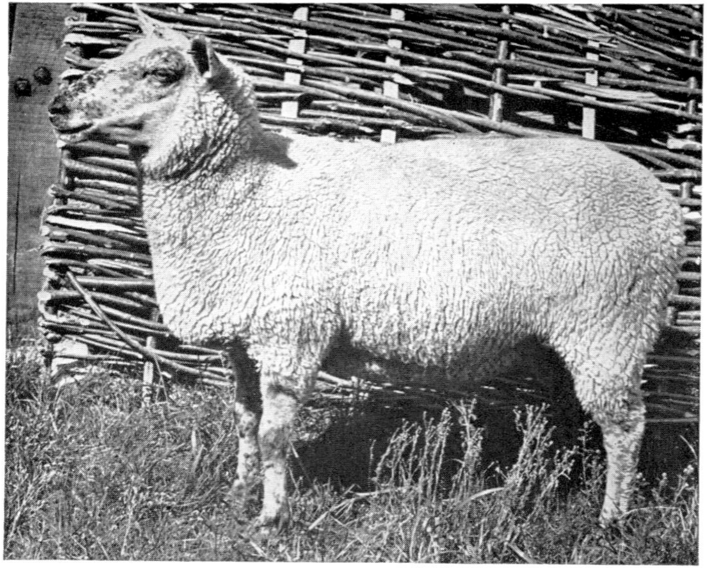

(above): A TC1 ewe : the first sheep to be sold in Britain under a brand name with no reference to the breeds in its pedigree.

(left): Dipping sheep, with a policeman looking on to see that the law is carried out. The Sheep Scab Order, 1938, is still held in reserve, though in England and Wales local authorities have not invoked it of recent years since the disappearance of the disease.

of 9 in. to 10 in. is adequate for mountain lambs while 12 in. to 14 in. is necessary for heavy lowland breeds.

'Sheep will only drink water which is absolutely clean, fresh and, above all, cold. Water that is only slightly fouled or warm will be rejected even to the point of death. The ideal is a supply running through a trough in the shed but this can seldom be achieved. The alternative is to have a trough continually being fed from a very slow running tap with a good overflow to an outside area. The trough should be so positioned as to cause the sheep to step up to drink as this helps to prevent fouling. A trough 1 ft. long is adequate for about 40 sheep.'

It is essential that sheep houses are very well ventilated, and ample use of Yorkshire boarding helps in this direction.

Where slatted floors are used, Mr. Williams recommends that the slats are laid parallel to the door openings. (*See also under* HOUSING OF ANIMALS.)

Traditional practice in the U.K. is described below.

The normal age for the first mating of female sheep is 19 months, at which age they are known as gimmers (north) or theaves (south). The first lamb is then dropped at two years of age. Lambs or tegs in forward condition will frequently take the ram, and conceive, at eight or nine months of age, and thus bear lambs when they are little more than a year old; but the drop of lambs produced in this way is small, and the development of the mothers is adversely affected. Ram lambs of the larger and earlier-maturing breeds are quite regularly used for breeding, although they must be allotted no more than about half the number of ewes allowed to mature sheep. The latter number varies from 30 or 40 on mountain grazings, where the ewes are widely scattered, to 60 as a normal and 80 or 90 as a maximum on enclosed land. Apart from Dorset Horns, which are peculiar, ewes of British breeds take the ram only during a particular part of the year, which varies from breed to breed, and according to the local climatic and food conditions. Hampshires will generally come on heat as early as July, while mountain ewes will begin to take the ram only in late October or in November. On arable land in the south, rams are actually put out as early as the middle of July, so that lambing may commence before Christmas, and be completed by the end of January. At the other extreme, the normal date to commence mating on blackface mountain grazings is November 22, so that the first lambs fall about the 18th of April. The practice in other flocks varies between these limits, being determined partly by the normal date of the advent of mild weather and spring growth, and partly by the amount of arable crops (roots, etc.) available as winter food. If ewes are in good thriving condition when put to the ram a majority will be tupped and will conceive within 3 or 4 weeks. After 6 weeks the rams are ordinarily withdrawn. Where provision is to be made for special care during the lambing season, a record is kept of the time of service of each ewe. This is accomplished by smearing the breast of the ram with colouring matter so that he may leave a mark on each ewe as she is served. At the end of generally each week, all the ewes that have been tupped are given a distinguishing mark, so that they can be separated out as they approach the end of their gestation period. The colour on the ram is changed after 15 days, and again after 30 days from the commencement of the mating period, in order that any recurrence of œstrum, in ewes that have been already tupped, may be noted. If any large proportion of ewes are seen to be marked with the second colour as well as with the first, another ram is procured as soon as possible. In large commercial flocks it is customary to run two or three rams, with a combined allotment of ewes, in one lot, so as to minimise the loss that would result if a particular ram should prove to be a non-breeder.

It is usual to 'flush' the ewes by feeding them, for a period of 2 or 3 weeks before they go to the ram, on specially nutritious and palatable food. (*See* FLUSHING, HORMONES.)

The feeding and management of the ewe flock during the winter period varies greatly according to conditions. The hardiest mountain breeds remain on the hill-sides, being, however, herded off any areas that are very high lying, or are liable to snow-drifting, during periods when severe weather seems probable. At the threat of severe storms the sheep are gathered to the lower ground in the vicinity of the homestead. No hand feeding was done except when, owing to the ground being covered with hard frozen snow, the sheep were unable to reach the natural herbage. Under such conditions, if they persist—it used to be argued—" hay

SHEEP BREEDING

must be fed, but the sheep are left to their own resources as long as possible. If hay feeding is commenced early the ewes cease to forage for themselves and, since the total quantity of hay that can be fed is very limited, feeding early in winter, and before real necessity arises, is not good practice."

On the other hand, work at the Hannah Dairy Research Institute has indicated the wisdom of hand feeding with starchy concentrates (rather than high protein or high roughage rations) to obviate the hill ewe burning up her own tissues in order to keep warm and alive during very cold weather. (*See under* Abortion.)

Lambing, etc.—On semi-arable farms the ewes run on pasture without any additional feeding, until perhaps the middle or end of December, after which time they receive a small but gradually increasing root ration—up to a maximum of 10 lb. A few weeks before lambing is due the ewes are given a ration of concentrates which is increased to about 1 lb. per day at lambing. The concentrates used may consist of oats, dried distillers' grains, cotton cake, peas, bran, etc., and a mixture of several materials is generally preferred. Good-quality silage may be fed —8 lb. before lambing, 12 lb. after. Dried grass is excellent.

On arable farms in the south where lambing occurs in winter, more intensive feeding is necessary, and it was usual to arrange for a succession of folding crops to cover the whole of the autumn and winter period—rape and white turnips followed by marrow-stem kale and swedes, with autumn-sown catch crops for early spring. Hay and often silage are also fed along with concentrates when winter pasturage becomes scanty.

Dipping is sometimes carried out in winter, generally at least a month before lambing is due to commence. Most flock-masters, however, prefer to dip in summer and again in autumn. (*See* Dipping.)

Mountain flocks were normally allowed to lamb on the hill, but lowland flocks are separated into batches, according to the date of service, and the batches are taken in succession to a well-sheltered lambing field where during the day they can be kept under supervision. At nights the ewes are confined within a lambing pen, consisting of a large central enclosure, which is kept well littered with straw, surrounded by a series of small pens into which the individual ewes are put as parturition commences. The regular shepherd and the temporary lambing man keep watch on alternate nights. A certain amount of redistribution of lambs has generally to be done, in order that all the ewes in milk may have at least one lamb and none more than two. Triplets are in some years quite frequent with certain breeds.

The 'crop' of lambs, which is generally estimated at the time of castration and docking (usually two or three weeks after the conclusion of lambing) varies greatly according to circumstances. Mountain flocks rarely give more than an average of one lamb per ewe, and eighty or ninety per hundred ewes is a fairly satisfactory average over a series of years. Lowland flocks may be expected to give from 130 to 160 lambs per 100 ewes, the last figure being exceeded in rare cases only, though 180 or 190 per 100 ewes is not unknown.

In the case of low-ground flocks, feeding of the ewes at and after lambing time must be fairly liberal, and must be continued until abundant pasture or a supply of spring forage crops becomes available. Where pasture forms the main summer food, the ewes are grouped, as far as the number of fields will allow, according to age and number of lambs, the two-year-old ewes with double lambs being given the best available pasture and older ewes with single lambs the poorest. Where much folding on arable forage crops is done, the lambs are allowed to run in front of the ewes, being given access to fresh sections of the field by means of open hurdles through which the ewes cannot pass. The ewes follow on to clean up what the lambs have not eaten. Where the lambs are intended for the fat market at an early age they begin to receive concentrated food soon after they are a month old. Normally the ewes are excluded from the enclosure that contains the feeding-boxes, as otherwise they are likely to become too fat. Where the ewes are being fattened off as well as the lambs they are of course fed together. Lambs will eat as much as ¼ lb. of mixed lamb food by the time they are six or seven weeks old and the quantity may be rapidly increased up to about a pound per day.

Clipping is carried out during May in the southern counties, early in June in upland semi-arable farms, and during July in mountain flocks. The date is determined by the natural 'rise' of the wool, which becomes apparent in a very few weeks after the advent of spring weather and abundant food. Non-breeding sheep are usually

SHEEP BREEDING

ready for the shears a week or 10 days before the milking ewes. In Britain only very early lambs are clipped during their first year of life. Summer dipping is ordinarily carried out 2 or 3 weeks after clipping, because at this stage, when there is just enough wool to carry the dip, parasites are most readily destroyed. A second dipping is given in the autumn. Lambs are weaned, with the exception of those to be sold fat off their dams, at 3½ to 4 months old. At weaning the ewes are transferred at once to the poorest available pasture in order to 'dry off' their flow of milk, while the lambs are transferred to the best and cleanest grass, or to fresh forage crops. On hill farms the lambs are kept enclosed while the ewes are herded out to the highest ground, and after the lapse of a week the whole flock is again thrown together. From June or July till September or October great numbers of lambs are sold by their breeders, and are purchased by other farmers for stock purposes or for fattening.

Drafting.—The next important business of the flockmaster is the culling and drafting of his ewe flock and its replenishment by young females (gimmers or theaves). In most flocks the ewes are drafted out at a fixed age, generally after having borne either three or four crops of lambs, and being therefore either 4½ or 5½ years old. Ewes so drafted, a majority of which will be still full in the mouth and healthy, generally go to form flying flocks on farms where permanent breeding stocks cannot be profitably maintained. Apart from the regular draft there will generally be a few among the younger ages that will have become unsatisfactory. These are sold separately, either fat or for fattening. The gimmers or theaves, which may either have been purchased or reared on the farm, join the flock after the draft has gone, the stock of rams is replenished if necessary, and everything is ready for the commencement of the next cycle of operations.

Fat Sheep.—In past times great numbers of sheep were kept until they were 3 or 4 years old before being fattened for the butcher. There are still to be found a few wether stocks, the animals being sold fat from the hills in autumn when they are 2½ years old. But the great majority of sheep, with the exception of such as have been used for breeding, now reach the butcher between the ages of 4 months and 2 years. Early lamb begins to come on the market in the South by April, and in the North by May. Wether lambs from the hills, weighing perhaps 40 to 50 lb. live weight, are generally available, in good seasons, from August onwards, and form at this season the supply of the choicest meat. The main autumn supplies consist of lambs of a great variety of breeds that after weaning have been folded on aftermaths, rape, and other catch crops, with generally an allowance, amounting to perhaps 1 per cent of the live weight daily, of cake and corn.

For winter fattening, roots form the basis of the ration. Hoggets or tegs (as lambs come to be called from the beginning of winter) may be folded on turnips for some time, but when folding has continued for a month or two (commonly during January) they begin to lose their temporary incisor teeth. When this occurs the roots require to be cut and fed in boxes. The change from grass or forage crops on to roots, particularly if the root ration is not restricted, is attended with a considerable amount of risk. Most flockmasters make the change as gradual as possible, either by folding the sheep for a gradually lengthening daily period, or by carting a limited amount of roots to the animals while still on pasture. A further difficulty arises if wet weather occurs, as the root land may then become very uncomfortable and the sheep become loaded with mud. This may involve temporary transference of the sheep back to pasture. Along with the roots it is usual to feed hay more or less *ad libitum*, the quantity consumed being usually small— ¼ to ½ lb. per 100 lb. live weight. To these are added a ration of cake, or grain, or both, which may vary from ¼ to 1 per cent of the live weight, depending on the rate of fattening that is desired. Tegs are, of course, still in active growth while being fattened and thus require a concentrate that is fairly rich in protein. Various oilseed cakes and dried distillers' grains are used when obtainable for younger sheep; apart from their general suitability, they are specially useful in the earlier part of the winter in counteracting the laxative tendency of the roots. Towards the end of the fattening process materials of higher energy value, such as flaked maize, linseed cake, etc., are generally added to the mixture.

Tegs of the mountain breeds do not adapt themselves readily to the process of winter fattening on roots. Hence those not fit for the fat market in autumn are often carried over the winter as stores, being fed largely on the winter pasturage of lowland farms. Ewe tegs destined to form part of mountain flocks are ordinarily dealt with in the same way. Ewe tegs of the lowland breeds, destined for the breeding flocks, are generally wintered with a certain amount of turnips and hay, but usually without cake or corn; in spring they are placed upon the poorer pastures, where they are joined by the ewes at weaning time.

The foregoing is no more than a very rough outline of the methods of sheep husbandry employed in Britain. There is great variation in methods from district to district, depending on the general system of farming—whether arable, semi-arable or pastoral—on the particular food materials that can be most economically produced, on the nature of the soil and climate, and on the special characteristics of the breed kept. For more detailed information the reader may be referred to Dr. Allan Fraser's *Sheep Husbandry* (Crosby, Lockwood & Son Ltd.).

(*See also under* STRESS *and* STOCKING RATES.)

SHEEPDOGS.—Sheepdogs are popularly regarded as exceptionally healthy, but a 1953 survey in Scotland showed that at least 11 per cent were suffering from Black Tongue (which see) as result of an inadequate diet. On average, this consisted basically of ½ lb. oatmeal, ½ lb. maize, and (by no means always) ½ pint of milk; the first two ingredients being made into a brose or mash by pouring on boiling water. The occasional rabbit, or piece of boiled mutton from a dead sheep, or—at lambing time—the afterbirths, were not sufficient to prevent Black Tongue.

Sheepdogs may walk or run 90 miles per day at lambing time and must have meat if stamina and health are to be maintained. Even fish-meal is of service—also dried blood—if meat or fish are unobtainable. (*See under* GID, RICKETS, *and* BLACK TONGUE.)

SHEEP DIPPING (*see* DIPS AND DIPPING).

SHEEP POX (*see* VARIOLA).

SHEEP SCAB.—This is the popular name for psoroptic mange, a Notifiable Disease in the U.K. (*See* PARASITES, p. 690.)

SHEEP, DISEASES OF (*see under* ABORTION; ACTINOBACILLOSIS; ANTHRAX; ARTHRITIS; BALANITIS; BLACK DISEASE; BLACK-QUARTER; BLINDNESS (*under* Eye, diseases of); BLOUWILDEBEESOOG; BLUE TONGUE; BORDER DISEASE; BRAXY; 'CAPPIE'; CASEOUS LYMPHADENITIS; ENTEQUE SECO; FOOT-AND-MOUTH DISEASE; FOOT ROT; GAS GANGRENE; HYPOMAGNESÆMIA; JAAGSIEKTE; JOHNE'S DISEASE; JOINT-ILL; LAMB DYSENTERY; LIVER FLUKE; LOUPING-ILL; MILK FEVER; MOREL'S DISEASE; OVINE EPIDIDIMYTIS; OVINE INTERDIGITAL DERMATITIS; PARASITES; NEMATODIRUS; 'PINING'; PNEUMONIA IN SHEEP; PREGNANCY TOXÆMIA; PULPY KIDNEY; 'REDFOOT'; 'RINGWOMB'; SCALD; SCRAPIE; SWAYBACK; TICKS; TOXOPLASMOSIS; UDDER, DISEASES OF; VISNA; 'YELLOWSES').

SHEEP, WINTER COATS FOR (*see* CLOTHING OF ANIMALS).

SHELTERS, NEED FOR (*see under* EXPOSURE; *also* STELL).

SHIGELLOSIS (*see* SLEEPY FOAL DISEASE on p. 343).

'SHIPPING FEVER'.—A disease of cattle caused by a virus or viruses. Secondary invaders (bacteria) may be involved. Immunisation has been tried using myxovirus parainfluenza-3 and *P. septica*, for example.

SHIVERING is a nervous disease of heavy horses chiefly, although it may also occur in light draught and saddle horses; it is characterised by spasmodic contractions of certain groups of muscles, particularly in the hind quarters and tail, although sometimes the muscles of the shoulder, neck, and head may be affected. It runs a slowly progressive course, and constitutes a definite unsoundness.

Cause—Heredity plays a part, for animals bred from mares or stallions thus affected usually show the condition when approaching maturity, or when adult.

Pathologically, there is found either a fibrosis of the nervous tissue of the spinal cord and sometimes an ankylosis of the vertebræ, similar to the ankylosis of ringbone, and according to some identical with the effects of articular rheumatism in man. These changes produce pressure on those motor nerve-cells or fibres associated with the control of the skeletal muscles. It may follow strangles, influenza, etc., when it is partly due to the action of the toxins.

Symptoms.—In the early stages it is often very difficult to detect shivering. In a well-marked case, the muscles of the hind quarters are seen to quiver or tremble when the horse is made to back, a process often difficult and occasionally impossible. At the same time, the tail is usually elevated and also shows the quivering movements. In advanced cases it may be difficult or impossible to pick up either of the hind feet, and shoeing is only accomplished with difficulty in stocks; occasionally only by casting the animal. When the hind-limb is raised from the ground during backing, in many cases it also quivers, or 'shivers', and in some instances one or both of the fore-limbs, or the muscles of the fore-quarter, exhibit the same feature. In time, horses become less fit for their work; hunters fail to jump as well as previously, draught horses cannot be made to back a load, though they may be quite able to pull straight forwards, and lying or rising from the ground becomes an ever increasingly difficult procedure.

Many methods are in vogue to exaggerate the shivering movements for purposes of diagnosis, among which the following are perhaps the most reliable and efficient: backing the horse as forcibly as possible over rough ground, cobblestones, etc.; turning the horse round in small circles; moving it from side to side in the stall. A repeated tendency in a good jumping hunter to strike with the hind legs when crossing an obstacle should be looked upon as suspicious of the commencement of shivering.

As a rule, shivering tends to become worse and worse with work, but rest and a run at grass results in improvement in most cases, though a complete recovery is rare. In some cases, regular, steady, slow work can be carried out for years without any appreciable increase in severity of the symptoms of shivering, but such horses are unfit for prolonged or strenuous work, and are liable at almost any time to develop signs of paralysis of the hind quarters, especially when they lie for a time after hard work.

Shivering in the dog may occur, especially in fox-terriers, for no apparent reason and may be unconnected either with cold or fear. At the prospect of a walk the dog may suddenly cease trembling.

SHOCK is the condition of collapse which may follow severe injury, surgical operations, excessive hæmorrhage, and other conditions that produce a deep impression upon the nervous system. Shock is essentially an abrupt fall in blood pressure; or acute hypotension, as it is technically called. The animal must be given a blood transfusion, plasma, stimulants such as coramine, or adrenalin. (*See* COLLAPSE, DEXTRAN, ARTIFICIAL. HIBERNATION.)

SHOE-GALL (*see* CAPPED ELBOW).

SHOEING OF CATTLE.—This may be undertaken to reduce weight bearing on an injured claw, especially where there is a fracture of a phalanx.

SHOEING OF HORSES.—From very early times horses used by man for working purposes have been shod with some form of iron shoe. It appears probable that previous to the use of an iron shoe the horse was shod with pads of straw, or with shoes made from the stout hides of wild animals, and to this day both these kinds of shoes are used by some races in the East. The early iron shoes were made in the form of a plate, in the middle of which a hole was cut, and this was held on by three nails on either side. A similar shoe is still used by Arabs and other nomadic races in Asia. The hole in the middle being to allow sand to escape, was found necessary to prevent collections of

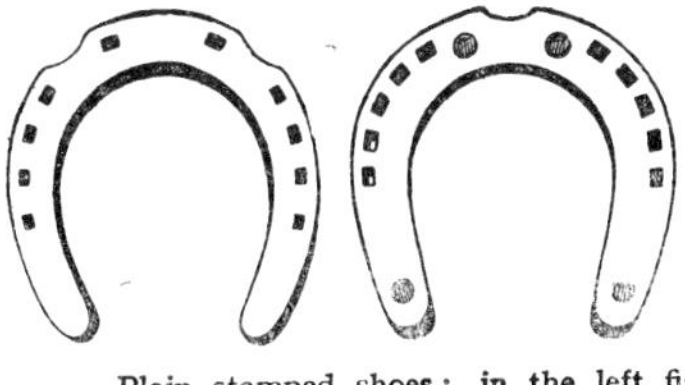

Plain stamped shoes; **in the left figure** there are two side-clips and two toe-nails, in the right figure there is one toe-clip, and holes have been drilled at toes and heels for screw-shanked frost studs.

sand from accumulating between the shoe and the sole of the foot. In later years, the shoe was made as a narrow rim of iron nailed round the lower edge of the wall by small nails, and, with modifications, this is the form which has become universal.

Objects of shoeing.—Horses are shod to prevent undue wear of the foot when working upon surfaces which, otherwise, would tend to reduce the foot by friction to the extent where lameness would occur.

Shoes are also necessary to prevent the wall from cracking and splitting, to afford the horse a better grip upon slippery surfaces, and to reduce a certain amount of the concussion which the foot would have to sustain were no shoes used. Some people look upon shoeing as a necessary evil; there is, however, no reason why it should be an evil at all if the feet are well cared for, well prepared, and the shoes are well made, fitted, and nailed.

Essentials of shoeing.—The essentials of a well-shod foot are: that the shoe shall be suitable for the purpose for which it is intended; that the foot shall be reduced to a proper bearing surface; that the shoe shall rest upon the bearing surface all the way round; that the outline of the wall shall be followed by the shoe without being wide or close, except at the heels where the shoe may be wider than the foot with some advantage; that the shoe shall be strong enough to last for a month, but not heavy enough to tire the horse unduly; that only a sufficient number of nails be used to keep the shoe in position, and that each nail shall be so driven that its point emerges from the wall at a proper height, and is clenched so that it obtains a proper hold; and that the toe-clip or quarter-clips are so made that they only require the removal of a minimum amount of wall below them, and while strong enough to prevent the shoe from shifting on the foot, are not unduly high, pointed, or coarse. Other important essentials are that the outer surface of the wall shall be untouched, except for the making of the 'beds' for the clenches, and that the sole and frog shall not be pared away with the knife.

Preparing the foot.—The growth of horn that has occurred since the last shoeing must be reduced in the first place. For this the toeing-knife, drawing-knife, and rasp are used. The wall must be reduced so that it remains level all round the foot, as much being taken from one side as the other, and the toes and heels of the foot being so reduced that the balance of the foot is preserved. The proper bearing surface for the shoe consists of the wall, the horn of the white line, and a margin of about $\frac{1}{16}$ of an inch of the outer part of the sole, all of which must be brought to the same level. Loose or overgrown portions of the frog and sole only are removed; there should be no endeavour made to increase the arch of the sole, or to reduce the frog so that it will not come into contact with the ground. (*See* FOOT OF HORSE.) The bars should not be cut away, nor should the connection between wall and bars (at the buttresses) be severed.

Preparing the shoe.—A suitable length of bar-iron (usually measured by adding the length of the foot to its width) is cut off and heated in the fire at its middle portion. It is then bent into a form like the capital letter '**V**'. Each branch is then heated respectively, and turned by hammering over the beak of the anvil. Next, the whole shoe is heated, and a groove or 'fuller' cut in the ground surface by the fullering iron. The fuller allows the heads of the nails to be slightly counter-sunk below the surface of the shoe, and gives the horse an extra grip on slippery surfaces, as well as tending to prevent the shoe from being sucked loose, or even coming off, when the horse travels over wet clay land. The nail-holes are next stamped in the depths of the fuller at the toes and quarters (nail-holes are only put in the heels for surgical purposes or in special shoes). The toe-clip is next drawn, and quarter-clips for the hind feet if necessary, usually on the outside quarter only. Thereafter, if calkins are used they are turned down from each heel, and if a toe-piece is desired it is welded across the toe of the shoe. After each of the nail-holes has been squared up with the pritchel, both from the ground surface (pritchelling) and from the foot surface (back-pritchelling), the shoe is ready to be fitted to the prepared foot. The pritchel is driven into the nail-hole at the outside toe (usually), and the shoe is carried to the foot. It has been brought to a dull red heat, and is held in position long enough to allow it to burn a slight bed for itself, and to ensure that it is a good fit all round. Any necessary adjustments are made, and the shoe is then taken to the cooler and cooled by being plunged repeatedly into cold water or oil. This sets the surface iron, and makes a harder shell, as well as rendering the shoe cool enough to be nailed on.

Nailing consists of driving one of the toe-nails firstly, wrenching off its tip after emergence from the wall, and then the opposite heel-nail follows. If the shoe shifts on the foot, as the result of driving the first nail, it must be tapped back into position before the second nail is driven. Thereafter the nails are put in, first on one side and then on the other.

When all have been driven the closed jaws of the pincers are put against the end of the nail on the wall, and the head is driven well home into the nail-hole. This causes the clench to turn over slightly. A small portion of horn is next removed from under each clench, to form the 'bed' for the clench, and with the closed jaws of the pincers against the head of the nail, the clench is properly turned over by the hammer. Finally, the edge of the rasp is rubbed round the junction between the lower border of the horn and the shoe, so as to form a slight groove, which prevents the edge of the wall from splitting, and shoeing is complete. (For further details works on shoeing must be consulted.)

SHOOTING (*see under* DESTRUCTION OF ANIMALS and EUTHANASIA).

SHORT-SIGHTEDNESS is a condition in which objects near at hand are seen easily, but those at any distance cannot be appreciated. The condition is technically known as 'myopia', and with the exception of certain sporting dogs and horses it is of little consequence among animals. Sometimes greyhounds are encountered which have great difficulty in seeing their quarry until they are quite close to it.

SHOULDER is the joint formed between the shoulder-blade or scapula and the upper end of the humerus. It is one of the typical 'ball-and-socket' joints of the body, which allows play in all directions, outwards, inwards, backwards, and forwards. The rounded head of the humerus fits into a more or less corresponding concavity on the lower end of the scapula, which is called the 'glenoid cavity'. The tendons of the biceps cross the shoulder, originating from an attachment above and towards the front of the joint called the tuberosity of the scapula, and, passing downwards through two deep grooves, merge into the fleshy belly of the muscle. Just to the outside and slightly behind the grooves for the biceps tendon there is a projection from the head of the humerus, called the 'external tuberosity of the humerus', which can easily be felt in the living animal, and which is called the 'point of the shoulder'. This forms an important landmark concerning the situation of the joint cavity, which is just above and slightly inside the projection. The joint is surrounded by a loose joint-capsule, which is strengthened at some parts by ligamentous tissue, but the main strength is derived from the massive muscles that run from the fore-arm to the scapula and the trunk. In spite of this fact, it is liable to dislocation, especially in young horses that are not in the best of condition. (*See* DISLOCATIONS.)

SHOULDER-BLADE (*see* SCAPULA).

SHOULDER-GALLS and SHOULDER TUMOURS are in most cases directly due to badly fitting collars in horses. When a horse wears a collar which is too large for it, at each step one or other shoulder tends to slip within the collar, and if this goes on for any length of time, the skin over the shoulder-joint, or sometimes over the spine of the scapula, becomes chafed and raw. This constitutes a so-called shoulder-gall. With palliative treatment, and with rest from friction with the collar, wearing breast harness if necessary, most simple chafes will heal. In a number of cases, however, the raw area becomes infected with the micrococcus *Botriomyces ascoformans*, the cause of botriomycosis. This gradually develops into a hard fibrous tumour-like swelling, which inter-

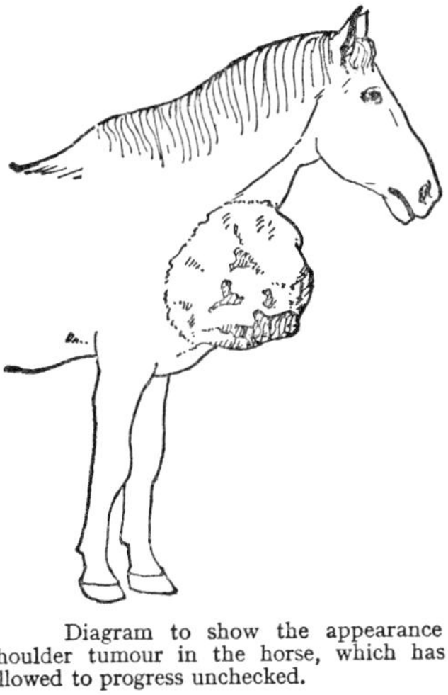

Diagram to show the appearance of a shoulder tumour in the horse, which has been allowed to progress unchecked.

feres with the work of the horse. (*See* BOTRIOMYCOSIS.)

SHOVEL BEAK.—A disease occurring in intensively reared chicks fed dry mash. It affects usually birds of 2 to 8 weeks old. The upper or lower beak (or both) may be deformed, with ulceration or necrosis. Infection with *Fusiformis necrophorus*, *Staphylococcus aureus*, or *Clostridium welchii* follows.

SHYING (*see* BOLTING).

SIALOGOGUES (σίαλον, saliva; ἄγω, I draw) are substances which produce a copious flow of saliva, *e.g.* pilocarpine and arecoline.

SICKNESS (*see* VOMITING).

SIDEBONES.—Ossification of the lateral cartilages of the horse's foot. (*See* LATERAL CARTILAGES.) When this occurs in a young animal it is looked upon as an unsoundness, not so much because of the immediate lameness and trouble it causes, but rather because it indicates a tendency towards new bone formation, which, when it occurs in other parts of the foot, is very much more serious. In old horses, all cartilages, not only in the foot, tend to become ossified as an almost natural course of events, and sidebones are accordingly not looked upon as so serious.

Causes.—Heredity is considered as a predisposing cause, but in many instances no such relationship can be shown. It has been suggested that a vitamin D deficiency in foalhood may be partly responsible. Concussion, such as is occasioned by work on hard streets when the foot carries a shoe which prevents normal frog-pressure, or when due to treads or other injuries on the coronets, may be an exciting cause. In other cases, sidebones appear to develop without any external cause, and, moreover, without any external signs of their formation. (*See* FOOT OF HORSE.)

Symptoms.—Ordinarily, the upper part of each cartilage can be felt at the coronet as a flexible ridge or edge, lying immediately below the skin, but when the cartilage has ossified, this ridge is no longer flexible, and is more or less thickened as well. In some instances the ossified cartilage assumes enormous proportions, and can be easily seen when the feet are viewed from the front. The condition is more common by far in the fore limbs, and may occur on the outside or inside, or in both places, on one or both of the fore feet. As a rule, when due to external injury there is only one sidebone at the seat of the injury, while when due to other causes the sidebones are often present in bilaterally symmetrical positions.

When sidebones have formed, there is no lameness, pain, heat, or other signs of inflammation, but when forming, there may be pain over the quarters involved, and lameness may be present. In contracted narrow feet, especially where the frog is of small size, there may be more or less permanent stiffness, due to the pressure exerted by the bony formation upon the soft sensitive tissues of the quarters. In the more severe cases, such as this latter, lameness may occur. It is usually characterised by the taking of a shorter step by the affected foot, and the tendency to do this may result in a peculiar short and long step. Pain is shown when the quarters are tapped by a hammer, or when the cartilages are firmly pressed from above.

Treatment.—As a rule, in horses with wide open feet and well-developed frogs, no treatment is required. The sidebone does not interfere with slow work of a regular nature, and many hundreds of heavy draught horses thus affected work every day without showing the slightest inconvenience. When the hoof is narrow and contracted the horse should be shod with a bar or round shoe, so that as much frog pressure as possible may be ensured, or if this does not result in any improvement, a rubber bar-pad should be worn with a shortened shoe. Easing the bearing under the sidebone, or fitting with a 'set-heeled' shoe, may assist during the stage when the sidebone is causing lameness. The operation of grooving, or hoof-section, may be necessary in cases where the contraction of the heels is so great that no relief accrues from the methods given above.

In those forms of sidebone complicated with ringbone, which are common when the horse is old and has led an active life on hard streets, the lameness is most often only ameliorated by the operation of median neurectomy. This operation, as also hoof-section, should only be undertaken with the horse under a general anæsthetic. (*See also* RINGBONES.)

SIDE-EFFECTS.—The side-effects of a drug are those produced in addition to that for which purpose the drug is given. Examples: deafness in humans following the administration of streptomycin, moniliasis after the use of aureomycin, aplastic anæmia after the use of chloramphenicol.

SILAGE, or ensilage, is a succulent food varying in quality according to the crops from which it was made, and the stage of growth at which these were cut.

Dr. H. Ian Moore has classified silage in three groups: Grade I containing 15 per cent and over crude protein, and made from young grasses—none in flower; clover, lucerne, or sainfoin in bud stage. Grade II containing 12 to 14·9 per cent crude protein, and made from grasses in their flowering stage, late autumn grass, clover passed full flower, marrow stem kale, pea pods, cereal-legume crops cut when cereal is 'milky'. Grade III containing less than 12 per cent crude protein, and made from seeding grasses, stemmy clover, maize, pea haulm and pods, sugar-beet tops, potatoes.

Grade I makes a substitute for cake, whereas Grade III is good enough only as a substitute for roots, straw, or low-grade hay.

Ensilage involves a fermentation process, in which the carbohydrates of the grass or other crop are broken down to carbon dioxide and organic acids; the proteins to amino-acids. Lactic, acetic and butyric acids are produced. In good silage, lactic acid predominates. Silage with a high butyric-acid content must be fed with caution, and may be recognised by its unpleasant smell and lighter colour—yellowish-green instead of dark brown.

The Dorset Wedge system of silage-making has enabled better quality to be achieved.

When silage is of good quality, and when the general management of the animals is good and their concentrates adequate, both fattening bullocks and dairy cows do well upon silage, maintain their condition, settle well, and give as good production results as on other forms of feeding.

Good silage alone can give daily live-weight gains of over 2 lb. with yearling cattle, and such results could be enhanced by using late-maturing crosses and bulls, which Mr. F. Raymond suggested should have a place in the EEC-orientated 1970s. Yearling cattle fed a ration of two-thirds silage and one-third dried grass have gained 2.2 lb. a day in several experiments. Over 2½ lb. per day liveweight gain has been achieved with steers fed on a diet comprising maize silage, urea, and dried lucerne.

Work at Hurley has not revealed any single factor which appears to account for the low intake of many of 90 silages. Consumer resistance, if one may apply this term to cows, was evident with silages of a low pH, probably due to the high acid content; whereas with those of a high pH the limiting factor was apparently protein breakdown.

Acetonæmia is often seen in cattle receiving large quantities of silage of low quality. Hay should be made available as well; also 2 oz. per head of bone flour with salt added.

When self-feeding of silage is practised, care must be taken that conditions underfoot do not become dirty and slushy to an extent where softening of the horn of the hoof occurs and foot troubles develop.

Silage must be free of ragwort. (*See under* RAGWORT POISONING.)

'SILENT HEAT' (*see under* INFERTILITY).

SILICONE SOLUTION.—An anti-coagulation solution used in connection with blood transfusion apparatus and syringes to prevent clotting.

SILVER SALTS are used in medicine both externally and internally. The chief salts are: the nitrate, which is a caustic when used concentrated, and an astringent in weak solutions; the proteinate, which is a compound of an albuminous substance with silver, also called 'protargol', and 'silver protein', and which has the advantage over the nitrate that it does not precipitate albumin; and in addition to these, there are other preparations that are less used, such as colloidal silver or collargol and argyrol. These may be solid, liquid, or ointments.

When given internally in large doses, silver salts act as irritant poisons, producing inflammation of the walls of any organ with which they come into contact, coagulating the protoplasm and causing sloughing. Externally, the chief uses are in the repressive treatment of warts, exuberant granulations, ulcers, and other diseased conditions where a caustic stimulant is required; in the treatment of corneal ulcers of the eye, when one of the protein compounds is most useful.

SIMMENTAL.—A dual-purpose breed of Swiss cattle, now to be found throughout Europe and in the U.S.A. In Germany the Simmental has been developed with emphasis on beef production.

SINUS (*sinus*, a hollow) is a term applied to narrow hollow cavities of various kinds, occurring naturally in the body, or produced as the consequence of disease. Thus the word is used to indicate the air-containing cavities which are found in the skull, and which communicate with the

SINUSES, DISEASES OF THE

nose. (*See* Sinuses of the Skull.) The term is also applied to dilatations of the venous system of the brain which provide for a free exit of the blood from this vital organ, and which in most animals are connected with similar sinuses in the base of the skull. There are also lactiferous or milk sinuses at the bases of the teats (*see* Milk Sinus); renal sinuses in the kidney; and urogenital sinuses. (*See also* Skull, Teeth, Fistula, etc.) In pathology, 'sinus' refers to a blind infected tract.

SINUSES, DISEASES OF THE.—The sinuses of the head are placed in a somewhat sheltered position, and as a consequence are not very frequently the seat of disease. They are lined with a membrane which is continuous with that of the nasal cavities, and which acts as a periosteal covering for the bone. As a result, when there is inflammation of the nasal mucous membrane there is a likelihood that it may spread to the lining of the sinuses.

DROPSY OF THE SINUSES.—In this condition a serous fluid exudate fills one or more sinuses. It is generally due to a general lack of tone in the whole body, or to a weak heart. It demands surgical methods for its elimination or cure, an opening being made on to the surface of the head by which the fluid is drained.

TUMOUR FORMATION. — Symptoms.— Little or nothing may be seen until the tumour has attained to a considerable size, and then the bone over the seat of the growth commences to bulge outwards. At the same time there appears a purulent discharge from one or both nostrils, according to whether one or both sides of the head is affected. On tapping over the swelling a dull sound similar to that given out by a muscle is emitted, instead of the normal resonant drum-like sound that should be obtained. When the condition is very bad there may be some interference with respiration. The tumour invades the tissues between the sinus and the nose, and partially or wholly obstructs the passage of air through the nasal passages. In other cases the bone itself becomes invaded by the tumour, and may become so soft as to yield to pressure by the fingers.

Treatment.—This is purely surgical, and depends upon the extent and variety of the tumour growth.

EMPYEMA OF THE SINUSES.—This is a condition in which the sinuses contain pus and in a number of cases blood. The mucous membranes are thickened and inflamed, and are frequently covered with granulations or growths of 'proud flesh'.

Causes.—The causes are varied. In the horse the cause of a collection of pus in a

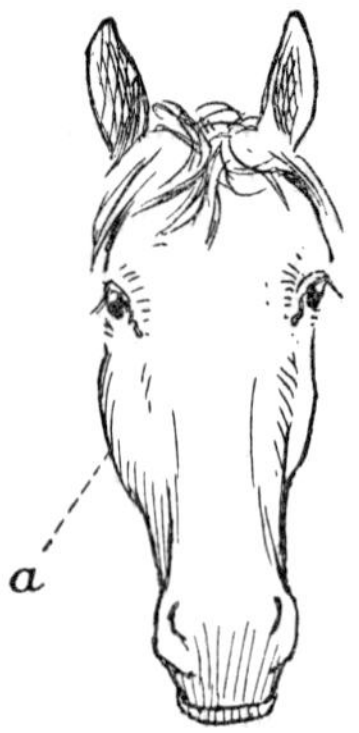

Diagram of a horse's head affected with suppuration in the right maxillary sinus, the result of inflammation of the roots of the upper cheek teeth. The bulging of the side of the face is seen at *a*.

sinus is often a diseased tooth, the root of which has suppurated and the pus burrowed through the thin plate of bone that separates the tooth socket from the sinus cavity. The pus in the sinus infects the membrane, and this in turn suppurates and produces more pus. In other cases, the pus is the result of a penetrating injury from the outside, such as is occasioned by a blow on the forehead which fractures the external plate of bone and allows the ingress of infection. Gunshot wounds are also a cause of pus in the sinuses, the pus not generally appearing for some time after the infliction of the injury. Animals living near the seashore or in sandy and windy localities are sometimes afflicted with collections of fine sand in the sinuses which have been inhaled and has settled in the lower parts of the cavity. The sand irritates the delicate membrane and pus is consequently formed. In sheep, and sometimes in the horse, sheep nostril fly larvæ of the *Œstrus* family may be found in the sinuses, and are generally associated with pus formation. In dogs especially, but also in other animals, tumour formation is often accompanied by the presence of pus in the sinuses, and in these animals a parasite called *Linguatula tænioides* sometimes affects the sinuses with the production of pus.

Symptoms.—The most prominent sign of the presence of any amount of pus in the sinuses is the usually slight, but continual, dribbling of discharge from one or both nostrils. This discharge is usually more marked when the animal lowers its head than otherwise. Horses or cattle feeding from the ground frequently contaminate their food with the discharge, and if fed from a low manger quantities collect in this, and are easily seen when the feed is done. If the peculiar odour of a diseased tooth is present, the cause of the trouble is most probably in the roots of one or other of the cheek teeth, and the animal has difficulty in chewing. The lymph glands on the same side of the head as the discharge are found to be swollen and painful to the touch. In cattle the purulent discharge is generally blood-stained, and may irritate the nasal membrane so as to cause some amount of sneezing. When the frontal sinus in any animal is affected there are often signs of giddiness, especially when the animal is made to turn round in a small circle. The head may be carried to one side, generally with the diseased side lower than the other. Only in long-standing cases is there any sign of thinning or bulging of the outer wall of the sinus, and then there is generally a complication by tumour formation.

Treatment.—This consists of opening the diseased sinus by trephining the bone over the surface, and irrigation and evacuation of the cavity. Penicillin or the sulphonamides may be indicated. The openings are made so that drainage from the interior is not interfered with, and no places are allowed to collect little pockets of pus. Where much pus or other débris is present, its removal by enzymes (*see* STREPTODORNASE) will facilitate treatment. When a tooth has been the primary cause of the condition it is extracted, and its cavity temporarily plugged with gauze until healthy tissue fills up the space between the tooth socket and the sinus. Parasitic inhabitants are removed, either by the injection of fluids that will kill them, or by picking each out separately with forceps. Chloroforming the animal will often kill such parasites, but is attended with some risks of suffocation if they are numerous.

SPECIFIC INFECTIONS.—In a horse that is suffering from strangles or glanders it sometimes happens that the infection reaches the sinuses by way of the membranes of the nose, and they become filled with purulent, yellowish or straw-coloured discharges due to the disease in question. In actinomycosis and botriomycosis affecting the head the sinuses are occasionally affected, and in such cases contain tumorous swellings similar to those characteristic of these diseases occurring in other parts. (*See under the respective headings.*)

SINUSES OF THE SKULL, also called the PARANASAL SINUSES, are directly or indirectly connected with the nose. There are four pairs: (1) maxillary; (2) frontal; (3) spheno-palatine, or sphenoid; (4) ethmoidal.

Horse.—(1) *The maxillary sinus* is the largest; it is situated on the side of the head immediately above the last three cheek teeth in the upper jaw. It is roughly quadrilateral in shape, its anterior wall corresponding to a line drawn from just anterior to the end of the facial ridge across towards the inner angle of the opposite eye, its posterior wall being the bony orbit of the eye; its lower wall is formed by the roots of the last three teeth; and its medial wall is along a line drawn from the inner angle of the eye on the same side of the head to the corner of the nostril. These lines are not always absolutely correct, as the extent of the sinus varies in animals of different breeds and even in animals of the same breed. Its cavity is divided into two parts by a line running in an upward and backward direction from about the anterior edge of the second last cheek tooth of the upper jaw. In the posterior part are two openings; the more posterior of these opens into the frontal sinus, while the other opens into the nasal cavity. Air is thus able to circulate from the nose into the sinuses, and discharges from the sinuses can escape into the nasal cavity and so to the outside.

(2) *The frontal sinus* lies between the eye of the same side and the median plane of the skull. It extends forwards an inch or so anterior to a line drawn between the anterior margins of the orbits of the eyes, and back to a plane joining the joints of the mandible with the temporal bone. Its lateral boundary is the bone forming the inner wall of the bony orbit of the eye, while in the centre line of the skull it is divided from its fellow-sinus of the opposite side by a complete septum or division. It communicates with the posterior part of the maxillary sinus, and receives air from the nose by this communication.

(3) *The spheno-palatine sinus* lies in the foremost part of the body of the sphenoid bone and in the posterior part of the

palatine bone. It communicates with the maxillary sinus.

(4) *The ethmoidal sinus* lies in the cavity of the ethmoid bone and in the posterior part of the upper turbinal bone. It also communicates with the maxillary sinus.

Ox.—(1) *The maxillary sinus* differs from that of the horse in that it is not divided and it extends slightly farther forwards. The floor of the cavity is irregular, and has the roots of the last three or four cheek teeth projecting into it.

(2) *The frontal sinus* is the largest in the ox and in the horned breeds of sheep. It extends almost completely over the forehead from the level of the eyes backwards and well into the horn cores when these are present. The cavity is very irregular, being divided and subdivided by numerous ridges and plates of bone. The openings are into the ethmoidal sinus and from there into the upper part of the cavity of the nose. This latter fact is of some importance, because, when an animal breaks its horn, the hæmorrhage appears at the nostril of the same side, the blood having flowed down through the frontal sinus into the back of the nasal passage.

(3) *The palatine and the sphenoidal sinuses* are separate in the ox. The palatine is excavated in the hard palate, and the sphenoidal is situated in the sphenoid bone; the former communicates with the maxillary but the latter does not.

Pig.—(1) *The maxillary sinus* is a small sinus situated over the side of the face and does not communicate with the frontal, but has a large irregular orifice leading into the nose.

(2) *The frontal sinus* is a huge excavation involving all the front of the face and reaching back over the cranium, as well as down on to the nose. The sinus is divided into a number of compartments by irregular septa.

(3) *The sphenoidal sinus* is also large, involving the body and the various processes of the sphenoid bone.

Dog.—(1) *The maxillary sinus* is small and in such free communication with the nose that it is often regarded as a recess of the latter rather than an actual sinus.

(2) *The frontal sinus* is of considerable size in the larger breeds of dogs, but in the smaller toy varieties it is small. It is always confined to the frontal bone, and is generally divided into a small anterior and a large posterior part.

SINUSITIS (*see under* SINUSES).

SINUSITIS, INFECTIOUS.—This is common in turkeys, and also in game birds. In turkeys it is sometimes a sequel to de-beaking. The cause is infection with P.P.L.O. organisms, which also cause Chronic Respiratory Disease in chickens. Symptoms include a swelling below the eyes, and sneezing. Treatment may consist of surgically draining the infra-orbital sinus and using antibiotics. Birds which recover often remain 'carriers' for a time.

Infectious Sinusitis in pheasants and partridges may be confused with 'Gapes', Fowl-Pox, Newcastle Disease, nutritional roup caused by vitamin A deficiency, aspergillosis, and perhaps with pasteurellosis. In artificially reared poults, the disease occurs mainly between 2 and 8 weeks of age. Mortality may be as high as 90 per cent.

SITFASTS (*see* SADDLE-GALLS).

SKELETON (σκελετός, dried up).—(*See* BONE, CARTILAGE, SKULL.)

SKIM MILK.—This is a valuable food, retaining, as it does, the solids-not-fat after most of the fat has been removed. These solids include the valuable milk-protein, the sugar lactose, valuable minerals, and vitamins of the B group. It is poor in the fat-soluble vitamins A and D; and also in vitamin E; and if given along with cod-liver oil to beef stores, may lead to cod-liver oil poisoning or muscular dystrophy (which see).

Skim milk is a useful food for pigs, but is not suitable on its own. It can be fed *ad lib.* to suckling pigs; weaners may receive 5 pints per day; fatteners from 14 weeks to slaughter, about 6 pints.

Skim milk is, if from infected cattle, a source of tuberculosis in pigs, and pasteurisation may be desirable in many countries.

For sows and piglets, skim milk should be fresh or completely sour; 0·1 per cent formalin is sometimes added to skim milk for fattening pigs.

SKIN is the protective covering of the body, and is continuous at the natural openings with the mucous membranes. It consists of two layers, which differ entirely in structure and origin. The outermost of these is the *epidermis, cuticle,* *scarf-skin*, or *epithelium*, which is formed from the outermost layer of the embryo; and the second is the *corium*, *cutis vera*, *true skin*, or *dermis*, which is a fibrous and vascular layer developed from the middle layer of the embryo.

The epidermis.—This is a cellular layer of non-vascular, stratified epithelium of varying thickness, covering the outer surface of the body, which presents the openings of the cutaneous glands and of the hair follicles. In animals it is divisible into two layers, the outer, hard, dry *stratum corneum*, and the deeper, softer, moist *stratum germinativum*. The cells of the latter are pigmented, and by their growth compensate for the loss by exfoliation or shedding of the surface cells from the stratum corneum, which forms the scurfy deposit upon an ungroomed horse. This inner layer consists of the part of the skin which is living, and is formed by several layers of cells set upon the corium and nourished by it. The cells continually multiply, and are slowly pushed upwards to replace the constant wear and tear which occurs on the cells at the surface. There are no blood-vessels in the epidermis, but there is a ramification of the surface sensory nerves which supply the skin with its delicate sense of perception. A *blister* is a collection of fluid separating the stratum corneum from the stratum germinativum.

The corium.—This consists essentially of a feltwork of fibrous tissue and elastic fibres. It is very vascular, contains the hair follicles, the sudoriferous (or sweat) glands, and the sebaceous glands, as well as a certain amount of involuntary muscle. The most superficial part is known as the *corpus papillare*, on account of the presence of numbers of tiny papillæ, which are received into corresponding depressions in the epidermis. These papillæ contain loops of blood-vessels, which nourish the epidermal cells, and numerous sensory nerves, which act as tactile organs, affording sensations of touch, pain, temperature, etc. The papillæ are most numerous wherever the skin is thin and sparsely covered with hair, *i.e.* on the lips, eyelids, vulva, anus, scrotum, etc. The true skin also carries the hairs, which penetrate the epidermis to appear on the surface of the skin, and the sweat and sebaceous glands, which have ducts which open into the hair follicles in the case of the sebaceous glands (except on the anus, vulva, lips, etc.), or on to the surface of the skin in the case of the sweat glands. These glands are situated partly in the deeper parts of the corium, known as the *tunica propria*, and partly below it in the layer of subcutaneous fibro-fatty tissue. In this deepest layer, which forms the bulk of the skin, or lying in the deeper part of the corium, there are certain tactile bodies, known as *Pacinian corpuscles*. The fibrous tissue of the skin consists of interlacing bundles of white fibrous tissue which form a dense feltwork. Here and there elastic fibres are mixed with them, and these serve to give the skin its pliability, and at the same time keep it in place and stretched reasonably tightly.

Hair.—Practically the whole of the body of each domesticated animal is covered by hair, except in the pig. Portions of the skin which appear to be bare are found on close inspection to be covered with very fine hair of delicate texture. The hairs are constantly being shed and replaced by others, while at certain periods of the year in the horse, and to a less extent in the other animals, they are cast off in great numbers, and constitute the 'shedding' or 'casting of the coat'. This normally occurs twice a year, once in the autumn, when it is more marked, and again in the spring with the first warm weather of the year.

Hairs are of several kinds: in the first place there are the ordinary hairs which, on account of the small amount of pigment that each carries, give the coat its characteristic colour; and there are different kinds of special hairs. Among these ordinary hairs scattered over almost the whole body are: *tactile hairs* of the lips, nostrils, and eyes; *cilia*, or *eyelashes*, growing from the free rim of the eyelids; *tragi*, in the external ear; and *vibrissæ*, round the nostrils. In addition to the ordinary and tactile hairs, certain regions carry specially long and coarse hairs, such as the mane (*juba*), the forelock or foretop (*cirrus capitis*), the tail, where the hairs (*cirrus caudæ*) are very large and long, and the 'feather' of the fetlocks and cannons (*cirrus pedis*), which gave the name to this region (fetlock=feet-lock—a lock of hair on the foot).

Each hair has a shaft, the part above the surface, and a root, embedded in the hair follicle. Below this is a little fibrous papilla possessing blood-vessels, which is capped by the expanded end of the hair root, and known as the hair bulb. The follicles are set somewhat obliquely in the corium, and at varying depths; the long tactile hairs reaching down to the underlying muscle. Most of the follicles have little bands of plain muscle attached to one side, known as the *arrectores pilorum*; these serve to erect the hairs during anger, fear, or extreme cold, and also to express from the sebaceous gland a small portion of sebaceous secretion. The follicles of the tactile hairs possess remarkably thick walls, which contain little blood-sinuses between their outer and inner coats, and surrounding these are the branching fibres of tactile nerves. In the herbivora these sinuses are crossed by little trabeculæ which give the sinus the appearance of erectile tissue.

Glands of the skin are of two kinds: sweat and sebaceous. The former are scattered over the body in nearly all animals, being most numerous in the horse, and least in the dog, where the largest are found only on the pads of the feet. Each sweat or sudoriferous gland consists of a long tube, usually greatly coiled in its inner part, which has a duct leading up to the surface of the skin. A watery fluid secretion is produced, in which there are quantities of waste material, salts, and excess water. (*See* PERSPIRATION.)

The sebaceous glands, except in certain places, open into the follicles of the hairs a little way below the surface. Each consists of a little bunch of small sacs, within which fatty or oily material is produced. This secretion is forced from the sacs by the contractions of the arrectores pilorum muscles, and during exercise it also escapes on to the shafts of the hairs. Its function is to keep these pliable and lubricated and prevent them from becoming brittle through drying. A copious secretion from the sebaceous glands results in a sleek shining coat, such as is associated with a well-fed and well-groomed horse.

Appendages of the skin.—In addition to hair, the skin possesses certain appendages, which in reality are modified hair only. Thus, horns, hoofs, claws, nails, ergots, chestnuts, and other horny structures, are closely packed epidermal cells which have undergone keratinisation or cornification; they can be compared to hair matted together into a solid mass by the intervening epidermal cells. They are formed from a specialised form of corium, to which the name *matrix* is applied. (*See* FOOT OF HORSE.) The hollow horns of cattle are of this nature, but the antlers of deer and the horns of the giraffe, as well as those of certain other animals, are composed of true bone. The horns of the rhinoceros are composed of densely matted hairs, growing from papilla instead of being sunk into follicles. Spurs of poultry are horny epidermal sheaths covering a centre of bony outgrowth from the metatarsal in the case of poultry, or from the carpus or metacarpus in the case of the spur-winged geese and screamers. The baleen of whales, which is in the form of long plates with frayed fibrous edges, and is used for straining purposes, is also an epidermal hair-like structure, developing similarly to the rhinoceros horn. Feathers are highly specialised scales. The down feathers of the chicken are simple, and consist of a brush of hair-like 'barbs' springing from a basal quill or 'calamus'. From the whole length of each barb a series of smaller 'barbules' comes off not unlike the branches of a shrub. The adult or 'contour feathers' are formed at the bottom of the same follicles that lodged the down feathers, which by the growth of the adult feather become pushed out of place. At first they are nothing more than enlarged down feathers, but soon one of the barbs grows enormously, and forms a main shaft or 'rachis' to which the other barbs are attached on either side. From the sides of the barbs grow the barbules, just as in the down feathers, and these, in the case of the large wing feathers ('remiges') and the tail feathers ('rectrices'), are connected by minute hooks so that the feather 'vane' has a more resistant surface for flight than in the case of the breast feathers, for instance. Moulting in birds occurs periodically, and the bird casts off the old feathers and gets a complete new set. It is comparable to the casting of the skins or scales in reptiles, and makes a considerable demand upon the body resources, birds being more liable to be attacked with certain diseases during the moult than otherwise.

Functions of the skin.—The main use of the skin is a *protective* one. It covers the underlying muscles, protects them from injury, and in virtue of its padding of fat prevents them from extremes of temperature. The hair, fur, wool, or feathers assist this heat-regulating mechanism more still, and usually the growth of the coat is determined by the temperature of the surroundings; for example, when horses are kept out of doors during winter they grow long thick coats, while when kept in warm stables and covered with rugs they assume a close sleek coat, and the same applies to other animals. The cuticle forms a highly impenetrable surface, its dense horny character and elasticity being well adapted to withstand wounds and prevent ingress by organisms, while the presence of sebaceous secretion makes it practically waterproof. Thus poisonous substances, drugs, etc., are not readily absorbed by the skin unless compounded with an oily base, or made in the form of an ointment and well rubbed in.

Secretion is another important function of the skin; perspiration and sebaceous material being produced in considerable amounts. Their functions have been referred to already, and further details are given under PERSPIRATION.

Heat regulation is one of the most important functions of the skin. The domesticated animals are 'warm-blooded', that is, their temperatures remain practically constant no matter what the temperature of the surrounding medium may be. In order to maintain this regularity it is obvious that an animal must possess some means of raising its body heat when the surroundings are cool, and of lowering it when the surroundings are hot. The main source of heat in the body is from muscular effort, each muscle, whether voluntary or involuntary, producing a certain amount of heat each time it contracts. The skin plays a very important part in the conservation of this heat. When cold air, water, or other cooling substances come into contact with a large area of skin, the numerous blood-vessels of the true skin immediately contract, reducing the amount of blood circulating in them, and therefore reducing the amount which will be exposed to the cooling action from outside. On the other hand, when the surrounding medium is at a higher temperature than the normal—*i.e.* when it is approaching body heat, or rises above it—the blood-vessels of the skin dilate, more blood is brought to the surface, and this stimulates sweating, or excretion, and when the perspiration evaporates, especially when the surrounding atmosphere is dry, considerable cooling of the skin surface occurs. In animals which do not sweat, as well as in those that do, the extra amount of blood circulating near the surface gives up heat, and in this way also cooling occurs. This alternate contracting and dilating of the skin blood-vessels is under the control of reflex nerve action, and is regulated by centres in the brain and spinal cord. When the temperature rises so high that no heat can be given off from the body, very serious results occur (*see* SUNSTROKE, *and under* BRAIN the sub-heading 'Heatstroke.') It can readily be understood why the body, human or animal, tolerates dry heat better than moist heat, since evaporation from the skin occurs much faster in a dry atmosphere than in a wet one, and the regulation can be effected more rapidly as a consequence.

Respiration.—Certain of the lower animals, such as the frog, expire as much waste material by the skin as by the lungs, and can exist by skin respiration alone. Gaseous exchange occurs in exactly the same manner as in the lungs, oxygen being absorbed and carbonic acid gas being given off. Exactly the same occurs in animals, though the skin in them is very much less important than the lungs. Varnishing the skin causes death in rabbits, due mostly to loss of body heat, rather than to retention of effete materials, as was formerly supposed. It is probable that a considerable amount of the characteristic odour of an animal building is due to the presence in the air of organic matter given out by the skin.

SKIN, DISEASES OF.—The majority of the commoner diseases of the skin in animals are due either to parasitic invasion, or to conditions of the nature of eczema. These are treated under separate headings —*e.g.* mange, of all varieties, is dealt with under PARASITES, p. 689; ECZEMA; URTICARIA; RINGWORM; ACNE, CONTAGIOUS, etc.; *see also* GREASE, MUD FEVER, NECROSIS (BACILLARY), IMPETIGO, VARIOLA, DISTEMPER, SITFASTS, MALLENDERS, HARNESS INJURIES, SPOROTRICHOSIS, GLANDERS, SWINE ERYSIPELAS, LIGHT SENSITISATION, etc., in all of which, as well as in other diseases, the skin is affected. In the treatment of several non-parasitic skin diseases in all animals vitamin A is often of service. (*See* HYPERKERATOSIS.)

SKIN, POISONING THROUGH (*see under* POISONING, HYPERKERATOSIS).

'SKIN TUBERCULOSIS'.—This is characterised by the appearance of swellings, varying in size from that of a pea to that of a tangerine, on the limbs and occasionally on the trunk of cattle. Lesions are often multiple and in the form of a chain. They are unsightly but appear to cause the cow no discomfort, and their economic importance lies only in the fact that they apparently sensitise the animal to mammalian and / or avian tuberculin, thus complicating the interpretation of the tuberculin test. This, indeed, may give

SKULL

rise to anxiety on the part of the owners of attested herds. A re-test after an interval of 30 to 60 days will, however, in the absence of tuberculosis, usually give a reaction justifying retention of the animal within the herd.

Microscopically, the lesions of 'skin tuberculosis' closely resemble those of tuberculosis, and acid-fast bacilli resembling *M. tuberculosis* are present in them. So far, however, attempts to grow the organisms in the laboratory, or to set up an infection experimentally, have failed.

SKULL is the collection of flat and irregularly shaped bones, which protects the brain and forms the skeleton of the face. These bones support the organs of mastication, keep patent the nasal and pharyngeal passages, hold the eye in its socket, give protection to the very delicate organs of hearing, and give the head of an animal its characteristic outline. The skull as a whole is not solid. Excavated in it at certain parts there are large irregular spaces known as 'sinuses', which act as air reservoirs, and also make the skull lighter than it would be if these parts were solid. (*See* SINUSES OF SKULL.)

General arrangement of the skull.—The skull is divided into two parts: (1) the *cranium*, and (2) the *face*. The former consists of the posterior part, which encloses the brain, while the face lies entirely to the front of the head. In the young animal's skull these two portions can be separated, but in the adult the whole skull, except for the lower jaw (mandible), is intimately fused together into a complete whole.

Most of the bones of the skull are flat bones developed from a structure which is partly cartilage and partly fibrous membrane. Centres of ossification appear in these during early life, and soon after birth the greater part of each bone has assumed its eventual outline, but is separated from its neighbours by an intimately dovetailed joint. These joints, none of which is movable, allow growth until the animal is adult, when bony fusion usually occurs, and the joints become obliterated. Many of these joints—'sutures', as they are called—can be felt in the skull of a newly born animal, particularly over the dome of the head in a foal or puppy, and for a time constitute especially vulnerable parts of the skull.

Bones of cranium.—The bones which enclose the brain and its membranes are ten in number—four single and three paired. They are occipital, sphenoid, ethmoid, interparietal (single), and parietals, frontals, and temporals (paired). The occipital lies at the posterior lower aspect of the skull, and forms the hinder wall of the brain cavity. Through it passes the spinal cord, which emerges by the 'foramen magnum', and to a roughened prominence above this foramen is attached the very powerful 'ligamentum nuchæ', which supports the head. On either side of the foramen are the 'occipital condyles' which articulate with the atlas—the first of the cervical vertebræ. The lower part of the occipital—the 'basilar part'—runs forward along the base of the brain to meet the body of the sphenoid bone. The inner surface is adapted to the cerebellum—the most posterior upper part of the brain, while above the basilar portion lies the medulla which is continued backwards into the spinal cord. The sphenoid lies at the base of the brain, and cannot be felt on the exterior of the living horse's head. It has the form of a body with two pairs of wings and one pair of projections. It is supposed to resemble a bird with two pairs of wings in flight trailing its legs behind it. The body is continuous with the basilar part of the occipital, and helps to form the base of the brain. The wings curve upward and outward, and also help to form part of the brain cavity. The ethmoid lies between the back of the nasal passage, whose posterior boundary it is, and the brain cavity. It consists of a 'cribriform plate'—a sieve-like partition between nasal passage and brain, through the perforations of which pass the nerves of smell—a 'perpendicular plate' in the median line, and two lateral masses, or 'labyrinths'. The interparietal bone, as its name suggests, lies between the parietals. It is a small bone, quadrilateral in outline, and has projecting from its inner surface the 'osseous tentorium', which serves to separate incompletely the cerebral hemispheres in front from the cerebellum behind. The parietals, one on either side, form the greater part of the roof of the cranium on either side of the interparietal. Each is quadrilateral in outline, and together they meet in the middle to form the 'median' or 'sagittal suture'. The frontal bones lie between the parietals behind and the nasal bones in front. Together they form the greater part of the expanse of the forehead. Each has a process which runs laterally to take part in the formation of the bony 'orbit', in which is lodged the eye. Internally, the frontal bones complete the roof and anterior wall of the cranium, occupying the space between the parietals and the ethmoid.

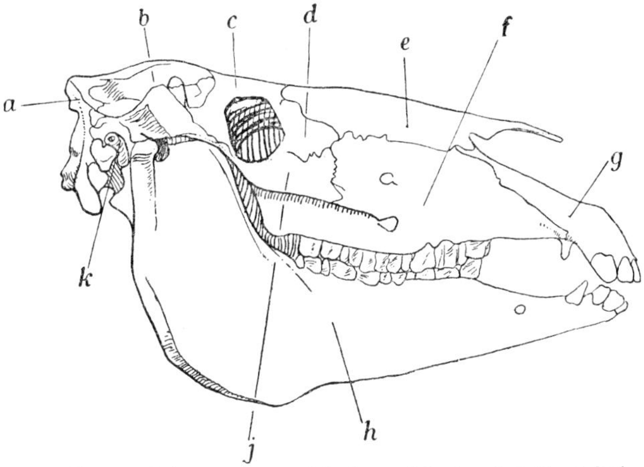

Diagram of the arrangement of the bones of the horse's skull. *a*, Occipital bone, to which is attached the ligamentum nuchæ; *b*, parietal, which forms the roof of the cranium; *c*, frontal bone; *d*, lacrymal bone, forming part of the bony orbit; *e*, nasal bone; *f*, maxilla, which forms the greater part of the upper jaw, roof of the mouth, and floor of nasal passage; *g*, incisive bone, carrying the upper incisor teeth; *h*, mandible, the lower jaw-bone; *j*, the zygomatic, or malar, which forms part of the bony orbit, and part of the zygoma; *k*, petrous temporal bone, showing the external bony canal through which the sound waves pass on their way to the middle ear.

Excavated in the frontal is the frontal sinus, one of the air sinuses of the skull. In the horned domesticated ruminants, ox, sheep, and goat, the 'horn core', which is a part of the frontal bone, projects outwards, assuming whatever shape is characteristic of the race and breed. The frontal sinus is continued into the hollow horn core for a considerable distance. Temporal bones are those which lie at the base of each ear, one on either side. Both bones, right and left, have two parts: a 'petrous' part—hard, dense, and stone-like, in which are excavated the tunnels where lie the delicate nervous structures concerned with the sense of hearing—and a 'squamous' or scale-like part, which forms part of the lateral wall of the cranium. The squamous part also carries the surface with which the mandible forms the joint of the lower jaw, and from this a process runs forward to form part of the 'zygomatic arch'.

Bones of the face.—The bones which form the face number 21, 9 being paired and 3 single. Their names are maxilla, incisive, palatine, pterygoid, nasal, lacrymal, zygomatic, upper turbinated and lower turbinated, which are paired; and vomer, mandible, hyoid, which are single. The maxillæ lie one on either side of the face, forming the greater part of the upper jaws, and touch almost all the bones of the face. They carry the upper cheek teeth, form the maxillary sinus, and through each passes the tear-duct of the same side. Projecting inwards from the body of each is a rigid plate, and these two plates form almost the whole of the basis of the 'hard palate'—the roof of the mouth and the floor of the nasal passage. On the outside the maxilla possesses part of the 'zygomatic' or 'facial crest', which in the living horse can always be felt as a ridge running forward below the eye. To this is attached part of the powerful masseter muscle, which is of supreme importance in chewing. The incisive bones lie in front of the maxillæ, continuing them forward, so to speak, and carry the incisor teeth. At the juncture with the maxilla lies the socket for the canine tooth of the corresponding side in the male. The palatine bones form the posterior part of the hard palate, and constitute together the greater part of the boundary of the posterior nostrils, which is completed by the thin bent pterygoid bones. The nasal bones form the ridge of the bridge of the nose and the roof of the nasal cavities. They lie anterior to the frontal bones. The two lacrymal bones are found along the anterior edge of the orbit, part of whose forward boundary they form. Each has a little depression for the lacrymal sac, at the commencement of the tear-duct which carries the overflow tears down into the nose. The zygomatic bones lie below the lacry-mal, completing the front and lower boundary of the socket for the eye. On each side each bone carries the posterior part of the facial crest, which is continued forward as the facial crest of the maxilla, which has already been mentioned. The four turbinated bones—two upper and two lower—are delicate scroll-like rolled bones, attached to the inside of the lateral walls of the nasal passage. During life these bones are covered with highly vascular membranes, which warm and moisten the air on its way to the lungs. The vomer, or 'plough-share bone', lies at the posterior and lower part of the nasal septum. It separates the two posterior nostrils from each other. The mandible forms the whole of the lower jaw, and is the only movable bone of the skull. It is composed of two bilaterally symmetrical halves, which in the horse, pig, and dog fuse at or soon after birth. In cattle and sheep, however, these two halves do not fuse until later, when the animal is adult, and in some cattle no bony fusion ever occurs. Each half carries the incisor, canine, and cheek teeth of the corresponding side, and immediately behind the last cheek tooth each branch takes an upward bend, forming the 'angle of the jaw', and ends at the squamous temporal bone, with which it forms the joint of the lower jaw. In front of the articular surface is situated an upward projecting process, for muscular attachment, known as the 'coronoid process'. The hyoid bone lies in the root of the tongue, supporting both it and the larynx. It is attached by a bar of cartilage to the petrous temporal on either side, and there is a similar attachment to either side of the larynx. In no place does the hyoid bone lie sufficiently near to the surface to be palpable from the outside.

The skull as a whole.—The most striking feature of the skull of horse, ox, sheep, or pig is the comparatively small size of the cranium compared to that of the face; but this is not so in the cat and the short-skulled breeds of dogs, such as the pug or bulldog. In these latter the proportions more nearly resemble those of the human being. This is explained to some extent by the difference in size of the brain, but to a greater extent by the more extensive development of mouth and masticatory organs. The more coarse and innutritious the food the greater is the provision that must be made for chewing, and therefore

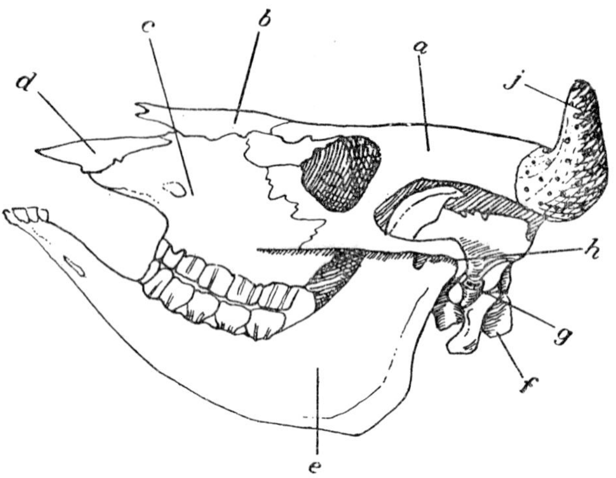

Diagram of the arrangement of the bones of the ox's skull. *a*, Frontal bone, which is continued outwards to form the horn core, *j*, of spongy bone; *b*, nasal bone; *c*, maxilla; *d*, incisive bone, slight and fragile, and carrying no incisor teeth; *e*, mandible, the lower jaw-bone; *f*, occipital bone; *g*, petrous temporal bone; *h*, mandibular joint.

the more extensive is the development of teeth, tongue, etc. In the carnivora the food needs less chewing, and the mouth and its contents are therefore smaller. (*See also under* BRAIN.)

In the horse and dog the skull appears to be considerably smaller than the head of the living animal would suggest, whereas in the ox and sheep the reverse holds good. This is explained by the greater relative development of musculature at the sides of the cranium and in the cheeks than in the ruminants, while in the horned breeds the presence of the horn cores, which are sometimes very large, makes the skull as a whole seem larger.

Another striking feature in ruminants is thecomparative smallness and weak appearance of the incisive bones, occasioned by the absence of upper incisor teeth.

In dogs the shape of the skull and its proportions differ according to the breed. The skull has been altered by artificial selection over a long period of time probably more than any other part of the skeleton. Two extreme types have been evolved. In one the length of the face and the narrowness of the skull have been exaggerated, and have reached their maximum in the greyhound, whippet, Borzoi etc.; in dogs of the other extreme the face has been foreshortened and the skull has increased in breadth to an extraordinary extent, while the cranium has become distinctly domed, as in the bulldog, pug, King Charles spaniel, etc. The term *dolichocephalic* is applied to skulls of the former type; *brachycephalic* is used to indicate skulls of the second type; while skulls which are more normal, between these extremes, are called *mesaticephalic*, such as those from fox-terriers, Aberdeen terriers, field spaniels, etc. These variations are sometimes expressed as the 'cephalic index', which is the breadth multiplied by 100 and divided by the length. Dolichocephalic skulls give a cephalic index of about 50 to 55, brachycephalic skulls of from 85 to 90, while most mesaticephalics give 70 to 75.

SKUNKS and foxes are now the two most important wildlife hosts of the rabies virus in the U.S.A.

SLATTED FLOORS.—These were tried in England in the last century and described in the *R.A.S.E. Journal* of 1860, and have been used for many years in Norway, before being re-introduced into Britain as a means of saving money on straw. The current practice is to sprinkle sawdust on the slats (of wood or concrete), but to use no straw. The use of slatted floors can hardly be regarded as anything but a retrograde step from the animal husbandry point of view, however attractive commercially. The animals obviously cannot rest as comfortably as on straw, and if strict precautions are not taken (as in Norway) they may be subjected to severe draughts with resultant ill-health and poor food conversion ratios. Teat and leg injuries, and injuries or abnormalities of the feet, may also develop in animals on slats.

A slatted dunging area and a bedded area are satisfactory. (*See also under* Sow Stalls *and* Slurry.)

SLAUGHTER (*see under* Destruction of Animals).

SLEEP.—The following is from an account by Sir Frederick Smith:

The actual cause of sleep is not known. The tissues require rest and repair, and these are effected during sleep; but no explanation which has been generally accepted has accounted for the loss of consciousness which occurs during this process of anabolism. The amount of sleep required by animals appears to be greater in the carnivora than in herbivora. The dog and cat spend a considerable time sleeping, but the herbivora less and only for short periods at a time. Neither class sleep with the same depth or intensity as man; it is not conceivable that the dog or cat would remain asleep during a considerable noise. The horse is such a light sleeper that the faintest footfall suffices to wake it up. It sleeps with eyes open or semi-open, and lies fully extended on its side. The ruminant sleeps with the head turned in to the side, and the nose tucked in to the flank, or with the head extended and the chin resting on the ground in front. The horse sleeps for short periods at a time; its immense weight does not allow of lying for any length of time on one side, for during this time the lower lung does no work and the muscles get cramped. Occasionally the horse will rise and turn on to the other side or may roll over; and at other times it will rise, feed for a time, and then lie down again on the other side. Horses require little sleep, but it must be of good quality, and hard-worked horses cannot do without it. They have the power of sleeping while standing, for which the limbs are provided with certain mechanisms, whereby the greater part of the strain of standing is taken, not by the muscles but by tendons or ligaments, or at least by muscles which possess a great deal of tendinous tissue. The horse that sleeps while standing drops the head below the level of the withers, the eyelids fall partially over the eyeballs, and the limbs are brought rather more under the body than usual. The extensor muscles of the limbs cannot be relaxed or the horse would fall; they must accordingly continue to have nerve impulses poured into them to maintain them in a state of contraction. Nor is this confined to the limb muscles; those which sling the body between the fore-legs must also have tone imparted to them if the standing position is to be maintained. The impulses concerned with body equilibrium and balance must also continue in operation. None of the mechanisms of the limbs which aid the muscles and tendons are in any way adequate to explain these facts. The extensor muscles, on which everything depends, receive assistance from the fascia of the arm and thigh. The muscles themselves are extremely powerful, and possess in their substance a large amount of fibrous material, such as is found in all muscles which are constantly in action. During sleep the horse is unconscious, and the muscles are therefore under no kind of cerebral control, yet they remain strong and in action without the knowledge of the animal. This is mainly due to the very highly organised reflex action controlled by the spinal cord (*see* NERVES), and partly to the influence of the cerebellum, which must remain in full operation to ensure standing; so that, asleep or awake, the muscular tone is kept up, not only in the limbs but also in the back, loins, and chest wall. The attitude of the bird sleeping on one leg is another instance of the maintenance of reflex balance, consciousness being in complete abeyance. The rest obtained by horses sleeping in an erect position is, actually, not sufficient for their needs. They require complete relaxation of their muscles, and this can only be furnished in the recumbent position. When from fear, ankylosis of vertebræ, or other cause a horse does not lie down, it should be placed in slings, or given some form of support, such as a rope between the heel posts upon which the hind-quarters may bear, so that it may obtain the requisite rest. When horses are not hard worked they may never lie down for years, but they are not then so fit for their work; on board ship, and for surgical or other reasons, horses may be kept standing without harm for considerable periods, but they should be exercised for a short while two or three times daily, in order that the muscles may be prevented from becoming stiff. Horses are liable to fall while standing asleep, and may, in rare cases, actually come to the ground through the relaxation of their extensor muscles; what happens more frequently is that they knuckle over on to their fetlocks, recovering themselves almost at once, but not before a slight injury has been inflicted to the skin over the joint. The fall always occurs in front, not behind, probably because of the extra weight carried by the fore-legs.

The respirations become slower and deeper, pulse-rate falls, the secretion of urine becomes lessened, and the production of carbon dioxide is lessened, while the loss of nerve control over heat production causes a fall in temperature. The essential physiological factor in sleep appears to be anæmia of the brain.

SLINGS.—A device whereby a large animal may be kept in the standing position for long periods without becoming completely exhausted. The apparatus consists essentially of a broad strong sheet which passes under the animal's chest and abdomen, supported by a block-and-tackle or other means to a beam overhead. Connected with this there are two strong straps, one passing round the front of the chest, and the other passing round the buttocks. These latter serve to hold the sling in position, and prevent the animals from struggling free. The whole is adjustable so that it may fit animals of different sizes. The sling is often made with a metal or wooden bar along each end of the sheet; these bars serve to distribute the weight of the animal along the whole width of the sheet, and afford a rigid means of attachment to the cross-beam of the slings, to which the chain or rope of the block-and-tackle is attached.

In addition to the above use, slings are one of the means of lifting a horse that has either fallen or lain down in a stable and is unable to rise. The horse is placed so that the slings may be pulled under it, or is rolled on to them, and after the chest and breeching straps are arranged the horse is lifted by the block-and-tackle high enough to be able to use his feet. It sometimes happens that if the horse has lain for a considerable time it refuses to support its weight on its feet, but hangs 'like a herring' in the slings. In such cases it may be necessary to startle the horse, when it will generally make a plunge and 'find its feet'.

Slings are employed in a variety of conditions: fractures, punctured wounds of joints or tendon sheaths; large deep wounds which might become soiled with litter, etc., if the horse lies down; cases of extreme weakness, where the animal might lie and be unable to rise; in some cases of azoturia, purpura hæmorrhagica, sprained tendons or ligaments, or ruptured muscles.

When slings are applied to an animal, they should not be fixed up so tightly that the animal is unable to walk a step or so in each direction. They are only required as a means of support for the animal when it so desires, and not as a suspensory apparatus which is always in use. The animal soon learns to lean on the slings and rest its feet. When they are drawn up so tightly that whenever the animal tries to move it is lifted off its feet, they are likely to defeat the purpose for which they were applied, as the animal gets irritated by not being able to move and is much more likely to start violent struggling in an endeavour to free itself from the encumbrance of the slings. The hand should be able to be passed under the sling webbing when the animal is standing immediately under the centre of the block-and-tackle, and neither the chest strap nor the breeching should be buckled up tightly. It is generally necessary to secure the head of the animal by a halter to restrict its movements, and to supply a suitable manger or other receptacle from which it may feed easily.

SLINK CALVES.—Immature or unborn calves improperly used for human food. The flesh of slink calves is often called *slink veal.*

'SLIPPED'.—A colloquial expression meaning aborted.

'SLIPPED' DISC (*see under* SPINE).

SLIPPED SHOULDER is a term loosely applied to at least two conditions: it is used by some to indicate dislocation or luxation of the shoulder joint; and it is employed by others, perhaps more commonly, to mean suprascapular paralysis. (*See* DISLOCATIONS *and* SUPRASCAPULAR PARALYSIS.)

SLIPPED STIFLE is the popular term for dislocation of the patella, which is liable to occur in young colts at grass, especially when in poor condition or running upon hilly ground. It may be partial, when the patella slides in and out of the trochlear depression on the femur with each step; or it may be complete, when the patella becomes fixed above the outer lip of the pulley-like trochlear surface, causing all the joints of the affected leg to become straightened, and the limb to be held pointing behind the horse.

Dislocation of the patella is a common condition in the dog.

'SLIPPED TENDON'.—A condition seen in chickens, turkey poults, and ducklings, in which there is displacement of tendons and an inability for the leg to support the bird's weight. It is due to a manganese deficiency, and may arise from feeding lime to excess.

SLOPE CULTURE.—A method of growing micro-organisms on solid media (*e.g.* agar) in tubes which are usually arranged in racks at the correct angle for the agar to solidify on cooling.

SLOUGH means a dead part separated by natural processes from the rest of the living body. The slough may be only a small part such as a piece of skin that has been burnt by heat or chemicals, or it may be a whole foot. (*See* GANGRENE.)

SLOW-MILKING COWS (*see under* MILKING MACHINES).

SLUGS.—The common field slug, *Agriolimax meticulatus*, is of veterinary interest as intermediate host of the sheep lungworm *Cystocaulus ocreatus*. (For the danger of **slug poisons,** see METALDEHYDE.)

SLURRY.—Deaths of pigs have been reported following agitation of slurry during the emptying of tanks or pits under the piggery slats. It is recommended that slurry should never be allowed to come within 18 inches of the slats, and that especially in hot weather emptying should be carried out at least every 3 or 4 weeks. Methane, hydrogen sulphide, ammonia, and carbon dioxide may all be given off as the result of bacterial action on slurry; giving rise to a mixture both lethal and explosive.

Cows, too, have been overcome by slurry gas.

For methods of slurry disposal see DAIRY HERD MANAGEMENT. See also under SALMONELLOSIS, PASTURE, SILAGE.

SMALLPOX IN ANIMALS (*see* VARIOLA).

SMEAR PREPARATIONS.—A film of blood, pus, etc., smeared on to a slide, fixed—and if necessary stained—for microscopical examination.

'SMEDI' VIRUSES were obtained from pig herds, in the U.S.A., having stillbirths (S), mummified fœtuses (M), embryonic death (ED), and infertility (I). The viruses were serologically of two groups: (a) swine picorna viruses, (b) related to Ontario polio-encephalitis and œdema disease viruses.

SMELL.—The sense of smell is situated in the nasal mucous membrane, and in the nerve centres of the brain which are connected with the nasal mucosa by the olfactory nerves. The power to appreciate smell depends upon the stimulation of tufts of hair-like processes found in certain cells in the nasal mucous membrane, by particles of matter given off by an odoriferous substance. These particles, either gaseous or solid, are dissolved in the secretion present, and so far as present knowledge goes, appear to act chemically on the nerve tufts. The act of ' sniffing ', familiar in the case of the dog especially, simply ensures that the particles are rapidly and forcibly drawn upwards into the nose. There are certain substances which act more quickly than others in particular animals : thus the smell of fish, blood, and offal has a remarkably stimulating effect upon the carnivorous animals, while grass, grain, and vegetable substances stimulate the sense organs of herbivorous creatures particularly. The odour of flesh, blood, etc., is repulsive to the herbivora, and may cause great nervousness and fright. Most of the wild grass-eating animals have remarkably well-developed powers of smell, and are able to locate their enemies at great distances : thus deer and antelope can detect a carnivorous animal which has recently made a kill at a distance of two miles if the wind is favourable. It is through the sense of smell that the male is attracted to the female during the season of ' œstrum ' of the latter ; the odour at this period is most persistent, and can be appreciated at great distances. Females recognise their offspring by their sense of smell, and dams whose young have died can often be deceived and persuaded into accepting other young animals by clothing these in the skins of the dead ones. This fact is made use of in the case of ewes which have lost their lambs.

SMELLS AS EVIDENCE OF DISEASE.—In certain cases the presence of a smell connected with an animal is almost a diagnostic feature of disease. Thus in caries of the teeth or decomposition of bone there is a characteristic smell which, when once it is appreciated, can never be forgotten, although it is difficult to describe. The breath, urine, and the milk of a cow suffering from acetonæmia have a characteristic sweetish sickly smell. Poisoning by certain drugs, *e.g.* carbolic acid, can be diagnosed to some extent by the smell of the drug that is left in the mouth or on the skin. Foul smelling clay-coloured fæces in the carnivorous animals indicate insufficiency of bile. The urine of the horse has the smell of violets after the administration of turpentine in large quantities. In gangrene of the lungs in horses, a putrid odour of the breath is the earliest symptom of the last stage.

SMOG.—This is the popular name for fog containing a dangerously high proportion of sulphur dioxide and other harmful gases derived from coal fires and factory chimneys. It has led to the death of cattle, *e.g.* at Smithfield Show, and in 1952 it killed over 4000 people in London. Urine-soaked litter, or a wick in a bottle of dilute ammonia solution, will give some protection.

SNAILS.—One or two species are of veterinary interest in connection with LIVER FLUKES and tapeworms.

SNAKE BITE.—In certain tropical countries snakes are responsible for a very heavy loss both of human and animal life. In Great Britain (excluding Ireland) and the major portion of Europe, harmful snakes are, however, not at all common, and deaths from their bites are rare. It is true that on some moorlands of England and Scotland adders (or vipers) are not uncommon among heather, and occasional losses from their bites do occur among sheep and dogs.

Animals susceptible.—Dogs are most frequently killed by snake bites, both at home and abroad, and sporting dogs suffer more than others. Sheep, cattle, and horses come next in frequency, whilst cats and pigs are only very rarely killed. The reasons for this appear to be that hunting dogs most often disturb snakes, and that grazing herbivorous animals, moving only slowly over a tract of country, disturb snakes less ; while the cat is not often attacked because of its greater caution when hunting, and because of its superior agility. Pigs apparently are least often killed because of the protection they possess in a hard tough skin, with a padding of fat immediately below it.

Identification of snakes.—Broadly speaking, those which have *two rows* of small solid, equal-sized teeth on either side of the upper jaw are non-venomous ; while those with *one row* of small teeth on either side of the upper jaw, and two or more large, curved, hollow or grooved fangs on the outside of the smaller teeth, should be considered venomous. These large fangs are important, since it is by a groove on the surface of the fang (cobra type), or a canal down its centre (adder type), that the venom is introduced through the fang wound into the victim. In a few instances, such as the Ring-hals in Africa, the poison may be squirted with uncanny accuracy for a distance of about 6 feet into the eyes of the victim, the snake rising and opening its mouth wide, with the whole head thrown back. The poison is produced by a poison-gland, at or near to the root of the fang, or situated along the upper jaw and communicating with the fang by a duct.

The majority of the venomous snakes inflict two comparatively small but deep wounds with their fangs, and two converging rows of smaller shallow wounds with the palatine or inner rows of teeth, and therefore the snakes can to some extent be identified by the nature of the wound made by the bite ; in the domesticated animals, however, owing to the covering of hair or wool, these wounds can only be seen when the skin is shaved.

Symptoms.—Two kinds of symptoms are produced, depending upon the kind of venomous snake involved. In those of the cobra type there is a period of excitement immediately after the bite, lasting only for a few minutes and followed by a period of normality. Then nervous excitement appears, convulsive seizures follow, and death takes place from asphyxia. If death does not occur at once, dullness and depression are seen and death or recovery takes place some hours later. There is usually but little pain at the site of injury, and practically no local reaction in rapidly fatal cases. The symptoms of bite by the viperine (adder) variety are similar in general, but there is local pain and considerable swelling at the seat of the bite. The skin becomes a livid colour, tumefied, and if in a limb there may be severe lameness. The animal does not usually show nervous symptoms, however, but stands dull and depressed, as though it had had warning of impending fate.

Treatment.—Where anti-venom sera are obtainable, the immediate injection of these is the most rapid and reliable method of treatment. Instructions for use are provided by firms supplying them. Otherwise immediate and free incision over the seat of the bite, ligaturing firmly above it, to prevent absorption of the venom into the circulation of the rest of the body, and the immediate insertion of crystals of potassium permanganate deeply into the wounds, should be undertaken without delay. Stimulants, such as hot strong coffee, tea, etc., may be given to dogs, and every endeavour be made to keep up the body heat.

SNEEZING means a sudden expulsion of air through the nostrils, designed to expel irritating materials from the upper air-passages ; the vocal cords being kept shut till the pressure in the lungs is high, and then suddenly released, so that the contained air is driven through the throat into the nose. Entrance to the mouth is prevented by the soft palate closing the exit from the mouth.

Sneezing is induced by the presence in the nose of particles of irritating substances, such as pungent odours, smoke, dust, spores of certain species of fungi, pollen from some grasses, etc. It is also the forerunner of chills, colds, influenza, etc., when it is usually accompanied by a running at the nostrils, and it is a sign of the presence of certain parasites, such as *Œstrus* larvæ in sheep and horses, and rarely *Linguatula* in dogs.

S-N-F. (*see* SOLIDS-NOT-FAT).

SNOOD.—The long, fleshy appendage extending from the front of a turkey's head over its upper beak.

'SNOW BLINDNESS' IN SHEEP (*see under* KERATITIS on p. 325).

SOAP is a substance made by boiling a fat or oil with an alkali. The most commonly used oil is olive oil, and the most frequently used alkali is caustic soda. In the process of manufacture the fatty acids of the oil separate out and unite with the alkali to form the soap, and glycerine remains behind. In soft soap, either green or black, caustic potash is used instead of soda. In marine soap cocoanut oil is used ; curd soap results from the use of tallow as a fat ; and many of the higher class toilet soaps have palm or almond oil. In the superfatted soaps care is taken that the fat is in excess so that no free alkali remains to irritate the skin, and in glycerine soaps a quantity of this substance is incorporated so as to exercise an emollient action.

Uses.—Soap is, of course, mainly used as a cleansing agent, although it is often employed in the preparation of balls, etc. As an enema soapy water is useful, but care is necessary that the soap does not contain any free caustic which may irritate or even blister the lining of the rectum. Soap liniment is a favourite and useful cooling application for sprained tendons or ligaments and for muscular stiffness. Liquid soap—20 per cent solution—is recommended for treating bites inflicted by animals suffering from rabies.

SOAPWORT POISONING is possible when the soapwort plant (*Saponaria officinalis*) grows abundantly in pasture. The plant contains a poisonous glucosidal substance called *saponin*, which causes frothiness when stirred in water. When saponin is introduced into the body it causes solution of the red blood-cells, stupefaction, paralysis, vomiting, and purging with the passage of large amounts of frothy fæces, which are mixed with blood and have an objectionable odour.

SOCIAL BEHAVIOUR (*see under* BUNT ORDER).

'SOD DISEASE'.—The name given in 1920 to a disease of poultry in the U.S.A. Blisters and scabs formed on the feet and legs, mainly in birds under a month old, occasionally in adults, which were ranging over unbroken prairie sod. Mortality: 20 to 90 per cent. A somewhat similar but less severe condition in Cardiganshire was described in 1952. It involved a batch of Light Sussex cockerels, which became lame, walked with a pronounced 'goose-step' with redness and swelling of the feet, and later blisters and scabs. There were no deaths. The condition could not be experimentally reproduced, and is thought to be of an eczematous nature.

SODIUM is a metal whose salts are white, crystalline, and very soluble in water. Common salt, or sodium chloride, is contained in the fluids of the body under natural circumstances, and therefore the salts of sodium, when used as drugs, act not through their metallic base but according to the acid radicle with which the sodium is combined. Generally speaking, the salts of sodium act in a manner very like corresponding salts of potassium (*see* POTASSIUM) but are better tolerated.

SODIUM CARBONATE, commonly called 'washing soda', has a softening action upon the skin, and is sometimes used dissolved in warm water to cleanse the skin and remove wax or fat from its surface. It is sometimes used to cleanse the outer ears of animals from waxy deposits. It is an irritant internally, and is therefore not given by the mouth.

SODIUM BICARBONATE, or 'baking soda', is very largely used as an antacid; it is added to stomachic powders for horses, cattle, pigs, and dogs, in combination with bismuth, vegetable bitters, etc. It is also much used dissolved in warm water as a soothing application to inflamed mucous membranes, such as those of the nose, mouth, vagina, etc., especially when it is desired to remove accumulated mucus and catarrhal deposit. It is sometimes used to irrigate the urinary bladder in inflammations of bladder and urethra, and it is also employed to irrigate the vagina before service, where acidity of the mucous membrane is suspected of causing sterility in cows and mares. The corresponding salt of potassium is also employed for this purpose.

The citrate, acetate, sulphate, and hydroxide of sodium are used in a similar manner to those of potassium. (*See* POTASSIUM.) SODIUM IODIDE has many uses and a solution of it can, if necessary, be given intravenously whereas an effective concentration of potassium iodide may prove fatal by this route.

SODIUM FLUORIDE is a useful and cheap anthelmintic for pigs, highly effective against ascarids, and not requiring previous fasting. The matter of dosage requires great care, however, and druggists' instructions as to its use should be followed meticulously. (The drug is best given as 1 per cent of a dry meal, the quantity of the latter being such as a group of pigs would eat in one day. The dose is actually 0·1 to 0·15 gramme commercial sodium fluoride per 1 lb. bodyweight. If the drug is given in a wet mash, the smaller dose should be used and the pigs *must* be weighed.)

Sodium fluoride has also been used as an anthelmintic in the horse.

SODIUM MONOFLUOROACETATE.—Also known as '1080', this is a rodenticide restricted in the U.K. to use in sewers only. In the dog symptoms of poisoning with '1080' include yelping, sometimes vomiting, and convulsions. This compound is sometimes used in wildlife rabies control operations against foxes, etc.

SODIUM NITRITE (*see under* NITRITE POISONING).

SODIUM PROPIONATE (*see under* PROPIONATE).

SOFT PALATE.—For a condition of this causing distressed breathing in the race-horse, *see under* PALATE.

SOIL-CONTAMINATED HERBAGE.—Experiments in Australia and New

Zealand with intensively grazed sheep were undertaken to investigate tooth wear in ewes and wethers at various stocking densities. It was found that 'tooth wear was low when soil content of fæces was low and they rose to a peak simultaneously'. Moreover, in the majority of cases, soil content of the fæces was highest where stocking rates were high; when stocked at nine adult sheep to the acre, the daily intake of soil per head could be as much as 13 oz. in the rainy season.

In Britain, a N.A.A.S. officer has suggested, July thunderstorms over first-year lays may—by a combination of splashing by rain and poaching by feet—produce a herbage that is seriously contaminated with soil. This could well irritate the sensitive lining of the gut in young lambs with consequent scouring, which is often seen among lambs believed reasonably free from parasitic worms.

SOLIDS-NOT-FAT.—These include the protein casein, milk, sugar, and minerals. In Britain, the average S-N-F content of milk has fallen by about 0·25 per cent during the past 25 years—a fact important in human nutrition in that it represents a decline in the protein solids such as casein.

In Britain, milk which contains less than the legal presumptive standard of 8·5 per cent solids-not-fat may not be accepted by the buyer, or, if accepted, may be paid for at a substantially reduced price.

Deficiencies of solids-not-fat lead to difficulties in processing the milk and render it unsuitable for manufacture into high-class products. Milk produced by a cow affected with mastitis, or by one approaching the end of a lactation, is particularly undesirable.

Maintaining the S-N-F percentage at a satisfactory level is a more difficult problem for the milk producer than rectifying variations in the butterfat percentage. The causes of S-N-F deficiency are not always apparent, and attempts at remedying them may have no rapid effect.

Factors involved include: breed of cow, her inherited capacity, age, stage of lactation, the season of the year, feeding, management, and attacks of mastitis.

The diet should contain adequate fibre as well as protein. There is some evidence suggesting that an all-silage diet may lower S-N-F, unless the silage is of the highest quality. Hay, as well, is desirable. (*See* WINTER RATIONS.)

The percentage of solids-not-fat is relatively high in October and November, after which time it begins to decline and falls to a minimum in February and March. It then starts an upward trend, reaches a high level in May, and may drop again in July and August.

Milk from cows of the Jersey and Guernsey breeds is relatively high in solids-not-fat. British Friesians, as a rule, give milk low in S-N-F. Inherited capacity is important.

The percentage of solids-not-fat in milk varies according to the stage in the lactation. It is high at the beginning, but falls rapidly to a low level in from 6 to 8 weeks after calving. Thereafter, it rises gradually if the cow is pregnant, while it tends to decline further if she is not again in calf. Towards the end of the lactation, when the cow is drying off, it may fall very low.

SOMATIC (σωματικός) means everything belonging to the body except the germ cells in the gonads.

SORES (*see* ULCERS).

SORE THROAT is a popular term for laryngitis or pharyngitis, which is often present during a common cold, strangles, influenza, etc. (*See* THROAT, DISEASES OF.) A cowman with a sore throat may pass his infection to a cow's udder, setting up mastitis.

SORGHUM.—Poisoning in horses has been recorded in horses grazing pasture containing sorghum species. Hindquarter weakness and paralysis of the bladder may result.

SORREL POISONING (*see* DOCKS, POISONING BY, *and* SOURSOB).

SOUND is a metal rod, either curved or straight, which is used for passing along a natural channel or duct of the body. Thus there are bladder sounds, for passing into the bladder by way of the urethra, teat sounds for the udder, uterine sounds for the uterus, etc. They are generally used to discover whether there are any hard or solid bodies present, such as stones in the bladder or milk sinus.

SOUNDS are made both normally and abnormally by some of the organs of the body. Thus during the heart-beat there can be distinguished two definite sounds normally. The first of these, known as the 'first heart sound', is a long booming noise, similar to the syllable *lūb*, which is heard when the ventricles are contracting and the atrio-ventricular valves are closing, and which is produced by these processes. The 'second heart sound' is a short, sharp, sudden sound, similar to the syllable *dûp*, and is heard at the end of the contracting period of the ventricles, when the semilunar valves at the bases of the pulmonary artery and the aorta are closing.

Respiratory sounds are also present normally. The sound made by the air entering the alveoli is generally called the *respiratory*, or *vesicular murmur*. It is a soft, low, quiet blowing sound, which can be imitated by the gentle blowing of air from a pair of bellows. In addition to the friction of the air in the alveoli there is also a sound produced by the air in its course down the trachea and along the greater bronchi, but as this is quite indistinguishable from the former the two are classed together.

The stomach and the intestines produce audible sounds, always of a very varied character, during the process of digestion.

During disease there are unusual sounds produced, especially by the organs in the chest: for these *see* RÂLES; RONCHI; HEART, DISEASES OF; LUNGS, DISEASES OF; etc.

SOURSOB.—The Australian name for *Oxalis cernua*, a member of the sorrel family, found in Australia, South Africa, the continent of Europe, and now the West of England. It has caused fatal poisoning in sheep.

SOW'S MILK.—The production of colostrum lasts for about 5 days during which time the milk composition changes rapidly to 'normal'. In reality, however, there is no such thing as 'normal' milk because its composition changes continually throughout lactation. 'The protein and mineral contents rise steadily, while lactose and fat contents fall.

'Sow's milk is particularly rich in fat having, on average, some 8·5 per cent, or 45 per cent of the dry matter. The fat percentage, although very erratic, tends to reach a peak around the third week of lactation and has been reported as high as 17·2. This sudden, very high fat level in the diet . . . may be of considerable significance in the incidence of piglet scours which frequently occurs at about 3 weeks of age.

'The diet of the sow, both quantitatively and qualitatively, affects the fat content of the milk. Weight loss during lactation, associated with high pregnancy and low lactation feed allowances, results in a reduced yield of milk but of higher fat content. It appears that milk of high fat content, and so of higher than usual energy value, has a depressing effect on the growth rate of the pigs.

'Apart from its inadequate iron level, sow's milk appears to be an ideal feed for young pigs, allowing as it does an efficiency of feed conversion on a dry matter basis of some 0·8 lb. feed per lb. of gain. Its failure is quantitative rather than qualitative; thus, an average yield is about 100 lb. milk per piglet suckled, or 20 lb. dry matter in 8 weeks which, at an efficiency of conversion of 0·8, is sufficient to allow a weight gain of 25 lb. With an average birth-weight of 3 lb. this would allow the production of 28-lb. weaners at 8 weeks, so a 40-lb. pig at this age must have consumed some 24 lb. creep-feed at an efficiency of feed conversion of about 2 : 1.

'Sow's milk has a crude protein content increasing from about 25 to 33 per cent of the dry matter as lactation advances; the major requirement, therefore, is for energy. This fact seems frequently to be overlooked in the compounding of creep-feeds which tend to have needlessly high protein levels. While an early-weaning diet requires to have a high protein content, which will vary with the age of pig to which it is given, this is not so for a creep-feed which is merely an energy supplement to milk—already higher than it need be in its percentage of protein.' (Dr. G. A. Lodge.)

SOW'S MILK, ABSENCE OF, following farrowing, may be due to prior feeding with excessive quantities of fodder beet, or to inflammation of the uterus (metritis). Another cause is an endocrine failure. Post-parturient fever (p. 741) is an important cause. Wet, cold floors and cold, draughty premises appear to predispose sows to mastitis and agalactia.

In Southern Rhodesia heavy losses of piglets have resulted from this failure of the sows' milk supply, and the cause was traced to the fungus ergot, parasitic on bulrush millet ('Munga'). (*See* PREDNISOLONE, POST-PARTURIENT FEVER *and* ERGOT OF MUNGA.)

SOW STALLS.—These are now widely used for dry and pregnant sows, and ensure that each animal obtains her fair share of food. However, in partly slatted stalls high culling rates have sometimes resulted from defective slats causing foot and leg injuries, leading in some instances to partial or complete paralysis of the hindquarters.

SOYA BEAN POISONING.—It is an unfortunate fact that chiefly through wrong usage the extremely valuable soya bean has been the cause of outbreaks of poisoning. These beans are very rich in proteins and fat, and when given first to an animal are frequently offered in much too large quantities. Scouring and indigestion of a very severe type follow, and death may occur in some instances. In addition to this, the beans are imported for the purpose of extraction for soapmaking, and a solvent known as trichlorethylene is sometimes used; thereafter the residue may be pressed into soya bean cake, and if a small proportion of the solvent remains in the cake it is liable to produce symptoms of poisoning. At present the cakes on the market are mostly safe, but they, soya beans, and soya bean meals, should be given to animals in very small amounts to begin with, and the maximum amount per head of cattle per day should not greatly exceed one pound. Used in this way the beans are perfectly harmless, and constitute a very valuable and rich food-stuff for growing animals, milking cows, and fattening bullocks.

SPANISH FLY is a popular name for cantharides, which is used as a blistering agent. (*See* CANTHARIDES.)

SPASM (*σπάσμα*, a convulsion) means an involuntary and, in severe cases, a painful contraction of a muscle, or of a hollow organ with a muscular wall. Spasm may be due to some affection in the muscle itself where the spasm takes place, or it may originate in the nervous areas that control the spasmodically acting muscles. Spasms affecting the whole body are spoken of as 'convulsions': those of a painful nature are called 'cramp' when they affect the skeletal muscles, and 'colic' when they affect the hollow muscular organs. When the spasm is a prolonged firm contraction it is called a 'tonic spasm', and when it occurs as a series of short twitches, or as alternate contraction and relaxation, it is known as a 'clonic spasm'. Spasm is a symptom of a great variety of diseases, and further information is given under ASTHMA; COLIC; CHOREA; CONVULSIONS; CRAMP; EPILEPSY; MUSCLES, DISEASES OF; SPINAL CORD, DISEASES OF; STRYCHNINE; TETANUS; TETANY; etc.

SPASTIC (*σπαστικός*, drawing) is a term applied to any condition showing a tendency to spasm, such as 'spastic gait'. It is specially associated with disease affecting the cranial part of the nervous system concerned in movement (*i.e.* the upper neurone) so that its regulating function is lost and the muscles are in a state of over-excitability.

In British Friesian cattle, an inherited spastic form of lameness may appear when the calf is six or eight weeks old, but sometimes not until it is six months old. Before long, the toe may not touch the ground as the calf walks, and the affected hind leg is held backwards. Later, the leg becomes shortened and useless. If, however, the case is treated early enough, a simple operation will correct the deformity and prevent these unfortunate sequels. But of course, that calf, grown to maturity, can transmit the deformity to a proportion of his offspring. The condition has also been seen in Shorthorns and Aberdeen-Angus crosses. (*See* TENOTOMY.)

SPAVIN (old French *esparvin*) generally means that condition of the hock which is more correctly called 'bone spavin', to differentiate between 'bog spavin' and the rarely used term 'blood spavin'. (*See* BONE SPAVIN, BOG SPAVIN, BLOOD SPAVIN.)

SPAYING is the term commonly used for the removal of the ovaries in the female. Ovariotomy, oöphorectomy, and female gonadectomy are other terms with the same meaning. Strictly speaking, the term 'ovariotomy' should be reserved for the removal of diseased ovaries, while 'oöphorectomy' should be applied to the removal of healthy ovaries. The word 'ovarohysterectomy' indicates the removal of the ovaries and the uterus.

Objects.—Healthy female animals are, in many countries, operated upon for the same reasons as males are castrated. The operation in the mare is carried out to prevent promiscuous breeding.

Also, mares to be used in cavalry regiments, or polo pony mares, as well as certain thoroughbred racing mares, where the occurrence of œstrum and its associated phenomena would interfere with the proper performance of work, and mares which are suffering from some definitely hereditary disease, are subjected to the operation.

In 'nymphomania', ovariotomy, when performed before the symptoms have been in existence for long, usually results in a complete cessation of the kicking, squealing, and fractiousness which generally render the mare unfit for work.

Cows are operated upon to enable them to continue to produce milk for long periods (sometimes for as long as four years) without the disturbances accompanying parturition. They usually give an increased flow of milk which has a better butter fat content than previously, and the flow remains practically steady for at least 18 months. In certain city byres, where the cows are kept purely for milk production, and where calves are not wanted, since there is no accommodation for them, the operation, carried out as soon after calving as possible, allows a more uniform supply of milk to be ensured, and at the same time encourages fattening, so that by the time the cow has fallen below the arranged productive standard (*e.g.* perhaps 3 gallons per day) she is usually ready for immediate disposal to the butcher. Such commercialisation of dairy cows offers very great advantages over the usual system of only milking the cows during a normal lactation period, and then selling them for beef. The flesh from a spayed cow is more tender and succulent, and the carcase more uniformly fattened than in ordinary dairy cows. On ranches where there are large numbers of cattle, in North and South America, the females are very commonly spayed to enable them to settle down in the herd more quietly, and to fit them to produce better quality beef.

In pigs the operation is very commonly performed in commercial fattening herds. Gilts are spayed at about 10 weeks of age, and the difference between those which have been operated upon and those that have not becomes noticeable in the course of 1 month or 6 weeks later. The spayed pigs fatten quicker; they are undisturbed by œstral excitement; castrated males can be fed with them, and their carcases are of better value.

Cats are spayed to prevent the extremely promiscuous breeding that would otherwise occur. The operation is almost invariably satisfactory, and involves few if any disadvantages.

Bitches are spayed to a less extent than cats. The operation may be requested by the owner on account of domestic difficulties or convenience, or it may be advised as a means of preventing pyometra or to overcome nymphomania, for example. It is desirable after fracture of the pelvis or in the treatment of 'sexual alopecia'. Joan O. Joshua, F.R.C.V.S., has advised (*see Vet. Record* for June 5, 1965) that the uterus should be removed as well as the ovaries, and that the operation should be delayed until after at least one 'heat' period; preferably more than one.

Operation.—The actual operation may be performed in one of two ways: after appropriate preparation, an incision may be made in the left flank, the cleansed hand inserted, and the ovaries secured and removed by an ecraseur; or the incision may be made in the roof or floor of the vagina, and the same procedure followed. With ordinary care no complications occur, though hæmorrhage in some cases may be somewhat alarming. In many parts of America, and in parts of Switzerland, where large numbers of animals are spayed annually, the operation is regarded as of no more consequence than castration in the male.

Kittens are best spayed when between 4 and 6 months old, under nembutal or ether anæsthesia. Ovariohysterectomy is performed, usually through a flank incision.

SPEARWORT POISONING (*see* BUTTERCUP POISONING).

SPECIFIC (*species*, a particular kind; *facio*, I make) is a term used in various ways. It is applied to remedies that have a definite curative effect on certain diseases, *e.g.* cobalt in pining or potassium iodide in actinomycosis. The term is also applied to certain diseases that have an identity of their own, are due to a definite cause, and do not consist of a group of symptoms; such as, for example, foot-and-mouth disease, etc. Those conditions which are vague, such as diarrhœa, enlarged glands, or dyspepsia, are not specific.

SPECTACLES, so-called, of plastic

material are sometimes used to prevent poultry from resorting to cannibalism, etc. 'Spectacles' for horses in mines are really eye-shields.

SPECULUM (*speculum*) is an instrument designed to aid the examination of the various openings of the body surface. Specula vary in shape and size according to the purposes for which they are intended, but they are either hollow, or else they consist of two or three blades which are inserted closed, and then are opened to separate the lips of the orifice to be examined. Many are provided with small electric lamps which illuminate the cavity under examination.

SPEEDY-CUT is the name given to the injury that results from a horse striking the inside of a fore or hind knee or cannon bone with some part of the inside of the shoe of the opposite foot. (*See* BRUSHING AND CUTTING.)

SPERMATIC. — Blood-vessels, nerves, and other structures that are associated with the testicle.

SPERMATOZOA.—The male germ cells. (*See under* REPRODUCTION *and* ARTIFICIAL INSEMINATION, and Plate 8.)

S.P.F.—Specific Pathogen-free. In Britain as in the U.S.A., S.P.F. pigs are available for repopulating farms where disease has become a problem. S.P.F. piglets are removed from the uterus by surgery in a sterile manner, reared in elaborate isolation premises, and immunised and prepared for a normal farm environment. (*See also* 'DISEASE-FREE' ANIMALS.)

SPHENOID (σφήν, a wedge; εἶδος, form) is a bone lying along the base of the skull in front of the occipital bone, and immediately above and slightly behind the throat.

SPHINCTER (σφιγκτήρ).—A circular muscle which surrounds the opening from an organ, and by maintaining constantly a state of moderate contraction prevents the escape of the contents of the organ. The muscle fibres forming the sphincter relax under nervous influence when the contents of the organ are due to be discharged to the outside past the sphincter. Sphincters close the outlet from the stomach, bladder, rectum, and regulate the escape of the contents from these organs. Under certain conditions the nervous mechanism which keeps these sphincters shut is liable to become upset, so that fæces and urine, for instance, can escape freely. This incontinence is one of the important symptoms seen in fracture of the spinal column, and in some forms of paralysis.

SPHYGMOGRAPH (σφυλμός, the pulse; γράφω, I write) is an instrument used for recording the pulse.

SPICA BANDAGE (*spica*, a head of grain) is a method of applying the ordinary roller bandage so that it will accurately fit a part that has a variation in its diameter at different places. (*See* BANDAGES.)

SPINAL ANÆSTHESIA (*see under* EPIDURAL ANÆSTHESIA, the form most commonly used in the domestic animals).

SPINAL COLUMN is the name given to the chain of bones reaching from the base of the skull along the neck and back to the tip of the tail. It is composed of the vertebræ, and forms the central axis of the skeleton. Through the spinal canal, formed by the arches of adjacent vertebræ, runs the spinal cord, which gives off the spinal nerves running to various parts of the body. (*See* BONES, NERVES, SPINAL CORD.)

SPINAL CORD is the posterior part of the central nervous system, which is situated within the spinal canal of the spinal column. It forms the direct continuation of the medulla of the brain, being usually arbitrarily held to commence at the *foramen magnum*, the large opening in the occipital bone at the back of the skull. Posteriorly, it ends about the middle of the sacrum, although in this region the cord has lost its original form, and consists of a bundle of nerves, the acutal termination being at about the level of the joint between 5th and 6th lumbar vertebræ, the continuation of bundles behind this being known as the *cauda equina*, owing to its supposed likeness to a horse's tail. The spinal cord is thus considerably shorter than the spinal column which houses it. During its course in the horse it gives off 42 pairs of spinal nerves, each of which takes origin by means of a dorsal and ventral root, which join each other, before emerging from the spinal canal. These spinal nerves, according to their position, are known as *cervical* (8), *thoracic* (18), *lumbar* (6), *sacral* (5), and *coccygeal* (5), although the last ones take origin, not from any cord in the sacral or coccygeal regions, but from the cauda equina. The cord itself is divided into cervical, thoracic, lumbar, and sacral parts.

In the greater part of the thoracic region the cord is of uniform thickness, but the cervical and lumbar regions are considerably enlarged. Like the brain the cord is surrounded by three membranes, the *dura mater*, *arachnoid*, and *pia mater*, from without inwards. The arrangement of the two outermost membranes is, however, much looser than in the case of the brain. In the spaces of the arachnoid is a quantity of cerebro-spinal fluid, and between the outside of the dura and the inside of the bony canal is a padding of fat and blood-vessels, which together prevent injury to the spinal cord itself during the movements of the spinal column.

On section the spinal cord is found to be composed partly of grey, but mainly of white matter. It differs from the arrangement in the brain in that while in the brain the grey matter is on the outside of the white mass, in the cord the white matter is superficial. The arrangement of grey matter, as seen in section transversely across the cord, resembles the capital letter H, each half of the cord possessing a thinner dorsal and a thicker ventral ' horn ', and the masses at each side are joined by a wide bridge of grey matter known as the ' grey commisure '. In the middle of this commisure lies the ' central canal ' of the cord, which communicates with the ventricles of the brain. The horns of grey matter reach practically to the margin of the section (*i.e.* surface of the cord), and opposite their extremities commence the dorsal and ventral branches of the spinal nerves. The white matter is divided almost completely into two halves by a dorsal septum and a ventral fissure, which project inwards from the surface of the cord. The white matter on the ventral side of the central canal, however, runs across from one half to the other as the ventral ' white commisure '. This arrangement divides up the white matter into three main columns, known as the ' dorsal column ', ' lateral column ', and ' ventral column ', on either side of the middle line.

Microscopic structure.—The *grey matter* consists greatly of ' neuroglia ' cells, the supporting scaffolding fibrous-tissue cells of nerve regions, and in the meshes formed by these cells lie the large multipolar motor nerve cells, and the fibres which spring from them and unite one cell to another, or pass out of the cord to form the fibres of the nerve trunks. The *white matter* is composed almost entirely of bundles of nerve fibres, most of which possess a medullary sheath, the white colour being due to the appearance of these sheaths in the mass. (*See* NERVES.) There is also in the white matter a certain amount of supporting tissue. Most of the nerve fibres run towards or away from the brain, so that on cross-section of the cord the appearance of the ends of the nerves is that of a multitude of dots, each surrounded by a clear space. Blood-vessels are found in both white and grey matter.

Functions.—The cord has a double function. In part it receives impulses of sensation and transforms them into impulses of movement ; and in part it acts as the highway of nerve stimuli passing to or from the brain. The presence of governing nerve-centres in the cord, which possess the power of dealing with sensory stimuli and initiating the necessary movements, can be proved in several ways. For example, it has been calculated that the number of nerve-fibres entering or leaving the cord by the spinal nerves is about twice as great as the total number of nerve-fibres in the upper segment of the cord, immediately behind the brain. Further, if the cord be severed in the thoracic region (by fracture for instance), the control of the bladder and rectum does not immediately cease. Again, if a portion of the hind foot of an animal be stimulated, as by a mild electric shock, the movement ofd rawing away the foot from the source of pain occurs before the pain sensation has had time to reach the brain (the rate of nerve transmission being known). Many of these nerve-centres have been located in certain parts of the cord, and the position of the centres which regulate the size of the arteries, which control sweating, and which govern breathing and se ual mechanics, are known to exist in the cord. Over most of these, if not all, the brain exercises a supreme controlling power, and it is probable that before any incoming sensation is registered by the conscious mind, a free passage must be provided for it right up to the brain. Many of the acts of the skeletal muscles of an animal, especially those which are lightning-like in their rapidity, originate entirely in the spinal cord, without control of the brain ; thus, the placing of the feet upon the ground after landing from a jump by a horse, and the initiation of the spring forward for the next step, occur without the complete knowledge of the brain until after the event.

Most of the spinal centres act in a rhythmical or *automatic* manner, while certain others act purely *reflexly*. (*See* NERVES for a fuller description.)

SPINE AND SPINAL CORD, DISEASES AND INJURIES OF.—These will be considered together, because the chief danger of injury or disease in the spine is that the spinal cord and its nerves may be simultaneously injured or diseased. Only some of the practically important conditions will be considered.

FRACTURE of the spinal column is probably the commonest severe injury that affects this part. It may be met with in any animal, but is probably commonest in the horse and dog. It usually occurs from external violence, such as falls, falling timber, running into stationary objects and other run-away accidents, in the larger animals, and in the smaller animals it is often occasioned by run-over accidents, kicks or blows from large animals, falls from great heights, etc. It may occur from powerful muscular contractions when a horse is cast, or falls in a loose-box, and cannot easily regain its feet; while suddenly pulling up during a gallop in a hilly field occasionally causes it in saddle-horses. Paralysis of the hind-quarters, with loss of sensation, and often local sweating behind the injury, are symptoms of fracture, in addition to severe shock, occasioned by the laceration of the cord. (*See also* PARAPLEGIA *and* PARALYSIS.)

CONCUSSION of the cord, occasioned by factors similar to but milder than those which cause fracture, is also common. Generally speaking, if the onset of the symptoms of paralysis occurs a day or two after the accident, instead of at the time, concussion, with or without hæmorrhage, should be suspected, and hope of recovery can usually be entertained so long as there is not much systemic disturbance.

INTERVERTEBRAL DISC PROTRUSION.—Each intervertebral disc, which has a soft, pulpy centre and a fibrous or gristly outer ring, acts as a shock-absorber between the vertebræ, and supports the spinal cord between them. The nature of the usual disc injury is one of partial or complete rupture' with compression of the spinal cord to a less or greater extent. The injury is most common in Pekingese, Dachshunds, Sealyhams, and Spaniels. It also occurs in cats.

Cause.—The chief factor would appear to be a gradual wear of the disc with age, and perhaps the extra strain on the spine which may be imposed upon the short-legged breeds. In some cases there is no history of violence; in others, a sudden muscular effort, *e.g.* in jumping to catch a ball.

Symptoms.—These consist of pain and weakness or paralysis of the hind-quarters, and may appear shortly after the dog has been observed to jump, slip, or fall, or they may appear in cases where the owner has not observed any violent movement whatever. For example, a dog apparently normal at night may be found paralysed in the morning.

The muscles which control the passage of urine and fæces may become paralysed.

Outcome.—In many cases natural recovery takes place within a fortnight, and this applies even to dogs with paralysis. Where this persists, the outlook becomes progressively less hopeful; though a complete recovery after twelve months is not unknown.

Treatment.—A 'fenestration' operation is occasionally performed to relieve pain by relieving pressure upon the spinal cord, but it is not of much use for paralysis. Other measures are for the treatment of paralysis generally. (*See also* NANDROLONE.)

ANKYLOSIS of the vertebræ is not rare in horses. It originates from diffuse inflammation of the spinal column, frequently due to rheumatic causes, and one after another of the vertebræ becomes fused to its neighbour in front or behind. In severe cases practically the whole of the thoracic and lumbar regions of the horse may fuse into a rigid bar. Such horses usually can perform straightforward work for some time, but are unable to carry any weight, to back heavy loads, or to lie down or rise with ease. They may develop into 'shiverers', but so long as the spinal cord is not compressed they may live for years.

PACHYMENINGITIS, or inflammation of the membranes of the cord, sometimes occurs in old dogs. It is called 'ossifying pachymeningitis' in these animals, because of the tendency for bone to be deposited in the dura mater. Like most conditions of the spinal column it cannot be treated.

ABSCESS in the cord, or in one of the vertebræ, is not an infrequent accompaniment of tuberculosis in thoracic or lumbar vertebræ of cattle and pigs, and sometimes in the cervical region of the horse (where it causes a stiff neck). (*See* TUBERCULOSIS.) Abscesses may also occur during the course of strangles, and even glanders, in horses. Very often the presence of the abscess is never suspected during life, and it is only in the slaughter-house or the knackery that it is found upon post-mortem examination.

CHOREA (*see* DISTEMPER *and* CHOREA).

SPIRILLUM (diminutive of *spira*, a twist) is a form of micro-organism which has a wavy shape. (*See* BACTERIOLOGY.)

SPIRIT (*see* ALCOHOL *and* SURGICAL SPIRIT).

SPIROCHÆTE (σπεῖρα, coil; χαίτη, hair) is one of the names applied to bacteria possessing a more or less spiral or wavy outline. Another term applied to this group is 'spirillum'. There are three genera which are important causal agents of disease: *Borrelia*, *Treponema*, and *Leptospira*. The first has large wavy spirals and is flexible; the second has regular rigid spirals, while the last has small spirals and one hook-like end.

Many spirochætes produce disease in man and animals, the best known among which are: *Treponema pallida*, the cause of syphilis in man; *Treponema pertenuis* or *I. pallidula*, which causes frambœsia or yaws; there are also certain other forms which produce relapsing fever and African tick fever in man, and the *Borrelia gallinarum* is responsible for a form of tick fever or spirochætosis affecting fowls in the Sudan, and is transmitted by the fowl tick (*Argas persicus*). *Leptospira canicola* causes nephritis in dogs and canicola fever in man; *L. icterohæmorrhagiæ* causes Weil's disease in man and jaundice in dogs. Leptospirosis also occurs in cattle and pigs.

SPIROCHÆTOSIS OF FOWLS.—Although this disease does not occur in Great Britain, it is a serious cause of loss in many parts of the world. It was first observed in 1891 by Sakheroff in geese in the Caucasus, and he named the organism *Spirochæta anserina* (now called *Borrelia gallinarum*). It was later observed in South America in fowls, and the organism was then called *Spirochæta gallinarum*. The disease is met with in Africa, Asia, West Indies, South America, Australia, and in Europe. It occurs in fowls, ducks, geese, and turkeys. Canaries and other birds are susceptible to artificial infection.

Transmission.—The disease is transmitted from diseased to healthy fowls by the tick, *Argas persicus*. This tick is commonly called the 'Fowl Tick' and is one of the most important parasites of poultry. It is also known as a 'Tampan'. The ticks are very active at night, and may travel long distances to reach a host. They remain hidden during the day in crevices in the hen-house, cracks in spars, and underneath the bark of trees. Myriads of these ticks may attack fowls on the roost, a large quantity of blood being sucked, the affected birds becoming weak and unthrifty and having ragged plumage; diarrhœa is often present.

If, however, the ticks have fed on a bird affected with Spirochætosis, they become carriers of this disease and may transmit the infection through the egg to the next generation of ticks.

Symptoms.—Affected fowls show diarrhœa, loss of appetite, loss of power of the head, and may die in convulsions. A more chronic course is also described, birds becoming paralysed and emaciated, and dying in about a fortnight.

Treatment.—Penicillin is very effective.

Preventive Treatment.—This consists in ridding the premises of ticks.

SPLANCHNIC (σπλαγχνικός) means anything belonging to the internal organs of the body as distinguished from its framework.

SPLAYLEG, CONGENITAL (*myobrillar hypoplasia*) of piglets may involve either the fore-legs or all four. Recovery from this defect can be expected if the piglet can manage to keep out of the sow's way. (*See* VITAMIN E.)

SPLEEN is an organ situated in the abdominal cavity, and lies on the left side of the body a short distance away from the greater curvature of the stomach in most animals, but applied closely to the outside of the rumen in the ruminating animals. It possesses a copious blood-supply, but has no duct leading from it, and no connection with any other organ, beyond folds of peritoneum which keep it in place.

It is a soft, highly vascular, plum-coloured organ, possessing a smooth surface formed by a dense fibrous capsule over which the peritoneum is closely applied.

Structure.—Beneath the outermost covering of peritoneum lies the dense fibrous tissue coat, from the inner surface of which numerous strands or 'trabeculæ' run into the organ. The fibrous coat and the trabeculæ possess elastic fibres and a fair number of plain muscular fibres. The trabeculæ branch and rebranch throughout the substance of the organ, and in the meshes so formed lies the spleen-pulp. This consists of delicate connective-tissue fibres passing between the trabeculæ, and enormous numbers of white and red blood corpuscles. Blood-vessels run through the trabeculæ and end in areas where the blood cells appear to be highly concentrated; these concentrations are known as 'Malpighian corpuscles' or 'bodies'. The blood escapes into the pulp of the spleen instead of travelling through capillaries everywhere as in other organs.

Functions.—These are at best only vaguely known. The organ appears to play some part in the formation of the white blood corpuscles, for a greater number of these are to be found in the splenic veins than in the splenic arteries, and if the spleen be stimulated by passing a current of electricity through it the number of white blood corpuscles in the splenic veins greatly increases above normal. There is reason for believing that the spleen also destroys the old worn-out red blood corpuscles, and in some animals it appears to be capable of manufacturing new red blood corpuscles. At the same time, the function of the spleen is not thoroughly understood, for if it be removed in most cases death does not occur. There is a compensatory increase in the lymph glands all over the body, and, after a period of adjustment, life continues without any apparent disadvantage.

The spleen is apparently concerned with bodily defence, and resistance to liver fluke infestation is reduced after removal of a sheep's spleen.

SPLEEN, DISEASES OF.—In fact it is usually only at post-mortem examination that spleen diseases are manifest. It may be affected with disease of a specific nature in common with other organs, but it usually does not show any characteristic symptom when diseased. In the horse it may be affected with the nodules of tuberculosis, and with glanderous abscesses or thickenings. In anthrax it becomes greatly enlarged, and possesses large numbers of the *B. anthracis*, which can be found in its substance. Tumours are sometimes found in connection with its capsule, or even in its substance; sarcomata, especially of the melanotic type, being the commonest. Echinococcus cysts may be found on its surface. In common with other lymph glands it may be greatly enlarged in Hodgkin's disease, but it shows no change in structure when examined microscopically.

SPLENECTOMY.—Surgical removal of the spleen.

SPLINTS are means whereby an injured or wounded part is supported. They are in most cases employed where a bone has been fractured, and are designed to take the strain that was formerly sustained by the bone, as well as to keep the fractured ends at rest and in contact. The weight of the body in the ox and the horse makes it impossible to adjust a splint to the upper part of a fractured limb in such a way that it may give support, for the splint would require to be fixed so tightly that the skin and softer tissues would be injured beyond repair. They are, however, employed for the fixing of the limbs of the smaller animals, especially dogs and cats. They are generally made from wood, poroplastic felt, cardboard. They are either made so as to conform to the shape of the limb, or else they are padded with layers of cotton-wool. Bandages are used to hold them in position. Plaster of Paris bandages and casts are often used together with, or instead of, splints. Splints may be improvised from anything of a stiff nature that presents itself, such as strips of cardboard or laths. (*See* FRACTURES *and* KIRSCHNER-EHMER SPLINT, *and* PLATE 7.)

SPLINTS IN HORSES are bony enlargements which occur upon the cannon bones, or in connection with the small metacarpals or metatarsals ('splint bones') as the result of localised periostitis or ostitis. They form most commonly in the limbs of young horses doing strenuous work upon hard or uneven surfaces, and only rarely after the horse has reached the age of six years. At or about this age fusion between the large central cannon bone and the smaller splint bones is generally complete.

Splints are found in the fore-limbs more commonly than behind, and on the inside oftener than on the outside of the limb. They occur in all classes of horses, though they are very rare in such breeds as the Shetland, Iceland, and Fells and Dales ponies. They may assume almost any shape, being either diffuse or discrete,

SPLINTS IN HORSES

prominent or otherwise, regular or irregular, and they may be placed high up towards the joint, being then known as 'knee splints', or they may be placed low down on the cannon. They may be situated towards the anterior aspect of the limb, or they may be found farther back where they may interfere with the freedom of play of the flexor tendons.

Causes.—Inflammation of the periosteum only, or of this and the bone below it, with subsequent deposition of lime salts, directly results in the formation of a splint. A vitamin D deficiency in the foal may possibly be partly responsible. The factors which contribute to this inflammation are numerous; they probably include the following:

Excessive concussion before the horse is mature, often occasioned by working young horses upon hard surfaces or at too fast paces; striking with the inside of the shoe of the opposite foot (*see* BRUSHING AND CUTTING); deformities of the knee (or fetlock) whereby the limb, when viewed from in front, is bent either inwards ('knock knees') or outwards ('bandy leg'), and extra strain is thereby thrown either upon the inside or the outside of the knee and cannon, and also upon the corresponding small splint bone; this causes the ligament which binds the small splint bone to the cannon bone (interosseous ligament) to become sprained and later inflamed, and the inflammation spreads to the covering periosteum and produces new bone tissue; in a similar manner, excessive pull by the outer or inner collateral ligament of the knee-joint may result in sprain of the interosseous ligament; a false step upon an irregular surface; continually straining the inside of one leg and the outside of the other, such as occurs when colts are kept upon hilly ground, and ascend or descend by paths worn obliquely across the face of the hill; and faulty shoeing, whereby the outer or inner heel or branch of the shoe is too high or too low, throwing added strain on outside or inside of the knee, are other causes. It is well established that heavy horses which are light in the bone, whereby the joint surfaces are smaller than normal, are more often affected than those with heavier, stronger bone. In other cases splints appear in horses that are well formed and rationally managed, and where no obvious predisposing causes have been in operation. In such instances, it is possible that heredity may exercise an influence.

Symptoms.—Very often splints may be found in a horse which has shown no lameness or other disability; in such cases it is probable that the normal process of fusion between the small splint bones and the cannon has gone too far, so to speak, but that acute inflammation has been entirely absent. More commonly, however, lameness appears before any bony enlargement can be seen or felt, although pressure over the region of splints causes pain. This lameness usually increases with exercise, and is worse on hard ground where concussion is greatest. The horse may walk sound, but trots lame to a surprising extent, considering the apparently sound walk. Continued trotting exaggerates the lameness, but after a rest it may not be seen until some little distance has been travelled. Later on, a soft putty-like swelling can be felt, and this becomes harder with time, until it can be finally recognised as bone. In knee-splint the leg is carried to the outside, and appears stiff. When the cause has been a blow or injury from the opposite foot the lameness is present from the start, and external signs of the injury can be seen. As a rule splints are not serious, since with rest and treatment the bony fusion becomes complete, and the horse goes sound. When they are placed high up, however, there is a danger that the new bone formation may involve the knee-joint, and when they are situated far back, so as to interfere with the tendons, they may produce permanent lameness and injury to the tendon. In a horse under six years old they should be looked upon as liable to cause future trouble, but in an adult mature horse over six years old they can be disregarded unless lameness is present.

Treatment.—Most mild cases require nothing further in the way of treatment than a rest from work, applications of cold water or cooling lotions, during the acute stage, and later a run at grass for a fortnight or so. When due to striking, the shoeing should be altered, a brushing or speedy-cutting shoe, with a knocked-up or feathered inside edge being used. Protective speedy-cutting boots may be worn by the horse, or rubber pads may be applied. Chronic cases may require the operation of median neurectomy (unnerving), and other cases must be dealt with according to circumstances.

SPONDYLOSIS.—Loosening or breaking down of a vertebra.

SPONGES.—In modern stables it is recognised that if a contagious disease breaks out, the sponge used for a number of horses is an important factor in the spread of the disease, and consequently a piece of flannel or other material which can be boiled is generally used instead for 'quartering' (*see* GROOMING).

SPONGY BONE is a term used in at least two distinct senses. It is used to indicate bone whose normal appearance is suggestive of a sponge, that is, bone which is perforated by multitudes of small and large holes, through which pass blood-vessels in the living animal, such as is found in the bone of the foot that is enclosed in the hoof. In another way spongy bone means the cancellous bone that is formed as the result of inflammation affecting what was previously a compact bone. This is well seen in certain diseases such as actinomycosis of the lower jaws of cattle, and in osteoporosis. (*See also* 'RUBBER JAW'.)

SPORADIC DISEASE is a disease occurring in single cases here and there, as distinct from disease occurring as an enzoötic, throughout a district, or epizoötic, through a country or large tract of land. (For SPORADIC BOVINE ENCEPHALOMYELITIS *see* BUSS DISEASE.)

SPORES.—Reproductive cells of protozoa, bacteria, and fungi, etc., usually able to withstand an adverse environment.

SPORIDESMIN.—A poisonous substance, isolated from the fungus *Pithomyces chartarum*, which causes Facial Eczema and liver damage in sheep and cattle in New Zealand and Australia.

SPOROTRICHOSIS is a disease of horses and man, caused by *Sporotrichum beurmanni*, which usually gains entrance through a scratch or small wound of the skin. It is characterised by the formation of nodules in the skin, and is unaccompanied by pain. Common sites of the disease are the regions of the insides of the fetlocks, coronets, inside of the cannons, and on the insides of the thighs, but it may also occur on the body, in positions which are liable to be abraded by the harness. The nodules commence as small swellings about the size of peas or a little larger; these slowly increase in size, and after a short time the surface of the skin in their centres becomes soft, and eventually a very small amount of pus is formed and escapes on to the hair around, which becomes matted and scaly. A raw-looking ulcerated surface remains behind, and is soon covered with a hairless scab. In from 3 to 4 weeks healing is complete, except for a small hairless area, but later on new nodules usually form at a little distance from the original lesion. Horses do not show any general disturbance.

The sporothrix may be transmitted to man, to the rat and mouse, and affected animals should be isolated.

Treatment.—Internal administration of iodide of potassium, together with external cautery by strong tincture of iodine (10 per cent strength), and later daily dressing with ordinary tincture of iodine.

SPOTTED FEVER (*see* ROCKY MOUNTAIN FEVER).

SPOTTED HORSE (*see under* APPALOOSA).

SPRAINED TENDONS is an extremely common condition both in the heavy and light draught horse. The flexors, superficial and deep, are mostly affected, but various other tendons may also be affected, such as those around the knee or hock, or the anterior extensors.

Causes.—The superficial flexor tendon is sprained during maximum weight-bearing by the limb, and the deep flexor becomes sprained at the period of thrust or push-off from the ground. While these statements are true in the majority of cases, it is probable that sprains can also occur from other causes, such as extreme tension when backing a load, during a slip, especially when the hind foot slides forward under the body, and when a horse makes a false step. Continued but mild strain, occasioned by allowing the toes of the feet to grow too long (as occurs when horses are allowed to wear their shoes for too long a period), colts running out on hilly pasture, over-training young animals, especially steeplechasers and hunters, and carelessness in jumping, are other causes.

Symptoms.—There are the usual signs of inflammation—heat, pain, swelling, and redness, although the latter may not be visible. Lameness is also present, but both it and the above signs vary in different cases. The swelling may only be slight, and localised to the upper, middle, or lower third of the back of the region of the cannon, or it may be diffuse and pronounced, causing an enlargement from the back of the knee or hock down to or even below the fetlock. Generally, the amount of lameness present is no indication of the severity of the situation of the sprain. A horse with a badly sprained deep flexor may walk almost sound, but goes pronouncedly lame when made to trot. A localised sprain of the check ligament and its insertion into the deep flexor tendon often produces acute lameness, but the condition is not so serious as a sprain of the tendons lower down. From an owner's point of view, however, differential diagnosis between the various forms and situations of sprain is not important.

Treatment.—The best mode of treatment of early sprains is to encase the injured part of the limb in an antiphlogistic dressing. Kaolin and glycerine paste, or the proprietary substance 'Antiphlogistine', spread with cotton-wool, and applied hot, being bandaged with an elastic bandage, fairly firmly, gives very good results indeed. The horse must be kept at rest, however, not being taken out of the stable for watering or exercise, or for any other reason, for about a week or 10 days, according to progress. Its shoes should be removed and a heel or calkin fitted to each, to ensure the horse standing level. The hair, if long, should be clipped away first, and the inflamed area may with advantage be massaged for 20 minutes previous to the application. After the heat and pain have to a certain extent subsided, the dressing may be removed, and cold stimulating and astringent applications substituted.

Generally a horse with a badly sprained tendon is not fit for work for from a month to six weeks, although it may be apparently sound before this time.

Chronic sprained tendons are often incurable, but good results have sometimes been obtained with diathermy. Efforts may be made to render the horse fit to do light slow work, and in some cases heavy work may be possible for a certain time, but eventually, when the shortening and thickening of the tendons has resulted in excessive knuckling, it becomes necessary to pension off the horse (mares being sometimes used for breeding), or to have it destroyed. (*See* DIATHERMY.)

SPRAINS are injuries in the neighbourhood of joints, consisting usually in the tearing of a ligament with the subsequent effusion of blood. The term is also applied to an inflammation of a tendon, generally the result of an excessive stretching of its fibres. Sprains usually occur in the limbs of animals as the result of slipping, stumbling, great muscular effort such as is necessary to start a heavy load, or other condition where the tendons are submitted to severe strain. Sprains may affect muscles in certain cases, such as in 'sprained back' or 'sprained neck'. In these conditions the injury is the consequence of violent effort on the part of the horse or other animal, and as there are no tendons of any size or importance which take the strain, all the stress is borne by the muscles themselves. Their fibres may be incompletely torn, or they may be only severely stretched, but the painfulness that follows is almost equally severe in the two instances, although an actual rupture of some of the fibres is much the more serious, and results in a considerable stiffness. (*See* SPRAINED TENDONS.)

SPRAY 'DRIFT'.—By this is meant droplets of spray liquid carried by the wind to fields adjacent to that which is being intentionally sprayed with some farm chemical for purposes of weed control, pest control, haulm destruction. It is a potential cause of poisoning in grazing animals. (*See* SPRAYS USED ON CROPS.)

SPRAY RACE.—A race which can be used for spraying sheep or cattle. Nozzles are arranged at intervals and fed with suitable parasiticide liquid by means of a pump.

SPRAYS, consisting of antiparasitic dressings, are sometimes used in the treatment of mange in cattle, horses, pigs, and sheep. (*See* BHC; DIELDRIN.)

SPRAYS USED ON CROPS include weedkillers such as DNOC, insecticides such as Parathion, and potato haulm destroyer such as arsenites. Such substances constitute a hazard to livestock which gain entry into fields. (*See* POISONING, INSECTICIDES, WEEDKILLERS, etc.)

'SPREADING FACTOR' (*see* HYALURONIDASE).

SPURGES, POISONING BY.—The various species of spurges (*Euphorbia* sp.) are, apparently, mostly poisonous, though not to the same extent. Animals are not extremely likely to eat them because of the acrid milky juice. Species which have been blamed for causing poisoning are as follows: Caper spurge, *Euphorbia lathyris*; Irish spurge, *E. hibernica*; Petty spurge, *E. peplus*; and the Sun spurge, *E. helioscopia*; and of these the first seems to be the most dangerous.

Symptoms.—Inflammation and swelling of the mucous membranes of the mouth and tongue, pains in the abdomen, coldness of the extremities of the body, dizziness, fainting, leading to unconsciousness and death in 2 or 3 days. In one of the South African spurges, *E. genistoides*, the topical symptom, in addition to these mentioned here, is an acute inflammation of the urethra, accompanied by frequent and painful attempts at urination. Cornevin states that where abundant sweating occurs during the course of the symptoms recovery will usually follow; when no sweating occurs death may be looked for in a few hours after fainting and unconsciousness become severe. Profuse superpurgation and symptoms of acute enteritis (inflammation of the intestines) also indicate a fatal termination.

Treatment. Skilled assistance should be sought at once, and since the milk of affected cows may cause illness to people drinking it, it should not be used either for human or animal consumption.

SPUR VEINS.—The veins liable to damage by the horseman's spurs.

SQUILL is the sliced bulb of *Scilla maritima*, a plant from the shores of the Mediterranean. It contains several substances which have an irritant effect upon the glands of the stomach and bronchial membranes, as well as on the kidney. In small doses these glands are stimulated to extra secretion, and the discharge of thick mucus or other material is hastened by the thinning action of the poured-out fluid.

Uses.—The syrup of squills is used mostly. It is given in cases of dropsy when there is reason to suspect the kidneys of sluggishness, and in cases of bronchitis when the secretion is very thick and difficult to dislodge and expel. It is useful in the case of old dogs on account of its stimulating action on the heart. (*See also* Red Squill.)

'STABLE COUGH' (*see* Equine Influenza).

STABLES.—Whenever possible stables should be arranged so that the horses' heads are all directed towards the outside walls, and with a wide passage behind them. It is customary to have the horses all against one wall, with the passage close to the wall behind them, in smaller farm stables, and this is undoubtedly the more satisfactory method of arrangement. Each horse should have its own stall, divided off from its neighbours by a good, strong, and ample stall-partition. The stable should be large enough to allow each horse a cubic space of 1000 cubic feet for heavy draughts, and 750 cubic feet for the cab-horse type. These figures are the minimum. In most modern stables there is accommodation at one or both ends for animals which will not settle satisfactorily in a stall, by providing one or more loose-boxes. So long as these are only used by horses which are healthy or are not affected with a contagious disease there is no objection to their situation, but when *contagious* or other troubles break out in a stable there is a great temptation to put the sick horse in this loose-box, instead of isolating it in a proper sick-box by itself.

Stalls.—The length of a stall from the facing wall to the heel-post of the stall partition should be 13 feet for large and 10 feet for average horses, and the width from 6 ft. to 6 ft. 6 in. Each horse should have its own manger and hay-rack, the latter preferably on the same level as the former, for when the racks are high up horses are very liable to get hay-seeds in their eyes and mane. The manger should be made of metal with a wide edge which the horses cannot grip with their teeth. It should be lined inside with some material which can be disinfected when necessary and which does not rust. The partition should be of 2-inch thick wood up to a level of about 4 feet from the floor, and of metal rails above this. At the front of the stall the height of the partition should be about 7 feet, and from this backwards it should drop until it is about 5 feet at the heel-post. At the front of the stall it is usual to have a cast-iron plate, back to a distance of about 5 feet from the wall, instead of railings, so that horses cannot see each other when feeding, and nervous animals will not be annoyed by their neighbours. Kicking plates of mild steel are often fitted on either side of the stall partitions, to prevent undue wear and tear of the wood of the partition towards the rear of the stall. The heel-post should not project above the rest of the partition, nor should it have any projections which may catch the reins of a horse which is being backed out of a stall. Opposite each stall there should be a window, or, at least, there should be a window between every two horses.

Floors should meet with the requirements specified previously, and should be provided with surface drainage. In each stall the surface is usually grooved in some fashion which will enable any urine passed, and any water used for washing, to flow to the back of the stall and into the shallow gutter which runs the length of the stable. At one end this gutter runs out of the building through a false brick, and discharges its contents into a gulley-trap, preferably connected to a liquid manure tank. The floor should slope sufficiently to assist the escape of fluid by these channels, *i.e.* in each stall there should be a fall of about 2 inches, and in the length of the stable there should be a fall of about 1 in 70. All corners should be filled in with a fillet of cement and rounded off so that no dirt may be collected.

Passages.—There should always be ample room in a passage, whether in a single-rowed or a double-rowed stable, for a horse to be backed out of its stall and turned round with ease and comfort. For this purpose a passage of about 8 feet for a single stable, and 15 feet for a double stable, is necessary. It is false 'economy' to 'economise' space by providing too narrow a passage, for with increasing narrowness the risk of accidents increases.

It is better to have no loft or store above the stable, for having a free air space above the animals the ventilation is always better, and, moreover, the presence of a loft, especially where hay is kept, is always a source of danger from fire—malicious or otherwise. Generally speaking, the stable should be in a situation where sunlight can fall direct upon it, and in a part where access to the stable is easy, and it should be convenient for the implement shed. The windows on one side should have a southern exposure in countries north of the equator. No other building should be nearer to it than about two and a half times the height of the taller building, but this requirement cannot always be ensured in towns and cities. Doors should open outwards. Harness should not be hung on pegs inside the stable, but should be accommodated in a harness-room at one end, and the corn-bin should be placed in a position where it will not interfere with the passage of horses entering or leaving.

Although some horses may never be inside a stable all their lives it is advisable, economical, and convenient to have a place where horses may be housed after their work, eat their food in comfort, and lie down to rest. In a good stable the essential points are that it should be light, well ventilated without being cold or draughty, be warm but never stuffy, have a floor which is impervious yet which gives a good foothold, have an efficient drainage system by which urine and water may escape to the outside before being received into a drain (surface drainage), have a roof which is absolutely rain-tight and which does not become cold in winter and hot in summer, and be built in a convenient position. The doors should be high and should not open in to the stables (good sliding doors are probably best); the windows should be out of reach of the horses' heads; the mangers should be made of iron and able to be cleansed with ease; the hay racks should not be above the level of the horses' heads lest hay seeds and débris get into their manes, ears, and eyes; the stall partitions should be such as will allow each horse to feed without fear of interference from its neighbours and yet not such as will interrupt the free circulation of air; and there should be no loft over the stable. (*See also* BEDDING.)

STABLE VICES AND TRICKS.—Horses which are shut in stables without exercise or work frequently learn vices and tricks which not only may be harmful to the animals themselves, but may be dangerous to persons who attend them. Perhaps the most objectionable is the habit of kicking when being approached. (*See under* KICKING, CRIB-BITING, WEAVING.) Eating the bedding may be merely an endeavour on the part of the horse to acquire a sufficiency of coarse bulky food when the ration is too concentrated, or it may be a bad habit. It can be prevented by supplying sawdust instead of straw, or peat moss litter, or tan bark, or another unpalatable kind of bedding material. (*See* BEDDING MATERIALS.) Chewing the head ropes, which is a bad habit often acquired by mules, can usually be stopped by soaking the rope in a mixture of spirits of tar and aloes for 12 hours, and then hanging it out to dry in the air. The objectionable taste of aloes and the smell of the tar combine to make the animal stop the habit. The use of a chain instead of a rope will prevent the animal from breaking loose, when the above measures fail. Refusing to lie is often the result of fear, nervousness, or physical inability, such as ankylosis of the spinal column. Horses may lie when housed in a loose-box instead of a stall, or a stout rope from one heel post across to the other may allow the horse to obtain some amount of rest. (*See* VICES, SLEEP, etc.). Gnawing the walls is usually a sign of the presence of worms, bots, a mineral or other deficiency, or indigestion, and appropriate measures should be taken to determine which condition is present, and to treat it accordingly.

STAG.—A male ox or pig castrated late in life, or a turkey cock (over one year old).

STALLION.—An adult male horse, uncastrated, over 4 years old. In Britain stallions over 2 years old must be licensed.

STAPHYLOCOCCUS (σταφυλή, a bunch of grapes; κόκκος, a kernel) is the name given to a micro-organism which under the microscope appears in small masses very like a bunch of grapes. The organism is found in pus and discharges from wounds or abscesses. (*See* BACTERIOLOGY.)

STARCH (*see* CARBOHYDRATES, DIETETICS, *and* DIGESTION).

STARCH EQUIVALENT.—This term is used to indicate the feeding value of a given food in terms of starch. For example, linseed cake has a starch equivalent of 74 per cent; *i.e.* 100 lb. of the cake has the same energy value as 74 lb. of starch. The S.E. of grass silage varies between 0·1 per cent and 12 per cent, according to the sample; that of kale is about 9 per cent. (*See also* PROTEIN EQUIVALENT.)

STARING COAT, A.—In the dog there are several causes of this, but one is lack of suitable fat in the diet. As a first-aid measure, offer bread and butter or dripping (but not margarine) for a few days as an 'extra'. (*See also under* WORMS.)

STARVATION.—Abstention from food or the taking of too little food for a sufficiently long period to induce a loss of condition of the body generally. It may occur gradually, as when an insufficiency of food is obtained, or it may result from a total deprivation of food, as when an animal strays from control in a part where there is no food suitable to its needs. (An abundance of unsuitable food may still give rise to malnutrition, which is really 'starvation' from a lack of certain essentials.)

When food and water are withheld from an animal for a considerable period, two definite changes take place in the body economy; the animal becomes rapidly lighter, as the result of using up its reserve stores of food, and its temperature falls. If water be given alone emaciation is very marked, but death does not take place so rapidly, nor are the sufferings of the animal so great. If the creature is compelled to undertake great efforts of a physical nature, without food or water, the loss of condition, from using up the natural stores of nourishment faster, is extremely rapid. If, in addition to the previous privations, it is forced to withstand great cold, the combination of adverse circumstances reaches its maximum, and life cannot be sustained for more than a few days. In spite of these facts, there are instances on record where animals have lived after being exposed to extreme conditions of starvation. Horses have been known to live without food or water for as long as 3 weeks; dogs have lived 4 weeks under the same conditions; sheep buried in the snow have survived for 8 weeks and 5 days, and have recovered afterwards; and a horse has lived for 30 days when allowed water but no food.

When animals have been starved for any length of time, it is unwise and unsafe to give large feeds for the first 3 or 4 days. To commence with only fluids should be offered, such as barley gruel and whisky, linseed tea, oatmeal drinks, and for the smaller animals preparations such as hydrolised protein, 'Benger's Food', 'Glaxo', 'Mellin's Food', etc. It is asserted that horses that have been completely starved for over 15 days although allowed water, will never recover no matter how they may be treated. This period does not, however, apply to other animals, as witness the sheep above mentioned. (*See* NURSING OF ANIMALS, FASTING.)

STASIS (στάσις, halt) is a term applied

to stoppage of the flow of blood in the vessels or of the food materials in the intestinal canal.

'STEAMING UP'.—A term used by dairy farmers to describe the practice of feeding a concentrates ration 6–8 weeks before calving in order to provide for growth of the fœtus and provide reserves against the onset of lactation.

STEATITIS.—A yellow discolouration of fat occurring in cats, mink and pigs fed mainly on fish scraps or tinned fish. Listlessness, tenderness over the back and abdomen, and a reluctance to move are observed. Treatment: administer vitamin E; also the B complex.

STEATORRHEA.—Fatty fæces.

STEER.—A young male ox, usually castrated, and between the ages of 6 and 24 months.

STEINACH'S OPERATION.—Occlusion of the *vas deferens*—a 'rejuvenation' operation in man. (*See under* CASTRATION.)

STELL.—A circular stone or corrugated metal shelter for sheep or cattle, built on moorland or hill, and affording good protection against snow drifts. Stells were in use in the early nineteenth century, if not earlier, but metal ones have now come on to the market.

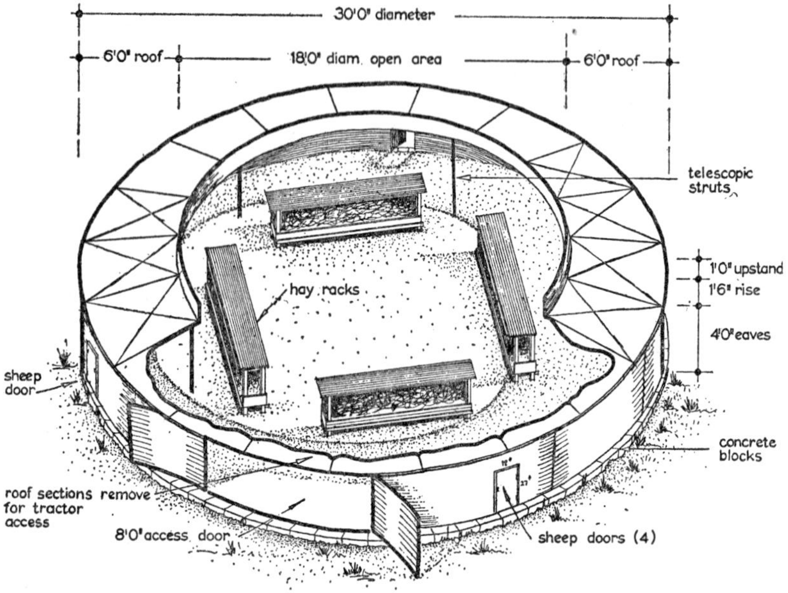

Of metal construction, on a base of concrete blocks, this modified Stell at the Rowett Research Institute, Aberdeenshire, was designed by Dr. E. Cresswell. Sheep doors and an 8 ft. doorway for tractor access are shown.

STENOSIS (στενός, narrow) is a term applied to any unnatural narrowing of a passage or orifice of the body. It is specially reserved for application to the heart valves, and to the opening through the larynx—the glottis—but is applied to any of the large arteries, as well as to the parotid ducts. (*See* HEART DISEASES, LARYNX, PAROTID DUCT, PYLORIC STENOSIS.)

STENSON'S DUCT is the duct which carries saliva from the parotid gland into the mouth. (*See* PAROTID GLAND.)

STEPHANOFILARIASIS.—A chronic skin disease occurring in cattle in parts of the U.S.A., and caused by the nematode worm *Stephanofilaria stilesi*. The intermediate host is the horn fly.

STERILISATION is a word used in two senses; it may mean the removal of the essential sexual organs—testes and ovaries —from animals, whereby they are rendered incapable of breeding (*see* CASTRATION; *also* SPAYING), or it may mean the process of rendering objects which come into contact with disease, or wounds, food, etc., free from infective organisms. The manner of rendering animal-buildings, which have housed diseased inmates, free from infection is given under the heading DISINFECTION; and the processes applied to instruments, dressings, skin surfaces, etc., is given under ANTISEPTICS, ASEPSIS, and WOUNDS. For most general purposes the best sterilising agent is boiling water. Boiling should be continuous and should last for at least 10 minutes in order to kill vegetative bacteria, viruses, and most other types of micro-organisms. Many spores withstand boiling for hours and some even for days.

STERILITY, or BARRENNESS, means failure on the part of an animal to breed. When this failure is temporary, the term 'infertility' is commonly used. (*See* INFERTILITY.)

STERNUM (στέρνον, the chest) is another name for the breast-bone.

STEROIDS.—Chemical substances closely related to the sterols. Examples: the sex hormones, hormones of the adrenal cortex, bile acids. (*See also* CORTICOSTEROIDS *and* DIABETES.)

STEROLS.—Solid alcohols, waxy substances derived from animal (and plant) tissues. Examples: cholesterol, ergosterol.

STERTOR (*sterto*, I snore) is a term applied to noisy breathing resembling snoring. It is met with in all animals, and in the short-faced breeds of dogs, such as bulldogs, pugs, King Charles spaniels, etc., it is often a normal accompaniment of breathing. It is a symptom of paralysis of the soft palate in the horse, sometimes met with in grass sickness, cases of strangles, or sore throat, and in other affections of the respiratory tract. Concussion of the brain may produce it in any animal; it may be due to apoplexy, suffocation, or poisoning during the administration of a general anæsthetic. It may be due to a lolling back of the tongue into the pharynx when anæsthesia is well established, and when the animal is lying on its back. To prevent the tongue falling back it is generally secured by the anæsthetist.

Stertor must not be confused with *stridor*, a crowing breathing, due to spasmodic narrowing of the larynx; nor to the prolonged *wheezing* breathing characteristic of asthma in old dogs; nor must it be mistaken for *puffing* breathing which is seen in certain forms of pneumonia in dogs, when the lips are blown out with each expiration and sucked in with every inspiration. Roaring, due to paralysis of the muscles which activate one or both vocal cords, must be differentiated, as must also whistling breathing (*See* ASTHMA, PNEUMONIA, ROARING. etc.)

STHENIC (σθένος, strength) is a term applied to certain diseases, especially fevers, to indicate that they are not associated with prostration. It is the opposite of asthenic, which is associated with great weakness.

STIFF LAMB DISEASE.—This is a mild disease occurring in East Anglia due to infection with *Erysipelothrix rhusiopathiæ*, the cause of swine erysipelas. The same name is also applied to Muscular Dystrophy, a condition similar to that occurring in cattle as a result of vitamin E deficiency.

' STIFF-LIMBED LAMBS '.—This is a hereditary condition affecting newly born lambs, to which the name *Myodystrophia fœtalis deformans* has been given. It is commoner among Welsh Mountain sheep than among other breeds, but has been encountered in Suffolks, Southdowns, Hampshires, and Dorset Downs, and it is possible that it may occur more rarely in other breeds. The condition is an arrest of the development of muscular tissue during fœtal life, and a replacement by fibrous tissue. This contracts and pulls the limb into an unnatural, stiff attitude, and gives rise to difficulty in parturition. The condition is bilaterally symmetrical in that, although the degree of deformity may not be identical on each side, one limb only is never affected. The muscle tissue of the diaphragm is absent or represented only by small strips, and the intercostal muscles are affected, in consequence of this, although the lamb may be born alive—since its heart is beating—it cannot breathe, and consequently dies within about 3 minutes.

The condition is a Mendelian recessive lethal, which is transmitted from both the sire and dam of an affected lamb. The parents, however, cannot be distinguished from normal sheep until they have actually produced a deformed lamb; that is, only a breeding test will serve to differentiate them.

The mode of inheritance may be illustrated as follows:

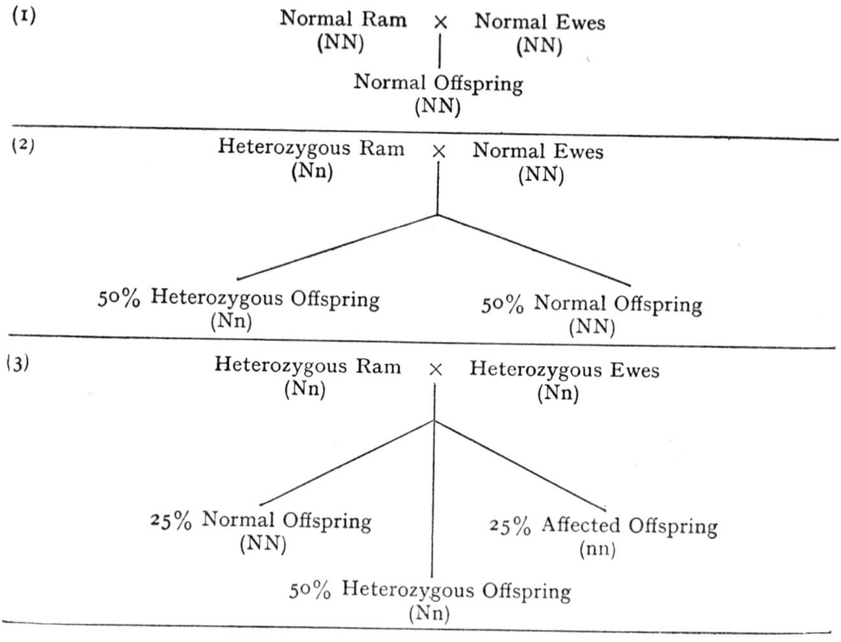

The condition has also been reported from Britain and America affecting cattle, but it is not at all common in them.

STIFF SICKNESS (*see* THREE-DAY SICKNESS).

STIFLE, THE.—The joint corresponding to the human knee. (*See* BONES *and* JOINTS.)

STILBŒSTROL (*see* HORMONES, HORMONE THERAPY).

STILLBORN PIGS.—Breeding stock should, of course, have access to pasture, but if for any reason this golden rule is going to be broken, then rations should be supplemented in summer as well as in winter, with vitamin A. In a group of 20 gilts which were suddenly switched from succulent feeding to dry, fibrous grazing late in pregnancy, severe constipation resulted, and there were dead piglets in 19 of the litters.

A survey carried out by the Veterinary Investigation Service in England and Wales showed a 4·8 per cent incidence of stillbirths out of a total of 4394 piglets born in 371 litters. The incidence varied widely from herd to herd, as would be expected; ranging from 0·4 to 12·9 per cent. Constipation appears to be a cause of stillbirths, and SENNA may be used.

There are several infections which give rise to abortion and stillbirths. Apart from swine fever and swine erysipelas, abortion may be caused by *Brucella abortus suis*—in Denmark, at least. Staphylococcal infections and *Coryne bacterium pyogemes* are other causes; likewise leptospirosis and toxoplasmosis. Mummification and absorption of the embryo piglets in the womb may occur in Aujesky's disease. (*See also* INFERTILITY.)

STIMULANTS (*stimulo*, I goad) are drugs or other measures which are employed to call forth special powers of the body or of a particular organ in order to effect some special purpose, or to offer increased resistance against an attack of acute disease. The use of stimulants presupposes a certain amount of resistance on the part of the body, or the organ stimulated, which is lying dormant or inert, and requires an appropriate stimulus before it can be brought to perform its special function. In fact, when the whole body is greatly depressed, as from severe starvation, a stimulus often proves too much for the overtaxed tissues, and death results.

Heart stimulants are probably the most typical examples of the class, and among the commonest of these may be mentioned caffeine, digitalis, camphor, strychnine, coramine, etc. Respiratory stimulants include carbon dioxide, minute doses of prussic acid and coramine.

STINGS (*see* BITES AND STINGS).

STIRK.—A young female bovine of 6 to 12 months old, sometimes a male of the same age, in Scotland.

STITCHING, or SUTURING (*see* WOUNDS).

STOCKING RATES.—During the peak of grass growth from early April to mid-June, 8 to 10 ewes and their lambs can be carried per acre. But this is a maximum figure for this period only. For cattle, continuous grazing, the figure is perhaps 1 to 3 acres; after two years of Rational Grazing, to use André Voisin's definition, the figure may become 1 to 2 acres.

In Britain, 'most grass is greatly understocked during the grazing season, chiefly due to the lack of capacity to carry more stock over winter.

'Good farmers, using intensive grass-farming methods, require 1½ acres or more per cow, even when winter feeding is supplemented considerably with concentrates.

'Estimates in New Zealand have suggested that dairy cows at 1·2 per acre may consume as little as 30 per cent of the available herbage.' (Director, Grassland Research Institute, Hurley, 1966.)

STOCKS are wooden or iron erections used to control the larger animals during minor operations, dressing wounds, rasping teeth, shoeing, etc. They consist of four strong uprights, usually sunk into concrete foundations, and united together by cross-bars. Provision is made for securing the horse's feet and head, so that it cannot do itself injury. Most are made so that the horse is led or backed between the posts, and when in position a cross-bar in front of the chest and behind the buttocks prevent exit. (*See* diagram *and also under* CRUSH.)

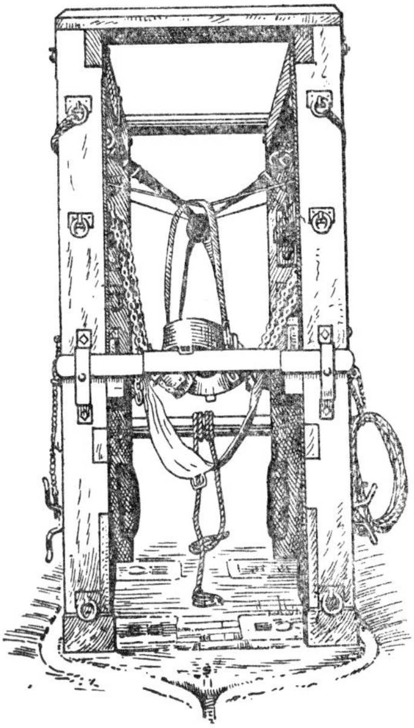

Drawing of a useful type of stocks for securing horses for minor operations, foot dressing, etc.

STOMACH.—The stomach is a dilated portion of the alimentary canal, provided with special digestive glands, and usually lying at the termination of the œsophagus. In ruminants, which are popularly thought to possess four 'stomachs', there are three dilatations of the œsophagus or gullet lying anterior to the true stomach. These act more as reservoirs for food than as active digestive organs, although certain mechanical processes and a considerable amount of bacillary digestion takes place in them before the food reaches the true stomach.

External appearance and relations.—Horse.—The stomach lies in the upper (dorsal) part of the abdominal cavity, behind the diaphragm and liver, and to the left of the middle line of the body. It lies between the level of the 13th to 17th ribs, moving backwards and forwards between these limits during inspiration and expiration.

It consists of a curved, somewhat flattened ovoid sac, arranged something like the letter 'U', with its entrance (the *cardia*) and its exit (the *pylorus*) close together. Between the cardia and pylorus, along the edges of the organ, there are the *greater* and *lesser curvatures*. The former

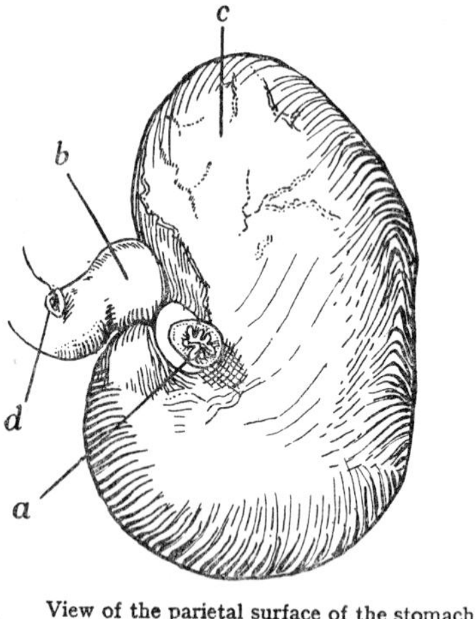

View of the parietal surface of the stomach of the horse. *a*, Cut end of œsophagus; *b*, commencement of duodenum; *c*, *saccus cæcus*, or blind sac; *d*, bile and pancreatic ducts entering the duodenum. (After Bradley's *Abdomen of the Horse*.)

of these is extensive, and the latter very small. The stomach possesses a 'parietal surface' lying close to the diaphragm; a 'visceral surface' related to the intestines; a 'left extremity', or *saccus cæcus*, which lies uppermost and to the left side, close to the base of the spleen and the pancreas; and a 'right extremity', or *pyloric extremity*, which becomes continuous with the duodenum—the first portion of the small intestine. At the cardia is a sphincter muscle which guards the entrance into the stomach from the gullet, and at the other end is the pyloric sphincter which regulates the passage of food material from the stomach into the small intestine. The capacity of the stomach is relatively small in horses, varying between 2 and 4½ gallons in horses of average size. It is attached by folds of peritoneum: to the diaphragm, by the *gastro-phrenic ligament*; to the spleen, by the *gastro-splenic ligament*; to the liver, by the *gastro-hepatic ligament*, or *small omentum*; to the colon and small

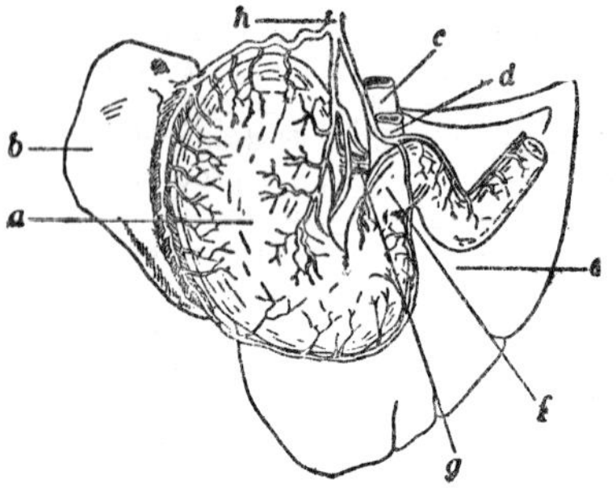

Diagram of the relations of spleen, stomach and liver in the horse. *a*, Visceral surface of stomach (*i.e.* the surface opposite to that shown in Fig. 282); *b*, spleen; *c*, caudal vena cava; *d*, portal vein; *e*, liver; *f*, pylorus; *g*, the cardiac end of the œsophagus; *h*, cœliac artery. (After Bradley's *Abdomen of the Horse*.)

intestine, by the *gastro-colic ligament*, or *great omentum*; and to the duodenum, liver, and pancreas, by the *gastro-pancreatic fold*.

Ox.—For convenience and to ensure continuity of description the three dilatations of the œsophagus will be described in addition to the stomach proper. Ruminating animals take in considerable quantities of food without thorough preliminary chewing. Provision is made for storing this material until time and circumstance will allow of deliberate and thorough chewing. This process is known as 'rumination' or 'cudding'. (*See* RUMINATION.) To enable the ox to store and prepare the large amount of bulky comparatively innutritious food, which forms its normal diet, three preliminary compartments have been provided: these are the *rumen*, 'paunch' or 1st stomach; the *reticulum*, 'honey-comb bag' or 2nd stomach; and the *omasum*, 'manyplies', 'book' or 3rd stomach. Lying behind and to the right of these is the *abomasum*, 'rede', 'rennet' or true stomach, or the 4th stomach.

Rumen.—The whole of the left side of the abdomen, except for a small portion occupied by the spleen, is taken up by the capacious rumen, which, when distended, reaches considerably over on to the right side of the median plane. It extends forwards as far as the space between the 7th and 8th ribs, and back to the pelvis. Its capacity varies between 20 and 30 gallons in small cattle; 25 and 35 gallons in medium-sized cattle; and up to 48 or 50 gallons in the largest cattle. Posteriorly the rumen is divided into an upper (*dorsal*) and a lower (*ventral*) *blind sac*, by deep depressions. The entrance of food into the rumen is by the termination of the œsophagus—where there is situated a structure known as the *œsophageal groove.* This actually lies in the wall of the reticulum, and food material from it gains the rumen by means of muscular movement which causes the end of the œsophagus (the *cardia*) to project very slightly from the reticulum through the *rumeno-reticular orifice*—a large oval opening between rumen and reticulum.

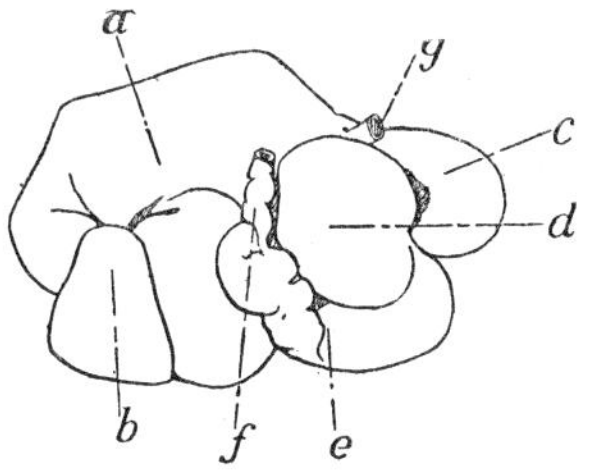

Diagram of the arrangement of the stomachs of the ox, viewed from the right side, with the animal's head facing to the right. *a*, Dorsal sac of rumen, inner face; *b*, posterior part of ventral sac of rumen; *c*, reticulum; *d*, omasum, which lies to the right of the middle line of the body; *e*, true digestive stomach or abomasum, from which the duodenum, *f*, takes origin.

Reticulum.—This is the smallest of the divisions, and the most anteriorly situated. It is placed immediately behind the diaphragm, practically in the middle line of the body, and in front of the rumen. Its entrance is by the *rumeno-reticular orifice*, and food material passes from it by the *reticulo-omasal orifice*, which lies at the lowermost part of the œsophageal groove. In its wall, as mentioned already, is situated the cardia and œsophageal groove. It is important to remember that a space of only about an inch separates the wall of the reticulum from the heart-sac (pericardium), and since sharp-pointed foreign bodies are very frequently swallowed by cattle, and almost invariably become lodged in the reticulum, the danger of such foreign bodies becoming forced through the wall of the reticulum, into and through the diaphragm, and so into immediate contact with the heart, is very considerable. (*See* HEART DISEASES.)

Omasum.—The 3rd stomach lies over to the right of the middle line of the body, between the level of 7th and 11th ribs, and comes into contact with the right abdominal wall between the 7th to 9th ribs. The entrance (*reticulo-omasal orifice*) and the exit (*omaso-abomasal orifice*) lie close together and at a lower level than the rounded or ellipsoidal bulk of the organ. In outline the organ is not unlike a laterally compressed football, and it lies between the rumen and the right abdominal wall, and mainly above the abomasum.

Abomasum.—The true digestive stomach of the ruminant is an elongated flask-shaped sac, lying for the most part on the right lower abdominal floor, to the right of the rumen and below the omasum. It has an upper short *lesser curvature* and a lower long *greater curvature.* It reaches from the 7th to the 12th intercostal space, and has an entrance from the omasum and an exit into the small intestine at the pylorus.

Sheep.—With certain minor differences the arrangement of the stomach in the sheep is similar to that of the ox in miniature. Its total capacity is about 4 gallons. The rumen is relatively larger than in the ox, and has not such extensive divisions. The reticulum is also larger in comparison, and lies more to the left of the middle line of the body. The omasum is very small, holding only about a pint, and is much compressed laterally. It is situated higher up in the abdomen, and does not come into contact with the right abdominal wall. The abomasum is relatively larger and longer than in the ox: it holds about half a gallon, which is practically twice as much as the reticulum.

Pig.—Like the horse and dog, the pig has a single stomach. It is of medium size, holding from 1½ to 2 or even 2½ gallons. It lies across the anterior lower part of the abdomen, touching both the right and left abdominal walls and reaching as far back as the umbilicus (navel). On the left side it is almost entirely under cover of the posterior part of the rib-cage, lying between the liver anteriorly and the spleen posteriorly, but on the right side it lies behind the rib-cage. It is characterised by possessing a small, flattened, conical, blind pouch (*diverticulum*) attached to the left extremity. Between the cardia and pylorus, which are not so close together as in the horse, is a lesser curvature uppermost, and a greater curvature in contact with the lower abdominal wall. The œsophagus joins the stomach very obliquely and practically in the middle line of the body.

Dog.—The dog's stomach is relatively large, holding about 2½ to 5 pints in animals of average size. It is irregularly pear-shaped, the larger end lying to the left side and the tapering pyloric end lying to the right. It lies behind the liver and diaphragm, while behind it are situated the pancreas, the left kidney, and the intestines, and the spleen lies along its left posterior surface. When the stomach is empty it is situated higher up in the abdomen, but when full it comes into contact with the lower abdominal wall, and the left abdominal wall over a considerable area.

Cat.—The stomach in the cat is very similar to, but smaller than, that of the dog.

Internal appearance and structure.—In all animals the stomach (or stomachs) is lined with *mucous membrane* lying above a *sub-mucous coat*. A thick *muscular wall*, with fibres arranged longitudinally, transversely or circularly and obliquely, and in some places irregularly, lies between the sub-mucous coat and the outer *peritoneal covering*. The muscular and peritoneal coats assume the form of the stomach, and, except that in the rumen of the ox and sheep there are thicker strengthening strands corresponding with grooves (*sulci*) on the surface, these layers call for no further description. The mucous lining, however, differs widely in the different animals. It can be divided into two types: the first possesses digestive, enzyme-secreting glands, and is known as *glandular mucosa*; and the second type possesses no glands, but is usually provided with a hard or horny ridged or papillated surface, and is known as *non-glandular mucosa*.

In the *horse* the interior of the stomach is lined by two kinds of mucous membrane: that which is found around the œsophageal orifice, and in the left sac generally, is white in colour, hard to the touch, devoid of digestive glands, and microscopically is covered by stratified squamous epithelium. This portion of the stomach appears to act as a reservoir in which a certain amount of food can be stored before being passed into the remainder of the stomach for digestive purposes. This non-glandular œsophageal portion ends abruptly along an elevated irregular line, which is known as the *margo plicatus*. Between this line and the pylorus the mucous membrane is glandular; it is soft, reddish-brown or pink in colour, has a velvety appearance, and usually has a certain amount of mucus adherent to its surface. At the pylorus and cardia there are *sphincter muscles*, which, when examined from the inside, are seen to cause the mucous membrane to be thrown into folds.

In the *ox* the rumen is lined by brownish mucous membrane except over the muscular ridges, where it is pale. It is non-glandular and thickly studded with large papillæ, which measure from ¼ to ½ an inch in length, and are of varying shape. Over the lips of the œsophageal groove the membrane is brown and wrinkled, but in the depths of the groove it is pale in colour and possesses longitudinal folds, while in the lower portion it carries a number of pointed horny papillæ somewhat resembling the claws of a bird. The reticulum is lined by a peculiar form of mucous membrane, being thrown into *primary* and *secondary ridges*. The primary ridges are about ½ an inch high, and enclose four-, five-, or six-sided pouches or *reticular cells*. These larger cells are further subdivided by the secondary ridges into secondary reticular cells, in the floors of which there are numerous pointed horny papillæ. The mucous membrane of the omasum is characterised by possessing large numbers of rounded horny papillæ carried upon about 100 large leaf-like folds or *folia*. These folia, about a dozen of which are very large and reach from the upper rounded portion of the organ (where they are attached) down to the neck, possess muscular fibres and have the power of contraction. As each folium contracts, its adjacent and contiguous neighbours, one on either side, remain stationary, so that food between any two folia undergoes a thorough process of grinding by the horny papilla. The action of the folia can be compared to rubbing the palms of the hands together to separate the grain from the chaff, etc., of an ear of wheat. The mucous membrane of the abomasum is glandular. In that part which is nearest the omasum there are about 12 large spiral folds, which provide a larger gland-carrying surface than would be the case if no folds were present. In the pyloric compartment, which is divided from the above by a constriction, the mucous membrane resembles that of the corresponding region in the horse.

In the *pig* the mucous membrane of the stomach around the cardia is œsophageal in character. It possesses no glands, is hard and white. This area, which only measures 3 or 4 square inches, is sharply separated from the rest of the lining, which is pale grey in colour, soft and velvety, and carries digestive glands. At the pylorus the glandular mucous membrane presents a number of folds and a remarkable ridge, which projects from the lesser curvature and decreases the size of the pyloric opening.

In the *dog* and *cat* the mucous membrane is wholly glandular. The œsophageal mucous membrane ceases abruptly at the cardiac orifice, and merges immediately into the glandular mucosa of the rest of the organ. The lining of the stomach is not folded or ridged as in some of the other animals, but the concentration of digestive glands is greater.

Functions of the stomach.—Broadly speaking, the function of the stomach is to store, warm, soften, and prepare food materials, and then to pass them on in regulated amounts into the intestine, where the more important digestive processes and absorption occur. The action of the gastric juice upon the food, and the processes which occur in the stomach, have been described under DIGESTION. The function of rumination in the ox and sheep has been described under RUMINATION.

Muscular movements of the stomach are of the greatest importance. In herbivorous animals particularly, where the natural food consists to a large extent of comparatively dry fibrous material (hay, for example), the muscular movements are of supreme importance to mix this dry material thoroughly in the stomach, and to incorporate amongst it water and digestive juices, including saliva swallowed from the mouth, so that the whole of the stomach contents is of a uniform consistency, and the drier food materials have fluids thoroughly distributed through them. In cattle, to a very large extent, these preparatory functions have been completed before the food reaches the abomasum, and they are, in these animals and sheep, of a very much more elaborate nature than they are in the other animals. (*See* RUMINATION.)

The movements, as seen by X-ray examination in the smaller animals, consist of a series of waves, occurring at different frequencies—usually faster in the smaller breeds of animals, and slower in larger breeds. When the stomach is only half-full or less the movement becomes sluggish, but when two-thirds full, or when reasonably full but not distended, the movements are most vigorous. Generally, during a feed, the food material left over from the last meal (a small amount of which always remains) is forced down into the pylorus and leaves the stomach before the meal has been completed. If the amount taken is large, especially in the horse, that which was eaten first has passed into the duodenum before the feed is finished. This is necessary in an animal with a comparatively small stomach. The horse in nature feeds at a slow but regular rate for a long period of time, and then rests for a short period, generally during the middle of the day, and resumes feeding again shortly afterwards. The ox, particularly in a wild state, apparently feeds rapidly, almost ravenously, for a comparatively short space of time, eating a large amount of material, and then lies down in some secluded part to ruminate in a slow, regular, and deliberate manner. These facts have important bearings upon the frequency of feeds that should be given to animals, and the time allowed to eat them. The horse does best when given three or four small feeds during the working hours of the day, and alar ger, bulkier feed at night, when there is plenty of time to eat it. Cows, on the other hand, do very well with three, or even only two, large feeds per day, always provided they are allowed a sufficiency of time to ruminate afterwards, and are not disturbed during the process—by milking or grooming, for example. In summer weather most of the feeding by herbivora is during the early morning and late at night; during the hottest part of the day, when flies are troublesome, the animals prefer to stand or lie under whatever shade is available. Animals which sleep in at night in the summer should therefore be turned out as soon after dawn as possible, and should stay out till dusk. In many cases better results can be obtained by allowing animals to sleep outside at night, taking them in during the day. For fuller information, works on comparative physiology and veterinary physiology should be consulted.

STOMACH, DISEASES OF.—Only the more common diseases of the stomach can be discussed here. The majority of them exhibit, as their most marked, and not infrequently their only symptoms, the characteristic signs of *dyspepsia*, and accordingly their differentiation is very often a matter of great difficulty, demanding the services of a skilled practitioner, and often requiring the use of X-rays to determine with accuracy their exact nature, particularly in the dog and cat. The following description refers only to the most prominent features which usually characterise gastric disorders. Reference should also be made to sections on BRAXY, CALCULI, COLIC, DISTEMPER, PARASITES ('Bots', p. 676; 'Stomach worms: ox, sheep, dog', etc., p. 659 *et seq.*), and various different poisons, in each of which the stomach is primarily or secondarily affected.

DYSPEPSIA (δυσ-, with difficulty; πέπτειν, I digest) means pain or discomfort associated with the function of digestion. Vagaries of digestion in the different domesticated animals are productive of symptoms of different sorts, sometimes not at all connected with the taking of food, and the whole subject is intricate and even recondite. The condition of the teeth is of importance. Under artificial management animals do not get the same time to eat their food, nor are they allowed to eat it to satisfy the dictates of appetite, with the result that they suffer from digestive derangements to an extent more or less roughly in ratio to the intensity of their domestication. Thus the dog, living in the closest association with man, partaking of its food, often cooked and greatly altered, and only fed according to the caprice of the owner in very many instances, suffers frequently from dyspepsia. It is, in fact, in the dog that dyspepsia proper is most troublesome. In the other domesticated animals impaction of the stomach with coarse, indigestible, fibrous materials, brought about partly by an insufficiency of water, is probably the most common digestive derangement, cattle suffering more than other animals.

Causes.—Some of the causes have been mentioned above; to them must be added the eating of decomposed, unwholesome, unsuitable, or poisonous food materials.

In highly strung temperamental animals, especially horses and dogs, great excitement before or after feeding may bring about a nervous form of dyspepsia, which is of a functional nature and usually disappears with rest and quietness. Thus after a railway or sea journey, a race meeting, a sale or show, or a great fright, animals may refuse food, or if they do eat may become attacked with colic, vomiting. Exhaustion following upon nervous or muscular exertion may give rise to another form of dyspepsia, due, in this case, to the exhaustion which affects not only the skeletal muscles and nerves, but also those of the involuntary systems. It is on account of this exhaustion of involuntary muscles (and nerves) that horses will very often refuse solid food for some hours after returning from a hard day's hunting. (*See* MUSCLES.) Those that are given a full feed and eat it at once, perhaps ravenously, are not infrequently attacked by colic, brought about by gastric and intestinal indigestion. In the chronic form of dyspepsia, which is of a milder but more prolonged nature, the cause is usually some contained irritation of the mucous membrane of the stomach. In horses the presence of large numbers of the larvæ (bots) of *Gastrophilus* sp. (the *horse bot-flies*) commonly give rise to dyspepsia, while conditions such as crib-biting, wind-sucking, eating the bedding, eating the dung, and the excessive use of spices and digestive stimulants, or coarse fibrous food-stuffs (*e.g.* straw), or even the use of very rich concentrated foods such as bean meal, barley meal or boiled barley, sainfoin, lucerne, etc., may set up chronic dyspepsia, with eventually great thickening of the stomach wall and impaired digestion. In cattle the functions of the stomach may be disturbed by the use of unsuitable food-stuffs; by swallowing indigestible foreign bodies, such as metal objects, stones, articles of clothing, after-births, etc.; and by the invasion of the walls of the 4th stomach by parasitic worms. This latter is also a common cause in sheep and goats. The presence of hair-balls, wool-balls, and other concretions in rumen, reticulum, or abomasum may also be associated with dyspepsia in young or old ruminating animals. There is a condition, called parturient dyspepsia, which commonly occurs from a week to a fortnight after calving (frequently about the tenth day) in dairy cattle, the cause of which is not established, but it is believed that it depends upon disturbance in the uterus. Dyspepsia in young calves being reared by hand is extremely common. In lambs, acidity of the ewes' milk, occasioned by a change on to rich pasture or concentrated food, and occasionally assuming serious proportions, is a very common cause of dyspepsia. It is accompanied by the formation in the

STOMACH, DISEASES OF

stomach of a very dense cheese-like mass of coagulated milk, which cannot be digested. In pigs the use of richly spiced foods; the excessive administration of 'worm-powders', some of which, made by commercial firms, have been known to contain small amounts of powdered glass which is exceedingly dangerous; continued feeding with house or restaurant refuse impregnated with common salt, saltpetre, etc.; parasitic worms, bristle-balls, etc.; are liable to set up irritation in the stomach, with consequent dyspepsia. In dogs, which are notoriously omnivorous, a multitude of different conditions are liable to cause dyspepsia. The eating of unsuitable food substances is almost a characteristic of the dog, and in view of its scavenging instincts it is not to be wondered at that stomach function is often disturbed. In the dog, however, vomiting is much less serious than in other animals, and constitutes a natural method of getting rid of harmful substances before they have had time to cause any serious trouble. It is usually only when vomiting is excessive or continued that it must be regarded seriously. (*See also under* FOREIGN BODIES · in this section.)

Symptoms.—The chief symptoms of dyspepsia in all animals are: absence or capriciousness of appetite; abdominal pain following feeding; dullness and general depression; vomiting in those animals which possess the powerof vomiting, the material voided being usually recognisable as food-stuff which has undergone little or no digestion; a foul odour from the mouth, and frequent eructation of gases. Thirst is usually in excess, and within limits should not be discouraged. Hiccough is seen in some animals, especially horses and dogs, and in the latter animals there is often a tendency to seek a cold spot, and to lie on it with the hind limbs fully stretched out behind. Rumination in cattle and sheep is generally suspended, or is incomplete.

In chronic cases food is eaten, but without any regularity. The animal sometimes eats ravenously, and at other times refuses ordinary food but shows a great liking for the most unusual and often repulsive substances. These generally increase the dyspepsia, and exaggerate an already serious condition. Bodily condition is gradually lost; the coat stares, and the skin loses its normal pliability and elasticity; the tongue becomes coated with a greyish deposit (often known as 'fur'), and there is a foul smell from the breath and fæces. Urine is voided copiously, and at frequent intervals (polyuria). Anæmia, denoted by paleness of the visible mucous membranes, weak heart action, and lessened fitness for work, become marked; and in this condition an animal is more readily attacked with some other chronic disease, such as tuberculosis, for example. Finally, emaciation becomes pronounced, and the animal, rapidly becoming weaker and weaker, eventually dies from exhaustion.

Treatment.—Drugs are of secondary importance; it is much better to put the animal on to very plain, wholesome, easily digested foods.

Owing to the serious consequences that often follow simple indigestion in the domesticated animals, it is always very advisable to call in veterinary advice early. (*See also* NURSING OF SICK ANIMALS.)

It will be convenient to consider the various other stomach complaints grouped according to the animals they affect, instead of describing the symptoms in each of the animals under the headings of each diseased condition. This is necessary because of the different arrangement of the stomach in the various animals.

Horse.—In view of the comparatively simple arrangement of the stomach, and the natural fastidiousness of the horse in the matter of food, stomach diseases are not so common as in some other animals.

GASTRITIS, or INFLAMMATION OF THE STOMACH, is usually brought about by the ingestion of irritant, poisonous, or otherwise harmful substances, or by the spreading of diseased processes from other parts of the body. Vegetable poisons in the food, or eaten by accident, such as yew, rhododendron, boxwood, equisetum, castor beans, laburnum, etc., produce active inflammation of the stomach, while laurel and some of the less active poisons cause intense congestion without actual erosion or acute inflammation. Lead, arsenic, corrosive sublimate, and powerful acids or alkalies, which may be taken inadvertently or given in mistake for common drugs, also produce gastritis. Mouldy hay, decomposed beans, peas, or oats, are said to be responsible for its production, but it is probable that only when taken in large amounts do they result in inflammation of the stomach.

Symptoms.—Attacks of violent abdominal pain, occurring shortly after feeding, or even before feeding is completed, indicate that the stomach is affected. Dullness and depression are noticed; patchy sweating may break out; food is refused; the temperature rises slightly in mild cases, and to as high as 106° F. in severe instances. Usually in from 2 to 3 hours after taking food the acute pain ceases, but the horse remains dull, and gives the impression that it is affected with a dull ache rather than with acute pain. Vomiting does not usually occur unless the stomach is ruptured or the œsophagus is dilated.

Treatment.—Withhold all solid food for 24 hours, using a muzzle to prevent the horse from eating its bedding. Violent purges should be avoided. Later, stomach sedatives, such as chlorodyne and sodium bicarbonate, salol, magnesium carbonate, and chalk, may be administered in the form of an electuary with treacle, syrup, or honey.

IMPACTION OF THE STOMACH is a condition in which engorgement of the stomach with food takes place. It may be due to lack of vitality (atony) in the muscular walls, to impaired gastric secretion, to the presence of large numbers of horse bots, or to narrowing of the outlet at the pylorus; and it may occur in a horse with a normal stomach feeding upon coarse, dry, fibrous or woody food-stuffs, or upon cereals or pulses which, swallowed whole, swell to a great size in the stomach under the influence of warmth or moisture. Insufficiency of water, greedy feeding, insufficient chewing due to irregular or diseased teeth, and eating large amounts of food after a fast, especially when the horse has undergone severe exertion, are other common causes.

Symptoms.—Signs of impaction may occur, suddenly or gradually. There is depression, uneasiness, and perhaps colic, in those cases where a horse overeats. Breathing becomes shorter and shorter, owing to the pressure of the engorged stomach on the diaphragm; gases may be eructated from the stomach, not usually in such quantities as in true gastric tympany, however, and in some cases not at all. If dilatation is pronounced, food material may be vomited through the nostrils. Temperature is unchanged, but the pulse gets soft and full. In some cases staggering movements, aimless wandering, or even great excitement, may be seen; while in others there is marked depression.

Sometimes a horse obtains relief by vomiting through the nostrils a quantity of the impacted material, which reduces the amount in the stomach so that the remainder can be dealt with in the usual way. At other times rupture of the stomach, leading to peritonitis and a fatal termination, may occur.

Prevention.—It is easier to prevent impaction of the stomach than it is to cure it. So far as is possible, those conditions which have been mentioned as liable to give rise to impaction should be avoided or prevented. Bots should be eliminated or prevented. (*See* PARASITES, p. 676.) Pasture grazing towards the end of summer and during autumn should be carefully supervised and changes made to younger, fresher grass as the old pastures get coarse and woody. Rough over-ripe hay and similar fodders of other kinds should be mixed with stuff of better quality. Whole beans, peas, wheat, or barley should not be used for feeding to horses. Horses should always be allowed as much water as they desire to drink, and should be watered before feeding in all cases. Diseased or rough and irregular teeth should be treated by extraction or rasping.

Medicinal treatment is often unsatisfactory. The rational method is to attempt to empty the stomach by washing it out with the stomach-tube, using large amounts of warm and cold water, saline solutions, etc., in turn. Hot packs to the abdomen relieve pain and soothe spasm; copious enemata of warm soapy water encourage safe peristalsis. Expert attendance is very desirable.

TYMPANY OF THE STOMACH.—When vegetable food ferments from any cause, gas is produced. Certain foods, especially when unsound, undergo fermentation in the stomach instead of digestion, and the gas so formed is liable to collect in that organ often under pressure producing great distension. Foods which ferment easily are: succulent green crops, clovers, lucerne, tares, rank growing wheat during spring or early summer, frosted or rotten roots, raw potatoes eaten in quantity, barley, wheat, or maize, especially if these are cooked first and fed in large amounts. Crib-biters and wind-suckers take into the stomach gulps of air, and if the habit is greatly indulged in, the air collects in the stomach and gives rise to colic and the symptoms of tympany.

Symptoms.—Distress usually commences about an hour after feeding, and gradually increases in severity. There is no remission of the pain, such as is usually seen when the intestines are tympanitic. Horses may roll, plunge, and paw the ground during the earlier part of the attack; later they cringe as though to lie, but do not do so. Respirations increase in rate, and become laboured. This is due to the pressure exerted upon the diaphragm by the distended stomach. Sometimes a certain amount of relief is obtained by quantities of gas escaping through the œsophagus into the pharynx, but, owing to the form and structure of the cardiac end of the gullet, it is not likely that all the gas contained ever escapes. The abdomen becomes tense and often swollen, and in many instances horses assume a crouching attitude with their hind-quarters, not unlike the way in which a dog sits. When the tympany is severe, unless relief is afforded by the passage of the stomach-tube, rupture of the stomach occurs, and death follows.

Treatment.—The stomach-tube should be passed as soon as the condition is diagnosed. For this operation the horse requires to be thoroughly under control, for otherwise, it may throw itself down with serious consequences. The hypodermic injection of atropine, which tends to reduce the tension of the cardia of the stomach, makes the passage of the tube easier both to the operator and the horse. A rush of gas occurs when the nozzle enters the stomach, and immediate relief follows. It is next necessary to prevent the formation of further gas by restoring the function of the stomach by stimulants, and by checking fermentation. For these purposes medicinal oil of turpentine may be used. Chloral hydrate also is good, as it tends to allay irritation, and acts as a stimulant to bowel movement.

RUPTURE OF THE STOMACH may occur from those several causes which have been mentioned earlier. It may also take place when a horse falls violently to the ground soon after a big feed, *i.e.* when the stomach is full.

Symptoms.—The distress characteristic of engorgement and tympany suddenly ceases when the stomach ruptures, and for a short time the horse appears so much better that the owner imagines recovery will result. After a short time, however, the more serious symptoms of peritonitis and shock occur. Profuse perspiration usually breaks out; the pulse changes to what is called a 'running down pulse', *i.e.* there are a few strong beats which gradually become weaker until they are almost imperceptible, and then a succession of strong beats return; this is repeated rhythmically. Ears and feet become cold and clammy to the touch; respiration is blowing; and the expression on the face of the horse is one of very great anxiety. Death occurs in from half an hour to several hours when the rupture is large, and in 24 to 48 hours when small. Vomiting is said to characterise rupture of the stomach, but it is probable that in most cases the vomiting occurs *before* the rupture takes place; the food material escapes into the abdominal cavity after rupture has occurred rather than up into the pharynx and nostrils. (Vomiting in the horse occurs through the nostrils because of the great length of the soft palate, which hinders the entrance of food from the pharynx into the mouth.)

Treatment is useless. Death invariably follows rupture of the stomach, and if the condition is positively diagnosed, immediate destruction of the animal is the most humane course.

Ox.—The rumen, reticulum, and omasum are, as already explained, concerned with the preparation of food for its proper digestion in the abomasum, and their diseases are of a more mechanical nature than those of the abomasum.

IMPACTION OF THE RUMEN is a condition in which a large amount of food material becomes packed into the organ so tightly that its walls are unable to contract, movement ceases, rumination stops, and the whole digestive system is thrown out of work. It is brought about by eating dry innutritious fodder, especially tough, coarse, dry grass stalks towards the end of summer and during the autumn and winter. Large amounts of straw, chaff, meals of various kinds (such as may be eaten when an animal escapes into a feeding-store, barn, etc), an insufficiency of water, deficient salivary secretion, and lack of power in the walls of the rumen in old weak animals, are other causes. In some parts of the country it is common in cattle at grass during the spring at the time when cocksfoot (*Dactylis glomerata*) is in flower. It seems that at this time the flowering heads are particularly attractive to cattle, and they eat them in large quantities, with the result that they become impacted into the rumen, and give rise to what is often called 'spring staggers', 'grass staggers', or that ubiquitous term —'stomach staggers'. Sudden changes from green feeding to dry indoor feeding may cause impaction, and turning young animals out for too long at first on to rich succulent grazings, such as young clover or rye-grass, may induce them to eat too much, producing BLOAT (which see). (*See also* LACTIC ACID.)

Symptoms.—As a rule, animals do not become ill suddenly. They usually lie down after a feed, and it is only when disturbed later that anything is seen wrong with them. At pasture the animal leaves the rest of the herd, and generally lies at the back of a fence or even in a ditch. Feeding ceases, no thirst is exhibited, but the animal becomes gradually more and more uneasy. It lies for a time, then rises. When made to move, the majority of cattle emit a groan or moan which is almost characteristic, and a number continue to moan even when left to themselves. They may kick at the abdomen, or turn and gaze at the flanks; great excitement is practically never shown, although in rare cases the animal may stagger round in aimless circles, or may turn and stare at some imaginary object. The breathing is always distressed after the impaction has become well established, and a grunt may accompany each breath. The animal stands with the back arched, the hind legs apart, or with its head uphill; pressure over the left side of the abdomen, especially in the hollow of the flank, causes pain, and in this region, which is no longer a hollow, but is filled out to the level of the surrounding structures, can be felt a firm putty-like mass. No sounds of movement can be heard with the ear applied over the left side of the abdomen, and the whole of that side is tense and, as it were, tightly stretched. In a number of cases the formation of gas complicates a simple impaction. This gas consists of methane, and other compounds of carbon. (*See* TYMPANY.)

Treatment.—In the first place, it is necessary to relieve any tympany that may be present.

By the mouth, a drench may be given consisting of 1 pint of linseed oil containing 2 ounces of turpentine, and, if available, 2 teaspoonfuls of chloroform. This acts by softening and penetrating the impacted mass in the rumen, and also stimulates the movements of that organ. Massage of the rumen, performed by thrusting the closed fists slowly but strongly into the left side of the abdominal wall 10 or 12 times per minute for 10 minutes, greatly assists the distribution of the mass. It should be carried out 3 or 4 times each day.

When impaction of the rumen occurs owners should seek skilled assistance in every case, for the veterinary surgeon by his training is enabled to interpret at their true value the different symptoms exhibited. Generally severe impactions take a surprisingly long time to disappear, even with the most active treatment, and the animal may be ill for a week or ten days.

The operation of rumenotomy, and the removal of about half the contents of the rumen by hand, is practised when other methods of treatment fail.

TYMPANY OF THE RUMEN, which is also called 'bloat', 'blown', or 'belly-struck', consists of a collection of gas in the rumen, filling it to distension, and producing paralysis of its walls and cessation of the normal movements of digestion. It may be caused by many of the factors which produce impaction, and frequently accompanies that condition. It is also due to eating frosted roots, cabbages, or potatoes, large amounts of green food, wheat, maize or barley, and it may occur through some obstruction to the natural eructation of gases by the mouth, such as may occur during choking, when an animal lies on one side for a long time, or when an enlarged lymph gland presses upon the œsophagus where it passes over the root of the lung. It is a common complication of milk fever in cows, and other diseases where there is temporary or permanent partial or complete paralysis.

Symptoms.—The most noticeable symptom of tympany is the distended condition of the abdomen, especially well seen on the left side in the hollow of the flank. The animal becomes rapidly uneasy; it stands shifting from one hind foot to the other, switches the tail, kicking at the abdomen occasionally, and turning and gazing at its sides. Breathing soon becomes distressed, each breath being short and jerky, and expelled somewhat explosively. The mouth is often held wide open and the tongue may be outstretched. If choking occurs as well there is a profuse discharge of saliva, and frequent attempts at swallowing. (*See* CHOKING.) Excitement may be seen in some cases, but usually after the distension has become severe any movement increases distress, and the animal stands quietly. Unless relief is speedily afforded tympanitic animals are very likely to die in a surprisingly short space of time from inability to breathe—actual suffocation. Temperature is usually normal, unless excitement causes it to rise; the pulse is normal at first, but becomes faster and fuller than normal after a short while, and a little later, as the distress increases, it gets weaker and softer, and finally becomes almost imperceptible.

Treatment.—It is of the utmost importance to provide for removal of the accumulated gases from the rumen at once. Half an hour's delay may be sufficient to cause death. The trocar and cannula should be used at once, if they are available. (*See* TROCAR *and* CANNULA.) If not, a gag may be placed in the ox's mouth, to facilitate expulsion of the gas by the mouth. It may be made of straw, or a suitable piece of wood may be placed between the cheek teeth and tied in position by a rope round the poll. Where a trocar and cannula are not available, a bold plunge forward towards the elbow of the opposite side, made with a knife with a blade of 6 inches or more, and possessing a sharp point, may give relief until a trocar can be obtained. Massage of the rumen after puncture will assist to expel the remaining gases and also stimulate normal muscular movements. As soon as the gas ceases to escape, 2 tablespoonfuls of medicinal turpentine may be poured direct into the rumen through the cannula. The trocar is then reinserted and the two instruments removed. Where an animal becomes tympanitic a second time (which may occur within a few hours of being relieved), it must be tapped a second time, and the cannula should be left in place, tied by a tape which passes round the abdomen.

It is very often a sound plan to examine carefully the other animals in a batch where one has become tympanitic, especially when at grass. (*See also under* BLOAT.)

INFLAMMATION OF THE RUMEN (*see also* RUMEN ULCERATION) may be due to ingestion of irritant poisons, either of chemical or vegetable origin, to penetrating foreign bodies, or to the spread of inflammatory conditions from other parts in specific diseases, such as malignant catarrhal fever, rinderpest, or even foot-and-mouth disease. The symptoms are indefinite and are usually masked by other general symptoms. They consist of pain on pressure over the left side of the abdomen, intermittent tympany, arching of the back, grunting, sometimes vomiting, and irregularity both of appetite and passage of fæces. The treatment depends upon the cause.

HAIR BALLS, etc., may be found in the rumen, as in other parts of the alimentary system. Hair is most likely to be swallowed by young animals, and especially by calves shut in calf-houses with an insufficiency of fibrous food early in life. Lambs frequently swallow wool from the ewes' udders, or pick loose portions up from pasture. (Hence the common practice of good shepherds to collect every small piece of wool during and after lambing.) The symptoms are those of recurrent indigestion, often associated with diarrhœa, flatulence, or impaction of the rumen. In both lambs and calves these balls are liable to obstruct the passage from the rumen into the other stomachs, and occasionally cause death from stoppage in this way. They may reach the abomasum, where they set up inflammation until, or unless, they become coated over with a deposit of salts, giving them a smooth glazed surface. In many cases they are apparently quite harmless, being found after death in animals that were slaughtered for food, or that died from some other cause. (*See also* WOOL BALLS.)

FOREIGN BODIES IN RETICULUM are of great importance in both young and adult cattle, because of the close proximity of this organ to the pericardium and heart. The reticulum, lying as it does immediately below the opening of the œsophagus, receives any heavy solid objects which have been swallowed; only rarely do they pass far enough back to enter the rumen, unless they happen to be of great length. In the reticulum two things may happen to them; they may fall to the lowermost part of the sac and remain there for an indefinite period, or they may slowly penetrate its wall and wander forwards through the diaphragm. Their subsequent course has been described under the section on HEART DISEASES, Sub-heading: *Traumatic pericarditis of cattle*, to which reference should be made. The sharp-pointed foreign bodies usually wander; while rounded, or short, thick bodies remain in the reticulum. They may consist of stones, pieces of wood, metal, or bone, nails, screws, pieces of wire, domestic cutlery, even the ribs of an umbrella, and in the famous 'Trojan bull case' the bull in question swallowed a piece of wire 22 inches long and almost ¼-in. thick. The foreign bodies which are most likely to wander forwards are usually about 2 to 3 inches long, pointed at one end, and fairly straight. Two- and 3-in. wire nails are common objects found causing traumatic pericarditis.

Symptoms.—Generally the symptoms produced by foreign bodies in the reticulum are vague, and consist of irregularity in feeding with attacks of indigestion, tympany, and abdominal pain. Arching of the back and grunting are noticed; the bowels are irregular, and purgatives which are ordinarily satisfactory often fail to act.

These symptoms may develop into the characteristic signs of traumatic pericarditis, or they may pass off. In the latter cases they often return at intervals, causing sometimes great wasting in condition, and resulting in the animals becoming 'piners'.

Treatment.—When, from previous history, a positive diagnosis can be made, the operation of rumenotomy and the removal of the offending objects is the only possible line of treatment. (*See also under* MINE-DETECTOR.) The cavity of the reticulum can be reached with a little difficulty from an incision in the rumen, and the foreign bodies are then removed by hand. If the foreign body passes forwards through the diaphragm there is little hope of saving the animal, and immediate slaughter for food becomes necessary. Occasionally, however, it happens that a foreign body does not pass into the heart. It may wander into the lung, and passing through it sets up pneumonia, and may eventually produce an abscess in the chest wall, which, on bursting, reveals the point of the object, which can be easily removed.

INFLAMMATION OF THE OMASUM is not common. It occurs usually when some powerful irritant poison has been taken into the stomachs, such as arsenic, corrosive sublimate, oxalic acid, rhododendron, yew, etc. Owing to the fact that other parts of the alimentary canal are also acutely inflamed in these cases, it is usually impossible to differentiate between the symptoms which are shown.

Treatment.—Surgical interference may be necessary if improvement does not follow the administration of an oil.

IMPACTION OF THE ABOMASUM.—This occurs in Britain but is perhaps not as widely recognised here as in Canada.

Symptoms.—Loss of appetite, constipation, sunken eyes, skin dull and dirty. The abdomen may become greatly extended.

INFLAMMATION OF THE ABOMASUM, abomasitis, or gastritis, is brought about by the ingestion of irritants, or by the spreading of specific diseases to the stomach, such as may occur in anthrax, rinderpest, or malignant catarrhal fever, but it is probably most commonly due to parasitic round worms. (*See* PEPTIC ULCER.)

Symptoms. — The symptoms usually commence suddenly. Animals which have eaten poisonous plants while at grass, separate themselves from the rest of the herd, stand with their backs arched, and show signs of abdominal pain. They cease to feed, rumination does not occur, and the temperature may be very high. Thirst is generally excessive.

Treatment.—At first, it is usually advisable to administer a gentle purgative. Large doses of powerful purgatives should be avoided. Salts should not be given, for their chief action is on the small intestine, not on the stomach. Later, stomach tonics and sedatives should be administered. Bicarbonate of soda, of magnesia, and of bismuth, mixed together and given in a quart of gruel or milk, makes a useful mixture. Where poisonous substances have been eaten the appropriate antidotes should be given at once. (For the causes, symptoms, and treatment of parasitic gastritis in cattle and sheep, *see* p. 693).

DISPLACEMENT OF ABOMASUM referred to above, and giving rise to symptoms of loss of appetite, loss of weight, and depression of milk yield, may sometimes be successfully treated by casting the cow and, with her lying on her back, rotating or rocking her through an angle of 45° from the vertical each way. Surgical treatment may be necessary.

PEPTIC ULCER is a condition by no means rare in cattle. It is sometimes associated with displacement of the abomasum, and may give rise to symptoms a few days after calving. Death follows perforation. Symptoms are similar to those given above. Ulceration is not uncommon in calves after weaning, giving rise to capricious appetite and sometimes evidence of abdominal pain. *Fusiformis necrophorus*, *Corynybacterium pyogenes*, and *Pasteurelle* organisms in other parts of the body may be associated.

Sheep.—The diseases of the stomachs of the sheep resemble in general those of the same organs in cattle. There are, however, certain conditions which are peculiar to sheep which require special mention.

BRAXY is characterised by a patch of acute inflammation in the wall of the abomasum, usually about the size of the palm of the hand, where the mucous membrane is to a large extent destroyed.

GASTRITIS IN LAMBS is responsible for numbers of deaths every year. It may be due to the irritation produced by wool balls, but it is very often due to changes in the ewe's milk. There is a form of this disease which is met with when the lambing flock is put on to pasture where there is a profusion of the acrid buttercup (*Ranunculus acris*). The ewes eat the acrid leaves with apparent impunity, but it causes an acid change in their milk, so that when the milk enters the lamb's abomasum it sets into a dense solid curd, closely resembling a hard cheese, some of the lumps of curd being almost as large as a walnut. The presence of these curds sets up an acute and rapidly fatal gastritis.

Treatment.—The flock should be immediately shifted to higher and drier pasture where there are few or no buttercups, until such time as the lambs are stronger, and the ewes should be put on to a mixture containing considerable amounts of bran, say about ¾ to 1½ lb. per head per day.

Another form of gastritis is due to parasitic worms in the young lambs. (*See* PARASITES.)

Pigs. — GASTRITIS. — Irritating or poisonous substances, specific disease, or parasites, are among the causes.

Foreign bodies (which are very liable to be eaten by young store pigs) causing gastritis, include such substances as stones, coal, pieces of wood or metal, and fabrics of various kinds. Salt poisoning is associated with gastritis, as are also poisonings by arsenic, copper, saltpetre, sheep dips, etc. During the course of swine fever, swine erysipelas, foot-and-mouth disease, and even tuberculosis, the wall of the stomach may become involved, and inflammation may result. (*See under* GASTRIC ULCERS.) Parasites may also cause this condition (*See* PARASITES.)

Symptoms.—Vomiting is the first and most important symptom of stomach disturbance, though it may not always be shown at the commencement of the illness. Affected animals suddenly become ill, perhaps soon after feeding. They stand by themselves with their backs arched, and usually with the head lowered. Great thirst is a noticeable feature, and if an animal is allowed access to water it will usually drink slowly for a considerable time, and then commence to vomit almost immediately afterwards. The vomited material is usually frothy and always brought up with ease, but the pig appears greatly depressed and miserable subsequently. Constipation is generally evident at first, but gives way to a blackish or red-stained diarrhœa afterwards. In pigs which are being fattened there is often a certain amount of skin discoloration, irregular patches of red or purple appearing along the belly, between the thighs, behind the ears, and in other parts where the skin is red. Convulsions and twitching of the limbs may be seen in young pigs.

Treatment.—All solid foods must be withheld, and soft light foods given instead. Whole milk is one of the best. Where it is believed to be due to poisonous substances the appropriate antidotes must be given. (*See* ANTIDOTES.)

Dog.—In the wild state the dog is able to eat and digest without ill effects the most varied and unwholesome kinds of food; under the artificial conditions of domestication, however, and probably because its food is to a large extent not natural, the stomach has become a more easily upset organ.

FOREIGN BODIES IN THE STOMACH may include: pieces of carpet, or other fabric, the rubber from a golf ball, the covers of tennis balls, bones, wool, pieces of wood, etc. In less common instances unusual material is found in great quantities in the stomach, such as parings from horses' feet and horse-shoe nails in the stomach of a farrier's fox-terrier, large numbers of corks in a chemist's dog, the wads of shot-gun cartridges in sporting dogs, etc. A depraved appetite may be due to hunger, a mineral or vitamin deficiency, or to bad habits.

Symptoms. — Ineffectual attempts to vomit, accompanied by painful retching, an arched back, salivation from the mouth, and signs of discomfort. Sharp-pointed bodies may cause perforation of the stomach walls, peritonitis, and death. These results are shown by excruciating attacks of pain, tenderness over the abdomen, great general depression, and high fever, leading rapidly to collapse and unconsciousness.

In small toy dogs it is quite usual for symptoms of acute nervous excitement to be shown.

Treatment.—An emetic of salt and water, mustard and water, or, better, of apomorphine given by hypodermic injection, will rid the stomach of the greater part of fibrous or soft ingesta, but where sharp-pointed foreign bodies have been swallowed, obviously it is unsafe to give emetics. To remove these and large rounded objects which cannot be easily vomited, operative measures may be necessary. When undertaken early the results are satisfactory but when perforation or ulceration has occurred, or when there is acute inflammation, the case is less hopeful.

GASTRITIS is probably less common than enteritis or nephritis, both of which may give rise to vomiting.

Causes.—In certain cases, the substance which causes the gastritis may be irritant or caustic ; for instance, in poisoning by arsenic or corrosive sublimate. In such instances the first effect is chemical destruction of the surface cells, and thereafter either death from shock, or the absorption of the poison together with, in the majority of cases, bacterial invasion of the tissues. In poisoning by arsenic, however, bacterial activity is not of great importance, for even some days after death the organs may appear quite fresh and little or no decomposition may be in evidence. Most, if not all, of the poisons which are taken in by the mouth produce gastritis, and it is on this account that many attacks of gastritis, which have nothing whatever to do with chemical or vegetable poisons, are immediately ascribed to these causes by the owners of the animals.

Ulceration of the stomach in dog and cat may be associated with gastritis—sometimes with tuberculosis, malignant growths, and actinomycosis. Ulcers similar to peptic ulcers in human beings, and leading to perforation, have been recognised in cats.

Symptoms.—As a rule, a severe attack of vomiting immediately after a feed, and refusal to touch food subsequently, is the manner in which acute gastritis commences, provided it does not complicate an attack of dyspepsia or the subacute form, in which case the two conditions merge into each other. Thirst is always excessive, and if gratified, vomiting usually follows. The irritability of the stomach becomes rapidly worse, until the slightest change of position or the gentlest handling of the dog causes an attack. The appearance of the vomit varies from a slimy, white, tenacious mucus, to a thin frothy, yellowish or green-stained fluid, usually possessing a foul, sour odour. In some cases, especially when the gastritis is very acute or hæmorrhagic, the vomit is blood-stained, or may appear to consist of pure blood. If capillary hæmorrhage occurs into the stomach, perhaps as the result of retching, the blood which slowly oozes from its walls, collects in the cavity of the stomach, undergoes partial digestion, and becomes changed into a brownish granular material, strongly resembling moist coffee grounds. This always has a most foul and objectionable odour. The dog itself becomes extremely miserable, dragging itself slowly from place to place, and showing preference for cold places where it may lie stretched out with its hind legs straight behind it, so that the lower wall of the abdomen is in close contact with the cold surface, *e.g.* a stone step, or linoleum in a passage. Constipation usually occurs unless the intestines become involved, when diarrhœa is noticed. The mouth becomes cold, although in the early stages it will usually be hot and dry, and the nose is invariably hot, dry, and often cracked. On the teeth and tongue a brownish or even blackish deposit forms, and not infrequently small ulcerated areas appear around the roots of the teeth. Pressure on the abdomen causes pain, and sometimes a dog lifted by the hand under the abdomen cries out. The temperature is raised at first.

Treatment.—In the first place the dog should be made as comfortable and warm as circumstances will permit. Hot packs applied to the abdomen soothe pain and relieve tension. A stomach sedative: one or other of the salts of bismuth—the carbonate, subnitrate, salicylate, or oxychloride—is usually best to commence with. (*See also* POISONING *and* ANTIDOTES.) Other drugs which may be used to check vomiting when the above fail, are: chloretone or chlorodyne. These are not always satisfactory. Dogs affected with gastritis should be under the charge of a veterinary surgeon, who will vary the treatment according to the circumstances.

At first food is better withheld and use made of normal saline. Later, what food is given should be light and easily digested, and should make no demands upon the stomach. (*See* PYLORIC, GLUCOSE, SALINE, HYDROLISED PROTEIN, etc).

STOMACH-TUBE is a rubber tube from 9 to 10 ft. long for horses and cattle, and about $\frac{1}{2}$ to $\frac{5}{8}$ths of an inch in diameter. It is used for introducing into the stomach (either through the mouth or more often through the inferior meatus of the nostril on one side), with a view to relieving tympany, or introducing medicines or solutions of salt, in the treatment of disease. A larger-sized tube which possesses two channels is sometimes used to attempt to remove from the stomach portions of poisonous plants which may have been eaten. Water is pumped down through one channel, and when the stomach is full it runs from the other carrying with it small pieces of the harmful material. It is not possible to empty completely the stomach by the double stomach-tube, but considerable amounts of the harmful material may be removed. In certain cases of impaction of the stomach a proportion of the impacted material may be removed in the same way.

The stomach-tube is extremely useful in those cases of colic which depend upon disturbances in the stomach, and if warm water is introduced by it in impaction of the large colon, peristalsis can often be stimulated. (*But see* DEHYDRATION.)

Its use demands care and a knowledge of the structure of the nasal passage, pharynx, gullet, and stomach, but in skilled hands it can do no harm. The small amount of capillary hæmorrhage which may follow its use in ponies and horses with small meati can be disregarded.

STOMATITIS (*στόμα*, the mouth) means inflammation of the mouth, and generally means such inflammation as produces small vesicles or abscesses, as the case may be, which on bursting leave shallow ulcerated areas. The condition is a symptom of foot-and-mouth disease, but is also seen in other cases where there is no infection or contagiousness. (*See* BOVINE PAPULAR STOMATITIS; FOOT-AND-MOUTH DISEASE; VESICULAR STOMATITIS; MOUTH, DISEASES OF.)

-STOMY (*στόμα*, mouth) is a suffix signifying formation of an opening in an organ by operation, *e.g.* gastrostomy and colostomy.

STONES (*see* CALCULI).

STOT (*see* STEER).

STRAIGHTS.—Single feeding stuffs of animal or vegetable origin, which may or may not have undergone some form of processing before purchase; *e.g.* flaked maize, soya bean meal, fish meal, barley.

STRAIN 19 VACCINE (*see* BRUCELLOSIS IN CATTLE, *where* STRAIN 45/20 *is also referred to*).

STRAMONIUM is the leaf of *Datura stramonium*, which is popularly known as the thorn apple or the Jamestown weed. It contains an alkaloid called *daturine*, which is almost identical in its actions with atropine.

The plant has caused fatal poisoning in pigs in Britain. The tincture of stramonium is sometimes used for the 'doping' of horses that are suffering from broken wind, when it conceals the symptoms. Its effects pass off in about 4 hours, and in many cases its action can be nullified by the injection of strychnine. Unscrupulous horse dealers who resort to this method of deceit generally demand immediate 'clinching' of a deal, as the horse will exhibit his defects when on trial.

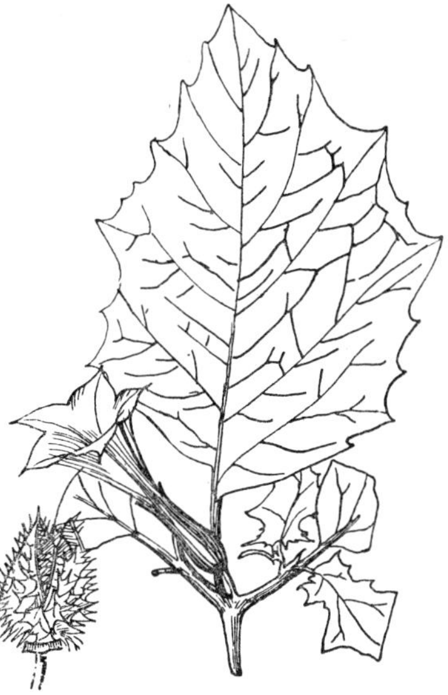

Thorn apple (*Datura stramonium*), which is also known as Jamestown, or 'Jimson', weed. On the left is a fruit capsule, and on the right is a flowering spray. (After Moussu and Dollar's *Diseases of Cattle.*)

STRANGLES is an acute contagious fever of horses, asses, and mules, which is characterised by catarrhal inflammation of the mucous membranes of the nasal passages and pharynx, accompanied in most cases by abscess formation in the submaxillary or pharyngeal lymphatic glands, and in occasional cases by abscess formation in other parts of the body.

Cause.—*Streptococcus equi*; but to the practical stockowner the well-established predisposing causes are even more important.

Predisposing causes.—(1) Age. Strangles is commonest and most serious in horses under 6 years of age. Mature horses living in a stable where an outbreak has occurred are frequently unaffected, even though every opportunity for infection exists. It is possible that an attack when young confers a certain degree of immunity which protects older horses from all but very virulent infections. (2) Bad ventilation is a very virulent contributing cause. (3) Overcrowding. (4) Overworking young immature horses. (5) The season of the year, for most outbreaks occur during autumn, winter, and spring, when the weather is variable. In summer weather the disease is rare. (6) Over-excitement, such as occurs in markets, fairs, sales, and shows.

The infection may remain in stables, loose-boxes, pens, etc., which have held cases of strangles, in spite of so-called 'disinfection', and healthy horses may subsequently become attacked when housed in such places. Similarly, utensils, food-stuffs, litter, public drinking-troughs, nose-bags, harness, etc., which have been contaminated, may act as agents responsible for the spread of the disease.

Symptoms.—There are two forms of strangles: the ordinary, or typical form; and the irregular, atypical, or 'bastard' form.

(1) *Typical attacks* commence with dullness, lack of appetite, rise in temperature to between 103° F. and 105° F., and injection of the visible mucous membranes, especially of the nose and eyes. The pulse is usually soft and sluggish, but not greatly increased in frequency, and the breathing is only a little faster than normal. Nasal discharge is at first thin and watery, but soon becomes thicker, and is eventually of a creamy yellow appearance, profuse, and issues from both nostrils. A more or less similar discharge may appear at the eyes. Two or 3 days after the first symptoms appear, one or both of the submaxillary glands, or perhaps one of the pharyngeal glands, becomes enlarged, hot, tense, and painful to the touch; there is usually a certain amount of diffuse swelling around the gland, which may fill up natural hollows in the vicinity. For 2 or 3 days more the affected gland increases in size, tensity, and painfulness, until a soft spot, usually over the most prominent part of the swelling can be detected. This indicates the 'pointing' of the abscess. Shortly afterwards the skin gives way, the strangles abscess bursts, and discharges a considerable amount (sometimes over a pint) of thick, creamy, yellowish-white pus, usually containing streaks of blood. This pus contains large numbers of streptococci and is highly infective, as also are the nasal and ocular discharges. Following the bursting of an abscess the horse improves greatly; temperature falls, appetite returns, and the animal becomes much brighter.

For some days the abscess cavities discharge a thick bland-looking pus, and gradually heal up from the bottom—the swelling slowly subsiding. If the pharyngeal glands are affected, the swelling, instead of being located in the characteristic position—just within the lower part of the angle of the jaw—is situated over the side of the throat, often nearly half-way up to the base of the ear. In this position swallowing and respiration may be obstructed, and the head may be held stiffly—as though the animal had a stiff neck—or the horse may protrude the nose forward into the position known as 'star-gazing'. The swelling is usually very much more diffuse, and since it occurs to the inside as well as to the outside—the wall of the pharynx being bulged inwards—swallowing may become impossible and the breathing may become roaring, leading perhaps to asphyxia, and even death from suffocation. Pharyngeal abscesses may burst inwards into the pharynx, whence the pus is swallowed or discharged through the nose, or they may burst outwards

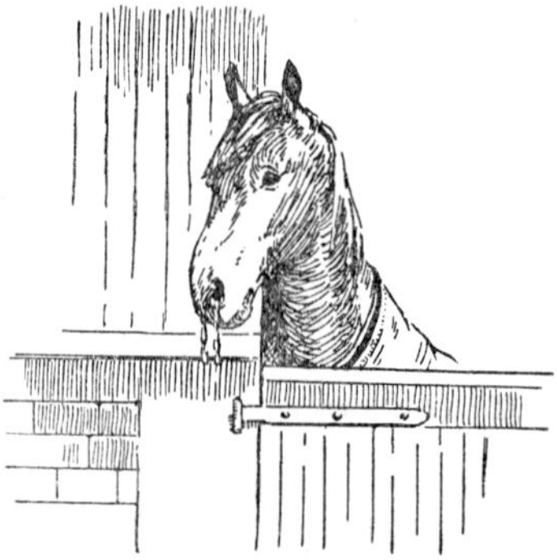

Horse affected with strangles, housed in a hygienic sick-box, with free access to fresh air, but protected by a rug from draughts. The discharge from the nostrils is indicated.

through the thickness of the parotid gland. After bursting or lancing great relief is usually obtained, the horse improving in general appearance even more rapidly than in the case of submaxillary abscesses.

Several different complications may occur during a typical attack of strangles. The inflammatory catarrh may spread from the pharynx down the trachea into the bronchi and lungs, causing bronchitis or broncho-pneumonia. A pharyngeal abscess may burst into the throat and the pus may be sucked into the larynx, trachea, bronchi, and so to the lungs, setting up a fatal septic pneumonia; or pus may be swallowed and liver or mesenteric glands become the seat of abscess formation. Inflammation may extend up the Eustachian tube and involve the guttural pouches or middle ear. If the blood-stream becomes infected through an abscess bursting into an artery or vein, or by other means, small abscesses (known as metastatic) are liable to develop in almost any part of the body, perhaps most commonly in lungs, liver, kidneys, spleen, or brain, and the symptoms produced vary according to the structures involved. Joints, or tendon sheaths, may become affected, abscesses forming and causing intense lameness and often irreparable damage. The udder in the mare may be infected, and from the pus in the milk the foal may contract strangles in an acute and very often fatal form, while half or the whole of the udder may be destroyed.

(2) *Atypical attacks* of strangles, consisting of a respiratory catarrh, but without the formation of abscesses in the submaxillary lymph glands, may occur.

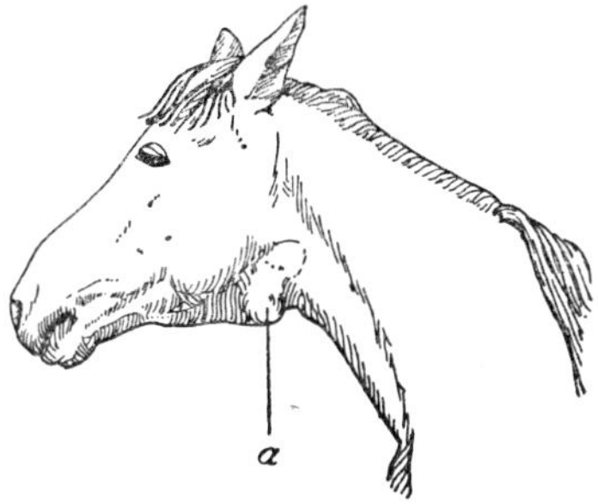

Strangles abscess on the off-side of the jowl, *i.e.* affecting the right submaxillary gland, viewed from the near side to show at *a* the place where the abscess is 'pointing'.

In other instances abscesses may form in some of the glands down the neck or at the front of the shoulder, and sometimes a large single abscess containing a gallon of pus may be found in this situation. At other times abscesses may occur in the skin of the face, in the pleural or pericardial cavities, or in the lungs, no respiratory catarrhal inflammation having been seen previously. Abdominal strangles, in which diffuse abscess formation may occur in the peritoneal cavity or in the mesenteric glands, is not uncommon. These glands may be infected secondarily from the pharynx in typical strangles, but in other cases no typical symptoms may ever be shown. The symptoms are generally vague, consisting of colic, abdominal pain, depression, constipation, complete absence of appetite or a capricious appetite, and a fluctuating temperature. Emaciation is generally rapid, and death from the bursting of an abscess into the peritoneal cavity, and subsequent peritonitis, usually occurs in from 1 to 3 weeks, although a chronic form lasting for from 2 to 3 months may develop. Rarely an abscess may cause adhesion of the bowels, may burst into the cavity of a portion of intestine, or actually out through the abdominal wall.

Relapses do not usually occur when horses are carefully nursed, but certain sequels are common in spite of all care. Roaring, whistling, purpura hæmorrhagica, and various inflammations of tendon sheaths, etc., are not at all uncommon. Adhesions between the inside of the chest wall and the outer surface of one or other lung, causing difficulty in breathing when exerted, and lack of staying power in fast light horses, may also occur.

Treatment.—Immediate isolation of affected horses is necessary. The box or stall where they stood must be disinfected as carefully and thoroughly as possible, and should be left vacant for 3 to 4 weeks afterwards. The sick horse should be clothed and made comfortable; rugs, hood, or bandages being applied according to the weather and circumstances. Clean dry bedding and clean cold water should be provided, and every care should be taken to ensure a plentiful supply of fresh air. Penicillin injections are of great value in lessening the severity of an attack and hastening recovery. Sulpha drugs are also useful. Laxative doses of salts to prevent constipation may be necessary. The feeding should be regulated so that the horse is tempted to eat at least a little each day. (*See* NURSING OF SICK ANIMALS.)

Owing to the great diversity of the symptoms in complicated and atypical cases, the owner should call in assistance, and be guided by the veterinary surgeon.

Prevention.—An efficient vaccine can be produced only if encapsulated *Streptococcus equi* is used (*i.e.* from very young cultures) and the capsule not destroyed by formalin and excessive heat. In older cultures, the capsule is lost and the organism no longer invasive.

STRANGULATION (*strangulo*, I choke) is an occasional cause of death of cattle in Africa, and has been reported from quarantine camps. A ligature is usually employed for the purpose. Unless human malice is suspected, deaths may be attributed to other causes.

It is also a term applied to the stoppage of the circulation in a piece of bowel, as the result of some pressure exerted on the bowel wall or on the mesentery which carries the blood-vessels of the section of bowel which is affected. The causes are varied: it may result from a hernia, from a twist of the bowel, or from the condition known as 'gut tie' in cattle. A dangerous result of strangulation is that when the blood-supply is cut off from a section of bowel the teeming millions of micro-organisms that are found in the bowel contents are able to invade and penetrate the wall of the bowel, whence they gain the peritoneal cavity, and set up a septic peritonitis, which is nearly always fatal. Moreover, supposing this does not occur, food material is unable to pass the inert bloodless piece of gut, and an obstruction to the passage of ingested food-stuff is the consequence. The risk that strangulation may take place at almost any time forms the chief danger of hernia. (*See* HERNIA; GUT TIE; INTESTINES, DISEASES OF.)

STRANGURY (*στραγγουρία*) is that condition in which there are constant attempts to pass water, accompanied by much pressing or straining, and resulting in the passage of only a few drops at a time. It is a symptom of an inflammatory condition situated in the kidneys, bladder, or urethra, as well as being often present in colics that are due to impaction of the double part of the colon. In this latter condition the pressure of the accumulated fæces is so great that it acts on the part of the bladder wall where sensations of fullness are received (*i.e.* the trigone), and gives the animal the false idea that its bladder requires emptying.

STRAUSS TEST for glanders consists in inoculating material from a suspected case in horse or man into the testis of a male guinea-pig. In positive cases there occurs in about 2 to 4 days a purulent condition of the tunica vaginalis and an orchitis from which the casual organism—*Pfeifferella mallei*—can be demonstrated.

STRAW.—References to this will be found under BEDDING, DAIRY HERD MANAGEMENT, DEEP LITTER.

Straw feeding of cattle.—The system originally was a strictly maintenance diet of 4 lb. each of barley and a low protein-mineral-vitamin concentrate with some 10–12 lb. barley straw.

This has since undergone several modifications: (1) the incorporation of the barley and the concentrate into a cube; (2) a re-adjusted cube of a higher rate of feeding to cover both maintenance and the first gallon of milk; (3) the use of potatoes or mangolds as a full or part replacement of the barley (or other cereal); and (4) the devising of a concentrate of about 15 per cent protein content, such that 7 lb. plus 10 lb. of straw would cover maintenance needs with a further 4 lb. for each gallon.

'STRAWBERRY FOOT-ROT'.—The colloquial name applied to a condition caused by the virus of Orf or *Dermatophilus pedis*.

STREAMS.—As a source of drinking water for cattle these should always be suspect, since they often carry infection from one farm to another, e.g. COCCIDIOSIS, JOHNE'S DISEASE, SALMONELLOSIS.

'STREET' VIRUS.—This term refers to the naturally occurring rabies virus, such as may be isolated from a rabid dog, as opposed to 'fixed virus' which is passaged through a series of animals, increasing in virulence for that species and giving rise to a shorter incubation period.

STREPTOCOCCAL MENINGITIS.—A disease of piglets 2 to 6 weeks old (though these age limits should not be taken as hard and fast). The disease has been recognised on the continent of Europe and in North America for several years, and more recently in Britain.

Cause.—A streptococcus.

Symptoms.—Loss of appetite, fever, a tendency for the piglets to bury themselves in the litter. Later, an unsteadiness and sometimes a complete loss of balance. The hindquarters sway and the piglets walk stiffly. The ears are often drawn back and held close to the side of the head. An inability to rise, and paddling with the hind legs precedes death in some cases. Some piglets recover; others die from pneumonia or from septicæmia associated with arthritis.

STREPTOCOCCUS (στρεπτός, a necklace; κόκκος, a kernel).—A micro-organism which under the microscope has much the appearance of a string of beads. It is responsible for a large number of diseased conditions, among which strangles, botriomycosis, mastitis, acute abscess formation, and certain forms of 'blood poisoning' are the chief. (*See* BACTERIOLOGY.)

STREPTODORNASE, STREPTOKINASE.—Enzymes used to dissolve pus, fibrin, and blood clot in infected wounds. They have also been used in the treatment of mastitis.

STREPTOMYCIN.—An antibiotic obtained from *Streptomyces griseus.* Active almost entirely against Gram-negative organisms, streptomycin has given promising results against infection with *C. pyogenes, Staph. pyogenes, C. renale, B. coli,* and *Past. septica.* It is of value in cases of calf pneumonia and calf scours, some types of bovine mastitis, acute nephritis, and complications of virus diseases in the dog, and in septic conditions in the cat. (In medical practice, streptomycin is regarded as one of the most toxic of the antibiotics in common use. It may cause deafness and vestibular disturbance in man.)

STREPTOTHRICOSIS.—Infection with streptothrix organisms.

In Britain, the name is applied to the disease in cattle equivalent to 'Lumpy Wool' or 'Wool Rot', caused by *Dermatophilus dermatonomus.* A scurfy, scaly condition of the skin is produced, and scabs come away with a bunch of hairs attached if plucked. The *Dermatophilus* parasite responsible for this condition is hardy in the sense that it can probably survive on a large scale in the vicinity of an infected animal. Anything which lowers the resistance of a hitherto healthy animal facilitates infection; and prolonged wetting, insect bites, thistle pricks, and other tiny breaks in the skin may all predispose to infection.

In the tropics, the name is applied to infection with *Dermatophilus congolensis.*

The disease may be concentrated on the back, especially behind the withers; or on the muzzle, lower limbs, tail and perineum; and it may become generalised, leading to emaciation and death in some cases.

The onset of the rains brings an increase in the incidence and severity of the disease, which is of great economic importance in central and west Africa. Flies, ticks, and thorn bushes appear to play some part in the production and spread of the disease. Zebu cattle, as exotic cattle, appear highly susceptible; while N'dama and Muturu humpless cattle are resistant. It seems that infection does not give rise to later immunity.

The disease is of great economic importance in central and west Africa. Treatment with antibiotics or sulphonamides offers most chance of success, but is impracticable in many areas. Local applications of sulphur in groundnut oil are less effective.

STREPTOTHRIX (στρεπτός, a necklace; θρίξ, hair) is the name of a group of pathogenic micro-organisms closely allied to the moulds. (*See above,* and SENKOBO.)

STRESS.—In human medicine it is now recognised that mental stress, anxiety, and frustration can exert a profound effect for the worse upon bodily health, and that many people who are now ill would become well again if only they could, before too long, recapture peace of mind. The minds and thoughts and emotions of domestic animals are undoubtedly far dimmer and simpler than our own, but not necessarily non-existent as some scientists would almost have us believe, and undoubtedly there is some equivalent of our peace of mind—call it a familiarity with surroundings, an absence of fear, or an absence of frustration.

Dr. Joseph Edwards has referred to a farm in New Zealand where theoretical considerations were all against high milk yields, yet where the yields were, in fact, extremely high. After a detailed investigation it was concluded that the reason could only be sympathetic handling at milking time by the owners—father, son, and daughter—who were strikingly 'in harmony' with their cattle.

By contrast, on another New Zealand farm where everything—staff, milking machines, and herd management—remained the same, the strangeness of a new milking shed was apparently the sole cause of a 15 per cent reduction in milk yield.

Stress is recognised as a predisposing

cause of disease in pigs, following the mixing of litters, castration, etc.; and in all species following parturition.

With sheep, problems arise in paddock grazing. The grassland breeds, says Stephen Williams, 'need a greater space, if they are to remain happy, than those of the Down breeds. The open flocking types of sheep reveal indications of stress and unhappiness under compression. They are the hedge-breakers and fence-testers. They "work away" at weak places with a will to escape. The answer is clearly strong, reliable fences and to meet this requirement the Thurgarton sprung (lightning) fences have been especially developed. If these types of sheep are overcrowded unhappiness is expressed, too, by their apparent nervousness. Even slight disturbance is greatly magnified as it passes through each flock. The sheep readily take fright or stampede in response to a strange sight or a strange noise.

There is much disappointment in the practice of intensive sheep management where a very large number of sheep are dealt with in one unit. It is peculiarly desirable, in our experience, to break up the flock of grass sheep into units of 80 ewes during the intensive management period at grass. To have more grass ewes in a unit is to magnify the psychological problems.' (*See also* BUNT ORDER, INTENSIVE LIVESTOCK PRODUCTION.)

STRICTURE (*strictura*) means a narrowing of one of the natural passages of the body, such as the gullet, bowel, or urethra.

'STRIKE'.—Blowfly myiasis, the condition resulting from infestation of the living skin of sheep by the larvæ of blowflies which, in certain circumstances, lay their eggs in the wool. The flies are, apparently, attracted by putrefactive odours, and strike accordingly most often occurs in the region of the hindquarters in sheep which have been scouring. Some cases of strike begin, however, in the clean wool covering the shoulders and loins; and other parts may be affected.

Where there is sufficient moisture the eggs hatch in about 12 hours and the resulting larvæ attack the skin with their mouths and secretions, causing raw areas. The consequent moisture favours the larvæ, and their excreta attracts further blowflies which give rise to further generations of larvæ.

Symptoms.—A characteristic twitching of the tail is seen when the hindquarters are affected. Tufts of white wool, discoloured wool, and the odour are indications of strike in other parts of the body. Death may occur within a week, and the mortality may be high among hill sheep especially, as the trouble may in them go undetected.

Treatment consists in the use of a dressing which will kill the larvæ and facilitate healing of the wounds, *e.g.* a BHC and acriflavine preparation.

Prevention.—*See* DIPS, INSECTICIDES.

STRINGHALT, or 'SPRINGHALT', is the term applied to a sudden snatching up of one or both hind legs of the horse when

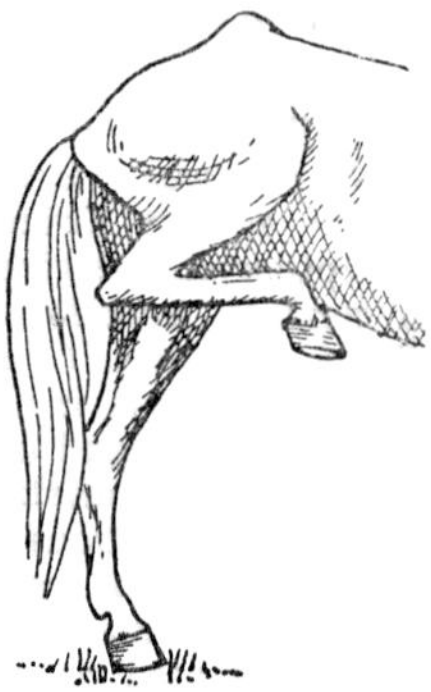

Stringhalt. The affected foot is vigorously snatched up from the ground, sometimes almost as high as the stomach, whenever the horse is made to turn sharply, or, in severe cases, during ordinary progression.

walking or, less often, when trotting. The condition is caused by an excessive contraction of the flexor muscles of the hock which brings the foot higher than normally, so that as the horse progresses the affected limb is seen to be moving much faster than the normal limb. The foot has farther to travel and must move faster. In most cases there is a very pronounced noise when the foot comes to the ground, so that it may be easily possible to detect stringhalt by hearing the footsteps of the horse only. The shoe wears faster, and the continual concussion weakens the foot and renders it liable to become affected with certain inflammatory conditions.

All classes and ages of horses may be affected, although it is perhaps commonest in older horses. It often appears about the time when maturity is reached—*i.e.* 5 to 6 years or a little sooner—after horses have been kept idle for some time in a stable or yard. In such cases the preliminary symptoms are mild, but the condition becomes aggravated with age and work, until a more or less stationary state is reached, after which there is no increase in severity.

Causes.—The cause of stringhalt is unknown.

An Australian form of stringhalt is seasonal in incidence, and possibly associated with plant poisoning. Several horses in a locality may be affected. Recovery occurs after weeks or months, but not in all cases.

Symptoms.—Stringhalt may appear suddenly in a horse of almost any age, or it may commence as a hardly noticeable jerk of the limb when turning, or after a period of rest; this becomes gradually more and more pronounced with the passage of time. Very often a horse may show slight signs of stringhalt, and then for a period may show absolutely no unusual action. Later, the characteristic jerky action and the snatch of the foot again become obvious and may persist, or may in turn be followed by another period of normal action.

The characteristic feature of stringhalt is an abnormal raising of the affected foot or feet, accompanied by excessive flexion of all the joints of the limb; it is as though the horse was stepping over some imaginary obstacle at each step. In severe cases the foot may even strike the abdomen, and in time causes a certain amount of bruising of skin and superficial tissues. The foot, as already mentioned, is placed heavily and noisily on the ground, and causes a kind of stamping action which tires the limb and renders the tissues more susceptible to the results of concussion. In well-developed cases the condition is not hard to recognise, but in the early stages, especially in young horses, or when it is not typical, it may be extremely hard to detect. Certain methods are employed to render more evident an occult case, and may be used in instances where stringhalt is suspected. In the first place, great care is required when dealing with hackneys and hackney ponies, which normally have extremely free flexion in the hind as well as the fore limbs, and which are trained so that this free action is accentuated even still more. In them particular care should be paid to uniformity between the flexion of the near and off fore limbs. When viewed from behind, each shoe should be seen to the same extent as the other during the walk and trot, and when viewed from the side the two hind limbs should rise to the same level above the ground. This can perhaps be best appreciated by holding an envelope in front of the observer's eyes, so as to obstruct the view of the horse's trunk but expose the view of the feet and limbs below. Comparisons between the level of the feet during the trot can then be made by noting how near they come to the level of the lower part of the envelope. This may be of assistance with horses of other classes. By resting the horse after exercise for 1 or 2 hours and then taking it out, watching each step it takes, and immediately causing it to be turned rapidly round in a very small circle, the characteristic snatch may be seen. Trotting a horse in a straight line, and then turning it suddenly, may elicit the characteristic lift of the foot. Backing a horse up an incline, either alone or yoked to a cart, as is sometimes done to bring out signs of shivering, assists also in the detection of stringhalt. Walking a horse in circles across ploughed land is a method recommended by some authorities, and others advocate giving the horse a drink of cold water and then immediately flicking it with a whip just as it finishes.

Treatment.—Those forms of so-called stringhalt which are occasioned by limb lesions usually disappear with recovery from the causal condition, whereas in the true form no improvement is seen after recovery from a possible co-existing lesion.

No treatment is of much avail in true stringhalt, although in the early stages a number of horses benefit from the operation of peroneal tenotomy. Otherwise, attention should be paid to the shoeing to diminish concussion. The affected foot or feet should be shod with thick leather soles (or soles of double leather), plenty of tar and tow being stuffed under the sole. A shoe made from thick bar iron should be used, for experience has shown that, within limits, the thicker the iron of the shoe the less is the concussion sustained by the foot. Heavy road haulage and trotting on causeway-sets should be avoided; the horse should work on the land only.

STRIP-CUP (*see* p. 540).

STRIP-GRAZING of cattle behind an electric fence tends to give greater production per acre, but it carries with it a risk of worm infestation under lush conditions unless a back-fence is brought up at 5-day periods, and 'resting pastures' avoided. The use of an electric fence for strip-grazing on 'early-bite' is valuable,

It induces the cattle to eat the whole plant instead of nibbling off the most succulent leaf-tips—which predisposes to Bloat.

STRIPPING (*see* pp. 540 *and* 557).

STRONGYLES (*see* p. 656 *and under* RED WORMS).

STRONTIUM (*see under* RADIO-ACTIVE STRONTIUM).

'STRUCK' (*see* ENTERO-TOXÆMIA).

STRYCHNINE is on of the two chief alkaloids of the seede of *Strychnos nux vomica*, an East Indian tree, the other being *brucine*, which is less powerful and not used medicinally, although its actions are similar to those of strychnine. Strychnine itself is a white crystalline substance, possessing an intensely bitter taste, perhaps the most bitter taste of any substance. It is used either as one of the salts of strychnine, or as a preparation of nux vomica such as the tincture, dry or liquid extract.

Actions.—In ordinary doses strychnine, whether given as nux vomica or otherwise, is a vegetable bitter which stimulates the secretion of gastric juice and assists digestion. Appetite is improved, and the tone of the stomach and intestines is raised. Upon the nervous system strychnine has marked effects. It has a special action upon the spinal cord; all the functions which the latter controls are more quickly carried out, and reflex action is increased; the muscles, both voluntary and involuntary, are kept in a greater state of tone, and the whole bodily activity increases. In the medulla somewhat similar changes are seen: the respiratory centre is stimulated, breathing becoming faster and deeper; the heart's action is strengthened; and blood-pressure is raised. In man it is said to increase the mental powers and sensibility, so that sight, hearing, and touch are rendered more acute.

Uses.—Strychnine is a useful tonic during convalescence from debilitating disease.

It is given as nux vomica, and is often combined with other vegetable tonic bitters and substances which aid digestion. In nerve conditions where paralysis is threatened it is valuable on account of its stimulating action on the spinal cord. In colic where there is absence of tone in the bowei wall, and collections of fæces causing obstruction in the intestines, it is sometimes prescribed along with carbonate of ammonia. In pneumonia and other respiratory disease it is given for its action on the respiratory centre and heart. In gastric derangements in cattle, as well as in cases of ante- and post-partum paralysis, it gives good results. For the dog it has similar uses, although great care is required because poisoning is caused with relatively small doses.

STRYCHNINE POISONING occurs mostly in the small animals, and particularly in the dog. It may arise from overdosage (*see* STRYCHNINE), from malicious use of poisons for trespassing dogs, from indiscriminate use of rat-poisons containing the drug, and from its cumulative effects when used in small doses for a long period. This latter effect must always be kept in mind, for the drug is excreted very slowly from the system, and it may still be found in the urine as long as a week after administration has ceased.

Symptoms.—In the larger animals the symptoms consist of convulsive seizures, characterised by a pronounced spasmodic contraction of the muscles of the limbs and trunk, and by a drawing back of the head and hollowing of the back (opisthotonus). This is followed by muscular quivering and then a period of complete relaxation, followed at a short interval by another severe convulsion. In the horse, the eyeballs roll and the eyelids are seen quivering and often becoming drawn back, exposing the white of the eye. In the smaller animals the same symptoms are seen, but the seizures are of a more violent nature, and the periods of relaxation are shorter. The symptoms are similar to those of tetanus, so far as the convulsions are concerned, the slightest noise or external stimulus being sufficient to produce a convulsion, but the characteristic 'locking of the jaws' is absent.

Treatment.—If a large dose has been taken, an emetic should be given to the smaller animals at once, preferably apomorphine given hypodermically; the larger animals should have their stomachs emptied as far as possible by the use of the stomach-tube. Tannic acid or strong tea is indicated. Thereafter, or when small doses have been taken over a long period, a large dose of chloral hydrate should be given, and the animal immediately afterwards anæsthetised. In no poison more than in strychnine is rapidity of action in giving antidotes more necessary. Once the drug has been absorbed and the effects on the nervous system have become obvious—*i.e.* when convulsions occur—attempts to remove the drug by emetics, etc., are futile, and may be dangerous. Expert advice should be sought without loss of time.

STUMPED-UP TOE is the popular phrase used to indicate that during shoeing of the horse the shoe has been set back too far on the foot, and the horn at the toe which projects has been cut away with the toeing-knife, so that the toe is shortened, and the bearing surface reduced. It is a very bad fault, and leads to weakness at the toe, with a risk of seedy-toe forming from pressure by the toe-clip upon the thinned horn. Moreover, it gives the horse's foot a foreshortened, stumpy appearance. The term is also occasionally applied to rolling the toe, which consists of bending the shoe slightly upwards at the toe, and reducing the foot to correspond. In this the toe does not rest on the ground when the horse is standing, but when the weight is moved forward, just before the foot is lifted from the ground, the foot as a whole rolls forward on to the toe. Rolling the toe is a useful method of shoeing certain horses which are liable to stumble when trotting.

STUNNING, ELECTRIC, OF CATTLE.—This is practised in Sweden and the Netherlands by means of the Elther apparatus (prior to Jewish ritualistic slaughter or otherwise). It is successful also for calves, sheep, and goats.

STUNNING, ELECTRIC, OF PIGS.—This has been practised extensively since the 1930s, and involves the use of brine-soaked electrodes, applied on each side of the pig's face, by means of which the electric current is passed. A voltage of not less than 75 is recommended by Dr. Phyllis G. Croft, and a current of not less than 250 milliampères, assuming 50 cycles-per-second alternating current. An electroplectic fit is caused, with anæsthesia lasting for about 60 seconds, *when conditions are satisfactory*. After 60 seconds, there may be a half-minute period of paralysis during which sensation is present. Therefore, the pig must be stuck *during the first* 60 *seconds*. If care is not taken and the apparatus be faulty or unsuitable, paralysis only, and not anæsthesia, may result; the pig being conscious when stuck.

STURDY (*see* GID, also PARASITES, p. 653).

STUTTGART DISEASE ('CANINE TYPHUS') is the name formerly given to a group of symptoms—notably, in the acute form: thirst, vomiting of coffee-coloured material, offensive breath, rapid loss of condition, a coppery colour of the tongue with ulceration at its tip and ulceration of the gums and inside of the cheeks, prostration, and death within 3 days—occurring in the dog. Stuttgart Disease was formerly regarded as a gastro-enteritis of unknown origin, but the syndrome described above is now known to be associated with kidney failure and uræmia, and probably in nine cases out of ten has its origin in infection with *Leptospira canicola*. (*See* LEPTOSPIROSIS.) In a few instances the syndrome may possibly occur during the course of a virus disease, while the mouth lesions alone may be set up by a nicotinic acid deficiency, which can be overcome by feeding yeast.

STYE (*see* EYE).

STYFZIEKTE is a name meaning 'stiff sickness', which is used to describe either the symptoms associated with chronic aphosphorosis, which is the forerunner of lamziekte in South Africa, or those associated with a mineral deficiency in certain parts of Northern Nigeria.

STYPTICS (στυπτικός, astringent) are applications which check bleeding, either by making the blood-vessels contract more firmly or by causing more rapid clotting of the blood. Some possess both actions. The use of styptics is discussed under HÆMORRHAGE and BLEEDING, ARREST OF.

SUB-CLINICAL.—A disease is said to be sub-clinical when the symptoms are so slight as to escape the notice of the animal owner. Examples: sub-clinical mastitis, which by lowering the milk yield of a herd of cows may be of considerable economic importance; similarly, a sub-clinical infestation with parasitic worms.

SUBCUTANEOUS (*sub*, under; *cutis*, the skin) means anything pertaining to the loose connective tissue lying under the skin, such as a subcutaneous injection, where the injected fluid is introduced below the skin. (*See* HYPODERMIC INJECTIONS.)

SUBLUXATION (*sub*, under; *luxatio*, a dislocation) means a partial dislocation, and is a term sometimes applied to a sprain of a tendon or ligament occurring near a joint.

SUCCUSSION (*succussio*, a shaking) is a method of examination of a patient by shaking the body in order to elicit splashing sounds, with a view to determining the presence of fluid or gas (or both) in the interior of a natural cavity, such as the thorax or abdomen.

SUCKING or **INTERSUCKING.**—This habit or 'vice' occurs among dairy calves. The M.M.B. has commented: 'If allowed to go unchecked, the practice may become habitual, involving a risk to the health of the calves, and, if persisting into adulthood, the welfare of the herd in general may be affected. A particularly severe case was encountered in a herd of 50 Friesian cows where the habit grew so pronounced that the herd became uneconomic and had to be dispersed. Cattle of all ages were involved and milk loss was considerable. Purchased calves acquired the same habits after a short while. Intersucking is a problem in only a small proportion of herds, usually those of above average size, where the calves are bucket fed, or where they are grouped at or shortly after birth.

The most effective remedy is to separate the calves after feeding, but if this is not practicable, mechanical devices or the provision of dry food are good alternatives. It seems that a useful preventive measure is to delay grouping calves until they are more than four weeks of age.

SUCKLING (*see* NURSE COWS, CALF REARING).

SUDORIFICS (*sudor*, sweat; *facio*, I make) are drugs and other agents which produce a copious flow of perspiration. (*See* DIAPHORETICS.)

SUFFOCATION (*see* ASPHYXIA and CHOKING).

SUGAR is a substance containing the elements carbon, hydrogen, and oxygen, and belonging therefore to the chemical group of carbohydrates. This group includes three main subdivisions as follows:

(1) Monosaccharides, or glucoses ($C_6H_{12}O_6$):
e.g. Dextrose or grape-sugar,
Levulose.

(2) Disaccharides, or sucroses ($C_{12}H_{22}O_{11}$):
e.g. Cane-sugar,
Lactose or milk-sugar,
Maltose or malt-sugar.

(3) Polysaccharides, or amyloses ($(C_6H_{10}O_5)n$):
e.g. Starch,
Glycogen (animal starch),
Dextrin and other gums.

Grape-sugar is found in various kinds of fruit, and is the form of sugar produced by the tissues and excreted in considerable amounts by the kidneys in diabetes.

Cane-sugar is very widely distributed through the vegetable kingdom, though it is particularly plentiful in the juice of the sugar-cane, sugar-beet, and maple. When taken into the body it is converted into grape-sugar by the digestive juices prior to absorption; this change is known as 'inversion'. Cane-sugar is a valuable food, being utilised in the production of heat and energy, though it is also a tissue-builder so far as fat is concerned, and this is one reason why fattening cattle are often given treacle in the ration.

Milk-sugar is found in milk, and it is to the fermentation of this sugar by bacteria, with the consequent production of lactic acid, that the souring of milk is due. Milk-sugar has little sweetening power when compared with cane-sugar, but it is sometimes used as a laxative and diuretic, and in making up certain poisonous drugs into pills it is used to give bulk.

Malt-sugar is produced by the action of the ferment diatase upon the starch contained in barley, and also by the ferments of the saliva and pancreatic juice, though it appears to be still further changed by the latter ferments into glucose before it can be absorbed into the body.

Starch is mentioned under a separate heading, and its use as a food-stuff is described under DIET AND DIETING.

SULPHA DRUGS (*see* SULPHONAMIDES).

SULPHADIMIDINE (*see* 'Sulphamezathine' *under* SULPHONAMIDE DRUGS).

SULPHAQUINOXALINE.—A yellow powder given to poultry, mixed in their food or in their drinking water, for the control of coccidiosis.

SULPHONAL is a hypnotic agent, of most use in the dog.

SULPHONAMIDE DRUGS are, to susceptible organisms (*e.g. streptococci*) bacteriostatic rather than bactericidal; that is to say, they prevent the multiplication of bacteria rather than killing them. Sulphonamide drugs are all synthetic and closely related to *p*-aminobenzoic acid, which is believed to be essential to bacteria, and which is absorbed by them; and it is believed that the sulphonamides are absorbed by the bacteria similarly, with the result mentioned above. Individual sulpha drugs do not have specific actions against specific bacteria; their differences lie in the differing concentration or level which can safely be obtained in the animal's blood-stream, and their excretion route.

Uses.—Sulphonamide drugs are extensively employed in veterinary medicine for dressing wounds, for the prevention of post-operative sepsis, and in the treatment of pneumonia, metritis, enteritis, 'joint-ill', foul-in-the-foot of cattle, and arthritis in young pigs, etc. They must be used in full dosage, or resistant strains of bacteria may be set up.

Toxicity.—Sulphonamides differ from penicillin in that they may have an adverse effect upon the host's cells as well as upon the invading germs. For this reason (and to avoid giving rise to resistant strains) sulphonamides should be used only under veterinary advice and not indiscriminately. Fortunately, however, domestic mammals, with the exception of the goat, show few signs of intolerance. Sulphanilamide is, however, highly toxic to birds.

Names of individual compounds.—The list of these is being continually extended, but mention may be made here of:

SULPHANILAMIDE.—Of value as a dry dusting powder for wounds, teat sores, etc. It may be combined with 1 per cent neutral proflavine sulphate.

SULPHAPYRIDINE ('M. & B. 693').—Gained a great reputation in human medicine in the treatment of lobar pneumonia. Has been used in calf pneumonia. More toxic than several other sulphonamides.

SULPHATHIAZOLE.—Has been used in the treatment of calf pneumonia and fowl coryza.

SULPHADIAZINE.—Has been used in the treatment of calf pneumonia, etc.

SULPHAMERAZINE.—Has been used in the treatment of calf pneumonia, etc.

SULPHAGUANIDINE.—Used in the treatment of White Scour of calves, necrotic enteritis in pigs, and enteritis in other animals. Readily taken in the food.

SULPHAQUINOXALINE.—Used in the control and treatment of coccidiosis in chickens and turkeys.

'SULPHAMEZATHINE' (Sulphadimidine).—Of value in 'Foul-in-the-foot' in cattle, pneumonia, enteritis. Is readily accepted in the food by all animals.

SULPHUR is a non-metallic element which is procurable in several different allotropic forms. 'Crude sulphur' or 'black sulphur' is obtained from deposits in volcanic districts, and from it is prepared 'sublimed sulphur' by heating. This sublimed sulphur is either run into moulds to form 'roll sulphur', or is allowed to deposit as 'flowers of sulphur'. Flowers of sulphur may be washed to free it from irritating impurities, when it is known as 'washed sulphur'. Again, the sublimed sulphur may be boiled with slaked lime and treated with hydrochloric acid, when the sulphur settles down as a fine greyish-yellow powder, known as 'precipitated sulphur' or 'milk of sulphur'.

Actions.—The action of sulphur given internally as the sublimed sulphur is due partly to the grittiness which, by irritating the mucous membrane of the intestines, causes a slightly greater secretion of fluid, thereby rendering the evacuations more soft, and partly to the formation of small amounts of the sulphide in the alimentary canal. Some of the sulphides are absorbed and stimulate the intestinal glands, and after passing through the circulation are excreted by the kidneys and skin, stimulating these also and having, in the latter case, an action against mange mites and lice.

Uses.—For sulphur fumigation, sticks or 'candles' of rock or roll of sulphur are burned in byres, stables, etc., which have first had the walls and floors sprayed or hosed with cold water. Windows, doors, and other apertures are closed, wet sacks being laid across spaces below doors, etc., and the pungent fumes are allowed to remain in the closed building overnight. The sulphurous acid gas unites with the water on the walls and floor, and the mixture exerts powerful disinfectant actions upon bacterial and insect life. As a parasiticide sulphur has been largely replaced by BHC, derris, etc., although proprietary *organic* preparations of sulphur are still used in the treatment of mange.

Poisoning.—Overdosage must be avoided—3 oz. of flowers of sulphur has killed cattle. Dosing by guesswork on the part of a shepherd killed 140 ewes in a single flock.

SULPHUR DIOXIDE.—A poisonous gas which is a constituent of Diesel engine exhaust fumes. (*See* SMOG.)

'SUMMER MASTITIS' (*see under* MASTITIS).

'SUMMER SORES' in horses are caused by infective *Hebronema* larvæ deposited in wounds by stable- or house-flies. They are very itchy. Eyelids may be affected. The infestation results in the formation of fibrous nodules which may later ulcerate. Summer sores are uncommon in Britain.

SUNBURN.—Some cattle with a white coat colour and pink skin, which have been bred in temperate climates, show a diffused superficial inflammation of the skin when imported into hot countries. Herefords are most often affected about the head, and especially around the eyelids, and so well known is this fact that for export purposes animals which have a red ring round each of the eyes are preferred to those which have pure white faces. (*See also* LIGHT SENSITISATION.)

SUNLIGHT (*see under* RICKETS, INFERTILITY, LIGHT SENSITISATION).

SUNSTROKE (*see* HEATSTROKE).

SUPER- (*super*, above) is a prefix signifying above or implying excess.

SUPERFŒTATION.—The presence in the uterus of fœtuses of different ages, due to successive services.

For example, a cow is got in calf at one service, comes on heat again, and settles to a further service ; in due course producing a calf as the result of the first mating, but more often than not having little or no milk. She later calves again, as the result of the second mating, and this time lactation begins. Calves born in this way are not, of course, twins. Although contemporaries within the dam, they are of different ages, and can have different sires !

An elderly cow which had always had single calves, was 'put to A.I. again and subsequently on three occasions at normal intervals, after which she appeared to hold'.

Presuming that she had held to the last service, her owners were very surprised to find her one morning two months before she was expected to calve, licking a full-term heifer calf which was 'quite obviously hers'. The milk yield was poor, and so the cow was left at grass to suckle her calf. Two months later she 'suddenly bagged up well and calved a live, full-term bull calf in circumstances that left no doubt it was hers also'.

Subsequent blood-tests, carried out in Copenhagen, showed that the first calf was not by the A.I. Centre's bull as stated. The second was.

The remarkable features of this example of 'double pregnancy' are that artificial insemination did not disturb a 2-month embryo ; and the stress and exertion of calving did not affect a 7-month fœtus, either.

SUPERINVOLUTION is the contraction of the womb after parturition when the shrinkage proceeds beyond the normal, and the organ is less in size than before conception. It may proceed to such an extent that the dam is subsequently unable to breed, or it may simply result in a reduction in size of the organ which is not very important. It is most commonly seen in highly nervous or excitable bitches or thoroughbred brood mares.

SUPEROVULATION.—The production of extra (mammal's) eggs. It can be induced by means of hormones. (*See* TRANSPLANTATION OF OVA, TWINNING.)

SUPERPURGATION (*super*, above=too much ; *purgo*, I cleanse) is excessive purgation which continues for some considerable time, and may end fatally. It is most serious in the horse, where it may follow the administration of aloes. (*See* ALOES.) It may also arise through the ingestion of food-stuffs which are unwholesome, such as sprouted potatoes, decomposed mouldy oats (when polyuria is usually also present), and other cases result from eating excessively large amounts of green luscious herbage, when the alimentary system has not previously been accustomed to this food ; *e.g.* it may result from horses breaking out from a stable and getting into a field of clover or lucerne.

Symptoms.—The most marked symptom is the evacuation, in large quantities, of fluid, and often frothy fæces, which may occasion straining. There is great thirst, weakness and depression, and the pulse fails to maintain its strength. Colic, shown by rolling, kicking at the belly, a crouched attitude, and boarding of the abdominal muscles, generally occurs, and there may be prostration, convulsive seizures, and death, unless relief is obtained.

Treatment.—It is always better, wherever possible, to call in skilled assistance as early as possible, for superpurgation may easily end in death.

SUPPLEMENTARY FEEDING. — For that of hill ewes, *see* p. 834. (*See also* FLUSHING OF EWES, CREEP FEED.)

SUPPLEMENTARY VETERINARY REGISTER (*see under* VETERINARY SURGEONS ACT).

SUPPLEMENTS.—Technical products for use at less than 5 per cent of the total ration, in which they are included, and designed to supply planned proportions of vitamins, trace minerals, one or more non-nutrient additives and other special ingredients.

SUPPOSITORY (*suppositorius*, something introduced beneath) is a small conical mass made of fat or glycerine, and containing drugs intended for introduction into the rectum. It may be a convenient way of giving an aperient, such as a glycerine suppository ; it may be intended to allay inflammation or irritation of the mucous membrane of the rectum, such as a belladonna or an opium suppository.

SUPPRESSION is the name applied to a failure on the part of the kidneys to excrete urine.

SUPPURATION (*suppuratio*) means the formation of pus. When pus forms upon a raw surface the process is spoken of as 'ulceration', while a deep-seated collection of pus is called an 'abscess'. For further information *see under* ABSCESS; INFLAMMATION; PHAGOCYTOSIS; WOUNDS.

SUPRARENAL BODIES (*see* ADRENAL GLANDS).

SUPRASCAPULAR PARALYSIS is a form of peripheral paralysis very commonly met with in young horses that are used for ploughing, but it may affect any horse which works in a collar. It is considered to be due to strain of the suprascapular nerve, or to actual separation of the nerve from the muscles which it supplies—supraspinous and infraspinous, *i.e.* the muscles above and below the spine of the scapula. The term 'slipped shoulder' is applied to the symptoms which are shown in a typical case. The two muscles mentioned above act as ligaments of the shoulder-joint, and when they are paralysed the shoulder slips outward each time the foot is placed upon the ground and when weight is put upon it. After the paralysis has been in existence for some few days two distinct hollows appear over the shoulder, due to atrophy of the muscles, and the spine of the scapula stands out prominently between these hollows. When viewed from in front the animal appears to have lost the symmetry of the two shoulder regions. In typical cases there is difficulty in bringing the limb forward, and often the leg appears to swing outwards with a circular movement. When the horse stands quietly, the affected limb is usually brought well under the body, and may even take up a position across the middle line of the body. At first there is lameness or difficulty in progression, but this soon passes, and the atrophy already mentioned, becomes obvious. The paralysis may rapidly disappear, and in 6 weeks the horse may be recovered ; but in more severe cases, especially those in which the symptoms have appeared after an accident, or after the horse has had a foot fast, or has been cast, as many as 18 months may elapse before the horse is fit for work. Treatment consists in applying soothing and relaxing fomentations, such as warm water containing soap liniment, until the acute symptoms subside ; thereafter giving the horse a run at grass generally results in improvement. Electric treatment is also employed by the veterinary surgeon but should not be attempted without professional advice.

SURAMIN.—A drug used against trypanosomes.

SURFACTANTS.—Surface active agents used in America and elsewhere to increase growth rate of poultry. They are less effective than antibiotics.

SURGICAL SPIRIT.—This commonly contains half a fluid ounce of castor oil per pint of industrial methylated spirit, together with a little methyl salicylate and brucine.

SURRA (*see under* PARASITES, diseases caused by trypanosomes).

SUTURE (*sutura*, a seam) is the name given either to the close union between two adjacent flat bones of the skull at their edges, or to a series of stitches by which a wound is closed. (*See* WOUNDS.)

SWABS.—Swabs are used for sampling mucus, etc., for diagnostic purposes; the material subsequently being cultured so that pathogenic organisms, if present, may be identified. For swabbing as a guide to infertility in the thoroughbred mare, *see under* UTERINE INFECTIONS.

SWAMP FEVER (*see* EQUINE INFECTIOUS ANÆMIA).

SWAYBACK is a disease of new-born and young lambs, characterised by progressive cerebral demyelination, which results in paralysis and often death. It occurs in many parts of the United Kingdom. Knowledge as to its cause is still incomplete, but prevention can be effected

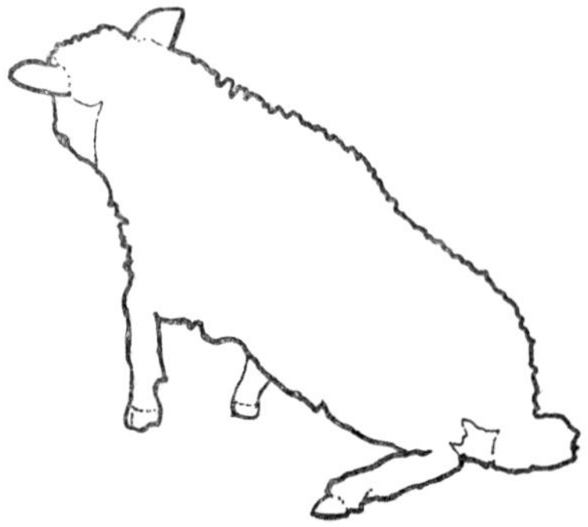

Swayback—a characteristic posture.

by the provision of mineral licks containing 1 per cent of copper. It has been suggested that Swayback has become more prevalent since nicotine, or tobacco, preparations with copper sulphate gave way to phenothiazine. Accordingly, copper salts have been added to at least one proprietary preparation of phenothiazine.

Symptoms.—A staggering gait or inability to walk. Severely affected cases all die.

Treatment.—None.

Prevention.—Allow the pregnant ewes access to copper licks.

SWEAT (*see* PERSPIRATION).

SWEAT GLANDS (*see* SKIN).

SWEAT HOUSE SYSTEM.—This is a method of keeping pigs in a building in which temperature is maintained at 75° F. and humidity at 80 per cent. The system, which is to be deprecated, was claimed to reduce respiratory infections, but in hot weather the humidity falls and bacteria can be expected to cause trouble. Suffocation or heat stroke may occur with cold weather ventilation. The liquid feed usually supplied is often associated with (sometimes fatal) ulceration of the stomach. The pigs are often brown from liquid fæces, and the fabric of the building deteriorates rapidly.

'SWEATING SICKNESS'.—This is a tick-borne disease of cattle in Southern Africa, affecting mainly calves. (Sheep can also become naturally infected.) There is a high fever. The disease takes its name from the characteristic moist eczema. Some calves die, others recover completely.

SWEDISH RED AND WHITE CATTLE.—This is the main breed of Sweden. The herdbook dates from 1928, when the Swedish Ayrshire and the Swedish Red-white breeds—similar in origin and characteristics—were amalgamated. Each was the result of breeding from old Swedish stock to which had been introduced some Dairy Shorthorn and Ayrshire blood.

It is a long-lived breed, with an overall milk yield average in excess of 950 gallons at 4·1 per cent butter-fat. The dams of all bulls sold at the 1958 Breed Society sales had averaged in all their recorded years (5·8 per cow) over 1,196 gallons.

There is very little white in the coat-colour; and some animals are entirely red.

'SWEET ITCH'.—An old-fashioned name for ECZEMA in the horse, especially that resulting from allergic reaction to some pasture plant.

SWILL.—The feeding of unboiled swill —a practice which is illegal—is a frequent source of swine fever and foot-and-mouth disease infections.

'SWIMMERS.'—The colloquial name for puppies showing the juvenile femoral rotation syndrome. They are unable to rise on to their hind legs at the usual age, due to the head and neck of the femur being wrongly positioned on the shaft. Sometimes the name 'Flat Pup' Syndrome is applied.

SWINE DYSENTERY.—For many years this was thought to be a specific contagious enteritis caused by *Vibrio coli*. It is now thought that a spirochæte may be responsible, but the cause remains an enigma, and experimentally no single infective agent has reproduced the disease.

About 1 in 3 pigs in a herd become ill, and the mortality rate is 10 to 60 per cent. Chronic scouring, without dysentery, may persist. The fæces are greyish. Treatment with arsenicals is effective.

SWINE ERYSIPELAS is an infectious disease of pigs and characterised by high fever, reddish or purplish spots on the skin, and hæmorrhages on to the surfaces of certain of the internal organs in acute cases; and by general debility, lameness, and difficulty in breathing in chronic cases. In these latter there are usually found characteristic cauliflower-like masses on the valves of the heart.

The disease may occur in man; also in chickens, turkeys, pheasants and grouse.

Causes.—The distribution of swine erysipelas is confined to the Old World. The disease is unknown in America. In Europe it is ordinarily very prevalent both in the acute form and in the chronic, but at times it assumes the nature of an epizoötic, sweeping throughout large territories, and leaving a high percentage of deaths in its wake. In Britain the chronic form is usually met with in small outbreaks in different parts of the country, but from time to time in certain areas, especially in East Anglia, and up to the east coast generally, and especially during the hot dry summer weather, it breaks out in a more menacing form, and large numbers of pigs become affected with the acute form, and considerable numbers die. These facts are apparently due to external conditions being suitable for the survival and spread of the causal agent—the *Erysipelothrix rhusiopathiæ*, which may also infect sheep at shearing or dipping time through small wounds or abrasions, and may cause mild illness in man as a result of infected cuts. (*See* ERYSIPELOID.) Adult sows which do not thrive well and are often chronically affected act as carriers, and from them the disease in the acute form is contracted by younger pigs.

Infertility, involving abortion, still-births, and mummified fœtuses, commonly results from erysipelas.

The organism also infects birds, especially turkeys.

Symptoms.—There are three recognised forms of swine erysipelas: the mild or subacute, the acute, and the chronic.

Mild or *subacute* attacks come on suddenly; there is high fever, loss of appetite, dullness, a tendency to lie buried in the litter, and when moved to do so reluctantly, and the skin over the thorax, neck, back, and over the thighs, becomes flushed at first, and soon changes to a red or purple colour. The outlines of the areas affected are often square, or they may be the shape of the playing-card diamond, from which the disease gets one of its names—'diamond disease'. The areas are usually raised above the level of the surrounding skin, are painful to the touch at first, but not so later, and, appearing about the second or third day of the attack, last for 4 days, and then disappear. Recovery is usually rapid, and in a week affected pigs may be apparently better. They are liable later, however, to be attacked by the chronic form, and may subsequently succumb. In some cases, pigs may show painful swellings of the knees and hocks, but this is not invariable. The affected areas may become gangrenous, but this is not usual. Young pigs between 3 and 5 or 6 months old are most commonly attacked; it is rare before 3 months, but may occur in older animals.

Acute type, or *septicæmic type*, is the type usually seen in large outbreaks. The animals often become exhausted, and die without showing other symptoms. They may hide in the straw, become apathetic, cease to feed, vomit, and are constipated at first, but the reverse later on. The eyelids are often swollen and a slimy conjunctivitis makes its appearance. The flushing of the skin may appear first upon the finer parts of the body, behind ears, inside thighs, and under elbows, etc., and later may spread over practically the whole of the body. In the early stages, the skin is extremely sensitive to the touch, but not so later ; gangrene of quite large areas may appear, and a certain amount of serous exudate may form over the flushed areas. The general disturbance is usually great ; breathing is laboured ; the visible mucous membranes are often livid ; the pulse is weak ; and the temperature is at first high, but falls to below normal just before death occurs, which may be at any time from the 4th or 5th day to a week or 10 days. Death in these cases usually results from septicæmia, the organisms being present in the blood-stream in enormous numbers.

Chronic type, which may follow recovery from one of the two forms above described, is the most insidious, and pigs affected with it are probably responsible for causing most of the outbreaks of the previous types, since, being bad thrivers, they are often disposed of through the open market and bought by owners of clean herds. They feed, but do not always finish their food ; they appear well, but do not thrive ; they have a normal temperature, but are easily distressed when made to take exercise. Breathing becomes shallow, and a cough generally develops. The pulse becomes thready, and if the heart be listened to, a flowing murmur can be heard over the left side of the chest. This is due to the vegetative (or verrucose) endocarditis, which is almost *the* characteristic feature of post-mortem examination of pigs dead from chronic swine erysipelas. The chronic form may last for several weeks, or even for 2 or 3 months, especially in strong robust young breeding gilts, but towards the end emaciation and prostration become very obvious.

Treatment consists in the administration of antiserum as soon as possible. Penicillin is also very effective.

Prevention consists in avoiding any pigs in the open market which appear to be thin and not thriving, especially sows and boars, or older pigs. Any showing wrinkling of the skin of the ears, or patches of flushing on the skin, those which have swollen joints, or those which have diarrhœa, should not be bought. Pigs showing extreme breathlessness upon mild exertion should be likewise avoided. After purchase of new pigs through a market, each lot should be quarantined for a period of 3 weeks or a month before being mixed with the general herd. At the same time, it must be remembered that the causal bacillus is a normal inhabitant of the pig's alimentary tract, and that pigs may contract the disease without any contact with outside animals at all. Protective inoculation gives good results but is somewhat costly. This confers a strong degree of immunity, which, if not lifelong, is at least long enough to protect fattening pigs. It is of most use in a district where there are enzoötic outbreaks of the mild or acute types.

Arthritis and heart disease may be a result of pigs becoming hypersensitised to the bacteria, and not the results of attack by the bacteria themselves. This must be borne in mind when prescribing the vaccine.

SWINE FEVER, hog cholera, pig typhoid, or ' the fever ', is a highly infectious and contagious disease of pigs.

Cause.—The cause of swine fever is a virus, which is associated with certain secondary invaders, *e.g. Salmonella suipestifer*, or *B. cholera suis*, and the so-called swine plague bacillus, or the bacillus of swine fever pneumonia—*Pasteurella suiseptica* ; and *Actinomyces necrophorus*. None of these secondary organisms is, however, necessary for the production of swine fever.

It inevitably happens that pigs harbouring the virus of swine fever, but not yet showing symptoms of the disease, are slaughtered for human food. Under such circumstances, the virus can survive in the skin and muscle for 17 days. In frozen pork the survival time has been quoted as over four years ; in bacon 27 days. No wonder that unboiled swill is responsible for so many outbreaks.

Apart from this difficulty, swine fever is spread through the acts of unscrupulous pig-owners who, when they suspect the disease in their pigs, attempt very frequently to avoid loss by selling them through the market or to the private buyer. At public markets, the urine of infected pigs so often drains into adjoining pens and alleyways. The urine may, too, get splashed on to men's clothing, boots, etc., and droplets of it find their way into lorries and on to farms. In 1953 about 30 outbreaks, spread over 10 counties, arose from the sale of a single infected pen at a large market.

It seems probable that the virus may be carried by rats and mice for short distances at least. Manure carts lifting dung from different piggeries may become contaminated and spread infection from place to place. Horse-flies can carry the virus, which—according to an American report—can be harboured by larvæ of the pig lungworm. These larvæ are, in turn, harboured by earthworms.

The use of antibiotics contained in feedingstuffs has had the effect of masking the classical symptoms of swine fever, and is sometimes said to have extended the incubation period.

There is an immunological relationship between the virus of swine fever and that causing mucosal disease of cattle.

Symptoms.—In young pigs the disease is usually acute or peracute, while in older pigs it tends to assume a chronic form, although they also may be affected with the severe rapidly fatal form.

Acute type.—Young pigs, either still suckling or recently weaned, are most commonly affected with this form of swine fever. They are acutely fevered; have a high temperature; refuse to feed; lie hidden or half-hidden in the litter all day and when forced to move do so peevishly, giving little annoyed whining squeaks, and only moving a few steps away. Their backs are arched; their tails are uncurled; and their whole appearance suggests acute misery and sickness. There is often a small amount of yellowish discharge from the eyes, and sometimes the eyelids are stuck together. Diarrhœa, usually of a greenish or brownish colour, and always possessed of a foul odour, is present. The skin often shows a reddish rash, not raised above the surrounding skin; being particularly common at the back of the ears and round the tail, it is generally easily seen. The breathing is distressed, and in an affected litter which has been disturbed and brought out from the straw there are always one or two of the little pigs attacked with a fit of coughing. Deaths occur about 3 days after the first symptoms are shown in the peracute type, although sometimes the finding of one or two dead pigs in a litter is the first indication of the presence of swine fever. In mixed piggeries, older pigs are usually not attacked at first, but where only fattening stock is kept, swine fever may appear in pigs up to 4 months of age or more. A number of pigs survive for from 1 to 3 weeks and then die, having become very emaciated in the meantime.

Pneumonia is a common *post-mortem* finding. 'Button ulcers' may not be present at all.

Chronic type.—In this form, pigs are dull, do not come readily to the troughs, burrow in the straw, uncurl their tails, occasionally vomit, and though to a casual observer the general health of the herd may appear to be good, when a few pigs are caught and have their temperatures taken a surprising number register 2, 3, or more degrees of fever, while one or two will be found to have a very high temperature, perhaps 106° F. or more. If moved about, one pig will be seen occasionally to stagger, and one or two are noticed to be weak behind, perhaps swaying when standing, or dragging their hind feet when made to walk. Some may be affected with diarrhœa; some may have a chronic cough; some may show a catarrhal conjunctivitis; and others appear ill without any very definite symptoms being seen. Occasionally, one or two pigs die. Pregnant sows frequently abort, or if they produce a full-time litter, become ill immediately afterwards, and usually lose all the young pigs within a very few days.

Infection of a pregnant sow can be followed by the presence of virus in her piglets, either stillborn or living. The sow is not a 'carrier' in the usually accepted sense, since after the birth of her piglets the virus—having crossed the placental barrier—no longer remains within her body. A period of 56 days may elapse between the last deaths on a farm and a recrudescence of the disease.

Treatment.—The best results are derived from hyperimmune serum. Sulpha drugs and antibiotics are not effective against the virus but combat the secondary invaders.

Prevention.—Crystal violet vaccine is no longer used in the U.K. It is absolutely necessary to ensure that all swill is boiled, for pieces of infected pig meat may otherwise give rise to an outbreak of the disease. Pigs introduced into a herd should be from premises known to be free from the disease. Visits by pig-dealers should be discouraged.

Control.—In Britain swine fever is notifiable and must be reported to the Local Authority, usually to a police constable in the first instance, and thereafter any outbreak is dealt with by a veterinary officer specially appointed by the Ministry of Agriculture.

A swine fever eradication programme, with compulsory slaughter, and compensation, was introduced in Britain in 1963. The disease was eradicated in 1966, but re-appeared briefly in Yorkshire in 1971.

SWINE FEVER, AFRICAN.—This disease, formerly restricted to the African continent, appeared in Spain and Portugal during 1960. Including animals compulsorily slaughtered, Spain lost 120,000 pigs and Portugal 16,000.

The disease is also known as Wart-Hog disease, as these animals besides bush-pigs are affected. In some parts of Africa, pig-raising has had to be abandoned on account of the disease, which is highly contagious, nearly always fatal, and gives rise to 'carriers'—those few that survive often transmitting the infection to other pigs for a year or more.

Cause.—A virus, which is resistant to heat, drying, and putrefaction, and which can survive in smoked or partly cooked sausage and other pork products. The virus attacks blood-vessel cells and the disease is accordingly characterised by hæmorrhages.

Symptoms.—After an incubation period of 5 to 15 days, there is fever; the pig running a temperature of 105° or so. There may be no other symptoms for about 5 days. Then the fever subsides, and there are more obvious signs of illness—followed by death within a day or two.

Control.—There was, in 1962, no vaccine available, and control depended upon compulsory slaughter, the banning of markets and movement of pigs, etc Since then, live vaccine has been used in Portugal and Spain, but has given rise to 'carriers'.

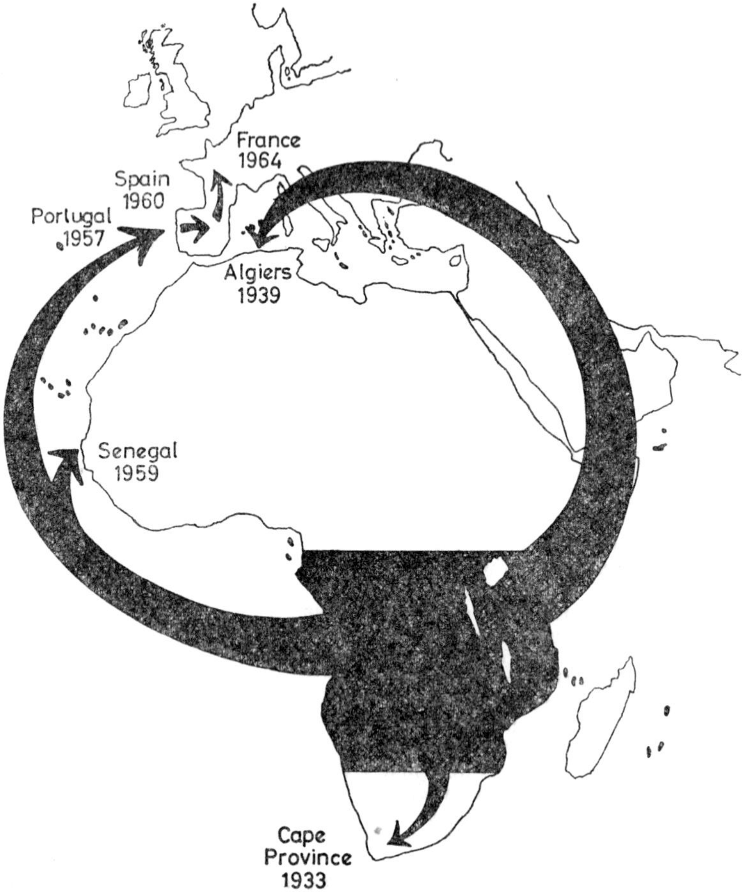

The spread of African swine fever.

SWINE INFLUENZA—A contagious disease of sucking and young store pigs, characterised by catarrh of the respiratory passages and broncho-pneumonia. According to the Ministry of Agriculture (1971) the swine influenza virus has not been isolated in the U.K. for many decades. (*See also* ENZOOTIC PNEUMONIA.)

Cause.—A myxovirus; important secondary invaders include: *Hæmophilus influenzæ suis, Pasteurella suiseptica, Brucella bronchiseptica*, and *streptococci*.

Symptoms.—Sneezing, coughing, and laboured breathing, temperature seldom above 104°. Delirium may occur. In the less acute form, unthriftiness and a persistent cough are noticed. Mortality: about 30 per cent. Recovery is seldom complete and 'carriers' may exist.

SWINE PLAGUE is the term applied to what in Britain is considered to be the pneumonic form of swine fever, but what in America and the continent of Europe is held to be a separate disease. (*See* SWINE FEVER.)

SWINE POX (*see* VARIOLA).

SWINE TYPHOID, TYPHUS.—Infecion with *Salmonella choleræ suis*.

SYMBIOSIS (*see* PARASITES).

SYMPATHETIC is a term applied to certain diseases or symptoms that arise in one part of the body as the result of disease or disturbance in another area. Thus inflammation may arise in one eye as the result of an injury to the other, generally owing to the spread of organisms along the lymph vessels connecting the two eyes; it is then called a 'sympathetic inflammation'.

SYMPATHETIC NERVOUS SYSTEM is that part of the nervous system from which most of the nerves that connect and regulate the actions of the internal organs appear to take their origin. It consists of scattered collections of grey nerve matter known as 'ganglia', united by a very irregular and complicated network of nerve fibres. Those parts where the ganglia are close together and the network of fibres specially dense are called 'plexuses'. The central part of the sympathetic system is formed by two cords running the whole length of the body, one on either side and slightly below the bodies of the vertebra, and possessing at regular intervals, corresponding with the nerve roots of the spinal cord, ganglia from which fibres pass out to the more distant parts of the body. (*See also* NERVES.)

SYN- (σύν, with) is a prefix signifying union.

SYNAPSE (σύν, with; ἅπτω, I touch) is the term applied to the anatomical relation of one nerve cell with another which is effected at various points by contact of their branching processes. The state of shrinkage or relaxation at these points (synapses) is supposed in some cases to determine the readiness with which a nervous impulse is transmitted from one part of the nervous system to another. Certain drugs also are supposed to act upon the nervous system through their effect in closing or widening these junctions.

SYNCHRONISATION OF ŒSTRUS.—**In the ewe.**—Syncro-Mate may be used. This is a polyurethane sponge impregnated with Cronolone, a new compound having an action like that of the hormone progesterone.

Syncro-Mate is used intra-vaginally, insertion being made with a specially designed applicator. Trials involving 17,000 ewes in Australia and 5000 ewes in Britain have demonstrated that during the breeding season œstrus can be synchronised effectively for two to three œstrous cycles following pessary removal. In late anœstrus Synchro-Mate will stimulate earlier synchronous cyclical breeding activity. Conception rates are highest (80 to 90 per cent) at the second synchronous œstrus after pessary removal and in the case of grassland ewes treated in late anœstrus, the number of lambs born per ewe is higher following conception at the second œstrus after pessary removal than following conception at the first œstrus after pessary removal. Ewes conceiving at either the first or second œstrus after pessary removal will lamb over a period of approximately 7 days.

In cattle.—The same technique may prove practicable.

In pigs.—The technique is to use methallibure. This is effective only in gilts which have shown œstrus. 100 mg. is fed daily for 20 days. The majority of treated animals will come into heat 4 to 9 days after treatment ends.

SYNCOPE (συγκοπη) is the scientific name for fainting. (*See* FAINTING.)

SYNDROME.—A group of symptoms.

SYNECHIA (*see* p. 326).

SYNERGISM is the opposite of antagonism. Synergism between drugs, *e.g.* penicillin and sulphathiazole, may be of practical value, for with the two it may be possible to obtain the required effect with a dosage of one which, if used alone, would be insufficient, but which cannot be increased because larger amounts would cause side-effects. Another advantage of using two drugs is the possibility that this would tend to prevent the multiplication of mutants resistant to one of the compounds.

SYNOSTOSIS (σύν, together; ὀστέον, bone) is the term applied to a union by bony material of adjacent bones usually separate. It may occur in the spinal column in old horses.

SYNOTIA.—The (virtual) absence of head in a stillborn animal.

SYNOVIAL MEMBRANE forms the lining covering the surfaces of the opposed articular cartilages, which enter into the formation of a joint. (*See* JOINTS.)

SYNOVITIS means inflammation of the membrane lining a joint. It is usually accompanied by effusion of fluid within the synovial sac of the joint. It is found in various injuries and inflammation of joints.

SYNOVITIS, INFECTIOUS.—This is a disease of chicks, of about 2 to 10 weeks old, and of turkeys; and was first diagnosed in Britain in 1959. It is believed to be caused by a virus. Symptoms include: reluctance to move, lameness, swelling of the joints. Many birds refuse to eat. Aureomycin has been used in America for treatment; also Terramycin.

The confined conditions under which broilers are raised appear to render them particularly susceptible to this disease. Mortality is low, but a third of the survivors may be downgraded, so that severe financial loss may be caused. Control depends upon hygiene, and being careful about the breeding stock.

SYRINGE (*see* INJECTIONS, *and* DETERGENT RESIDUE).

SYRUP, which is composed of a mixture of sugar and water, is a fluid frequently used for the administration of drugs, either to detract attention from the unpleasant taste of these, or else to prevent changes taking place in their composition which would otherwise occur were the ingredients exposed to the air. Among common syrups used for animal administration may be mentioned the following: syrup of chloral, syrup of codeine phosphate, Parrish's syrup, syrup of buckthorn, syrip of squills.

SYSTEMIC INSECTICIDES are those which are absorbed by a plant and kill insects feeding on the sap. Some of the systemic insecticides contain organic phosphorous compounds which are poisonous to farm livestock. (*See under* WARBLES.)

SYSTOLE (συστολή) means the contraction of the heart as opposed to the resting phase, which is called 'diastole', and which alternates with the former contracting period. In the cardiac cycle systole takes about one-third, and diastole about two-thirds, of the whole period of the heart-beat. (*See* HEART.)

T

TACHYCARDIA (ταχύς, rapid ; καρδία, the heart) is a disturbance of the heart's action which produces great acceleration of the pulse.

TÆNIA (*tænia*, a ribbon) means a tapeworm. (*See* PARASITES.)

TAIL, AMPUTATION OF (*see under* DOCKING, WELFARE CODES.)

TAIL-BITING.—In pigs this 'vice' can be of great economic importance. (*See* TAIL SORES.)

TAIL SORES IN PIGS.—These may follow tail-biting by one or two pigs out of a large batch, and if untreated can lead to pyæmia.

In six months, out of 135 pig carcases condemned in an Oslo abattoir, 56 were affected with pyæmia—and of these 43 had tail sores.

Feeding only concentrates is regarded as a contributory factor in tail-biting. Boredom, absence of bedding, and floor space of less than 5 square feet per pig, are also regarded as conducive to tail-biting. High temperature and humidity are possible causes. Bitten tails require amputation or dressing if pyæmia is to be prevented.

TALFAN DISEASE.—This is a disease of pigs, and its cause is a virus. Experimentally, the incubation period is stated to be 12 days. Piglets 3 weeks old and upwards are affected. The disease has also been seen in pigs aged 8 months, but this is rare. By no means all piglets in a litter or on a farm become ill and the mortality is usually low. The main symptom is weakness or paralysis of the hind legs. There is little or no fever or loss of appetite. Recovery occurs in a proportion of animals which are hand fed. The disease is present in Britain to a small extent. (*See also under* ENCEPHALOMYELITIS, VIRAL, OF PIGS.)

TANNIN, or TANNIC ACID, is a non-crystallisable white or pale-yellowish powder, which is very soluble in water and glycerine. It is prepared from oak-galls. Tannin is also found in strong tea or coffee. When brought into contact with a mucous surface, tannin causes constriction and stops or diminishes secretion. It coagulates albumin, and acts as a styptic when brought into contact with a bleeding surface (this action is due to the encouragement it gives to clotting of the blood). When brought into contact with many poisonous alkaloids it renders them temporarily inert by forming the insoluble tannate, and thus is a valuable antidote to vegetable poisons of an alkaloidal nature. In most cases, however, it becomes split up, and the poisonous principle is again liberated ; it is accordingly necessary to administer a purge or an emetic immediately after giving tannin, so that the tannates may be eliminated before they are again split up.

Uses.—The most common use of tannin is in the form of gall and opium ointment, which is employed to soothe irritated conditions of the rectum and anus, such as in hæmorrhoids in the dog, inflamed anal glands, after the return of a prolapse or eversion, and in certain itchy conditions of an eczematous nature. It is employed in diarrhœa and dysentery in young animals, either as pure tannin, or more often as catechu or kino, two vegetable drugs which contain a large amount of tannin. It is often administered as the first step in the antidotal treatment of poisoning by vegetable substances containing an alkaloidal active principle. For this purpose it may best be given as a drench of strong black tea or coffee, which may be boiled for a few minutes instead of made in the usual way.

Tannalbin, tannigen, or tanocol, consist of tannin in chemical combination which is not destroyed in the stomach, and in these forms tannin gives better results in the treatment of diarrhœa. Tannoform consists of tannin and formalin in combination ; it is used internally for the same purposes as is tannin, and combines with its astringent action certain antiseptic powers. Externally, it is astringent and antiseptic. Tannic acid jelly is a very valuable burn dressing, and tubes of this should be included in every first-aid kit. It lessens the absorption of break-down products from the burned area and hence diminishes the secondary effects of a serious burn. It is not suitable for large areas owing to the danger of liver damage if large quantities are absorbed.

TAPEWORMS belong the the class of parasites known as *Cestoda* (*see* p. 650). Their life-cycle requires two hosts, sometimes three. The presence of the adult worm may give rise to few if any symptoms or, on the other hand, to anæmia, indigestion, and nervous symptoms—or even to blockage of the intestine. The cystic stage of tapeworms may involve the brain. (*See* GID.) With some tapeworms it is possible for adults and infective larvæ to occur within the same host, but this is not usual. Tapeworms are of considerable public health importance. (*See* MEASLES IN BEEF, MEASLES IN PORK, *and under* PARASITES.) The broad tapeworm of man may attain a length of 60 ft.; in the dog, it is not so long. For species, life-histories, hosts, etc., *see* p. 652 onwards. (For flea-borne tapeworms, *see under* FLEAS.)

In pigs, cattle, and sheep cysts of the tapeworm *Tænia hydatigena* (which infests the dog and may occasionally attain a length of 16 feet) may be so numerous in the liver that the latter ruptures, causing death.

TAPPING is the popular name for the withdrawal of fluid from body cavities, or the subcutaneous tissues of the body. (*See* ASPIRATION.)

TAR is the thick, oily, strong-smelling, black liquid which is obtained by distillation from shale, coal, and wood. Tar from the roads is a common cause of irritation between a dog's toes, causing the animal to lick or bite the part. The tar must be removed with a bland fat or oil. Crude tar, *e.g.* from a gasworks, should never be used on an animal's skin.

Wood-tar, which is also known as 'pix lipuida', is obtained by the destructive distillation of various species of pine tree. It is prepared in large amounts in Sweden and Russia, and, exported from Stockholm and Archangel, is commonly known as 'Stockholm tar' or 'Archangel tar'. Wood-tar is slightly soluble in water, and more readily in alcohol, oils, and strong alkaline solutions. It resembles turpentine in its actions though it is less powerful, being prepared from the same source.

Uses.—Externally, Stockholm tar is used as a preservative for horn and hoof. (*See also* PITCH POISONING.)

TARSUS.—The hock. (*See under* BONES.)

TARTAR is the name given to the concretion that often forms upon the crowns and upon the necks of the teeth, as well as upon exposed portions of the roots. The material is of a brownish, yellowish, or greyish colour, and consists chiefly of phosphate of lime which has been deposited from the saliva, with which are mixed numerous food particles. The whole mass is always swarming with bacteria of a harmful nature. Tartar is most often seen in the mouths of dogs and cats, although the herbivorous animals may also be affected at times.

It is important that accumulated tartar be removed from time to time, for if it is allowed to collect for an indefinite period the gums shrink before the advancing deposit, the root becomes exposed and ultimately affected, and the tooth loosens and falls out. In addition to this, there are generally signs of systematic disturbance, such as a bad smell from the breath, indigestion from inability to feed properly, and in bad cases, great irritability and loss of condition. In the worst cases, pus is formed around the roots of the teeth.

TARTAR EMETIC, which is also called 'tartrated antimony', or antimony potassium tartrate, is a white crystalline substance, once popular as a medicine. It is poisonous in large doses and has been largely replaced by safer drugs. It is a specific in Leishmaniasis and is also used in the treatment of certain forms of trypanosomiasis.

TASTE is one of the special senses, and is situated in certain papillæ found on the tongue. There are several varieties of papillæ, those associated with taste being known as fungiform, vallate, or foliate, according to their shape and situation. In the crevices of the papillæ there are certain small organs which are called 'taste-buds', and it is in these buds that the sensations are first received. Each of these buds possesses a number of minute projections from its free surface; these are the endings of nerve-fibres which receive impressions from dissolved food or other material which is present in the mouth, and convey them along the main nerve branches from the region to the brain. The taste-buds are not limited to the tongue alone; a few are found in the palate, epiglottis, and even in the larynx, but the great majority are on the tongue. It has been estimated that in one single vallate papilla of the ox there are as many as 1760 taste-buds, and when it is stated that there are from 20 to 30 papillæ, it will be understood that the main sense of taste lies in the tongue. It is necessary for the purpose of taste that the substance should be dissolved in a fluid, and it seems that this is one of the functions of the saliva. The sense of taste is closely associated with the sense of smell, and, although little is known of either of these senses in animals, it seems that sense cannot exist without smell, or *vice versa*. (*See* TONGUE, SMELL.)

TATTOOING.—This is done, by means of a special pair of forceps, etc., for the purpose of indentifying farm live-stock. On black skins, tattooing is not an effective method, and the use of NOSE PRINTS has been tried for cattle.

Tattooing is not entirely free from the risk of introducing infection, *e.g.* black-quarter, tetanus.

TAXIS (τάξις, an arranging) is the name given to the method of pushing back into the abdominal cavity a loop of bowel which has passed through the wall as the result of a rupture or hernia.

T.C.E. (*see* TRILENE).

TEARS (*see* EYE. For 'soapy' tears *see* ALGÆ POISONING).

'TEART PASTURES, SOILS' (*see under* MOLYBDENUM).

'TEASER', A (*see under* VASECTOMISED).

TEAT CLUSTERS.—In 1961 Mr. C. D Wilson, Weybridge, stated: 'The disinfection of teat clusters in a bucket-plant is not practicable since the time-honoured method of dipping the clusters in disinfectants is well recognised to be ineffective'. He did, however, refer to the use in the parlour of a method still under investigation—in which cold water is run through the milk tubes and teat cups for 30 seconds before each cow is milked. The N.I.R.D. is investigating also the automatic treatment of teat cups and milk tubes with steam at 85 degrees Centigrade for 6 seconds—in experimental units.

TEAT DIPPING.—First practised by a veterinary surgeon in 1916, this has proved a most useful measure for the control of mastitis in cattle. The liquid chiefly used for the purpose is an iodophor; but excellent results can be obtained with hypochlorite teat dips containing 1 per cent available chlorine. (*See under* MASTITIS.)

TEATS, COW'S (*see under* MAMMARY GLAND; *also* VIRUS INFECTIONS OF COW'S TEATS, MASTITIS).

TEAT SYPHONS are metal tubes used for the purpose of withdrawing milk from the mammary gland, when, owing to some inability, it will not flow readily through the teat. The diameter of the tube should be such that it will not fall out of the teat canal when inserted, and will not injure the sphincter muscle of the teat when introduced. The end which is inserted is solid and rounded off, so that it may be easier to introduce, and at a short distance from it is an elliptical opening by which milk in the canal enters the tube. At the other end is a metal ring (often double) which allows a piece of tape to be used to prevent the loss of the syphon if it should be knocked out of the hand.

Method of use.—The syphon and tape must be boiled upon each occasion before use, if the danger of introducing infection into the udder is to be avoided. The teat should be cleansed with soap and a weak solution of antiseptic, using a little cotton-wool to swab the whole of the teat. The point of the syphon is gently inserted through the sphincter and for a distance of about 1½ to 2 inches into the canal. Milk will immediately flow through the syphon, and by gentle massage the quarter can be practically stripped. It is of the utmost importance to ensure that the boiled syphon should not touch anything except the teat canal, when it is being inserted. If it accidentally falls, touches a sore on the teat, or becomes otherwise infected, it must be disinfected and boiled again.

Teat syphons should only be used under the instruction of the veterinary surgeon.

By careless use, a cow may be rendered useless for further milk production if the udder becomes infected through the use of a dirty syphon setting up acute mastitis, or if the teat sphincter is damaged by the use of too large a syphon, or by its too frequent use, so that it becomes relaxed, and unable to retain the milk in the udder. (*See also* MAMMARY GLAND.)

TEETH are hard, white, or yellowish-white organs, which are developed in connection with the mucous membrane of the mouth, being actually calcified papillæ. They are implanted in sockets or ' alveoli ' in the upper and lower jaws, being only separated from actual contact with the bone by a layer of ' alveolar periosteum '. They serve to enable the animal to secure, bite, and chew its food, and in some cases they are used as weapons of offence or defence. They are divided into three main classes, according to their situation in the mouth : viz. incisors, canines, and molars. The *incisors* are implanted in the incisive bones of the upper jaw, and in the anterior part of the mandible ; they are situated in the front of the mouth, are purely prehensile organs in all animals, and are absent from the upper jaw of the ox, sheep, and goat, as well as other ruminating animals. The *canines* are situated behind the incisors, and are used mainly for fighting purposes, being most developed in carnivores and omnivores. They are useless to the domesticated herbivorous animals, and in them are usually of small size. They are not present in the upper jaws of ruminants, and in the lower jaws have moved forward and assumed the shape and function of incisors. The *molars* are the remaining teeth, situated farther back in the mouth. They are used for chewing purposes, and are specially adapted for this purpose by having broad strong irregular tables or grinding surfaces. The term ' cheek teeth ' is often applied to these teeth, since, strictly speaking, they are composed of ' pre-molars ', which are represented in the milk dentition, and ' molars ' which are not so represented. (*See* DENTITION.)

Each tooth has a portion covered with enamel, the ' crown ' ; a portion covered with cement, the ' root ' ; and a line of union between these two parts known as the ' neck '. A constriction occurs at the neck in the temporary incisors of the horse, in the incisors of the ruminants, and in incisors and molars of the dog and cat ; in the remaining teeth there is no such constriction. The free surface, which comes into contact with a tooth or teeth in the opposite jaw, is known as the ' table ' or ' grinding surface '.

Structure.—Teeth consist of four tissues. In the middle of the tooth is the ' pulp ', occupying the ' pulp cavity '. It is soft and gelatinous, well supplied with blood-vessels and nerves, and is large in the young tooth. It nourishes the remaining tissues, and forms dentine for so long as the pulp cavity is open. In later life it is small or absent, the pulp cavity having filled with dentine formed from the pulp. The ' dentine ' forms the greater part of the tooth. It is hard, yellowish, or yellowish-white in colour, and is surrounded in the crown by enamel, and in the root by cement. The ' enamel ' consists of a comparatively thin layer of a brilliant white colour and extremely dense and brittle, which forms a cap to the dentine, or is arranged in layers through it. The ' cement ' is always the outermost layer of a tooth, being formed on the outside of the dentine in the root, and filling up the irregular spaces and hollows of the crown. It forms an outermost soft cap on the unworn virgin tooth, but when wear commences it soon disappears except where it is protected. Its structure is very similar to bone but without any Haversian canals, unless where the cement is very thick in the root of the tooth. The implanted part of a tooth is fixed into the socket by a layer of vascular fibrous tissue, which serves as the periosteum both of the tooth root and of the lining of the alveolus. It is known as the ' alveolar periosteum '.

The microscopic structure of teeth is important to explain certain phenomena connected with disease. Dentine is composed of a mixture of animal matter and lime salts, pierced by innumerable tiny tubules which run in a wavy manner outward from the pulp and give off branches before they end immediately under the enamel. Each tubule contains a tiny nerve fibril in the deeper part of the dentine, which supplies the tooth with a certain amount of sensation. Enamel is the hardest tissue in the body, and consists mainly of phosphate of lime. It is composed of prisms placed side by side, with one end resting on the dentine and the other end towards the free surface in a simple tooth, such as the canine of a dog. A thin surface skin of horny material covers the surface of the enamel of the unworn simple tooth, known as ' Nasmyth's membrane ', but this soon wears off when the teeth come into use. It is the remains of the ' enamel organ ' which produces the enamel before the tooth cuts through the gum. The enamel is entirely insensitive in all animals, and contains only an extremely small amount of animal matter. Cement is practically of the same structure as bone, without possessing Haversian canals.

Arrangement and form (*see* DENTITION).

Development.—In the fœtus the mouth cavity is at first devoid of teeth, and the mucous membrane covering the ridges of the gums is smooth. The first stage in the formation of a tooth is the infolding of a groove of thickened epithelium along the line of the gum, forming a narrow plate of cells, and known as the 'common dental germ'. At regular intervals along this germ plate there is further thickening and a budding out into the mucous membrane. Each little bud or rudiment is to form one of the milk teeth, and is known as a 'special dental germ'. A vascular papilla lies below each germ, and assumes the shape of the crown of the tooth. The special germ slowly grows into first of all a flask-like shape, and later becomes cut off from connection with the epithelium of the mouth, and surrounded by a vascular membrane—the 'dental sac'. The papilla becomes transformed into the dentine and pulp of the future tooth, while the cap of epithelium from the mouth (*i.e.* the original dental germ) becomes transformed into the 'enamel organ', and forms the enamel. The root of the tooth and the cement covering it is formed at a later period when the tooth commences to grow upwards into the mouth. Alongside each of the germs which form the milk teeth there is developed a second germ which in a similar manner eventually forms the corresponding permanent tooth. The permanent teeth which are not represented in the temporary dentition are formed from dental germs in exactly the same way as are the other teeth. The tooth is chiefly pushed out from the gum into the mouth by the growth of its root, which is comparatively rapid. When the time comes for the replacement of the milk tooth by the permanent tooth, the root of the former is gradually absorbed by pressure from the crown of the permanent tooth, which in the horse and ox lies immediately below the root of the milk tooth, and when no further absorption is possible the remaining crown falls out of place, or is rubbed or knocked out by the movements of the tongue. Once the way is clear for the development of the permanent tooth it very quickly grows up into place, until its further progress is checked by the opposed tooth of the other jaw. (For times of cutting of the various teeth, *see* DENTITION.)

TEETH, DISEASES OF.—Disorders of the teeth are of great importance, because, in the first place, the digestive system, to function correctly, must have the food suitably prepared in the mouth, and if the teeth are abnormal, proper chewing does not take place and digestion suffers as a consequence; and, secondly, most diseases or disorders affecting the teeth are associated with pain or discomfort, which results in absence of appetite, capriciousness in feeding, or other disturbances. Only the commoner diseases will be mentioned here; reference should also be made to TARTAR, LAMPAS, PYORRHŒA; FLUORINE; SINUSES, DISEASES OF; MOUTH, DISEASES OF; etc.

IRREGULARITIES. — In certain cases, the incisor or molar teeth develop out of their normal positions in the jaw, with the result that perfect apposition between the upper and lower teeth is not possible, and the rate of wear is not uniformly distributed over the tables of the teeth. In other instances, extra or 'supernumerary' teeth are formed; in the incisor region these are usually placed behind the arch of normal teeth, while extra molars may be found as projections from the gums on the inside or the outside of the line of normal teeth.

When the temporary teeth are shed, it sometimes happens that the permanent teeth erupt irregularly to one side or behind the temporaries, and are distorted accordingly. This frequently happens in puppies, and to a less extent in the herbivora. In the former, trouble is likely to be experienced between 3½ and 5 or 6 months, and in young horses at 2½ and 3½ years of age. In such cases it is necessary to extract any temporaries which persist, so that the permanent teeth can arrive in their proper places in the mouth.

In dogs frequently, in sheep sometimes, and in other animals less commonly, there may be a discrepancy in length between the upper and lower jaws. When the upper jaw is too long, the condition is known as an 'overshot jaw', and when the lower jaw projects too far forward, it is popularly spoken of as an 'undershot jaw'. In bulldogs, pugs, and other breeds of dogs with very short upper jaws the undershot condition is practically normal, while in certain breeds with extremely long upper jaws, such as the greyhound and show collie, overshot jaws are very common. In the herbivorous animals, which have to graze on pasture, both of these malformations are great disadvantages, since they hinder proper cropping of grass. Animals so affected do not usually thrive so well as others which are normal in this respect, and since the condition is definitely hereditary, they should not be used for breeding purposes.

Symptoms.—In very many cases irregularities of development of the teeth do not produce any definite symptoms, and it is only by accident that they are discovered. As a rule, the nature of the irregularity determines whether the condition is serious or not. In animals with supernumerary teeth, chewing may not be affected until the extra teeth have grown to a large size and even then they only cause difficulty in chewing when situated where they interfere with the closing of the jaws, or the movements of the cheek or tongue. These remarks also apply to teeth which are developed out of their normal positions in the mouth. Difficulty in chewing may also be brought about by persisting temporaries. Young animals which are changing their teeth (*see* DENTITION) often show a sudden loss of condition, and cease to feed with normal relish. Hoggs and other sheep at the age of 10 months to about a year are notorious in this respect, so much so that in most districts it is common practice for shepherds to cut turnips for them when folded, as they are unable to bite the roots whole. Overshot and undershot jaws have been mentioned earlier.

Treatment.—In most cases the offending tooth (or teeth) requires to be extracted. In the case of temporaries no anæsthetic is needed, but where permanent teeth have to be removed general anæsthesia makes the operation easier to perform and less of a shock to the animal.

ABNORMAL WEAR, which is due to malformations of the jaws to excessive softness of the teeth, or to the direction of the teeth, is another mechanical cause of tooth disorder. (*See* SOIL-CONTAMINATED HERBAGE *with reference to sheep.*)

Abnormal wear varies in different cases, and is productive of some well-known conditions, as follows: (1) *shear mouth,* in which the molar teeth of the upper and lower jaws wear so that in time they appear like the blades of a pair of sheep-shears, the upper row being worn away on its inner border, and the lower one along its outer border; (2) *step mouth,* where the cheek teeth, instead of being all at the same level, are arranged with some higher than others, somewhat like steps, a high tooth in the lower jaw being opposite a short one in the corresponding upper jaw; (3) *overhanging* upper jaw, which is where the first upper cheek tooth on either side is placed too far forward in the mouth, and does not come into accurate apposition with the tooth immediately below it, causing the formation of a hook. At the same time the last lower cheek tooth is situated too far back and also forms a hook; (4) *curved tables,* where the line of cheek teeth in the upper jaw shows a convexity in its centre, and a corresponding concavity exists in the lower row.

Symptoms.—In most of these instances the animal affected (almost always a member of the horse tribe), instead of

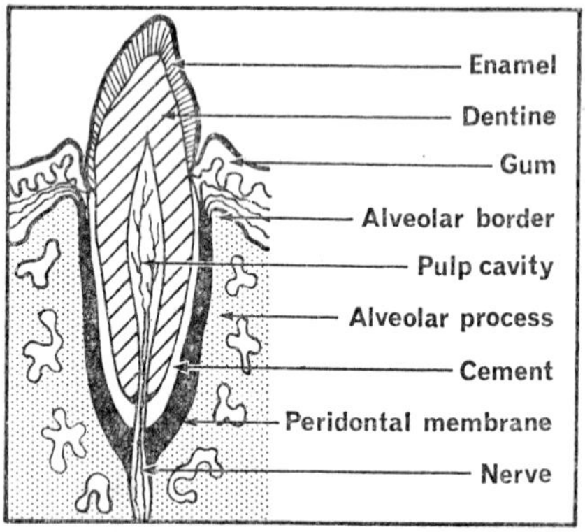

Tooth structure. (From de Coursey's *The Human Organism,* McGraw–Hill.)

chewing its food and swallowing it in the usual way, rolls it round and round in the mouth until it collects into a sodden mass, often about the size of a couple of fingers, and puts it out of the mouth instead of swallowing it. This is known as 'cudding' or 'quidding', and the mass is known as a 'cud' or 'quid'. Salivation and dribbling of saliva from the mouth are also seen, especially when the irregularities in the teeth cause pain from bruising or scratching of the mucous membrane. Loss of condition eventually becomes marked, although many horses only lose condition slowly. In certain cases, hard foods may be refused, the animal eating grass, but leaving its oats and chaff untouched. Large hard grains, such as whole oats, beans, peas, etc., may pass through the intestinal canal without digestion, and be recognisable in the fæces, and in these also can be recognised particles of hay, chaff, or grass, etc., about an inch or an inch and a half long, having been swallowed without sufficient chewing. Pain may be shown when the hand is passed along the outside of the cheek, especially when pressure is put upon the line of teeth.

Treatment.—Rasping the teeth by means of a special tooth-rasp will reduce smaller irregularities, and bring the teeth back into their proper function.

CARIES of the teeth consists of a destruction of the hard structures which form the teeth by micro-organisms. It is not very common, especially among the carnivores, this being probably due to the fact that caries does not readily attack intact enamel, and in the carnivores the enamel forms a complete covering over the dentine and cement, whereas in the other animals it does not. The condition is often present in the mouth of an animal for a very long time before it is suspected, and then it practically only shows signs of its presence by the extremely foul and persistent odour it produces. In advanced cases, however, proper chewing of the food becomes eventually impossible, and quidding is noticed. Sometimes a horse will suddenly stop feeding, and change the food to the other side of the mouth, and then resume. In other cases, a drink of cold water will cause a horse to snatch its head suddenly away from the trough, and commence working its jaws, as though to dislodge some offending particle of food from between the teeth. (*See* FLUORINE.)

Treatment consists in the removal of the diseased tooth or teeth by extraction.

INFLAMMATIONS OF THE PERIOSTEUM lining the root cavity of a tooth are common. They may be due to small particles of food getting forced down into the socket of the tooth, to fractures or fissures of the teeth, to caries, tumour formation, depositions of tartar, and to certain specific diseases, such as actinomycosis, etc.

Symptoms.—These vary from a slight redness of the gum around the root of the tooth, which is painful when pressed by the finger, to a large suppurating tract running alongside the root of the tooth down into its socket, and perhaps through the skin to the outside or into one or other of the sinuses. Abscess formation in the tooth socket may take place, and the abscess may burst into the mouth, to the outside through the skin, or up into a sinus. In many cases there is a distinct bulge of the surface above the diseased tooth, which may give to the face a one-sided appearance.

Treatment.—The affected tooth or teeth must be extracted, and the areas of suppuration cleansed and curetted if necessary. The cavity usually has to be packed with antiseptic gauze afterwards for a few days until it begins to fill by healthy granulation tissue.

PARADONTAL DISEASE is a name for chronic infection of the peridontal membrane. It is one form of inflammation of the periosteum, or alveolar periostitis. It causes loosening and shedding of the teeth, pain, failure to masticate, and loss of weight.

ODONTOMATA are tumours formed in connection with teeth. They may occur in connection with the root of one tooth, or they may be found in the jaw, sinuses, or even involving part of the nasal passage, and be composite or compound, when multitudes of small rudimentary teeth are present. They cause swelling and bulging of the surface of the face, and can only be treated surgically.

PORPHYRIA gives rise to a pink or brown discoloration of teeth. (*See under* BONE, DISEASES OF.)

TOOTHACHE is most spectacular in the dog, which rubs its mouth along the ground, paws at its nose or mouth, works its jaws, salivates, and may whine or moan.

A veterinary surgeon will offer a diagnosis and initiate the necessary treatment.

'BROKEN MOUTH' is important in hill sheep. (*See under this heading.*)

TEM.—Triethylenemelemine, a gametocide which, in America, has been used in field trials for the control of birds. The chemical is mixed with corn, and has the effect of making the male bird infertile. The birds continue to defend their territories and nest, but do not produce any young.

TEMPERATURE, AIR (*see under* HOUSING OF ANIMALS).

TEMPERATURE, BODY, is of the greatest importance, both as evidence of good health, and as one of the basic signs of fever.

Animals are generally divided as regards their temperature into two classes, viz. *cold-blooded animals*, including invertebrates, reptiles, amphibians, and fishes, whose temperature, within certain limits, varies according to the temperature of their surroundings; and *warm-blooded animals*, including mammals and birds, whose temperature remains practically constant, no matter how the surrounding temperature rises or falls. In warm-

TEMPERATURE, BODY

blooded animals, this constancy of body temperature is effected by a perpetual balancing of the various factors which produce heat and which give off heat. The chief heat producer in the body is the oxidising action that takes place on muscular contraction, and the chief cooling agents are the skin and the lungs, which act by the exposure of blood circulating in them to the air, and by the evaporation of water vapour from their surfaces. The temperature of different warm-blooded animals varies considerably, being highest in birds (from 105° F. to 107° F.), and lowest in man (98·4° F.), although it is said that the hibernating bear's temperature may fall to as low as 94° or 95° F. Even in a healthy animal (or person) the temperature is not stationary; it is almost continually rising or falling, being usually lowest in the morning and highest in the evening. The chief reasons for these variations are to be found in the different conditions of activity at different times of the day. In the morning the body has just completed a period of comparative inactivity, and in the evening a period of bodily activity is ending. The temperature also varies in different parts of the body, being lowest in the skin and highest in the liver, the difference being between one and two degrees. In areas of the body which have a poor blood-supply, such as paralysed limbs, the temperature may sink very low, and the part may feel distinctly cold to the touch.

Normal temperatures of animals.—Averages between the considerable limits through which a healthy animal's temperature may vary have been drawn up to represent the 'normal temperatures'. It must not be imagined that there is any hard and fast rule; the temperature may be found a little higher or a little lower than the figures which follow without there being any abnormal condition present; generally speaking, it is only when there is an elevation of 2 degrees or more above normal that an animal should be considered to be ill.

For ordinary practical purposes the usual average temperatures of animals are given as follows :—

Horses . . .	100·5° F.
Cattle. . .	102·0° F.
Sheep. . .	104·0° F.
Pigs . . .	103·5° F.
Dogs . . .	101·0° F.

In the table the figures in brackets are on the Centigrade scale, the others being Fahrenheit.

Animal.	Normal variations.	Remarks.
Horses .	100·4° to 100·8° (38° to 38·2°)	Higher in youth. Lower in old age
Oxen . .	101·8° to 102·4° (38·7° to 39°)	Higher in cows in full milk
Sheep .	101·3° to 105·8° (38·4° to 41·0°) Commonly between 103·6° and 104·4° (39·7° and 40·2°)	Higher in hot weather, and when in full fleece
Goats. .	As for sheep.	
Pigs . .	100·9° to 104·9° (38·2° to 40·5°)	
Dogs . .	100·9° to 101·7° (38·2° to 38·7°)	
	Average.	
Cats . .	100·4° (38·0°)	
Rabbits .	100·8° (38·2°)	
Fowls .	106·9° (41·6°)	
Small birds	108 6° (42·5°)	
Elephants (Steel)	97·6° (36·4°)	
Camels (Steel)	99·5° (37·5°)	

Method of recording temperature.—Temperature is measured by a thermometer, those which are used for clinical purposes usually possessing a rather long, narrow bulb, made from very thin glass, and an index scale reading from 95° F. to 110° F., and being so constructed that the column of mercury does not fall back into the bulb until forcibly shaken down. This allows the correct temperature of an animal to be read without alteration through the cooling of the bulb and the return of the mercury to it. A small 'trap' is arranged below

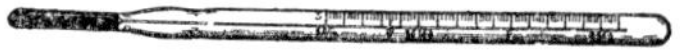

Clinical thermometer.

the level of the lowest reading, and the mercury contracts into the bulb from there only.

There are two scales in use, although in Great Britain and the United States the Fahrenheit is used almost exclusively for clinical purposes. In France and on the continent of Europe generally, the Centigrade scale or the Celsius scale is used.

The difference consists in this, that in the Centigrade scale the freezing-point of water is marked 0° and the boiling-point 100°, while in the Fahrenheit scale these are 32° and 212° respectively. Accordingly 100 divisions on the Centigrade scale are equivalent to 180 divisions on the Fahrenheit scale, and 1 degree equals 1·8 degrees Fahr. To convert from degrees Fahr. to degrees C. the following formula may be used :—

$$n^\circ \text{ Fahr.} = [(n-32)\times\tfrac{5}{9}] \text{ C.},$$

and to convert from degrees C. to degrees Fahr. the following :—

$$n^\circ \text{ C.} = [(n \times \tfrac{9}{5}) + 32] \text{ Fahr.}$$

For examples :—

$$98{\cdot}6^\circ \text{ Fahr.} = [(98{\cdot}6 - 32) \times \tfrac{5}{9}] = 66{\cdot}6 \times \tfrac{5}{9} = 37^\circ \text{ C.}$$

$$38^\circ \text{ C.} = [(38 \times \tfrac{9}{5}) + 32] = 68{\cdot}4 + 32 = 100{\cdot}4^\circ \text{ Fahr.}$$

As to the part of the body where the temperature is taken, by far the most satisfactory place is within the rectum. In females the thermometer may also be inserted into the external part of the genital canal ; as a rule, the vaginal temperature is about half a degree higher than the rectal temperature, so that when a series of temperatures is to be taken, one site or the other should be selected. For horses, a twitch may be necessary, or it may be sufficient to have one of the fore limbs picked up by an assistant. In cattle, little or no restraint may be needed unless the animals are loose. Sheep can be held by an assistant, and pigs will often lie quiet while their temperatures are being taken if a short piece of stick is used to rub along their backs. With dogs and cats, one person should hold the animal, preferably on a table, while another inserts and holds the thermometer. In each animal, after the bulb of the thermometer has been lubricated with a little soap or vaseline, etc., the tail is raised vertically by the left hand, and the thermometer is inserted through the anal ring and into the rectum, by a screwing movement if any resistance is encountered. It is held in position for ½, 1 or 2 minutes, according to the make of the thermometer, and is then withdrawn. With a piece of cotton-wool any adherent fæces are wiped away, and the temperature is read off. Subsequently, the thermometer should be washed in cold water, and a *cold solution* of disinfectant should be used to disinfect it.

For purposes of temperature stress research, American scientists use a special ear thermometer in cattle. As in similar medical research, this tympanic thermometer is more reliable than the rectal thermometer, and can sense changes as small as $\frac{1}{50}$ ° F.

Temperature in disease.—A high temperature is one of the classic symptoms of fever, and in greater or less measure accompanies practically all acute cases of disease. A comparatively steady rise in temperature is as a rule, succeeded by a correspondingly steady fall, and is to be looked upon as a more favourable sign of the natural course of a disease than when the temperature rises and falls with great suddenness. The reduction of temperature in simple fevers is in almost all cases much slower than the rise. A wavering temperature, which shows little tendency to come down to normal, generally indicates that there is some active focus of disease, such as an abscess, which the body cannot overcome. Sudden rise in temperature in an animal which has shown a steady fall previously is an indication of a relapse or recurrence of the disease.

Fall of temperature may be occasioned by great loss of blood, starvation, collapse, or coma ; it is characteristic of certain forms of kidney disease. Certain chronic diseases in which emaciation is marked are also associated with a subnormal temperature.

Temperature near calving time. — A healthy cow—even though showing the familiar signs—is unlikely to calve during the next 12 hours if her temperature is 102° F. This is a useful guide to herdsmen.

See also under FEVER, HOUSING, etc.

TENDERNESS is pain that is only felt when a diseased part is handled.

TENDON (τένων) is the dense, fibrous, slightly elastic cord that attaches the end of a muscle to the bone or other structure upon which the muscle acts when it contracts. Tendons are composed of bundles of fibrous tissue, white in colour, and arranged in a very dense manner, so as to be capable of withstanding great strains. Some are rounded ; some are flattened into ribbons ; others are arranged in the form of sheets ; while those of a fourth variety are very short, the muscle fibres being attached almost directly on to the bone or cartilage which they actuate. Most tendons are surrounded by sheaths lined with membrane similar to that found in joint cavities, *i.e.* synovial membrane. In this sheath the tendon glides smoothly over surrounding parts. The fibres of a tendon pass into the fibres of the periosteum covering a bone, and blend with them. One of the largest tendons in the animal body is the '*tendo Achilles*', which runs from the large muscles at the back of the stifle down to the point of the hock ; it is often called the 'hamstring', and is the structure that is injured in the condition known as 'hamstrung'.

TENDONS, DISEASES AND INJURIES OF.—(*See also under* MUSCLES, CONTRACTED TENDONS, SPRAINED TENDONS.) Tendons are of the greatest importance in horses and dogs, which become practically useless unless able to move about without lameness. In the horse, owing to the elongation of the digit (from knee and hock downward), and owing to the fact that only one digit is functional, these structures, which transfer the insertion of a muscle to a point distant from its fleshy belly, are more liable to be sprained or strained than in other animals where there are several digits (each possessing its own set of tendons, which take a share in the work of the limb), and where the life of the animal does not put such great demands upon the limbs.

In most cases the injuries to which tendons are liable are in the nature of minute lesions in which fibres have been torn across through over-extension of the tendon as a whole. Accompanying these there are often slight hæmorrhages or extravasations of blood into the substance of the tendon, and the tendon itself is thickened at the injured part or, when severe, practically over the whole of its length. At the same time, a certain amount of damage has usually been sustained by the tendon sheath, or by its lining, and an unusually large amount of the lubricating synovial fluid is thrown out, which fills the tendon sheath to the point of dilatation, causing it to stand out on the surface of the limb. In this way it will be seen that there are certain features which can be recognised from the outside, viz. pain on pressure over the injured portion, swelling or thickening of the tendon, and in many instances dilatation of the tendon sheath by a collection of synovial fluid.

When recovery occurs, the swelling subsides, fluid is absorbed, and the broken ends of the fibres become attached by strands of fibrous tissue to other intact fibres near by, pain disappears, and the animal becomes sound. In certain instances, however, when the amount of injury has been insufficient to cause such severe results, but where it is repeatedly occurring, a condition of permanent thickening results. The tendon which is continually subjected to over-exertion, such as occurs when the toes of the foot are not properly reduced at each shoeing, or when the heels are too much reduced, becomes chronically thickened. To some extent this is Nature's way of strengthening the part. The increase in size is due to the extra amount of connective tissue (fibrous tissue) laid down in the tendon, but, unfortunately for the animal, connective tissue of this nature always tends to shrink

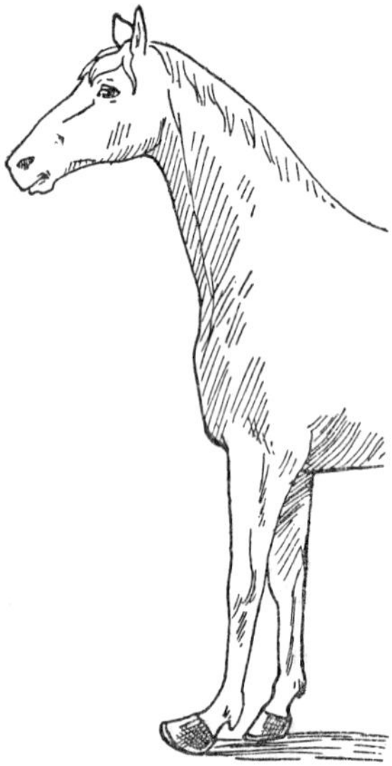

Rupture of both deep and superficial tendons of the near fore limb. The fetlock descends and the toe of the foot tilts upwards so that the weight rests entirely on the heels. Compare with the next figure, where the tendons are intact.

as time goes on, until eventually the tendon shortens in length. For instance, when the deep flexor tendon is affected with chronic sprain there comes a time when the horse 'knuckles at the fetlock'

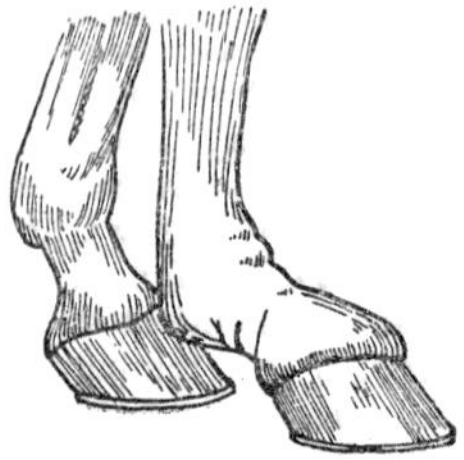

Rupture of the suspensory ligament (interosseous muscle) in the off fore limb. The normal near fore is also shown for comparison. The characteristic sinking of the fetlock is well shown. Note that the foot remains in the normal position on the ground.

due to the shortening of the deep flexor, which lifts the fetlock joint forwards. (*See also* KNUCKLING.)

Certain of the tendons of the horse's limb are liable to become ruptured when subjected to great or sudden strains. In most cases a more or less characteristic deformity of the limb is the consequence. Little can be done for such cases, but suture of the ruptured ends of the tendon

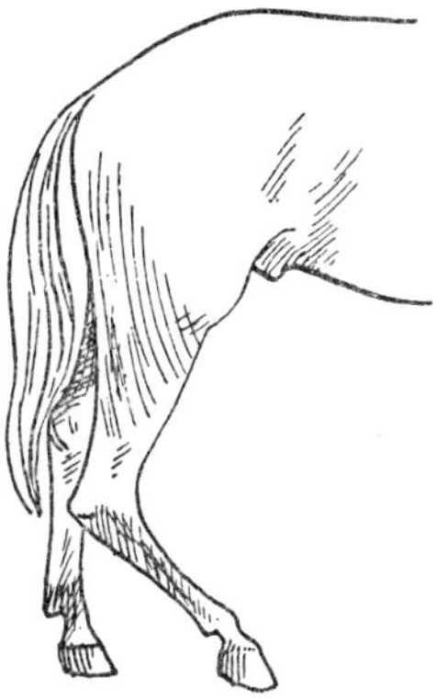

Rupture of the Achilles' tendon. The hock sinks whenever weight is put upon the foot, and the limb is, in consequence, quite useless. Practically speaking, this is the same condition as 'hamstrung'.

has given good results when performed early, and when a sufficient amount of support can be provided by splints or other means. The commoner forms of rupture are shown in the diagrams.

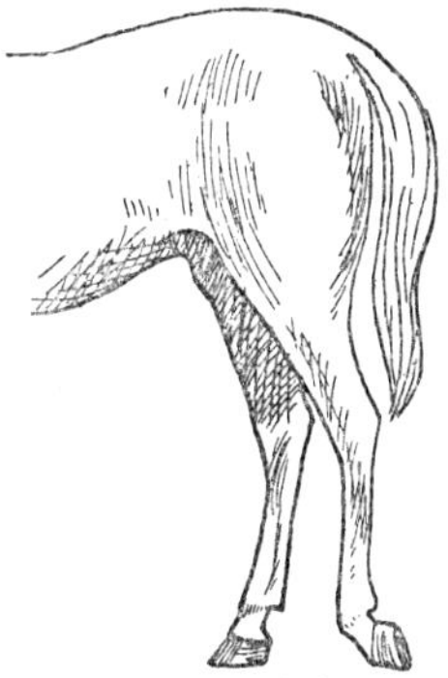

Rupture of the anterior long extensor tendon. In this condition there is great difficulty in advancing the limb, the foot cannot be extended, and unless it is placed forward by hand the limb assumes the above position and weight cannot be borne.

Other conditions affecting tendons are usually of the same nature as those that affect fibrous tissue in other parts of the body, and call for no further mention here.

TENESMUS (τεινεσμός) is a symptom of disease affecting the posterior part of the large intestine, such as impaction, diarrhœa, etc. It consists of continued but futile efforts to pass fæces, *i.e.* straining. A little blood or mucus may be evacuated, but there is little other result.

TENOTOMY (*τένων*, a tendon; *τέμνω*, I cut) means an operation in which one or more tendons are severed by a surgical incision under the most strict aseptic precautions. It is not of extensive application among animals, but the flexor tendons of the horse are sometimes divided in chronic cases of thickening and contraction, which produce deformity of the lower part of the limb, and one of the tendons below the hock is sometimes divided for the alleviation of stringhalt.

TEPP.—Tetra-ethyl pyrophosphate, used in agriculture as a pesticide, is a potential danger to livestock. A Texas rancher diluted 1 gallon of TEPP with water to make 120 gallons, and sprayed 20 head of cattle. All were dead within three-quarters of an hour. Symptoms of poisoning in a puppy comprised drowsiness, muscular inco-ordination, and vomiting. The antidote is atropine sulphate.

TERATOMA (*τέρας*, a monster, or monstrosity; *-oma*, meaning tumour) is a developmental irregularity in which the embryo, instead of growing normally in the uterus, develops into a monster. Such monsters are comparatively common in cattle, and give rise to difficulty at parturition. 'Teratology' is the study of monstrosities. (*See also under* TUMOURS.)

TERRAMYCIN.—A brand name for the antibiotic oxytetracycline, relatively non-toxic, and readily absorbed after oral administration. Apparently useful for any condition in which penicillin, aureomycin, or chloramphenicol is effective, and in the treatment of bacterial complications of distemper, respiratory infections, ear infections, urinary infections, infectious feline rhinitis, and secondary bacterial complications of feline panleucopenia. It appears to be of value in certain types of enteritis in all animals, and against F. necrophorus infections and Foot-Rot. The dosage for small animals is 25 to 50 mgm. per lb. per day by mouth, in three or four divided amounts, or 5 mgm. per lb. per day by mouth, in three or four divided amounts, or 5 mgm. per lb. per day intravenously, also in three or four divided amounts, for 2 to 4 days. (*See* ANTIBIOTICS.) (*See also* TETRACYCLINES.)

TESCHEN DISEASE.—A virus disease of pigs, first recognised in Czechoslovakia, and now known to occur in Germany, Switzerland, Yugoslavia, and France.

Symptoms.—Fever, excitement, paralysis. Death occurs in about 50 per cent of cases. In the others recovery is often incomplete, paralysis persisting.

Treatment.—None.

(*See also under* ENCEPHALOMYELITIS, VIRAL, OF PIGS.)

TESTICLE, or TESTIS (*testis*), is the essential male generative gland or gonad, which, along with the epididymis and its associated structures, lies in the scrotum in each of the domesticated animals. In certain of the wild animals, such as the rat, and in many tropical animals, *e.g.* the elephant, the testes are found in the abdominal cavity, either permanently or temporarily between periods of sexual activity. In all mammals the testes are first developed high up near the roof of the abdomen, not far behind the kidneys. From this position they gradually descend, reach the internal inguinal ring, pass into the inguinal canal, and through it into the scrotum. In the foal the testes appear in the scrotum usually very soon after birth, but they are subsequently drawn up into the abdomen, and do not reappear until between 5 or 6 months and 10 to 12 months. In a certain proportion of cases the testes are retained in the abdomen until 2 years of age, and then descend into the scrotum; in a number of cases they do not descend at all. The name 'rig', or 'cryptorchid', is applied to such animals, and the condition is known as 'cryptorchidism'. (*See* CRYPTORCHID.)

The testes consist of a dense fibrous coat, the 'tunica albuginea', containing a certain number of microscopic tubules, which are held in place and supported by fibrous tissue. Blood-vessels, nerves, etc., run throughout the fibrous tissue and nourish the cells of the tubules. These latter are lined by layers of specialised cells which form the spermatozoa, or male germ cells. The tubules, known as 'seminiferous tubules', are connected with each other near the centre of the testes, and communicate with the coiled tubes of the epididymis, from which springs the 'vas deferens' connecting with the urethra at the opposite end. The epididymis appears to act as a storage place for spermatozoa until such time as they are required for fertilisation of female germ cells. The 'spermatic cord', which consists of the vas deferens, spermatic artery, veins, and nerves, enclosed in the layer of serous membrane (tunica vaginalis), passes upwards through the inguinal canal and enters the abdomen, whence it runs back to the region of the neck of the urinary bladder, opening finally into the urethra. Along its (*i.e.* urethra's) course are the openings of the ducts from the secondary sexual glands—seminal vesicles, prostate, and bulbo-urethral glands—which pour out a secretion which mixes with, nourishes, and protects the masses of spermatozoa coming from the testes.

Externally, the testicle is covered by a layer of serous membrane, lying immediately outside the tunica albuginea, and known as the 'tunica vaginalis propria', which also covers the epididymis. On the outside of this tunic is the 'tunica vaginalis communis', or the parietal layer. Outside this is a fairly thick layer of scrotal fascia, in which is deposited the 'cod-fat' of the bullock and wedder. A strong reddish, fibro-elastic 'tunica dartos' forms the next outermost layer, and provides the septum between the right and left pouches of the scrotum. Finally, on the outside, there is the practically hairless, thin, elastic, oily-feeling skin of the scrotum.

Functions.—The essential function of the testis is to manufacture the male germ cells—spermatozoa. These are formed by an elaborate process of cell division in the seminiferous tubules, undergoing a distinct metamorphosis before they become recognisable as fully-formed spermatozoa. It seems that the process of manufacture continually goes on during the active sexual period of the life of the animal, and that the formed sperms are stored chiefly in the ducts themselves and the epididymis until such time as a call is made upon them. It has been estimated that between 60 and 80 million sperms are discharged at each copulatory act by the stallion at the beginning of the breeding season. Since a stallion may serve more than 100 mares during the season, many of them upon two separate occasions, it will readily be understood that the testes are extremely active organs, and make a considerable demand upon the vitality of the body generally. The necessity for a recuperative period in breeding males will also be obvious. As a rule, there comes a time when the store of sperms is exhausted, and unless a period of complete rest from sexual activity is provided, those females served when the stores have failed will include many barren ones among their numbers.

The other function of the testis is that associated with the elaboration of the male sex-hormone ('proviron'), which is concerned with exercising upon the system certain trophic and other effects, resulting in the production of the secondary sexual characteristics, such as the arched neck and great body size of the stallion, the broad forehead, massive development of horns, and deep voice of the bull, the horns of the ram, and the tusks of the boar, etc., as well as the instinctive desire for sexual intercourse. (*See under* HORMONES.) Its effects can best be seen when the testes are removed by the operation of castration; male characteristics are not shown in the gelded sexless product. (*See also* REPRODUCTION, DUCTLESS GLANDS, STERILITY, ARTIFICIAL INSEMINATION.)

TESTICLE, DISEASES OF.—During service, an irritable mare may kick a stallion and rupture one of the testes, or seriously injure it. Damage may also be occasioned to these organs by the bites of dogs when fighting, by gores from cattle, or by injuries from the tusks of boars, etc.

ORCHITIS, or acute inflammation of the testis, is usually the result of injuries in which there is a wound which admits organisms from the outside, such as arises from pricks from thorns, nails, incised injuries, etc. It also arises occasionally during the course of a specific disease, such as strangles, influenza, distemper, etc., and it is said to have been met with in cases of orf in rams. The testis, being enclosed in a fibrous, comparatively non-elastic capsule, is not able to swell to any great extent, although the loose tissues of the scrotum often swell to an enormous extent. The scrotum becomes reddened in animals which have unpigmented skin in the inguinal region, and the whole area is very painful to the touch.

Treatment consists in applying soothing warm fomentations, poultices, packs, etc., when the skin is not broken, and hot and cold antiseptic douching, or irrigation, thereafter enveloping the scrotum in cotton-wool, gauze, etc., and applying a suspensory T-bandage over the loins and through between the hind limbs. Expert advice should, in every case, be obtained. (*See also under* STERILITY.)

ORCHITIS, INFECTIOUS.—This is a virus infection of bulls, and occurs in Czechoslovakia.

HYDROCELE is a local dropsy affecting usually one tunica vaginalis, and distending that side of the scrotum with fluid. It is met with in the dog mostly, although it may affect other animals. It is treated by tapping the fluid and douching with a mild solution of iodine in water.

HYPOPLASIA (*see under* STERILITY).

TUBERCULOSIS of the testicle is not uncommon in cattle and pigs during old age, and is extremely important from the breeder's point of view, because there is evidence that when bulls affected in this way are allowed to serve cows, not only may they spread the infection to the female genital passages, but the calf is likely to be born with congenital tuberculosis. Unfortunately, it does not show any external signs of its presence until very advanced.

TUMOUR FORMATION is not uncommon either in the testicle, epididymis, or scrotum. In the latter the tumour is usually either a fibromata or a papillomata, but when affecting the testicle, tumours are often malignant, either carcinomatous or sarcomatous.

TESTOSTERONE (*see* HORMONES *and* HORMONE THERAPY).

TETANUS (*τέτανος*) ('LOCKJAW') is a specific disease of the domesticated animals and man, caused by *Clostridium tetani*, which obtains access to the tissues through a wound. Horses are most commonly affected. The organism is present in most cultivated soils, especially such as receive heavy dressings of farmyard manure, in which it is extremely plentiful.

In certain districts tetanus is so common that it is usual to take precautions by inoculating horses with antitoxin whenever they receive even comparatively slight wounds, and always before castration or major operations. Lambs are lost each year after docking and castration, or before the umbilicus (navel) has closed after birth, from tetanus.

Causes.—The tetanus bacillus is an anærobe, *i.e.* it thrives only in an absence of oxygen. It gains entrance into the tissues below the skin through a wound, but instead of invading the circulation, as do many germs, it remains localised near its point of entrance. Its serious effects are produced by the elaboration of a toxin, which is absorbed into the general circulation, and exerts its effects upon the nervous system of the brain and spinal cord. This toxin is one of the most powerful known. Tetanus may occur in an animal which has had a slight wound which appeared to heal without any complication. It may follow tattooing.

The commonest situations of wounds which become affected with the organisms are in the feet and lower parts of horses' limbs, around the anus, and in the inguinal region. Deeply punctured wounds, from which oxygen is excluded, are much more serious than even large superficial wounds, the surfaces of which are exposed to the action of sunlight and fresh air. Picked-up nail wounds, cracked heels, injuries from the prongs of stable-forks, etc., are examples of wounds which often become contaminated with tetanus germs. As already mentioned, castration and docking wounds are well-known sources of infection, and the disease may also occur from infection of the uterus by unclean hands, ropes, or instruments. Cases are met with where no wound can be found on the surface of the body, nor is there any history of an accident; such cases are held by certain authorities to be due to the injuries inflicted by worms in the intestinal wall, or to slight scratches from unusually hard or rough herbage.

Symptoms.—In the early stages the symptoms are usually indefinite; the animal is stiff, disinclined to move about, becomes slower than usual while at work,

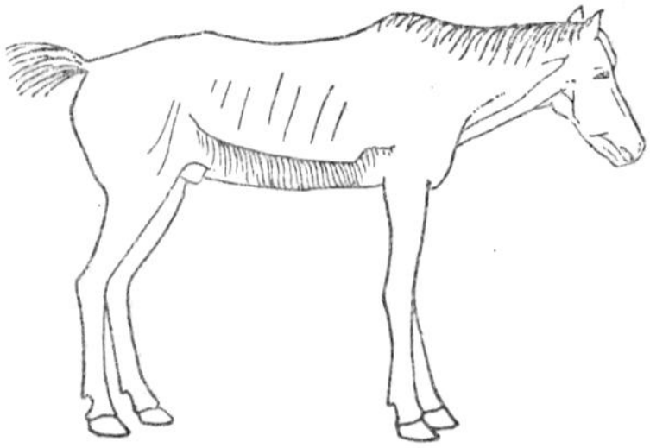

Diagram of the attitude assumed by the horse affected with acute tetanus. The elevated tail, tense appearance of the muscles of the neck and jaws, as well as the distinct costal arch, are characteristic features of the disease.

may drag the toes along the ground, and usually carries the head higher and more rigidly than normally. If the horse is compelled to keep working, breathing becomes distressed, and the nostrils get trumpet-shaped. The expression on the face is one of anxiety or extreme nervousness, and the ears are continually moved backwards and forwards. Later, perhaps after 24 hours, the stiffness increases, and an unusual excitability will be noticed. There is difficulty in turning the head round to the side, and the fore-legs are splayed outwards as though to enable the unfortunate animal better to retain its balance. Areas of the body may break out in patchy sweating, or practically the whole of the trunk may be bathed in perspiration. Any sudden movement, or any sharp or loud noise, causes a painful and lengthened spasm of a group or groups of muscles, usually about the head or neck to begin with, and later involving practically the whole of the skeletal muscles. This is known as a 'clonic spasm', in distinction to a 'tonic spasm', which is sudden but of short duration. In this state a horse stands with the head raised higher than normal, the nose points well forward, the lips are stretched backwards exposing the teeth in a saturnine grin, the ears are often fixed with their points turned in towards each other, and the two jaws are 'locked'. The masseter muscles, which normally close the jaws, are thrown into a state of continuous contraction, and it is beyond the power of the animal to relax them.

If the head be lifted sharply up, by placing the hand under the chin, the 'haw' or third eyelid (nictitating membrane), is seen to flicker across the eye to an extent much greater than usual. So marked is this feature that it is looked upon as a reliable, though rough, clinical test for tetanus. Fixity of the jaws, or 'trismus', which has been reponsible for the popular name given to tetanus (*i.e.* 'lock-jaw'), is not always in evidence in the early stages of an attack, and is not seen at all in a small proportion of cases in horses, although there is always a certain amount of stiffness of the jaws.

Salivation, frothing of saliva between the lips, due to the movements of the tongue, accompanies trismus, and often first points to the mouth as the seat of some abnormality (even before the typical symptoms of tetanus have become established). In the majority of cases, the tail and hindquarters are affected. They are seized with violent, muscular, spasmodic contractions, usually accompanied by pain, whenever the horse attempts to move, and particularly when an effort is made to turn or back. The tail is held out stiffly quivering, a little more over to one side than the other, and the muscles of the quarters can be felt either hard and board-like, or rippling under the flat hand. The spinal column may be twisted, arched, or hollowed. When it and the trunk generally are bent to one side or the other, the condition is known as left or right 'pleurosthotonos', according to the side upon which the concavity is present. When the head and the tail are raised and drawn toward each other, so that the back is hollowed, the word 'opisthotonos' is used. When the head and tail are drawn downwards producing arching of the back, the term 'emprosthotonos' is applied to the condition.

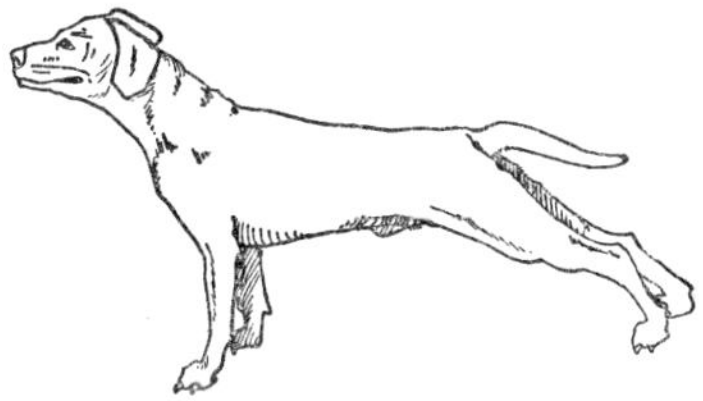

Diagram of attitude assumed by a dog affected with tetanus. The hind limbs are kept well out behind the body, the tail is held rigidly or quivering, and the muscles of the face are drawn into a sardonic grin—the '*risus sardonicus*' of ancient authors. Closure of the jaws is not always in evidence.

During the course of an attack, fæces and urine are usually withheld, and digestive disturbances may occur. sometimes resulting in fatal collections of gas in the large intestines. Daylight and unusual sounds sometimes disturb the horse with tetanus; all perceptions being extremely acute, and the animal hypersensitive. So much so is this that ordinary sounds which pass unnoticed, such as the slamming of a door, are sufficient to throw the horse into violent spasms. Every sensation of sound, sight, smell, touch, etc., is enormously magnified by the time it reaches the suffering horse's brain, and the reactions are correspondingly increased. To this excessive sensibility the term 'hyperæsthesia' is applied.

Complications, such as choking or pneumonia from fluids or saliva entering the trachea owing to the paralysed condition of the throat, and digestive disturbances, are not uncommon, and usually result in death after a very short while.

The symptoms in cattle are very similar to those in horses, trismus and protrusion of the jaw being well-marked. Muscular stiffness is usually severe; flatulence and tympany are noted, and the tail may be outstretched. Tetanus in cattle is not, however, at all common. In sheep, standing is generally impossible; the affected animals lie on their sides, rapidly become tympanitic, and die after a very short illness. In lambs after castration or docking, the disease is very rapid in its effects, and several are affected at the same time. The symptoms shown are essentially the same as those given for the horse. In pigs the head and neck are very commonly affected, and frothing at the mouth is always marked. In dogs, where tetanus is not common, all that the owner may notice is 'something peculiar about the eyes and mouth', and either stiffness or recent lameness. Later, the limbs are usually stretched out as far from each other as possible, and opisthotonus is seen. Squinting and grinning are common, but closure of the jaws is not always in evidence. When it is present it is complete, and death practically always follows. Hyperæsthesia is also very marked.

Treatment.—If possible, the site of the wound by which the organisms have gained entrance should be sought out and carefully disinfected, preferably with compounds rich in oxygen, such as potassium permanganate, sodium permanganate, hydrogen peroxide, Condy's fluid, etc. Wounds in the feet of horses, especially if deep, must be pared out, and strong antiseptics should be packed in afterwards. (*See also under* WOUNDS.)

If showing signs of the hyperæsthesia already referred to, farm animals should be placed in a darkened loose-box. The regular attendant should carry out his duties quietly and slowly so as not to disturb the animal. If the animal is quiet, on the other hand, he may be treated while out at grass—especially if a sedative is given.

Although tetanus antitoxin is very reliable for administration as a preventive before symptoms have appeared, it is of less use after the animal has become ill. It must be given in very large doses, and repeated frequently. Hexamine has been recommended for its apparent property of rendering the damaged tissues more permeable to the antitoxin. Muscle relaxants such as promazine—which obviate exhaustion and may save life—may be required in addition to serum or antitoxin treatment.

Prevention.—Few if any methods of preventing disease are so uniformly attended with good results as the use of tetanus antitoxin. In districts where the disease is common it is the usual practice to give a dose of this before every operation, especially castration, and foot operations, and to administer a large dose whenever a horse is injured or sustains a wound which may become infected. It is very advisable, where wounds are long in healing, to give a second injection about a fortnight later, since the effects of a single dose usually wear off in from 10 days to 3 weeks.

A longer period of immunity can be obtained by means of vaccination. It is practicable to vaccinate pregnant mares so that later their new-born foals will be protected against tetanus infection via the navel. (*See last paragraph under* IMMUNITY *and* PLATE I.)

TETANY (Fr. *tétanie*, from τέτανος) is a condition in which localised spasmodic contractions of muscles takes place. There may be twitching or convulsions. Tetany occurs when the level of blood calcium falls below normal. (*See also under* GRASS TETANY, TRANSIT TETANY, 'MILK FEVER'.)

TETRACHLORETHYLENE.—A drug used in dogs and cats against hookworms. It is given in capsules. It should not be given during pregnancy, fevers, or disease of liver, kidneys, or lungs.

TETRACYCLINE. — The common chemical nucleus of chlortetracycline (Aureomycin) and of oxytetracycline (Terramycin). Tetracycline is also known as Achromycin.

Tetracyclines cause fluorescence in bone and teeth. In late pregnancy or in young growing animals, high dosage can result in teeth discolouration and can interfere with the formation of enamel.

TETRAIODOPHENOLPHTHALEIN is a substance used as an aid to diagnosing various abnormal conditions of the gall-bladder. After administration it is excreted into the gall-bladder and causes an opaque shadow to be thrown upon a fluorescent screen by X-rays. Similarly, an X-ray photograph can be taken of the organ, and abnormalities such as over-distension, constrictions, tumour formation, etc., can be determined. It also serves to denote the position of the gall-bladder in relation to other organs.

TETRAMISOLE.—An anthelmintic (trade name: 'Nilverm') for use in sheep and cattle against gastro-intestinal roundworms and lungworms. It can be given to very young lambs and to in-lamb ewes with safety. Effective against nematodirus.

TEXAS FEVER (*see* PARASITES, p. 637).

T.G.E.—Transmissible gastro-enteritis of pigs.

THALLIUM.—Thallium sulphate is used in poison baits to destroy rats, ants, and other pests, and accidental poisoning in domestic animals may occur. Thallium poisoning in dogs gives rise to gastro-enteritis, profuse vomiting, and severe pain. If death does not immediately follow, there may be a brick-red discolouration of lips skin of groin or axilla. Hair begins to fall out.

THEAVE (*see under* SHEEP).

THEILERIOSIS.—Infection with tick-borne parasites of the *Theileridæ*. (See EAST COAST FEVER, ETC., p. 637, and TZANEEN DISEASE, CORRIDOR DISEASE.

THEINE is the alkaloid which gives its stimulant properties to tea. It is almost identical with caffeine. (*See* CAFFEINE.)

THEOBROMINE is the alkaloid upon which the stimulant action of cocoa and chocolate depends.

THERMOLABILE.—A term meaning that a certain property or attribute is lost on exposure to a certain degree of heat.

THERMOMETER (*see* TEMPERATURE).

THIABENDAZOLE.—A new chemical which became available in Britain in 1962 for use against parasitic worms. At least 13 species of gastro-intestinal roundworms in sheep are stated to be susceptible to the drug, which is palatable and can be given in the feed. It does not stain the fleece. The margin of safety in dosing is very wide. Effective also against strongyles in horses, and useful in combination with piperazine against worms in pigs. Also of value for 'Gapes'.

THIALBARBITONE SODIUM.—This barbiturate is used as a short-acting anæsthetic, mainly for dogs, cats, and sheep. It is useful for euthanasia if followed by Scheele's hydrocyanic acid. A 10 per cent solution of the drug is used, given intravenously or intraperitoneally. It has a less depressing effect on respiration than other barbiturates.

THIAMIN, THIAMINE. — Thiamine hydrochloride, or vitamin B_1. A secondary deficiency occurs in bracken poisoning and horse-tails poisoning in horses, and in carnivores eating too much raw fish.

'THIN SOW' SYNDROME.—Groups of sows or gilts lose weight, usually in the middle or later stages of pregnancy, and remain emaciated for perhaps six months or more. Prolonged under-feeding may eventually result in some sows being unable to cope with adverse conditions encountered at time of stress, *e.g.* weaning. It has also been suggested that infestation with the stomach worm *Hyostrongylus* or with the nodular worm *Œsophagostomum* may be a cause. The use of sow stalls, in which animals cannot move away to escape draughts, is another possible cause.

THIOURACIL.—An antithyroid agent which lowers the rate of metabolism. It reduces the food intake and at the appropriate dosage it increases bodyweight. It has been used for fattening pigs, but results have not been favourable.

THIOUREA.—This is naphythyl antu, a rat poison which causes dropsy of the lungs. It is dangerous to domestic animals and birds.

THIRST, like appetite, is an instinctive craving for something necessary for the maintenance of bodily activity. When there is a deficiency of water in the system, evaporation of moisture takes place, in addition to other situations, from the back of the mouth and throat and the sensation of thirst is referred to these parts. The most generally accepted theory of the cause of thirst is the drying of the sensory nerve-endings which lie at the back of the mouth, but it is probable that thirst is general rather than local.

Thirst is a symptom of fever, is present in cases of diarrhœa, kidney disease, diabetes, severe hæmorrhage, salt poisoning, and great exhaustion. It is commoner in hot weather, and when the food is excessively dry. Animals producing large amounts of milk, most particularly dairy cows, show greater thirst than males or non-lactating females.

THORACIC DUCT is the large lymph vessel which collects the contents of the lymphatics proceeding from the abdomen, hind limbs, part of the thorax, etc., and which discharges its contents into the left innominate vein. (*See* LYMPHATICS.)

THORACOCENTESIS (*θώραξ*, the chest; *κέντησις*, a pricking) means tapping of the fluid found in certain diseases of the chest. (*See* ASPIRATION.)

THORACOTOMY.—A surgical operation involving opening of the chest cavity. It is occasionally performed in the dog in cases of œsophageal obstruction which cannot be relieved by other means, and in cases of rupture of the diaphragm.

THORAX (*θώραξ*) is another name for the chest.

THORN-APPLE (*see* STRAMOMIUM).

THOROUGH-PIN, or **THROUGH-PIN,** is a distension of the sheath of the deep flexor tendon where it passes over the arch of the tarsus (hock). It is characterised by swellings one on either side of the hock, about the level of the 'point of the hock' (summit of the tuber calcis), and lying in front of the strong Achilles' tendon. The contents of these swellings consist of synovia from the sheath of the deep flexor tendon, which collects as the result of sprain or stress communicated to this tendon by some unusual exertion of the limb, such as backing heavy loads on slippery ground, excessive service by stallions, drawing up suddenly when galloping, especially on soft ground, rearing or kicking violently, and other conditions where the hind limbs come far forward under the belly.

The above applies to true thorough-pin, but there is another condition, called 'articular thorough-pin', which is formed by a pouch of the capsule of the true hock joint bulging on the inside, lower down on the side of the hock, practically at the level of the angle formed between the tibia and the shank of the calcis. It is usually associated with bog spavin, and pressure upon the distension of the bog spavin causes more pronounced bulging of the articular thorough-pin. A corresponding swelling may be present in a similar position on the outer aspect of the joint in severe cases.

The name 'thorough-pin' is a corrupt form of the older word 'through-pin', so-called because pressure on the swelling on one side causes the fluid to pass *through* to the opposite side and increase the swelling there.

Thorough-pins vary in size in different cases; they are usually larger when the horse is working, and decrease with rest; they are generally smaller in winter than in summer; in young horses they may suddenly appear and as suddenly disappear without treatment, but in mature horses once they become established they remain; and when horses are newly shod (particularly with high heels) thorough-pins may decrease in size, but gradually increase again as the shoe wears.

Lameness is seldom present unless the condition is severe and the flexor tendon has been sprained as well.

Treatment.—Except for the blemish which results from the swellings thorough-pins are not usually serious conditions, except that they denote a certain weakness. They constitute unsoundnesses, not so much on account of any disability they cause, but because they are generally looked upon as hereditary, the inherent weakness being transmitted to the hocks of progeny. Shoes with calkins, or better with a patten-bar, which reaches across from one calkin to the other, are sometimes used. Aspiration of the fluid under strict aseptic precautions gives good results in certain cases.

THREAD-WORM is a popular term for *oxyuris* worms (*see* PARASITES, p. 658).

THREE DAYS' SICKNESS OF CATTLE, which is also called STIFF SICKNESS, EPHEMERAL FEVER OF THE OX, DENGUE FEVER OF CATTLE, is an acute, infectious, and transient fever of the ox, characterised by sudden onset and a high temperature, and is accompanied by muscular pains, and lameness which has a tendency to shift from limb to limb. The disease was first described in South Africa in 1867 and has been seen in Rhodesia, Egypt, Australia, Malaya, and India. The disease apparently does not occur in cold climates, and it is doubtful if it has occurred in Europe. In 1967–68 considerable economic loss was caused by an outbreak among beef and dairy cattle in northern and eastern Australia.

Cause is a virus. The disease usually commences suddenly and attacks a large percentage of the cattle in affected districts, taking the form of an acute epizoötic; then, in a few weeks, it dies down again as quickly as it arose. The disease is probably propagated by the bites of some insect or other parasite. The incubative period is short, probably 2 or 3 days.

Symptoms.—The disease is ushered in by a suddenly occurring rise of temperature which may reach 107° F. This is accompanied by loss of appetite, cessation of rumination, rapid respirations, a quick and full pulse (which, however, may become very weak later), and a staring coat. The affected subject stands with head down and ears dropped; the eyes have a 'glassy' appearance, and there may be some lacrimation. The attitude of the patient is rather characteristic, the four legs being placed far under the body and the back arched, suggestive of the position of a horse suffering from laminitis. The animal may occasionally lift up one foot, but as a rule is disinclined to move at all. One or more legs may be so affected. The muscles of the shoulders, flanks, and hips are held stiffly, and muscular tremors or twitchings may be seen over these areas. The hind-quarters sway from side to side. The neck is often very stiff, which adds to the difficulties of walking, and at the same time makes swallowing difficult. The belly appears 'tucked up'; the chest is held stiffly, and there may be a double heave of the abdomen in expiration, similar to that seen in a broken-winded horse. At first, constipation may be a noticeable symptom, but later the fæces may be loose, and it is not uncommon to see masses of mucus or even clots of blood mixed up with them.

In milking cows, the milk yield is much diminished, but abortion is not a common complication. Many animals prefer to lie down rather than remain on their feet, and once down are most reluctant to get up again. The symptoms along with the elevated temperature continue like this for about three days—hence the name. There is usually a considerable loss of condition.

A small percentage of cases die as the result of gastro-enteritis or heart-failure, but more commonly deaths are due to congestion of the lungs, or pneumonia, brought on by the administration of drenches which the animals cannot properly swallow. Not more than 3 per cent, but usually less, of the animals die. Calves are more likely to die than adult cattle.

Animals which have recovered only retain an immunity for a few months following an attack, and have been known to suffer from a second one after about six weeks. This, however, is rare, as epizoötics do not usually last very long in any one district, nor do they follow one another at such short intervals.

THREE-QUARTER SHOE is one used for horses which have some painful or diseased condition in the heel, and consists of an ordinary shoe with the heel on the affected side cut off at the quarter. Pressure is relieved from the heel, bar, and the seat of corn. In a 'three-quarter bar shoe' the iron of the intact heel is drawn across the foot to form a bar over the frog.

THROAT is, in popular language, a somewhat vague term applied indifferently to the region behind the angles of the lower jaw, to the jowl, to the part of the pharynx lying behind the mouth cavity, to the larynx, and even to the posterior part of the nasal passages. Correctly used, the word throat applies to the pharynx. (*See* PHARYNX.) Information will also be found under LARYNX, NOSE AND NASAL PASSAGES, MOUTH.

THROAT DISEASES.—Most of these will be found under separate headings such as STRANGLES; GLANDERS; CALF DIPHTHERIA; TUBERCULOSIS; CHILLS; EQUINE INFLUENZA; ACTINOMYCOSIS; ANTHRAX; CHOKING; MOUTH, DISEASES OF; LARYNX, DISEASES OF; ROARING; WHISTLING; TONSILLITIS.

SORE THROAT is a fairly common condition among horses kept in badly ventilated stables, or after exposure to unfavourable climatic conditions. It is very often the first symptom of an attack of strangles or influenza, but in other instances it only exists as a local affection. Animals with sore throat, from whatever cause, usually hold their heads forward with the nose pointing ahead, giving an appearance as though the animal was looking upwards, and called in popular language 'star-gazing'. Food is usually refused, and fluids, if taken, are frequently returned through the nostrils. Coughing is generally present and distressing. At first the cough is harsh, dry, and painful, but later it abates in severity. There is no elevation in temperature in simple cases, and the horse usually appears quite bright. (For further details of treatment, *see under* CHILLS AND COLDS, *and* LARYNX, DISEASES OF.)

THROMBOSIS (*θρόμβωσις*, a curdling) means the formation of a blood-clot in the heart or the vessels during life. The process of clotting depends on the same factors as in clotting of the blood after death, or when outside the body. (*See* PROTHROMBIN.) The indirect cause of thrombosis is usually some damage to the smooth lining of the blood-vessels brought about by inflammation, by injury or disease, or it may be due to other conditions in the walls of the vessels, such as atheroma. The blood is also liable to clot during some general diseases.

Thrombosis may occur in the heart and terminate a chronic wasting disease; it also may take place in the arteries of the brain and cause apoplexy; it may arise from the blockage of an artery by a piece of diseased tissue, or by a collection of bacteria, all of which are called *emboli*; it is not an uncommon condition in the iliac arteries of the horse following some injury to the back, during foaling, or after a severe fall; and it may arise in an aneurism when the coagulated blood tends to strengthen the weakened walls of the vessel, and, after invasion of the clot by fibrous tissue cells, the dilatation of the vessel practically disappears. Aortic thrombosis is apparently not uncommon in the cat, and give rise to shock, loss of use of hind legs, and sometimes pain. Thrombosis of the iliac and femoral arteries has been reported in the dog. (*See under* THROMBOSIS ANTI-COAGULANTS.)

THRUSH is a degenerative condition of the horn occurring in the central cleft of the frog of the horse's foot, which is produced as the result of a catarrhal inflammation of the glands in the sensitive frog. Thrush is a fairly common condition in the hind feet of heavy draught horses, especially when the heels are insufficiently pared down when the horse is shod, or when normal wear does not occur in the posterior half of the foot through the use of very high calkins. Upon lifting the foot a characteristic foul odour is noticed, and the horn in the cleft is soft, black on the outside but white inside; a thick fœtid discharge can be seen oozing up from the depths of the cleft and extending almost to the junction between skin and horn at the back of the foot.

Treatment.—The soft degenerated horn must be all pared away in the first place, until a clean surface of solid, rubber-like, healthy horn is obtained. In doing this it sometimes happens that the degeneration appears to have advanced over the surface of the bulb of the frog on one side or the other, constituting canker. (*See* CANKER.) Afterwards, the surface should be dressed with antibiotics or sulpha drugs or iodoform.

THYMUS GLAND (*θύμος*) is a temporary structure situated in the anterior part of the chest cavity, which attains its largest size during early life and thereafter gradually dwindles away. Its function is not definitely known, but it appears to have a retarding effect upon sexual development. It may also be associated with calcium metabolism. Very occasionally it is found to persist throughout the life of the animal. (*See* LEUKÆMIA.)

The gland consists of a collection of nodules bound together by connective tissue, closely resembling lymph nodules upon microscopic examination. Scattered through the lymphatic tissue are peculiar 'nests' of flattened cells, known as 'Hassall's corpuscles', which are not found anywhere else in the body. The gland is copiously supplied with blood from several large vessels, and with lymph by many lymphatic vessels.

THYROCALCITONIN.—A hormone produced by the thyroid gland and having the effect of lowering the plasma levels of calcium and phosphate, apparently by increasing the deposition of these in bone. It might be useful in the treatment of osteoporosis.

THYROID CARTILAGE (*θυρεοειδής*, shield-shaped) is the largest cartilage of the larynx, and forms a well-marked prominence at the upper end of the trachea. It gives attachment to one end of each of the vocal folds, which are concerned in the production of voice. (*See* LARYNX.)

THYROID GLAND (*θυρεοειδής*, shield-shaped). This is a very highly vascular organ situated in connection with the upper extremity of the trachea (windpipe). It is of a reddish-brown colour, and consists of two lobes and a connecting isthmus (sometimes absent in dogs) in the majority of animals, although one, two, three, or even four accessory thyroid glands may be present in some animals. In adult horses and dogs the isthmus is usually small, and often it is rudimentary or absent altogether.

Minute structure.—Each lobe is enveloped in a thin capsule of fibrous tissue, strands from which pass into the organ, dividing it into lobules. Each lobule is composed of a number of closed vesicles, lined by epithelium, and containing a quantity of a thick yellowish (colloid) fluid. Around each vesicle there is a dense network of fine capillary blood-vessels, while extremely fine lymphatic vessels communicate with the interior of each vesicle.

Function.—The colloid substance contains an active principle, known as *thyroxine*, which exerts a profound action upon the nutrition of the body. It has been prepared synthetically, and a standard preparation is recognised officially as *thyroxinsodium*, which has the same therapeutic actions. Thyroxine contains a certain amount of iodine, which is essential to the body metabolism, and the various extracts of the thyroid gland which are on the market at the present time afford a means whereby deficiency in thyroid secretion may be made good. (*See* THYROXINE ; HORMONES ; *also under* MYXŒDEMA.)

Lying embedded within each lobe of the thyroid gland or in close association with it, is a little pale, soft body, known as a 'parathyroid gland'. In some animals there are two glands on each side. They consist of masses of cells closely packed and resemble embryonic thyroid tissue. In certain diseases the parathyroids become disorganised, and in consequence muscular spasms known as 'tetany' occur. Extract of parathyroid is sometimes used for chorea, epilepsy, and certain forms of spasmodic contraction of muscles, with varying results.

THYROID GLAND, DISEASES OF.—Originally the thyroid gland of the sheep was used for transplantation, either in whole or in part, into human beings who were affected with atrophy of the thyroid, but later it was found that the same results could be obtained by eating the fresh gland, and more recently, a glycerin extract of the dried gland. Atrophy of the gland produces a condition which in young animals is known as 'cretinism', and in adults as 'myxœdema', and these conditions, though not at all common in animals, can be controlled to some extent by the administration of fresh thyroid or extracts of thyroid. (*See also* ENDOCRINE GLANDS.) Enlargement of the thyroid is known as 'goitre' (*see* GOITRE), and when associated with nervous conditions and protrusion of the eyeballs is known as 'exophthalmic goitre'.

Cases in which there is a minor insufficiency of thyroid secretion, with modified symptoms of myxœdema, are known as *hypothyroidism*, while a mild degree of overaction of the thyroid gland produces a train of symptoms in which nervousness, tremors, palpitation of the heart, and irritability are marked, and constitute the condition which is known as *hyperthyroidism*. The latter can to some extent be treated by the administration of iodine internally, while for the former the treatment is the same as for myxœdema.

In addition to these uses of thyroid or thyroid extracts, beneficial results are often derived from administration of thyroid in cases of extreme fattiness in old dogs or cats, in animals which are losing their hair from an unknown cause, in the later stages of pregnancy when bitches (especially) become markedly sluggish and lazy, in eclampsia, pregnancy toxæmia, and for the treatment of certain skin diseases.

It has been shown that the thyroid is to some extent involved with the proper growth of horns, hair, and wool, for if it be removed artificially these structures among others do not develop in the normal manner.

THYROXINE is a crystalline substance, containing iodine, isolated from the thyroid gland and possessing the properties of thyroid extract. It has been used instead of the extract of the gland in cases of defective function of the thyroid, such as goitre, cretinism, and myxœdema. Experimentally, synthetic thyroxine (and, more recently, iodo-casein) has been used to increase the milk yield of cows. Thorbeck (Denmark) found that the addition of 25 gm. of iodised casein to the daily ration of cows during the period of declining lactation, increased the milk yield by up to 54 per cent. But although the animals were given additional food sufficient to cover this increased milk production they lost weight (10 to 17 per cent), while the pulse and respiration rates were increased by about 40 per cent.

The above emphasises the dangers and snags in what is at present a purely laboratory procedure and not yet ripe for exploitation in the sphere of animal husbandry.

However, 'I' Thyroxine has been used in New Zealand to stimulate the growth of more wool of better quality by sheep. (*See also* THIOURACIL.)

TIBIA (*tibia*) is the name of the larger of the two bones which lie between the stifle and the hock. In animals which possess less than five digits in their hind limbs the tibia has become modified so that it sustains the greater part of the weight borne by the limb, the fibula, its complementary bone, having become reduced in size and importance. The tibia lies just below the skin on the inside of the limb, in such a position that it is liable to be injured by kicks, blows, etc., and in this connection is of more importance than those bones that are surrounded by massive muscles which afford some protection. It is not uncommon for the tibia to become fractured, but the parts remain held together by the very dense and strong periosteum that covers the bone. If the animal be rested and taken care of when in this state, the fracture generally mends, and no permanent damage is sustained. On the other hand, however, if the beast is allowed to lie down and rise, or if it be subjected to hard or fast work, a sudden twist to the limb results in the complete separation of the pieces of bone, and destruction is necessary. This applies in particular to the larger animals, such as the horse and ox. In the smaller animals the setting of the fractured bone is practicable. (*See* BONES, FRACTURES.)

TICKS.—These are among the most serious parasites of domestic animals. In the tropics they transmit numerous protozoal and viral diseases ; in the U.K., tick-borne fever and louping ill.

Some cause illness by means of a toxin, while all feed on the host's blood—which can result in a serious anæmia. Large numbers of ticks also 'worry' the host, and cause unthriftiness. Suppurating wounds may also result.

Transmission of disease.—When an tick feeds infected upon a calf, it transmits the parasites—or causal organisms—of the tick-borne disease in question. The calf soon becomes ill, and either dies or recovers. As a rule, recovery is associated with immunity. This means that under natural conditions that animal will not again become ill with that particular disease. However, dipped cattle may lose their immunity ; and relapses may occur in animals thought to be immune to Redwater, for example.

Except with ticks of the *Boophilus* species, larvæ hatching from a tick's eggs will not immediately be infective because these larvæ have not yet fed on any host ; but as soon as they start feeding they may ingest the causal organisms of a tick-borne disease. When they moult and become nymphs, they may then be capable of transmitting disease. Similarly, when the nymph, on moulting, becomes an adult tick, it will be infective if there were already parasites in its blood.

Not all tick vectors will transmit all causal organisms ; and, of course, not all species of host are susceptible to the same causal organisms.

An infective three-host tick feeding on a non-susceptible host 'cleans' itself of infection and will not transmit disease in the next stage of its life cycle. This fact provides a useful control measure.

The specific diseases transmitted by the ticks are not passed on mechanically, but must undergo a special development in the tick. This is easily understood when it is realised that any one stage in the life-history of a hard tick bites only one animal. Accordingly, a tick infected in one stage must be capable of producing the disease in some succeeding stage, which depends on the tick.

A. Young larvæ, whose mothers have sucked infected blood, transmit the disease, *e.g.* :
   Boophilus. Texas fever.
   Rhipicephalus spp. Texas fever, Spirochætosis, Anaplasmosis.

B. Nymphs from infected larvæ, or adults from infected nymphs, *e.g.* :
   Rhipicephalus evertsi Nuttalliosis, Theileriosis.
   Amblyomma . Heart-water.

C. Adults from infected larvæ, *e.g.* :
   Amblyomma . Heart-water.

D. Adults descended from infected females, *e.g.* :
   Hæmaphysalis leachii Canine Babesiosis.

Some ticks infect in more than one way, *e.g.* :
   R. sanguineus can infect in three ways :
      Nymph from infected adult.
      Adult from infected nymph.
      Adult from infected adult.

Control of ticks.—In many tropical countries energetic measures for the regular and frequent dipping of cattle and sheep are necessary. In order to achieve absolute control of the tick-borne diseases, it is important that 'hand-dressing' of certain parts of the body should be carried out in addition to the weekly dipping or spraying. This applies to inside the ears, around the base of the horns, around the eyes, anus, etc.

The acaricides, or tick-killing chemicals, comprise chiefly (1) arsenical compounds, (2) chlorinated hydrocarbon compounds, and (3) the organo-phosphorus compounds. Products based on pyrethrum are also used.

Dipwashes containing arsenic are unsuitable for spraying because of the danger of pasture contamination. Although cheap, stable, and soluble, arsenic compounds are very poisonous. Another disadvantage is that some species of ticks acquire a resistance to arsenic preparations. If these are used in greater strength, severe burning of the skin of cattle will be caused.

Ticks may become resistant to BHC. This is cheap, far less poisonous than arsenic, but is insoluble and has other disadvantages in use. DDT is expensive but very effective against *Boophilus* species. Toxaphene is a very useful acaricide.

Organo-phosphorus compounds tend to be expensive, and are used mostly against ticks resistant to other acaricides. (*See below and* PARASITES.)

If Ticks are Resistant to :	*Change to :*
Arsenic	BHC
BHC	Arsenic (dipping tanks only)
Arsenic BHC	Toxaphene
Toxaphene	Arsenic (dipping tanks only) *or* Organo-phosphorus—*e.g.* Delnav.

TICKS IN BUILDINGS, such as quarantine premises, kennels in the tropics, private houses, etc., can be eradicated by placing a block of 'dry ice' on the floor and closing all doors and windows. Adults, nymphs, and larval ticks will be found, after a time, clustering around this source of CO_2 and can then be easily collected and destroyed. (Captain B. J. Thompson, R.A.V.C., 1969).

TICK-BITE FEVER of man in Africa is due to a Rickettsia. Local reactions, swelling of lymph glands, occur in some individuals. So far as is known, tick-bite fever is not fatal. The bont tick, bont-legged, blue tick, yellow dog tick, and the brown tick—all common in East Africa—transmit this disease. It can be transmitted to the guinea-pig by inoculation of blood.

TICK-BORNE FEVER OF CATTLE.—Cases of fever in England have been

COMMON TICKS IN EAST AFRICA*

Tick Species	Number of Hosts	Preferred Site of Attachment	Animal Affected	Parasite	Disease Transmitted
Brown-ear tick (*Rhipicephalus appendiculatus*)	3	Ears, base of horns, around eyes, tail brush, and heels	Cattle Cattle Cattle Cattle Sheep and goats Sheep, cattle, and goats Man	*Theileria parva* *Theileria lawrencei* *Thieleria mutans* *Babesia bigeminum* *Virus* *Virus* *Rickettsia*	East Coast Fever Corridor disease Mild gall-sickness Red-water Nairobi sheep disease Louping-ill Tick-bite fever
Red-legged tick (*Rhipicephalus evertsi*	2	Larvæ and nymphæ in ears. Adults perineal region	Cattle Cattle Cattle Horses Cattle, horses, sheep, and goats Lambs	*Babesia bigemina* *Theileria parva* *Theileria mutans* *Babesia nuttalli* } *Babesia cabailli* } *Spirochæta theileri* *? Tick toxin*	Red-water East Coast Fever Mild gall-sickness Biliary fever Spirochætosis ? Paralysis
Yellow dog tick (*Hæmaphysalis leachi*)	3	Whole body	Dogs Man and animals Man	*Babesia canis* *Virus* *Rickettsia*	Biliary fever 'Q' fever Tick-bite fever
Blue tick (*Boophilus decoloratus*)	1	Face, neck, dewlap, and sides of the body	Cattle Cattle Man Horses, cattle, goats, and sheep	*Babesia bigeminum* *Anaplasma marginale* *Rickettsia* *Spirochæta theileri*	Red-water Gall-sickness Tick-bite fever Spirochætosis
Bont tick (*Amblyomma spp.*)	3	Larvæ and nymphæ on head and ears. Nymphæ and adults on perineum, udder, scrotum, and tail brush	Cattle/Sheep/Goats Sheep Man and animals Man	*Rickettsia ruminantium* *Virus* *Virus* *Rickettsia*	Heartwater Nairobi sheep disease 'Q' Fever Tick-bite fever
Bont-legged tick (*Hyalomma spp.*)	2 or 3	Adults on perineum, udder, scrotum, and tail brush	Cattle, sheep, goats, and pigs Man and animals Man Man	*Tick toxin* *Virus* *Tick toxin* *Rickettsia*	Sweating sickness 'Q' fever Tick paralysis Tick-bite fever

caused by a Rickettsia, demonstrable in the white blood cells. The disease causes loss of milk yield for a time and probably a lowered resistance to other diseases. In the United Kingdom, ticks infect cattle with two other diseases: Red-water caused by *Babesia bovis* and Louping-Ill, and transmit *Theileria mutans*. (*See* p. 637.)

TICK-BORNE FEVER OF SHEEP is a disease transmitted by the tick *Ixodes ricinus*.

Tick-borne fever is a mild febrile disease of sheep in which the essential symptom is a rise in temperature occurring after an incubation period of 4 to 8 days, and lasting about 10 days, when it subsides. During this period (which may be prolonged) there is dullness and listlessness, and a considerable loss of weight may occur. Death occurs in only a small percentage of cases; most sheep recover unless some other complicating condition such as louping-ill supervenes. Abortion is an important result of infection in many instances, and may affect 50 per cent of breeding stock introduced from tick-free areas.

Rickettsia can be demonstrated in the polymorphonuclear white cells of the blood.

The importance of tick-borne fever is that it is capable of rendering the vasculo-meningeal barrier of the central nervous system vulnerable to the virus of louping-ill, while without its presence, though the louping-ill virus may be introduced into the blood-stream (by the bite of a tick) it cannot pass this barrier to attack the nerve cells and so produce the typical nervous symptoms. It has been shown that both infective agents—that of tick-borne fever and of louping-ill—frequently exist together in ticks found on animals on farms where louping-ill is common, and it is probable that under natural conditions the great majority of adult

* Reproduced by courtesy of Cooper, McDougall, & Robertson (East Africa) Ltd.

sheep on such farms have been infected with tick-borne fever infection and have recovered.

A pyæmia of lambs, due to *Staphylococcus aureus*, is also transmitted by tick-bites. Abscesses occur in the joints and elsewhere, causing lameness, unthriftiness, and death.

TICK PARALYSIS is a form of paralysis affecting man and the sheep, which has been recorded from Africa, Australia, and various districts in the north-west of North America, especially British Columbia and adjacent states. It is caused by the presence on the animal of various species of *Ixodes* (especially the dog tick) in South Africa and Australia, and *Dermacentor* in America. In E. Africa, the bont-legged tick (*Hyalomma spp.*) and possibly the Red tick (*Rhipicephalus evertsi*) cause paralysis.

The paralysis is associated with the peculiar habit of the ticks in showing preference for attaching themselves to the base of the neck in man and along the line of the vertebral column in sheep. It is suggested that the cause of the paralysis is an irritant substance, present in the salivary secretion of the tick, which is injected into the wound made by the mouth parts at the time of biting, and which specifically affects the motor nerve centres.

In human beings, 3 or 4 days after the ticks attach themselves, paralysis of the limbs occurs, then paralysis of the arms takes place, later the chest and neck become involved, and ultimately the heart and respiratory centres are attacked. In the sheep, the parts are affected in the same general sequence.

This form of paralysis is peculiar in that symptoms disappear in from 2 to 6 days after the ticks are removed, and recovery takes place subsequently. Individual lambs, for example, can be reinfected and recover more than once, if the ticks are removed by hand. They are usually not easily seen unless a deliberate search is made in the wool over the vertebral column from the base of the skull back to the tail.

TIMBER TONGUE, or WOODEN TONGUE (*see* ACTINOBACILLOSIS).

TINCTURE (*tinctura*, a dye) is an alcoholic solution, generally of some vegetable substance. Most tinctures are made with different strengths of alcohol or with rectified spirit. Among the best-known drugs from which tinctures are made are the following: belladonna, digitalis, hyoscyamus, nux vomica, opium, squills.

TINEA (*tinea*, a moth) is a technical name for ringworm. (*See* RINGWORM.)

TINNED FOOD.—Feeding dogs for a period of six months or so exclusively on tinned meat may give rise to a thiamine (Vitamin B_1) deficiency, associated with myocarditis and heart failure. (*See also* CAT FOODS, STEATITIS.)

TIPS are half-shoes, covering the anterior half of the foot only, which are used for shoeing colts and young horses, to prevent their feet from cracking, and are also applied to hunters, brood mares, and other horses running at grass in the summer, or to polo ponies during winter. They are also useful for certain diseases of the feet, such as contracted heels, or some cases of sidebone, etc., when frog pressure is desirable; and in bilateral corns they are sometimes applied to relieve the posterior part of the foot from contact with the shoe. Tips or half-shoes are also used with rubber bar-pads.

TISSUE CULTURE VACCINES (*see* VACCINES).

TISSUES OF THE BODY are the simple elements from which, on microscopic examination, the various parts and organs are found to be built. The entire body results from the union of a male and a female cell, and the subsequent division and subdivision of the single cell thus formed; but as growth proceeds, the new cells produced form tissues of varying characteristics and complexity. As the result of this early differentiation it is customary to divide the tissues into five groups:

(1) *Epithelial tissues*, including the cells covering the skin, those lining the alimentary canal, those forming the secretions of the internal organs, etc. (*See* EPITHELIUM.)

(2) *Connective tissues*, including fibrous tissue, fat, bone, and cartilage. (*See* these headings.)

(3) *Muscular tissues* (*see* MUSCLES).

(4) *Nervous tissues* (*see* NERVES).

(5) *Corpuscular tissues*, which are present in the blood- and lymph-streams. (*See* BLOOD, LYMPH.)

Many of the organs of the body are formed of one of these tissues alone, others are formed mainly of a single type with an admixture of another kind of tissue (such as fibrous tissue or cartilage) for supporting purposes; while other structures that are widely distributed are formed of two or more simple tissues in varying proportions; such are: blood-vessels (*see* ARTERIES, VEINS), lymphatic vessels and glands (*see* LYMPH AND LYMPHATICS), serous membranes (*see* SEROUS MEMBRANES), synovial membranes (*see* JOINTS), mucous membranes (*see* MUCOUS MEMBRANES), secreting glands (*see* GLANDS, SALIVARY GLANDS, THYROID GLAND, etc.), and skin (*see* SKIN).

TITRE.—The extent to which an antibody-containing biological substance can be diluted before losing its power of reacting with a specific antigen. 'High titres' indicate, in practical terms, that a patient's blood serum contains high levels of antibody e.g. to the rabies virus.

TOADS have a defensive venom which is secreted by skin-glands and by the parotid salivary gland. The principal toxic substance is BUFOTALIN (which see). Symptoms of poisoning in the dog are profuse vomiting followed by the emission of ropy saliva and by loss of consciousness, which may persist for a couple of hours. Adrenalin has been used in treatment.

TOBACCO (*see* NICOTINE).

TOE-PIECES are bars, square in cross-section, which are welded across the front of the shoe just behind the toe; they are chiefly employed in the northern parts of Britain. They are used for heavy draught horses, along with calkins at the heels.

TOES, CURLY ('CURLY TOE DISEASE', 'CURLED TOE PARALYSIS') is a condition arising in chicks from a deficiency of riboflavin. The toes curl underneath the feet. (*See* VITAMINS.)

TOES, TWISTED ('CROOKED TOES').—A condition also seen in chicks; one or more toes twisting inwards or outwards. There is, at least, a hereditary disposition to this abnormality, but it may occur in *temporary* and *reversible* form where infra-red brooders are in use.

-TOMY (τομή, a cutting) is a suffix indicating an operation by cutting.

TONGUE (*see also* MOUTH) is a muscular and fibrous organ, richly supplied with blood-vessels and nerves, and covered with a highly specialised mucous membrane. Its shape varies in the different animals, but in all it consists of a free part or 'tip',

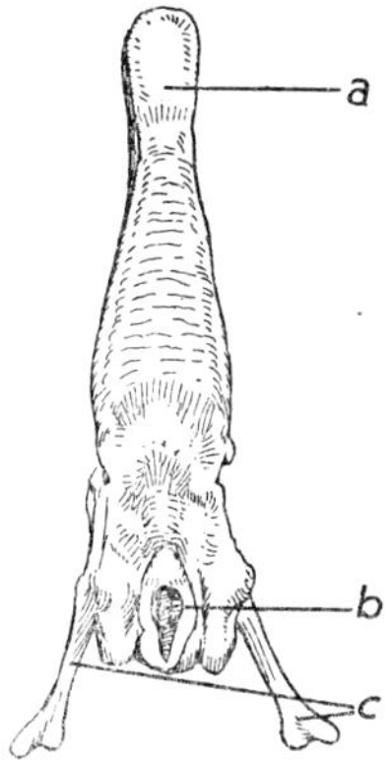

The tongue of the horse removed from the mouth. *a*, The free tip; *b*, the opening into the larynx; *c*, the two branches of the hyoid bone by which the tongue is supported.

a middle part, the 'body', and a hinder part, the 'root'. In the horse the tongue is long and spatulate, with a blunt tip, freely movable, and there is a definite narrowing just behind the tip. In the ox the tip is short, and pointed or conical; mobility and pliability are not so great; and on the upper surface is a hump-like eminence or 'dorsum', divided from the tip by a distinct, deep, transverse groove. The dorsum is of the greatest use in swallowing, and in bringing the small balls of cud from the back of the mouth forward for chewing by the cheek teeth. In the sheep, pig, and dog the tongue resembles that of the horse. Only a small dorsum is present in the sheep and goat; the pig's tongue is short or long according to the shape of the head and the length of the snout; in the dog the tongue is long, thin, and very mobile, and can be protruded a considerable distance from the mouth, especially when the dog is panting.

There is no bony skeleton in the tip or body of the tongue, but in the root the tongue rests upon the hyoid bone. This composite bone possesses little power of movement other than is afforded by the elasticity of the cartilages which unite it to the squamous temporal bone, but, nevertheless, the root of the tongue is regularly raised and lowered during swallowing movements.

Structure.—The greater part of the substance of the tongue is composed of muscle-fibres running in various directions; between them is a small amount of fibrous tissue which forms a freely movable scaffolding. The muscles are so arranged that the tongue can be moved in practically every possib e direction, and can assume practically every possible curve, within the limits of the mouth, and to a certain extent beyond it, as, for example, when the ox inserts the tip of its tongue into its nostril. In addition to these intrinsic muscles, the tongue has other muscles which attach it to surrounding structures, such as the lower jaw, the larynx, palate, and the base of the skull.

The *mucous membrane* is intimately adherent to the underlying muscles, except on the under surface. It is very thin below the tip, thicker at the sides, and very thick over the upper surface in all animals. Uniting the tip to the floor of the mouth is a fold of dense membrane, known as the 'frenum', and containing the edges of two muscles which help to protrude the tongue. Uniting the posterior part of the tongue with the soft palate there is, on either side, a fold of mucous membrane known as the 'anterior pillar of the soft palate'. Over the general surface of the upper part of the tongue there are numerous small finger-like processes, known as 'papillæ', and of four kinds in the horse —filiform, fungiform, vallate, and foliate. The *filiform* are distributed over the upper surface of the body and tip, and are fine pointed projections. The *fungiform* are mushroom-shaped, and are found chiefly at the sides of the body and scattered thinly over the upper surface. The *vallate* papillæ are two in number, although a third may be found in some cases. They are roughly circular in outline and a little less in size than a threepenny piece. They are found on the upper surface far back, about half an inch on either side of the middle line. Each is situated in a little depression surrounded by a trench in the walls of which open the ends of the taste-buds. *Foliate* papillæ are found just anterior to the anterior pillars of the soft palate, where they form a little rounded eminence marked by transverse fissures. Taste-buds are found in each variety of papillæ except the filiform, the purpose of the papillæ being to support the end organs of the sense of taste and protect them from injury. In the ox, vallate papillæ number between 20 and 30 and foliate papillæ are absent. In the other animals all four varieties are found.

Functions.—The main uses of the tongue are of three kinds: (*a*) to control the food during mastication, working it between the teeth, and moulding it into a bolus for swallowing; (*b*) as a delicate sensory organ, which possesses not only an acute sense of touch, but also the faculty for tasting the food; and (*c*) to play a certain part in the production of voice. In the ox it also has a prehensile use, gathering the food before it is cropped up by the lower incisor teeth and the dental pad, and in this animal it also serves to keep the nostrils free from obstruction. In the ox, dog, and cat the tongue is also used for toilet purposes, to lick over the greater part of the body; in the two latter animals it is used for lapping, and in all the domesticated animals, as well as in most wild creatures, the tongue is of great service for cleansing and drying the coat of the newly born young. Many animals lick wounds with their tongues, and in popular parlance are said to 'keep the wounds clean' by so doing. Actually, the cleansing action is little more than mechanical removal of pus, or discharges, while clean wounds may easily become contaminated if licked by the tongue, especially in the carnivores where particles of decomposing flesh swarming with organisms are found in crevices of the mucous membrane, teeth, etc. In the cat, where the tongue is covered by a large number of rough, horny, backwardly directed papillæ, licking may so irritate a wound as to prevent healing, or greatly retard it.

TONGUE, DISEASES OF (*see under* MOUTH, DISEASES OF; *also* ACTINOBACILLOSIS; CALF DIPHTHERIA; FOOT-AND-MOUTH DISEASE; BLUE-TONGUE; MUCOSAL DISEASE; 'BLACK TONGUE', RANULA; 'CURLED TONGUE').

TONICS (τόνος, strength) are remedies which help to restore to strength and vitality the muscular system (both voluntary and involuntary), the nerve-cells, and various body organs, from a lax and sluggish state occasioned by disease, lack of exercise, or insufficiency of food. The term, like the name 'stimulants', is very vague, but while stimulants cause an immediate increase in activity, tonics act more slowly and their action remains in evidence for a longer period of time.

Varieties.—There are many types of tonics acting in different ways, though all require time in order to exert their full beneficial action. Among them may be mentioned nux vomica and strychnine, cinchona and quinine.

Various bitters such as ginger, gentian, and malt, stimulate appetite.

Liver extracts, iron compounds, and certain phosphates are used as tonics in anæmia and debility. Turning out to grass is in itself a tonic to animals which have been confined indoors.

Uses.—There is probably no class of drugs more abused by the owners of animals than 'tonics'. In a large number of cases a tonic is believed to be a panacea for any and all ills of an obscure nature.

Unrestricted use of tonics is harmful and may be dangerous. Many of the most useful contain small doses of powerful poisons, and if used over too long a period of time, cumulative poisoning may result. In addition, the continual stimulation of a jaded system by tonics is likely to result in a condition of the body in which the administration of a tonic becomes a permanent necessity, enabling an animal to remain in apparent health for so long as it gets the tonic, but doing nothing towards effecting a cure of the disease.

Although tonics form a valuable class of remedies, their employment demands not an indiscriminate rule-of-thumb system of administration, but careful consideration of all aspects of the case, judicious selection of the drugs likely to be most useful, and continual supervision during the time of their administration.

Generally speaking, tonics are most useful when given during the convalescent stages of debilitating diseases, high fevers, and during recovery from starvation, exhaustion, overwork, hæmorrhage, etc. (*See also* PROTEIN, HYDROLISED; VITAMINS.)

TONSILS (*tonsillæ*) are collections of lymphoid tissue, situated between the anterior and posterior pillars of the soft palate at the back of the throat. In the horse there is not a compact tonsil, as in man, the dog, etc., but a diffuse collection of lymphoid tissue, mucous glands, etc., causing elevations on the surface, in which are seen the numerous depressions or crypts which characterise the tonsil and differentiate it from other lymphoid tissue. In the sheep the tonsil is bean-shaped and does not project into the throat, as in most other animals.

The tonsils appear to be concerned with the production of numbers of lymph corpuscles which escape into the saliva and discharge some important function in connection with digestion, and they also probably help to protect the body from harmful bacteria or germs taken in with the food. In some cases they become affected with actinomycosis in cattle, and in pigs they are sometimes the seat of tuberculous lesions.

TONSILLITIS.—Inflammation of the tonsils, a symptom of, *e.g.* canine virus hepatitis.

TOOTHACHE (*see* TEETH, DISEASES OF).

TOPICAL APPLICATIONS of a drug are those made locally to the outside of the body.

TOPPING OF PASTURES.—This practice is beneficial from a veterinary point of view in that it is unfavourable to the survival of parasitic worm larvæ.

TORSION (*torsio*) means twisting, and is the term applied to the process by which tumours, organs, etc., which are attached to the rest of the body by a limited neck or 'pedicle', become twisted so that their blood-supply is in danger of being cut off. The term is reserved to a great extent for the twisting that occurs in the gravid uterus. (*See* UTERUS.)

Torsion is also applied to the twisting of the smaller arteries to check bleeding during an operation. The cut ends are grasped with a pair of artery forceps, and turned round repeatedly until the artery has curled to such an extent that its lumen is obliterated.

TORTICOLLIS (*tortum*, twisted; *collum*, the neck) is another name for 'wry-neck'.

TORTOISES are sometimes a source of Salmonella infection causing illness in children. About 250,000 spur-thigh tortoises were imported into Britain from Morocco during 1959. Only 1 per cent can be expected to survive their first year in Britain.

TOUCH, according to popular idea, is the fifth sense, distributed all over the body, by which an animal is made conscious of its surroundings, otherwise than by the four special senses of sight, smell, hearing, or taste. The sensations imparted from the surface of the body to the central nervous system are, however, not of one kind only; when investigated they are found to consist of five different kinds as follows:

Touch sense proper, by which touches or

strokes are perceived, such as the lightest sensation caused by a fly settling on the skin ; the size and shapes of bodies in contact with the skin which are not seen is also appreciated by this sense ; and associated with it is the second form, known as

Pressure sense, by which the weight of heavy objects and their hardness can be determined, such as the presence of a man in the saddle of a riding horse ;

Heat sense, by which the heat of the surrounding atmosphere, or of bodies in contact with the skin, is appreciated as being above that of body temperature ;

Cold sense, by which an animal perceives that a body, gas, or fluid in contact with the skin is cold ;

Pain sense, by which painful impressions, whether from slight pricks, or from severe wounds, is appreciated.

For convenience it is usual to add to these the following, which are recognised in human physiology :

Muscular sensitiveness, by which the painfulness of a squeeze is perceived. It is possibly due to direct pressure upon the nerve-endings in the muscles ;

Muscle sense, by which the weight of an object can be tested, and the amount of energy necessary for an effort can be gauged ;

Sense of locality, by which, without using the powers of vision, the attitude and position of any part of the body is known.

The distribution of the sense organs which are concerned with the reception of these sensations is very widespread. There is no part of the surface of the body, except the horns, hoofs, and claws, which can be cut without giving evidence of pain, and there is no part, including horny structures, which is insensible to touch. Heat spots, which register sensations of heat, are not so widely distributed over the body as are cold spots ; this would suggest that it is more important that an animal should be able to recognise that it is too cold than that it is too hot. (It should be remembered that a feeling of hotness or coldness only indicates that the skin, and not the body generally, is too hot or too cold.) The seat of pressure sense is mainly in the hair follicles, around each of which there is a fine nervous ring. These rings are most developed at the bases of the long tactile hairs around the muzzle, on the face, and above the eyes ; they serve most important functions of acquainting the animal of its proximity to stationary objects, sensations of touch being conveyed to them through the long stiff hairs. In the fine skin of the muzzle of the horse, where the hairs are few and small, there are numbers of tactile corpuscles, which serve to acquaint the horse with the nature of its food, and also of objects with which it is not familiar. The sense of touch in this part is extremely delicate, and is trusted by a horse much more than its eyesight. An example of this is seen when a nervous animal meets an unusual object on the highroad, or when it sees a known object in an unusual place or position, such as a stooping man, a recumbent person, a log of wood, piece of paper, even a bundle of straw. If it is led up to the object, and is allowed to smell it, or, better, touch it with its muzzle, all signs of fear disappear at once. In the foot there is also an important seat of the sense of touch. By it the animal is made acquainted with the nature of the surface over which it travels, and is thereby enabled to exert greater caution when necessary.

Disorders of the sense of touch occur under different conditions, and in association with various diseases.

Hyperæsthesia (more correctly called ' hyperalgesia ') is a condition in which a mere touch results in an exaggerated response. It is seen most markedly in a horse suffering from well-developed tetanus. Certain inflammatory conditions of the spinal cord may produce it, especially immediately above the level of the disease. It is present in so-called ' acute muscular rheumatism ' in dogs, and is also seen in the very early stages of wet eczema, before the actual raw area appears, and rabies.

Anæsthesia, or a diminution of the sense of touch, producing numbness, is present in most conditions where the continuity of the sensory nerves has been destroyed or upset. It is seen in broken back, beyond the level of the fracture ; it is present in paralysis of those peripheral nerves which are partly or entirely sensory ; and it may be produced by the use of most local anæsthetics. (*See also* NERVES, SKIN.)

TOURNIQUET (Fr.) is an appliance used for the temporary stoppage of the circulation in a limb or appendage of the body, so that hæmorrhage may be controlled. In emergencies, a handkerchief may be tied round the part, the knot being arranged above the principal artery, and a rigid object, piece of wood, penknife, etc., used to twist the loose part up tightly.

In applying a tourniquet it must always be fastened tightly enough to stop the circulation completely. If applied only tight enough to stop venous circulation but leave the arteries open, the bleeding is made worse. A tourniquet must not be left in position round a limb for longer than is absolutely necessary, or gangrene of the lower part will result. Occasionally, a circular bruise may occur under a tourniquet, especially in the limbs of horses; this, after healing, leaves a ring of white hair marking the place where the tourniquet was applied. Such a circular mark is due to a destruction of the pigmentary apparatus of the hair follicles. (*See also* BLEEDING, ARREST OF.)

TOXASCARIS (*see under* TOXOCARA).

TOXÆMIA (τοξικόν, poison; αἷμα, blood).—The presence of toxins in the bloodstream. The term is used to indicate the presence of those poisons in the blood which should, in the ordinary way, have been eliminated by the various excretory organs. Toxæmia may also involve the presence of bacterial toxins.

TOXAPHENE.—An insecticide which remains active for a long time on the hair of cattle, and of value against ticks also.

'TOXIC FAT SYNDROME' of broiler chickens, mainly between 3 and 10 weeks old, has occurred in the U.S.A. and Britain. It is associated with dropsy of the pericardium and abdomen, a waddling gait, squawking, laboured breathing, and sudden death. Mortality may reach 100 per cent. Recently it has been seen in chicks only a few days old.

This condition has to be differentiated from Roundheart disease, which usually occurs sporadically among older birds and is not associated with the feeding of fat-supplemented rations.

TOXICOLOGY (τοξικόν, poison; λόγος, a discourse) is the science dealing with the study of poisons, their symptoms, and their antidotes. (*See* POISONS.)

TOXINS (τοξικόν, poison) are poisons produced from animal tissues, generally by the action of bacteria. It appears probable that particular strains of certain organisms are able to produce toxins from the materials upon which they develop whether of animal or vegetable origin, and from their own bodies; the latter are called 'endo-toxins', and the former type are called 'exo-toxins'. (*See* BACTERIOLOGY, IMMUNITY, SERUM THERAPY, SNAKE BITE.)

TOXOCARA CANIS.—A roundworm parasite of the dog and fox. It is of Public Health importance because its larvæ have been found in human tissues, giving rise to *visceral larva migrans* which has rarely caused death and occasionally blindness. *T. cati* and *Toxascaris leonina* may also cause the condition.

The eggs are sticky, and there is a danger to children, especially, if they handle a bitch with a litter of puppies or a newly bought puppy which has not received adequate treatment to remove such worms. The animal's coat, box, blanket, etc., may all be contaminated with the eggs. It has been advocated that dogs and cats should not be kept in households where there are children; and that dogs should not be allowed to defæcate on children's playing fields. Worm larvæ have been found in rodents and, therefore, cats which hunt should be dosed periodically. 'Once every six weeks is not too frequent.' (Animal Health Trust.)

Toxocara canis is chiefly a parasite of the young puppy. It is acquired prenatally from the bitch, arrives in the gut within three days of birth, and matures at around the ninth day of life. Bowel obstruction due to *Toxocara* has been observed as early as the seventh day in heavy infestations. Egg production begins when the puppy is about two months old. The adult worm virtually disappears from dogs over 12 months of age, and eggs are rarely detected on routine fæcal examination in adult animals. It is impossible experimentally to produce intestinal infestation with *Toxocara* in dogs over three weeks old by feeding eggs, possibly because of immunity resulting from prenatal infections. In older dogs the larvæ are distributed throughout the tissues of the body.

Toxascaris leonina is not common in puppies but occurs most frequently in dogs up to two years old; after which age the incidence rapidly diminishes. Larval migration in the bitch and prenatal infection do not occur. The most efficient anthelmintic is piperazine.

Diagnosis.—Immunofluorescent techniques are useful.

TOXOID.—A toxin which has been rendered non-toxic by physical or chemical means, while retaining its antigenic properties.

TOXOPLASMOSIS.—This is a disease of man, cattle, sheep, pigs, dogs, rabbits, and can be transmitted from one species to another. A cross-infection from and to birds is probable. Toxoplasmosis has been diagnosed in medical practice in Britain, but very infrequently. On the other hand, infection without illness is evidently commonplace, and as a result of blood tests it has been suggested that, in various parts of the world, millions of people become infected during their lifetime. Having 'come to terms' with the organism they are apparently none the worse.

There is little or no evidence as to the extent to which toxoplasmosis occurs in farm livestock, dogs, cats, etc., in Britain, but it has been recognised here in pigs, sheep; and in dogs as a complication of Distemper.

Cause. — A single-celled parasite, *Toxoplasma gondii.* It has been isolated from the milk of bitches, cows, ewes, and sows, and it has been shown that the young of these may be born already infected. The parasite can live in ticks and lice, so that the spread of toxoplasmosis by these is not unlikely. For a differential diagnosis, laboratory techniques are essential.

Symptoms.—These include loss of appetite, scouring, coughing, mastitis, distressed breathing, emaciation, muscular tremors, and death. Young may be stillborn. In dogs, encephalitis is caused.

In an outbreak of toxoplasmosis among piglets in Worcestershire, recorded in 1961, the main symptoms were laboured breathing and wasting. The parasite was recovered from the sow's brain.

A serological survey in Yorkshire (recorded in 1961) suggested that toxoplasmosis may be a common cause of abortion and stillbirths in sheep.

Several species of Toxoplasm are recognised, including *T. hominis*, *T. musculi* (of mice).

TRACE ELEMENTS are those of which minute quantities are essential for the maintenance of health in animals (or plants). They include: iron, manganese, iodine, cobalt, copper, magnesium, zinc, selenium. (*See under* HYPOMAGNESÆMIA, PIGLET ANÆMIA, PINING, IODINE, HYPOCUPRÆMIA, PEROSIS, ZINC, SALT LICKS.) Calcium and phosphorus are also needed, but in much larger quantities than is the case with trace elements.

TRACHEA (τρα ύς, rough) is another name for the windpipe. (*See* AIR PASSAGES.)

TRACHEOTOMY (*trachea* and τέμνω, I cut) is the operation in which the trachea (windpipe) is opened from the surface of the neck, so that air may be, so to speak, 'short-circuited' direct into the lower air passages without having to pass through the throat and nasal canals. The operation is undertaken when, through obstruction in some part higher up, an animal is in danger of suffocation from an inadequacy of air being inspired. It is indicated when some foreign body has gained entrance into the trachea or larynx and hinders the flow of air; it relieves breathing when an abscess develops at the back of the throat in strangles in horses, and threatens to occlude the passages; it is also undertaken in œdema of the glottis, in roaring when a horse must run a race or perform some other violent exertion; and it is sometimes necessary to perform tracheotomy when the glottis is stenosed from tumour formation, actinomycosis (in cattle), choking and in other conditions.

An incision is made into the trachea, through the skin and muscles, usually in the middle line (in cattle sometimes at the side), and a tracheotomy tube is inserted and fixed in place. Where a horse has to wear a tube for any length of time, it is necessary that it should be removed, cleansed, lubricated with Vaseline or oil, and replaced, at frequent intervals; otherwise discharges and clotted serum collect and tend to obstruct breathing, or to become sucked into the windpipe and set up bronchitis or even pneumonia. The atmosphere of the stable must be kept as clean and free from dust as possible, and during foddering or bedding operations a plug should be put into the hole to prevent pieces of chaff, hay seeds, etc., from getting drawn in by the inspired air.

TRACHOMA (*see* EYE, DISEASES OF.)

TRAINING (*see* MUSCLES, EXERCISE).

TRACK LEG.—A condition seen in the racing greyhound. There is a swelling of the triceps muscle or the semitendinosus muscle—due to sprain. Prolonged rest is necessary.

TRANQUILLISERS.—This term usually implies drugs which reduce anxiety without inducing sleep or drowsiness. They include phenothiazine derivatives ('Pacatal' and 'Nutinal' are proprietary examples) and are used in veterinary practice to calm or restrain vicious or nervous animals; to obviate travel sickness; and to facilitate the induction of anæsthesia. Their use is not permitted at Kennel Club shows.

In human medicine, some tranquillers which were stated to be safe have been proved dangerous in practice, *e.g.* methylpentynol and meprobomate, thalidomide.

In the U.S.A., and Australia, amongst other countries, tranquillisers have been administered to cattle by firing a hypodermic syringe from a crossbow. (*See also* SEDATION OF PIGS, ROMPUN.)

TRANSFERABLE RESISTANCE (*see under* ANTIBIOTIC RESISTANCE).

TRANSFERRINS.—These are also known as beta globulins, constituents of blood serum. Transferrin typing is discussed under ELECTROPHORESIS.

TRANSFUSION OF BLOOD (*see under* BLOOD TRANSFUSION).

TRANSIT OF CALVES ORDER, 1963, lays down certain rules concerning the humane treatment of calves and the standard of vehicles used.

TRANSIT TETANY is a condition not uncommon in lactating mares which are sent long distances by road vehicle or rail to be served by a stallion. It is especially likely to occur in very warm weather and if the mare is in œstrus or is subjected to excitement or fatigue. It occurs less commonly in other horses, but has been observed in young, unbroken colts or fillies sent to sale-yards in cattle trucks. It is also seen in cattle.

Symptoms.—Transit tetany is associated with a lowering of the blood calcium, sometimes to a marked degree. The animal is usually found in a state of distress; sweating is profuse, respirations are rapid and laboured, pulse is hard and strong, and temperature may be raised 2 or more degrees. On removal from the conveyance, the horse may stumble and stagger; the feet are lifted in a stiff, unnatural manner, and spasms of tetanic muscular contractions affecting the muscles of the jaws, neck, and shoulders are exhibited. The condition bears some resemblance to tetanus, but is less severe.

Treatment.—Measures should be taken to remove the horse from all sources of excitement or fear. It should be housed in a loose-box and made comfortable. Clean cold water in copious amounts should be available, and thick bedding provided. The injection subcutaneously of 50–80 c.c. of calcium gluconate solution (5 per cent) repeated in an hour usually serves to terminate an attack. If untreated, the horse usually falls to the floor of the horse-box and injures itself—often seriously—in its endeavours to regain its feet. It may pass into a state of coma and die.

TRANSMISSIBLE GASTRO-ENTERITIS OF PIGS (T.G.E.).—This virus disease was first recognised in the U.S.A., and in Britain has caused a great many deaths of piglets 3 weeks old or under. The stomach becomes severely inflamed, sometimes with ulceration and bleeding.

In the first East Anglian outbreak of 1957–58, many pregnant sows became ill at farrowing—with resultant agalactia and also with the piglets being involved, too. Severe diarrhœa was the principal symptom—fæces of piglets being greenish. Some piglets vomited. Mortality was 90 per cent during the first week of life. Fattening pigs survived but their growth rate was greatly reduced during the scouring. The disease is periodically of considerable economic importance.

The disease does not occur during the summer months.

In the U.S.A. a live and virulent transmissible gastro-enteritis virus has been given by mouth three weeks before sows farrow. This provides passive immunity for the piglets during their first few weeks of life, but the method is not without risk. For example, the infection may become established and spread to other herds.

In Canada dogs have been shown to have antibodies to a T.G.E.-associated virus, and rectal swabs from dogs have led, when fed to pigs, to the latter's death from T.G.E.

TRANSPLANTATION OF MAMMALIAN OVA.—This technique is in its experimental stages. Briefly, it consists in stimulating super-ovulation—the production of a number of eggs at one time—by the female; removing these eggs from the female; keeping them alive for the necessary length of time; and in introducing one such egg into another female. By this means it should be possible to obtain a first-class calf from a 'scrub' cow, or indeed, a pedigree Jersey out of an Aberdeen-Angus. The technique is being developed at Cambridge, where it has already been successfully carried out in sheep—ewes having produced young of which they were not, in the full sense, the mothers. Up to the end of 1958, it had been found possible to collect living eggs from a cow without any surgical interference, but no calves had been produced as a result of transferring the eggs to other cows. (*See* Plate 15.) Sheep eggs have been exported from England to South Africa in a rabbit, and used to produce lambs whose true parents had never left England. Fertilised pig eggs, obtained in Canada, have produced a litter of three in a sow at Weybridge.

TRAUMA, TRAUMATIC (*τραῦμα*, a wound) are terms used to indicate disorders that are the result of violent injury.

TRAUMATIC PERICARDITIS is the name given to inflammation of the outer coat of the heart sac caused by an object which inflicts an injury. In cattle, in which this condition is commonest, it is often produced by a sharp foreign body wandering from the second stomach, through the diaphragm, and so into the pericardial sac. (*See* HEART DISEASES.)

TRAVEL SICKNESS is observed in dogs and cats—some individuals being particularly susceptible—and may be relieved by the administration of chloretone or a tranquilliser prior to the journey. Fitting a chain to a car so as to act as an 'earth' has been recommended. (*See also* TRANSIT TETANY.)

TRAVELLER'S JOY, or *Clematis vitalba*, is said to cause poisoning when any part of the plant is eaten by stock. During spring, donkeys and goats can eat the plant with impunity, but later in the year it produces violent purgation, dysentery, polyuria (an excessive excretion of urine), and occasionally death.

TREADS are injuries inflicted at the coronet of the horse's foot, either by the shoe of the opposite foot, or, when horses are worked in pairs, by the adjacent horse. In winter, when frost-studs, frost-nails, or other sharpened projections are worn to prevent slipping, treads are usually more serious than at other times of the year. As a rule, the injury is superficial, but when inflicted by a sharp-pointed object it may involve the coronary matrix and result in hindrance to hoof formation and

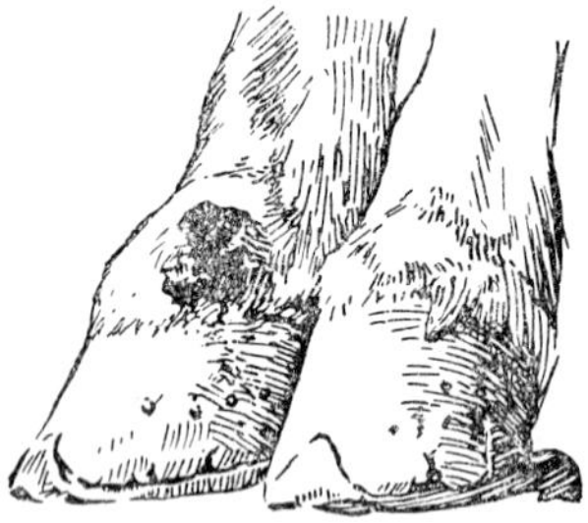

Diagram to show the position of a tread caused by careless turning. The shoe of the opposite foot in this case inflicted the injury.

considerable deformity. When situated in the posterior half of the foot the upper free edge of the lateral cartilage may be damaged and a quittor result.

Treatment.—The area should be clipped free from long hair in the first place, and cleansed with an antiseptic solution. If it be deep it may be plugged with a piece of gauze soaked in acriflavine, which is renewed every day; if superficial, ordinary dry wound dusting-powder is usually satisfactory. Where there is much suppuration, which does not decrease with treatment, expert advice should be sought without delay.

Allowing horses plenty of time when turning at their work, tying horses wider apart when in double harness, and the use of a thick rubber ring round the pastern, are methods of preventing treads from occurring.

TREFOIL is a cause of Light Sensitisation in Australia.

TREMBLING IN DOGS (*see under* SHIVERING).

TREMBLING IN PIGS.—A condition occasionally seen in young pigs. The whole litter may be affected with a spasmodic twitching. A few piglets may die within 48 hours of birth. It appears to be an inherited condition which the survivors outgrow, although it has also been suggested that Swine Fever virus of low virulence may be responsible.

'TREMBLINGS' IN EWES (*see* 'MOSS-ILL').

TREMORS (*tremor*).—Very fine jerky contractions of a muscle or of some of the fibres of a muscle. They are often seen in nervous animals when frightened, and they are one of the signs of viciousness in a horse when seen on the quarters, especially when the horse is 'watching out of the corner of his eye'. They are, however, met with in certain nervous affections, such as shivering in horses and chorea in dogs. (*See also* 'CRAZY CHICK' DISEASE.)

TREPHINING (τρύπανον, a trephine) is an operation in which a small disc of bone is removed from the cranium to permit of the elevation of a depressed portion, or to allow access into the brain cavity; for example, in gid or sturdy in sheep the cranium is trephined so that the cyst stage of the worm—*Tænia cœnurus*—which is the cause of gid, can be removed. (*See* PARASITES, p. 653.) In certain purulent conditions of the air sinuses of the horse's head trephining may be required to give drainage for the pus, and when teeth have to be punched out of their sockets the plate of bone covering their roots must be first trephined.

TREPONEMA.—A genus of spiral organisms of the family Treponemaceæ, which includes also *Borrelia* and *Leptospira*. (*See* PARASITES.)

TRICHIASIS (τριχίασις) means a diseased condition of the eyelids, generally the result of old-standing inflammation, in which the eyelashes grow inwards towards the eye so as to cause great pain and irritation during the movements of the eyelids. (*See* EYE.)

TRICHINOSIS (τρίχινος, hair-like) is the name given to an infestation of the muscles of the pig, man, dog, etc., with the larvæ of *Trichinella spiralis*, a small roundworm. Pigs become infected by eating infected rats or raw swill or garbage containing pieces of infected pork. Trichinosis constitutes a serious problem among sledge-dogs in the Arctic and may follow the eating of walrus, bear, seal, or foxmeat. In 1941 an outbreak of trichinosis occurred among human beings at Wolverhampton, when 500 cases were reported. There have been several smaller outbreaks in Britain since the Wolverhampton one, and infested rats represent a constant threat to public health—with the pig in the rôle of intermediary. The disease is far rarer in meal-fed pig than in those fed on swill. A temperature of −15° C. for 20 days is needed to kill the larvæ. (*See* PARASITES, p. 664.)

TRICHLORPHON. — An organophosphate insecticide used against warbles, and applied as an external dressing to the backs of cattle. It is important that cattle should not be treated with anthelmintics during the fortnight before or after its application as a warble dressing.

Toxicology.—Sudden deaths of steers have been reported from 16 to 52 hours after dressing with Trichlorphon; and even up to a fortnight afterwards. Muscular weakness was followed by coma, which did not respond to atropine treatment. *Post-mortem* findings included inflammation of all internal mucous membranes, with hæmorrhages. Effervescing blood was seen on taking a sample from the ear vein.

TRICHOCEPHALUS (θρίξ, hair; ϰεφαλή, the head), or WHIP-WORM, is the name of a worm that infests the cæca of various animals. (*See* PARASITES, p. 661.)

TRICHOMONAS.—A protozoan parasite. *T. fœtus* is a cause of inferility in cattle. *T. rumentium* inhabits the rumen and appears not to be pathogenic. Perhaps the former has its origin in the latter. (*See under* PARASITES, p. 635, *and under* INFERTILITY *and under* MANURE.)

TRICHOPHYTON (θρίξ, hair; φυτόν, plant) is the name of the vegetable parasite that causes one variety of ringworm. (*See* RINGWORM.)

TRICUSPID VALVE is the valve lying in the heart between the right atrium and the right ventricle, which possesses three cusps or flaps. (*See* HEART.)

TRIGEMINAL NERVE is the fifth of the cranial nerves. (*See* NERVES.)

TRILENE.—A proprietary name of trichlorethylene (T.C.E.), an anæsthetic used in small animal surgery. Induction is slow as Trilene is not very volatile. It is less toxic than chloroform.

TRIPLOID.—An animal having one and a half times as many chromosomes in its cells as a normal (*i.e.* diploid) animal. (*See* COLCHICINE.)

TRISMUS (τρίζω, I grind the teeth) is another name for the locking of the jaws, which is characteristic of tetanus.

'TRIVETRIN.'—An antibacterial drug containing trimethoprim and sulfadoxine intended for use where antibiotics are contra-indicated or ineffective, and stated to be efficacious in treating calf diphtheria, salmonellosis, *E. coli* infection.

TRIXYLPHOSPHATE.—A substance used in the manufacture of plastics. Poisoning of cattle has occurred through contamination of molasses with this substance. Symptoms included diarrhœa, coughing, unsteady gait, partial paralysis. Over-extension of a hind leg was observed, also pain on micturition in some animals.

TROCAR AND CANNULA are the instruments used for the relief of tympany or the collection of gas in the rumen of the ox, and for the withdrawal of fluid or gas from other parts of the body. The trocar is a sharp-pointed stilette which fits closely inside a metal tube, its point projecting about half an inch beyond the tube The two parts of the instrument are pushed through the skin, abdominal muscles, peritoneum and wall of the rumen, with a quick vigorous stab, the stilette is withdrawn from the cannula, which is left in position so that the gas may escape. The site selected for the introduction is a point midway between the last rib, the point of the haunch-bone, and the projecting processes of the lumbar vertebra on the right side of the body, and the instrument should be directed towards the opposite elbow. The cannula may be safely left in position for some hours, so that gas formed subsequent to the operation may escape instead of causing a second collection. (*See under* STOMACH, DISEASES OF ; *also* BLOAT.)

TROCHANTER (τροχαντήρ, the round head of the thigh-bone) is the prominence that lies above and slightly behind the head of the femur in the living animal. It can be felt moving under the skin when an animal walks if the hand be placed flat over the region of the hip-joint. It serves as a place of attachment for some of the powerful muscles of the quarter.

TROCHES (τροχός, a disc).—Another name for lozenges.

TROMBICULOSIS.—Infestation with *Trombicula autumnalis*, the harvest mite.

TROPHIC (τρέφω, I nourish) is a term applied to the influence that nerves exert upon the tissues to which they are distributed, from the point of view of healthiness and nourishment. When nerves of a part become diseased or injured, this influence is lost and the muscles waste, the skin loses its healthy appearance, the hair falls out, and ulcerated areas are commonly seen. In cases where the operation of neurectomy has been performed in the limbs of horses, there is always a possibility of such changes taking place below the seat of the operation ; in fact, the whole hoof may slough off in occasional instances.

TROPICAL CANINE PANCYTOPAENIA.—A disease of dogs, characterised by hæmorrhages, especially from the nose, and probably caused by *Ehrlichia canis*. (*See also* ' HÆMORRHAGIC DISEASE ' OF DOGS.)

TROPICAL DISEASES include a number of diseases which occur in temperate countries, but are more common or more severe in hot latitudes, in addition to those diseases which are only normally encountered in the tropics. The most common are described under their appropriate titles, as follows : *see* BARBONE ; BLUETONGUE ; HORSE SICKNESS, AFRICAN ; CATTLE PLAGUE ; CONTAGIOUS BOVINE PLEUROPNEUMONIA ; RABIES ; EAST COAST FEVER ; ANTHRAX ; GLANDERS ; HEARTWATER ; THREE-DAY SICKNESS ; BURSATEE ; KALA-AZAR ; FOOT-AND-MOUTH DISEASE ; CASEOUS LYMPHADENITIS OF SHEEP ; HÆMORRHAGIC SEPTICÆMIAS ; SUNSTROKE, etc., and under the PARASITES, p. 624 *et seq.*, are described those diseases due to organisms of a protozoal nature, such as the trypanosomes piroplasms, anaplasms, etc.

TRYCHOPHYTON (*see* RINGWORM).

TRYPANOCIDE.—A drug which will kill trypanosomes within the host's body.

TRYPANOSOMES (τρύπανον, a gimlet ; σῶμα, body) are small single-celled parasites that are found in the blood-stream in certain diseases that are classed together as the ' trypanosomiases '. (*See* PROTOZOÖN PARASITES, p. 631.)

TRYPSIN is the name applied to the chief protein ferment of the pancreatic secretion. It changes proteins into peptones and forms the main constituent of pancreatic extracts used for digestion of food. It is often helpful in cases of non-specific diarrhœa in dogs.

TSETSE FLY is the insect vector which is of such importance in the spread of trypanosomiasis of various kinds to man and animals. A description of the various species of tsetse fly (belonging to the genus *Glossina*) will be found under PARASITES.

Much information has been acquired during the last few years regarding the *biome* of the tsetse fly by the Department of Tsetse Research of Tanganyika. The biome is the study of all living creatures found within a fly-belt with a view to elucidating the inter-relationships of the tsetse fly, vegetation, and animal communities. The fly-belts referred to are tracts of bush country, sometimes stretching for miles in extent, within which no living animals are found except such usually inferior ones as have contracted trypanosomiasis (often Nagana) and have achieved a degree of immunity, tolerance, or *premunition*, sufficient to enable them to survive being continually reinfected with trypanosomes by the bites of the fly.

The question of the control of tsetse, and therefore of the trypanosomiases which are fly-carried (including ' sleeping sickness ' of man), is vast and cannot be discussed in detail here. Ruthless methods of cutting down all bush and timber, and of destroying all wild game in the ' fly-belts ', which were ill-advisedly advocated some years ago, are now known to be unsatisfactory and most undesirable, even if they were possible. A more enlightened view is that cattle should be concentrated upon the fly-free areas, which with adequate methods of husbandry are quite capable of sustaining the necessary cattle population, while the wild game should be allowed to populate special game reserves provided in fly-free areas. Spraying with DDT from the air has been extensively practised in one or two game reserves, but is not altogether effective. A more recent method is the subject of study, namely the sterilisation of tsetse flies by the chemicals tepa or metepa, or by gamma radiation, and the release of sterile males. This would be complementary to the use of insecticides. A difficulty at present is the rearing of tsetse flies in sufficient quantities.

TUBERCLE (*tuberculum*, a little lump) is a term used in two quite distinct senses. As a descriptive term in anatomy a *tubercle* means a small elevation or roughness upon the surface of a bone, such as the tubercles of the ribs. In a pathological sense a *tubercle* is a small mass, barely visible to the naked eye, formed in some organ as the starting-point of the disease which has been called after the tubercle, viz. *Tuberculosis*. The name of *Tubercle bacillus* is given to the micro-organism that causes the disease. The term *tubercular* is applied to any symptom, localisation, etc., of the nature of, or connected with, tuberculosis, such as *tubercular cough*, *tubercular glands*, *tubercular pleurisy*, etc. The term *tuberculous* is applied, in the stricter sense, to any diseased organ which is full of these tubercles, such as a *tuberculous udder*, a *tuberculous joint*, or a *tuberculous lung*, etc.

TUBERCULAR (*see under* TUBERCLE).

TUBERCULIN TEST.—We owe the tuberculin test, the original form of which came into use in 1890, to Koch, who grew his tubercle bacilli on broth. To-day a special Purified Protein Derative (' P.P.D.') is used for culturing the bacilli : a feature which adds to the reliability of the test. Tuberculin is prepared by killing and filtering off the bacilli from the culture medium. To the liquid which remains trichloracetic acid is added. This precipitates tuberculoprotein, which is poured into cylinders to form a sediment, is centrifuged, diluted to a standard strength, and bottled.

Tuberculin has in the past been used by instillation beneath the lower eyelid of one eye (the ophthalmic test) ; by subcutaneous injection (the subcutaneous tuberculin test) ; and by injection with a special syringe into the thickness of the skin of a defined area (the intradermal test). To-day, in this country, the test used is the intradermal Comparative Test. Two different tuberculins are used—one mammalian and one avian. This follows the discovery, made some years ago, that the reaction following the injection of tuberculin prepared from the tubercle bacilli of birds may differ from that following the injection of mammalian tuberculin.

A fold of skin is measured with special calipers before the injection, and again 70 hours later. Interpretation of the test is based upon the resultant swelling of each injection site.

The reaction is a complex process not yet fully understood, but it is believed that certain cells in the body become sensitised by anti-bodies produced by *e.g.* tubercle bacilli, and that the action of tuberculin upon such sensitised cells gives rise to toxic substances which result in the reaction at the site of injection.

Bovine tuberculosis is not the only disease which can bring about this sensitisation. Human tuberculosis and tuberculosis of birds will also do it; so will so-called skin tuberculosis and Johne's disease. Hence the advantage of the Comparative Test which helps the veterinary surgeon to distinguish between these various possible causes of a positive reaction.

The human tubercle bacillus is of very low virulence for cattle. It does not constitute a menace to the herd, except that it may confuse the issue by causing animals to react to the test when they are not affected with bovine tuberculosis. They will cease to react a few months after the infected person has gone away.

So-called 'skin tuberculosis' (see under this heading) may also cause confusion. A re-test after an interval of 30 to 60 days will, however, in the absence of tuberculosis, generally give a reaction justifying retention of the animal within the herd. (*See also* JOHNE'S DISEASE *vaccine*.)

If cattle are running on the same land as poultry, and some of these happen to be infected with tuberculosis, the cattle may react when tested with the avian tuberculin. There will not be a significant reaction at the site where the mammalian tuberculin was injected, however; hence the value of the Comparative Test. Avian tubercle bacilli are not virulent for cattle, which usually cease to react within a few months of the infected birds being removed. Reaction to avian tuberculin may also occur in an animal suffering from Johne's disease.

It will be seen, therefore, that the detection of bovine tuberculosis in cattle is far from being a simple matter. Nevertheless, the Comparative Test is of supreme value in the eradication of tuberculosis from our herds, is an improvement upon former tests, and will serve us well until such time as more specific tuberculins are available; and work is going on all the time to produce ones which will differentiate sharply between these five diseases.

TUBERCULOSIS. — Synonyms: Consumption, Phthisis, Pearl Disease, Grapes, 'T.B.', etc. Tuberculosis is a chronic contagious disease of man, all the domesticated animals, many wild animals in captivity, birds, fishes, and reptiles. It is caused by *Mycobacterium tuberculosis* (bovine, human, or avian strains). It is characterised by the formation of nodules or tubercles which tend to undergo cheesy degeneration in almost any or all of the organs or tissues of the body. The specific bacillus can be recovered from the tubercles in every case by appropriate measures. (*See also* 'SKIN TUBERCULOSIS'.)

History.—Tuberculosis is one of the oldest diseases known. It seems to have been recognised as at least a dangerous disease in food animals as early as the fifth century, and some writers hold that many of the prohibitions concerning meat, and the laws governing sacrifices, given in the Book of Leviticus, were directed towards decreasing the spread of this disease to the human subject. The laws of the Church of the Frankonian parts of Germany in the eleventh century forbade the use of tuberculous meat for human food, and King John of France in 1363 decreed letters patent against flesh affected with tuberculosis. At Munich in 1370 the sale of tuberculous flesh was forbidden, and other German towns soon followed suit. From this time onwards both public and medical opinion fluctuated sometimes in favour of, and sometimes against, the use of tuberculous meat for human food, but it was not until the middle of the 19th century that real light was thrown upon the subject by various workers, and the causal organism discovered by Robert Koch in 1882. This epoch-making discovery placed the hitherto only partly accepted theory of the contagious character of tuberculosis upon a firm basis.

Occurrence.—The prevalence of tuberculosis in animals bears a direct ratio to the intensity of the methods of agriculture in an area. Cattle kept in fair numbers, intensively reared, forced to early maturity for milk or meat production, markets, or shows, and housed to a great extent in buildings, are much more often affected than are those living a free open-air life. The cattle in the prairies of North America, on the tablelands of Central Africa, and in the steppes of Eastern Europe, are almost entirely immune from its ravages, while it is unknown in many islands (Iceland, Sicily, etc.). Large town dairies suffer more than do small herds belonging to farmers in mountainous regions. Pigs are affected in parallel circumstances to about the same degree. Where the young stores of large piggeries are fed upon dairy refuse—skimmed milk, products of creameries, buttermilk, etc.—and live together in numbers, it is much more prevalent than in those herds where pigs are kept in the open air.

Bovine tuberculosis affecting cattle herds has been virtually eradicated from Finland (1949), Denmark (1952), the Netherlands (1956), Switzerland (1960), Britain (1960), and from the U.S.A.

Animals affected.—Among the ordinary domesticated animals, cattle and pigs are much more commonly affected than are other species. Cats and dogs are not uncommonly affected, especially the former. Horses, sheep, and goats appear to be more resistant. Asses and mules are only very seldom attacked.

Age is an important factor. Young animals (calves and little pigs especially) are not as a rule extensively affected, but they are least resistant. As the prime of life is reached, the resistance increases, but the number affected rises, and the percentage of cases among old animals is very high. At the same time it is seldom that old animals which have passed the tuberculin test after they became mature, become affected, even although they are exposed to conditions favourable for infection. The body has established immunity. The following table illustrates incidence according to age. Of 9046 cattle examined and found to be diseased the ages were as follows :

Age.	Numbers.	Age.	Numbers.
3–4 weeks	3	3 years	81
5 months	1	4 ,,	118
7–9 months	4	5 ,,	326
1 year	12	6 ,,	1223
2 years	39	7 and over	7239

Sex bears a certain influence upon the incidence of tuberculosis. It is much more prevalent among cows than bulls or bullocks. In fact, in some herds of dairy cattle the percentage of the cows and heifers that react may be as high as 75 per cent, and in the bulls it is seldom more than 15 per cent.

The conditions under which animals are kept are of the greatest importance. Those that are housed in byres or in buildings that are damp and dark, or where there is an inefficient ventilation, are far more often attacked than those living in hygienic buildings, and beasts that are poorly fed, or suffering from some other concurrent disease, as well as those that are being intensively milked, succumb more readily than more naturally kept stock.

Methods of infection.—Cattle are infected in two chief ways : (1) by the respiratory system, and (2) by the digestive tract. They are susceptible to infection from humans suffering from bovine tuberculosis and serious ' breakdowns ' in attested herds have been traced to cowmen suffering from the disease. Cattle are also susceptible, to a lesser degree, to tubercle bacilli of the human type. (*See also under* COMPARATIVE TEST *re* avian tuberculosis.)

Sometimes tuberculosis may be contracted through a wound (*e.g.* after de-horning) or by direct introduction into the tissues of a penetrating instrument, and an infection of the udder may easily occur through the teat canal. When sputum from a case of tuberculosis is coughed out it may be deposited upon the walls, floors, troughs, etc. of the byre or cow-house, and here it gradually dries up. Later on it may be disturbed, and the dried, but by no means killed, tubercle bacilli are stirred up and disseminated through the air of the byre. Moreover, cattle with tuberculous lungs are continually exhaling a mixture of the bacilli with particles of water vapour, and these, floating in the atmosphere, may be inhaled by neighbouring cattle. Cows, either standing near the source of the disease (*i.e.* an already tuberculous cow) or at some distance from it, inhale this germ-laden air, and the bacilli settle in the air passages or in the lungs themselves. Sputum may contaminate the food of the cattle, so that when it is eaten the bacilli gain entrance to the digestive system. When once they have gained entrance into the body the bacilli are transported either by the lymph or blood-stream, and, continually multiplying, they invade new organs or tissues.

Further, it happens that in some cases of the disease the primary lesion is situated in one organ or set of organs, and the contaminated material which leaves that region gets carried to hitherto healthy tissues and infects them. For example, swallowed sputum from infected lungs may spread the infection to the intestines.

Some of the bacilli swallowed are probably destroyed by the juices of the digestive system, others may attack the walls of the stomach or intestines, some find their way to the lymph glands in the mesenteries, or to some part of the peritoneum (where they set up the condition called 'pearl disease'), some may travel to the liver, where they form abscesses, and others yet are discharged in the dung. When large numbers of organisms are being swallowed, and when the dung is heavily infected with these germs, it is obvious that it is an important factor in the spread of the disease, and consequently should be disposed of in a safe manner.

Tuberculosis of the vagina occurs in cows, and the disease may be spread from them to healthy cows through the medium of service by the bull or by the use of infected instruments.

Dehorning of adult cattle constitutes a slight risk.

Nature of the lesions.—Wherever tuberculous infection occurs in the body there are certain more or less definite changes that result. If the germs are deposited upon a mucous membrane surface or in an area of lymphatic tissue, they begin to multiply, irritate the part, and produce a slow, mild inflammation and an increase in the amount of fibrous tissue, which is followed by the production of a *tubercle*—a small nodular swelling whose centre contains either pus or dry yellowish cheesy material. Some of the bacilli may be killed or carried to other parts of the body, where they set up a fresh focus of infection and similar changes. Occasionally the disease remains localised to the area of its first infection and does not spread. In other cases the defensive forces of the body overcome and destroy the whole of the germs present, and the animal becomes spontaneously cured.

Wherever, in the body, there are living tubercle bacilli there is always the elaboration of a toxin which is absorbed into the general circulation, and if present in large amounts causes a certain degree of fever, with a rise in the temperature.

In some cases tubercle bacilli gain entrance into the body and, instead of causing any disturbance, lie dormant. They are not dead, however, for when any lowering of the vital resistance of the body takes place, such as the calving of a cow, a chill, cold, or when some other disease commences in the body, they become vigorous and produce their usual effects. In this way an animal which was thought to be quite healthy until it received an injury, etc., may appear to become suddenly tuberculous, and the factor which produced the lessened resistance is often blamed for the subsequent illness instead of the real cause—the tubercle bacillus.

Diagnosis.—*See* TUBERCULIN TEST, and below.

Symptoms are very varied, and only a general average description is possible.

1. **Cattle.**—As a rule a considerable period of time elapses between the infection of an ox with the germs of tuberculosis and the appearance of the first symptoms, no matter in what part of the body the disease becomes localised.

Tuberculosis of the lungs—the commonest type—manifests itself by a hard, dry, short cough in the early stages. This sometimes disappears for a time, but it is always liable to reappear whenever the animal is in low condition. It is specially noticeable when the air is cold or dusty, and after a drink of cold water on a cold day. As time goes on—perhaps after months—the cough becomes more frequent and painful. It is usually dry, but a good deal of purulent yellowish-white sputum may be coughed up at times. This may either be swallowed or discharged on to the ground. It is best seen first thing in the morning lying in the feeding trough, before that has been cleaned out or before it has been filled with food. As the cough progresses in severity the breathing becomes more rapid and laborious, and is accompanied by a definite 'lifting' of the chest-walls. It is particularly distressing when the animal is made to hurry out of doors, either at exercise or work.

It is about this time or very soon after that the appetite becomes affected. On some days the animal eats heartily, and on others it only picks at its food or leaves it altogether. Swallowing may cause pain, and a fit of coughing frequently follows the eating of the first few mouthfuls of a meal. When feeding becomes capricious the bodily condition rapidly falls away. If there is any pleuritic affection at this period the animal shows pain when its sides are pressed or when it is made to turn sharply. If the pleurisy is severe the beast may grunt or groan.

The mucous membranes of the eyes, nose, and mouth, etc., become pale and anæmic; the skin loses its elasticity and is firmly adherent to the underlying structures, producing the condition that is called 'hidebound', and the coat is hard, dry, and 'staring'. The eyes lose their lustre and are sunken in their sockets, the expression of the face is woeful and worried-looking. The appetite gets worse, attacks of diarrhœa are common, and the body becomes more and more emaciated.

Towards the termination of the disease the respiratory distress becomes increasingly more pronounced. The animal stands for long periods with its head lowered and refuses to move from the spot; any forced exertion causes it to gasp and blow. The cough is now weak, pain is frequent, and can be easily induced by pressure on the throat or back of the animal. Any discharge which may have been formed earlier on, and licked away from the nostrils by the animal's tongue, is now disregarded, and is easily seen. Later, the animal goes down since it has not the strength to remain standing, and usually dies in 2 or 3 more days.

The alimentary canal is sometimes invaded by the germs, generally as the direct result of the swallowing of tuberculous sputum, or from eating food contaminated with discharges in the trough. The bowel wall may be invaded, and a profuse watery diarrhœa follows, in which mucus can often be seen; the lymph glands in the mesentery of the intestine may be attacked, with consequent formation of tubercular abscesses in them; the peritoneal lining of the abdominal cavity is often affected, with the result that its surface becomes studded with little nodules, about the size of a pea ('pearl disease'). In many of these cases there are no external signs of the presence of tuberculosis in the abdominal region, and the disease is not discovered until the animal has been slaughtered and its carcase dressed for human food. In other cases the existence of a profuse diarrhœa along with the cough before described, and the presence in the mouth or throat of either ulcers or lymphoid swellings, allows of a fairly definite diagnosis of tuberculosis beiformed.

Whenever there is an extensive infection with tuberculosis there is always the chance that some of the superficial lymph glands of the muscular areas of the body may be attacked and become enlarged. Those at the back of the throat or at the corner of the lower jaw, or the glands of the neck, shoulder, or stifle, may be so much swollen that they can be easily seen bulging under the skin. This feature is most often met with in old tuberculous cows that are badly infected.

Tuberculosis of the udder—which is all-important from the milk standpoint—begins with the exhibition of little or no change that can be considered definite. The gland slowly becomes diffusely thickened, and more solid to the touch than normally. After milking, it does not feel quite so collapsed and elastic as it should, and in some cases distinct hard nodules can be felt. When only one or two quarters are affected the changes in them can be most readily appreciated by comparing them with the remaining healthy quarters. In practically no case does the udder appear to be painful when handled, and there is no inflammation or vascular congestion such as is seen in an ordinary mastitis (inflammation of the udder). The most easily seen feature of the disease is the absence of symmetry and uniformity between the affected and the unaffected quarters, but this does not become definitely developed until the disease has progressed to a considerable extent. The lymph gland of the udder—the supra-mammary—which lies high up between the buttocks at the most posterior part of the organ, is almost always elongated and enlarged, either on the right or the left side, when the disease has attacked the udder. In some cases it is quite definitely swollen before there are any marked changes in the rest of the mammary gland, but its appearance is not always characteristic. So far as the production of milk is concerned, there is, at first, practically no change either in quantity or in quality. This is very unfortunate, for it tends to induce a sense of false security, and the milk, perhaps teeming with millions of living tuberculosis organisms, continues to be sold for human consumption. As time goes on, however, the amount of the secretion diminishes, until it finally ceases altogether in the affected quarters. These are never so fully collapsed after milking as are the healthy, and while the size of the udder may appear to be unchanged when it is full, it is usually the case that when empty the more fleshy and 'full-feeling' tuberculous quarter can be easily noticed. It frequently happens that owners of such animals are advised of their condition and warned to get rid of the cows, and, knowing that the discrepancy in size between the quarters cannot be so easily detected when the udder is full, they send them to the market without first having them milked. Such cows have all the appearances of being good milkers, and are often bought by unwary buyers who only discover their mistake when it is too late to rectify it.

(**Tuberculoid** mastitis. Over 700 cases of this, due to rapidly growing acid-fast organisms other than *M. tuberculosis*, occur in the U.K. annually—mainly due to not cleaning the teats before introducing antibiotics.)

When the disease affects the main secretory or excretory organs of the abdomen, *i.e.* the liver, pancreas, or kidneys, there is usually no definite changes discoverable in the living animal until the beast has become seriously attacked. Even then the symptoms are often obscure to all but the trained observer. The disease is so insidious that the tissues are able to accommodate themselves to the presence of the germ for a considerable time without having their functions greatly modified.

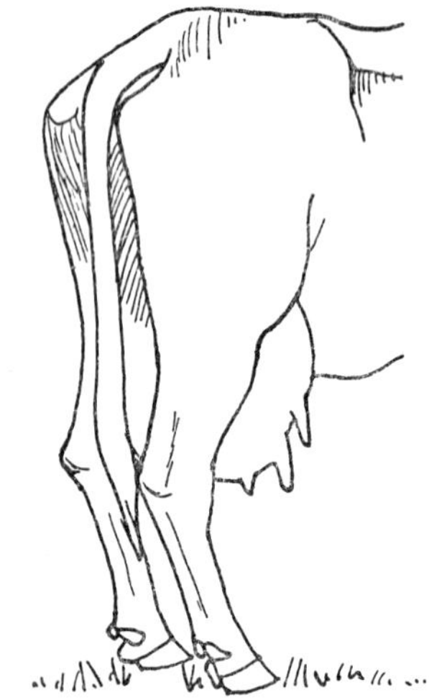

Appearance of an advanced case of tuberculosis of the udder, all four quarters of the gland being affected.

In the central nervous system tuberculosis may show a definite series of symptoms, but more often they are vague and inconclusive. There may be an unsteady swaying gait, signs of fear, severe epileptiform convulsions, partial or complete paralysis of limbs or of groups of muscles, squinting or blindness in one or both eyes, stiffness or twisting of the head and neck, and a slow, irregular pulse. Frequently these symptoms terminate in death a few days after their first appearance. In other cases the animal may show great restlessness, becomes greatly excited, and passes into a stage of delirium or raving madness, with violent and spasmodic contractions of the limbs and head. Unconsciousness soon follows, and the animal goes down into a stupor from which it never rises. These variations all depend on the seat of the lesions in the brain—whether in the fore or the hind part, deep or superficial, diffused or localised, or upon tuberculosis affecting the spinal cord.

Tuberculosis of the bones and joints is not uncommon. These tissues become affected in as slow and chronic a manner as other tissues; so much so that in the great majority of cases the presence of the disease is only confirmed upon the post-mortem examination of the animal's carcase. Sometimes, however, when there is a tuberculous condition in some other part of the body and a joint begins to swell in a dull, slow manner, with gradually increasing pain and inflammation, and a greater or lesser amount of lameness which does not respond to ordinary treatment, the presence of tuberculosis in that joint may be definitely suspected.

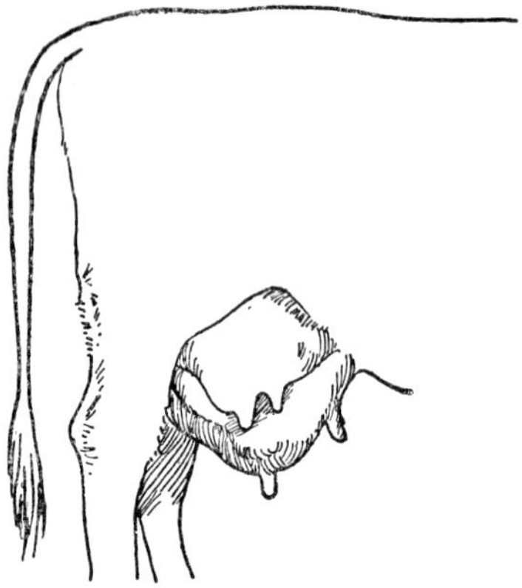

Diagram to show the characteristic asymmetrical appearance of the udder of the cow when only one-half is affected with mammary tuberculosis. The affected side is the larger and does not collapse after milking. It appears to be fleshy when handled.

In the skin there occasionally develop hard tumours, about the size of a hazelnut (*see also* 'SKIN TUBERCULOSIS'), which, if they be opened, are found to contain cheesy or mortar-like masses in their centres. These may burst of their own accord, or they may be accidentally opened, and develop into tubercular ulcers showing no tendency to heal even with appropriate treatment.

'Galloping tuberculosis' is a term applied to the disease when, although it has remained in a chronic state in the body for perhaps quite a long time, it suddenly becomes very acute. This is due to a heavy invasion of the blood-stream by tubercle organisms, and the consequent formation of multitudes of small abscesses, about the size of a millet-seed (hence 'miliary tuberculosis'), in any or all of the organs of the body, but particularly in those of a glandular nature and in the lungs. An animal in this condition becomes highly fevered, goes off its food, its pulse becomes fast and weak, its respirations are laboured and generally very fast, and death occurs in the course of a week or 10 days. (*See* BREAKDOWNS.)

2. **Sheep and Goats.**—A distressing painful cough, always present, but most noticeable upon exertion, a gradual, but quite definite, loss of condition, with progressing weakness, are the main symptoms observed in these animals. Sheep are very rarely affected, but milking goats kept in the vicinity of infected cattle not uncommonly develop tuberculosis. There is nearly always a marked anæmia, pneumonia, sometimes diarrhœa, and occasionally an infection of the udder corresponding to that found in cattle.

3. **Horses.**—Tuberculosis in the horse is not very common, but there are certain symptoms which should always lead one to suspect its presence. Briefly, these may be stated thus: a gradual emaciation in spite of good food and without any other established possible cause; a slight fluctuating increase in the temperature; an occasional moist weak cough, especially on commencing work in the morning; a lack of spirit and a disinclination for heavy or sustained work; a tucked-up appearance of the abdomen, or in some cases (where dropsy exists) a heavy pendulous condition, 'Pot-bellied'; and occasionally symptoms of slight colic. Thirst becomes increased, and the amount of urine passed is greater than normal. (This is often wrongly considered to be diabetes by the attendants.)

Cases in which the abdominal organs are affected sometimes terminate by lung complications—*i.e.* miliary tuberculosis sets in—the animal becomes highly fevered, distressed in its breathing, refuses all food, and generally dies in a few days. Tuberculosis may also become localised in the skin, lymph glands, brain, or udder, but these are not common. It is comparatively often found that sooner or later some part of the skeleton (the bones of the neck being a very usual situation) becomes the seat of a tubercular condition. When a horse becomes thus affected it experiences a difficulty in walking (when the limb bones are diseased), or it is unable to eat from the ground (when the bones of the neck are affected). A slight amount of inflammation sets in round the particular joint, some new bone is deposited, and the freedom of movement is lessened. In the case of the neck bones the horse develops a 'stiff neck', its eyeballs become more mobile than usual, and it has the appearance of watching its surroundings 'out of the corner of its eye'. Finally it becomes impossible to get a collar over the head, and the neck sets almost rigid.

Occasionally, tuberculosis in the horse may be caused by the human or avian type of the tubercle bacillus.

4. **Swine.**—When tuberculosis affects the pig it may be due to feeding with infected whey from cheese-making establishments and creameries, or with infected and unboiled swill from sanatoria. Between 1952 and 1968 80 per cent of routine isolations of the causal organism at the Central Veterinary Laboratory, Weybridge, were avian; the remaining 20 per cent being bovine. (*See* AVIAN TUBERCULOSIS.) Tubercular poultry, or wild birds such as wood-pigeons, are a not uncommon source of infection.

It is only when there are open tubercular lesions, or definite swellings of the surface lymph glands of the body, that tuberculosis is suspected during life, as a rule.

A diagnosis may be established by means of the tuberculin test.

When the swelling of these glands progresses to any great extent, the skin sometimes ruptures over their surfaces, and open, indolent, ulcerous sores result. They discharge a thick, purulent or cheesy-yellow material, and they show no tendency towards healing. When the tubercle bacilli invade the digestive organs a progressive loss of condition that is due to faulty digestion results, and intermittent attacks of diarrhœa are frequent. The pigs—generally young stores—mope and stand about with their backs arched; their tails uncurl (always a sign of illness in the pig), and the animals spend much time sleeping half-buried in the litter of the sty. The appetite usually holds good at first, but becomes fastidious later on. In tuberculosis of the lungs in the pig there is at first a dry, short, half-suppressed cough, and an increase in the rate of respiration. The cough gradually becomes more frequent and distressed, and in later stages it may excite attacks of vomiting. The condition of the body suffers, as in all other cases of this disease, the usual rotundity of the pig giving way to gaunt-ness and even emaciation. Anæmia is common. As in horses, the bones of the pig are especially vulnerable to attack by the bacilli. The ribs, vertebræ, and the joint surfaces of the limb bones are common seats of the disease, and it depends upon the bones affected as to what symptoms will be exhibited—stiffness, lameness, swelling of joints, or painfulness on manipulation.

Lesions which, to the naked eye, appear identical with tuberculosis, may be caused by infection with *Corynebacterium equi*. Even the use of a microscope sometimes fails to differentiate between the two infections.

5. **Dogs and Cats.**—Owing to their close relationship with man these animals are liable to become infected with tuberculosis, either as the result of receiving tubercle-containing milk, or as the result of infection from sputum or discharges from a human case. Objectionable as it is, this fact must be faced, for not only may dogs and cats contract the disease from man, but they may be dangerous sources of infection to healthy human beings, and especially to children.

As in other animals, the symptoms are somewhat vague until the disease is well established. The first signs may be no more than a capricious appetite, slight loss of condition, general weakness, and exhaustion when at work or exercise, but in the great majority of cases either the lungs, pleura, or abdominal organs become attacked. Pulmonary tuberculosis, usually begins with a short dry cough, and vomiting follows in many cases. Later, the cough becomes more frequent, and may be accompanied by a yellowish or whitish discharge from the nostrils. The respiration becomes more and more distressed, and is accompanied by râles or gurgling sounds, often quite audible from a distance. In the lungs themselves solid tuberculous areas develop, in which the slow chronic inflammatory change so characteristic of the disease is at work. The disturbance of the appetite and emaciation result in death from exhaustion at a later stage. Pulmonary tuberculosis is less common in these animals than the abdominal form. (*See* BREAKDOWNS.)

Tuberculosis of the abdominal organs is indicated by impaired nutrition and anæmia, attacks of diarrhœa and constipation alternating with each other. The mesenteric lymph glands are very often the seat of tuberculous abscesses, and since the blood-vessels which supply the intestines pass along the mesenteries, they are liable to become pressed by the developing abscesses, and circulation to the intestines is hindered. Disturbance of the abdominal circulation results in a passive congestion of the capillaries and the exudation of a fluid serous material. This collects in the cavity of the abdomen and results in dropsy, which is an extremely common symptom of tuberculosis in the cat, and to a less extent in the dog. Emaciation is very rapid in these cases, and death follows in a variable time. During the course of an attack, the temperature rises and falls in a very irregular manner. On some days it may be normal or only slightly elevated, while at other times it may be 2 or 3 degrees higher than normal. Immediately before death it often falls as much as 4 or 5 degrees below normal.

Joints and sinuses of the neck may be sites of infection in the cat.

Treatment.—The treatment of tuberculosis in the domesticated animals is not attempted, for four reasons: (1) because of the nature of the disease; (2) because of the ever-increasing danger to human beings who have to attend affected animals; (3) economic conditions would forbid it in all but the most valuable breeding stock; and (4) humanitarian ones. In zoological gardens animals are sometimes treated. (*See* P.A.S. *and* I.N.H.)

Prevention.—There is probably no disease which illustrates the wisdom of keeping animals under hygienic conditions with a view to prevention of disease better than tuberculosis. It is essentially a trouble of indoor life, being most prevalent where animals are crowded together and where fresh air is limited. The freedom from tuberculosis of young cattle living in hilly or mountainous districts, or upon great ranges, well illustrates this fact. Consequently, with a view to preventing the ravages of this disease in all animals, they should be kept outside as much as possible, and given an adequate supply of fresh air when indoors, and overcrowding should be avoided.

Cow-sheds should be so built that there is ample air-space per cow, and a thorough ventilation. They should be thoroughly and frequently cleansed with water and a disinfectant (at least once a week), and every day the byre should be flushed out with water from a hose-pipe under pressure. Particular attention should be paid to the troughs and the walls near the cows' heads. In this connection it should be noted that continuous feeding or watering troughs in byres favour spread of the disease.

Tubercle-free herds.—The building up of a herd of cattle for breeding or dairy purposes absolutely free from tuberculosis, and its maintenance in this state, is an undertaking not easy to carry out. Theoretically it ought to be possible to select a number of perfectly healthy cattle, and, by gradually replacing the old cows by young heifers bred on the premises, to maintain the herd free from tuberculosis. But there are two important factors which are antagonistic: the first of these is the elusiveness of the disease, and the powers of latency and great resistance possessed by the germs; the second is the fallibility of the tuberculin test.

History of Control in Britain.—It was not until 1928 that measures to control bovine tuberculosis were introduced by the Government. In that year the Tuberculosis Order, enacted in 1915, came into force, and the attempt to control the disease by the detection and elimination of 'open' cases began. In 1935 the Attested Herds Scheme carried control measures a stage further.

'Before a herd is eligible for inclusion in the Register of Attested Herds, two tuberculin tests must have been carried out with an interval of not less than 60 days and not more than 12 months between the tests, and there must have been no reactors at either test. The herd is then tested once again by a whole-time veterinary officer of the Ministry of Agriculture, and if no reactors are found, the Certificate of Attestation is granted.'

Much progress had been made under the Attested Herds Scheme, but it was still too slow if we were to see this country rid of bovine tuberculosis within a reasonable number of years. So we came to the third stage—Area Eradication—which began in 1950, and meant, at first, an extension of the Attested Herds Scheme on a voluntary basis, and then the compulsory slaughter of reactors within the prescribed areas. At June 30th, 1958, there were about 7·8 million cattle in Attested Herds and Attested Areas in Great Britain as against 3·9 million 5 years, and 1·4 million 10 years, previously.

In October 1960, the whole of the U.K. was declared one Attested Area; bovine tuberculosis being virtually eradicated from all herds of cattle.

In 1962, the incidence of bovine tuberculosis in herds in England and Wales was 0·14 per cent. The number of reactors slaughtered was 8,846. About £538,000 was paid in compensation. In 1967, the incidence was 0·049 per cent, and 3,047 reactors and 326 contacts in 1,316 herds were slaughtered.

During 1968 5,854,915 cattle were tested in 108,452 herds and as a result 2,170 reactors (including 2 'affected' animals) and 202 contacts in 1,040 herds were slaughtered. The percentage of reactors was 0.037 per cent compared with 0.049 per cent in 1967, but in more than half of the reactors, no macroscopic evidence of tuberculosis was found. Once again there was a reduction in the number of herds with reactors from 1,316 in 1967 to 1,040 in 1968. The number of herds with 'open' cases totalled 119 which is the same as the 1967 figure.

The Tuberculosis Orders, 1964, provide for the notification and slaughter of cattle found to be affected with certain forms of tuberculosis—*i.e.*, tuberculosis of the udder; giving tuberculous milk; tuberculous emaciation; chronic cough accompanied by clinical signs of tuberculosis; or found to be excreting or discharging tuberculous material. Two animals were slaughtered in 1968 as being 'affected' as defined in these Orders.

Interval Between Tests.—In Denmark, where herds were freed of bovine tuberculosis in 1952, testing was at first done at two-year intervals, but is now done at three-year intervals.

In 1959, 0·018 per cent of cattle reacted in Denmark, and a human source of infection has proved by far the most common cause of the reappearance of tuberculosis in cattle.

Insurance.—Lloyd's Underwriters offer a T.B. Reactor Insurance Scheme.

THE RELATIONSHIP OF TUBERCULOSIS IN ANIMALS AND MAN.—**Bovine Tuberculosis.**—This is not a pedantic way of saying 'tuberculosis in cattle', but indicates that one is referring to disease set up by the bovine strain of tubercle bacillus as opposed to the human strain or the avian strain. Man may become infected by any one of the three strains. The bovine strain of the tubercle bacillus is particularly pathogenic for children under 16 years of age.

In considering statistics dealing with incidence of bovine tuberculosis in humans, it must be borne in mind that bovine tuberculosis can be spread from one person to another, just as it can be from animal to man.

Human infection with tuberculosis may also arise from eating infected meat, but this risk is, in civilised countries, not great owing to (*a*) meat inspection services, (*b*) cooking of the meat. But in 1949 the British Veterinary Association issued a warning to the public against buying uncooked meat at 'pet food stores'. Some of this meat may have been condemned as unfit for human consumption on account of its being affected with tuberculosis or other disease. There is an obvious danger of dogs and cats becoming ill from this cause unless the meat is thoroughly cooked, but there is also a danger to animal owners handling such meat before it is cooked, and so contaminating their hands and kitchens.

As previously mentioned, tuberculosis in human beings may arise also from infected dogs, cats, poultry and other birds. (*See* BREAKDOWNS.)

TUBERCULOSIS, AVIAN (*see* AVIAN TUBERCULOSIS).

TUBERCULOUS (*see under* TUBERCLE).

TULARÆMIA is a disease of hares (*see* HARES), ground squirrels, rabbits, and rats, caused by the *Pasteurella tularensis*, and spread mechanically either by flies or ticks, or by direct inoculation; for example, into the hands of a person engaged in skinning rabbits. In man, the disease takes the form of a slow fever, lasting several weeks, with much malaise and depression, followed by considerable emaciation. It was first described in the district of Tulare in California, but is found widely spread in North America, also in parts of Europe and Japan. Sheep and pigs are attacked and many die. Streptomycin may prove effective in treatment.

TUMBU FLY (*see under* SCREW-WORM FLIES).

TUMOUR, or TUMOR (*tumour*), means literally any swelling, but, by usage and common consent, the term is held to include only such solid swellings as are produced without inflammation or association with specific diseases, and are of the nature of neoplasms, or new-growths, parasitic in a measure upon the body in which they grow.

Tumours are usually separated into two great classes, being either *malignant* or *benign*.

Malignant tumours are those which tend to grow and spread rapidly, destroying neighbouring tissues and infiltrating the healthy structures near by, so that after apparently complete removal the growths appear again. They are liable to ulcerate through the skin when superficial, are usually soft in consistency, are non-encapsulated, and may spread to distant parts of the body by the blood- or lymph-stream, giving rise to secondary tumours there. To the typical class of cancers in human beings, often known as 'gnawing tumours', Hippocrates gave the name of 'Carcinoma' (καρκίνωμα), but not all the. malignant tumours are carcinomatous (Further information upon malignant tumours appears under the heading CARCINOMATA AND SARCOMATA.)

Benign, simple, or benignant tumours are those which, growing slowly at one place, press neighbouring parts aside, but neither invade nor destroy them, only seldom ulcerate through the skin or mucous membrane, have usually a capsule of fibrous tissue surrounding them, and when once completely removed by surgical excision or other means, do not recur.

While this classification serves in a measure to differentiate typical varieties into two classes, it is by no means absolutely satisfactory. There are certain kinds of normally benign tumours which may remain comparatively small and circumscribed for a number of years, and then, under the influence of some unknown factor, suddenly become malignant. There are others that have all the naked-eye and microscopic appearances of typical malignant cancers, but remain of the same size and localised to the same spot for the duration of the animal's life. In fact, it may be said that tumours generally conform to few if any of the laws of the body, and are bound down by few laws of their own. Thus, a lipoma (fatty tumour) may grow in a thin emaciated animal; a rapidly growing fibro-fatty tumour in the dog has been known to develop to a size actually larger than the dog upon which it was parasitic; a myoma (muscle tumour) may develop in a uterus the muscular tissue of which is greatly atrophied. Some tumours may mimic gland tissues so closely that it is almost impossible to differentiate them from the normal tissue, and occasionally they may actually produce a secretion very similar to that of the normal gland tissue, which may even be available for use by the body. This is especially so in the case of some tumours of the thyroid gland and the liver. While normally all tumours tend to increase in size—either slowly or rapidly—some grow to a certain size, remain stationary, then decrease in size, and a few may even disappear completely.

SIMPLE TUMOURS. — ADENOMA is a tumour growing in connection with a gland, and composed of gland-like tissue. It is relatively benign, though in the horse's kidney a malignant form is found not uncommonly. A secretion similar to the normal product of the gland may be formed, but since no ducts are present to carry it away, it collects and forms pockets of fluid in the tumour, which when large give the cystic appearance which is usual in old-standing adenomata, and is responsible for the name 'cystic adenomata'. Among animals, adenomata are found in the mammary gland (bitch), ovary (mare and cow), adrenal gland, liver (ox, sheep, and dog), kidney (horse), anal gland (dog), thyroid, salivary, and lacrymal glands.

ANGIOMA is a tumour formed by a mass of small blood-vessels, or spaces in which blood or lymph circulates. This type is commonly found in the livers of cattle, where it exists as a 'cavernous hæmangioma', *i.e.* an angioma formed of spaces in which blood circulates. The nævus, 'port-wine mark', or 'birth mark', which is not uncommonly seen on the skin of the face or neck in man, is also of this nature. In another form—lymphangioma—instead of blood, lymph circulates in the tumour spaces. This form is rare except in dogs, where it is not infrequently found under the jaw, causing a fluctuating swelling, which may rupture and give rise to a troublesome and persistent flow of lymph.

CHONDROMA is a tumour mainly composed of cartilage. Two varieties are recognised—hyaline and fibrous—and in some cases a chondroma may be formed of these varieties mixed together. Chondromata are very liable to undergo a change into fatty tissue, or they may become calcified or ossified. They have been found in the testicle, parotid gland, and ovary, but are perhaps more commonly found in the mammary gland of the bitch, where they enter into the composition of those complex tumours, varying between the size of a marble and a walnut (or larger), which are so often met with in old bitches which have been bred from, and which have had previous uterine complications of an inflammatory nature. Chondromata are, however, more typically found in connection with bone or cartilage in some part of the body where these normally occur.

FIBROMA is a tumour which mainly consists of fibrous tissue. Fibromata may be either hard or soft, and are the commonest kinds of tumour met with in the domesticated animals, especially in horses. They may occur anywhere in the body where fibrous tissue is normally found, but are particularly common under the skin. They are extremely common in the inguinal region of the horse, especially in geldings, where they may be found in the prepuce (sheath), scrotum, inside of the thighs, and between the buttocks. In these situations the tumours are multiple, rounded, well defined from each other, loosely attached under the skin, and able to be moved about within limits. When removed and sectioned they have the colour and general succulent appearance of slices of pineapple, when seen by the naked eye. They are usually benign, but may be confused with spindle-celled sarcomata, which are highly malignant. Fatty, mucoid, or calcareous degeneration may occur in a fibroma, with consequent alteration in size and consistency. A variety of fibroma, known as a 'cheloid' or 'keloid', is found upon rare occasions in connection with the car tissue in a healed wound, while in the abdominal wall another variety—known as a 'desmoid'—is sometimes encountered.

GLIOMA is a tumour which is rare in the domesticated animals, though the commonest tumour met with in the brain. It is developed from the spider-like cells of the supporting neuroglia tissue of the brain or spinal cord. Gliomata are benign tumours, but they tend to invade surrounding tissues, and are liable, according to the part of the brain where they occur, to cause paralysis of limbs, or areas of the surface of the body, or where the vital centres in the medulla are involved, to result in death.

LIPOMA is a tumour chiefly composed of fat, or adipose tissue. It is not an uncommon tumour among animals, especially the horse, where it is found in connection with the omentum, or under the peritoneum of the bowel wall. In the dog it is sometimes seen under the skin of the abdomen, thighs, or shoulders. Lipomata are usually single, well defined, possess a stalk or pedicle, and are extremely soft to the touch during the life of the animals; upon excision, or after death, they harden considerably. They are sometimes mistaken for a slowly developing chronic abscess. In most cases they grow to about the size of an apple, but in dogs they frequently attain an enormous size, and have been known to weigh more than the dog itself. In occasional cases a diffuse tumour-formation may occur around some organ or organs of the abdominal cavity in the ox. The rectum, or the bowel immediately in front of it, may become surrounded by a cylinder of fat, sometimes measuring as much as 4 inches thick. This is not an uncommon condition in adult beef shorthorns artificially fed for show or sale purposes. The condition is known as 'diffuse lipomatosis'.

MELANOMA is a somewhat special variety of tumour occurring in grey horses, and in other animals. Melanomata are quite common in grey horses, but hardly ever occur in horses of other colours, even roans. They generally arise after middle life, and are usually found below the skin around the anus, at the root of the tail, or in some part of the head or neck. They are usually about the size of an orange, or less, of definite outline, firm to the touch, and when cut they are coal-black within. They consist of various kinds of cells loaded with black pigment from the hairs, called 'melanin', so that their outlines are obscured. Fibrous tissue cells are common and give rise to the name sometimes used, viz., 'melanotic fibromata'. The pigment is derived from the colouring matter of the coat, and the tumours are usually found at the stage in the life of the horse when its coat colour begins to turn lighter. In cattle they are infrequently met with on hocks, elbows, or lips, and are seen in red or red and white animals. Melanomata may be very malignant, many tumours being then present in the same animal; removal of some hastens the growth and activity of those that remain.

MYOMA is a tumour composed mainly of muscle fibres, usually of the plain unstriped variety, though occasionally striped fibres may be found. They are most commonly found in the female genital tract, often in connection with the wall of the uterus, but they may also arise in the urinary tract, or in the stomach or intestines in dogs. They are not common among animals, though of great frequency and importance in human beings.

MYXOMA is a tumour made up of embryonic connective tissue, very similar to what is found in the umbilical cord. They are found in different situations in animals, are commonest in young immature subjects, and only occur rarely (in the eye and heart) in old adults. When cut their inward structure strongly resembles the flesh of a skate or other similar fish, and they contain a large amount of fluid which exudes from the cut surface and causes the tumour to shrink. One peculiarity of this variety of tumour is that under certain circumstances sarcomata and other species of tumour may degenerate into myxomatous growths; the reason for such degeneration is not understood. They are occasionally met with after injury to the point of the haunches in cattle, where they may attain to a large size, and in horses they show a predilection for the palate or other part of the mouth.

NEUROMA is a growth composed of nerve tissues. A 'false neuroma', which appears to be commoner, is composed of fibrous tissue growing upon a nerve, and generally causes pressure and some pain. Both these varieties are probably comparatively rare among animals, but they may be more common than would appear, since they may easily be overlooked during post-mortem examination. The so-called 'amputational neuroma', which consists of a tangled mass of nerve fibres and connective tissue on the cut end of a nerve (*e.g.* after plantar or median neurectomy in the horse, or amputation of a limb in the dog), is not a tumour, according to the general view. It is merely an irregular regenerative or reparative process.

ODONTOMA is a tumour composed of the tissues which go to form the teeth. Several varieties of odontomes are encountered, all in the horse. These are, 'epithelial odontomes', which arise from the epithelial cap of a tooth; 'composite odontomes', which arise from the cap, dental papilla, and alveolar cavity of a tooth, and usually result in the formation of growths bearing some resemblance to a normal tooth; 'compound odontomes', which arise in connection with the germ of a tooth, and possess a cavity lined with a membrane in which are embedded very large numbers of rudimentary teeth; and 'connective tissue odontomes', which arise from the connective tissues of a tooth or its cavity, and may contain masses of dentine, cement, fibrous tissue, and even partially formed teeth. In the horse's upper jaw, usually in connection with one or other of the cheek teeth, or its root, is the common situation of odontomata, but a special variety also arises in colts in connection with the petrous temporal bone. This is usually about the size of a turkey's egg, firmly embedded in the bone or loose upon its surface, and generally characterised by the presence of a sinus opening on to the surface of the skin about the base of the ear. (Some authorities consider that this form is not an odontoma, but is a teratoma—a tumour composed of a twin inclusion.) At the bottom of the sinus there is usually found a mass of hard material, which has great similarity to a normal cheek tooth.

OSTEOMA is a tumour composed of bone. A pure osteoma is exceedingly rare, but tumours containing bone tissue mixed with other kinds of tumour tissue are only comparatively rare. These are usually called 'compound osteomata'. Osteomata have been found in the testes of horses, in connection with the ribs, in the brain, pericardium, omentum (sheep), lungs and aorta. They are of irregular shape, and painless unless or until they press upon some sensitive soft structure around. (An exostosis, such as ringbone in horses, is not an osteoma: it is practically always produced as the result of inflammation of the periosteum, while an osteoma never is.)

PAPILLOMA is a tumour composed of connective tissue elongations covered with epithelium, and arising on the surface of the skin or mucous membrane. The core of fibrous tissue may be like a single finger, or branched and re-branched like the fingers of the hand, giving an appearance suggestive of a cauliflower. In papillomata of the skin (warts) the covering epithelium may soften and degenerate, and the tumour is then liable to bleed upon slight injury; in other cases, especially in the sheep, the surface cells may become keratinised, and a horny covering is formed, giving rise to a so-called 'cutaneous horn'. Papillomata are extremely common in animals, and when small can be disregarded. They are found along the lower line of the abdomen in cattle, especially such as are shut in courts, standing knee-deep in manure; they occur commonly in connection with the scrotum or udder, about the eyelids and lips, on the ears, etc., in horses, where they are called 'angleberries'. In the dog they are commonly met with in the mouth, but in this situation they are not of the same nature as those on the skin of other animals. These are capable of transmission from one animal to another, can often be cured by administration of strong alkaline drenches or by the use of tonics which contain arsenic by the mouth, and in some cases suddenly disappear without apparent cause. Microscopically, however, they have all the appearances of papillomata met with elsewhere. On the surface of the penis of the male dog, and in the vulva and vagina of the bitch, another form of papilloma is not uncommon. These usually possess no epithelium, and are not unlike sarcomata, in that they are of rapid irregular growth, and are capable of being spread from one sex to the other during service.

Other varieties of tumours, much less common than those which are given above, are *adamantinoma*, which develop at the roots of teeth; *psammomata* (a word which in veterinary pathology has a different meaning from that in human pathology) are tumours found in connection with the lining of the ventricles of the brain, containing not sand as in man, but almost 50 per cent of a substance called cholesterin; *chordoma*, which is a very rare tumour originating along the spinal column in the remnants of the embryonic notochord, and sometimes causing nervous disturbances. Mention must also be made of the *teratomata*, which term is usually considered to include monsters or monstrosities of a developmental nature. In this sense it includes many of those extraordinary and often weird-looking objects which result from some irregularity in intra-uterine growth, such as two-headed calves, eight-legged lambs, foals with only one median eye, etc. The word is also used to include those growths of otherwise perfect individuals where a twin, or a portion of a twin, is included within the body of the first individual. Thus, in the horse's testicle, and sometimes in ovaries, there may be found a collection of skin, hair, teeth, and other irregular tissues, enclosed within a covering envelope. These growths are not of the nature of neoplasms (new-growths).

Symptoms.—The symptoms of a tumour are as varied as the situations in which they are found. When on the surface of the body they cause no further symptoms than the presence of the swelling. The only other symptoms, apart from pain in fast-growing tumours, are those of an accidental nature, due to pressure upon surrounding organs, interference with the patency of a canal or cavity, obstruction to vital processes, and special inconveniences when situated in peculiar positions.

Treatment.—Removal by complete surgical excision, wherever that is possible. (*See also* CARCINOMATA *and* WARTS.)

TURKEY SYNDROME '65.—The provisional name given to a group of symptoms seen in turkey poults 3 to 6 weeks old: reduced growth rate, loss of appetite, broken feathers with discoloration. Sometimes there is deformity of the hock and metatarsal bones, giving the bird a bandy-legged appearance. 'Depraved' appetite may occur.

A report in 1971 stated that a similar condition could be reproduced with *Mycoplasma gallisepticum.*

'TURKEY X DISEASE'.—This was the provisional name given in 1960 when in Britain 150,000 turkey poults died from what is now known to be poisoning by aflatoxin. (*See* GROUNDNUT MEAL.)

TURKEYS.—Diseases include: Blackhead, Coccidiosis, Erysipelas, Fowl Pest, Moniliasis, Pullorum disease, Rupture of the aorta, Sinusitis, Synovitis (and see also above and Arizona disease).

Overseas, diseases include virus hepatitis (U.S.A.) and turkey meningo-encephalitis (Israel).

TUP (*see under* SHEEP).

TURBINATE BONES (*see under* NOSE).

TURNIPS—Like kale, these contain a goitre-producing factor, and if fed in large amounts to pregnant ewes are liable to cause abortion—unless iodine licks are provided. (*See* VAGINA, RUPTURE OF.)

TURPENTINE, MEDICINAL OIL OF.—Turpentine is the oleo-resin which exudes from various members of the pine family, especially the *Pinus Australis, Pinus tæda,* and *Pinus sylvestris.* The oil distilled from this oleo-resin is known as oil of turpentine. The natural turpentine is not used in medicine, as it is highly irritating, and when the word *turpentine* is employed the oil of turpentine is indicated.

Action.—Externally, turpentine is a blistering agent if applied in a concentrated form and if its evaporation is hindered or prevented. It is vigorous in its action, and the vesicles that are produced are painful and slow to heal. It is a common constituent of stimulating liniments. Internally, it possesses stimulating, antiseptic, hæmostatic, diuretic, and anthelmintic actions. It acts as a stimulant to the muscular wall of the stomach and bowel, causing vigorous contractions, and tending to cause expulsion of any accumulated gases. It exerts a disinfecting action upon fermenting material in the alimentary canal, and it checks bacterial activity in the ingesta. It is rapidly absorbed and distributed round the system, and is excreted by the kidneys, stimulating their action, by the skin, intestines, and through the glands of the bronchi, whose secretion it increases. A peculiarity of turpentine is that it gives to the urine the odour of violets when given to the horse in ordinary doses.

Uses.—In any condition in which there are collections of gas in the abdominal organs medicinal turpentine is useful. It is given in tympany in horses and cattle. Large doses are liable to irritate the stomach and kidneys.

Turpentine should *never be given* when an animal is suffering from congestion of the kidneys, nephritis, inflammations of the bladder, stomach, or bowels, as its active irritant action only increases the already existing inflammation.

'TWIN LAMB' DISEASE.—A colloquial name for PREGNANCY TOXÆMIA.

TWINNING, ARTIFICIAL.—In the interests of increased beef production, attempts were begun in 1959 to exploit commercially an experimental technique for the production of twin calves. A suitable dose of pregnant mare's serum (P.M.S.), injected subcutaneously at a suitable time, *e.g.* 4 days before œstrus, will on average give twins; but there will be some triplets and singles. The follicle-stimulating hormone (*see* page 427) contained in the serum causes an extra follicle to mature and shed an extra egg with resultant twinning. Over-dosage, however, leads to undesired quadruplets etc.; or to numerous eggs which pass quickly down the Fallopian tubes without being fertilised—result—no calf at all. There is a risk of stillbirths and of strain on the dam.

TWINS (CALVES).—Twins tend to run in families. For example, one cow had three pairs of twins, her daughter four pairs, and a grand-daughter two pairs. That might be called twinning at its best. Of course, there is sometimes trouble. Perhaps the condition of the dam is pulled down; or perhaps the 'cleansing' is retained, becomes infected, and infertility follows.

In strains not noted for twins, twinning may occur on farms where there is a herd infertility problem; as though Nature were preparing in advance for a uture dearth of calves. That is a less happy side to twinning.

Identical twins—always of the same sex—result from the division of the fertilised egg into two; whereas ordinary twins are produced as the result of the fertilisation of two eggs.

These two eggs may come from the same ovary, when the two fœtuses may develop in the same horn of the womb. Sometimes they also share the same blood circulation. If, under these conditions, they are of the same sex, all is well; but if one is a male and the other a female, the male's sex hormones will influence and alter the female's reproductive system, and make her a sterile freemartin.

On the other hand, twins may arise from two eggs each shed by a different ovary, and the fœtuses will then usually occupy separate horns of the womb. Even if of different sex, no freemartin will result. Dr. Joseph Edwards once related the experience of a Swedish research worker which shows that there is evidently, with cattle, a close affinity between identical twins—as there undoubtedly is with human beings. **Six pairs of twins were split at birth and reared separately, for fifteen months. At this age they were all put into a field together. Within a few days each twin had found and paired off with its sister.** (*See* ERYTHROCYTE MOSAICISM; *also* SUPERFŒTATION *and* TWINNING *above*.)

TWINS (FOALS).—In the mare, the presence of twins in the uterus is a common cause of abortion. About 3 per cent of pregnant mares conceive twin fœtuses, but the birth of healthy twins is exceedingly rare—about 0·01 per cent.

TWINS, MONOZYGOUS. — Identical twins, from the same ovum.

'TYING-UP' SYNDROME.—Also known as set-fast, this condition in racehorses appears to be identical with azoturia. Symptoms include stiffness, a rolling gait, blowing and sweating and, if exercise continues, the adoption of a crouching attitude. Pain is evident. The animal may lie down and be unable to rise. (*See* AZOTURIA.)

'TYLAN' (*see below*).

TYLOSIN.—An antibiotic which gives effective control of vibrionic enteritis in pigs, and of C.R.D. in poultry.

TYMPANITES (*tympanites*) is a name applied to the drum-like condition of the abdomen, which results from distension of the stomach or bowels with gas, as the result of fermentation, decomposition, constipation, or of simple obstruction. (*See under* STOMACH, DISEASES OF; INTESTINES, DISEASES OF; BLOAT.)

TYMPANY is distension of a hollow organ with gas. (*See* TYMPANITES, BLOAT.)

TYPHLITIS (τυφλός, blind).—Inflammation of the cæcum or first part of the large intestine, into which the termination of the small intestine opens.

TZANEEN DISEASE.—This is a tick-borne infection with *Theileria mutans* in cattle, the African buffalo, and the Indian water buffalo, and often occurs simultaneously with other infections. There may be only a mild fever or, less commonly, serious illness, and death. Anti-malarial drugs are of use.

U

UDDER (*see* MAMMARY GLAND).

UDDER TOWELS (*see* MASTITIS).

UDDER INFLATION is a method formerly much used in the treatment of 'Milk Fever' (which see), but one which has long been replaced by the more rational treatment of injections of calcium borogluconate. Inflation of the udder was obtained by the use of a simple pump, a cylinder of CO_2 or a compressed air container. Udder inflation is effective, but the risk of setting up mastitis through the use of teat syphons is an objection.

The udder and teats are washed with an antiseptic solution, especial attention being paid to the tips of the teats, and a clean towel is laid under the whole organ to prevent soiling. The teat syphon should be boiled immediately before use, and should be protected from contamination before and during use.

Milk is removed from the udder, and the undermost teats are inflated first until the air begins to escape from the distended teat, and then are clipped to prevent loss of air. When all have been inflated, the quarters of the gland are massaged by hand to distribute the air throughout the udder substance. The clips are removed and the cow is made comfortable. She should be propped up on her sternum by bags filled with straw or by bales of hay, and thereafter turned over on to the other side every three or four hours. As a rule she will rise to her feet within four hours after inflation, but some take longer than this. Occasionally a case requires to be reinflated. Little or no milk should be taken from the cow during the 12 hours subsequent to her regaining her feet, and she should not be milked dry during the next two or three days.

UITPEULOOG ('Bulging Eye Disease').—A recently described oculo-vascular myiasis of domestic animals in South Africa.

ULCER (*ulcus*).—A breach on the surface of the skin, or on the surface of any mucous or other membrane of a cavity of the body, which does not tend to heal. The process by which an ulcer spreads, which involves the death of minute portions of the healthy tissues around its edges, is known as 'ulceration'. Ulceration and abscess formation are in some respects similar, being inflammatory processes, but while the latter takes place in a cavity from which its pus cannot escape until the abscess bursts, the former occurs upon a surface from whence the pus can discharge almost as soon as it forms.

An ulcer consists of a 'floor' or surface which, in consequence of the loss or destruction of tissue, is usually depressed below the level of the surrounding healthy structures, and an 'edge' around it where the healthy tissues end. The floor of a healing ulcer consists of 'granulations', which are masses of cells engaged in forming connective tissues and richly supplied with capillary blood-vessels that give the ulcer a bright-red appearance; while the edge usually shows as a darker line (the so-called 'blue-line') of growing epithelial cells, which are constantly spreading inwards. In the process of healing, the fibrous connective tissue formed by the granulations contracts and thus draws the edges of the ulcer together, and gives a puckered appearance to the scar that is left. This shows as a star-shaped outline to the scar some time afterwards, and is responsible for the name of 'stellate scar' that serves to distinguish such a lesion from that left by an incised wound, to which the name 'lineal scar' is applied.

Simple ulcers have a shallow and reddened floor, with a distinct dark line at their edges. They have a slight purulent discharge and no smell. They are usually not serious, but may be found in any part of the body. Treatment consists of removing any pieces of dead tissue on the surface of the ulcer and treating the raw under-surface with stimulating healing lotions or dressings, such as weak tincture of iodine, iodoform powders, sulphanilamide, etc., and protectively bandaging where there is a risk of irritation or injury.

Inflamed ulcers are those in which, as the result of the presence of bacteria, or owing to continued external irritation, there is a tendency to spread. The floor of such an ulcer is very red, often deeply sunken below the level of the surrounding tissue, and bleeds easily, while there is a copious and thick white discharge from its surface. The skin around is swollen, and parts of it are liable to die, and so the ulcer spreads. If such an ulcer is large and if it is heavily infected with germs, it may cause the death of the animal.

Callous ulcer is the type of chronic ulcer that is often met with in horses and dogs, when there is any pressure or irritation that interferes with the blood-supply but does not necessarily cause immediate destruction of the skin. In most cases it is covered by a hard leathery piece of dead skin from under which escapes a fluid with an offensive smell. Sometimes they are dry, and though persistent do not cause a great deal of inconvenience to the animal, but at other times they are painful, especially when some part of the harness presses upon them. When they occur upon the backs of horses under the saddle they are usually called 'sit-fasts'. Bed-sores in all animals are of this nature, as well as those ulcers that are sometimes seen on the elbows, stifles, and hocks of heavy dogs that spend much of their time lying upon the ground.

Corneal ulcers appear upon the normally clear anterior wall of the eye as little whitish or greyish areas about the size of a large domestic pin's head or somewhat larger. They are the result of some local injury, such as a scratch, blow, or laceration from grit, dust, or a small thorn. When examined carefully they are seen to possess an eaten-out central pit, and are surrounded by a zone of milky-white opacity.

Internal ulcers may occur in the mouth (*see* MOUTH, DISEASES OF), in the stomach (*see* STOMACH, DISEASES OF), in the bowels (*see* INTESTINES, DISEASES OF), and in other parts.

Glanders ulcers, which are typically met with in the mucous membrane of the nostrils, and have a 'punched-out appearance.

Foot-and-mouth disease 'ulcers', which are seen in the mouth affecting almost any part that is covered with membrane, at the junction between the skin and horn of the feet, and on the teats of the udder in females; actually these lesions are not ulcers, but are the remains of burst blebs or blisters.

Lip-and-leg ulcers, which occur in sheep affected with the condition known as 'orf'.

Rodent ulcers or *malignant ulcers*, which are simply the names that are given to either cancer or tuberculosis affecting the skin, after the surface has broken down and a red discharging sore remains.

'Button' ulcers, which are found in the cæca of pigs that are affected with the chronic form of swine fever, etc.

In addition to these, ulcers may appear during the course of many other diseases; for fuller details see under the specific diseases mentioned above, and also ULCERATIVE CELLULITIS, URÆMIA, EPIZOÖTIC LYMPHANGITIS, DISTEMPER, STOMATITIS, ACTINOMYCOSIS, PURPURA HÆMORRHAGICA, BURSATEE, and CALF DIPHTHERIA, MUCORMYCOSIS, etc.

Causes.—Generally speaking, they are produced when there is any agent at work that irritates the surface, and by its presence prevents healing. Any condition that lowers the general vitality of the animal, such as old age, chronic disease like tuberculosis, rickets, etc., malnutrition, defective circulation, or chronic constipation, will act as a predisposing cause. Among the commonest of the direct causes may be noted bacterial agents gaining access to slight wounds and escaping destruction, constant irritation from badly fitting harness, pressure of bony prominences upon hard floors insufficiently provided with bedding (*see* BED-SORES), irritation of wounds by discharges pent up under dressings that are too seldom changed, and the application of too strong antiseptics to wounds.

Treatment.—In many cases, especially in the specific diseases, general treatment is followed by healing of the local ulcer. In other cases, three objects must be kept in view: (1) To remove the cause of the ulceration; (2) to render the floor and the edge of the ulcer healthy so that healing may commence; (3) to assist the healing process and ward off any further irritation.

(1) **Removal of the cause.**—Under this head it must be remembered that any constitutional cause should be remedied as well as the direct local cause. Thus, in badly nourished horses that are overworked as well, it is necessary to rest the animal and feed it upon good food. A run of a few weeks at grass will often do quite as much towards effecting healing as local treatment. In the smaller animals halibut-liver oil may be indicated. Penicillin or one of the sulpha drugs may be used (*and see* YEAST).

(2) **Rendering the ulcer healthy** aims at converting the ulcer into what virtually becomes an ordinary open wound. The surface is treated with some suitable antiseptic, such as gentian violet, 'T.C.P.', acriflavine, etc. If one or two days of such treatment does not result in a clean,

bright-red, odourless wound, or where there are shreds of dead tissue adherent to the surface, it may be necessary to scrape the surface so that the dead cells may be separated from the healthy below them.

After the surface of the ulcer has been rendered as healthy as possible it is necessary to cease from further use of strong or powerful agents, as these retard healing by the destruction of surface tissues. The use of what are often referred to as 'heroic measures' is in itself a possible cause of ulceration.

(3) **Assistance of the healing process.**—Some simple dressing, such as would be used for an ordinary open wound, is all that is required after the pus and dead tissue have been removed. (For other details *see under* WOUNDS.)

ULCERATIVE LYMPHANGITIS, also called ULCERATIVE CELLULITIS, is a contagious chronic disease of horses and other members of the horse tribe, which is characterised by inflammation of the lymph vessels and a tendency towards ulceration of the skin over the parts affected. It most commonly attacks animals that are already suffering from some parasitic skin disease, or those with wounds of the skin. As it may sometimes affect tissues other than the skin, such as the lungs, it must be regarded as a serious condition.

Cause.—The cause is usually a small bacillus which cannot be differentiated from that causing caseous lymphadenitis in sheep, called the *Preisz-Nocard bacillus* or *Corynebacterium ovis*. It gains access through injuries of the heels, such as cracked heels or mud fever, or by abrasions that result from scratching when the legs are affected by lice or mange. Infection may be carried by grooming tools, harness, utensils, etc., from one horse to another.

Symptoms.—The commonest seat of the disease is the fetlock of a hind leg. This part becomes swollen and slightly painful. Small buds or abscesses appear, varying in size from a pea to a walnut; after a few hours they burst and discharge a small amount of thick pus, which, later, turns to a yellowish sticky blood-tinged fluid. An ulcerated area remains and heals over in from 10 to 20 days. Other ulcers appear in the vicinity, and the condition gradually spreads up the leg. A horse may be affected for months, or even years, before any severe general disturbances arise; and as a rule lameness is only noticed when the lesions are in close proximity to a joint. Occasionally the disease appears in other areas of the body, such as inside the thighs, on the shoulders or fore-arms, and sometimes in the lungs and kidneys. In these more severe instances, or where the lesions are very numerous, there may be some wasting, rise in temperature, absence of appetite, and even death in very bad cases.

Treatment.—As a rule the lesions can usually be induced to heal by surgically opening the buds as they appear, evacuating the contained pus, scraping the cavities, and dressing with such lotions as acriflavine, eusol, or aqueous solution of iodine, potassium permanganate. It must be remembered, however, that as lesions heal up others are liable to develop, and that when a case is considered better, there may still be a relapse or a recrudescence at some future period. Encouraging results have followed the injection of Terramycin. Disinfection of the stable is necessary, and the burst buds should be protected from the attacks of flies in the summer.

ULCERATIVE SPIROCHÆTOSIS OF PIGS.—This has been reported in the U.K., Australia, New Zealand, South Africa, U.S.A. It may give rise to footrot in pigs, ulceration of the skin, and scirrhous cord.

ULNA is the inner of the two bones of the fore-arm. The shaft has gradually become less and less in size in ratio as the number of digits has decreased, so that while the ulna is a perfect bone in the dog and cat, in the horse its shaft has almost completely disappeared and the bone is only represented by the olecranon process which forms the 'point of the elbow'. The shaft of the ulna is liable to become fractured from violence to the fore limb, but the commonest seat of an ulnar fracture is the olecranon process. This occurs from a fall in which the fore limbs slip out in front of the animal, and the weight of the body comes down suddenly on to the point of the elbow. (*See* FRACTURES.)

ULTRA HIGH TEMPERATURE TREATMENT of milk involves heating it to between 275° and 300° F. for a few seconds. Suggested in 1913, this process is used to produce 'Long-keeping' milk, on sale in Britain from 1965 onwards.

The process does not affect the calcium nor the casein, but destroys some vitamins and probably some serum proteins (immune globulins). Calves grow less well on it than on raw or pasteurised milk.

ULTRA-VIOLET RAYS are used in the treatment of various skin diseases, etc., and in the diagnosis of ringworm and porphyria and in the fluorescent-antibody test for various infections including rabies. (*See* LIGHT TREATMENT.) Ultra-violet ray emitters are used in piggeries, dairies, etc., in order to reduce sources of infection, but levels of irradiation that are effective in killing bacteria may cause skin burns or damage to sight, and so are not suitable for pens or rooms.

UMBILICAL CORD, CUTTING THE (*see* p. 702).

UMBILICUS (*umbilicus*) is another name for the navel, the area of the abdominal wall at which the fœtal vessels and membranes enter, emerge, or are attached. When the umbilical cord dries up and falls off, which should take place soon after the birth of the young animal, a scar remains which can always be easily seen, and forms a valuable guide to the surgeon when operating in the region.

UNCONSCIOUSNESS is a condition depending upon some abnormality, disorder, or disease of the brain. There are many varieties, ranging from sleep, which is a natural form of unconsciousness, through grades up to coma, in which there is a state of complete oblivion to external things, and a nearness to death. In 'syncope' or fainting, the brain ceases to act for a time either owing to bloodlessness from an impaired heart's action, or due to some form of shock. In certain forms of epilepsy the animal is unconscious of its surroundings, but it is able to perform familiar and reflex acts, such as walking or running. 'Stupor' is the name given to a partial state of unconsciousness from which the animal may be roused by powerful stimulants, such as the inhalation of ammonia. 'Apoplexy' is that form which results from a severe injury to the brain itself or to the membranes within the skull. 'Narcosis', another form of unconsciousness, follows the administration of narcotic drugs, such as barbiturates, etc.

UNDECYLENATE OINTMENT. — A fungicide, used in the treatment of ringworm, etc.

UNDULANT FEVER IN MAN is caused by *Brucella melitensis*, the cause of Mediterranean fever in goats; *Brucella abortus suis*; or *Brucella abortus*. The latter organism is responsible for 'contagious abortion' (brucellosis) of cattle, and it is probable that most cases of undulant fever in man caused by *B. abortus* arise through handling infected cows or from drinking their milk. Infection can readily occur through the skin. Numerous cases have occurred in veterinarians, following mishaps with Strain 19 vaccine; *e.g.* accidental spraying into the eyes. In America, *Brucella abortus suis* is an important cause of undulant fever in man.

Symptoms are vague and simulate those of influenza except that undulant fever lasts for a much longer time, even up to 4 months. Temperature is generally raised but fluctuates greatly; there are painful manifestations in the limbs and trunk, and one or more joints may swell. Constipation is a prominent feature, and in some cases more specific symptoms are shown, indicating that one or more organs are particularly affected. The organisms are present in the blood-stream and in the spleen. Death occurs in about 2 per cent of cases.

Prevention.—The disease is serious, not so much because of its mortality (1 to 2 per cent), but because of the loss of work occasioned by its long duration. Aborting cows on farm premises should be looked upon as potentially infective agents, and after handling them the worker should take precautions to disinfect his hands and arms. Pasteurisation safeguards milk. (*See* BRUCELLOSIS *and* CHEESE.)

UNSTABLE SUBSTANCES (*see under* INJECTIONS).

URÆMIA (*οὖρον*, urine; *αἷμα*, blood) is the condition which results when the poisonous materials that should be excreted into the urine are retained in the body through some diseased condition of the kidneys, and are circulated in the blood-stream. Blood-urea is in excess. The condition is very serious and nearly always fatal. It may produce death in a few hours, or it may act more slowly, and is preceded by convulsions and unconsciousness. In the slower types there is usually a strong urinous odour from all the body secretions. In acute cases a laxative is indicated, together with the administration of glucose saline subcutaneously. Withdrawal of a quantity of blood may be helpful (provided saline is given). (*See* URINE, ABNORMAL CONDITIONS *and* LEPTOSPIROSIS, KIDNEY, *also* STUTTGART DISEASE, etc.)

URATES (*see* URIC ACID).

UREA (*οὖρον*, urine), or CARBAMIDE, is a crystalline substance of the chemical formula $CO(NH_2)_2$, which is very soluble in water and alcohol. It is the chief waste product discharged from the body in the urine, being formed in the liver and carried by the blood to the kidneys. The amount excreted varies with the nature and the amount of the food taken, being greater in the carnivora, and when large amounts of protein are present in the food. It is also increased in quantity during the course of fevers.

Urea is rapidly changed into ammonium carbonate after excretion and when in contact with the air, owing to the action of certain micro-organisms.

Determination of the blood urea level is an important aid to the diagnosis of kidney failure.

Urea feeding.—As long ago as the beginning of the century it was known that some of the micro-organisms which inhabit the rumen could synthesise protein from urea, and it was accordingly suggested that urea might be substituted for protein in concentrates fed to cattle. This has since been referred to as the protein-sparing effect of urea.

In recent times, the emphasis has shifted more, perhaps, to the value of urea in increasing the intake and aiding the digestion of low-quality roughages, and it has been widely used as a dietary supplement for cattle and sheep on poor pasture in many parts of the world.

The published results of much experimental work leave no doubt that urea can be very effective in increasing the voluntary intake by ruminants of low-quality roughage, sometimes by as much as 40 per cent, and that it speeds the breakdown of cellulose.

In the ruminant animal any injudicious feeding of urea will give rise to poisoning by ammonia, since it is this which the rumen bacteria convert urea into. An excess of ammonia in the rumen can cause death. It is essential, therefore, that urea is taken in small quantities over a period, and not fed a large amount at a time. 'Ideally,' Dr. E. C. Owen, of the Hannah Research Institute, emphasises, 'urea must be intimately mixed with the carbohydrates or fibrous part (or both) of the ration,' and for this reason he would strongly deprecate the direct sale of pure urea (as opposed to a commercial mix) to farmers. On the other hand, farmers who use a proprietary preparation of urea in the way advocated by Dr. M. H. Briggs should have no fears about poisoning.

Dr. R. C. Campling, of the National Institute for Research in Dairying, comments: 'When the crude protein content of the diet is about 10 per cent or over, the addition of urea would not be expected to be beneficial.' Dr. Owen agrees: 'If the ration is already adequate in protein equivalent, there will be little response.'

The crux of the matter, therefore, seems to be whether farmers can get good enough results from a ration containing urea but under 10 per cent crude protein. At the present time, many farmers seem convinced that they can, and in addition to its use in beef and sheep rations, urea is also being used as a supplement for dairy cows on a high barley diet.

There are several proprietary preparations of urea on the market; for example, Promax, Rumevite, Mozine molasses meal. Dr. M. H. Briggs writes:

'Promax is a solution of urea in mineralised molasses. It is fed in special, inexpensive ball-valve feeders which allow single licks but prevent its being drunk to excess. By this method the animals receive the urea in small amounts over a long period; and it is just these conditions that allow the maximum use to be made of the urea by the animal. Tests have shown that cows can be fed large amounts or urea in this manner with no ill effects.

'Under practical farming conditions, where optimum animal production is the aim, only 15 to 30 per cent of the dietary protein is replaced by urea.

'Urea is not merely a protein-replacer for ruminants. It also stimulates the production of cellulose-digesting organisms in the rumen, with the result that the animal can eat and efficiently digest much more cheap roughages than a protein-fed animal.'

More recently Dr. A. Eden has stated: 'Urea can be toxic if used too freely or if it is not uniformly incorporated throughout the ration. A 1 per cent usage (22 lb./ton) has not only been shown to be quite safe and, together with a cwt.

of barley, can replace a cwt. of ground nut meal in a ton diet, but also will sustain yields and milk compositional quality equal to those on more conventional feeding. Such usage may also reduce the cost of a dairy production ration, depending on the make-up of the latter and the extent to which purchased foods are being used. There appears, as yet, little evidence to show whether urea-containing diets are as fully satisfactory with really high-yielding cows.

'There is no doubt that urea has higher potentialities in the diets of fattening cattle fed virtually *ad lib.*, because this scheme of feeding lessens the risk of suddenly flushing the rumen with urea (and hence leading to ammonia poisoning) than is likely to occur in the dairy cow given large quantities of concentrates twice daily at milking times. Moreover, the protein needs of fattening cattle are less than those of the dairy cow and in the finishing diets of such cattle the level of urea can be raised to 3 per cent (67 lb./ton).'

Symptoms of urea poisoning include salivation, excitement, running and staggering, jerking of the eyeballs, and scouring.

URETER (*οὐρητήρ*) is the tube which carries the urine excreted by a kidney down to the urinary bladder. Each ureter begins at the pelvis of the corresponding kidney, passes backwards and downwards along the roof and walls of the pelvis, and finally ends by opening into the neck of the bladder. It pierces the wall of the bladder in an oblique manner so that while there is no impediment to the escape of the urine into the bladder, it is impossible for the urine to travel upwards and back to the kidney when the bladder is distended. The wall of the ureter is composed of a fibrous coat on the outside, a muscular coat in the middle, and this is lined by a mucous membrane consisting of cubical epithelium.

URETHRA (*οὐρήθρα*) is the tube which leads from the neck of the bladder to the outside, opening at the extremity of the penis in the male, and into the posterior part of the urino-genital passage in the female, and serves to conduct the urine from the bladder to the outside.

URETHRA, DISEASES OF.—Owing to its extreme shortness in the female the urethra is not subject to the same diseased conditions as in the male, where the tube is considerably longer. In fact, disease of the urethra in the female hardly ever arises except as a complication of either disease of the bladder, on the one hand, or of the vagina on the other.

Inflammation (urethritis) and stricture are the chief conditions of importance in animals.

URETHRITIS is usually brought about by a spreading of some inflammatory condition from the bladder (cystitis).

Causes.—The most frequent cause is damage by the passage of small concretions which have been formed in the bladder or kidney, and are of such a size that they are apt to be washed along the tube when urine is passed. These concretions, or calculi, often have sharp edges or projections that abrade the lining mucous membrane. Organisms obtain access and set up a painful inflammation. Septic inflammation of the walls of the bladder, brought about by various causes, may spread along the tube and involve its walls, and sepsis introduced from the outside, *e.g.* from the uterus after parturition, or from the passage of dirty instruments into the bladder, may similarly attack the urethra.

Symptoms.—In most cases of urethritis there are signs of pain and distress whenever urine is passed or when the parts are handled. The dog and cat, in which animals the condition is commonest, arch their backs, press or strain, and may emit cries. The urine, instead of coming away freely, is passed in jets or else in drops, and the act takes much longer than normally. In very severe cases there is some difficulty or stiffness when the animal walks, and the hind limbs may be straddled. The dog may lick himself, and if the orifice of the urethra be examined a small amount of blood-stained pus may be seen. In nervous animals the pain occasioned may be sufficient to cause the animal to retain its urine for long periods until the pressure in the bladder makes it imperative that micturition shall take place. In such, the distended organ can be felt through the lower posterior part of the abdominal wall. The larger animals show similar but milder symptoms.

Treatment.—This varies with the cause of the inflammation, but in all cases the administration of bland fluids, such as milk, barley-water, linseed and hay teas, is of advantage in order to flush out the urethra. Many cases that arise through the action of calculi must be treated surgically by making an artificial passage to the outside as near to the neck of the bladder as possible, and evacuating any calculi that are found in the bladder, after removing those that are lodged in the passage. Local injections, carried out by a special syringe, are of benefit when the inflammation is due to bacterial activity.

STRICTURE is an abrupt narrowing of the calibre of the tube at one or more places.

Cause.—In almost all cases of true stricture there has been some injury to the urethra or penis, resulting in the formation of scar tissue, which eventually contracts and decreases the lumen of the tube. A few cases, however, especially in the horse, are produced as the result of the pressure on or around the passage of a rapidly growing tumour.

In sheep, the injudicious use of hormones to increase liveweight gain, has killed lambs, apparently as the result of urethral obstruction. In one outbreak in the U.S.A., 2,000 out of 9,000 lambs died after receiving 12 mg. stilbœstrol by injection.

Symptoms.—If the stricture develops slowly there may be no symptoms beyond the noticeable fact that the animal takes an increasingly longer period of time to effect the passage of its water. The stream of urine gradually becomes smaller and smaller till finally it is only a mere dribble. Little or no pain is noticed, but the animal may grunt or moan in a satisfied manner after the act. If a tumour be the cause it can generally be determined by its size and position. Stricture due to the injury caused by small concretions in the urethra is accompanied by urethritis (see above), and shows symptoms as given under that heading.

Treatment.—The cure or alleviation of stricture in animals is often attended by great difficulty. Surgical procedures, consisting in the passage of bougies to dilate the narrowed parts, or in the provision of an artificial opening above the stricture, are often tried, but very often they are only temporary measures, since they themselves are productive of irritation that may result in fresh strictures at other places. Where tumours press upon the tube they are removed if they are in such a position as will allow of operation. Amputation of the penis may be necessary in rare instances.

INJURIES TO THE URETHRA may follow a severe crush or blow which causes fracture of the pelvis or of the os penis in the dog. They are usually obvious when the injury has involved the surface of the body, and may be suspected if there is an inability to pass urine, or if the urine contains blood or pus following upon a severe injury to the hind quarters of the body. The great risks of urethral injuries are abscess formation around the urethra and consequent stricture at a later period.

URIC ACID (*οὖρον*, urine) is a crystalline substance, very slightly soluble in water, white in the pure state, and found in the urine of flesh-eating animals in normal conditions. It is found in the urine of birds and reptiles, but in the vegetable feeders it is not present, or only to a trifling extent, except when the animal is being starved and is therefore living upon its own tissues. It is present in the urine of the young suckling. It is found in greatest amounts in carnivores when the diet contains foods rich in nuclein, such as sweetbreads, the roes of fishes, or other glandular substances, and in foods rich in purin bases, such as meat extract. Owing to its great insolubility, when dogs and cats are fed upon these foods to excess the uric acid is apt to become deposited as urates of sodium and potassium, and these give rise to the formation of concretions in the kidneys, bladder, or urethra. In birds fed upon a diet too rich in protein, with a view to increasing the egg-production, the uric acid is sometimes deposited in the joints, upon the surface of the liver and other abdominal organs, where it may give an appearance resembling hoar-frost, and gives rise to a goat-like condition.

URINARY ANTISEPTICS include hexylresorcinol, mandelic acid, hexamine (for acid urine; not effective in alkaline urine), buchu. (*See also* PENICILLIN.)

URINARY ORGANS (*See* KIDNEYS, URETERS, BLADDER, URETHRA.)

URINE (*urina*) is the excretion produced by the kidneys, and consists chiefly of waste substances resulting from the activity of the body, which are dissolved in water. The function of the kidneys consists almost entirely in separating these substances from the blood-stream, their actual formation taking place in the liver, muscles, etc. Urine and perspiration are to an extent interdependent in most animals, though this does not apply to the dog and cat. At the same time, the salts that are excreted by the skin are not the same as those that are found in the urine, except during disease of the kidneys. (*See* KIDNEYS.)

Most poisons taken into the body are eliminated from the system by way of the urine ; thus, quinine, morphine, chloroform, carbolic acid, iodides, and strychnine can be recognised in the urine by means of appropriate tests, while there is abundant evidence to show that during bacterial diseases the kidneys eliminate toxins.

Specific gravity.—The specific gravity of the urine of animals varies between wide limits ; for average purposes the following figures are given, though much stress cannot be placed upon gravities outside these limits unless other factors are also considered :

	Lowest.	Average.	Highest.
Horse . .	1014	1036	1050
Ox . .	1006	1020	1030
Sheep . .	1006	1010	1015
Pig . .	1003	1015	1025
Dog and Cat.	1016	—	1060

The great variation in specific gravity depends upon many factors such as temperament, exercise, food, etc., that it is necessary to enquire into the mode of life of the animal before attaching importance to such physical examination.

Reaction.—As already stated, the urine of the herbivorous animals is usually alkaline, and that of the flesh-eating animals is acid. The alkalinity in those animals of the former class is due to the salts of the organic acids that are taken in with the vegetable diet, such as malic, citric, tartaric, and succinic ; these acids are converted into carbonates in the body, and these latter are excreted in solution. In the case of some foods, such as hay and oats, an acid urine may be produced when they are fed to the horse, due in the first place to the formation of hippuric acid, and in the latter instance to the absence of vegetable organic acids in the oats. In the carnivorous animals the acidity is due to sodium acid phosphate. The pig's urine may be acid or alkaline according to the nature of its food.

Generally speaking, the acidity of the urine is increased when mineral acids are given, and the alkalinity is increased when organic acids are given, or when mineral salts are taken in larger amounts than normally.

Amount.—The quantities of urine excreted depend upon many factors, among which may be noted : season, diet, amount of water consumed, condition of the horse (horses that are in 'soft' condition perspire easily and eliminate more waste products by the skin than those that are fit ; consequently the urine in unfit horses is less than in the fit), nature of the work, secretion of milk, pregnancy, age, and size of the animal. (*See* PREGNANCY DIAGNOSIS TESTS.)

The following are average figures of the amounts taken during 24 hours :

Horse .	5	to 20 pints,	aver. 9 pints.
Ox .	10	„ 40 „	„ 22 „
Sheep .	0·5	„ 1·5 „	„ 1 „
Pig .	2·5	„ 14 „	„ 8 „
Hog .	0·75	„ 1·75 „	„ 1·25 „

Composition, colour, odour, etc.—Horse.—In this animal the urine is usually thick and turbid-looking, often having the appearance of linseed oil that has lime suspended in it. In mares during œstrum it may be almost as tenacious and sticky as the white of an egg. The odour is aromatic and characteristic, but sometimes has a faintly ammonia-like smell. In colour it is either yellowish-white, yellowish-red, or brownish.

	Rest.	Work.
Quantity . . .	8·69 pints	7·88 pints
Specific gravity .	1036	1036
Total solids . .	8·11 oz.	8·19 oz.
Organic solids . .	5·15 „	5·37 „
Inorganic solids .	2·94 „	2·82 „
Urea	3·47 „	3·47 „
Ammonium carbonate as urea . . .	0·46 „	0·46 „
Ammonia . . .	0·09 „	0·19 „
Benzoic acid . .	0·23 „	none
Hippuric acid . .	none	0·55 „
Phosphoric anhydride . . .	0·04 „	0·06 „
Sulphuric anhydride	0·37 „	0·54 „
Other sulphur compounds . . .	0·26 „	0·27 „
Chlorine . . .	1·12 „	0·77 „
Calcium oxide . .	0·12 „	0·06 „
Magnesium oxide .	0·10 „	0·09 „
Potassium oxide .	1·29 „	0·95 „
Sodium oxide . .	0·09 „	0·06 „

The table above from Smith's *Veterinary Physiology* gives the composition of equine urine during rest and work.

Ox.—In many respects the urine of the ox resembles that of the horse. It has an aromatic odour, is clear, yellow in colour, except in the working ox, where it is turbid. As a rule there are larger amounts of urea present, especially when the diet contains foods such as beans, peas, and clover hay. Hippuric acid is found in large quantities when the diet contains much cereal straws, and in working oxen. Sucking calves excrete an acid urine which is poor in solids.

Sheep discharge urine that is rich in hippuric acid, and in which the urea is in proportion to the hippuric acid in the ratio of 3: 2.

Pig.—In the pig the urine simulates a typical herbivorous urine when the diet is mainly vegetable, and a carnivorous urine when the diet contains much animal protein.

Dog.—Owing to the great variety in the diet of the dog it is not possible to give an average composition of the urine. When animal flesh is fed, uric acid appears in the urine, but on giving vegetable diet it is not found. Hippuric acid is only present in small amounts ; indican and phosphoric acid are regularly found ; glycuronic acid is often present, and a pigment or colouring matter, called bilirubin, which originates in the liver, is capable of demonstration.

Abnormal substances.—Many unusual substances are from time to time excreted in the urine, but as the detection of them is only possible in a laboratory by using expensive apparatus, they will only be mentioned here. *Albumin*, a protein compound which is normally circulating in the blood-stream, may be excreted when there is some disease of the kidneys or other organs. This gives rise to a condition known as albuminuria, which if it persists may be very serious, owing to the elimination of large amounts of albumin. *Blood* is present when there has been some injury to a part of the urinary system. *Sugar* is found in diabetes—a condition that results from disturbance of the insulin-producing mechanism of the pancreas, and it is also found in smaller amounts after an animal has been fed on a diet that is too rich in sugar. In this latter case—known as 'glycosuria'—the sugar disappears when the feeding is corrected. *Pus* and *tube-casts* are the signs of inflammation or ulceration in some part of the urinary system. Pus alone usually denotes bladder trouble only, but when casts are present the kidneys are involved. *Bile* in the urine is a sign that there is some obstruction to the outflow of bile into the intestines, and that the bile is being reabsorbed into the blood-stream and excreted by the kidneys.

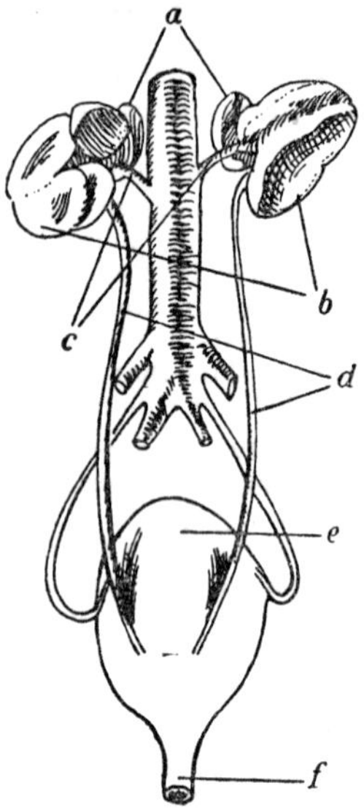

Diagram of the relations of the urinary organs of the horse. *a*, Adrenal glands ; *b*, kidneys ; *c*, renal arteries ; *d*, ureters ; *e*, urinary bladder ; *f*, commencement of urethra. The termination of the abdominal aorta is also shown lying between the kidneys.

URINE, ABNORMAL CONDITIONS ASSOCIATED WITH.—Oliguria means a diminution in the amount of urine secreted. It may be due to kidney disease, heart disease—in which the blood-pressure falls and the amount of blood passing through the kidneys is less than usual, impeded kidney circulation—from pressure of tumours or other tissues upon the renal vessels, or from great withdrawals of fluid from the body generally—as in dropsy, severe hæmorrhage, diarrhœa, etc.

Anuria is absence of urine. It may be *obstructive*, when some structural or diseased condition blocks the urinary passages—such as a calculus in the urethra—or *suppressive*, when the actual secretion of urine does not occur, through some severe diseased conditions in both kidneys, or in acute poisoning by turpentine or phosphorus. In both varieties of anuria the serious exigency of uræmia may supervene unless relief is afforded. (*See* 'Uræmia' *and* 'Retention of Urine', both under this section.)

Polyuria signifies an increase in the secretion of urine, especially as regards its water content. It occurs when a larger amount of blood than usual passes through the kidneys, when the blood-pressure is high, when the amount of water taken into the body is greatly in excess of the requirements, when the renal cells are influenced by certain chemical stimulants, such as medicinal doses of spirits of ether, turpentine, resin, etc., in some obscure nervous diseases, and in diabetes. The term is sometimes applied to the condition which results from the eating of mouldy or mow-burnt hay, but the term 'diabetes insipidus' is more correct. In this condition the excessive discharge of urine coincides with the feeding of damaged food-stuffs, and usually ceases when they are discontinued. In the more severe form of diabetes (called 'diabetes mellitus'), which is due to a disturbance in the pancreas, the quantity of urine secreted is not influenced in the same way by the feeding. The fact that the urine in diabetes mellitus contains sugar, while in diabetes insipidus it does not, is responsible for the preference shown by flies for the urine passed during attacks of the former disease.

Albuminuria, which means that albumin is present in the urine, is indicative of kidney disease, but it is most probable that some cases are physiological, especially in the dog and the pig. It is certain that it may occur in almost all animals and man during great muscular fatigue, but it is transitory in such cases. Otherwise, persistent excretion of albumin denotes some lesion of the kidney tissues. Normally only salts and water are excreted by the kidneys, and the colloidal substances are retained in the circulating blood. (The mucus present in urine is added by the glands in the ureters, bladder, and urethra.) When some inflammatory condition occurs which involves either the glomeruli or the epithelial cells of the tubules, albumin is allowed to pass out from the blood into the urine and becomes lost to the body. Among other diseases than those affecting the kidneys may be mentioned internal hæmorrhage, spinal or cerebral meningitis, myelitis, and many of the bacterial diseases in which poisons are produced in the system. In azoturia a certain amount of albumin can be demonstrated in the urine, but there still remains some considerable doubt as to the method of its production and its importance.

Hæmaturia signifies the presence of blood in the urine. (It must not be confused with the red colouration of urine which follows the use of phenothiazine.) It may be produced during such diseases as piroplasmosis and purpura hæmorrhagica; it is often seen in morbid conditions of the kidneys, ureters, bladder, and urethra, especially when there is acute inflammation or injury by stone or gravel; it follows the administration of large doses of carbolic acid, turpentine, or cantharides; and it may occur when the kidneys are infested with parasites. The urine varies from a smoky brownish colour to a deep dark porter colour. In some cases where the hæmorrhage has occurred into the bladder blood-clots may be passed, and in most cases when the urine is allowed to stand in a glass vessel a deposit consisting of red blood-cells and cell envelopes is thrown down.

Hæmoglobinuria is the condition in which the red blood pigment—hæmoglobin—is present in the urine. It is due to a breaking down of the red blood-cells in the blood-stream. It occurs in trypanosomiasis, piroplasmosis, and azoturia, as well as after the giving of large doses of potassium chlorate, phenacetin, etc. The urine is red, brownish-red, or porter-coloured, and shows a heavy brownish-red sediment on standing, but contains no red blood-cells or cell envelopes. (It must be distinguished from the red colouration of urine which follows the administration of phenothiazine.)

Pyuria is the name that is given to the presence of pus in the urine. It occurs when there is abscess formation or some purulent condition in the urinary tract.

Glycosuria means sugar in the urine. (*See* DIABETES MELLITUS.)

Oxaluria means an excess of oxalic acid in the urine, and occurs during indigestion and emaciation.

Phosphaturia means an excess of phosphates in the urine, and seems to be associated with certain bone diseases, such as rickets, in which, although the food contains quantities of phosphates, the body is unable to make use of them, probably on account of the absence or deficiency of vitamins.

Lipuria means fat in the urine. It occurs in fatty degeneration of the kidney.

Uræmia (*see under* this heading).

Retention of the urine is the phrase that is used to mean the condition in which urine is duly secreted by the kidneys but is retained in the bladder for some reason.

When the kidneys fail to produce urine the term 'suppression of the urine' is used.

Causes.—Urine may be retained in the bladder because its walls are too weak to expel it, or because there is some obstruction in its passage to the outside. Inability of the walls of the bladder to contract is usually due to some injury or disease of the spinal centres that govern micturition, though when total paralysis occurs the opposite condition 'incontinence' is generally evident. In this latter condition the muscle that should close the passage at the neck of the bladder is paralysed and the sphincter lies flaccid, offering no hindrance to the exit of the urine. Retention may also follow operations in the vicinity of the bladder, when the sphincter is thrown into a state of spasmodic contraction and refuses to dilate. This is particularly seen in nervous highly strung animals. It may occur during conditions of stress—such as travelling by rail, long confinement in unfamiliar surroundings, etc.; or from pressure by neighbouring structures—such as inflammation and enlargement of the prostate gland, impaction of the rectum with hard dry fæces, and during prolonged parturition in females. In other cases the urethra becomes blocked—either by tumour or calculus, or from contraction of the fibrous tissue that is formed after inflammatory conditions of this part—a contingency known as 'stricture'. (*See* URETHRA, DISEASES OF.)

Symptoms.—These vary in almost every case. In many animals no symptoms beyond a general dullness, disinclination for movement, and signs of discomfort in the abdomen, can be discovered. In others acute pain may be evinced whenever the region of the bladder is handled, while in the most severe cases uræmic symptoms may appear. (See earlier in this section.) Accurate diagnosis depends upon the manipulation of the posterior part of the abdomen from the outside in small animals, and upon rectal examinations of the pelvis in the larger creatures. In both instances the greatly distended bladder will be felt as a pear-shaped fluctuating but tense mass in the situation mentioned. If it be gently pressed the animal may cry out in pain.

Treatment.—Cases in which the bladder is unable to expel its contents are treated by the passage of a catheter along the urethra and into the cavity of the organ. It may be necessary to repeat this procedure at 4-hourly intervals until the tone is restored to the muscular walls. Where obstructions in the urethra are concerned they are removed or corrected. (*See* URETHRA, DISEASES OF.) Constipation should be relieved by enemata of warm soapy water. Enlargement of the prostate requires the passage of the catheter immediately, and subsequent unilateral or total castration. In other cases, hot packs or fomentations over the lower posterior part of the abdomen, or the administration of belladonna to relieve spasm. Professional advice should always be sought promptly.

URINOMETER (*οὖρον*, urine; *μέτρον'* measure) is an instrument designed for the estimation of the specific gravity of urine.

UROLITHIASIS.—The formation of stones or sandy material in the urinary system. (*See* CALCULI, *and* p. 964 under STRICTURE.)

UROTROPINE (*see* HEXAMINE).

URTICARIA, or 'NETTLE RASH', is a disease of the skin in which small areas of the surface become raised into weals of varying sizes. It occurs in horses, cattle (when it is often called 'blaines'), pigs, and dogs.

Causes.—The condition is not necessarily specific. It may follow exposure to the leaves of the stinging nettle (hence one of its names); insect bites may produce it; it is associated with dietetic errors in which too much protein is fed and an insufficiency of exercise is provided; it may occur during the course of certain specific conditions, such as purpura, dourine, influenza, etc., and it is sometimes seen in fat horses that are called upon to perform some more vigorous exercise than usual, become heated, and are suddenly cooled by a shower of rain. Urticaria is sometimes of an allergic nature. Indigestion and salt poisoning are also blamed for its production in swine. Factitious urticaria, common in the dog but not recorded in the cat, is a term for an abnormal tendency for the skin to weal when rubbed or scratched.

Symptoms.—As a rule there is little to be seen beyond the local swellings on the skin. These may vary in size from a pea to a walnut, and are generally more or less almond-shaped. They are not irritable unless caused by bites or stings, are painless to the touch, show no oozing discharge, are scattered irregularly over the whole body, and sometimes involve the skin of the eyelids, nostrils, throat, and perineum.

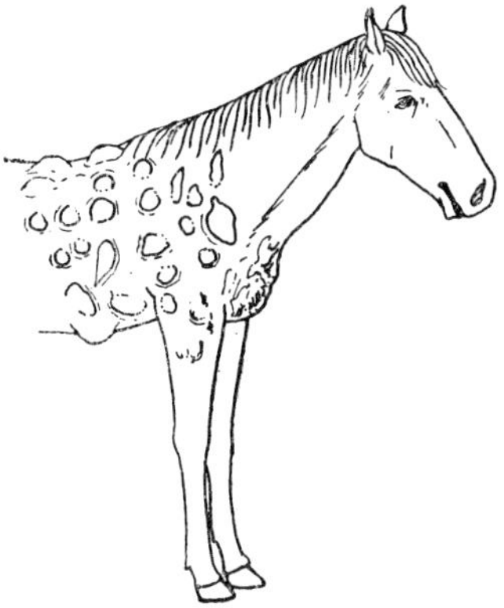

Diagram of a horse severely affected with urticaria. In the majority of cases the swellings are not so large as those shown in the diagram, but they are more numerous.

In cattle especially they may attain a great size in the throat region and produce difficulty in breathing.

Prevention.—Horses that are not in full work, and those that are given a holiday, should have their corn rations decreased. It may be necessary to give fat horses some exercise when they are not at work.

Treatment.—Consists in the use of antihistamines (which see), a laxative, a light diet, and gentle exercise. An antibiotic may be used to prevent infection occurring.

UTERINE INFECTIONS.—These are discussed under UTERUS, DISEASES OF and under INFERTILITY. A list of the principal organisms which infect the uterus in the various species is given under ABORTION; but in the **mare** a survey carried out in 1964 by Lord Porchester's Veterinary Committee, for the Thoroughbred Breeders' Association, showed the following results:

	Barren	Foaling	Maiden	All Mares
	1208	2162	258	3628
Negative swabs	912 (75·6%)	1784 (82·2%)	238 (92·2%)	2934 (80·8%)
Positive swabs	296 (24·4%)	378 (17·8%)	20 (7·8%)	694 (19·2%)

	Per cent	Approx. percentages of all Mares Swabbed
Beta-hæmolytic Streptococcal infections	49	9·3
Klebsiella pneumoniæ	8	1·6
Escherichia coli and coliforms	16	3·3
Pathogenic staphylococci	11	2·0
Corynebacterium sp.	3	0·6
Mixed infections	10	1·9
Fungal infections (all types)	3	0·6

Abortion caused by the virus of Equine Rhinopneumonitis has also occurred in the U.K. for several years; most outbreaks being associated with imported or visiting mares.

UTERUS, also called 'womb', 'calf-bed', etc., is the structure that in the female receives and nourishes the developing young. It is a Y-shaped hollow muscular organ consisting of a body and two horns or 'cornua', and is lined by an elaborate mucous membrane which presents special features in different species of animals. The uterus lies in the abdomen below the rectum and at a higher level than the bladder. It becomes continuous with the vagina posteriorly. Its most posterior portion, known as the 'cervix', usually lies partly in the pelvis. From the tip of each horn to the ovary on the corresponding side runs the Fallopian tube or oviduct, which conducts the ova from the ovary into the uterus.

In the human female the body is large, and horns for practical purposes do not exist. In rabbits the two horns open into the vagina separately. The uteruses of domesticated animals are intermediate between these types. (See later.) The walls consist of three coats—a peritoneal covering on the outside continuous with the rest of the peritoneum; a thick muscular wall arranged in two layers, the fibres on the outside being longitudinal and those on the inside circular; the innermost coat is mucous membrane. This latter is very important, since it is by its agency that the ovum and the sperms are nourished before they fuse, and it is through the mucous membrane that nutrients and oxygen are conveyed from dam to fœtus, and that much of the waste products leave the fœtal circulation to pass into the maternal blood-stream. It consists of epithelial cells, amongst which lie the uterine glands which secrete the so-called 'uterine milk' which serves to nourish the newly fertilised ovum.

The most posterior extremity of the uterus is called the 'os uteri', and this forms the opening into the 'cervix uteri', which is a thick-walled canal guarding entrance into the cavity of the body of the uterus. Normally this is almost or completely shut, but during œstrum it slackens, and during parturition it becomes fully opened to allow exit of the fœtus. The uterus is held in position by means of a fold of peritoneum attached to the roof of the abdomen, which carries blood-vessels, nerves, etc. This is known as the 'broad ligament'; it is capable of a considerable amount of stretching.

The Mare.—The shape of the uterus of the mare most nearly approaches that of the human being. It possesses a large body and comparatively small horns. During pregnancy the fœtus generally lies in horns and body to an equal extent. The mucous membrane is corrugated into folds.

The Cow.—The body is less in size than the horns, which are long, tapering, and curved downwards, outwards, backwards, and upwards to end within the pelvis at about the level of the cervix. The fœtus lies in the body and one horn in single pregnancy, and when twins are present each usually occupies one horn and a part of the body. The mucous membrane presents upon its inner surface a large number (100 upwards) of mushroom-shaped projections, called 'cotyledons'. The fœtal membranes are attached to the dome-like free surface of the cotyledons, in which are a large number of crypts, which receive projections called 'villi' from the outer surface of the chorion.

The ewe's uterus is similar to that of the cow except that it is smaller and that the cotyledons are cup-shaped. In the sheep, where twin pregnancy is the rule, one lamb lies in one horn of the uterus and the second in the other horn.

The pig has a small uterine body and a pair of long convoluted horns that resemble pieces of intestine. The mucous membrane is ridged but has no cotyledons. The young lie in the horns only.

The bitch and cat have uteri with comparatively short bodies and long straight divergent horns that run towards the kidneys of the corresponding sides.

Functions.—The uterus is concerned entirely with the production of young. It nourishes the ovum until it has been fertilised by the sperm from the male, and thereafter it gives protection and nourishment to the developing fœtus until such time as it is ready for expulsion, when, by powerful contractions of its muscular walls, it expels the young and the membranes.

During pregnancy the walls are greatly thickened and distended, and after parturition they rapidly return to their normal size by a process known as 'involution'. (*See* PARTURITION.)

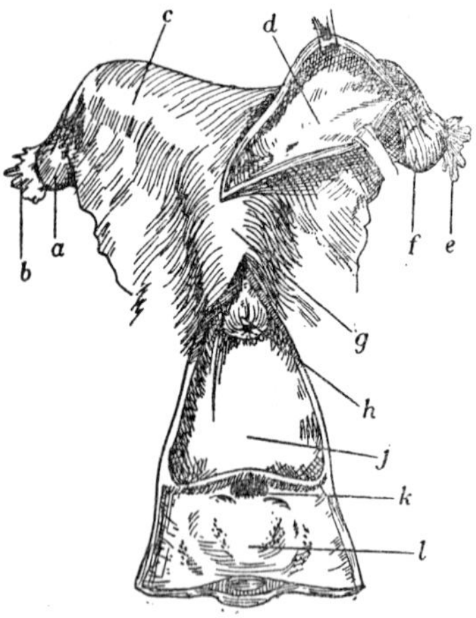

Diagram of the generative organs of the mare, seen from above. The vagina and vulva have been laid open by an incision along their upper parts, and the right horn of the uterus has been incised. *a*, Left ovary; *b*, fimbriated end of left oviduct; *c*, left horn; *d*, right horn of uterus laid open; *e*, end of right oviduct; *f*, right ovary; *g*, body of uterus; *h*, cervix; *j*, vaginal interior; *k*, opening of urethra from urinary bladder; *l*, interior of vulva.

UTERUS, DISEASES OF.—Since the uterus is connected with the vagina which has a direct opening to the outside of the body it is liable to become infected with pathogenic organisms. This is particularly the case during and after difficult parturitions, where *manual* assistance has had to be rendered; and when the fœtal membranes, not becoming expelled in the normal manner, undergo disintegration and decomposition. The walls of the organ are consequently susceptible to sepsis and its consequences. Moreover, owing to the strenuous part it plays during pregnancy and parturition, it is apt to become diseased, displaced, or injured as the result of the weight of the body of the fœtus.

INFLAMMATION OF THE UTERUS; Metritis; Puerperal fever. This may be either *acute* or *chronic*. It may involve the whole organ, or be localised to the cervix only (*cervicitis*). It may affect the mucous membrane only (*endometritis*); it may attack this and the muscular walls (*mesometritis*); it may be localised to the peritoneum (*parametritis*), or all three coats may be inflamed (*polymetritis*). Large amounts of pus may collect in the cavity of the organ as the result of chronic inflammation, when the term *pyometra* is used. (*See also* WHITE HEIFER DISEASE.)

A list of uterine infections giving rise to infertility and abortion in the various species will be found under ABORTION.

Inflammations of the uteri of the domesticated animals and their treatment demand such precise knowledge and special skill that little more than a general description can be given here.

The Mare.—ACUTE METRITIS. This may occur either before or after foaling. When it takes place prior to the act it is usually associated with the death of the foal and its subsequent abortion, with or without discharge of the whole or a part of the membranes. In such cases the inflammatory condition may persist in an acute form and cause the death of the mare, or it may assume a chronic form after the abortion and render the mare incapable of further breeding; other cases are followed by recovery. Acute metritis occurring after normal foaling may arise through the conveyance of septic material into the uterus by the arms or hands of the attendants, or by the ropes, instruments, or other appliances that are used to assist the birth of the foal, or it may be the direct result of retained membranes that undergo bacterial decomposition. In this connection it should be noted that it is very often the placental membrane that occupies the non-pregnant part of the uterus that is retained, while the remainder separates and is expelled to the outside in the normal manner. Since the membranes are all in one piece, the large mass that occupied the pregnant part hangs to the outside attached to the portion that is still retained in the non-pregnant part of the uterus. After a time the movements of the mare, along with the great weight of the extruded portion, cause a rupture between these parts; the pendant bulk falls to the ground, while the unseparated portion remains inside. This latter soon putrefies, and septic material from it finds its way into the rest of the organ, where it easily sets up inflammation. This can be more readily understood when it is remembered that there is a large area of uterine mucous membrane (15 to 20 square feet) which has been recently denuded of placental membrane, and which virtually possesses no protective epithelium. Septic and necrotic material lying upon such a surface rapidly infects the living tissue and produces an intense inflammation. The importance of this occurrence cannot be over-estimated, for the discharge of a large bulk of fœtal membrane induces in the layman's mind a sense of false security; he is apt to consider that no membrane remains behind, and therefore to under-estimate the gravity of succeeding phenomena.

Symptoms.—Acute metritis is a severe and often fatal condition. Within 24 to 48 hours of the commencement of the inflammation, the mare becomes greatly distressed and loses all interest in the foal. She lies most of the time and refuses food; her temperature is usually very high when taken in the vagina, but lower in the rectum owing to the admission of cold air through a slack anus; the pulse is full and fast in the early stages, but soon becomes soft and weak. A variable amount of dirty greyish blood-flecked discharge escapes from the vagina and soils the tail and hind-quarters. After a day or two, or sometimes simultaneously with the appearance of other symptoms, the mare becomes tucked up in her abdomen and stands with her back arched. When made to move she is seen to be very stiff and awkward, and has difficulty in raising her feet from the ground. When this happens it indicates that inflammation of the sensitive laminæ of the foot has taken place—a condition known as 'parturient laminitis'. (*See* LAMINITIS.) A mare affected in this way has little chance of recovery, and death usually terminates such a case in from 2 to 6 days. Complications, such as peritonitis, pneumonia, inflammation of the bladder, vagina, rectum, or udder, abscess formation in neighbouring organs, etc., are liable to develop, and serve to militate against recovery. Some uncomplicated cases recover when they are treated with penicillin and/or sulpha drugs in the early stages, and when the mare possesses great powers of resistance. A certain percentage pass into the chronic types and persist for weeks.

Prevention is of much greater importance and application than actual curative treatment. During foaling and after the act the greatest attention should be paid to the cleanliness of everything that is to come into contact with the genital tract of the mare. The attendant's finger nails should be trimmed short, and his hands and arms should be well scrubbed with soap and water containing some disinfectant, such as Dettol or Jeyes' fluid. Finally the hand and arm should be lubricated with a suitable preparation marketed for this purpose. All appliances that are to be used should be boiled and kept in a pail of hot water when not actually in use. It is most inadvisable to allow any one whose hands and arms are not cleansed and disinfected to handle instruments that are to be used within the passages of the mare. It should be remembered that the litter, mangers, walls, etc., in a loose-box—although they appear perfectly clean to the naked eye—are invariably contaminated with germs and dust.

One other factor is of the greatest importance. After a mare foals the fœtal membranes should be given attention. Normally they are discharged by means of a few comparatively mild labour pains within an hour of the birth of the foal. If they are retained for longer than this period the person in attendance should suspect that something may be wrong and give continual attention to the mare. It may happen that they will come away by themselves in a short while, in which case they should be laid on the ground and disentangled as far as possible so as to ensure that they are complete. In other cases a series of violent pains may commence, when the bulk of the membranes are passed to the outside, where they hang suspended. Should this happen a sack or sheet should be placed under the dependent mass, and held by two men so as to support the weight and relieve the tension on that portion that is still retained in the uterus. This is necessary lest the weight of the external membranes causes a tearing away from the non-separated part. *Gentle traction* should now be exerted upon the imprisoned portion, and as a rule it will gradually detach itself and come to the outside. If no progress is made, veterinary assistance should be sought promptly. Injections of pituitrin or stilbœstrol may obviate manual removal of the fœtal membranes. When this has to be done and veterinary assistance is not available the hand should be cleansed, dis infected, and lubricated, and the external parts of the mare washed with soap and water. The hand and arm are gently inserted, and explore the cavity until the place of non-separation is discovered. The membranes should now be gently separated from the uterine wall by the closed fingers used as a kind of lever. This operation demands the greatest care, and should only be undertaken by the unskilled in places overseas where veterinary assistance is not available. Any force or violence may result in severe hæmorrhage or even rupture of the wall of the uterus—two very serious contingencies. Regarding complete retention of the fœtal membranes—when only a very small portion is seen hanging from the vagina—measures for their removal, as indicated above, should be undertaken if there is no sign of any attempt at expulsion within from 4 to 6 hours after foaling, Generally speaking, membranes that have remained in position for 8 to 12 hours are commencing to decompose, and decomposition means bacterial infection of the uterus (*i.e.* metritis) in almost every case.

Treatment.—The case must be considered most serious. The use of antibiotics or one of the sulpha drugs is indicated. The treatment also aims at keeping up the strength and vitality of the mare, and removing purulent and necrotic material from the uterus by means of douching and syphonage. The mare is housed in a warm, dry, well-ventilated loose-box, provided with plenty of clean litter and water to drink. One or two rugs should be applied, and a hot salt bag, or a blanket wrung out of hot water, may give ease when applied over the loins and quarters. The foal may be left with the mare so long as it does not annoy her by trying to suck the empty udder, but it will need hand-feeding every three or four hours. The food of the mare (provided she can be tempted to eat) should be light and easily digested. In spite of this ideal, if she can be induced to eat other heavier foods she should be given small amounts of these, rather than that she be allowed to fast. Strychnine or caffeine, given by hypodermic injection, will stimulate a sluggish heart and overcome depression. Any retained portions of fœtal membrane must be removed from the uterus by hand and as much discharge as possible cleared out. A solution of acriflavine, proflavine, or brilliant green, 1 part in 1000 of boiled water, or some other suitable non-irritant antiseptic solution at blood heat, is douched into the cavity of the uterus by a length of rubber tubing, and, after allowing it to act for 2 to 5 minutes, is syphoned off. A special two-way tube is sometimes used for this purpose—the solution entering by one channel and leaving by the other. When all the fluid has been removed a pessary of iodoform may be inserted. When complications such as laminitis or pneumonia co-exist, they must receive separate attention. (*See* LAMINITIS, PNEUMONIA, etc.)

CHRONIC METRITIS.—Under this heading are included a number of more or less similar conditions which vary in some respects, but have a common feature in that they are all associated with the production of large or small quantities of muco-purulent discharge. This may either collect in the cavity of the uterus, causing distension of that organ, and a consequent enlargement of the abdomen, or it may escape by way of the cervix and vagina to the outside—perhaps almost continually, or perhaps periodically. In some cases abscesses are formed in the walls of the organ.

Causes.—Chronic metritis may originate as a sequel to an acute attack in some cases, but more commonly it is directly due to an injury or infection which is not sufficiently severe to produce an acute attack. At any rate, pus-forming organisms gain entrance into the uterus, and, by multiplication and tissue destruction, form greater or lesser quantities of pus. In certain cases the death and consequent maceration of the fœtus may produce chronic metritis.

Symptoms.—Individual cases show variations in the symptoms they present. As a rule there is a general unthriftiness following upon foaling. The mare's appetite is capricious, but her thirst is unimpaired. The temperature fluctuates a degree or two above normal. There may or may not be a dirty, sticky, grey, or pus-like discharge from the vagina, which causes irritation and frequent erections of the clitoris. Urine is passed in small amounts at frequent intervals, and is sometimes accompanied by arching of the back and straining. The mare resents handling of the genital organs, but if the lips of the vulva are gently separated the mucous membrane is seen to be inflamed and swollen. In other cases the pus collects in the cavity of the uterus and is retained there through closure of the os. This eventually leads to a distension of the organ, and if the condition is severe the abdomen becomes enlarged. During such a case it sometimes happens that after the pus has collected for a certain period the os suddenly opens and a gallon or more of pus is discharged. The os then closes once more; no further evacuation takes place until at some future time, when, the pressure having again risen, the process is repeated. The intervals between these evacuations may vary from a few days to 3 or 4 weeks. The mare's general condition shows an improvement immediately following a sudden discharge of pus, but as it re-accumulates she relapses into her former chronic state. Chronic metritis may get gradually worse, and the mare dies. Cases taken in time usually recover with treatment, but further breeding is often impossible.

Treatment.—It is necessary to attempt to keep up the strength and vitality of the mare by a suitable variety and quality in the food offered. In this connection cows' milk—especially newly calved cows' milk, which contains colostrum—is very useful. It is sometimes the only nutritive food that the mare can be tempted to take. Otherwise she should be offered food that is nutritive, laxative, and easily digested, and in small amounts at a time. An unlimited quantity of clean cold water should be supplied. The loose-box should be warm, well ventilated, and thickly littered. One or two rugs are required to keep up the body heat and prevent chills when the weather is cold and the mare's temperature is high, but in mild weather they can be dispensed with. An early opportunity should be taken to evacuate the pus from the uterus, by douching and syphonage, or by irrigation as already described under acute metritis. Sulpha drugs or antibiotics may be used. Small doses of salts are necessary to ensure elimination of effete materials by the bowels and kidneys.

If the foal is alive it may be kept with the dam provided it does not annoy her, but as her milk secretion invariably falls off in quality and quantity it will be necessary to hand-feed it.

It must be emphasised that no one line of treatment is equally applicable to all cases of chronic metritis; as in all serious inflammatory conditions, expert advice should be sought at the earliest opportunity.

The Cow.—Inflammations of the uterus of this animal are essentially the same as those of the mare, but there are certain differences that must be noted. In the following brief account much of what has been said in relation to the mare must be understood to apply to the cow as well, and only the main differences will be stated.

ACUTE METRITIS.—In some cases where birth of the calf has taken place easily and naturally, metritis supervenes in the course of the first week or ten days after calving, but in the majority of cases there has been some injury or infection at, or shortly after, parturition. Retention of the fœtal membranes, which is so much more common in the cow than in other animals, is very often the contributory factor to an attack of acute metritis. The dismemberment of the fœtus prior to birth—a difficult and often dangerous procedure—is another common cause. Inertia of the walls of the organ, exposure to chills and draughts before involution has occurred, and the conveyance of infection from an already existing case to other parturient cows by the hands and arms of the byre attendant, in his capacity of accoucheur, are other causes.

Symptoms.—The cow generally becomes obviously affected between the second and eighth day after calving. The vulval lips swell and are painful when touched, the lining membrane of the vagina is intensely reddened and swollen. There are frequent and painful attempts at the passage of urine, the temperature rises to 107° F. or 108° F., the appetite is lost and there is a gritting of the teeth, rumination is suppressed, the pulse is hard and fast, the milk secretion falls off or stops altogether, and the udder becomes soft and loose; the horns and feet are hot and the membranes of the eye are intensely injected with blood. The cow may lie in the early stages, but when the inflammation is at its height she stands continually. She paddles with her hind feet, may kick at her belly, and often turns and gazes at her flanks. Lameness may appear in one or both of the hind feet. A discharge appears at the vulva; this is at first clear and sticky, but soon becomes yellowish, reddish, and finally chocolate-coloured. In the later stages it is very thick, and has a persistent and objectionable smell. Relapses are common, and the cow may be almost better when she suddenly takes a turn for the worse, and dies after severe shivering fits and great depression.

Treatment.—Acute metritis in the cow should be looked upon as a contagious disease and all precautions taken to prevent infection being conveyed to other cows that are soon due to calve. The litter, discharges, membranes, etc., from a case should be burned or buried away from the byre. As a preventive, scrupulous cleanliness should be observed by attendants giving assistance at calving, as given under previous heading for the mare.

Actual treatment is similar to that as applied to the mare. Retained fœtal membranes are removed, the uterus is cleansed by douching and syphonage, etc., and penicillin and/or sulpha drugs administered, and antiseptic pessaries may be inserted. Hot fomentations to the abdomen may be useful to check undue straining and severe pain. The bowels must be kept loose. The strength of the patient should receive every attention, and internally medicines to promote increased heart action, peristalsis, and antisepsis, may be given.

CHRONIC METRITIS very often follows an acute attack in the cow. The animal partially recovers, the more acute symptoms subside, and there is apparently little or no pain. The general health, however, remains indifferent. Milk secretion does not continue, flesh is lost, there is either a constant or an intermittent discharge from the vulva, which soils the tail and hind-quarters, and has in many cases a putrid smell. Chronic metritis in the cow may be due to infection with *Brucella abortus* (*see* CONTAGIOUS ABORTION), *Trichomonas fœtus*, *Corynebacterium pyogenes*, or *Vibrio fœtus*, amongst other organisms.

Another form of chronic metritis that attacks cattle is seen in virgin heifers that have never bred.

Pyometra may arise in cases of trichomoniasis.

Treatment of chronic metritis in the cow is much the same as that in the mare, but *see also under* HORMONE THERAPY.

The Ewe, Sow, and Goat.—What has been said in respect to the larger animals applies to these animals to a great extent. It should be remembered that flesh from an animal that is suffering from a severe inflammatory condition, such as metritis, is not suited for human food. (*See also* SOW'S MILK, ABSENCE OF.)

The Bitch and Cat.—In these carnivores, owing to the diffused placenta, and to the consequent sudden stripping bare of protective covering of a large surface, inflammation of the uterus is very prone to follow protracted or difficult parturition, especially when manual assistance from unskilled persons has been undertaken. As in other animals, an acute and a chronic form are recognised.

ACUTE METRITIS.—This is as common as the chronic form, which is, however, the more spectacular. Acute manifestations follow exposure to chills and draughts, difficult or prolonged whelpings, and retention of one or more fœtal membrane. The membrane most commonly retained is that which belonged to the fœtus that was born last and occupied the extremity of one of the horns of the uterus.

Symptoms.—The onset of inflammation of the uterus generally occurs within a week after whelping, but some cases are delayed a little longer than this, especially in cats. As in other animals, there is a painful swollen condition of the vulva, and the animal—as a response to the pain stimulus—licks itself. After a short time signs of general fever appear ; these are denoted by a rise in temperature, increased pulse and respiration rates, dullness, disinclination for movement, and an absence of appetite. Cats and dogs seem to get ease from the pain by sitting crouched in an upright position on their hocks and elbows, and this posture is almost continually assumed. A discharge appears at the vulva ; sometimes this is white or grey like pus from a wound, sometimes it is blood-stained, and at other times it is dark brown and contains particles of decomposing membrane ; in most cases it has an objectionable putrid smell. Vomiting may occur. The secretion of milk ceases and the puppies or kittens become clamorous for food. The sides of the abdomen are held tense and rigid, and any attempt at handling these parts is resisted. The animal may groan or grunts if the flanks are firmly pressed between the hands. Severe constipation is very common and important in the carnivores. The passage of fæces is always a very much more deliberate and prolonged process than in herbivores, and necessitates a characteristic position and a certain amount of abdominal effort. Both of these factors cause an increased pressure upon the inflamed uterus, and the animal will often forgo the act rather than suffer the acute agony it occasions. Quantities of fæcal material collect in the large intestines, and the absorption of waste products begins. The illness increases and she becomes rapidly exhausted by the vomiting. Death usually ensues in such cases. It is preceded by a considerable rise in temperature ; a fall follows, coma (unconsciousness) sets in, and in a short time the animal expires in convulsions. In cases that progress favourably any carelessness or oversight on the part of the attendant is liable to be followed by a severe relapse.

Treatment.—The use of antibiotics or sulphonamides is important. The uterus is syringed out with non-irritant antiseptics such as acriflavine solution and pituitrin or ergotin given hypodermically. Pessaries of iodoform or chinosol may be introduced into the uterus. The feeding must receive great attention. Failure to retain foods upon the stomach points to absorption of toxins, or to constipation. (*See* NURSING, NORMAL SALINE, ANTIBIOTICS.) The puppies or kittens should be removed from their mother, and may be reared either by hand or through the agency of a foster-mother.

CHRONIC METRITIS is very common in the smaller animals, and is sometimes the sequel of an acute attack that has never completely cleared up. The cervix remains closed in most cases, so that the uterus becomes filled with pus (PYOMETRA) and the abdomen consequently enlarges. It is this increase in size that first draws attention to the condition, as a rule. The animal is often thought to be pregnant, or dropsy is suspected. A manual examination usually reveals the true condition. There are some cases in which periodic or continuous discharges take place from the vulva, and the uterus does not fill. In other respects chronic metritis resembles what is seen in the other animals, and what has been already described.

Treatment.—In cases of pyometra where some pus is coming away a course of pituitrin injections may be useful and it may be tried even where the cervix is closed. (*See* PITUITRIN.) Stilbœstrol is an alternative. (*See* HORMONE THERAPY.) A two-way catheter may be used to wash out the pus. Penicillin or acriflavine may be used for irrigation of the uterus, and antibiotics or sulphonamides systemically. Success has been reported following the use of quinine by mouth. Ovario-hysterectomy is indicated in a number of cases but should not be postponed until toxæmia is far advanced or the animal too weak to stand the operation. Shock is severe.

STRICTURE OF THE CERVIX is one of the results of an inflammatory condition of this part. When inflammation has been severe a certain amount of fibrous tissue is laid down around the canal, and, after recovery from the more primary inflammation, this contracts and causes a narrowing of the passage. The stricture may be so acute as to completely occlude the lumen of the cervix, and therefore to prevent conception ; or, in less serious cases, it may only offer actual hindrance when the fœtus is being born. (*See* 'RINGWOMB'.)

Treatment is surgical, and consists in forcible dilatation with special instruments, or, in bad cases, in making a series of incisions into its walls.

TUMOURS of the uterus are not common in the domesticated animals. When present they may cause no symptoms until parturition is imminent, when they may partially or completely obstruct the birth of the young animal. Their treatment depends upon their situation. If far forward and not large they may be left alone. If pedunculated (provided with a stalk) and situated in the posterior parts they are usually easily removed. Occasionally, when malignant tumours are present in the smaller animals, it may be advisable to remove the whole of the uterus. This, however, is unfortunately often followed by the rapid growth of a new tumour in some other part of the body. The varieties that have been found include carcinoma, lipomata, myomata, and papillomata.

PROLAPSE of the uterus, inversion, or procidence, means a partial or complete turning-inside-out of the organ, in which the inside comes to the outside through the lips of the vulva and hangs down, sometimes as far as the hocks. When the displacement is only slight nothing may be seen at the outside—as *e.g.* when one horn only is inverted into the body of the uterus. It is most common in ruminants, less frequent in the mare, and not often seen in the bitch or sow.

Causes.—In many instances it is not possible to point to any causal factor. The displacement may have occurred in animals that have given birth normally and without undue straining, as well as in those that have had a difficult parturition. It occasionally takes place during the birth of the young animal, but is more often seen a short time afterwards. Injudicious traction upon retained fœtal membranes when the uterus is in a flaccid and dilated state, by an attendant who attempts to hasten their expulsion, is one cause.

Symptoms.—With an incomplete inversion, the uterine horn that carried the fœtus becomes turned in upon itself like the finger of a glove, but it remains inside the passages, and nothing is seen to the outside. The animal is distressed for a time, paws the ground, stamps, lies and rises from the ground frequently, and a series of mild or violent labour pains occurs. She may settle down in a short while, but in a few hours she generally has a repeated attack, when the bulk of the uterus will be expelled to the outside of the body. In the early stages of such a case the real nature of the condition is seldom suspected. On the other hand, the animal may present a picture of great extremity. Hanging from the vulva is a large pear-shaped mass, or tumour, covered with intensely inflamed purple coloured mucous membrane, wounded and torn in parts, with a dirty putrid discharge upon its surface, and with pieces of litter, fæces, and rubbish adhering to it. The animal is highly fevered, strains continually and violently, and rapidly passes into a state of exhaustion which is but the prelude to unconsciousness and death. Between these two extremes there is every variety in the appearance and intensity of the symptoms.

The state of the mucous membrane lining of the uterus, which in the prolapse is of course on the outside of the mass, serves as a rough guide to the length of time that has elapsed since the accident occurred. For the first two or three hours the mucous membrane appears moist and of a reddish or brownish colour over the whole surface in the mare and sow. It usually shows small abrasions and excoriations where it has received damage during parturition or after the prolapse. In the cow, sheep, and goat, the general surface is red or pink, but the cotyledons show as deep-red mushroom-like eminences scattered over the outside of the tumour. In the bitch and cat there is a wide dark-brown zone. Later, the surface becomes dry—owing to its exposure to the air—and becomes deep reddish, violet, or purple, according to the amount of congestion and strangulation. If the animal has been violent there are dark torn areas, and even gangrenous patches, where damage has been sustained, and particles of bedding, dung, etc., are adherent to its surface. In the cow the whole of the outer upper surface may be covered with the fæces that are passed as the result of the severe straining. In all animals—but especially in ruminants—parts of the fœtal membranes may be adherent to the outer surface of the mass, and can be easily recognised. The surface is not sensitive to the touch, but any manipulation of the mass is provocative of further straining. In later stages still, *e.g.* where the animal has survived for

2 or 3 days, the tumour is in an advanced state of decomposition, and has a putrid odour, and the animal presents a greatly distressed picture to the observer, as already described.

Various complications may occur. The vagina is always displaced when the prolapse is complete; this obstructs the urethra, and dams back the urine. The animal's suffering is increased, and there is a risk of rupture of the bladder. Perforation of the wall of the uterus, by external damage, may expose the peritoneal covering to contamination from the outside, and peritonitis is certain to follow. Parts of the small intestines may insinuate themselves into the pear-shaped sac, and obstruction or strangulation of the bowel results. In other cases the neighbouring organs—rectum, bladder, and perhaps intestines—may be displaced from their normal positions, and their normal functions are upset.

Treatment.—Prolapse of the uterus is always an extremely serious condition in any animal, and in the mare and sow very often proves fatal. A good percentage of cows and ewes recover, when the prolapse is replaced *without loss of time*, and when there are *no complications*. There is scarcely any doubt that the inversion and prolapse of the uterus is a condition which must end fatally unless immediate human assistance is rendered. The organ cannot possibly become replaced spontaneously, and gangrene and decomposition must occur when exposed to the air for long. In many cases death takes place within 24 hours of the accident occurring, and sometimes it is more rapid than that, but in most instances the animal will live for 2, 3, or 4 days.

When treating a case—in whatever animal—it is absolutely necessary to comply with certain essentials as follows:

(1) *The prolapsed uterus must be protected from further damage.*—To ensure this the animal must be secured at once, and a large sheet or blanket—which has been previously dipped in mild antiseptic solution—must be placed under the mass, and held by two men so that the tension is relieved from the neck, and so that it cannot be further contaminated or injured.

(2) *The surface of the organ must be carefully cleansed.*—For this purpose a clean pail containing a warm solution of potassium permanganate and common salt (one teaspoonful of the former and ¼ lb. of the latter to the gallon of water) or diluted Dettol may be used. All the larger particles of straw, débris, etc., are picked off, and the smaller pieces removed by gentle washing. Care must be taken not to make the surface bleed.

(3) *The prolapsed portion must be replaced.*—To effect this the larger animals may require epidural or general anæsthesia to prevent the powerful expulsive pains that otherwise accompany the process, and make return difficult. When the animal has been anæsthetised the hind-quarters are raised as high as possible by building up the floor with straw bales, by hoisting the hind legs, or by other means. When the protruded mass is very large and has a distinct neck, the main bulk is raised to a slightly higher level than the external passage, and a process of 'tucking in' is begun near the vulva. This is carried out by the two hands—one at either side—using the hands half closed, so that the middle joints of the fingers come into contact with the uterus. The finger tips should not be employed owing to the danger of laceration or even puncture of the walls. When as much has been returned as is possible by this method, or where the prolapse has not been large, the mass may be further returned by placing the closed fists against the most prominent part of the tumour and pressing strongly forwards. The resistance is gradually overcome and the mass is forced along the passages back into the pelvis. It must not be thought that the return of an inverted or prolapsed uterus is an easy matter; it is a labour that often makes great demands upon the strength and endurance of the operator, and frequently takes an hour or more to effect. Moreover, when once the organ has been returned, unless it is straightened out into its normal position, it may be reinverted a second time.

(4) *Measures must be taken to retain the uterus in position.*—These measures are of two varieties: the animal may be given a sedative or narcotic to deaden pain and lessen the chances of subsequent straining; or appliances may be employed that offer a mechanical hindrance to a recurrence of the condition. Very often a combination of these two methods answers best. The hinder parts of the stall or stance are banked up to the extent of about 18 inches or 2 feet, so that the animal is compelled both to stand and lie with the hind-quarters raised above the level of the fore-quarters. This throws the abdominal contents forwards, and

helps to maintain the uterus in place. It is, of course, mainly applicable to mares and cows. Pessaries are not well suited for application to domestic animals since they are resented, and, being usually rigid, are liable to cause serious injury should the animal attempt to remove them. Sutures are not always satisfactory, but are occasionally used; they are inserted across the lips of the vulva. They are painful, and very liable to tear when straining is severe. Moreover, they always produce a certain amount of inflammation and infection, and occasionally result in sloughing. Trusses or bandages are usually the most satisfactory means to adopt. Overseas, in remote places where no veterinary assistance is available, a loop, made in the middle of a rope, may be placed round the animal's neck and the two ends are carried back to the root of the tail, where they are attached to each other by a knot. They then pass down, one on each side of the vulva. across which a lacing of bandage passes from one rope to the other, bend forward between the udder and the thigh, and are eventually attached to the original loop round the neck. They must be applied tightly for the first day or two, but they may be slackened after that.

After-treatment consists in giving gentle exercise daily, preferably in a field where a little grass can be eaten, and general nursing. The temperature must be taken frequently, as metritis is very liable to follow prolapse, and it is usually heralded by a sudden rise in temperature on the second or third day. (*See* INFLAMMATION OF UTERUS under this section.)

Amputation of the prolapsed uterus becomes necessary when all attempts at its reduction are futile, when the organ has received so much injury or has become so decomposed and gangrenous that it would be certainly fatal to return it to the abdomen, or when prolapse occurs time after time in spite of its repeated reposition, and in spite of all attempts at retention.

HERNIA OF THE UTERUS (*see* HERNIA).

HÆMORRHAGE FROM UTERUS (*see* BLEEDING, ARREST OF, PITUITRIN, HORMONE THERAPY).

DROPSY OF UTERUS—Hydrops uteri—consists of a collection of serous or mucoid fluid in the uterus. This results from injuries inflicted at parturition which have not become septic, and in which there has been a gradual oozing of fluid from the blood-stream and uterine glands into the cavity of the organ, and some obstruction to its evacuation, such as a closed cervical canal; or the condition may follow the breaking down of a monstrosity or mole, where a type of liquefaction takes place, as well as from other causes. Fluid accumulates in the cavity of the uterus, causing its dilatation, and later on the abdomen increases in size and may give rise to the belief that the animal is pregnant. At intervals there is an evacuation of fluid when the os opens, and as much as 4 or 5 gallons may be discharged. After this the abdomen partially collapses, but as the fluid re-forms it refills. Sometimes the walls of the organ are themselves dropsical, fluid being found among the muscle fibres, and they may be as much as 6 or 7 inches thick.

Treatment.—The cervix must first be forcibly dilated and the fluid syphoned off with all aseptic precautions, and the uterus subsequently irrigated with antiseptic and astringent fluids. Tonics are given, and the animal is exercised and fed on nourishing but laxative foods. The chief danger of this condition is that the contents may become infected with organisms, when a septic metritis is produced.

RUPTURE, either involving the uterine wall or the vagina or vulva, may occur before or during parturition in any animal, during the reduction of a torsion or prolapse, and occasionally it arises spontaneously when the wall of the organ is diseased. When it occurs in the uterus there is always a grave danger of peritonitis and death, and when it occurs in the vagina or vulva it can generally be treated as an ordinary open wound.

TORSION, or TWISTING, of the uterus is commonest in the cow and other ruminants, and very rare in other domestic animals. This accident consists of a partial or complete rotation of the uterus around its long axis, and usually involves the neck of the organ.

Causes.—It seems to be mainly produced by slipping and falling during the latter part of pregnancy, but it may also result from rolling on the ground, hard work, travelling rapidly up or down steep hillsides, violent movements of the unborn fœtus, and from turning up in-lamb ewes for purposes of dressing their feet, udders, etc.

Symptoms.—A a rule there is no indication of the presence of the displacement until parturition is due to commence. The animal is then seen to prepare herself in the usual way, but the preliminary labour pains are exceptionally feeble and separated by long intervals. After the lapse of some hours—when the 'water-bag' and other signs of the approaching act should have become evident in an ordinary case—nothing happens. The animal is slightly disturbed, shows an occasional pain, walks round aimlessly, may feed spasmodically, but does not appear to be greatly distressed. This condition may persist for as long as 48 hours. In other cases the animal is very much upset. It has spasms of violent and painful uterine contraction, is distressed and restless. In the course of a few hours these manifestations either become urgent, or else the animal appears to settle down. In cases such as the latter the symptoms recommence in from one to six days, and it becomes very evident that there is some obstruction to delivery of the fœtus.

Treatment.—The treatment of torsion simply involves the untwisting of the twisted uterus. An examination is made to determine whether the torsion is right-handed (clockwise) or left-handed (counter-clockwise). In partial cases it may be possible to pass the hand through the twisted part and feel the fœtal membranes, but generally this is not possible. When the direction of the twist has been decided upon an endeavour may be made to correct it manually if it is but slight. Otherwise more radical measures must be employed. The most successful method is the rotation of the body. The udder is stripped of its milk to obviate injury, especially in the cow, and the animal is cast upon the ground in an enclosure where there is plenty of room. The four legs are tied together and the animal is rolled over and over in the same direction as the twist. Thus in a left-handed twist the animal is rolled in a counter-clockwise direction. During rolling the hand is kept in the vagina to determine progress. Generally when the twist has been corrected there is a flush of amniotic fluid and the protrusion of the fœtal membranes (water-bag) from the vulva, and if no other obstruction exists the act of parturition continues.

In some cases laparatomy is performed, and the twisted organ is righted by hand.

UVEITIS.—Inflammation of the uvea (iris, ciliary body and choroid coat of the eyeball).

UVULA (*uvula*) is the small downward projection that is found on the free edge of the soft palate of the pig. It is not present in the other domesticated animals.

V

VACCINATION (*vacca*, a cow) is the taking of lymphatic material from an animal (usually a calf) affected with cow-pox (variola vaccinia) and inoculating it into another animal (or man), with a view to protecting it against an attack of its own special form of variola or pox. Thus calf-lymph from a calf suffering from cow-pox will protect against small-pox when inoculated into the human being.

The word 'vaccination', however, is greatly used to indicate the inoculation of an animal with any product which contains living or dead antigens, with a view to its protection against attacks of some specific diseased condition. The preparation of the antigen is called a 'vaccine'.

Mass vaccination of poultry has been successfully carried out against Newcastle Disease by dispersing finely divided particles of vacine over the heads of the birds with simple dust pumps.

Simultaneous vaccination of animals against a number of diseases is now practised. For example, sheep can be simultaneously immunised against Pulpy Kidney disease, Lamb Dysentery, Braxy, Blackleg, Black disease, Struck, and Tetanus.

VACCINE (*vacca*, a cow), strictly speaking, means a preparation from an animal affected with cow-pox (*see under* VACCINATION), but it is also used to include almost any antigen. The antigen may be living and virulent bacteria, living but attenuated bacteria, dead bacteria, viruses in minute doses or after attenuation, tissue pulp containing virus, toxins, or aggressins.

When an animal is inoculated with a vaccine as protection against a specific disease, *e.g.* blackleg, this is carried out with the object of producing 'antibodies' in its system, which will confer immunity against future attack by the blackleg organisms. In some cases immunisation against one particular disease will also immunise against other diseases of a similar nature; thus, a human being can be immunised against severe attack by small-pox, by inoculation with material from *cow-pox*. In a similar way, poultry can be rendered immune to chicken-pox by the use of pigeon-pox virus.

Vaccines are sometimes used for treatment as well as for prevention of a particular disease. 'Strangles' in the horse is sometimes treated by inoculation of attenuated cultures of the organism that is found in the lesions—*Streptococcus equi*—into the horse in increasing doses at definite intervals. In this connection the process is carried out with the intention of stimulating the body resources to increased production of antibodies. The attenuated organisms that are introduced are easily killed by a proportion of the antibodies that they excite, so that a superabundance of antibodies is released for the destruction of those unattenuated germs that were originally responsible for the disease. Such vaccines may be prepared from a case and kept in stock for the treatment of other cases, in which instances they are known as 'stock vaccines', or they may be prepared from the actual case for which they are intended to be used; they are then known as 'autogenous vaccines'. Vaccines that are used for protective purposes are necessarily of the stock variety. 'Phylacogen' is the name given to an extract of a culture from which the bacteria have been filtered out so that only their products remain.

Some of the chief diseases which may be controlled by using a vaccine for protective purposes among animals are: anthrax, blackleg, contagious abortion of cattle, braxy, lamb dysentery, rinderpest, swine fever, contagious pleuropneumonia of cattle, blue-tongue, strangles, and distemper. (*See* PLATE 10.)

Tissue vaccines have been used in the treatment of benign skin papillomata (warts) of cattle. Use is made of a glycerol-saline growth suspension. As several strains of virus may be involved, autogenous vaccines are preferable.

X-irradiated worm larvæ vaccine is used in the prevention of HUSK (*which see*). A similar vaccine has been used against *Hæmonchus contortus* in sheep in recent experiments carried out at the University of Glasgow Veterinary School. Similar vaccines have been prepared for use against gape-worms in birds and hook-worms in dogs.

It is important that, in the commercial production of live vaccines involving the use of chicken embryos (or of tissue cultures derived from them), contaminant viruses are eliminated. For example, the avian leucosis virus has contaminated distemper vaccine and would represent a risk to vaccinated poultry if contaminating vaccines for them.

VACCINIA VIRUS.—This term may refer to the virus of naturally occurring cow-pox, or to the virus of small-pox which has undergone mutation through passage of rabbits or calves. 'Vaccination' of human beings is the application of the vaccinia virus to a small scarified area of skin.

VAGINA is the passage that leads from the termination of the uterus to the level of the opening of the urethra in the female. It is part of the genital canal through which the young animal must pass at the act of birth, and is followed by the vulva. It receives the extremity of the penis during service. An artificial vagina is used at A.I. centres for the collection of semen. Vaginal mucus is altered in character during pregnancy, a fact which is made use of in pregnancy diagnosis.

Rupture of the vagina, with protrusion of the intestine and rapid death, occurs not uncommonly in ewes of a large breed, of mature age, carrying a twin—a week or two before lambing is due. Bulky foods—swedes, turnips, kale—are often involved.

VAGINITIS. — Inflammation of the vagina. (*See under* INFERTILITY—Diseases of the Genital Organs in Female; *also* 'WHITES', 'EPIVAG', VULVOVAGINITIS, PROLAPSE.)

VAGUS, THE (*see under* PNEUMOGASTRIC NERVE, GUTTURAL POUCH DIPHTHERIA).

VALVES are found in the heart, veins, lymph-vessels, etc., and serve the purpose of ensuring that the fluids will only circulate in one direction. (*See* HEART, VEINS, ILEOCÆCAL.)

VALVULAR DISEASES (*see* HEART DISEASES).

VAMPIRE-BAT (*Desmodus etc.*,) transmits the paralytic form of rabies in parts of South America, the West Indies, etc. The bat is about 4 inches long, and laps blood from the wounds inflicted with its upper incisor teeth on cattle, horses, etc. Other species of vampire-bat are also encountered, and in Mexico their activities have made necessary the preventive inoculation of 800,000 cattle a year. In Yugoslavia and U.S.A. ordinary insect-eating bats have carried rabies.

VARIED DIET (*see* DIET, AMINO-ACIDS, CAT FOODS).

VARICOCELE (*varix*, a dilated vein; κήλη, tumour) is a condition in which the veins of one or both testicles are greatly distended. It is met with in old animals.

VARICOSE VEINS (*varix*, a dilated vein). (*See* VEINS, DISEASES OF.)

VARIOLA (*varus*, a blotch on the face), or Pox, is the inclusive term that is employed to indicate a series of eruptive fevers of animals and man, in which the skin eruption takes the form of a 'pock'. Variola is due to a virus. The disease attacks man (small-pox), the horse, ox, sheep, pig, camel, and dog (horse-pox, cow-pox, sheep-pox, etc.).

It is now established that all poxes can be artificially transmitted to other species, and that they all will revert to cow-pox. There is a cross immunity, by which the virus of any one pox can be made to immunise an animal against the others.

Typical Lesions.—In typical cases five stages of the skin lesions can be recognised. At first an area of skin is reddened and inflamed, and appears similar to a flea-bite; this is called the *Roseola stage*. After a time small hard elevations or papules arise on this area—constituting the *Papular stage*. An exudation of lymphatic fluid forms under the outer covering of skin around the papules, a vesicle filled with fluid arises, and the *Vesicular stage* is reached. The vesicles may be numerous, small and discrete, or, in severe cases, they may be fewer, larger, and confluent. At a later stage the contained fluid becomes cloudy and pus-containing—the *Pustular stage*. Finally the pustules burst and the contained material dries into a yellowish or pinkish crust or scab, which becomes detached from the skin, leaving a shallow crater-like 'pock mark'. This is called the *Desquamative* or *Crustaceous stage*. The pustules very often do not burst, but their contents undergo desiccation and scab-formation in the same way. Small pustules may leave no permanent pock mark behind them, but the larger incrustations have a permanently depressed scar when they fall off. As a rule, there is an interval of from 2 to 4 days between each stage and the next, but this varies with each attack.

COW-POX — Variola vaccinia — is so called because it is commoner in cows than in other oxen, though all are liable to attack. It is transmissible to horses, sheep, and goats, and to man. It is spread from one cow to another by the contamination of the hands of the milkers, and may be contracted by the latter in the same way. Outbreaks may be introduced into a herd by a recently vaccinated person. The period of incubation varies from 1 or 2 days, when a scratch or wound is contaminated, to 6 days in other cases. True cow-pox, in the U.K., is now regarded as a rare disease.

Symptoms.—The typical lesion is an eruption upon the skin of the udder, and teats of cows, but the lips, perineal region, insides of the thighs, and the scrotum of the male may also be attacked. The first indication is often a tendency to kick while being milked, in an otherwise quiet cow.

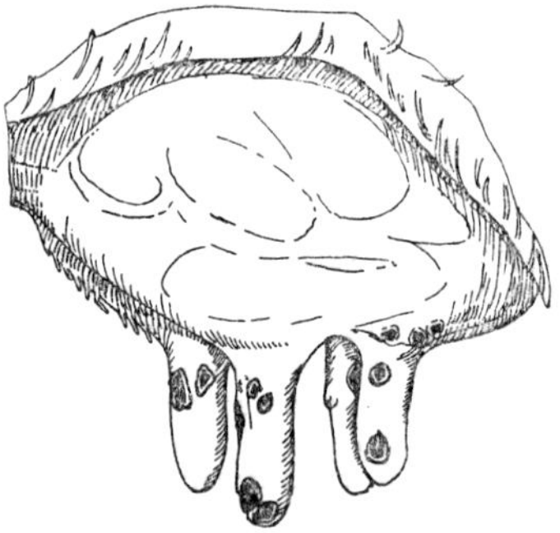

The lesions of cow-pox on the teats and skin of the udder. They are in the early desquamative stage, the dried scales having fallen off. Little shallow crater-like pocks remain.

The teats are found hard and swollen, and small nodules may be discovered upon them. In a few days these develop into the typical vesicle, which varies in size from a threepenny piece to a shilling. They are generally circular when on the udder and eliptical on the teats. Those on the udder run the usual course, but upon the teats the vesicles get ruptured by the milkers, and pass to the scab stage without the formation of pustules. If no re-infection takes place the condition disappears in about 2 to 2½ or 3 weeks, but where fresh areas of the skin become continually re-infected it may persist much longer. A slight degree of fever and some loss of appetite are noticed, and there is a falling off of the milk supply. The milk in some cases may be ropy, and it does not keep well in warm weather.

Treatment.—Since the infection may be contracted by human beings great care must be taken by those who handle and milk the affected cows. The animals are better separated from healthy ones where accommodation will allow, and should be looked after by separate attendants. In other cases where this is not possible, the affected cows must be left till last, and the hands, etc., washed in a disinfectant solution subsequently. The disease is a comparatively mild one in uncomplicated cases, and if the lesions are kept clean and anointed with an astringent ointment, such as zinc oxide ointment containing salicylic acid, before milking, and are dusted with sulphanilamide powder after milking, little else is required. Powerful antiseptic agents, such as carbolic acid, cresyl preparations, iodoform, etc., are unsuitable, as they taint the milk. If the milk is healthy in appearance it may be used for consumption by calves, lambs, or pigs, etc., after boiling or pasteurisation, but it is unsuitable even foran imal food if it is ropy or stained, and it is not advisable to use it for human consumption as long as the lesions are open or peeling. This applies particularly to children that have not, and to those that have recently, been vaccinated. (*See also under* MILKER'S NODULE.)

HORSE - POX —Variola equina — is a mild variola that attacks horses of all ages and both sexes. It is spread by grooming tools and feeding utensils, as well as by the hands of attendants. The blacksmith has been known to transmit it, and it may be rarely spread by coition.

Symptoms.—The lesions are usually seen on the skin of the hollow of the heels; the insides of fore-arms and thighs, lips, nostrils, and vagina are less often affected. The typical stages occur, but are not easily recognised owing to the covering of hair. The mucous membranes of mouth and nose may also be affected. In these parts the vesicle leaves a red shallow ulcer which heals up rapidly. They cause a good deal of salivation, smacking of the lips, dribbling of water when drinking, and may interfere with feeding. When lesions are present in the nostrils they produce a yellowish nasal discharge. Occasionally the genital organs may be affected when the eruptions occur on the penis of the male and on the vulva of the female.

Treatment.—Affected animals should be

isolated at once. Separate attendants should be provided, and the utensils, grooming tools, etc., should be all thoroughly cleansed and afterwards separate lots kept for the diseased and the healthy. The stalls, mangers, harness, litter, and other materials that may have become contaminated, should receive a thorough disinfection before they are considered free from infection. The food should be sloppy and easily swallowed when there are lesions in the mouth. Simple saline laxatives and diuretics, such as Glauber's salts and nitre, should be added to the water or food, and the lesions may be painted with alum in water. Eruptions on the skin may be dressed with tincture of iodine solution. The disease usually runs its course in less than three weeks, and that interval should be allowed to elapse before affected horses are returned to the stable to mix with other horses. Animals that have been attacked should not be allowed to come into contact with public horses for at least a month after the first appearance of the disease.

SHEEP-POX — Variola ovina — is the most virulent of the poxes that affect domesticated animals. It is highly contagious, and is spread by direct and by indirect contact. The virus is highly resistant to external conditions, and will survive where other viruses would be killed. It gains entrance in the system by inhalation, ingestion, and by inoculation. Young animals are more susceptible than adults, and both sexes are attacked. The period of incubation is from 2 to 7 days in the malignant type, and from 10 to 20 days in the milder form. It is always shorter in hot than in cold weather.

Symptoms.—Two forms of the disease are recognised: *malignant* or *confluent*, and a *benign* or *discrete*. In the former the lesions have a tendency to coalesce, and the mortality is often as much as 75 per cent of the infected; and in the latter the lesions remain separate, and the mortality is less than 10 per cent.

The first symptom is usually a fevered condition which appears before any lesions are visible. The sheep are greatly depressed and stop feeding. They are easily distressed in their breathing when made to move. The pulse is fast and full. The affected animals separate themselves from the rest of the flock, stand with their heads down, or lie with their mouths open, panting. In 24 to 48 hours after these preliminary symptoms the local typical lesions appear upon the skin of those parts that are not covered with wool. The five typical stages are well illustrated, the final crustaceous stage being the most severe. Large areas of the surface skin slough off attached to the scabs, and a necrotic ulcer remains behind. The sheep becomes very weak and emaciated if badly affected, and usually succumbs before the whole of the scab areas are cast off. Similar eruptions may occur in the mouth, causing salivation; in the throat and bronchial tubes, causing coughing and bronchitis; in the eyes and nostrils, causing discharges from these parts; and sometimes in the digestive system, setting up a profuse diarrhœa. In the mild form the disease runs its course in from 3 to 4 weeks, and one attack confers a lifelong immunity; in the malignant form it may be twice this period before the successive crops of eruptions have ceased spreading.

Treatment.—In Great Britain sheep-pox is one of the diseases scheduled under the 'Diseases of Animals Act', and all affected sheep are slaughtered. Even in countries where treatment is allowed it is found most economical to kill all the affected animals, and to watch carefully the others for the first symptoms, during outbreaks where the majority of the cases are of the malignant type. Where the cases mostly conform to the benign variety, the sheep are sheltered in an airy shed, provided with litter, water, and soft easily digested foods. Overcrowding is avoided, and the local lesions are dressed with lotions of alum, or some other mild astringent antiseptic.

Prevention consists in the prohibition of the export of infected sheep from infected countries, and the careful official supervision of outbreaks that occur from other sources. Measures for strict disinfection of infected premises, and the placing of infected fields, slaughter-houses and markets, etc., under control, are also necessary.

A process of protective inoculation, or 'ovination', is carried out in some countries where the disease is common.

GOAT POX—In the tropics (India and S.E. Asia) goats may suffer from Stone Pox or Goat Dermatitis, which has a mortality of 50 per cent or more. Symptoms include high fever, sneezing, a discharge from eyes and nose, head shaking, and pain.

The ordinary Goat Pox, which has almost a world-wide distribution, is characterised by milder fever and discharges. Death may occur from a secondary bacterial pneumonia.

SWINE - POX — Variola porcina, or Variola suilla—is not uncommon in piglets between 3 and 6 weeks of age. Although it can prove fatal, it usually occurs in a mild form. There is some evidence that piglets harbouring skin parasites, especially lice, are more likely to contract this infection and that these parasites may also be involved in spreading the virus between pigs. Isolation of infected pigs and routine use of anti-parasitic skin dressing, especially of bought-in pigs, should reduce risk of this infection.

Local lesions, which develop on the skin of the abdomen, flanks, head, and behind the ears, are similar to what are seen in the other animals. They show the five typical stages, an interval of about three days occurring between each stage and the next. General symptoms, similar to those seen in other animals, are noticed at the commencement of an attack.

Cow-pox may occur in the pig, and be indistinguishable from swine-pox.

Treatment.—Immediate slaughter of the affected and the in-contacts is the only rational method of dealing with an outbreak. Where treatment is to be adopted it should follow the same lines as for the sheep.

Variola also occurs in dogs, poultry, etc.

VASCULAR.—Consisting of, or containing a high proportion of, blood-vessels.

VAS DEFERENS (*see under* TESTICLE).

VASECTOMISED.—A male animal in which the *vas deferens* has been cut. Such an animal is sterile though it retains its libido and may be used for the detection of œstrus (*e.g.* in cattle).

VASOMOTOR NERVES are the small nerve fibres that lie in or upon the walls of the blood-vessels and connect the muscle fibres of the middle coat with the nervous system. By the continuous action of the nerves the muscular walls of the vessels are maintained in a moderate state of contraction. Any continuous and generalised increase in this action results in a raising of the blood-pressure of the body, while a diminution produces a lowering of the pressure. Such vasomotor nerves are called vaso-constrictors, but there are vaso-dilators as well. These latter are able to dilate the vessels, and cause either a general or a local fall in the blood-pressure, along with an increased supply of blood to the part.

VEGETATION is the term applied to the roughenings or accumulations that appear upon the valves of the heart, usually as the result of some inflammation in the valve wall, or of serious disturbance of the circulation, such as the presence of bacteria, tumour cells, strongyle larvæ, or pieces of free tissue in the blood-stream. They are very common in the chronic form of swine erysipelas, when they often are the direct cause of death.

The presence of vegetations on the heart valves results in a narrowing of the passage through which the blood passes, in an inefficient closing of the valves, and consequently to a general insufficiency of the heart's action. (*See* HEART DISEASES.)

VEINS are the vessels which carry the blood back to the heart after its circulation in the tissues of the body. With ne or two exceptions the veins lie alongside or near to the corresponding arteries —thus the renal vein brings back blood that has been carried to the kidney by the renal artery and lies alongside it. The veins are, however, more numerous and more irregular in their courses than are the arteries, especially on the surface of the body. In certain regions, such as the cheeks, brain meninges, and in the abdomen and thorax, there are veins arranged quite irrespective of the distribution of the arteries.

Structure.—A vein is a thin-walled tube which possesses a structure similar to that of an artery, and consists of three coats, viz. an outer fibrous, a middle composed of muscular and elastic fibres, and an inner coat composed of an elastic membrance and flattened epithelial cells. If an ordinary vein be split open along its length there are seen to be a number of flap-like valves attached to its inner surface. These are like little pockets, and are so arranged that they offer no resistance to the blood when it is flowing in the right direction, but they prevent any back-flow. These valves are most numerous in the veins of the limbs, where gravity would naturally tend to produce a back-flow, and least numerous in the veins of the internal organs.

Chief Veins.—The arrangement and relations of the veins are very different in animals of varying species, and even in different individuals, so that only a general description can be given here.

Pulmonary veins—as many as 8 or 9 in the horse and fewer in other animals—return the oxygenated blood from the lungs to the left auricle of the heart. They possess no valves. Opening into the right auricle are four veins; these are: (1) coronary sinus; (2) anterior, and (3) posterior vena cava; and (4) the azygos vein. The *coronary sinus* is a short thick trunk that discharges the blood used by the heart walls back into the general circulation. The *anterior vena cava* drains the blood from the head, neck, two fore-limbs, and much of the chest wall. It is formed by the confluence of the *jugulars* and the *brachial veins*, and receives other branches from the neck, vertebral region, and the chest wall. The *posterior vena cava* drains all the remainder of the body except the region of the diaphragm, the posterior intercostal areas, the œsophagus, and the bronchial tubes; the blood from these parts being collected into the *azygos vein* which joins the right auricle separately in most animals. The posterior vena cava is formed under the lumbar region by the union of the right and left *common iliac veins*, which drain the blood from the pelvis and hind-legs, and which are distributed in a more or less similar manner to the corresponding arteries of these parts. From here it passes forward below the lumbar muscles in company with the abdominal aorta, until at the level of the last thoracic vertebra it passes downwards and forwards, past the pancreas, and reaches the liver. Its further course is partly embedded in the liver substance until it arrives at a special opening in the diaphragm, called the *foramen venæ cavæ*, by which it gains the thoracic cavity. From here it passes along in a groove in the right lung to reach the right auricle. Its main tributaries are as follows: (1) *lumbar veins*, which empty blood from the lumbar muscles, etc.; (2) *internal spermatics* in the male, and *utero-ovarian veins* in the female, from the generative organs in either sex; (3) *two renal veins*, one from each kidney, satellites of the corresponding arteries; (4) several large *hepatic veins*, which return not only blood carried to the liver by the hepatic arteries, but also that which comes from the digestive organs by the *portal vein* to undergo a second capillary circulation in the liver (*see* PORTAL VEIN); and (5) the *phrenic veins* returning blood from the diaphragm.

In the venous system, even more so than in the arterial system, there is an intricate arrangement of anastomoses by which, when one vein becomes damaged or diseased, lateral branches from it may enlarge and carry away the excess blood into other veins so that no great hindrance to the return flow of the blood to the heart may be occasioned. If this were not so, the circulation might be easily upset from quite minor causes.

VEINS, DISEASES OF.—Like arteries, veins are not subject to a large number of diseases. Those lying near to the surface are frequently injured along with other tissues when contusions or lacerations have been sustained, but so extensive is their communication with neighbouring veins that it is usually possible for these latter to enlarge and undertake the functions of the damaged vessels, and thereby prevent serious consequences when a section is actually filled with coagulated blood and its walls are bruised. The deeper veins are protected from all but the most severe, and usually fatal, injuries.

INFLAMMATION of a vein, or PHLEBITIS, is usually due to the entrance and activity of organisms, which arrive either through a wound in the skin or by the blood-stream. In some cases inflammation in the organ drained by the vein may cause phlebitis, such as in pneumonia, or metritis. This condition may follow the collection of blood samples from the jugular when unclean instruments have been used, or when the resulting skin wound has not received attention. In almost all cases the contained blood coagulates and forms a venous thrombus. This may clear away and leave the vessel but little affected, or it may become colonised by fibrous tissue cells (a process known as '*organisation*'), when its lumen becomes blocked up, and it either persists as a hard cord, or else in time becomes opened up again by the absorption of the organised clot. In some cases the area drained by the vein becomes swollen and congested, owing to the damming back of the return flow, but more generally the blood is diverted into other veins in the region. Treatment, beyond the usual anti-inflammatory measures, is unnecessary, and, in fact, often impossible.

VARICOSE VEINS are produced as the result of some impediment to the circulation which is not sufficiently severe to inhibit all flow of blood. In this connection the affected veins—which are nearly always on the surface of the body—become enlarged and generally tortuous in their courses. With the exception of the so-called 'blood spavin' in the horse the condition is extremely rare in the lower animals. (*See* SPAVIN.)

VELD SICKNESS (*see* HEART-WATER).

VENA CAVA (*vena*, vein; *cava*, hollow).—Each of the two large veins that open direct into the right auricle of the heart. (For further details *see under* VEINS.)

VENEREAL DISEASES. — Animals, with the exception of the monkey, are not subject to infection by the two great human venereal scourges—syphilis and gonorrhœa, but there are several important contagious diseases that can be transmitted from animal to animal by coition. These include brucellosis, trichomoniasis, *vibrio fœtus* infection, and infectious vaginitis of cattle, venereal granulomata or venereal tumours of dogs (*see* VENEREAL TUMOURS), and dourine or 'Mal du coit' of horses (*see* PROTOZOÖN PARASITES).

VENEREAL TUMOURS, or INFECTIVE GRANULOMATA, are the outward signs of a contagious disease of dogs that chiefly affects the mucous membrane of the vagina of the females and the sheath and penis of the male.

Symptoms.—The tumorous vegetations are most commonly seen on the surface of some part of the genital tract, but they may also occur upon the lips (probably from licking) and the skin of other parts of the body. In the female the original tumour is a warty excrescence which soon grows and becomes cauliflower-like. In advanced stages there is a large mass of pinkish or greyish-red tissue, which easily bleeds when touched, occupying the greater part of the vaginal passage and often causing a bulging and swelling of the perineal region. No epithelium is found over these growths, which to some extent resemble sarcomata. A dirty sticky blood-stained discharge accompanies the condition, and the animal's general health suffers. In the male the warty growths usually have a distinct stalk, and are attached to the skin or mucous membrane of the sheath, or to the penis. (*See also under* WARTS.)

VENESECTION (*vena*, a vein; *seco*, I cut).—The operation of phlebotomy. (*See* PHLEBOTOMY.)

VENEZUELAN EQUINE ENCEPHALOMYELITIS.—A strain recognised in the 1930s. A severe outbreak occurred in Venezuela and Colombia in 1962–64, when thousands of horses died and about 30,000 people were infected. A later outbreak spread to Mexico in 1970 where 6,000 or more horses died, and then to Texas, U.S.A.

VENOMOUS BITES (*see* BITES).

VENT GLEET.—This condition in poultry is an inflammation of the cloaca, with which is associated a thin yellowish watery discharge which has a characteristic and particularly unpleasant odour. The cloaca and adjacent skin appear swollen and congested, and the bird exhibits signs of irritation. Other birds attracted by the reddening of the region may peck at the vent; this leads on to cannibalism.

Egg production drops, and in some cases egg binding and impaction of the oviduct result.

Treatment.—Thorough washing and injection of a mild antiseptic, such as acriflavine, is often successful. Acriflavine ointment has also been found of value. If the case does not tend to clear up, the bird should be destroyed. Care should be taken by the operator in handling birds, since cases of severe infection of the eyes of poultry-keepers treating this condition are not uncommon.

VENTILATION.—The problem of ventilation may be summed up as 'the measures necessary to rectify the pollution of the air in a building and that without the production of a draught'. It can be readily understood that whenever living animals are enclosed in a confined building they gradually use up the oxygen and discharge into the air quantities of carbon dioxide, water vapour, and effete particles of organic matter, until, if no fresh air be supplied, the percentage of oxygen decreases below the amount required for satisfactory respiratory function.

Necessary air space in cubic feet.—

Cow, Horse (Byre or stable)	200
(Loose-box or Yard) .	600–1200
Bacon pig . . .	60
Poultry	
(layers on slats) . .	6
(,, deep litter) .	12

The required amount of air for each animal must be continuously brought in from the outside, and an exit must be provided for an equal amount. This is arranged for by the provision of *inlet* and *outlet* ventilators.

Inlets.—These include windows, direct

inlet pipes, perforated bricks and gratings, and propulsive mechanical fans. Windows, of which the Sheringham Valve type is the most common and useful, serve the dual purpose of lighting and ventilation. Those on the lee side of a building serve as outlets when the wind is strong. In the Sheringham Valve windows the incoming air is deflected upwards by the hopper-like flap that falls inwards, so that it is spread over a greater area than is the case with other openings. Several varieties of inlet pipes are used, often in conjunction with windows, to ensure a supply of fresh air in the region of the animals' heads. These may be merely short lengths of clay piping let through the wall, or Tobin's Tubes may be used. These latter have an iron grating low down on the outside of the wall and a tube running either on the inside of the wall or else within it, to an opening higher up into the building. In this way the air enters low down and escapes at a higher level than the animals' heads. In other cases a brick may be made with a large number of perforations by which air can pass directly through it, or a brick space in the wall is fitted with an iron grating. These are usually at a low level so that the air enters below the animals' heads, or they may be placed just under the eaves. They may be single, or a continuous row may be built in.

Ventilation rates—(maximum)

	Changes of air per hour	*Cubic feet per hour*
Bacon pig .	20	200–1200
Broiler chicken	40	240
Laying birds .	30	360

Outlets.—These include an open ridge, Findlay's Ventilating System, roof windows or sky-lights, extraction cowls, louvre-board ventilators, outlet shafts, open eaves, exhaust fans, and other devices. The most satisfactory outlet is undoubtedly an open ridge along the whole length of the building. The heated impure air rises and is drawn through the open space by the suction of the wind. The disadvantages of this system are that the open space will allow entrance to a certain amount of rain or snow in bad weather, and that the system is inapplicable to buildings possessing lofts. In Findlay's System the space in an open ridge is closed by a long narrow window of glass on either side of the ridge, which may either be kept shut or may be allowed to remain open according to the weather. The glass provides a most excellent lighting, but the adjustable windows are apt to be closed when rain or snow is falling, and the attendant, quite humanly, forgets to open them subsequently. Roof windows and sky-lights, which are often fitted with an adjustable quadrant shutter, are useful when used along with cowls, but are not sufficient by themselves. Moreover they are liable to cause ' down-draughts ' when they are open in windy weather. Extraction cowls are devices fixed along the ridge of the roof which allow exit of the hot air as it rises, or which exert a suction upon the contained air by virtue of an arrangement of vanes, etc. They are not always satisfactory—especially when they possess moving parts, such as revolving tops, which get out of order after a time. Louvre-boards are good and effective when properly constructed. A louvre-board ventilator consists of a framework or box placed at the ridge of a building and provided with slates set at an angle of about 50° to the horizontal along two or more of its sides. The spaces between the louvre boarding allow exit for air, and the angle at which the boards are set deflects direct wind upwards as it passes through the box and produces a suction upon the air in the building. Outlet shafts are provided in buildings that are of two or more stories when animals are housed upon the ground floor. The shaft passes either straight from the ceiling of the ground floor to the roof of the building, or it may turn at a right angle and run along between floor and ceiling to the outside wall, where it turns at another right angle upwards to the roof.

Extraction area—
(Necessary with natural ventilation).

	Outlet : sq. ins. per beast
Cowhouse . . .	144
Farrowing house . .	15
Fattening ,, . .	10
Calf ,, . .	10
Poultry (adult) house .	2

Mechanical ventilators may be either of the *plenum* or in-forcing type, or of the *vacuum*, exhaust, or out-forcing variety. In the former a larger power-driven fan is enclosed in a chamber with communication to the outside of the building, and is connected by ducts or shafts with all parts that are to be ventilated. In the exhaust variety one or more electric fans are enclosed in turrets placed along the ridge of the roof. (*See also* HOUSING.)

VENTRAL (*venter*, the belly) means pertaining to the belly in the strictest sense, but is the term used in Comparative Anatomy to indicate that a particular organ or structure is situated towards the abdominal surface of the body, as distinct from the spinal or dorsal aspect. (*See* NOMENCLATURE.)

VENTRICLE (*ventriculus*, the stomach) is the term applied to the two larger cavities of the heart, and also to the hollow spaces found in the brain. (*See* HEART, BRAIN.)

VERATRUM (*see* HELLEBORE).

VERMES is the name of a great class of animals, called a *Phylum*, to which all the parasitic worms belong. (For a description of the parasitic worms *see* PARASITES.)

VERMICIDES and **VERMIFUGES** are substances which possess the property of killing or of expelling worms. (For the names of these drugs, *see under* ANTHELMINTICS.)

VERMINOUS ANEURISM is the diseased condition that results from the activity of the larval forms of *Strongylus vulgaris* in the anterior mesenteric artery of the horse. (*See* PARASITES, p. 658.)

VERMINOUS BRONCHITIS is a bronchitis due to worms living in the bronchial tubes. In cattle and sheep this condition is called ' husk ', and in poultry it is known as ' gapes '. (*See* HUSK, GAPES.)

VERMINOUS DERMATITIS (*see* STEPHANOFILARIASIS).

VERMINOUS OPHTHALMIA (*see under* EYE, DISEASES OF).

VERRUCOSE (*verrucosus*) means covered with warts or vegetative growths. In pigs a verrucose endocarditis is recognised, the growths being found on the heart valves. The condition may be associated with swine erysipelas or be caused by staphylococci or streptococci. There are no observable symptoms.

VERSION, or TURNING, means the changing of a presentation at parturition so that some other part of the fœtus than that which was presented originally comes through the pelvic opening first. For birth to be possible in the domestic animals it is necessary that the long axis of the young and that of the dam should be in the same direction. Consequently, when the long axis of the fœtus lies across that of the dam version is necessary. It is essential in all cases of this operation that all parts of the young animal shall lie within the abdomen since there is not sufficient room in the pelvis for altering position. Any parts that are presenting in the posterior passages are therefore first repelled back into the cavity of the uterus. This can be effected by hand when straining can be controlled, and when the bulk to be moved is not great. In other cases it may be necessary to use an instrument; one end of this is placed against the most suitable part of the fœtus, and the other end against the operator's shoulder or chest. In each case the unwanted parts are pushed back and the pelvic passage is left free for further manipulations. The next stage is securing of the fore or hind limbs, according to whichever are the more conveniently placed for delivery. A soft rope is placed round each fetlock in the form of a noose. The ends of the ropes are left outside the passage for assistants to pull upon. When arranged, a certain amount of traction is exerted upon the secured limbs and the fœtus is brought nearer to the pelvic inlet. It may happen that this manœuvre will result in a bringing forward of the whole body of the fœtus in such a way that the unwanted limbs block the passages; should this occur, repulsion is carried out as before and as often as necessary. Eventually the body of the young animal is arranged in the same axis as that of the dam, and delivery can be effected. In some powerful or fractious animals, especially young mares and heifers, it may be necessary to administer an anæsthetic.

It is better to bring the hind part forward rather than the fore part in most cases, as there are three extremities to provide for at the fore end of the body and only two at the hind end. It should be remembered, however, that in posterior or breech presentations it is more difficult to deliver a living fœtus than in anterior presentations.

In such procedures as this, as in all obstetric operations, it is necessary to observe the strictest cleanliness, both of the apparatus used and of the hands and arms of the operator. (*See* PARTURITION; UTERUS, DISEASES OF.)

VERTEBRA (*vertebra*) is one of the irregularly shaped bones that together form the spinal column of the vertebral column. (*See* SPINAL COLUMN.)

VESICAL (*vesica*, a bladder or blister) is the term applied to structures connected with, or diseases of, the bladder. (*See* BLADDER.)

VESICANTS (*vesica*, a blister) are blistering agents. (*See* BLISTERS.)

VESICLE (*vesicula*, a little blister) means a small collection of fluid in the surface layers of the skin or of a mucous membrane. The fluid is, in the majority of cases, derived from the blood serum, but it may contain some of the secretion of the sweat or other glands. Vesicles are present in a great number of diseases, and according to their location, some assistance is afforded for diagnostic purposes. Thus, in foot-and-mouth disease the vesicles are present in the mouth and on the feet, in cow-pox they are found on the teats, udder, and other parts.

VESICLES, SEMINAL.—These secondary sex glands, like the prostate, have openings into the urethra and are situated close to the neck of the urinary bladder.

At a bull-rearing unit four yearlings appeared fit and well. Their appetite was good and they showed no signs of pain or discomfort. When, however, samples of their semen were taken, clots of pus were noticed. This finding led to a careful examination of the bulls being made, and it was then discovered that each had a hard, painful swelling of one of their seminal vesicles. Inflammation was found to be due to infection with *Actinobacillus actinoides*. Other organisms sometimes involved include: tubercle bacilli; *Brucella abortus*; *streptococci*; *C. pyogenes*.

VESICULAR EXANTHEMA.—A virus disease of pigs (and rarely of horses but not of cattle) which has to be distinguished from foot-and-mouth disease. It was eradicated from the U.S.A. in 1959 and has never been recorded elsewhere.

VESICULAR STOMATITIS of horses resembles in some respects foot-and-mouth disease but is caused by a separate virus. The disease may also affect cattle and pigs. In Canada in 1951, foot-and-mouth disease was mistaken for vesicular stomatitis with serious consequences. It has become important in cattle and pigs, and occasionally affects sheep. It is a disease of the summer, and mainly of the Western Hemisphere, especially in the Caribbean area. An insect vector is likely, and the virus has been isolated from mosquitoes.

In man the disease is influenza-like, with fever, sore throat, and several days' malaise.

Two strains of the virus are recognised—the New Jersey and the Indiana. Experimentally, numerous mammalian species can be infected—likewise ducks.

VESICULAR VAGINITIS (*see* VAGINITIS, CONTAGIOUS GRANULAR).

VESICULITIS (*see* VESICLES, SEMINAL, *above*).

VETERINARY DEGREES are obtainable in the U.K. at the universities of Cambridge, London, Liverpool, Bristol, Edinburgh, and Glasgow, and lead to membership of the Royal College of Veterinary Surgeons. Higher degrees—M.Sc., Ph.D. and D.Sc. or equivalent—are obtainable after postgraduate study.

VETERINARY PRACTITIONER.—Someone on the Supplementary Veterinary Register; *not* a M.R.C.V.S. (*see below*).

VETERINARY PRODUCTS COMMITTEE.—The Agricultural Ministers established, in 1970, under the Medicines Act 1968, a new advisory committee, to be called the Veterinary Products Committee, to give advice with respect to safety, quality and efficacy in relation to veterinary use of any substance or article (not being an instrument, apparatus or appliance) to which any provision of the Medicines Act 1968 is applicable; and to promote the collection and investigation of information relating to adverse reactions for the purpose of enabling such advice to be given.

VETERINARY PROFESSION.—This comprises those engaged in private practice, in the Animal Health Division of the Ministry of Agriculture, the Royal Army Veterinary Corps, the Colonial Veterinary Service, in research and teaching at the universities, and also at A.R.C. research establishments, and those of the Ministry of Agriculture, etc., in food inspection and other municipal services, in A.I. Centres, in research and advisory appointments with, *e.g.* F.A.O., and commercial undertakings.

In Britain, the veterinary profession continues to grow. At the beginning of 1966, the register of the Royal College of Veterinary Surgeons contained a little under 7,500 names—about twice as many as there were in 1935. Allowing for 1500 overseas, this left about 4800 veterinary surgeons in the U.K. Of these, 3000 or so were in general practice; a little over 1000 in research, advisory, teaching, and other posts. In 1969 the total rose to over 8000.

'In Great Britain, there is one veterinarian to every 30 sq. miles, in the United States, one to every 270 sq. miles. In South Africa, there is one to every 1700 sq. miles and in Canada, one to every 1900 sq. miles, while in an underdeveloped region, such as East Africa, there is only one veterinarian to every 5000 sq. miles.'—Dr. K. L. Kesteven, Director of F.A.O.'s Animal Production and Health Division, 1960.

VETERINARY SURGEONS ACT, THE, 1966.—This relates to veterinary education, the management of the profession and the registration and professional conduct of veterinary surgeons and practitioners. The practice of veterinary surgery continues to be limited to veterinary surgeons and practitioners whose names appear on the registers maintained by the Royal College of Veterinary Surgeons. Unregistered persons may carry out only the very limited treatments, tests, or operations specified in section 19 of the Act, any exemption orders made thereunder, or Schedule 3.

The Supplementary Veterinary Register was established under the 1948 Act.

VIABLE is a term applied to a newly born animal to indicate that it is capable of living separately from the dam. It is also used in connection with the survival of bacteria, etc.

VIBICES are long tapering markings that sometimes occur on visible mucous membranes during certain diseases, such as purpura hæmorrhagica and pernicious anæmia of horses.

VIBRIO (*vibro*, I quiver) is a bacterium of a curved shape. *Vibrio coli* is a cause of enteritis in pigs, especially after weaning. (*See* SWINE DYSENTERY.)

VIBRIO FŒTUS is the cause of abortion in cattle and sheep. Recent work suggests that there are two types of *V. fœtus*; called (a) *venerealis Florent*, and (b) *intestinalis Florent*. The first attacks the genital organs of cattle, but does not produce disease in sheep; the second inhabits the intestines of cattle and is a cause of abortion in ewes. This means that it may be safe to have cattle on the same land as ewes which are aborting, whereas healthy cattle carrying *Vibrio fœtus* in their intestines could give rise to abortion in ewes.

VIBRIO FŒTUS INFECTION IN CATTLE.—An important cause of infertility in dairy herds. (Its ability to cause abortion in cattle and sheep was demonstrated by British workers.)

The disease is a venereal one, transmitted either at natural service or by artificial insemination. Many cows served by a particular bull fail to conceive, although usually a few become pregnant at the first mating. The genital organs of the bull, and his semen, appear normal. Following service the cow may have a slight redness of the vagina near the cervix, which is usually slightly swollen with an increase of mucous secretion—appearances not very different from those of a cow on heat. In a cow which has been infected for some time these appearances are altogether absent.

One infected bull was brought into an A.I. centre in the Netherlands, and of 49 animals inseminated with his semen only three became pregnant. Of these three, two aborted and *Vibrio fœtus* infection was diagnosed in them. Of the remaining 46 cows, 44 were inseminated with semen from a healthy, fertile bull; and it required six or seven inseminations per cow before pregnancy was achieved. These and many other experiences have led to the conclusion that infertility from this cause is temporary—cows developing an immunity some three months after the initial infection. Bulls, on the other hand, do not appear to develop any immunity and may remain ' carriers ' for years. On the average, abortion due to *Vibrio fœtus* seems to occur earlier than that due to the germ of brucellosis (' contagious abortion '), but later than that due to *Trichomonas*.

In an infected herd investigated in England, infertility was associated with retained afterbirth, vaginal discharges after calving, stillbirths, weak calves which later died, and a low conception rate. It was also found that abortions occurred between the fifth and eighth month of pregnancy—and not during the first months of pregnancy as quoted above.

Confirmation of diagnosis is difficult, and at present entirely dependent upon laboratory methods. A mucus agglutination test devised at Weybridge is of service except when the animal is on heat.

Treatment.—Aureomycin has proved effective.

VIBRIO JEJUNI is the cause of 'winter dysentery' of cattle. (*See also under* SCOURS.)

'VIBRIONIC SCOURS' IN PIGS.—(*See* SWINE DYSENTERY.)

VICES and VICIOUSNESS.—A definition comprehensive enough to include 'bad habits'.

See TAIL-BITING (in pigs) *and* FEATHER-PICKING, CANNIBALISM (in poultry). What follows here concerns the horse.

'Bad habits', mild vices, or whims.—These usually involve no bad consequences, imply no evil intent, and never entirely prevent the utilisation of the horse, but they are, at least, objectionable. It is perhaps necessary to indicate how they arise. When a horse is compelled to spend much of his time tied up in a stable, probably in solitude (especially if he has previously had his freedom), and with no occupation save such as he can devise, it is natural that he should search for something with which to occupy his attention. He has at hand a limited number of objects with which to amuse himself. The most obvious of these is the manger or some part of its fittings. He may play with the ring through which passes his halter rope, he may lick or nibble the edge of the manger or the wall in front, he may rest his head on the manger, or rub his poll along its lower surface. In other cases the clothing of the horse or his head collar may provide him with a plaything. He may tear his blanket or rug, bite or chew his headrope or halter shank, may slip his fastenings and get loose, or may scratch his head with a hind-foot. Sometimes a horse will persistently rub himself against the stall partition, or turn so that he may rub his tail and damage the hair. Occasionally a horse may rest one hind-foot upon the other and lacerate the coronet, and rarely a horse may be met with which trots in the stall. Pawing in the stable may be only a sign of impatience or loneliness; then it is not important, but sometimes it develops into a vice of such persistency that it entails great wear of the shoes, and may result in the production of holes in the stable floor. It should be remembered that pawing is sometimes a sign of abdominal pain (colic).

More serious vices.—It frequently happens that a horse that is naturally intelligent or impressionable will either carry any of the above mild vices to an extreme, or will copy the vices of other older horses with which he is stabled. In either of these ways may arise wind-sucking or crib-biting, weaving, kicking in the stable, bolting the food, extreme destructiveness to clothing, biting while being groomed, etc.

Another form of vice, which is important from the owner's point of view, is a disinclination to lie in the stall. A horse that shows this tendency does not get a sufficiency of rest and is consequently unfitted for a maximum amount of work. The condition usually originates through young nervous animals being frightened or injured when they first lie down in a stable. The custom of using 'bales' instead of complete stall partitions in large stables, which render the legs of a recumbent horse liable to be trodden upon by a neighbour, is one of the most important causes of this condition.

When an animal shows an ungovernable temper under the pressure of sexual disturbances, it is unfair to consider it vicious.

Other vices are jibbing, bolting in harness, backing in harness, intractability during shoeing, harnessing, or grooming, hostility to man, shown by kicking with fore or hind limbs, or biting, certain forms of shying, and aversion to special objects.

Backing in harness is a vice which is not commonly seen now.

Horses are sometimes met with which lay their ears back, switch their tails, and commence progressing backwards whenever they are annoyed. Sometimes the performance is accompanied by kicking, and the animal only ceases when he has damaged and perhaps cleared himself from the vehicle. It occasionally results from sore shoulders. A sore mouth, which makes the horse afraid of 'going up to his bit', has also been blamed.

Intractability during one or more of the common procedures to which horses are subjected is often the result of unwise or brutal treatment when the horse was young. Grooms that are themselves timid or nervous occasionally affect a loud-voiced hectoring attitude when handling young or unbroken horses. They use unnecessary harshness, and the animal comes to regard the particular process, whether it is grooming, harnessing, shoeing, or even only approaching, with distaste and finally

VICES AND VICIOUSNESS

resentment. Once the horse has learned that by showing a dislike he can avoid work, etc., he is likely to become a confirmed nuisance. The early treatment of horses that are ticklish or irritable should be pursued with kindness and patience, and when these fail, with uncompromising firmness, but not brutality, and the teasing of a sensitive animal should be dealt with in the severest manner at all times.

Hostility.—(*a*) ***Rearing and striking with the fore-feet*** is a dangerous vice that is more common among the light horses than among the heavy draught. Sometimes the animal merely rears from a desire to get started his work; sometimes he will not allow himself to be held by the head when in harness, but rears and strikes out at anyone approaching him; at other times he may strike out without rearing. A saddle horse, when rearing, may with his head strike the face or chest of his rider and unseat him, and may so lose his balance that he falls over backwards and perhaps crushes the rider. This vice may be remedied by the use of a short halter shank when in the stable, and by the use of a martingale when in the shafts or mounted.

(*b*) ***Kicking with the hind-feet.***—'With a kicking horse, pass in front', is a proverb that it is well to remember when dealing with the horse that uses his hind-feet for kicking. The hind-feet can be used to strike an object within a radius of from 4 to 6 feet *all around them*. It is a well-known fact that a mule can deliver a kick with his hind-feet to a person standing at its shoulder, and there are many horses able to do likewise. Two methods of kicking with the hind limbs are commonly employed; in the first, which is the horse's natural method of defence and offence, the head is lowered, the body is lifted from the withers backwards, and both the hind limbs are suddenly extended as far backwards as possible with tremendous force; in the second, the horse lifts one hind-foot and deals a short vicious backward or sideway kick without always fully extending the limb. Each method is productive of equally disastrous results to the person or animal within range. In addition to these there are 'cow kickers', which project one hind limb forwards, outwards, and backwards, so that they may reach a person standing as far forward as the shoulder. These are especially dangerous. The cause of kicking in a horse is not always ascertainable. It may result from a bad education, from nervousness and a tendency towards self-protection, from ticklishness, from jealousy against another horse, from getting the reins underneath their tails when in shafts, from resentment against the whip or spur, and from sheer bad temper. In single harness it may be corrected by the use of a kicking strap, running from one shaft, across the croup, and affixed to the other shaft, but in double harness, either as leader or wheeler, it is impossible to eradicate, and a horse showing this vice should be considered unsafe for double work. In the saddle it is a more difficult matter to deal with, but the experienced horseman will usually contrive by judicious management and the avoidance of undue use of whip or spur to break a horse from the vice. (*See also* KICKING.)

(*c*) ***Biting*** is commonest among stallions, and the remarks at the beginning of this section on *Serious Vices* should be noted. As a rule a biter may be cured by the use of the whip when he exhibits the warning signals of ears laid flat, lips retracted, teeth snapping shut, and tail switching. Sometimes a horse is so sudden in its attack that there is neither time nor opportunity for the use of the whip, and with such it is well to take precautionary measures, such as muzzling while grooming, tying up short, using double head ropes, one to either side of the stall, etc.

Shying.—In many cases where horses suddenly stop, plunge to one side, snort, tremble, attempt to turn in the opposite direction and run away, when confronted by some unusual sight, sound, or smell, the same causes as occasion bolting are operative. The horse does not trust his eyesight, is unable to interpret an unusual sound or smell, and consequently loses his head. Among the many objects at which horses are liable to shy may be mentioned the following: pools of water shining in the sunlight, fluttering pieces of paper, clothes hung out to dry, dogs, cats, fowls, and other small animals darting into the roadway. The odour of wild beasts, and the smell of blood and offal, that an animal perceives when passing a menagerie or a knackery or abattoir, are also likely to frighten it and cause it to shy.

Aversion to special objects.—Occasionally a horse is encountered which has an absolute horror of some special, usually quite harmless, common object; for example, pieces of white or coloured paper or rag, cock turkeys, pigs, goats, donkeys, small white inanimate objects of any nature, etc. Grey horses have been known to attack bay horses, and a brown-bay horse, light grey horses.

VILLUS (*villus*, a hair) is the name given to one of the millions of minute processes which are present on the inner surface of the small intestine. These are structures concerned in the taking up of fat. (*See* DIGESTION, INTESTINE.)

VIRAL.—Relating to viruses.

VIRAL HEPATITIS in dogs. (*See* CANINE VIRUS HEPATITIS.)

VIRAL PAPILLOMATOSIS.—A chronic disease (colloquially known as Angleberry) characterised by a proliferation of cutaneous warts and polypi of the genital organs.

VIRGINIAMYCIN.—An antibiotic which may be included in livestock rations.

VIRION.—A mature virus; the ultimate phase in viral development.

VIRUS B. (*see under* B. VIRUS).

VIROLOGY.—The study of viruses.

VIRUS DIARRHŒA OF CATTLE.—First reported in New York State, it is also known as Virus Diarrhœa. It is common in Britain, and varies from a mild to a severe illness with a 90 per cent mortality. It appears to bear some resemblance to Malignant Catarrh, but diarrhœa is not usually associated with the latter.

There may be a heavy mucous discharge hanging from the muzzle to the ground, diarrhœa, fever, and ulceration of the mouth. Lameness is common in infections due to the Indiana strain. (*See* 'MUCOSAL DISEASE.')

VIRUS HEPATITIS OF DUCKLINGS.—This is a Scheduled disease which attacks ducklings under 3 weeks old. Death occurs suddenly, and on *post-mortem* examination the liver is seen to be enlarged, with hæmorrhages. The Virus Hepatitis Order, 1954, refers.

VIRUS INFECTIONS OF COWS' TEATS.—These include *cow-pox*. Nowadays, true cow-pox is (in the U.K.) considered to be a rare disease. Another infection common to man and cattle is **pseudo-cowpox** or **milkers' nodules.** The skin disease in cowmen is indistinguishable from that in shepherds who have been handling sheep suffering from orf. It is now thought that the milkers' nodules virus very closely resembles the or virus, but that they are two distinct entities.

In 1965 two medical men in Dorset, had seven patients with milkers' nodules and with the aid of a veterinary colleague they found that the six dairy herds in which the men worked all had some cows with pseudo-cow-pox (or milkers' nodules) lesions on the teats. There are two types of this infection: one is described as benign or chronic, this lasts for months, it is painless throughout, and starts with a mild redness of the teats, followed by the formation of many scabs which get rubbed off at milking. The second, or acute, form involves pain before scabbing begins, but not afterwards. First there is reddening, then blisters which burst, then very large scabs form. So-called proud flesh is formed beneath the scabs. When these drop off, a characteristic horseshoe-shaped ring of minute scabs at the circumference is left. All this takes 7 to 10 days. What looks like a wart remains for several months.

This pseudo-cow-pox differs from true cow-pox in that the latter infection is associated with more pain, fewer scabs, quicker development of them and recovery within 3 weeks.

The virus which causes pseudo-cow-pox or milkers' nodules may be identical with, or closely related to, that of **bovine papular stomatitis** (BPS). According to research workers at Pirbright, this may well be a common disease in southern England. A disease clinically indistinguishable from BPS has been seen in Devon steers used at the Animal Virus Research Institute. In June, 1964, 14 typical cases were observed in a group of 64 animals.

Raised, roughened, brownish plaques were seen on the muzzle, and there were lesions on the lips and inside the mouth.

An ulcerative infection of the teats of dairy cows has recently been described in Scotland, and given the name **bovine ulcerative mammillitis.** It is caused by a herpesvirus, and was seen in eighteen herds. In these, 50 per cent of the milking stock showed symptoms, and of these 22 per cent developed mastitis.

The disease has been seen only in early winter, and lasts for up to 15 weeks. In severe cases it was of sudden onset, often appearing between milkings; the whole teat being swollen and painful. Blue discoloration was common. 'The resultant ulcer covered most, if not all, the teat.' In a less severe form (and six forms were described) vivid red discoloration was noted.

On account of the impossibility of milking cows with badly ulcerated teats, and because mastitis often followed, several animals had to be slaughtered.

The same disease has been the subject of another report from south-west England where the onset 'appeared to follow a prolonged period of wet weather. If the virus is of the herpes type it may be that it is endemic in the cattle population and produces lesions only under conditions which result in devitalising of the tissues.' Another possibility is that biting flies transmit the infection. (*See also under* FOOT-AND-MOUTH DISEASE.)

VIRUS PNEUMONIA OF CATTLE (*see* infections listed under CALF PNEUMONIA).

'VIRUS' PNEUMONIA OF PIGS (*see* ENZOÖTIC PNEUMONIA).

VIRUSES.—These are minute entities which can be differentiated from bacteria on account of the fact that they cannot multiply except in living cells. This is the most important characteristic of viruses, and means that their structure can be very simple, since they rely entirely upon their host's metabolic processes. For their multiplication to occur they must first attach themselves to living cells, enter these, and—to quote Dr. J. B. Brooksby*—'divert the normal cell metabolism in such a way as to produce new viral material, to assemble this, and then to leave the cell. . . Free virus resulting from this process need only survive in the environment outside the cell until some of the enormous number of particles that have been produced attach to uninfected cells and repeat the process.'

At the present time, any definition of viruses is likely to be challenged, for the subject is still controversial. Mr. R. A. Huck, B.SC., M.R.C.V.S., stated in the *Veterinary Annual*, 1965, that the most useful definition of viruses was suggested by Lwoff (1957). 'Viruses are infectious, potentially pathogenic, nucleoprotein entities with only one type of nucleic acid, which reproduce from their genetic material, are unable to grow and divide, and are devoid of metabolic enzymes.'

This definition eliminates the psittacosis group of agents, which possess both ribonucleic (RNA) and deoxyribonucleic (DNA) acids. (*See also* MYXOVIRUSES, ARBOVIRUSES, ADENOVIRUSES, etc.)

Viruses produce disease in man, animals, and plants. They give rise to antibodies in the animal's serum in the same way that bacteria do. They can be transmitted from one animal to another reproducing the same disease. Viruses will pass through porcelain filters which hold back nearly all bacteria but this is true of other organisms and hence no longer regarded as entering into the definition of viruses.

Viruses are mostly invisible under the microscope but have been photographed by means of the electron microscope. However, the larger viruses, such as those of the poxes, can readily be seen, when stained, under the ordinary microscope.

Viruses vary considerably in size. One of the smallest, that causing foot-and-mouth disease, is only 10 mμ. or ·00001 mm. in size; while a herpes virus may measure 180 mμ. (staphylococci measure about 1000 mμ.).

'Slow-acting' is a term used to describe viruses that do not cause overt disease for months, or even years, after they have infected a host. Examples: multiple sclerosis in man; scrapie and transmissible mink encephalopathy (TME) in animals.

VISCERA (*viscus*, the bowels) is the name given to the larger organs lying within the chest and abdominal cavities. The term 'viscus' is applied to each of these individually.

VISCERAL LARVA MIGRANS.—A syndrome produced in Man by the larvæ of *Toxocara canis*. Occasionally it is the cause of death. (*See* TOXOCARA.)

VISION (*see also* EYE). The capacity for being able to appreciate the position of objects in the outside world primarily depends upon the conversion of rays of light (vibrations of the ether, really) into nerve impulses, and the transmission of these to special centres in the brain. The process of conversion is effected in the retinæ of the eyes, and the impulses then travel by the optic nerves to the optic

* (*The Veterinary Annual 1962*, Wright, Bristol; 42s.)

centres of the brain. The functions of the eye are those of an optical instrument which brings the rays of light to a sensitive area and registers them there. Rays of light pass, in the first place, through the cornea, then through the aqueous humour that fills the anterior chamber of the eye. The light then enters the hinder part of the eye, through the pupil, a round, slit-like, or elliptical hole in the iris, which can be automatically narrowed according to the strength of the light rays that are passing through it. Immediately behind the iris lies the crystalline lens, a cl ar structure arranged in layers someweat like an onion, which also by automatic alterations in its curves, brings the rays to a focus upon the retina after they pass through a second clear jelly-like humour —the vitreous humour. The retina is the innermost of the three coats of the eyeball, and consists of the specialised terminations of the fibres of the optic nerve. The rods and cones, minute nervous structures in the deeper parts of the retina, seem to be the essential light-perceiving sensory endings. The rays of light fall upon these rods and cones and cause some molecular change, not well understood, and the resulting impulse is carried to the reception centre in the brain.

For obvious reasons the qualities of perception of outside objects by the eyes of animals are not well known, but, generally speaking, it appears that the soaring birds (eagle and hawk, etc.) are provided with the most acute vision, the carnivorous animals have the next most acute sight, and the herbivores—animals that are hunted and can utilise perceptions of hearing and smell more to their advantage than they can those of sight—have the least visual acuity. Whether the explanation of this lies in a greater number and a greater contiguity of rods and cones in the keen sighted than in the less keen-sighted animals, or whether the former possess vastly greater powers of accommodation centred in the more mechanical parts of the eye (cornea, lens, pupil, etc.) has not yet been definitely decided. Animals that prowl by night have often been credited with the power of being able to ' see in the dark ', but this is not strictly true; it will be immediately granted that they are *better able* to see in a *dim* light than man, but sight essentially depends upon at least faint rays of light falling upon the retina.

Monocular and binocular vision.—In animals whose eyes are laterally placed in the head it is impossible for both eyes to look at an object directly in front of them. One eye only can be focused upon an object at any one time, while the other eye sees a completely different picture. This is called ' monocular vision '. When the eyes are placed towards the front of the head so that they can both be concentrated upon an object, as in man, horse, and dog, each eye sees a slightly different picture, but the two ranges of vision overlap. This is called ' binocular vision '. It is partly owing to the fact that in binocular vision each eye sees slightly ' round the corner ' of the object, that a sense of depth and distance is conveyed to the higher brain centres. The two pictures are not quite superimposed, and the previous experience of the animal enables it to judge distance by this difference in superimposition. This is technically known as ' stereoscopic vision '. It is in the horse and dog, of the domestic animals, that eyesight is of most importance, and it seems probable that each possesses the power of using either monocular or binocular vision according to varying circumstances. When all a horse's concentration is brought to bear upon a single particular object situated directly in front of it, the two eyes are turned slightly inwards in an internal squint, each ear is pricked forwards, and the horse sees the object with both eyes. On the other hand, when a horse casually watches an object either behind or at the side of it, one eye only is employed. The head is slightly inclined towards the object, the corresponding ear is usually pricked, and the horse uses monocular vision only. In this latter case, where a stereoscopic effect is not possible, distance is probably judged by the amount of accommodation that occurs in the one eye to enable it to focus the object. This is, and must remain, largely a matter of conjecture, however.

A striking point in connection with the eyesight of animals is that, although many of them have their visual powers obviously very highly developed, they seldom *trust* their eyes in matters of emergency. The visual images alone do not convey to the mind the reality of the external world. It becomes necessary that the animal shall verify his visual impressions by tactile or olfactory impressions. In practically every case the fear of a harmless object may be immediately or shortly dispelled by allowing the animal to smell and examine it by touching it with the nose.

VISION, DISORDERS OF.—Disorders of vision, as distinct from diseases of the eye, are difficult to detect and usually impossible to correct in animals. Certain disorders, recognisable in man, and which may affect animals include:

Astigmatism.—This means that the curvature of the anterior surface of the cornea is not the same in the vertical as in the horizontal meridian, which it would be if the surface were accurately spherical. Measurement shows that in most horses the horizontal meridian is flatter than the vertical. So far as we are able to judge this does not appear to interfere with the horse's sight, however; it is probable that the brain centres have learnt by experience to disregard any distortion of the image cast on the retina due to astigmatism.

Emmetropia.—Eyes which possess the power of seeing objects distinctly both close at hand and at very great distances are called 'emmetropic'. A small percentage of horses' eyes appear to be emmetropic.

Myopia.—When the eyeball is too long, so that the image falls slightly in front of the retina, the condition is one of myopia, or short sight. According to Smith's observations on the eyes of horses 90 per cent show this defect.

Hypermetropia.—If the eyeball is too short and the image falls behind the retina, so that while all objects at a distance are clearly seen those close at hand are blurred, the condition is one of hypermetropia, or long sight. A small percentage of horses' eyes, and the eyes of nearly all wild animals are hypermetropic.

VISNA.—A disease of sheep, stated to be distinguishable from scrapie. It occurs in Iceland.

VITAMINS (*vita*, life; *amine*, related to ammonia) are substances present in natural foods, essential for health, and which exercise an influence in nutrition out of all proportion to the amounts consumed. Several vitamins are synthesised in the animal body, some being thus available independent of the diet, but it is important to note that a vitamin synthesised in the *lower* part of the alimentary canal may be available to an animal only if it eats its own droppings. (Nocturnal coprophagy is a regular practice with rabbits.) The chemical nature of many vitamins is now known, and many are obtainable commercially, though it is seldom practicable or necessary to administer them in the pure state.

Animals when feeding under natural conditions, with a free choice from a wide range of food-stuffs, consume, as a rule, all the vitamins they require. But under the influence of domestication, and especially of intensive rearing, animals often have no choice in the matter and suffer from vitamin deficiencies (which see) either because their artificial diet is too restricted, or because vitamins naturally present have been destroyed in the preparation of the food.

Deficiency of vitamins in the young, especially when in conjunction with limited exercise and restricted sunlight, produces marked body changes, which may handicap the subject for the rest of its life.

The principal vitamins are at present considered to be:

Vitamin A is a substance called *carotene*; it is found in carrots, green vegetables, egg-yolk, fish roe, liver, cod-liver oil, and in the livers of certain other varieties of fish. It is present in certain marine algæ, and from them passes by way of various marine animals and small fish to the cod. It is also present in some fats, but is not found in pig's lard if the pig has been fed on diets lacking it, or if the lard has been refined. This vitamin is either absent or only present in very small amount in vegetable oils, such as sunflower seed oil, maize oil, cotton-seed oil, arachis (peanut) oil, linseed oil, coco-nut oil, etc.

This vitamin is necessary for the growth and general well-being of the young animal in particular. By withholding it from the diet of young rats, at first there is a period of normal growth, when presumably the body makes use of its reserve supplies, but as soon as these are exhausted growth practically ceases. Soon afterwards the majority develop a characteristic eye disease, to which the name xerophthalmia' has been given.

VITAMIN B_1 (Aneurin, thiamin). Water-soluble. Present in yeast and liver.

VITAMIN B_2 complex, water-soluble, includes: riboflavin, nicotinic acid, pantothenic acid, choline, biotin. Most of these are present in yeast and liver.

Vitamins B_1 and B_2 are present in plant seeds, egg-yolk, and in some vegetables and fruits; they are chiefly found in the germ of seeds, such as wheat and rice, but the richest supply is from yeast. Ox liver and to some extent red flesh contain them, and there is a good supply in peas and lentils. Deficiency of Vitamin B_1 causes beri-beri in man, polyneuritis in birds; and is associated with bracken-poisoning in horses, cattle, and sheep. Lack of B_2 causes pellagra. These diseases are caused by feeding on a restricted diet of degermed and decorticated grain, *e.g.* wheat or rice. The vitamins are chiefly located in the germ or embryo and in the aleurone or vitamin layer of the pericarp, and since both germ and pericarp are removed in the manufacture of white bread it follows that white bread is made from 'devitalised' flour. When the pericarp or cuticle is removed from rice the germ also comes away, as it is superficially placed at one end. Beri-beri became prominent in the East when the custom of removing the cuticle or bran coat, to make the grain look more attractive, became prevalent; naturally beri-beri only occurs when milled rice forms the main portion of the diet and other potential sources of Vitamin B are withheld. Vitamin B_{12} is the anti-pernicious anæmia factor of importance in human medicine, and is associated with the Animal Protein Factor (which see).

Vitamin C.—This is ascorbic acid; it is found in the juices of most fruits and vegetables, and its absence causes scurvy such as occurred in the days of long voyages on sailing ships when no fresh vegetables were available and the diet mainly consisted of pickled meat and biscuits. The anti-scorbutic vitamin is found in nature associated with living tissues in which metabolic processes are still proceeding. When these cease or are greatly reduced, as in seeds, the anti-scorbutic 'vitamin' also disappears. In the case of seeds it is created anew during germination. The distribution of this factor thus presents a marked contrast with that of the anti-beri-beri factor, of which one of the principal sources is found in dry seeds. The anti-scorbutic vitamin is found in abundance in raw swede juice, tomato, orange, and lemon juice; meat and milk contain very little. Easily destroyed by cooking.

Vitamin D.—This is now identified as radiostol or irradiated ergosterol. It is the anti-rachitic principle found in cod-liver oil, meat juice, cow's milk, and egg-yolk. The absence of this vitamin causes rickets. There is an intimate association between the presence of this vitamin, the action of sunlight or the artificial irradiation by ultra-violet rays, and the mineral balance in the body. Sunlight falling on to cholesterol in animal cells, or on to phytosterol in plant cells, appears to endow the atoms of these substances with energy. In the case of animals during irradiation, either with sunlight or the ultra-violet rays emanating from a mercury-vapour quartz lamp, or even, to a less extent, from a carbon arc, the skin appears to become activated and the cholesterol present in it absorbed.

With its help salts of calcium and phosphorus, instead of being eliminated from the intestinal canal, are absorbed into the system and made use of in the calcification of bone. Thus rickets in both children and animals can be cured with a great degree of certainty, provided that they are not too far advanced. For children the somewhat spectacular artificial 'sun baths' are employed, but with animals results nearly as satisfactory can be obtained by exposing them to sunlight as much as possible and providing them with cod-liver oil—which is rich in Vitamin D. *Too much* D is harmful to pigs.

Vitamin E (fat-soluble).—This accessory food factor is found particularly in the germ of wheat and in red meat. It is necessary for fertility, and its absence from a diet has been shown to cause sterility in rats, by inducing firstly the death, and later the absorption, of the embryos.

Vitamin E could with advantage be added to all compound feeds as a precautionary measure; and at higher levels if the feed contains polyunsaturated fatty acids. Less vitamin E is absorbed from the intestine if the latter are present. Some feeds contain vitamin-E antagonists —present in lucerne and beans. The activity of vitamin E may be reduced by a high nitrate content in feed or drinking water. Animals which do not receive an adequate supply of the trace element selenium need extra vitamin E, because selenium has a vitamin-E sparing effect. Application of fertilisers rich in sulphates inhibits the absorption of selenium by plants from the soil, and in these circumstances grazing animals will require extra vitamin E.

Vitamin E content of feeds/crops may be reduced to a dangerous level on storage. (*See also* MUSCULAR DYSTROPHY.)

Vitamin H.—Used in treating eczema, alopecia.

Vitamin K.—A fat-soluble vitamin present in alfalfa, spinach, fish *meal*. It is associated with PROTHROMBIN.

VITAMIN K complex, mostly fat-soluble. Concerned with the formation of PROTHROMBIN (which see), and hence might be regarded as 'the anti-internal-hæmorrhage factor'. Present in spinach; synthetic preparations available for therapy.

While the study of accessory food factors has attracted the attention of scientists the world over, and much important information has been obtained regarding these interesting substances, which have a profound influence on the nutrition of people, and of children in particular, knowledge as to the significance of vitamins for live-stock is not yet complete. If the stockowner feeds and manages his animals on rational line she need not concern himself unduly about vitamins. He should expose his stock to as much direct sunlight as possible, give them a mixed and varied diet, and allow a regular and sufficient supply of fresh green food. Special attention should be given to the feeding of stall-tied cattle (particularly dairy cows), sty-reared pigs, poultry kept on the intensive system and calves reared on artificial foods, especially if the animals are confined in houses so constructed that direct sunlight cannot enter. It is only when through some unavoidable circumstance, rickets, unthriftiness, failure to grow or some other vitamin-deficiency disease appears amongst the young stock, that the stockowner should seek to discover wherein his ration is deficient, and so add the necessary vitamin-rich substance accordingly. From what has been already said regarding the results produced, he may obtain guidance, but it should be remembered that cod-liver oil (containing A and E), yeast (containing B), wheat bran (containing B and E), and green hay, lucerne, or clover (containing D), when fed in appropriate amounts will supply each of the known vitamins in adequate amount, as a rule.

Vitamin Deficiencies.—These may occur as the result of a vitamin-deficient diet, or a failure—in some instances—to synthesise a particular vitamin within the body. 'Secondary' or 'conditioned' deficiencies may also arise from any disease which impairs absorption from the alimentary tract, injuries to the liver, infections (which increase the consumption of vitamins), metallic poisoning, and as the result of some enzyme which destroys or inactivates a vitamin. (For examples of the last-mentioned cause, *see* CHASTEK PARALYSIS.)

The best way of avoiding primary vitamin deficiencies is to rear animals under as natural conditions of feeding as possible, with access to sunlight, and to avoid a restricted, artificial diet. Just as there is an 'endocrine balance' so it is probably true to say that there is a 'vitamin balance'. Hence it is important in correcting, or seeking to prevent vitamin deficiencies, not to be too heavy-handed. An *excess* of yeast fed to pigs as a Vitamin B supplement will induce severe rickets.

Anti-vitamin E factor may be present in barley as well as fats of animal origin.

Horses.—Vitamin A deficiency is unlikely to occur except in town horses denied adequate green food. Deficiency symptoms are stated to include night-blindness, hoof lesions, corneal lesions, respiratory symptoms, and reproductive difficulties. Some of the B vitamins are synthesised by adult horses, but backward foals have sometimes been stated to benefit from yeast. Infertility in the mare may sometimes be associated with a Vitamin C deficiency. It has been suggested that splints, sidebones, ringbones, spavins may be associated with a Vitamin D deficiency.

Cattle.—Vitamin A deficiency leads, in cattle denied adequate green food, to abortion or the birth of weak, blind calves, or of those suffering from diarrhœa which die within a few days. Corneal lesions and blindness may also result in growing cattle. (*See also* HYPERKERATOSIS.) Vitamins of the B complex are mostly synthesised in the rumen, but in the new-born calf a deficiency may occur and benefit be derived from the feeding of yeast. Vitamin C is apparently synthesised by adult cattle, but some cases of infertility may, it is believed, be due to a deficiency, and some cases of 'navel-ill' benefit, it is said, from Vitamin C treatment. In some parts of this country pasture or fodder crops contain too little Vitamin D, while sunlight during the winter months is insufficient to enable the shortage to be made good within the animal's body; the result is rickets. Vitamin E deficiency is associated with muscular dystrophy.

Pigs.—Vitamin A deficiency results in failure to grow in piglets and infertility in adult pigs, paralysis of the hind-quarters. A nicotinic acid deficiency gives rise to a condition simulating necrotic enteritis and poor growth. Yeast supplements will correct deficiencies of the

B complex, but excess may result in rickets. (*See* PLATE 2.)

A vitamin E deficiency in newborn piglets can result in their sudden death after being given iron injections to prevent anæmia. It is advisable to delay the injections until the piglet is a week old, when it is more tolerant of iron. Gilts' rations low in vitamin E or high in fatty acid predispose to this condition in the offspring.

Dog and Cat.—Vitamin A has been used with success in the treatment of diarrhœa in kittens. Corneal lesions, even blindness in extreme cases, and sometimes deafness, have also been attributed to a Vitamin A deficiency. Vitamin B (thiamin) deficiency results in fatigue and loss of appetite, and may be associated with cramp. Yeast may prove effective in cases of 'depraved appetite' and chorea. 'Black-tongue' in the dog and an ulcerative stomatitis in the cat are seen in the U.S.A. in naturally occurring cases of nicotinic acid deficiency. Lack of riboflavin is associated with eye lesions and skin disease. Rickets results from lack of Vitamin D, especially in the larger breeds.

Poultry.—Vitamin A deficiency will occur only in birds deprived of adequate green food. Maize and cod-liver oil (which must not be rancid) are alternative sources of this vitamin. Lack of it leads, in chickens, to drowsiness, weakness, staggering, stunted growth, and often a discharge from the eyes. Adult birds become dishevelled looking, weak and emaciated, and show a watery or cheesey discharge from eyes and nostrils. Deficiency of riboflavin (Vitamin B_2) in the diet is not uncommon, particularly in wire-floor battery brooders, in which the chicks have no access to droppings. (On solid floors chicks may correct the deficiency by eating their droppings, which contain riboflavin synthesised by organisms in the lower part of the gut, but not otherwise available to the body.) Symptoms are leg weakness and a curling inwards of the toes in chicks; decreased egg production and poor hatchability; the more advanced dead-in-shell showing curled toes. This vitamin is present in skimmed milk and yeast. A yeast supplement will also make good any deficiency of biotin. Lack of this may be suspected when the dead-in-shell have twisted legs or partly webbed feet. Thin egg-shells, reduced hatchability, and sometimes a temporary paralysis after laying, are indications of a Vitamin D deficiency. Chicks are unthrifty, walk with difficulty, and later show typical symptoms of rickets. Bone deformity and softening of the beak occur in adult birds. Sunlight, green food, and the judicious use in winter of cod-liver oil overcome this deficiency. Vitamin E, necessary for hatchability, is present in whole grain and, to a lesser extent, in greenstuff. The latter also contains ample Vitamin K, a deficiency of which leads to anæmia as a result of internal hæmorrhage.

VITELLUS, or **VITELLUM,** is the Latin name for yolk of egg.

VOICE (*vox*).—By the term voice is meant the sound produced in man and the higher animals as the result of the vibration of a column of air forced through the larynx by contraction of the respiratory muscles. The means by which this is produced are analogous to those by which sound is produced in a reed instrument, except that in the living animal the pitch of the voice can be altered at will. This is accomplished by the amount of tension exerted by muscular action upon the vocal cords; the more tense these are the higher is the pitch of the voice. In the majority of mammals the vibrations are produced when a blast of air is expelled from the chest, but in the ass the higher notes of the bray result from inspiration of air, and the lower notes from expiration.

The character of the voice can be altered to some extent by changes in the resonating chambers of the nose, mouth, pharynx, etc.; thus, the false nostrils of the horse are used to produce the 'snort' of fear or excitement, the nasal cavities transmit the whinny and neigh of pleasure, and the mouth and pharynx furnish the character of the neigh of impatience, loneliness, and sometimes the challenge of anger of the jealous stallion.

Neighing or *whinnying* in the horse is an expiratory act produced partly through the mouth and partly through the nose; the *bray* of the ass is expiratory for the low notes and inspiratory for the high; *bellowing* in the ox, *bleating* in the sheep, *barking* in the dog, and the *mew* of the cat, are all produced by expiratory efforts.

Animals use their voices upon widely different occasions. It seems probable that they make the greatest use of this faculty for the purposes of enabling the young to recognise their dams from a distance, and to maintain cohesion of herds or flocks. Stragglers getting left behind, or separated from their special companions, can be heard calling for long distances, and the calls are sure to be answered by other members of the company. In addition to these uses, male animals of many breeds will give forth a challenge or a warning upon the approach of newcomers or danger. Some animals cry out when fighting, but the majority engage in combat silently. Females generally produce little cries or screams when attended by males during periods of œstrum, or when making acquaintance with their newly born progeny. Almost all the domestic animals emit cries when suffering pain. In the horse tribe the sounds are often merely grunts or groans, especially when the pain is abdominal, but some highly strung animals endure the greatest pain in silence. In other cases horses will scream out with high-pitched piercing cries when they are suddenly subjected to acute pain, or to very great fright. The scream of an anguished horse can never be forgotten. Cattle and sheep in agony behave similarly to horses; they usually groan, but cows, ewes, and heifers may issue a long drawn-out bellow or bleat during difficult parturition. The pig has a range of notes from the satisfied grunt of a suckling sow, to the frightened squeals and screams of those that are being handled by man. The dog has a note for all occasions; he generally expresses all the emotions of which he is capable by differences in his bark. (*See also* LARYNX *and* MUTING.)

In rabies the character of the voice may be changed. In the 'dumb' form, barking is suppressed.

VOLAR.—At the back of the fore-limb.

VOLVULUS (*volvo*, I twist).—An obstruction of the bowels is produced by the twisting of a loop of bowel round itself. It is usually due to some spasmodic contraction of the muscular coat, or to the presence of gas, and is very dangerous owing to the great risk of strangulation of the blood-supply and consequent necrosis. (*See* INTESTINE, DISEASES OF.)

VOMICA (*vomica*, an abscess).—A cavity in the lung tissue produced by disease. Vomicæ are most commonly met with in cattle suffering from either tuberculosis or contagious pleuro-pneumonia.

VOMITING (*vomo*, I vomit) is an involuntary expulsion of the contents of the stomach through the mouth or nostrils. It is not merely a contraction of the stomach walls and a dilatation of the gullet, but it is a complex act in which the abdominal muscles, the diaphragm, the muscles of the chest and larynx, and those of the lower part of the neck all play a part. In certain cases there is an attempt at vomiting by an animal but no material is expelled; this is called *retching*, but the process is virtually the same as in vomiting.

Before the act there is usually a profuse secretion of watery saliva which serves to lubricate the passage of the stomach contents. The animal appears uneasy, and will usually seek a secluded spot. Soon rhythmic contractions of the abdominal muscles commence and culminate in the ejection of a quantity of frothy material. The diaphragm is generally fixed, and there is a powerful closing of the glottis to prevent any fluids from gaining access into the trachea.

The dog and cat vomit with great ease and frequency. The act seems to be one of Nature's safeguards against the possibly harmful effects of the ingestion of unsuitable food-stuffs or other materials. The dog is able to induce vomiting by eating portions of the green shoots of couch grass (*Triticum repens*), ingestion of which brings on vomiting in from 5 to 10 minutes. The cat also possesses this power but does not use it so frequently. The pig vomits when it has eaten some irritant substance, but the process is more exacting than in the carnivores. Cattle and sheep may vomit occasionally, but the act is an unusual one, and generally points to serious stomach trouble. The horse vomits upon rare occasions, and then when suffering from some extremely serious internal complaint. The act is frequently associated with collections of gas in, or a rupture of, the wall of the stomach, and when it occurs it should be considered a very grave symptom indeed. The material always escapes through the nostrils in the horse, and may have come from a dilated œsophagus rather than from the stomach in some cases.

Causes.—It will be sufficient to deal with vomiting under the headings as follows:

Travel sickness (which see).

Simple indigestion.—When the stomach has received either a quality or a quantity of food-stuff with which it is unable to deal the process of digestion does not proceed, or only proceeds up to a point. The material brought up is recognisable as food, but it is mixed with quantities of frothy mucus, water, and perhaps may be stained brownish from bile. It has a faintly sour smell which is greater the longer the process of digestion has been enabled to proceed. The ejecta is generally easily brought up, and the animal soon settles down and becomes normal.

Indigestion from foreign bodies.—When some foreign material has been swallowed by dogs or cats little or nothing may be noticed until the animal takes food. Then, in from a few minutes to half an hour the meal is returned. There is usually considerable distress, and retching may occur for some time after the stomach has been emptied of its food. Finally, however, the animal becomes bright and easy, assumes its normal life, and no further symptoms are seen until food is again eaten. Once more the food is vomited, and with each attack the symptoms become more and more exaggerated. If the foreign object be rough or sharp, such as a stone or piece of coal, there may be a small quantity of bright red blood in the vomit. In cases where the material is soft, such as wool, fabrics, fur balls, etc., some food can be retained, and vomiting is only marked when a large meal is taken.

Gastritis.—The walls of the tomach are inflamed and thickened, the mucous membrane is swollen and painful, and the nervous system is in an irritable state. Whenever food or water enters the organ vomiting immediately takes place. The vomit consists of the solid material swallowed, coated on the outside with mucus and froth. If liquids have been taken they are returned almost unchanged. When the inflammatory condition is very severe there are quantities of blood that has undergone partial digestion and has an appearance not unlike coffee-grounds, seen in the vomit. In such animals there will be a very offensive smell both from the ejecta and from the mouth of the patient.

Pyloric stenosis, which may be congenital, is said to give rise to 'projectile' vomiting.

Enteritis is associated with vomiting similar to the above, but there is diarrhœa as well.

Impaction of the rectum, whether from particles of undigested bone, or hair, hard fæces, etc., generally induces vomiting in which not only does the stomach expel its contents, but there are masses of bowel content as well. This vomiting of fæces is characterised by a most offensive fæcal odour, and is called 'stercoraceous vomiting'.

Acute nephritis is an extremely common cause of thirst and vomiting in the dog.

Pyometra in the bitch, cat, sow is frequently accompanied by vomiting. Vomiting may also occur reflexly during difficult parturition.

Accidents.—Direct injuries to the walls of the stomach, which lacerate them but do not produce rupture, are accompanied by vomiting. Sometimes the shock of a severe burn or accident will cause it, although the injuries have not been inflicted upon the stomach itself. In other cases, where the head has been injured, the area in the case of the brain which controls the act of vomiting becomes disturbed and the animal evacuates its stomach.

Poisons.—Very many irritant substances will produce vomiting, either when taken into the stomach, or when entering the general circulation by other means. Of the commonest may be mentioned—tartar emetic, mustard, salt, carbolic acid, areca-nut, castor oil, etc.; and of substances less common, but more drastic, the following are examples—strychnine, arsenic, phosphorus, apomorphine, croton oil, zinc and copper sulphates, and many of the metallic salts. Some of these have special characteristics; *e.g.* phosphorus vomit is luminous in the dark, copper sulphate vomit is greenish-blue, etc.

Diseases.—The symptom of vomiting is common to many other diseased conditions—meningitis, peritonitis, nephritis, leptospirosis, 'vomiting and wasting' syndrome in pigs, etc.

Treatment.—Before rational treatment can be undertaken the cause must be ascertained as nearly as possible. After this the principles consist in (1) relieving the source of the irritation, and (2) soothing the nervous centres. In the dog and cat the use of normaline saline or glucose saline by injection is frequently indicated as an alternative to giving food (liquid or otherwise) by the mouth during an illness (such as nephritis, uræmia, enteritis) in which vomiting is persistent. Diagnosis is all-important. Where impaction or stoppage of the bowels has taken place, an enema of warm soapy water must be given, and the collected matter removed; subsequently a laxative may be required.

'VOMITING AND WASTING' SYNDROME.—This occurs in piglets five days old and upwards, and is characterised by vomiting, depression, loss of appetite, constipation, emaciation, and a hairy appearance. It is probably caused by a virus. (*See also* 'ONTARIO ENCEPHALITIS'.)

V.P.P.—Virus Pneumonia of Pigs (Now generally known as Enzoötic Pneumonia).

VULVA is the term applied to the ultimate part of the female genital canal, and also to the external parts. It reaches as far forward as the opening of the female urethra, and consequently serves as the termination of the urinary passage.

VULVOVAGINITIS, GRANULAR.—Also known as nodular venereal disease, it was first described in 1887 as a cause of abortion and infertility in cattle. It has been reported in the U.K. and many countries overseas.

Cause.—This is now, following successful experimental transmission, believed to be *Mycoplasma bovigenitalium.*

Symptoms.—Granular elevations appear on the epithelium of vulva and vagina. A muco-purulent discharge is often seen.

This disease (G.V.V.) may be distinguished from INFECTIOUS PUSTULAR VULVOVAGINITIS (I.P.V., caused by a virus) as follows:

Clinical Features	I.P.V.	G.V.V.
Rise in body temperature	104·0 to 106·0° F.	None
Lesions: Appearance after experimental infection	1 to 2 days	3 to 22 days
when palpated	Soft, can be ruptured	Firm, translucent when small
Vaginal discharge	Straw-yellow colour	Whitish-yellow colour and frequently sticky
Epithelial cells of the vaginal smears contain intra-nuclear inclusion bodies	Yes	No

(from *Veterinary Record* for April 9, 1966)

'WALKABOUT DISEASE' (*see* KIMBERLEY HORSE DISEASE).

WALL-EYES in horses are met with when the greater part of the face, or that portion around the eyes, is white. The condition consists of an absence of colouring matter in the iris. The pupil of the eye appears to be encircled by a ring of bluish or greyish white, and the expression of the horse's face is consequently unusual. It is not necessarily a sign of vice, nor a serious defect except in tropical countries where the light is very intense.

'WANDERERS'.—Thoroughbred foals suffering from the blindness and aimless wandering stage of the condition described under 'BARKERS'.

WARBLES are swellings about the size of a marble or small walnut occurring upon the backs of cattle in spring and early summer caused by the presence in them of the maggot of one of the warble flies—*Hypoderma bovis* or *Hypoderma lineata*. (*See* PARASITES, p. 677.) These are of very great economic importance. The adults — especially *Hypoderma bovis* —

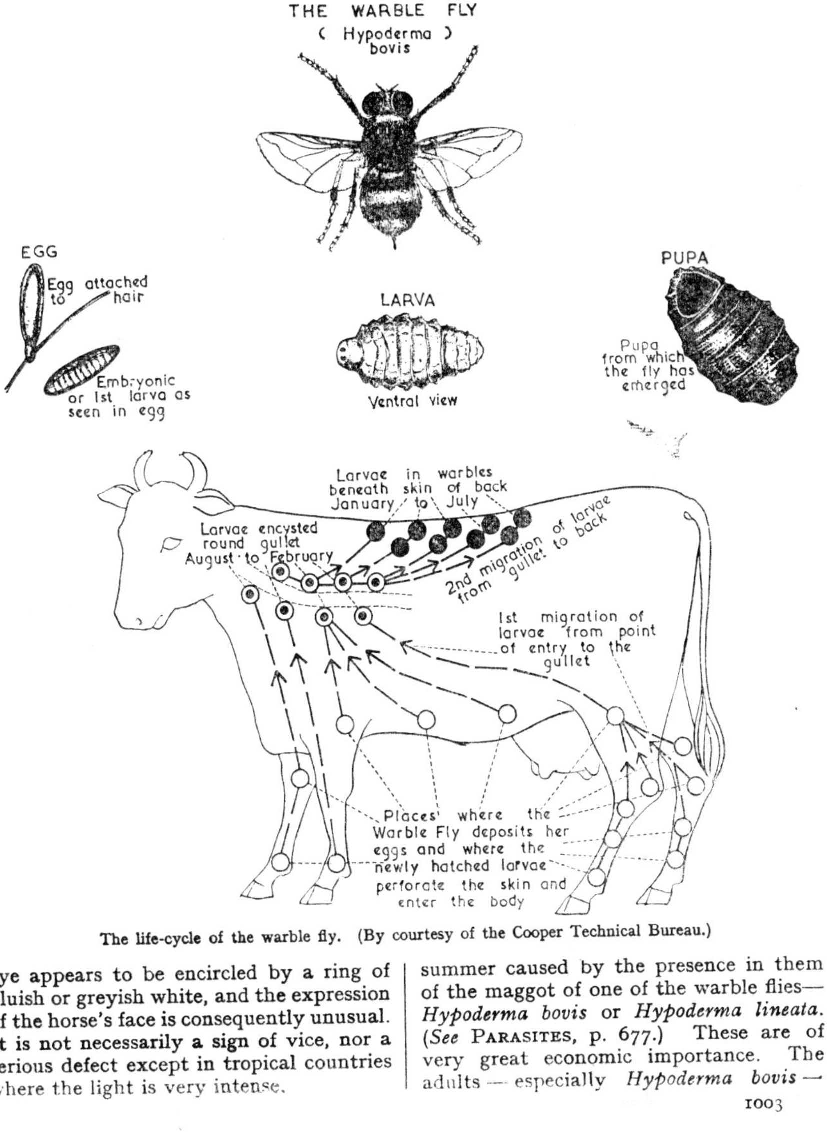

The life-cycle of the warble fly. (By courtesy of the Cooper Technical Bureau.)

 WARBLES

cause great annoyance to stock during the period when eggs are being laid. Not only does this result in injuries, animals rushing madly around to avoid the buzzing 'attacks', but the milk yield is reduced, sometimes by as much as 25 per cent, and condition is impaired.

These losses are slight, however, compared with the injuries produced by the larvæ. The young forms, newly hatched from the eggs, produce local sores at the points where they enter the skin; this may amount to a 'hypodermal rash'—especially in the case of *H. lineatum*. The same species in its migration through the body irritates the gullet; and both species may injure the spinal cord. The warbles on the back are really so many small abscesses which not only reduce condition very considerably but may, when many are present, result in the death of young animals. Fattening is difficult, and milk yield is reduced. The accidental crushing of a number of the larvæ in these cavities may cause the rapid death of the animal.

In the carcases there is considerable destruction of valuable meat around the warbles; 'Butchers' Jelly' or 'Licked Beef' is an œdematous, straw-coloured, jelly-like substance, which infiltrates the tissue near the grubs. The holes which the grubs produce in the hides reduce their value; heavily infected hides are often useless for leather.

Warbles are most frequent in young animals, in which loss of condition is most serious; but they have been found in small numbers in animals up to 15 years old. They are sometimes found in young horses. The larvæ occasionally enter the spinal canal and produce very serious lesions. Horses are attacked mostly by *Hypoderma bovis* larvæ, which affect the area of the saddle chiefly; but brain involvement has been once reported in the horse.

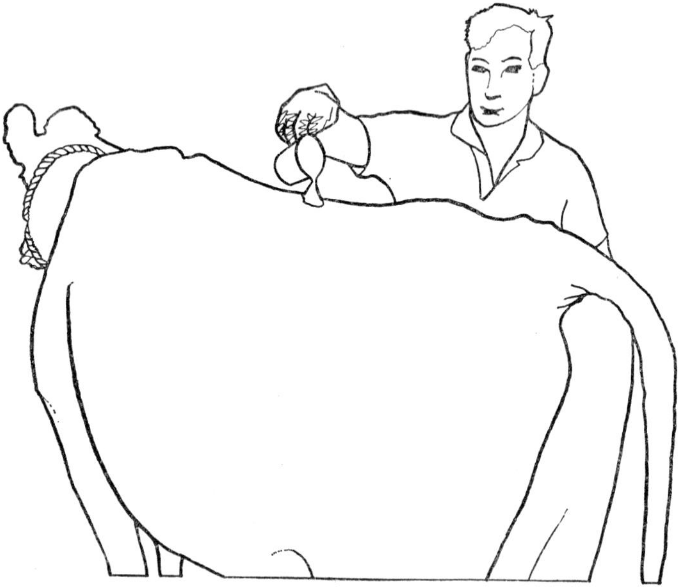

Dressing against warbles: applying 'Ruelene' to a cow's back.

The damage done by these flies and their larvæ in the United States is estimated at from fifty to one hundred million dollars yearly; in the United Kingdom it is conservatively believed to be several million pounds annually. This damage, in most districts, is entirely preventable, but it must be done by collective effort.

Methods of Control.—Satisfactory control depends on artificial interference with the life cycle. In Britain, the Warble Fly (Dressing of Cattle) Order of 1948, requiring that 'all visibly infested' cattle must be given Derris treatment on three occasions between March 15 and June 30, was revoked in June, 1964.

Previously, farmers were advised to purchase Derris soap mixture from a reliable firm rather than to make up their own solutions from materials of unknown potency and stability. Since a solution of *rotenone* in soap tends to lose its potency on exposure to the air, the solution should be made just prior to use, and any mixture remaining unused should be discarded.

The dressing may be applied in various ways. A stout syringe—such as a motor cycle oil-squirt—is both efficient and economical in applying the solution directly to the warble. Alternatively, a cloth (not a flannel cloth which quickly picks up hairs) may be dipped in the dressing and placed on the warble; the outer scab is removed by a twist of the cloth, the dressing from which is then squeezed into the hole. The solution is poured on to the skin before it is rubbed because it froths very easily and is then difficult to get close to the skin because of the hair.

Dressing should not be applied in wet weather as the rain washes much of it off. It should probably be applied at least four times during the season, the first occasion being determined by local circumstances and the remainder being about a month apart. Animals with living warbles in their backs should not be turned out to pasture, as even a single warm day may cause the larvæ to emerge and pupate. The average cost of the dressing is about threepence an animal.

The conventional treatment of warbles with derris has the great and obvious disadvantage that it kills the larvæ only after they have already caused much pain and tissue damage—to say nothing of ruined potential hides. A systemic insecticide, on the other hand, will kill a high percentage of larvæ *before* they complete their migration and penetrate the back.

Systemic insecticides, so well known to horticulturists, have come into use against parasites of farm live-stock. These insecticides are truly 'systemic', for in the same way that they are absorbed by the leaves of a plant and enter its sap, so they circulate within the animal body. Given by mouth, they will be excreted by the skin and, applied to the skin in a suitable manner, they will be absorbed and circulate in the blood-stream; though the same method of administration is not recommended for all.

The two most commonly used systemic insecticides in Britain against warbles are crufomate ('Ruelene') and trichlorphon. Both may be applied by pouring on to the animal's back.

When using organic compounds of phosphorus, such as these insecticides are, one has to bear in mind two potential dangers—that from residues in the carcase to people eating the meat; and the danger of the cattle being rendered ill by the dose. However, these compounds have been the subject of extensive trials both in Britain and overseas.

Crufomate poisoning as a result of over-dosage results in distressed breathing and a staggering gait; also a tendency to remain lying down. Atropine is an antidote. (*See also* TRICHLORPHON.)

In 1965 the British Veterinary Association supported the use of organophosphorus systemic dressings, recommending application between October 1 and November 15 or between mid-March and the end of the warble season (but *not* between mid-November and mid-March 'because of the location of the parasite in the host').

In 1968 a warbles eradication scheme covering a central zone of 50 square miles, surrounded by a 5-mile outer zone, was reported. Between 85–90 per cent of the cattle—over 17,000 in all—were sprayed annually with coumaphos and crufomate. The average number of warbles per animal were reduced from 13.7 to nil in two years. After five years the average incidence was 0.8 warble per head. Poisoning was not observed with either drug.

The warble fly has been eradicated from the Isle of Man, Cyprus, and Denmark.

The tropical warble fly of Central America is *Dermatobia hominis*, which lays its eggs on an intermediary vector—fly or mosquito—which it catches for the purpose.

WARFARIN.—An organic rat poison approved by the Ministry of Agriculture and internationally known. It is an anticoagulant, its use leading to death of rats and mice from internal hæmorrhage. In the strengths used, 0·005 per cent and 0·025 per cent, it is considered that properly prepared baits will not prove dangerous to live-stock if used with ordinary care. Cases of accidental poisoning have occurred, however, in the dog and the pig; and food contaminated by rodents' urine may be dangerous where Warfarin is used. Vitamin K is indicated as an antidote before internal hæmorrhage occurs.

WARTS are small solid growths arising upon the surface of the skin or mucous membrane. They belong to the class of tumours, and are technically known as 'papillomata'. They are composed of fibrous tissue cores covered over with a thick layer of epithelial cells similar to those of the region in which they are situated. They bear a great resemblance to overgrown skin papillæ when they occur upon the surface of the body, and are not unlike mucous membrane papillæ in other parts. They occur with great frequency in all the domestic animals, and are probably the commonest of all the tumours. When not complicated with other conditions they are non-inflammatory, painless except when they interfere with the movement of some part of the body, benign, and seldom sufficiently numerous to cause death. In size they vary from that of a pin's head to as large as an orange, but most often they are not larger than a pea.

Around the mouth they interfere with feeding, and when occurring about the nostrils they may obstruct the breathing. Soft warts in the œsophagus sometimes make swallowing difficult, and upon the penis or in the urethra they may hinder the passage of urine.

Horse.—The commonest situations in this animal are the skin of the udder or sheath, the lips and nostrils, the eyelids, outer and inner skin of the ears, the region of the breast, the insides of the limbs, and the face generally.

Ox.—In cattle the commonest seats of warts are the teats of cows. Young cows in winter are often affected about the skin of the eyelids and along the lower line of the abdomen, but the growths often drop off spontaneously from these positions when the young animals are turned out to grass in the early spring. Otherwise warty growths are found as in the horse. (*See* VIRAL PAPILLOMATOSIS.)

Warts on the teats may be of three kinds: (1) globular warts; (2) flat warts; and (3) cylindrical warts. The first and second of these are whitish or yellow in colour, hard to the touch, painless, and shaped according to their description. The globular variety are very often deeply embedded in the substance of the teat and may extend through its wall into the milk duct. They are generally about the size of a large pea, but sometimes they may be considerably larger. The flat type has a short stalk as a rule, and is somewhat scale-like. Cylindrical warts are the commoner kind. They are similar to the ordinary variety in other situations. They are often a dark colour near their free extremities, and are intimately attached to the skin. Sometimes they appear as single thorn-like projections, but more often they are multiple. In rare cases they have a thin stalk and are cauliflower like. (*See under* REMOVAL OF WARTS *below*.)

Dog and Cat.—In the dog especially, less so in the cat, warts are exceedingly common in almost every situation in the body. Single small warts with a cauliflower-like extremity or with a rounded top, are commonly found about the eyelids, lips, ears, paws, etc., as well as upon the general surface of the body. They usually grow very slowly and may be present for years without causing any pain or inconvenience. In other cases warts appear in connection with the gums, tongue, and insides of the cheeks; in these positions they arise in clusters and grow very rapidly. In the course of two or three months a dog's mouth that was previously quite clear may be studded with hundreds of growths of varying sizes, to such an extent that feeding is almost impossible on account of mechanical interference with the closing of the jaws. Cases such as these are usually accompanied by a great amount of salivation and a fœtid discharge from the mouth.

Removal of Warts.—Multiple warts in cattle have been successfully banished by means of intra-muscular injections of Anthiomaline (lithium antimony thiomalate). After a few injections the globular type of warts can then be 'shelled out' easily. (*See also under* VACCINE.) Otherwise removal of this type must be effected under local anæsthesia.

WASHING OF ANIMALS (*see* BATHS).

WASHING SODA.—Sodium carbonate (not to be confused with sodium bicarbonate or baking powder) is useful in emergency as an emetic for the dog—a small piece being given like a pill. (*See also under* DISINFECTION.)

WASP STINGS (*see under* BITES).

WASTING (*see* ATROPHY).

WATER AND WATERING OF ANIMALS.—Without a sufficiency of fluid, animals are unable to make good the loss of water that occurs through the secretions of milk, saliva, digestive juices, or the excretions of the skin (sweat) and kidneys (urine), and consequently they become unable to exercise their maximum powers of production—whether of flesh, milk, or work. Moreover, lack of water is not tolerated so easily as lack of food; animals can live for weeks without food, but they only exist for days when water is withheld. In addition to this it is essential that such water as is supplied shall be as pure as possible, for an impure water supply may be a source of disease. Not only may water serve as an intermediate agent in the spread of contagious diseases, but if it contains harmful products, such as excess of lead in solution, sewage or seepage from manure heaps, or quantities of decomposing vegetable matter, it may set up disease in animals drinking it. (*See* WATER SUPPLY.)

Amounts required.—The quantity of water needed per day by the various domestic animals depends upon the nature of the food they receive, the climate, and the size and the activity of the animals themselves. When very dry food is given, such as hay, bran, oats, etc., more water is required than when roots or growing grass is eaten. The safest method of watering animals is to allow them to have water regularly and let them drink as much as they desire. It is seldom that their sense of thirst will err if they are in good health otherwise. Roughly speaking, a horse needs 6 to 8 gallons of water per day under ordinary conditions; less than this will be taken when grass or roots are fed, and more than this will be required when the weather is very hot, when the horse perspires greatly, when the food is exceptionally dry, and in the case of the *pregnant* and the suckling mare. Cattle take more than this amount as a rule. It is usual to consider that a cow in full milk needs about four times as much water as the number of gallons of milk she produces; thus, a cow giving 4 gallons of milk per day should receive about 16 gallons of water.

In up-to-date byres continuously filled automatic drinking bowls are fitted, so that the cows may drink when and as much as they desire. The beneficial effects upon the health of the cows and upon the amount of milk they produce are remarkable. Bullocks fed upon roots will drink much less water owing to the high water content in the roots (as much as 90 per cent in the case of freshly pulled swedes). Calves require much more water after they are weaned than before; a common mistake is often made in not supplying plenty of water when the milk is being cut down, the calves receive a check to their growth, which they may never make up. Pigs take about a gallon of water for every 100 lb. live-weight, but the larger sows and boars will not require quite as much as this. Much of the water is supplied to pigs in the form of wet sloppy mashes, so that the actual amount of water they will drink is often less than would be expected. Under methods of dry meal feeding they should always be provided with as much water as they can drink. The benefits of creep-feeding may be lost if the piglets are denied water.

Sheep have shown symptoms suggestive of twin-lamb disease, and died, after being removed from a field where they had access to a stream and placed on pasture where the ball-valve of a drinking trough had been tied up.

Dogs, cats, and poultry should always be allowed an unlimited supply of water so arranged that they are unable to foul or upset the drinking vessels.

There can be no doubt that much of the intestinal trouble in animals is due, directly or indirectly, to an insufficiency of water. Lack of water directly leads to stiffness of the mass of ingesta, the digestive juices are unable to penetrate through the mass, fermentation takes place at its centre, gas is evolved, and its collection gives rise to the train of symptoms that are usually associated with tympany. (*See also* DEHYDRATION.)

A point that should never be lost sight of in connection with watering of horses is that wherever possible *water should be given before the food*, or not for 1 to 2 hours after feeding. The horse's stomach is small, and cannot contain a full feed and several gallons of water simultaneously.

Finally, animals of all kinds obtain the most benefit from their food if the water is given at regular intervals. A large amount given at one time is liable to be harmful, and the results of drinking too liberally when very thirsty may be fatal.

WATER-BED is the popular name for the whole of the fœtal membranes and their associated fluids, which are discharged either with or soon after the young animal is born.

The term is also applied to the part of the chorionic sac which appears at the lips of the vulva just before the real act of parturition begins, which is filled with fluid and has the function of dilating the passages and to some extent lubricating them, in readiness for the discharge of the fœtus; this is also sometimes called the 'water-bag'. (*See* PARTURITION.)

'WATER BELLY' (*see* TOXIC FAT DISEASE).

WATER-DROPWORT, *Œnanthe crocata*, a weed of marshy places, ditches, and other wet spots, is considered to be one of the most dangerous and poisonous of the commoner plants found in Great Britain, and many cases of poisoning, not only among animals but also among human beings, have been recorded. It is a member of the same botanical class as Cowbane, Hemlock, and Fool's Parsley, and like them the poisonous principle is found in all parts of the plant. In its leaves it has a great similarity to celery, and its rootstock has been mistaken for parsnip. The active toxic principle is called *Œnanthotoxin*, and is most abundant in the root. Owing to its luxuriant growth in marshy places to which animals have access it is often eaten when other green food is scarce.

Symptoms.—The symptoms appear very quickly after the plant has been eaten, and death follows in from 1 to 4 hours when large amounts have been taken. Cattle become very depressed in general appearance, and their respiration is fast and laboured. The mucous membranes become congested, the eye rolls, the pulse is weak and fast, and there is a certain amount of foaming at the mouth. Later there is colic and spasmodic contractions of the limbs and jaws. The animal may bellow, falls to the ground where it still moves its limbs, and soon becomes unconscious, and expires in violent convulsions. In some cases that are not fatal one or more of the limbs remain paralysed. In the horse the appearance of the symptoms and the course of the illness are much more rapid and the nervous symptoms are exaggerated. In the pig the poison is quickly eliminated by vomiting if the quantity swallowed has been small, but where large amounts have been eaten death occurs very rapidly.

Treatment.—Where one has reason to suspect that only small amounts of the plant have been eaten, the affected animals should be secured, and endeavours made to remove the portions eaten by use of the stomach-tube or by immediate rumenotomy wherever conditions are suitable. Where time allows, the animals should be given a dose of gruel containing strong coffee and opium or laudanum, but medicinal drenches are often out of the question.

The recognition and the careful elimination of the plant from marshy land to which cattle have access, is the most rational method of avoiding loss from water-dropwort.

WATER-FLEAS.—*Daphnia pulex*, a brown water-flea found in British ponds, is the intermediate host of the roundworms of ducks, *e.g. Acuaria uncinata*.

WATERHAMMER PULSE.—The peculiarly sudden pulse that is associated with incompetence of the aortic valves of the left side of the heart, and suggests the philosophical toy after which it is named.

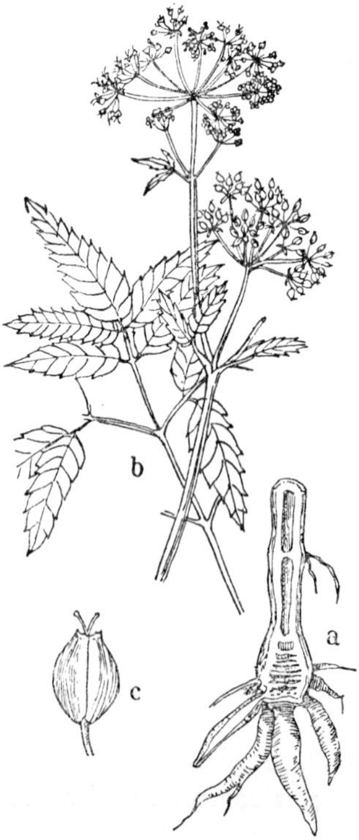

Water Hemlock or Cowbane (*Cicuta virosa*), showing at *a*, a portion of the tuberous root which may be mistaken for parsnip or celery by unwary persons; *b*, the foliage and flowering umbels; *c*, a seed capsule enlarged. The root contains the greatest amount of toxic principles, especially in the springtime.

WATER HEMLOCK is a common plant of damp marshy places in all parts of the Northern hemisphere. It has a short, stout hollow rootstock, and large much-divided leaves set on strong stems. The inflorescence is composed of minute white flowers with the tip of each petal turned back. (*See* p. 1008) The umbels measure from 4 to 5 inches across and before ripening are flat-topped. (For symptoms of poisoning, treatment, etc., *see under* COWBANE POISONING.)

WATER, LOSS OF, from the tissues—a serious condition—is referred to under DEHYDRATION. It occurs especially during the course of diarrhœa.

WATER ON THE BRAIN is a popular name for hydrocephalus. (*See* HYDROCEPHALUS, MENINGITIS.)

WATER ON CHEST is the popular designation of pleurisy with effusion. (*See* PLEURISY.)

WATER ON HEART is the popular name for pericarditis with effusion. (*See* HEART DISEASES.)

WATER SUPPLY. Sources.—*Rainfall* forms the primary source of all water supply. If collected under careful conditions, the vessels in which it is received being free from contamination and filth, it constitutes the purest and softest of waters, containing only such impurities as it has washed down or dissolved in its course through the atmosphere. In its passage through the air it becomes highly aerated, and, except in the neighbourhood of towns and densely populated districts, where factories abound and the pollution of the atmosphere may be considerable, it is practically pure. Where piped water is not available, rainwater may be collected from roofs by the gutters, which should be regularly cleaned. These conduct the water to specially prepared cisterns or tanks, preferably formed of slates, or bricks set in cement, or of concrete. Galvanised iron tanks are used in many parts and form useful receptacles, but care must be taken that the insides of these are kept clean, and that the galvanising is not chipped or broken, thereby allowing oxidation or 'rusting' of the iron and consequent deterioration. If paint is used to preserve the insides of the tanks it should be free from lead or other harmful substances that may become dissolved out by the oxygen contained in the water. All tanks used for the storage of water should be regularly cleaned out after the leaves have fallen from the trees in autumn, and should be provided with a cover to keep out dust, straw, and insects in the summer. Leaden cisterns are unsuitable for the storage of rain water because of the tendency of soft water to dissolve lead. (*See also* ZINC POISONING.)

Springs.—The portion of the rainfall which percolates through the soil absorbs carbonic acid gas from the lower levels of the air, and is thus enabled to dissolve many of the inorganic salts found in the soil. As it percolates still deeper it is slowly rendered clear and bright by the purification it undergoes by travelling down through the various strata on the surface of the earth's crust. This natural filtration is sufficient to remove most of the organic matter (particles of decomposing vegetable and animal matter, liquid manure, etc.) which the water has absorbed from the upper layers of the soil, always provided the distance that the water percolates is great enough.

As the water from springs may be contaminated at the point of issue, the spring should be walled in and provided with a discharging pipe that passes for some distance below the surface of the ground to the actual outlet, so that fouling by animals, and from storm waters in rainy weather, may be avoided.

Wells are of two main types—' shallow ' and ' deep ', a special form of the latter being known as '*Artesian*'. Shallow wells are liable to become polluted by soakings through the soil from leaking cesspools, liquid manure tanks and drains, from surface washings and manure, from animal and vegetable débris spread upon fields, and from other causes. Shallow wells are not usually of sufficient depth to allow of natural purification. Deep wells, in which the water is usually brought to the surface by pumping, tap the same kind of water as main springs, and yield an excellent wholesome supply. To protect them from pollution from surface and subsoil waters, they should be lined with bricks embedded in cement down to the depth of the first impermeable layer of clay or rock, etc., and their tops should be walled round and built up to such a height as will prevent any washings from the surface of the ground. Artesian wells pass through an upper impermeable layer to reach a store of water in a water-bearing stratum lying

WATER SUPPLY

upon a second impermeable formation. The water-bearing permeable stratum has its 'outcrop' at a higher level than where the well has been sunk, and consequently the water in its endeavour to find its own level rises up the well and issues at the top.

River water.—The quality of water derived from rivers differs according to the nature of the source from which it is obtained. Thus, water from near the source of a river, high up among granite-bound hills, may be perfectly pure and wholesome, but if it is obtained from the same river at lower levels after it has received the washings from manured fields, the soakage from cesspools, the sewage from hamlets and small towns, or the industrial refuse from factories, it may be highly unsuitable for drinking purposes. Every river in its course tends to purify its water. The sewage is diluted, the grosser particles are broken up against stones, or are scavenged by fish, and the oxygen which the moving water absorbs from the air decomposes the organic matter into harmless substances. This natural purification may be considerable where there is a large volume of water in the river, but in such cases there is almost always further contamination from other towns, etc., at lower levels, and the water is considered unfit for general use.

Upland surface waters.—The water contained in natural or artificial lakes, in hill streams, or from rivers near their sources, closely resembles rain water in composition, because it contains but little solid matter in solution, while any organic matter is of vegetable origin. These waters are usually highly palatable and pure, with the additional advantage of being soft. Peaty matter is frequently found in such upland surface waters, giving a slightly yellow discolouration and imparting a peaty taste, but this does not interfere with its usefulness, and the peaty matter can be removed by filtration where excessive. It should be noted, however, that peaty waters may possess a power of dissolving small amounts of lead by virtue of the peat acids they contain, and may be unsafe after passing through lead pipes. Only minute amounts of lead are taken into the systems of animals drinking such water, but lead is cumulative in the body, and the aggregation of these small quantities results in the production of the symptoms of chronic lead poisoning.

Quality.—Apart from actual badness, or a tendency to convey disease (see below), water may be either 'hard' or 'soft Hardness may be either temporary or permanent. The former is due to the presence of carbonates of calcium or magnesium held in solution by carbonic acid gas (CO_2), which may be driven off by boiling the water. This gas may also be got rid of by adding slaked lime to the water, which causes the production of stil more carbonate of lime, and the whole of this, *i.e.* what was originally present as well, settles down as a precipitate, and thus the temporary hardness is removed. Permanent hardness is due to the sulphates of calcium and magnesium, as well as to iron and aluminium, which cannot be got rid of by boiling. The Rivers Pollution Commissioners have classified the hardness of waters according to their sources, as follows: *Softest,* (1) rain water; (2) upland surface water; (3) water from cultivated lands; (4) river water; (5) spring water; (6) deep-well water; and *hardest,* (7) shallow-well water. Shallow wells may also contain soft water where there is but little depth of soil through which the water can percolate, and where there is no time for the solution of inorganic salts by the water.

Excessively hard water taken by animals for a considerable time is liable to upset digestion, and predisposes to the formation of calculi in the intestines or bladder. It is said that hard water produces a hard staring coat and sometimes constipation. Soft waters have been blamed for the production of rickets, owing to the deficiency of lime salts, but this is questionable. For all ordinary purposes a medium hard water should be chosen, but for washing purposes and for the making of dipping solutions a soft water is best.

Storage.—Where farms are situated close to towns the water supply for animal use is taken from the general town supply, and is usually of a high standard of purity. In other cases farms may have to depend upon individual supplies, which may be either wells, springs, ponds, or small artificial reservoirs made by damming up part of the course of a small stream, hollowing and widening the banks above, and providing regulating apparatus. In other cases, where the land is flat and does not allow of such measures, water is frequently pumped up from a deep well by means of a wind- or power-driven pump, and stored in tanks built at such a height as will allow of a sufficient head of water to rise through pipes to the highest part of the steading. Watering troughs are provided in yards, reeds, cattle-courts, and sometimes in the pastures, each being provided with a ball-cock regulating apparatus which maintains the supply at a fixed level. They should be built into the brickwork of the trough to prevent freezing in winter. The storage tanks for such systems are usually made of galvanised iron, and should be provided with a cover and some means of ventilation. The tanks should be cleaned out once a year, but vigorous scrubbing is to be avoided, as it removes the protective coating and allows of rusting.

Diseases spread by water.—Apart from illness that is actually caused by some inorganic substance dissolved in the water, such as lead from lead pipes or tanks, arsenic from contamination with sheep-dip, water-borne infection may cause disease in a generalised form. Among diseases that can be distributed in this manner are the following: Anthrax, from water used in tanneries or wool-washing premises, or when a carcase has been buried near a stream; Johne's disease and coccidiosis in cattle, from contamination of streams, ditches, and ponds with fæces from an infected cow; swine fever, from the drainage from infected piggeries; foot-and-mouth disease, from infection with buried carcases or from living animals in open fields, etc.; glanders, from public watering-troughs; influenza in horses, from watering-troughs or infection of streams, ponds, etc.; and probably also contagious pleuro-pneumonia of cattle, rinderpest, some of the parasitic worm infestations of calves, sheep, colts, and older horses. (*See also* SALMONELLOSIS, WATER AND WATERING OF ANIMALS.)

'WATERY MOUTH'. — A disease caused by *E. coli,* affecting new-born lambs in Britain. The lambs appear strong and healthy but on taking milk from the ewe they soon show signs of abdominal pain, and a watery fluid drips from the mouth. There may be scouring. Death soon follows as a rule.

WEALS are raised white areas of the skin which possess reddened margins. They may result from sharp blows or from continued pressure against some hard object. They are only visible upon the skins of pigs, as the hair of the other domestic animals hides the actual skin surface. (*See* URTICARIA.)

The term weal is also used in surgery in connection with the use of local anæsthetic solution. A primary weal is made, and when the local anæsthetic has taken effect, the needle of the syringe may be re-introduced into the now insensitive area and further injections made painlessly in order to anæsthetise a given area.

WEANING is a critical period in the life of the young animal unless carried out with care. Individuals sometimes require special precautions when they are weak or backward from disease or other cause, but generally speaking, it is necessary to accustom the young growing animal to a diet in which its dam's milk takes a more and more secondary place for some weeks before actual separation occurs. In the case of dairy cattle there is an exception to this rule, in that newly born calves are often taken away from their mothers as soon as they are born and have had some of the first-secreted milk containing colostrum, and are reared from a pail. Sudden changes in the diet are to be avoided at all times, and the change from a milk to a herbivorous or omnivorous diet should be gradual, for obvious reasons. In modern pig husbandry, creep-feeding is practised before weaning. More details will be found under the respective headings, such as CATTLE, BREEDS OF; PIGS, BREEDS OF; etc.

Early weaning of calves.—This is an alternative procedure to that of rearing dairy or beef calves on the bucket, using milk substitutes. The principle of early weaning is to provide an acceptable dry food which the calf will eat as early as 4 days of age. The rumen is thereby stimulated to growth and activity, and by the time the calf is 3 weeks old, the rumen is functioning—2 or 3 weeks earlier than under normal conditions. By 5 weeks, bucket feeding can be dispensed with, and the calf reared on solid food only—together with a liberal supply of water. Kale or silage can be introduced at this period in small amounts.

The advantages of the system are that, from the farmer's point of view, 5 or 7 weeks' bucket-feeding is dispensed with—and that means less labour and adherence to special feeding times. Moreover, it is claimed that the risk of scouring is less, and that the earlier rumen development makes for sturdier calves, able to go on to an adult diet sooner.

On the other hand, early weaning has

ed in some instances to illness and death as a result of the imperfect functioning of the immature rumen and abomasum. Technically known as gastric dyspepsia, the main symptom is often persistent scouring. After several days' depression and lack of appetite, the calf dies. There may be staggering or fits, but hypomagnesæmia and not dyspepsia may be the cause of these.

Diagnosis is difficult and even at *post-mortem* examination may have to be based largely upon circumstantial evidence. Lead poisoning and salmonellosis have to be ruled out, while with inflammation of the abomasum due to infection with *E. coli* excessive straw eating may be the *result* of so-called depraved appetite, and not the cause of the illness.

Early weaning of piglets 10 to 14 days old is now regularly practised on many farms. It obviates the marked loss of condition which befalls sows which suckle their piglets to eight weeks. Other advantages—from the farmer's point of view—are a quicker turn-round in the farrowing house, and consequently less accommodation needed; and the attainment of more than four litters in two years. Food costs per piglet are higher by this method, but weight at 8 weeks can be appreciably higher. The sow must be taken from the piglets, not *vice versa*, and housed out of earshot, as she will fret. Proprietary mixtures containing Vitamin B_{12} and an antibiotic are on the market.

Early weaning at 7–10 days, and transfer to cages for dry feeding at a temperature of 79–81° F., is a system introduced commercially into Britain in 1971. Except during twice-a-day feeding, the piglets are kept in darkness. On reaching about 15 lb. weight when three weeks old, they are moved from the three-tier cages which hold 9 piglets, to single-tier ones holding 6, and remain for about five weeks (50 lb. weight) when they are transferred to normal pens.

Under the HOHENRADENER system of pig keeping, devised by a German farmer, Heinrich Biehl, piglets are weaned when 4 days old. Removal from the sow takes place, therefore, while colostral immunity is high. In 1968 Biehl's company was handling 120,000 pigs a year.

The piglets are weighed and placed in individual battery cages in houses which hold 560 pigs and are maintained at 70–75° F. They are fed nine times daily on liquid sow milk substitute based on skim milk and added fat. Specially designed troughs allow a feeding time of 120 seconds, falling to 100 and finally 90 seconds at each of the nine feedings.

2. After 24 days in batteries, the pigs are transferred to individual pens in the main rearing houses each of which holds about 2500 pigs on steel slats. The pens just allow pigs to stand up, eat and lie down.

3. After about three days the pigs are grouped in pens of 20 at a stocking rate that still permits them only the movement to stand up to eat and lie down. Feeding periods are cut from nine to four per day.

The liquid diet is fed in specially designed troughs which are available to the pigs at intervals for a limited time. A hooter signals the beginning and end of feeding. The instant response of the pigs to the hooter means that within half a minute of cessation of feeding they are all lying down again.

After three years of use of the system no major health hazards had been reported. It is possible that the intensity of the stocking might not be acceptable under U.K. animal welfare regulations.
(*See also under* SOW'S MILK.)

Early weaning of lambs.—*See* SHEEP BREEDING.

WEATINGS.—The particles finer than bran of the husk of wheat, containing not more than about 6 per cent crude fibre. They are also known as offals and middlings, and much confusion exists between these various terms.

WEAVING is a habit of horses—swinging the head and neck and the anterior parts of the body backwards and forwards, so that the weights rest alternately upon each fore-limb. Sometimes the feet remain upon the ground all the time, but in bad cases each foot is raised as the weight passes over on to the other.

Causes.—Weaving appears to be most common in the lighter breeds of horses, and especially in those that are stabled for long periods in idleness. It has been expressed as 'the horse gets bored with his own company', and finds that movement, no matter how useless, is better than standing still. Certainly idleness at least predisposes to weaving, and once acquired it is extremely difficult to control. Unevenness of the stable floor has been blamed as a cause of weaving; the horse is unable to find a comfortable place for each of his feet, and consequently rests first upon one, and then upon the other.

Bad effects.—The principal effect is a useless fatigue of the muscles of the anterior part of the body, and a future tendency to stumble when at fast work. Like other bad habits it is likely to be imitated by other young horses in a stable, and in some cases has been known to spread to all the horses under the same roof. When the weaving horse is fastened with a chain the noise that results from the rattle of the chain through the manger-ring disturbs other horses and is objectionable to human beings.

Amelioration.—Weaving may be prevented by tying the horse with double head-ropes, one on either side, tightly enough to prevent a lateral movement but not so tight as to stop vertical movements of the head. Young horses should not be left for long periods without exercise or work; it is better to turn them out to grass rather than keep them idle in a stable. After the vice becomes confirmed in an older horse, it is advisable to house it in a loose-box away from others that may copy the habit. Unevenness in the floor of the stable should be corrected.

Weaving starts as a habit, develops into a vice, and eventually becomes a nervous disease, so that it constitutes a radical unsoundness for which a warranted horse may be returned to the seller.

WEDDER (*see under* SHEEP).

WEEDKILLERS used in agriculture include: DNOC, DNP, PARAQUAT, DIQUAT. Hormone weedkillers: M.C.P.A., Agroxone 4, and 2, 4-D. M.C.P.A. renders, it is claimed, pasture more palatable and has no ill effects upon cattle or their milk. Ragwort and buttercups also become more palatable, due to a temporary increase in their sugar content, and poisoning may consequently arise.

WEIGHTS OF CATTLE.—At birth, calves of the larger breeds weigh 80 to 120 lb. (170 lb. has been recorded). The averages for heifer calves are about: British Friesian, 86 lb.; Dairy Shorthorn, 80; Jersey, 56. Bull calves weigh about 5 lb. more.

WEIGHTS OF HORSES.—At birth, a Shire or Clydesdale foal averages $1\frac{3}{4}$ or 2 cwt.

WEIGHTS OF PIGS.—Averages in Britain are as follows: at birth, 2 or 3 lb.; at 3 weeks, 12 or 13 lb.; at 8 weeks, 36 or 37 lb. (*See also* 'BACON WEIGHT'.)

WEIL'S DISEASE (*see* JAUNDICE, LEPTOSPIRAL, OF DOGS).

WELFARE CODES FOR ANIMALS.—Codes for cattle (including calves), pigs, domestic fowls, and turkeys were approved by Parliament in 1969, and published in 1970. A regulation to prohibit the docking of cattle, the dewinging of poultry, surgical castration of poultry, and the attachment of 'spectacles' (blinkers) to poultry was proposed in 1971 (*see also under* BRAMBELL).

WESSELSBRON DISEASE.—Caused by a virus, probably transmitted by mosquitoes, and communicable to man, this infection was first reported in South Africa in 1955. It caused death of lambs, abortion, and some deaths of ewes; persistent muscular pain in man. It resembles Rift Valley fever.

WETHER (*see under* SHEEP).

WETTING AGENTS.—Substances which lower the surface tension of water, so that the latter spreads out over the surface rather than remaining in the form of drops. Good wetting ability is necessary for detergents, which play such an essential part in the disinfection of vessels, pipes, glassware used for milk, fats, etc.

WHARTON'S DUCT is the name of the tube by which saliva secreted by the submaxillary gland reaches the cavity of the mouth. It opens in the floor of the mouth almost opposite to the canine tooth in the horse.

WHARTON'S JELLY, or WHARTONIAN GELATINE, is the name of the embryonic connective tissue that forms the basis of the umbilical cord in the fœtus. In its substance are found the umbilical vessels and the other structures that constitute the umbilical cord.

WHEEZING.—(*See* BRONCHITIS *and also* BROKEN WIND.)

WHELPING (*see under* PARTURITION, in the bitch).

WHEY.—This can be a source of infection with tuberculosis in the pig. (*See* TUBERCULOSIS.) (*See also* HÆMORRHAGIC GASTRO-ENTERITIS.)

WHIPWORM is the popular name for a variety of worm that is found in the cæcum of the pig and the ox. (*See* PARASITES.)

WHISTLING is a defect affecting the respiratory system of the horse. In many respects it is similar to roaring, but the note emitted is higher pitched, usually more easily heard, does not tend to become exaggerated with age so far as the intensity of the note is concerned, and is not so likely to affect adversely the horse's general condition. Like roaring, it is due to a partial obstruction to the intake of air through the larynx, though sometimes it may be heard during expiration; it may be artificially produced by the compression of the throat-lash; it may be hereditary; it may appear after some respiratory disease; or it may arise spontaneously; and it is likely to endure for the rest of the horse's life. A whistler may develop into a roarer, but the converse does not hold. It is less serious than roaring, but it constitutes an unsoundness. What is said under ROARING with regard to symptoms, treatment, etc., applies to a great extent to whistling. (*See* ROARING.)

WHITE CELLS (*see under* BLOOD. For white cells in milk, *see under* MASTITIS).

WHITE DIARRHŒA, BACILLARY (*see under* PULLORUM DISEASE).

WHITE HEIFER DISEASE.—A condition that is reputed to be most common in white heifers—usually Shorthorns—in which there is a rubber-like sheet of fibrous tissue and membrane stretching across the posterior part of the vagina. This is called the 'hymen', and the above condition is spoken of as 'persistent hymen'. The rubber-like sheet may be partial or complete; in the latter case it is known as 'imperforate hymen'.

White heifer disease is not a very common condition, but when present it may be the cause of sterility by preventing service. In certain cases an imperforate hymen prevents the escape of secretions, shed epithelial cells, etc., from the uterus and vagina, and when the hymen is ruptured, either naturally or artificially, there is an escape of the pent-up material. A discharge occurs for a few days, but with free exit to the outside, and provided there is no infection with organisms, it soon disappears. In some cases the walls of the vagina are adherent to each other, and the results are similar. In other cases there is under-development of the uterus, which may be quite rudimentary.

Treatment.—The genital passage is made patent surgically. Where much débris has accumulated behind the membrane it may be necessary to irrigate the passage, using aseptic instruments and a boiled solution of 2 teaspoonfuls of common salt to the pint of water. For hypoplasia of the uterus nothing can be done.

'WHITE MUSCLE DISEASE' is another name for the result of Vitamin E deficiency. (*See* MUSCULAR DYSTROPHY.)

WHITE LINE is the margin of horn that runs round the outside of the sole, between it and the wall, in the horse's hoof. This strip of horn is usually lighter in colour and more elastic than the horn of the sole, but not so tough and dense as the horn of the wall. It acts as a kind of slightly pliable cementing material between wall and sole. It is important as a guide to the shoeing smith, since it forms a line inside which it is unsafe to drive a nail without risk of pricking the sensitive parts of the foot, and outside of which a nail is apt to split the wall of the foot and obtain an insecure hold. Nails should be driven *through* the white line in shoeing a normal foot.

'WHITE PIG DISEASE'.—This provisional name was given in 1963 to a condition seen in Eire among pigs on premises where floor feeding was practised, and characterised by anæmia, ulceration of the stomach, and hæmorrhage. It was believed to be associated with iron poisoning due to the concrete being made with sand of a high iron content.

WHITE PRECIPITATE is the popular name for ammonio-chloride of mercury.

'WHITES' is another name for leucorrhœa, and is a term popularly used in connection with *C. pyogenes* infection in cows. (*See* LEUCORRHŒA; UTERUS, DISEASES OF; VAGINITIS.)

WHITE SCOUR IN CALVES

WHITE SCOUR IN CALVES is a contagious bacterial disease affecting calves within the first 3 weeks of life in which the chief symptoms are severe whitish diarrhœa, great dullness, and a progressive emaciation and weakness. The disease is usually a rapid one. In the acute case the calf may be found dead or dying; in other cases death occurs in from 3 to 10 days after symptoms are first noticed. White scour almost always indicates bad management of one kind or another.

Cause is usually *E. coli*, but other organisms may be involved, including *Proteus vulgaris* and *Pseudomonas pyocyanea.*

Predisposing causes include exposure to cold and damp; deprivation of colostrum; sudden changes in diet; overfeeding; dark, dirty, badly drained, and badly ventilated calf-houses, where the young animals stand upon a considerable depth of decomposing dung; feeding calves with unsound milk or mouldy calf-meals from unclean utensils; allowing cows with unclean udders (*e.g.* when contaminated with fæces or liquid manure) to suckle calves; overcrowding; and housing healthy calves in pens or boxes that have previously contained cases of the disease and have not been carefully disinfected afterwards.

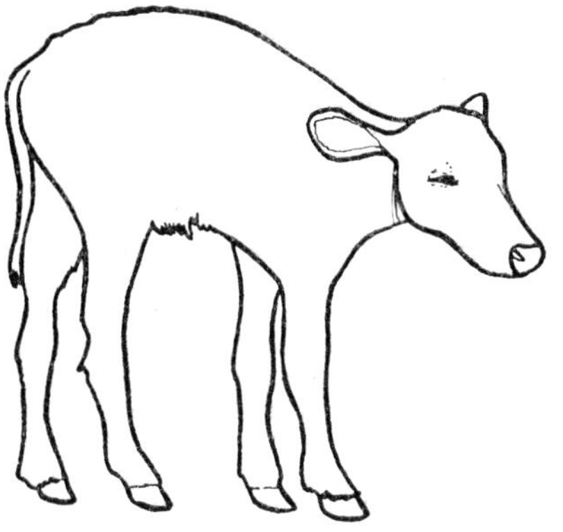

An arched back is characteristic of White Scour, also a dejected appearance.

Symptoms.—There is loss of 'bloom' and sometimes a disinclination to suckle. Diarrhœa may begin a few hours after birth, when the view is held that infection occurred during calving—maternal fæces having contaminated the calf's mouth, or it may not appear until the calf is about a week old. In the former cases the symptoms run a very acute course, and death occurs in from 24 to 48 hours. In the latter cases the diarrhœa becomes very profuse and usually of a yellowish- or greyish-white colour; it is frothy, contains flocculi, and is possessed of a most offensive odour. There is a great deal of very painful straining and moaning; the calf refuses food, or only takes small quantities; the eyes become sunken in the head, and the expression is one of great misery; the abdomen is 'tucked-up', the back is arched, and the skin becomes hard and does not move freely upon the underlying muscles (hide-bound). The temperature rises at first, but as weakness and prostration become more pronounced, it falls to below normal. In the final stages the calf lies in a semi-comatose condition, and death soon follows, sometimes in convulsions. Frequently, cases of white scour are complicated with a necrotic pneumonia or with brain lesions, and an acute diffuse peritonitis is not an unusual post-mortem finding.

Treatment.—White scour is one of those diseases in which curative measures are of less importance than preventative measures: providing the young calves with as hygienic surroundings as possible. There is no doubt that the rearing of calves is most successful in the open air, so long as shelter is provided against severe weather, but out-of-door rearing is not always possible from the economic point of view; it takes more labour, special arrangements of cropping, and necessitates a moderately equable climate all the year round. White scour is very rare in beef cattle at pasture.

Calving-boxes should be disinfected and well littered before the pregnant cattle occupy them, and if the animals themselves are very dirty their hind-quarters should be washed with disinfectant. The navel of the newly born should be protected from sucking by other calves. Many recommend the use of antiseptic dressings, particularly upon premises where the disease has existed before. Subsequently, the greatest care should be taken to ensure cleanliness of the surroundings, of the food-stuffs, etc., of the young calf. A protective serum has been used with encouraging results. Where bucket-feeding is adopted, colostrum must not be withheld.

Curative measures comprise the use of *E. coli* antiserum, sulphamezathine, or one of the other sulpha drugs, and in some cases the inclusion of yeast in the diet. Serum from the dam has been given by subcutaneous injection in default of colostrum.

WHITESIDE TEST.—This has been used for the detection of subclinical mastitis, by indicating an abnormally high white-cell count of the milk. A modified version consists in placing 1 drop of 4 per cent caustic soda and 5 drops of the milk on a glass plate, and stirring with a glass rod for 20 seconds or so. The presence of flakes indicates a positive result; a viscous mass at the end of the rod suggests a strong positive result. (For further details of this, the California Mastitis Test, and the Negretti Field Test, see *Veterinary Record* of September 22, 1962).

WILD BIRDS.—For unintended poisoning of these, *see under* GAME BIRDS. *See also* TEM.

WILTING of sugar beet tops is highly desirable before feeding in order to avoid poisoning, and with a lush crop of grass on a new ley, cutting and allowing to wilt may obviate Bloat.

WINDBREAKS (*see under* EXPOSURE).

WIND GALLS.—Distensions of the joint capsules, or of tendon sheaths, in the region of the fetlock. There are two recognised varieties: (1) articular wind gall, in which the actual joint capsule is distended with synovia, and in which the swellings appear on either side of the fetlock joint spreading in a forward direction; and (2) tendinous wind gall, where the swelling occurs in the so-called 'great sessamoid sheath', which runs up from the joint to about the beginning of the middle third of the cannon, and in which the swellings appear to run up the back of the limb between bone and tendons.

Sometimes the swellings produced are only just perceptible, and at other times they may be as large as goose eggs. They are very common in old horses, and generally cause no interference with work, nor do they produce lameness. They result from either sudden or sustained strain thrown either on the tendons at the back of the leg, or else upon the surroundings of the fetlock joint itself (*i.e.* upon the joint capsule). In certain cases they appear to be of a hereditary nature.

WIND-SUCKING (*see* CRIB-BITING).

WINTER DYSENTERY.—A disease of cattle caused by *Vibrio jejuni*. (*See under* SCOURS.)

WINTERGREEN (*see* GAULTHERIA).

WINTER DIET.—It is often wise to incorporate 5 per cent of animal protein in the winter rations of dairy cattle, which otherwise may be getting too little protein and give milk low in S.N.F. Succulent food such as silage or kale forms a high proportion of the winter diet for cattle, which may be receiving too little carbohydrate. On self-fed silage, the N.I.R.D. have recorded a 33 per cent reduction in dry matter intake compared with a diet of hay and concentrates.

'WINTER INFERTILITY' (*see* INFERTILITY).

WIRE (*see* FOREIGN BODIES IN RETICULUM, p. 885). Barbed wire is responsible for many small wounds of the cow's udder which predispose to mastitis, and for accidents in the hunting field.

WIRING (*see under* FRACTURES).

'WOBBLER'.—The name given to a horse which shows the following symptoms: a slight swaying action of the hindquarters, or stumbling, with worsening of the condition until, after 6 to 9 months, he cannot trot without rolling from side to side and falling. The cause is unknown, but possibly a spinal cord injury gives rise to these symptoms—seen in yearlings and two-year-olds; occasionally three-year-olds.

WOLF'S-BANE (*see* ACONITE).

WOMB (*see* UTERUS).

WOOD-ASH, EATING OF, by cattle is suggestive of a diet deficient in salt, calcium or magnesium.

WOOD PIGEONS (*see* TUBERCULOSIS in pigs; *also under* GAME-BIRDS, PIGEONS).

WOOD PRESERVATIVES.—Some of these are a source of arsenical poisoning; others, containing chlorinated naphthalene compounds, of hyperkeratosis. Creosote and pentachlorophenol are very liable to cause poisoning in young pigs.

WOODEN TONGUE, or WOODY TONGUE (*see* ACTINOBACILLOSIS).

WOOD'S LAMP is used in the diagnosis of ringworm; diseased hairs, etc., appearing fluorescent.

WOOL BALLS IN LAMBS.—On opening a lamb's stomach after death from some unknown disease, if a mass of wool and greyish or greenish softer material is found in the first or fourth stomach and no other readily obvious symptoms are noticed, the shepherd or owner is very prone to reach the conclusion that the cause of death was this mass of wool. In some districts, so-called 'wool balls' may be held to account for a high mortality among lambs, when the real cause is often lamb dysentery.

There is no doubt, however, that wool balls do kill lambs.

It is noticed that deaths from typical symptoms are more common in dry seasons or when ewes have for some other reason a reduced flow of milk. The hungry lamb withdraws all the milk available, but when it reaches the age of 2 to 4 weeks or so, this proves insufficient to satisfy its needs. It empties first one teat, then the other, and finally, searching for a further supply, it finds a small tag of wool on the udder or near to it and sucks at it. The somewhat salty taste of the contained wool grease may possibly be pleasing, and in time the lock of wool comes away and is chewed and swallowed. Another lock is found, sucked, and also swallowed. The wool so taken is collected by the rolling movement of the fourth stomach into a spherical mass amongst which are entangled curds of milk, grass, or other fibrous matter. Lambs may also nibble and finally swallow pieces of shed wool.

The mass of wool, which in young lambs is nearly always found in the fourth stomach (though in older ones it may be present in the first), induces a certain amount of stomach irritation and indigestion, which may lead to a desire to eat dung or more wool or other foreign material. I only a small amount is present it may pass through the alimentary canal to the outside, or may be expelled with the aid of castor oil. More often, however, it remains and increases in size. Diarrhœa or constipation results, inflammation of the stomach may occur, or actual blockage of the outlet from stomach to small intestine (pylorus). The lamb is noticed ill. Its back is arched, it grunts or groans when handled, it ceases feeding, and may only follow its mother slowly and half-heartedly. It may die suddenly or linger for a few days.

In such cases the wool ball is usually about the size of a bantam's egg (though more elongated), or even larger. It is dense in consistence, and may be firmly wedged in an inflamed pylorus. The stomach wall always shows a reddened or actively inflamed surface, and there may also be enteritis.

Prevention.—The removal of shed wool from the pastures, the 'udder-locking' (clipping all wool from the udder before or at lambing) of ewes, providing the lactating flock with adequate supplies of water during dry weather and salt.

WOOL ROT (*see under* LUMPY WOOL).

WOOLSORTER'S DISEASE is another name for anthrax in the human being.

WORKS CHIMNEYS (*see* FACTORY).

WORM EGG COUNTS.—The use of fæcal egg counts as a means of estimating the degree of infestation can be misleading. With *Ostertagia* worms in calves, for example, the pattern of fæcal egg counts tends to be the same whether the worm burden is large or small, increasing or decreasing. Counts increase fairly rapidly to an early peak from which they decrease according to a logarithmic curve. This means that the egg count at any one point in time bears a constant relation to the egg count a given number of days before. The limit to total egg output evidently depends on the host's degree of immunity.

WORMS.—Parasitic worms include round worms, tapeworms, and flukes. (*See* TAPEWORMS, ROUND WORMS, *and under* PARASITES.) (*See also* EARTHWORMS.)

In cattle and sheep, parasitic gastroenteritis and bronchitis (Husk) are important diseases caused by worms. (*See also* LIVER FLUKES, NEMATODIRUS.)

In horses, strongyle worm larvæ may give rise to a verminous aneurism with fatal results.

In dogs in Britain the worms usually encountered comprise: ascarids, hookworms, whipworms, and tapeworms. (*See also* ANTHELMINTICS.)

In pigs Ascaris worms in the intestine reduce growth rate, while their larvæ, migrating through the lungs, may give rise to pneumonia and the symptom known as 'rhumps'. Metastrongylus lungworms cause bronchitis and sometimes pneumonia. (See also THIN-SOW SYNDROME.)

WOUNDS.—A wound may be defined as a breach of the continuity of the tissues of the body produced by violence. (*See also under* BRUISES.)

Varieties.—Wounds may be classified according to the nature of the effect produced, viz. *incised, punctured, lacerated*, and *contused*.

Incised wounds are usually inflicted by some sharp instrument which leaves a clean cut; the tissues are simply divided without extensive damage to the surrounding parts. Bleeding from an incised wound is apt to be very profuse for a time, but it soon stops and is easily controlled.

Punctured wounds or stabs are inflicted with a pointed instrument. These wounds are certainly the most dangerous for animals, for not only may they involve some deeply seated organ or tissue, but hæmorrhage from them is hard to check, the provision of drainage is difficult, and they often heal over on the surface, thereby imprisoning dangerous germs. It is on account of the latter fact that a healed wound sometimes breaks open again and discharges large quantities of pus; moreover, tetanus is much more likely to become a future complication where the bacilli have been enclosed below the healed skin for some period, than where the wound has remained open to the action of the oxygen of the air. (A dose of tetanus antitoxin or toxoid is indicated in punctured wounds, especially in the horse, cow, and dog.) The wounds produced by a modern nickel-sheathed bullet, by a stable- or pitch-fork, by the horn of an ox, by the points of a reaping-machine or self-binder, by the canine teeth of dogs, etc., are all punctured wounds, and should be considered serious until the opposite has been proved.

Lacerated wounds are those in which great tearing takes place. They are usually very painful for a few days, but owing to the extensive nature of the injury drainage is generally good and the wounds heal up eventually. They sometimes do not bleed, owing to the tearing and twisting of the arteries that has occurred. Such wounds as these possess a good deal of damaged tissue, and suppurate before they heal. They are usually followed by disfiguring scars when extensive.

Contused wounds are those accompanied by much bruising of the surrounding tissues, as in the case of blows from heavy articles, kicks from shod horses, and from falls when in harness. There is usually little bleeding from the wound itself, but blood may be extravasated into the tissues around its edge, and healing is rendered slow.

Any one of these forms of wounds may become infected with pus-forming organisms, and develop into a suppurating, *septic wound*. (For other information *see under* ACCIDENTS, INJURIES; etc.)

First-aid treatment.—Generally speaking, the aid should consist of (*a*) securing the animal, and preventing it from doing itself further injury (*see under* RESTRAINT); (*b*) arresting hæmorrhage (*see* BLEEDING, ARREST OF); (*c*) cleansing the wound and applying dressings, etc.

Cleansing the wound.—The hair around the edges of the wound, along with any torn or lacerated portions of skin or other tissue, should be clipped away with a pair of sharp, preferably blunt-pointed scissors, the cavity of the wound having previously been packed with cotton-wool (wrung out of warm boiled water) to prevent further contamination of the raw surface. Finally the surface of the skin around the area is washed with water containing an antiseptic such as Dettol, T.C.P., acriflavine, etc. (*See* ANTISEPTICS.) If the wound is in such a part as can be bandaged a dressing of antiseptic dusting powder, or a swab soaked in a solution of acriflavine, may be applied, and a protective bandage fixed over all. (*See* BANDAGES.) It is always advisable to use a layer of cotton-wool over the wound so that pressure may be as evenly distributed as possible, and so that any bleeding may be encouraged to check itself by coagulation in the meshes of the cotton-wool.

Afterwards the animal should be kept as quiet as possible. The best plan is to give the animal a small feed and leave it by itself. If it is not too badly injured it will almost certainly commence feeding and remain quiet so long as the food lasts. It may be necessary in some cases to apply measures of restraint to prevent an animal from licking, biting, or scratching at a wounded part. The horse may be fitted with 'beads' or 'cradles', the ox may need tying up in a stall, and the dog may require muzzling. If the bandage seems comfortable, and if the bleeding has been stopped (or has almost stopped) the wound may not require any attention until the next day.

Where a large open wound has been inflicted it is usually advisable to draw the edges together to some extent by suturing. A procedure such as this is best left to the veterinary surgeon; the skin of the horse, ox, and pig, especially, is extremely thick, and often difficult to pierce with an ordinary needle; the animal strongly resents the stitching of a wound; and it is often difficult to get apposition of the edges. Where it becomes necessary for the untrained owner of an animal to insert sutures, it should be remembered that (1) the animal should be adequately controlled; (2) the materials should be boiled, and the hands carefully washed; (3) the needle should be inserted into the edge of the skin which is farthest away from the central nervous system first; and (4) as few sutures should be used as will gain the desired end of bringing the edges of the wound together, and they should not be applied too tightly lest they cut through the skin or prevent the escape of discharges.

The healing of wounds may be delayed by cortisone, and influenced by insulin. Vitamin A is used to promote or hasten healing of wounds.

Healing by first intention.—In a clean incised wound, such as is made during the course of aseptic operations, the immediate effect is bleeding from the ends of the vessels which have been cut. A small quantity of blood remains between the divided edges and clots. The blood-vessels round the incision dilate, the blood flow is slowed, and there passes out from the blood a fluid known as 'lymph', which coagulates upon the surface of the wound, forming a sticky layer of fibrin which, if the injured surfaces are in contact, causes them to adhere to one another. This forms the temporary scaffolding within which the process of repair will be carried on, and possesses the valuable property of being strongly germicidal to any organisms which come into contact with it. White blood cells pass out from the dilated blood-vessels and wander through this exudate in the wound. These white blood corpuscles absorb and destroy any foreign or dead substances which have to be removed to allow the process of repair to proceed (*see* PHAGOCYTOSIS), particularly minute portions of killed tissue and blood that has oozed into the deeper parts of the wound cavity. Following the entrance of the white blood cells, which occurs within 24 hours after the infliction of the wound, there comes an invasion by hosts of cells produced by multiplication of the cells in the tissues around the wound Some of these possess the power o. 'phagocytosis', and others, called 'fibroblasts', become transformed into a delicate network of fibrous tissue. Simultaneously with the formation of this network, minute buds shoot from the capillaries at the edges of the wound and form tiny blood channels, which pass from side to side of the gap, or form loops where the distance across the wound is large. The tissue so formed is now called 'granulation tissue', because, when its surface is closely examined, it has a red granular appearance. This is due to the loops of immature capillaries, each one covered by the masses of cells mentioned previously. The same form of tissue is seen in a rapidly healing ulcer. Epithelial cells from the skin now begin to grow over and cover the wound, the whole process being completed in about a week where the skin edges have been accurately apposed. In such a case in a part covered by hair no new hair follicles are formed, but the scar marking the line of incision is so thin that hairs from each side of the wound grow across it and hide it. It is still possible to recognise the situation of such a scar if the hair be rubbed the wrong way, or if the skin surface be shaved. The delicate tissue of the newly healed wound is gradually replaced by denser, firmer fibrous tissue, until in a few months the healed wound is only represented by a thin linear inconspicuous scar. With modifications, this process of repair takes place in all healing wounds.

Healing by second intention takes place where the granulation tissue remains exposed to view. It occurs in wounds which have broken down owing to suppuration, where there is an ulcer, where a large area of skin has been removed, or has sloughed off without poisoning, and in other cases. A larger, wider, thicker, and more noticeable scar remains after healing. This is by far the commonest method of healing of wounds among animals.

Healing by scab formation occurs where the lymph dries into a crust on the surface of the wound, and the healing process is carried on under the outer hard cake. Sometimes a wound begins to heal by scab formation, but thick white pus is produced under the scab, and unless exit is provided it may burrow under the surrounding skin and so enlarge the area that must heal.

Healing of infected wounds.—The germs in it dissolve the fibrin covering and destroy many of the cells engaged in repair. The reaction of the tissues becomes intense, and the inflammation of the wound is so evident that such are popularly called 'inflamed wounds'. As a result of the destruction many of the cells are discharged as pus. Granulation tissue is gradually formed around the site of infection in the depths of the wound, the bacteria are gradually cast off in the pus, and healing slowly proceeds by second intention. Antibiotics and/or sulphonamides may be used either locally or by injection, and enzymes (*see* STREPTODORNASE) may be used to dissolve pus and other débris.

After-treatment.—There now remains to be considered the treatment that is necessary after the wound has received first aid. Where hæmorrhage has been very extensive it is sometimes wise not to disturb the dressings for 30 or 36 hours after application. This allows the blood clots to become firmly established in the cut ends of the arteries, and does away with the risk of what is usually called 'secondary hæmorrhage'. In other cases the wound may be dressed again the day after infliction. The bandages are carefully removed, the surface blood clots are wiped away with clean cotton-wool, and a fresh dressing is applied. It is unwise to do more than this at an early stage, unless there are particles of damaged tissue to be removed, or unless large particles of foreign materials which have escaped removal at the first dressing can be easily taken away. Watery dressings are used for washing over the wound, or syringing into its depths. They may consist of proprietary antiseptics used according to the maker's directions. The dry dusting powders (*e.g.* sulphanilamide powder) are dusted on to the wound after it has been first cleansed by washing with some antiseptic lotion, or they may be spread on to cotton-wool and bandaged over the wound. Simple irrigation may be carried out by arranging a quantity of solution at a higher level than the animal, leading it down into the wound through a rubber-tube, and allowing it to ooze into the wound for hours at a time at a very slow rate. Solutions used include saline and acriflavine.

Whatever method is selected it is necessary to observe strict cleanliness of the dressings, of the attendant's hands, and of the bandages, wool, etc., that come into contact with the wound surface, and to dress the parts regularly once a day (except in special cases), until the cavity of the wound has filled up to near the level of the surrounding skin.

Other points that should be noted are: (1) that stitches should be removed if they commence to suppurate, and in any case after being in position for a week, after which they serve no useful purpose; (2) that if pus burrows under the skin surrounding a wound it must be given drainage by incision below the level of the most dependent burrowing or by drainage tubes; (3) that if the granulation tissue (*i.e.* 'proud flesh') rises to a higher level than the skin around, it must be repressed by cautery with a crystal of sulphate of copper or nitrate of silver; and (4) that in cases of injury to special parts, such as the eyes, nostrils, lips, genital organs, feet, etc., it is essential to seek skilled advice rather than to persist in rule-of-thumb methods which often lead the enthusiastic amateur astray, and cause the animal unnecessary distress. (*See also* BLEEDING, ARREST OF; FRACTURES; GRANULATION TISSUE; ULCER; *and* ANTISEPTICS; ANTIBIOTICS; SULPHONAMIDES; *and also under* ACCIDENTS, INJURIES, *and* CORTIOSNE.)

WRY-NECK, which occurs in foals particularly, is the name given to a lateral deviation of the head and neck to the right or left side of the body, usually so marked as to hinder or prevent foaling. The nose of the foal is tucked round into the flank, the neck being so rigidly curved that it defies all manual efforts to straighten it out into such a position as will allow of delivery. In fact, it is sometimes impossible to rectify the curvature after the foal has been born, in those cases where parturition *can* be effected. The bones of the skull and neck are frequently distorted, and the ligaments, tendons, and muscles on the inside of the curve are shorter than those on the outside. This is probably because the development of the fœtus has taken place with the neck permanently curved.

The condition is commonest in the progeny of young mares foaling for the first time, but may also be met with in older breeding mares, and it has been described in cattle.

Treatment.—In some cases, where the foal is small, delivery may be effected by strong traction upon the limbs, but in most cases it is necessary for the obstetrician to amputate the head or neck at whatever site is most convenient, and perhaps one of the fore-limbs as well. It is seldom that a foal with wry-neck is born alive, and when this does occur it is unwise to allow it to live, since it can never become a useful member of the stud.

X

XANTHOSIS is a yellowish brown pigmentation of meat, generally affecting the heart and the tongue. It gives the meat an objectionable colour, but is quite harmless.

X-RAYS.—The X-rays, or Röntgen rays, were discovered in 1894.

X-rays are radiations of the same nature as ordinary light rays, but of very much shorter wave-length, produced by the sudden stoppage of the negatively charged electrons in a special discharge-tube. The tube is so arranged that a stream of cathode rays impacts upon a target of plantinum or tungsten. These rays are given off from a concave aluminium cathode, converge in their course, strike the target upon which they are focused, and are shot off through space. They possess the power of acting upon sensitised photographic paper in the same way as light rays, but unlike these latter they are not stopped by any but the most dense substances. It is owing to this that radiography is possible in ordinary daylight. The photographic films or plates are enclosed in wrappings which are light-proof, but which are easily penetrated by the X-rays. The X-rays possess the further quality of acting upon certain compounds and making them luminous. Thus if the rays are allowed to pass through, say, the limb of a dog, and are then cast upon a fluorescent screen which has been specially prepared (e.g. with crystals of barium-platino-cyanide, zinc-blende, willemite, etc.), certain areas of the screen show a bright luminosity, where the rays falling upon them have passed through non-absorptive substances, such as flesh, and other areas show darker shadows, where the rays have been partially absorbed by opaque objects, such as bone or cartilage.

X-rays are capable of passing through considerable thicknesses of many substances which are opaque to ordinary light without undergoing material absorption, but other substances, even in very small thicknesses, are able to absorb the great majority of the rays: thus, flesh, wood, wool, cotton, paper, and most substances of vegetable origin (but not all) are very transparent; aluminium and ordinary crown glass are less transparent; healthy bone is fairly opaque, and the majority of the heavy metals, such as lead, iron, copper, and nickel, are very opaque, and stop almost the whole of the rays. Guard screens of lead glass, rubber impregnated with lead, or sheet lead, are used to protect the operators of radiographic apparatus, and precautions are necessary to shield the testes and ovaries of young persons and animals from the sterilising effects of the rays.

Precautions.—1. Persons under 16 years must not take part in radiological procedures. 2. Fluoroscopy or radiotherapy should not be carried out except under expert radiological guidance. Hand-held fluoroscopes must not be used under any circumstances. 3. Personnel radiation monitoring devices, such as film badges, must be worn by all persons who take part routinely in radiological procedures. 4. The animal should, if possible, be anæsthetised or tranquillised for radiography, and all persons should withdraw as far as practicable from the useful beam. 5. If it should be necessary to hold the animal for radiography, lead-protective gloves and aprons must be worn. Whenever possible, holding should be done by the owners, unless they are under 16 years or pregnant. 6. Persons should not expose any part of their bodies to the useful beam even when wearing protective clothing. 7. The useful beam should be restricted to the area being examined by means of a beam limiting device.

The chief use of X-rays is for diagnostic purposes. They are, as yet, mainly applicable to the smaller carnivora and to the limbs and heads of the larger animals, for, owing to the large mass of tissue in the trunks of these latter, an apparatus capable of producing rays powerful enough to penetrate is extremely costly.

The production of a radiograph of the internal structure of a small animal is a comparatively simple matter once the difficulty of control is overcome. The animal is arranged upon the table in such a position as will allow the rays to pass down through the part and become registered upon a sensitive plate placed flat upon the table immediately below. The animal may lie upon its back, on one or the other side, or on its chest and abdomen with the legs pulled out from under it. To maintain this position it is always advisable to administer an anæsthetic, *e.g.* nembutal. The discharge tube is best arranged immediately above the animal in such a position as will allow the rays to fall perpendicularly down through the body on to the plate. (For screening, the tube must be below the table, and the screen held or supported above the animal.) The period of exposure to the passage of the rays varies according to the tissues, according to the softness or hardness of the tube, to the distance of the tube from the plate, and to whether or not an intensifying screen is used.

Indications for X-ray use.—There are many conditions in which the actual extent of injury or disease can be accurately discovered *only* by the use of X-rays, but the most important and spectacular are the diseases and injuries of bones. Fractures of the limb bones are well shown up, and their extent is better realised than is possible by palpation. Exostoses (overgrowths of bone) can also be clearly indicated, while tumour formation (usually sarcomatous) shows as a thinning and enlargement of the bone tissue. Where only one limb is affected it is advisable to arrange the animal so as to include a picture of the normal limb for comparison. Foreign bodies—especially needles, pins, nails, and other metallic substances—which have been swallowed are best shown by a profile view of the abdomen. Pieces of game bones (which are especially dense and show up well) can also be seen in the stomach or intestines, and are very often surrounded by gas, which, in the negative, appears as a dark shadow, the bone itself appearing light. Internal tumours can very often be diagnosed. They appear as more or less discrete pale areas in positions where a radiograph from a normal animal is denser under the same conditions of exposure, etc. A method has been devised whereby certain tumours can be made to show up well by giving the animal medicinal doses of a lead salt for a few days before taking the plate. Some of the lead becomes deposited in the tumour and intensifies the contrast. Where some displacement, stricture, or dilatation of the stomach or of part of the intestinal canal is suspected, the animal is given a feed or a draught containing an emulsion of bismuth or barium carbonate, or some other harmless metallic salt, or has some of the same material injected into the rectum. After waiting until the salt has become suitably distributed, a radiograph of the abdomen is taken, and the outlines of those organs to which the salt has been carried by peristalsis, can be made out as pale areas in the negatives.

Other conditions in which X-rays are useful are as follows: stones in the kidney, urinary or gall bladder; calcified tubercular glands in the lungs or mesentery; ringbones, sidebones, splints, spavins, and other bony conditions affecting the limbs of horses; dilatation of the heart; solidification of a portion of a lung; fluid pleurisy—when the lung floats above the fluid (this requires a horizontal instead of a vertical passage of the rays); brain tumours, and the worm cysts that constitute sturdy in the brain of sheep.

X-ray therapy has been applied to a limited extent in the treatment of certain tumours in the dog. The necessary apparatus is cumbersome and extremely costly. (*See also under* VACCINE.)

Further information on X-rays and their use will be found in *Carlson's Veterinary Radiology* (2nd edition, 1968, Baillière, Tindall & Cassell, 666 pages, £10).

XEROPHTHALMIA.—A disease of the eye associated with a vitamin A deficiency. Blindness may be produced.

XYLAZINE.—The active ingredient of 'Rompun', a sedative used to render farm livestock easier to handle.

XYLOTOX.—A stable, non-irritating and non-toxic local anæsthetic, stated to be more powerful in action than procaine hydrochloride. It is more readily diffusible than most other agents and its action is therefore very rapid.

Y

YARDED CATTLE.—Before yarding cattle in the autumn, it is wise to make a gradual change from sugar-poor autumn pasture to things like roots. Otherwise digestive upsets are very likely to occur.

Similarly, in spring it is a mistake to turn calves straight out on to grass. This means a sudden change from protein-poor food to the rich protein of the early bite, and the resulting effect upon the rumen will set them back. It is best to get them out before there is much grass for a few hours each day ; let them have hay and shelter at night to protect them from sudden changes of weather. Hypomagnesæmia, too, is far less likely under these circumstances. (*See also* Housing of Animals.)

Boss cows can be a nuisance in yards, but the provision of yokes for feeding overcomes the main difficulty.

When self-feeding of silage is practised, precautions are necessary in order to prevent foot-troubles. (*See* Silage.)

Yarded animals fed on cereals, sugar-beet pulp, straw, and hay—but with little or no greenstuff—may go blind as a result of a vitamin A deficiency.

YEAST is a valuable source of Vitamin B, but should not be fed in excessive amounts to pigs or it may give rise to rickets unless adequate Vitamin D is simultaneously available. Yeast has proved successful in the treatment of tropical ulcers in humans, and success has been reported in a limited number of cases in horses in the tropics. The human patients were mostly those whose diet was deficient in Vitamin B, a deficiency further increased by sweating. The yeast is applied direct to the ulcer, and a small quantity given internally also. (*See also* Bacteriology *and* Plate 2.)

YELLOWS, THE.—This is a popular name for ordinary jaundice in animals (*see* Jaundice), and it is also applied to infectious jaundice of dogs, due to the parasite *Leptospira icterohæmorrhagica*. (*See* Leptospiral Jaundice.) 'Yellowses' is a popular name for Light Sensitisation accompanied by jaundice in sheep. It occurs in parts of Scotland during June and July. The plant responsible has not been identified, though the bog asphodel has been suspected.

YELT.—A female pig intended for breeding, up to the time that she has her first litter.

YERSINIOSIS.—Pseudo-tuberculosis.

YEW POISONING.—All varieties of the British yew trees are poisonous, but owing to its more frequent cultivation, the common yew (*Taxus baccata*) is most often responsible for outbreaks of poisoning among animals. The Irish yew (*Taxus baccata*, var. *fastigiata*) and the Yellow yew appear to contain less of the poisonous principle, which is called *Taxine* and is an alkaloid. The bark, leaves, and seeds all contain the active toxic principle, the leaves usually being the parts eaten. The older dark green leaves, and especially if these have been cut off and left to wither for some hours, are more dangerous than the fresh green young shoots, which cattle have been known to eat in small amounts without harm. Cases of poisoning have been noted among horses, asses, mules, cattle, sheep, goats, pigs, deer, rabbits, and even pheasants, but the majority of cases occur in young store cattle and in dairy cows which have access to the shrubberies, graveyards, etc., where the yew trees are most common.

Symptoms.—In many cases cattle drop dead without showing any preliminary symptoms at all. They may fall while cudding almost as suddenly as if shot. In other cases where less has been eaten, or where the stomach is already full and absorption slower, the animal shows signs of gastric irritation and narcosis. There is excitement, then slowing of the pulse and respiration rate, and finally the animal becomes prostrate. Its extremities are cold ; it requires vigorous measures to rouse it ; the stomach becomes tympanitic with gas ; and sometimes retching or even vomiting is noticed. In horses, there are quivers and tremors of the surface muscles, the intestine becomes paralysed, and death occurs in convulsions. Pigs often bury their heads in their litter and sleep, their sleep being interrupted by attacks of vomiting and groaning. It must be remembered, however, that it is more common to find that no symptoms have been shown at all. Cases have been noted in which the animals fell dead ten minutes after having eaten the branches cut from a yew tree during pruning operations. In others, they finished feeding, wandered away a short distance apparently normal, commenced cudding, and then fell dead.

Treatment.—It will be obvious that in many cases there is no time for the carrying out of any remedial measures. Antidotes: as for alkaloids.

As preventive measures, yew trees growing in parts to which cattle, or other animals, have access, should be protected by railings, or their branches may be trimmed so that they cannot be reached. All trimmings, whether from pruning or from dead or broken branches, should be disposed of by burning before cattle can get at them.

YOHIMBINE is an alkaloid prepared from the bark of the Yohimbehe tree (*Corynanthe Yohimbi*), which possesses marked aphrodisiac actions; that is, it stimulates sexual appetite among animals.

YOLK SAC INFECTION (*see* OMPHALTIS).

YORKSHIRE BOARDING.—Vertically arranged boards with a gap between each, used for partial cladding of a livestock building. (See Plate 3.)

Z

'ZANIL'.—A drug for use against liver flukes in cattle and sheep. Extensive trials have shown it to be of low toxicity, and safe to use in pregnant animals and those in poor condition.

ZEBU.—*Bos indicus*, the cattle of India, E. and W. Africa, and S.E. Asia. The American name is Brahman; in South Africa, the Afrikaner.

ZERO GRAZING.—Taking cut fodder to yarded cattle, or to cattle in exercise paddocks. Zero grazing has a place on heavy land, with high stocking rates, and large herds. It obviates poaching and the spoiling of grass, and a given acreage zero-grazed can provide more grass than if grazed. It means, however, cutting grass every day, and mechanical failures can upset the system. It is not yet considered economic for sheep.

ZINC is a metal, several of the salts of which are used in the treatment of animal diseases. Of the salts used, the oxide and the carbonate, both of which are almost insoluble in water, the sulphate and the chloride, both of which are soluble, are the commonest.

Zinc is a trace element, and a deficiency has occurred in pigs. (*See* PARAKERATOSIS.) A zinc supplement to prevent or correct this condition must be used with care, as 1000 parts per million can cause poisoning. It seems that a high calcium intake by pigs aggravates a zinc deficiency.

Actions.—The oxide and the carbonate are astringent and desiccant when applied to broken wet surfaces of the skin or a mucous membrane. They are either made up as a powder with other substances, or they are incorporated in ointment form. The sulphate of zinc is used for internal administration for almost the sole purpose of inducing vomiting in the dog, cat, and pig. It is a safe emetic for these animals, as it is immediately eliminated from the stomach, and has no opportunity to produce any irritant action. Externally it is stimulant and astringent to both the skin and to mucous membranes. Chloride of zinc is a powerful caustic acting by coagulating the albumin of the tissues and extracting water. It is an irritant poison when given internally.

Uses.—The insoluble salts—oxide and carbonate—are mainly employed in the treatment of eczematous conditions of the skin, such as mud fever, cracked heels, mallenders, sallenders, weeping eczema in the dog. The sulphate is employed as a solution in water for purulent inflammations of the eyes or the eyelids, especially after the acute stages have passed; for this purpose it should never be used in stronger solution than 2 or 3 grains to the ounce. It forms one of the constituents of the familiar 'white lotion', which is used for surface inflammations, and for swabbing clean open wounds when healing is slow. The uses of the chloride are confined to the repression of exuberant granulations, warts, etc., when its caustic action is employed.

ZINC BACITRACIN.—Official clearance has been given for the use of zinc bacitracin without veterinary prescription as a 'feed' antibiotic, following the Government's acceptance of the Swann Committee report. Zinc bacitracin may now be included in feeds for growing pigs and poultry at approved levels of up to 125 g/ton.

In 1971 the permitted use of zinc bacitracin was extended to growth promotion in lambs and calves up to six months of age, up to 125 g/ton. (*See* ADDITIVES.)

ZINC PHOSPHIDE is a black powder, slightly soluble in water and having an odour like that of garlic. It is used as a rodent poison, baits being made up of 2.5 or 5 per cent zinc phosphide. Symptoms include: loss of appetite, tympany and pain in cattle, lethargy, coma. Respirations are increased after a few hours.

ZINC POISONING.—Chronic zinc poisoning has been reported in a dairy herd as a result of contaminated drinking water—the result of inter-action between copper pipes and newly galvanised tanks. The main symptom was chronic constipation throughout the herd, and a diminished yield from the cows in milk. (*See* above.)

Fatal zinc poisoning has occurred in dairy cattle fed on dairy nuts to which zinc oxide had been added instead of magnesium oxide. The first death occurred after three weeks.

'ZOALENE'.—A drug used in the control of coccidiosis of poultry.

ZONDEK-ASCHEIM TEST (*see* PREGNANCY DIAGNOSIS TESTS).

ZONULAR PLACENTA is one in which there is an annular zone round the middle of the chorion of the fœtus-carrying numerous villi, as distinct from other forms of placentæ which may be 'diffuse' as in the mare and sow, or 'cotyledonary' as in ruminants. Zonular placentæ occur in the bitch and cat, and in the carnivora generally.

ZOONOSES.—Diseases communicable between animals and man. Information about them will be found under the following headings: ANTHRAX, B VIRUS (from monkeys), BRUCELLOSIS, CAT-SCRATCH FEVER, CHAGAS' DISEASE, EQUINE ENCEPHALOMYELITIS, EQUINE INFECTIOUS ANÆMIA, FOOT-AND-MOUTH DISEASE (very rare in human beings), GLANDERS, HYDATID, LEPTOSPIROSIS, LISTERIOSIS, LIVER FLUKES, LOUPING ILL, LYMPHOCYTIC CHORIOMENGITIS (from mice), NEWCASTLE DISEASE, ORNITHOSIS, ORF, Q FEVER, RABIES, RAT-BITE FEVER, RIFT VALLEY FEVER, RINGWORM, ROCKY MOUNTAIN DISEASE, RUSSIAN SPRING-SUMMER VIRUS, SALMONELLOSIS, SCABIES, SCHISTOMIASIS, TAPEWORMS, TICK-BITE FEVER, TICK PARALYSIS, TOXOCARA, TOXOPLASMOSIS, TRICHINOSIS, TUBERCULOSIS, TULARÆMIA, VESICULAR STOMATITIS, MARBURG DISEASE, WESSELSBRON DISEASE.

A lengthier list of zoonoses will be found in WHO technical report no. 378, 1967.

It should be added that typhus and plague may be transmitted, by flea-bite, from rats; and, in jungle areas, yellow fever, by mosquito-bite, from monkeys.

(*See also under* MONKEYS, INFLUENZA.)

Among skin diseases, the parasite of follicular mange may occasionally infest the human eyelid.

ZOOTECHNY.—Animal management.

ZYGOMA (*ζύγωμα*).—The bridge of bone which runs from near the base of the ear to the lower posterior part of the eye-socket. It protects the side of the bony orbit, forms part of the support of the outside of the joint of the lower jaw with the rest of the head, and serves as a base of attachment for part of the strong masseter muscle which closes the mouth and is important in the chewing of the food. The zygomatic arch (another name for the zygoma) is formed by projections from the temporal, zygomatic, and maxillary bones.

ZYGOTE.—The body that results from the fertilisation of a female germ cell by a male germ cell.